ROBERT C. GROTZ, M.D.

D0225197

YEAR BOOK's
MEDICAL LICENSURE REVIEWS
BASIC SCIENCES

Anatomy/Physiology/
Biochemistry/Microbiology/
Pathology/Pharmacology/
Behavioral Sciences

YEAR BOOK's MEDICAL LICENSURE REVIEWS

BASIC SCIENCES

Anatomy/Physiology/
Biochemistry/Microbiology/
Pathology/Pharmacology/
Behavioral Sciences

Alfred Jay Bollet, M.D.

Clinical Professor of Medicine
Yale University School of Medicine
Chief of Medicine
Danbury Hospital
Danbury, CT

Year Book Medical Publishers, Inc./Fleschner Publishing Co.
Chicago • London • Boca Raton/Woodbridge, CT

Copyright © 1989 by Year Book Medical Publishers, Inc. All rights reserved. No part of this publication may be reproduced, stored in a retrieval system, or transmitted, in any form or by any means—electronic, mechanical, photocopying, recording, or otherwise—without prior written permission from the publisher. Printed in the United States of America.

1 2 3 4 5 6 7 8 9 0 M F 92 91 90 89

Library of Congress Cataloging-in-Publication Data

Bollet, Alfred J.
    Basic sciences: anatomy, physiology, biochemistry, microbiology, pathology, pharmacology, behavioral sciences / Alfred Jay Bollet.
        p.   cm. — (Year Book's medical licensure reviews)
    Includes bibliographies and index.
    ISBN 0-8151-1021-9
    1. Medical sciences—Examinations, questions, etc.
2. Medicine— Examinations, questions, etc.   I. Title.   II. Series.
    [DNLM: 1. Medicine—examination questions. W 18 B691b]
R834.5.B65   1989
610'.76—dc19
DNLM/DLC   88-40
for Library of Congress   CIP

Sponsoring Editor: Richard H. Lampert

CONTRIBUTORS

Isidore Danishefsky, PhD
Chairman, Department of Biochemistry
New York Medical College
Valhalla, NY

Joan C. Fung-Tomc, PhD
Instructor, Laboratory Medicine
University of Connecticut School of Medicine
Farmington, CT

Frank Pastore, MD
Director of Undergraduate Education in Psychiatry and Behavioral Sciences
New York Medical College
Valhalla, NY

Margaret A. Reilly, PhD
Department of Pharmacology
Nathan S. Kline Institute for Psychiatric Research
Orangeburg, NY

Ira Schwartz, PhD
Associate Professor of Biochemistry
New York Medical College
Valhalla, NY

David Smith, MD
Former Associate Dean
Tulane University School of Medicine
New Orleans, LA

Richard Tilton, PhD
Professor of Laboratory Medicine
University of Connecticut School of Medicine
Farmington, CT

Michael Wang, PhD
Associate Professor of Physiology
Temple University School of Medicine
Philadelphia, PA

Thomas A. Weidman, PhD
Associate Professor of Anatomy
Medical College of Georgia
Augusta, GA

Richard Yeasting, PhD
Professor of Anatomy
Medical College of Ohio
Toledo, OH

ABBREVIATIONS

ADP   adenosine diphosphate
ATP   adenosine triphosphate
ATPase   adenosine triphosphatase
b.i.d.   twice daily
bpm   beats per minute
BUN   blood urea nitrogen
CNS   central nervous system
CPR   cardiopulmonary resuscitation
CSF   cerebrospinal fluid
CT   computerized tomography
DNA   deoxyribonucleic acid
DNase   deoxyribonuclease
ECG   electrocardiogram
EDTA   ethylenediaminetetraacetate
EEG   electroencephalogram
GI   gastrointestinal
GU   genitourinary
ICU   intensive care unit
IM   intramuscular(ly)
IV   intravenous(ly)
NPO   nothing by mouth
PCO_2 partial pressure of carbon dioxide
PO   by mouth
PO_2 partial pressure of oxygen
q   every
q.i.d.   four times daily
RNA   ribonucleic acid
SC   subcutaneous(ly)
SGOT   serum glutamic-oxaloacetic transaminase
SGPT   serum glutamic-pyruvic transaminase
t.i.d.   three times daily

INTRODUCTION

Year Book Medical Publishers has prepared a two-volume examination study aid that is intended to assist students and resident physicians to prepare for medical licensure examinations, such as the National Board of Medical Examiners and FLEX examinations. This volume is devoted to the clinical sciences, and the other to the basic sciences. The material covered provides a relatively quick review of essential points in each field, with sufficient depth to be valuable preparation for these licensure examinations, for undergraduate medical school examinations, and for preparation for discussions during teaching rounds. Each chapter contains a group of questions like those on the National Board and FLEX exams to provide experience with the formats used in these examinations as well as assistance in review of subject material.

In preparing these volumes, the authors assumed that readers had a basic familiarity with each subject, and the material is presented concisely since it is primarily intended for review purposes. Although a great deal of factual information is provided in most subjects areas, concentrating on salient points most likely to be covered on examinations, these volumes are not intended to serve as reference texts. Sufficient explanation is given to help in the understanding of the factual material presented, and therefore in its retention in memory, but these aspects are not discussed in the depth to be expected in a standard textbook. At the end of each chapter, a few basic references are provided to aid readers in selecting sources for exploring topics in further depth.

Each chapter on clinical subjects includes sections covering the factual information needed for decisions that candidates must make in answering patient management problems, which are a standard part of such examinations. These decisions cover diagnostic tests and therapeutic principles. Emphasis has been given to the facts in each subject pertinent to these decisions. Such information is important for multiple-choice questions as well, since such decisions are often the point of such questions.

In the clinical subjects, students are expected to bring information from many different basic science and clinical disciplines to bear on clinical problems. Although the examinations no longer divide the time into specific subject areas, mixing the clinical disciplines throughout the test, we have kept these subjects distinct in this volume for ease of review and in order to make the material more useful during undergraduate clerkship experiences. Students should remember, however, that on National Board and FLEX exams questions on these subjects are intermingled.

Some factual material obviously is more appropriate for specialty board examinations, since certified specialists in the field will be dealing with the type of clinical problem requiring application of that information. It is not appropriate to ask primary care physicians or physicians who are just finishing undergraduate training and entering residency programs to be responsible for such information. The authors tried to keep this in mind in preparing the review book. The chapters are aimed at undergraduate students and house officers who are taking licensure exams, not specialists taking advanced certifying board exams.

In selecting subject material for these volumes, the authors had in mind the philosophy of the examining boards regarding the type of information to cover on these exams. In general, this is the type of information that undergraduate medical students and junior house officers will need to function at the next level of their training. Graduates entering the first year of residency training usually have to work in emergency departments as part of their training; they may be faced with patients presenting with a wide variety of clinical problems and must be able to recognize the nature of the problem, take immediate action when necessary to prevent progression of the disease process, and know when to call for help. The committees that make up the National Board examinations have this function in mind; they wish to evaluate whether students are ready for the additional responsibilities that are needed to function in their further training. Thus, questions are directed at the most important points about the clinical problems an intern may face in the emergency department or as sudden developments in sick, hospitalized patients. In addition there is heavy emphasis on primary care problems the candidate is likely to experience in outpatient settings on rotation through various specialties. These subjects should be stressed by candidates in preparing for these examinations.

House officers must also know enough about problems appropriately treated by subspecialists to know when to refer, to be able to advise patients on appropriate courses of action, or to explain to such patients what is likely to happen to them as workup and treatment progress. Knowledge of subspecialty-level medical problems cannot be ignored, therefore, in undergraduate education or in preparation for licensure exams.

Students and house officers, in considering the importance of specific subjects when studying for examinations, should therefore consider whether they might be faced with such a problem as a first-line physician in an emergency room or in an outpatient setting, and what they must know to function properly as an intern or resident. Study for that function and you will be studying for these licensure examinations as well as for your needs in the immediate future.

For example, in evaluating a patient with anemia, house officers and therefore candidates for licensure should know how to distinguish folate for B_{12} deficiency from iron deficiency, appropriate types of therapy for each, how to identify a patient with an autoimmune hemolytic process, and what types of drugs are likely to be used and their major side effects. But such candidates need not be expected to know the appropriate dosage of immunosuppressant agents or choose among them.

With antibiotic choices, candidates are expected to know the types of drugs that should be used but not necessarily the exact ones that are the drugs of choice today, since rapid developments in many fields cause frequent changes in the specific drugs of choice. Remember that these examinations are prepared almost 2 years before they are given, and the subject committees know that much detailed information can become outdated by the time the examination is given.

In general, therefore, details of dosage are rarely asked, but it is expected that candidates will know major principles of drug use, major side effects to watch for, important drug interactions, and pharmacokinetic principles that are related to major categories of drugs. Similarly, for surgical procedures, students are expected to know indications, likely complications, and what the patient is likely to experience, as well as the usual duration of recuperation and disability.

POINTERS TO REMEMBER WHILE TAKING LICENSURE EXAMINATIONS

When taking multiple-choice tests such as those given by National Board of Medical Examiners and FLEX, candidates should bear certain useful principles in mind.

First, be familiar with types of questions used in National Board and FLEX examinations and practice answering them. Examples are provided after each subject in this volume. When taking the examination, read the instructions carefully and be certain you understand them before proceeding; this is especially important for matching questions, where each item may be used once, more than once, or not at all. In these exams, K-type questions are another source of confusion, since the correct response depends on the pattern of the answers rather than an answer to each individual item. Keep instructions in view; you might write them on the front of an exam book so you can have ready reference after each question. The general pattern is as follows:

Answer A if responses 1, 2, and 3 are correct.
Answer B if only 1 and 3 are correct.
Answer C if only 2 and 4 are correct.
Answer D if only 4 is correct.
Answer E if all are correct.

This format allows the answer sheet to have the same response pattern as in the "one best out of five" (A-type) questions; only one response is given, even though four true-false decisions are made.

My advice in taking these questions is to write T or F next to each statement in the exam book, thinking about them individually, then go back and determine the pattern and select the appropriate response. If you are sure one item is true or false, this obviously can help in a decision with another item because of the restricted number of possible patterns, but do not concentrate on getting help from the patterns or you will spend time worrying about patterns and not the correct answers.

Do not look for "tricks" in the questions. They are intended to be straightforward. If a trick or misleading clue inadvertently slips in, it will cause confusion that will be evident when the pattern of responses is checked after the exam is scored. An aberrant pattern of answers to a specific item in comparison to how candidates did on the remainder of the test will result in the item being eliminated from scoring. These examination questions are prepared by experienced committees helped by professionals in evaluation, and a sincere effort is made to avoid ambiguities and statements that might mislead candidates. The obvious answer is the one wanted, not a subtle possible alternative that applies to relatively few instances of the phenomenon. These questions are generally phrased better than questions prepared by individual faculty members, such as undergraduate medical school exams. I am sure, for example, that you will never see the words "never" or "always" in National Board of Medical Examiners or FLEX exams.

Some useful specific pointers follow:

1. If the question starts out with a lot of information (a long stem), skip to the end and start reading the specific answers at the end, then go back and read the long stem. This way you will know what points in the stem are pertinent to the answers that are given and will not have to reread the stem after you know the thrust of the answers.

2. Keep track of the time. Check the total number of questions in the part of the exam you are doing, how long you have, and therefore when you should be one-quarter, one-half, and three-quarters through. Do not get hung up on items you are unsure of, losing time you will need to answer questions you do know near the end. Mark questions you are uncertain about, keeping a list on the front of the exam book, and after you finish all the items you know, go back and reconsider the uncertain ones. That way you will get through the exam at least once and will be sure to get all the credit for the things you do know.

3. If you are unsure of an answer, guess. There is no penalty for guessing wrong, and remember—on true-false items, you have a 50% chance of guessing right.

4. Spot check periodically to be sure you are answering at the correct place on the answer sheet. Be sure you avoid a systematic error, marking all answers at the wrong place.

5. After you finish going through the exam once, go back and recheck the questions you marked for reconsideration during the first run through the exam. Do not go over answers you were sure about the first time; you will be tired at the end and less likely to make the correct decision on these items. Stick with your first choice. Recheck only the questions you did not answer, guessed at, or felt uncertain about, having marked them as you went through the exam the first time.

ADVICE FOR STUDYING FOR EXAMS

1. Keep in mind the level of information that the committee that drew up the question is expecting; they are not seeking a subspecialist's level of information about rare phenomena. Concentrate on the material you will need to function on your next level of training, and you will be preparing for that function and for the examination at the same time.

2. To make exam study books such as this one most useful, mark the pages with a highlighter or a pencil; write key points in the margin. Remember that importance is a personal matter: Mark what is most important to you, generally noting only points that you are not sure you know.

3. If a point is of critical clinical importance but you are sure you know it, do not mark it. You are not preparing a textbook listing important points for someone else to study; you are preparing a guide for review purposes to suit your own needs. If you know a fact, it is not important to review it for preparation for an exam, no matter how important it is clinically.

4. Keep a notebook handy as you study, preferably one with dividers for subjects. When studying, write *questions* or topic headings in the notebook, not factual answers. The questions can be brief, just enough to remind you to think of the point you want to be sure you have learned, such as "Tests for iron deficiency." Write the *location of the answer* next to the question (e.g., the page number) and highlight the answer in this book. Similarly, questions or topics can be written in the margin of this book, with the answers underlined, rather than rewriting the facts that are in the text in your marginal notes or in your notebook.

5. When reviewing, go through the questions in your notebook or those in the marginal notes you marked in this book. Stop and think of the answers or write them down briefly on separate sheets of paper (or another section of your notebook). Then check the answer your highlighted or underlined in the text. If you are satisfied that you know the point, put a check mark through the question (but do not obliterate it, so you can recheck if you want to). Mark in your notebook (e.g., with an asterisk in the margin) items you missed or are still unsure about; return to those points later and repeat the process until you are satisfied that you know the answers to all the points you marked in your notebook. Mark again any that you are still unsure about, so that when you are reviewing for the last time before the exam you can concentrate on those few points.

6. If your style is to write factual points in your notebooks and you do not want to change your habits, write them all on one side of each page, putting the questions or topic heading on the other side. When reviewing, keep the book folded so you only see the questions, think about the answers, and then look at your notes to check yourself. When reviewing, do not just read facts, but always be checking yourself to see if you know them.

7. Keep importance of the material in mind in a negative sense only: Ignore points that are not important enough to spend time on, in view of purpose and expected level of the exam and the facts you are sure you know.

ADDITIONAL INFORMATION

For more information regarding National Board Exams, write to
National Board of Medical Examiners
3930 Chestnut Street
Philadelphia, PA 19104
For FLEX exams, write to
The Federation of State Medical Boards of the United States, Inc.
Attention: Guidelines
2630 West Freeway, Suite 138
Fort Worth, TX 76102–7199;
For ECFMG exams,
3624 Market Street, Philadelphia, PA 19104–2685
Be sure you have read and understand all the informational material sent to you regarding these exams.

The authors and publishers of this study guide feel that the efforts they have expended to make this book useful to you were well spent. We hope that in using it you agree. And good luck on your examinations.

CONTENTS

1

ANATOMY

Thomas A. Weidman
Richard Yeasting

ORGANIZATION OF THE BODY

The human body is composed of four levels of structural and functional organization: cells, tissues, organs, and systems.

CELLS

Cells are the smallest of the basic structural and functional units of the body. They range in size from approximately 8 to 200 μm in diameter. Cells possess various shapes, dependent on their location within the body and concomitant function. All cells regardless of size or shape are living units and demonstrate similar basic physiological properties. Each cell obtains oxygen and other nutrients from its surrounding microenvironment, metabolizes the materials, and excretes waste products into the surrounding microenvironment. The microenvironment is composed of extracellular fluid, tissue fluid that is produced at the capillary level of the cardiovascular system. The extracellular fluid is continually being renewed as a part of the normal physiological maintenance of the homeostasis of the body. The substance of the cells (protoplasm, categorized in eukaryotic cells into cytoplasm and nucleoplasm) is separated from the surrounding microenvironment by an external cell membrane or plasmalemma. There is no cell wall as found in plants and some microorganisms. The nucleoplasm (nuclear material) is segregated from the cytoplasm by means of a fenestrated, two-layered nuclear envelope composed of plasmalemma material. Many of the functional units of the cytoplasm, organelles (small organs), are segregations of chemical microenvironments into protected, specialized units. The basic, general properties of cells include the following:

1. Motility
   a. Protoplasmic streaming
   b. Amoeboid activity
   c. Ciliary and flagellar activity
   d. Contractility
2. Irritability
3. Metabolism
   a. Anabolic
   b. Catabolic
4. Reproduction

TISSUES

A group of cells with similar morphological and functional properties is known as a tissue. The four basic tissue types are epithelial tissue, connective tissue, muscle tissue, and nervous tissue.

Epithelial tissue is a cellular tissue found as a covering of a body surface or a lining of body cavities. The glands of the body and their respective ducts are developed from epithelial tissue. A major function of the nonglandular epithelia is protection, in that the epithelial layer is in the position to determine what materials will enter or leave the general body. The epithelial tissues also have secretory and excretory functions, among others.

Connective tissue is a tissue that is composed of cells and an extracellular matrix, which consists of amorphous ground substance and connective fibers. The major function of the connective tissues is to interconnect and support other tissues.

Muscle tissue is a cellular tissue in which the individual cells are highly modified to accentuate their contractility and irritability. The major function of muscle tissue is to contract, thus producing movement in the cell and ultimately in the organism.

Nervous tissue is a cellular tissue that contains highly modified cells known as neurons. The neurons accentuate the basic properties of irritability (response to a stimulus) and conductivity (the ability to conduct an ionic, electrical impulse along extended cell processes). The neural tissue is also composed of cells that have the function of supporting and partially protecting the neurons.

ORGANS

An organ is a collection of several of the basic tissues to perform a special function in the overall economy of the body. The basic properties of the individual tissues are not altered within the organ but, in fact, combine to produce the characteristic morphological and physiological characteristics of each organ. The skin, for example, has components derived from the epithelial tissue (epidermis and its appendages), connective tissue (dermis), muscle tissue (arrector pili muscles), and nervous tissue (encapsulated and nonencapsulated sensory nerve endings).

SYSTEMS

An organization of organs that together cooperate to perform the various complex functions of the body is a system or organ system. The ten systems are muscular, skeletal, cardiovascular, respiratory, lymphatic, digestive, reproductive, endocrine, urinary, and nervous.

The **muscular system** is composed of muscle and connective tissues. The system produces movement of the body and of materials within hollow organs of the body. In the process of producing the movement, the system generates a portion of the body heat.

The **skeletal system** is composed of connective tissues. It provides protection for many of the internal organs of the body, serves as a lever system for the muscular system to work on, and serves as a reservoir for minerals within the body. It also provides a protected location for blood cell production.

The **cardiovascular system** is a tubular organ system composed primarily of muscle and connective tissues with a lining of a special epithelium, endothelium. It contains blood, which can be considered to be a very specialized form of connective tissue. The cardiovascular system functions to distribute oxygen and other nutrient materials and substances throughout the body and in so doing also collects waste materials and transports each class of materials to the appropriate locations for utilization or elimination.

The **respiratory system**, composed primarily of connective tissues and epithelium, allows atmospheric gases to be conveyed into an inner aspect (lungs) of the body, where a transfer occurs between the atmospheric gases and the gases absorbed in the blood of the cardiovascular system.

The **lymphatic system** is composed of lymphatic vessels, nodes, the spleen, and the thymus. It serves to return excess tissue fluid to the cardiovascular system, to filter the blood to remove degenerating cells and foreign materials, and to protect the body against foreign substances.

The **digestive system** is a long tubular system that has several major glands (liver, pancreas) attached to it. It is composed of epithelial, muscular, connective, and neural tissues. It provides the means by which food is transported into the inner aspect of the body, broken down (digested), and absorbed. It also serves as a means of eliminating nonabsorbed materials and other products of metabolism.

The **reproductive system** is composed of epithelial, connective, and muscular tissues to form the gonads and the ducts of the system. It serves as the site of production of gametes, the required nutritive substances, and in females the site of development of the fetus.

The **endocrine system** comprises a series of glandular structures composed of epithelium supported by connective tissues. The endocrine glands are unique in that they secrete substances (hormones) that are ultimately absorbed into the blood and circulated throughout the body instead of being released onto a surface of the body. The hormones control many of the physiological and biochemical activities of the body.

The **urinary system** is a tubular system that contains epithelial, muscular, and connective tissues. It serves to cleanse the blood, removing waste materials and moving the urine to the urinary bladder for storage and elimination.

The **nervous system** is composed of neural tissue and is supported by connective tissues. The major function of the nervous system is to coordinate the activities of the other systems and to allow the body to function within the external environment.

The organ systems work together to attempt to produce an internal environment that is limited in its range of temperature, pH, fluid content, etc. This process is producing homeostasis.

CELL STRUCTURE

The basic unit of the human body is the cell. It is constructed of protoplasm, which consists of two major types: (1) **nucleoplasm**, which is found in the nucleus and includes such components as DNA, various types of RNA, and "nuclear sap," and (2) **cytoplasm**, which is extranuclear in location. The cytoplasm contains the structural elements of the cell, the membrane-bound organelles, and the general molecular makeup of the cell. Because the genetic material is sequestered to a degree in the nucleus and does not lie free within the general cytoplasm of the cell, the human cell is described as being **eukaryotic** (true nucleus) as compared with more primitive cells such as bacteria (**prokaryotic**, before nucleus), in which the genetic material is in direct contact with the general cytoplasm and is not segregated within a nucleus.

The functional components of the eukaryotic nucleus can best be demonstrated in the interphase cell—that is, a cell that is not actively undergoing cell division. The components usually described as being intranuclear are the chromosomes, the nucleoli, and the surrounding nuclear envelope.

NUCLEAR COMPONENTS

Nuclear envelope

The nuclear envelope is composed of membranes similar to the typical unit membranes forming the plasmalemma and other membranous organelles. The nuclear envelope consists of two concentric membrane layers that are separated from each other by a space of approximately 25 nm. The inner membrane of the envelope has a portion of the nuclear fibrillar matrix and the chromatin associated with it. The outer membrane of the envelope is continuous with the endoplasmic reticulum of the cell and will often be studded with ribosomes, thus functioning as a rough endoplasmic reticulum (RER), with the space between the inner and outer membranes of the envelope serving as the lumen to receive the synthesized product.

Nuclear pores

Nuclear pores are produced by the joining of the two concentric membranes. The pores range in size from 30 to 100 nm in diameter and are spaced roughly 100 to 200 nm apart. The nuclear pores are maintained by nuclear pore complexes and may contain a fibrillar diaphragm. The nuclear pores allow the transport of macromolecules from the nucleus to the cytoplasm and vice versa, and the largest macromolecular complex that may pass through the pore is approximately 15 nm in diameter.

Nuclear matrix

The nuclear matrix serves as a structural framework for the nucleus. The matrix consists of two major portions. One of the portions, the **fibrous (nuclear) lamina**, is a thin, uniform layer of tightly intermeshed fibrillar material that is most evident as it adheres to the inner membrane of the envelope. The nuclear pore complex appears to be a portion of this peripheral material. The function of the fibrous lamina is to shape and reinforce the inner membrane of the envelope, to strengthen and secure the nuclear pore complexes, and to anchor chromatin material to the inner membrane. A second component of the nuclear matrix is a **fibrogranular network** that extends into the central portion of the nucleus from the peripheral fibrous lamina. A third component of the matrix is the framework of the **nucleolus**. The three components of the nuclear matrix are believed to play a major role in the overall structure and function of the interphase nucleus. Thus it is most likely involved in gene transcription (DNA to RNA) and in gene replication (DNA to DNA).

Chromatin

Chromatin is the material that composes chromosomes. Obviously, the DNA is a major portion of the chromatin. However, the DNA is further organized and modulated by the presence of proteins known as **histones and nonhistone proteins**. A small amount of RNA is also associated with the chromatin. The associated proteins cause the DNA double helix to assume a configuration that consists of a linear series of spherical structural subunits known as **nucleosomes**. The histones and nonhistone proteins are thought to be important in the regulation of gene expression. The formation of nucleosomes by wrapping the DNA strands around the histone proteins and other orders of supercoiling, looping, and winding produces an apparent 10,000-fold shortening of the DNA molecules, which are actually several centimeters in length, to microscopic chromosomes.

The chromatin exists in two phases in the interphase cell. One is known as **condensed**, or highly coiled chromatin, which in that form is genetically inactive. Condensed chromatin or **heterochromatin** (different chromatin) thus contrasts with the other physical form of chromatin (**euchromatin**, or true chromatin). Euchromatin has become uncoiled and is thus more available to interact in the processes of replication and transcription. Condensed chromatin is associated with the nuclear envelope (peripheral chromatin) and with the nucleolus (nucleolar-associated chromatin). The two types of condensed chromatin may be devoid of usable genetic material and serve a structural or configurational role. They may be said to be **constitutive heterochromatin**. Other heterochromatin or condensed chromatin is transcriptionally inactive and thus may be termed **facultative heterochromatin**. This chromatin is available for transcriptive use by certain triggering events playing on the cell. Except for replication of the cell cycle, approximately 90% of the chromatin in the cell may be in the condensed form.

Nuclear DNA and RNP

Nuclear DNA is composed of two long strands (polynucleotide chains) that are wound together to form a double helix. Both strands contain a backbone of alternating phosphate and deoxyribose groups. Attached to each of the sugar groups is one of four nitrogenous bases: adenine, thymine, cytosine, or guanine. The apposed nitrogenous bases link the two strands together with an obligatory pairing of the adenine and thymine groups and the cytosine and guanine groups. Group-

ings of the base pairs encode information that can later be used to produce the appropriate amino acid sequences within a polypeptide molecule. These groupings can be called **genes**. A broad definition of a gene is "a stretch of DNA that encodes for a particular RNA molecule." (The RNA molecule then encodes and organizes other molecules to synthesize a product for use within or outside the limits of the cell.) the process of encoding RNA from DNA (**transcription**) occurs within the nucleus. The RNA molecule then leaves the nucleus and enters the cytoplasm of the cell. There the RNA will organize (**translate**) amino acids into the appropriate polypeptides and other materials. In the eukaryotic cell, the process of transcription thus occurs within the nucleus and the process of translation occurs within cytoplasm of the cell.

During **replication** of DNA in the interphase nucleus, it appears that loops of interphase DNA will pass through replication complexes that are attached to the nuclear matrix. Replication thus is not a random process.

The **role of the nucleic acids** (DNA and RNA) is to organize and direct many of the synthetic activities of the cell, especially those related to polypeptide and protein synthesis. The essential differences between ribonucleic acid (RNA) and DNA include the following: (1) The sugar groups in RNA are D-ribose instead of 2-deoxy-D-ribose and (2) in RNA the nitrogenous base uracil replaces the thymine base of DNA. The obligatory pairings then consist of (DNA to RNA) G–C, C–G, T–A, A–U. There are three types of RNA: messenger RNA (mRNA), transfer RNA (tRNA), and ribosomal RNA (rRNA). In the production of a polypeptide or protein, the appropriate genetic code found as a part of the DNA is transcribed to a nucleic acid sequence known as mRNA. The transcription process occurs within the nucleus. Before the mRNA leaves the nucleus via the nuclear pores, it is modified to eliminate any of the unnecessary or spurious segments. When it is in the general cytoplasm of the cell, the mRNA will come into contact with rRNA, found in the large and small segments of ribosomes. (The RNA is originally transcribed in the nucleolus and migrated out of the nucleus into the cytoplasm, where it becomes associated with ribonucleoprotein to produce the structure known as a ribosome.) As the mRNA passes through the ribosomes it encodes them to interact with the appropriate tRNA molecules that bring the appropriate amino acids into the region, interact with the rRNA to assemble the amino acids into sequences, and then separate from the amino acid in order to attach to another amino acid molecule and begin the interaction with the rRNA again. The RNA molecule may be long enough that it will connect several ribosomes together to produce a synthetic unit known as a **polysome**. If the substance being synthesized is destined to be used within the cell, the ribosomes or polysomes will remain free within the cytoplasm. If the substance being synthesized is destined for secretion from the cell, the mRNA will contain an initial signal sequence. The initial signal sequence will cause the associated ribosomes to become attached to the membranes of the endoplasmic reticulum. The product that is synthesized at these ribosomes is then shunted into the lumen of the endoplasmic reticulum, where it is modified and transported to the Golgi apparatus. There it undergoes further modification and is ultimately released from the cell. Most mRNAs are short-lived; tRNAs and ribosomes are longer lived and are reutilized to produce more than one polypeptide or protein.

Nucleolus

The nucleolus is formed under the control of at least five different chromosome pairs. Although each of the five pairs of chromosomes could produce their own separate nucleolus, usually only one larger nucleolus exits in the cell nucleus because of the association of the nucleolar organizer regions of the chromosomes. The rRNA molecules that are transcribed from the nucleolar genes become associated with ribosomal proteins that have moved into the nucleus. This association takes place within the region of the nucleolus. The ribonucleoprotein particles leave the nucleus through the nuclear pores and are united into ribosomes within the cytoplasm. The nucleolus contains three major types of material. One of the types of material included in the nucleolus is the nucleolar organizer region of the chromosomes that bear it. The nucleolar organizer regions are surrounded by fibrillar centers that merge with the pars fibrosa. The pars fibrosa most likely is composed of newly transcribed rRNA. Other areas of the nucleolus are designated as the pars granulosa, which most likely is composed of ribosomal subunits in various stages of formation.

CELL MEMBRANES

The cell is separated from its surrounding microenvironment by the cell membrane, or plasmalemma. The material found within the nucleus is partially segregated from the remaining cytoplasm of the cell by the membranous nuclear envelope. Further, the various energy-producing and metabolic enzyme-containing organelles are functionally compartmentalized by cell membranes, which thereby segregate the functional, active molecules from the general cytoplasm. The organellar membranes also provide a structural substratum for the organization of functional entities that must be in a correct spatial arrangement in order to function properly.

The plasmalemma is one of the most important components of the cell. The plasmalemma, often described as being a unit membrane, serves as a semiselective barrier that determines what may passively enter or leave the cell. Special regions of the unit membrane play a role in the active or energy-using transport of materials across the membrane to enter or leave the cytoplasm. Channels or pores that penetrate through the membrane often selectively allow various ions to pass through the membrane. These pores and other activities that momentarily alter the nature of the unit membrane are often controlled by the interaction of molecules that are intrinsic to the membrane or attached to it with "messengers" in the microenvironment surrounding the cell. If the integrity of the plasmalemma is interrupted, the homeostasis of the cell is disrupted as the intracellular contents are allowed to come into contact with elements of the outside environment. The usual consequence of plasmalemmal disruption is cell death. The unit membrane also is found as the limiting membrane for the membrane-bound organelles. Here again, the membrane serves to organize enzymes and other constituents for proper relationships, allowing efficient operation of various chemical reactions. The membrane also segregates potentially harmful enzymes or other substances from the remainder of the cell cytoplasm. Disruption of the membranes of the various organelles will usually result in intracellular injury and often cell death.

The cell membrane of mammalian cells exhibits thicknesses that range from 7.5 to 10 nm, thus it is visible only with the electron microscope. When examined with the electron microscope, the membrane appears to be a trilaminar entity. When investigated further, the membrane is found to consist of a mixture of phospholipids, glycolipids, lipids, and proteins. The molecules are arranged so that the hydrophobic portions are oriented toward the center, or middle, of the membrane and the hydrophilic ends of the molecules are oriented outwardly. The deposition of osmium on the hydrophilic portions of the molecules produces a darker-staining layer on either side of a clear central region. Thus two molecules with hydrophobic and hydrophilic terminals arrange themselves in a bilayer in such a way as to produce a seemingly trilaminar structure. Protein molecules may be located directly within the lipid bilayer as integral proteins or may be attached to the surface of the layers, in which case they are known as peripheral proteins. The integral proteins tend to extend through the entire thickness of the bilayer and thus serve to define the boundaries of channels or pores that allow water-soluble materials such as ions to pass through the plasmalemma. Extensions of the integral proteins and glycolipids as carbohydrate moieties reach into the space external to the membrane and thus participate in the formation of the glycocalyx or cell coat. The various molecules that compose the plasmalemma are not locked into place by strong chemical bonding but are able to shift around to a degree. Thus the membrane is sometimes described as being a fluid mosaic.

Some ions (Na^+, K^+, and Ca^+) are able to pass through the plasmalemma via the protein channels or pores. Water is also able to diffuse across the membrane. Larger ions and molecules, however, are not able to pass through the membrane but must be "packaged" to be moved into or out of the cell. The process of packaging material to bring substances into the cell is known as **endocytosis**. One form of endocytosis is termed **fluid phase endocytosis** or **pinocytosis** (cell drinking). Small invaginations of the membrane are formed. They ultimately pinch off from the plasmalemma to form small vesicles containing extracellularly derived fluid. These pinocytotic vesicles may be transported through the cytoplasm to another surface of the cell, where the vesicle is capable of fusing with the cell-limiting membrane and opening in such a manner as to release the vesicular contents to the outside. In this manner, fluids and other substances may be transported across a cellular layer. The other major form of endocytosis is known as **receptor-mediated endocytosis**. In this type of uptake of extracellular substance, material that will ultimately be taken into the cell binds with an outward-extending receptor portion of various membrane molecules. The binding causes the receptor-bearing molecules to aggregate, if they were not previously aggregated. The aggregation of molecules induces the formation of coated pits as clathrin accumulates on the cytoplasmic side of the membrane. The clathrin directs the enlargement of the pit into a vesicle that separates from the limiting membrane through the action of reformation of the clathrin molecules. The resultant structure is known as a coated vesicle because of the presence of clathrin on the outside (cytoplasmic) surface. This vesicle may move through the cytoplasm of the cell and join with another cellular organelle or it might serve as a transport vesicle to another outer cell surface. A third form of endocytosis known as phagocytosis (cell eating) involves the incorporation, within vesicles, of particulate material into the cell.

ORGANELLES

Mitochondria

Mitochondria are membrane-bound organelles in which most of the cell's energy is produced. The mitochondrion consists of two membranous vesicles, one placed inside the other. The membrane of the inner vesicle, the inner membrane, is thrown into ridge- or finger-like projections, cristae, that extend into the intercristal space or luminal area of the inner vesicle, which contains an amorphous material known as the mitochondrial matrix. The coenzymes, cytochromes, and other components of the electron transport system of the citric acid cycle (Krebs cycle) are located in a relatively sequential order on the inner surface of the inner vesicle membrane, adjacent to the matrix. The enzymes for the citric acid cycle and fatty acid beta-oxidation are found within the mitochondrial matrix. A small cleft separates the inner mitochondrial membrane from the outer membrane. The surface of the outer membrane is not amplified in the manner of the inner layer. The amorphous mitochondrial matrix contained within the mitochondria is rich in protein and contains small amounts of (mitochondrial) DNA as well as the three types of RNA (messenger, transfer, and ribosomal). The matrix also contains granules that are rich in calcium and magnesium. The number of the mitochondria tends to be constant for any given cell type. The number and configuration of the mitochondria per cell are directly related to the metabolic activity of the cell. There also seems to be a correlation between the synthetic activity of the cell and the configuration of the cristae.

Ribosomes

Ribosomes are small electron-dense cytoplasmic particles composed of RNA. They measure approximately 20×30 nm and are composed of four types of rRNA and almost 80 different proteins. The proteins and RNA are organized into two subunits, one small and one large, that together compose a ribosome. The ribosomes may be found as individual units scattered throughout the cytoplasm of the cell, may be joined together by mRNA to form polyribosomes (polysomes) that are free within the cytoplasm, or may be found attached to the membranes of the endoplasmic reticulum. The free ribosomes and polysomes synthesize proteins that are destined to remain within the cytoplasm of the cell or become a portion of the unit membrane that composes many of the organelles of the cell. Proteins that are destined to be segregated from the cytoplasm or secreted from the cell are synthesized by the ribosomal units that are attached to the endoplasmic reticulum. The free and attached ribosomes essentially are chemically identical.

Endoplasmic reticulum

The endoplasmic reticulum is composed of a network (reticulum) of tubular, vesicular, or saccular membranous (unit membrane) structures. The primary functions of the two forms (smooth-walled and rough-walled) of endoplasmic reticulum are (1) segregation of newly synthesized proteins that are destined for secretion from the cell or must be sequestered from the cytoplasm, (2) proteolysis (alteration) of newly

synthesized proteins, (3) core glycosylation, (4) posttranslational modification of amino acids, (5) assembly of multichain proteinacious compounds, (6) lipid synthesis, and (7) degradation of endogenous and exogenous substances.

Rough endoplasmic reticulum (rER) is prominent in cells that are specialized for protein synthesis and secretion, such as fibroblasts, plasma cells, and pancreatic acinar cells. The rER is characterized by the presence of ribosomes and polysomes being attached to the cytoplasmic surface of the reticular membranes. The rER functions to segregate protein destined for the outside of the cell from the cytoplasm. The substance that enters the cisternae of the rER is not necessarily identical with the substance that is ultimately released from the cell because of events that occur within the rER. As noted before, these include glycosylation of glycoprotein, synthesis of phospholipids, assembly of the chains of multichained proteins, and posttranslational changes of polypeptides. It should be noted that protein synthesis is initiated on polysomes and then interrupted by the insertion of a signal sequence of amino acids. Ribophorins then bind the ribosomes and attached amino acid sequences to the cytoplasmic surface of the endoplasmic reticulum. The ribophorins also serve to form hydrophilic channels through the hydrophobic membrane so that the proteinaceous substance being synthesized on the cytoplasmic surface of the endoplasmic reticulum may enter into the cisternae or lumen of the reticulum. Once the polypeptide being assembled on the polysomes is injected into the lumen of the endoplasmic reticulum, the signal sequence of amino acids is cleaved from the major unit by an enzyme known as signal peptidase, which is found on the luminal surface of the reticulum.

Smooth endoplasmic reticulum (sER) differs from rER in two ways: (1) It does not have associated ribosomes or polysomes on its surface, and (2) the membranous reticulum tends to be more tubular in profile than the usually flattened, stacked profiles of cisternae of rER. The membranes of the sER are synthesized in the rER. The sER functions as the site of location of the enzymes essential for synthesis of steroid hormones and thus is plentiful in steroid-producing cells. The smooth membranous reticulum is also the site of oxidation, conjugation, and methylation (metabolic breakdown or neutralization) of hormones or toxic substances as seen in liver cells. It also functions in the metabolic processing of glycogen in the liver cells. (It should be noted that the microsomal portion of cell homogenates represents disrupted fragments of the sER. A form of sER is used in muscle cells to assist in the control of the contractile activity of the cell and has become known as the sarcoplasmic reticulum.)

Golgi apparatus

The Golgi apparatus or Golgi complex is a portion of the membranous cytoplasmic organelle system that is especially important in modifying the products that are synthesized in the rER and sER. This function is most evident in cells that are producing products for secretion from the cell.

The main structural unit of the Golgi complex is the **Golgi saccule**. This membranous unit does not bind ribosomes. The Golgi saccules are usually combined to produce a **Golgi stack**. The saccules within the stack are joined at their periphery by anastomotic tubules. If the cell contains more than one Golgi stack, the stacks are united by tubules also.

The functional correlations to the morphology of the Golgi complex are as follows. Transfer vesicles containing material synthesized in the RER move from the endoplasmic reticulum to the convex *cis* face of the complex. Here the membranes of the complex and vesicle merge and the vesicular contents are released into the lumen of the complex. Within the Golgi complex the secretory products may be chemically modified by the processes of glycosylation and sulfation, to name two. It is apparent that there is an orderly processing of the product as it passes through the Golgi complex, in that the various enzymes responsible for the chemical alteration are situated in definite locations in the complex, not randomly distributed. The material that is being processed may be transported from region to region within the complex either by the anastomosing tubules connecting the various saccules and/or by vesicular transport. As the Golgi complex functions, it sorts the products that it ultimately releases in two major groups. One group is the material that will ultimately be secreted from the cell. This group of compounds is packaged into secretory vesicles. The other major group of compounds that is released by the Golgi apparatus and packaged into membranous vesicles is the acid hydrolases that are used within the cell and are stored in the form of lysosomes.

The membranes of the endoplasmic reticulum transfer vesicles, and other vesicles are usually added to the *cis* face of the Golgi complex. The *trans* face of the complex is a site of vesicle formation and thus represents an area of net loss of membrane from the complex. It is possible that during the normal functioning of the complex that new saccules are being formed on the *cis* face of the stack as transfer vesicles accumulate. As new saccules are added, the preexisting saccules are shifted, relatively, toward the *trans* face. The oldest saccules, located at the *trans* face, serve as the source of membrane to form secretory vesicles, lysosomal vesicles, and other intermediate vesicles derived from the Golgi. In this way, the Golgi complex serves as a center for recycling or reutilization of a good portion of the membranes of the cell. There has been additional speculation that the Golgi complex may also serve to modify or repair some of the constituent portions of the membranes within the cell.

Secretory vesicles are formed by the *trans* face of the Golgi and contain the product that has been processed by the complex. When the secretory vesicles are first formed, the contents are relatively less electron dense than older vesicles. The difference in the electron density between the two stages of vesicles and the size of the vesicles can be partially explained by the extraction of fluid from the storage vesicle. The earliest forms of vesicles are thus known as condensing vesicles. The secretory vesicles ultimately are carried to the surface of the cell. At this time, the plasmalemma and vesicular membranes fuse. The plasmalemma opens at the point of fusion, and the contents of the vesicle are released to the exterior of the cell.

Lysosomes

Lysosomes are membrane-bound vesicles that segregate hydrolytic enzymes from other components of the cytoplasm, thus preventing digestion and degradation of the cell from the inside. The enzymes contained within the lysosomes are used by the cell to digest any exogenous particulate material or macromolecular components that might have been ingested from the immediate environment. The enzymes may also be used by the cell to digest or break down macromolecular components or organelles that are no longer useful to the cell. A lysosome that has not been involved in a digestive process is known as a primary lysosome. A secondary lysosome is produced by the fusion of a primary lysosome with a vesicle containing ingested material or intracellular material or organelle to be degraded, thus producing a larger vesicle in which the digestive process will occur.

Coated vesicles

Coated vesicles are predominantly used in the process of receptor-mediated endocytosis. The protein clathrin is found to collect on the cytosol (inner) surface of the plasmalemma. As it does so, the clathrin and other lower-molecular-weight proteins initially produce a hexagonal lattice composed primarily of three-armed subunits known as **triskelions**. Some of the triskelions form pentagons as well. Under appropriate stimuli, the proportion of pentagonal arrays within the lattice increases and the lattice shifts from a planar form to a curved form, with the associated cell membrane following suit. The process of coated vesicle formation may also take place with the plasmalemma without the initiation of receptor activation, as well as in conjunction with the Golgi complex and the endoplasmic reticulum.

Cilia and flagella

Cilia and flagella are cellular organelles that allow a cell to move in relationship to its environment. Cilia also allow a cell to move portions of its immediate environment in relationship to a stable cell, the more common situation in multicellular organisms. The cilia are also utilized by certain specialized cells to function as sensory transducers. Cilia are motile, hairlike processes that are approximately 10 μm long and about 0.2 μm in diameter. They extend from the apical surface of the cell and thus form a layer on the cell surface. A cell thus may have many cilia on its surface. Each cilium has a basal body at its attached, cytoplasmic end. The basal body is very similar to a centriole in structure and, in fact, is most likely formed under the direction of the centrioles. In preparation for the formation of cilia, the centrioles form centriolar organizers near the original pair of centrioles. The centriolar organizers in turn direct the formation of numerous procentrioles. The procentrioles migrate to the cell surface and become basal bodies. Microtubules growing outward from the basal body produce the microtubular skeleton of the cilium. The basal body also generates inwardly growing microtubules that are known as rootlets and laterally extending tubules known as the basal foot.

The microtubular framework of the cilium is slightly different from that of the centriole or basal body. The microtubules of both the cilium and the basal body are composed of tubulin dimers; but where the basal body has nine peripheral **triplets** of tubules, the cilium has nine peripherally located **doublets** of tubules. The microtubular doublets in the cilium also possess side arms composed of **dynein**. The basal body does not have a well-formed axial element, but the cilium contains a pair of singlet microtubules forming an axial structure. Thus the shaft of the cilium, the axoneme, consists of nine peripheral doublets and two central singlets of microtubules surrounded by the plasmalemma, whereas the basal body consists of nine peripheral triplets and no definite central microtubular array surrounded by cytoplasm. Under the ATP-ase activity of the dynein sidearms of the doublets, a sliding movement occurs within the doublets to produce the intrinsic beating of the cilium and interactions of the peripheral doublets while the central pair of singlets apply the forces necessary to forcefully bend the axoneme. Each cilium produces an effective stroke in which it is straight and relatively rigid and a recovery stroke in which it bends and regains the starting position. A **flagellum** is basically very similar to an individual cilium, only much longer and usually limited to one per cell.

CELL DIVISION

Mammalian cells usually increase their numbers by the process of cell division known as **mitosis** (Fig. 1-1). In this process there is a duplication and subsequent segregation of genetic material that is then followed by division of the cytoplasm of the original cell into two daughter cells, each of which will contain the proper amount and type of genetic material. Although mitosis is a continuous process that normally occurs within the cell cycle, for descriptive purposes it can be divided into four sequential phases. These phases have been named **prophase, metaphase, telophase,** and **anaphase.** The process of mitosis usually requires approximately 1 to 1½ hours to complete.

Before the process of mitosis can be initiated, several events must occur within the cell. One of the events takes place during the **S phase** of the cell cycle preceding the mitotic division. At this time, the individual chromosomes (s-chromosomes, single chromosomes) replicate themselves so that the premitotic cell contains 46 d-chromosomes (double or replicated chromosomes). During the division process, half of the complement of chromosomes will move to one cell, the other to the other half, so that each newly forming cell will receive an identical set of chromosomes. The other event that must occur before mitosis can take place is the replication of the centrioles. During the

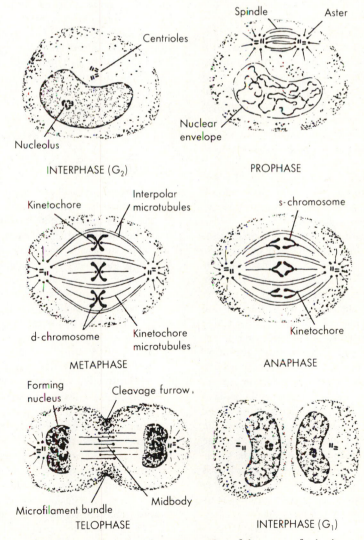

Figure 1-1.   Diagrammatic representation of the stages of mitosis.

nonmitotic phases of the cell cycle, each cell contains a pair of small, closely associated structures known as **centrioles**. These structures are 0.5 μm long and 0.25 μm in diameter. The centrioles are composed of nine longitudinal bundles of microtubules. The microtubules of the centrioles are composed of dimers of the protein tubulin. Each of the nine peripheral bundles of tubulin are composed of three microtubular structures. The so-called triplet microtubules are embedded in a very fine fibrillar material. The nine peripheral triplet bundles are organized around an axial component and seemingly are attached to it by the fibrillar material.

During **prophase**, the two pairs of centrioles separate and migrate to opposite ends (poles) of the cell that is about to divide. There the centrioles initiate the formation of microtubules that begin to radiate away from the centrioles. The early grouping of microtubules being organized by the centrioles is known as an aster (star). This early stage of microtubular development is occurring as the centrioles move apart from each other. As the centrioles continue to separate, the microtubules that are developing connect the pairs and become known as interpolar or continuous microtubules and soon constitute a spindle-shaped mass known as the mitotic spindle. At the same time as the spindle is being formed, the chromosomes are condensing and thus becoming more apparent. As prophase proceeds, the nuclear envelope and nucleolus disappear. The condensed d-chromosomes become associated with the mitotic spindle, especially with a second set of microtubules that is developing from the centrioles. This second set of microtubules does not pass from one centriole to the other, but extends from the end of the spindle to the kinetochore region of the chromosomal centromeres. The kinetochore or chromosomal microtubules create a dynamic equilibrium that arranges the d-chromosomes in an equatorial ring relative to the mitotic spindle.

The next phase, **metaphase**, is characterized by the organization of the chromosomes into a ring-like structure known as the metaphase plate, in which the chromosomes are randomly positioned in a single ring.

With further development, the cell moves into **anaphase**. This phase is characterized by the splitting of the centromere that has been holding the d-chromosomes together, and thus the s-chromosomes are free to move independently toward the opposite ends of the mitotic spindle. Although the exact mechanism producing the separation is uncertain, several facets of the spindle activity are known. One facet is that at this time the kinetochore microtubules are undergoing a net disassembly at the centriolar end and are thus becoming shorter. At the same time, the interpolar microtubules are continuing to be synthesized and thus are undergoing a net lengthening. This lengthening moves the two centriolar ends of the spindle farther and farther apart. The lengthening of the interpolar microtubules producing a further separation of the centrioles, which are serving as anchoring points for the shortening chromosomal microtubules, thus separates the s-chromosomes that were forming the mitotic ring. The process continues until one set of s-chromosomes has ultimately migrated (been pulled) to each end of the mitotic spindle. Thus the s-chromosomes are segregated from each other.

At the end of anaphase or the beginning of **telophase**, a constriction begins to form in the middle of the elongated, dividing cell. This constriction is oriented transversely in relationship to the mitotic spindle. This cleavage furrow is most likely produced by the interaction of actin that is associated with the cell membrane and other contractile proteins within the cytoplasm. For a short time, the two separating cells remain united by a midbody that consists of the interpolar microtubules passing through a very restricted intercellular connection produced by the ever deepening cleavage furrow. When the cells ultimately separate, the midbody may remain with one of the daughter cells.

After the two daughter cells have separated, the chromosomes begin to extend and chromatin granules appear. The nuclear envelope is reassembled, and the nucleolus is reconstituted. The cell then begins to synthesize cytoplasmic components to reestablish the usual size and nuclear/cytoplasmic ratio for the type of cell.

It should be noted that DNA replication may take place without a subsequent cell division, thus producing a polyploid cell. It should also be noted that it is possible to have DNA replication followed by nuclear division without subsequent cytoplasmic division (karyokinesis without cytokinesis). This is one means by which multinucleated cells may be produced.

The process of mitosis may be affected by ionizing radiation and by drugs. Ionizing radiation may produce changes within the individual chromosomes or by altering the structure and function of the centrioles and mitotic spindle. The synthesis of microtubules found within the mitotic spindle may be inhibited by durgs such as colchicine and vinblastine (vincristine). Because of the antimitotic activity of the drugs, they have been used extensively in attempts to control the mitotic activity of neoplastic (cancer) cells.

TISSUES

EPITHELIAL TISSUE

Epithelial tissues are composed of closely aggregated polyhedral cells that have very little intercellular substance between them. Intercellular connections are numerous and important in the function of the tissues, as the cellular sheets cover the surfaces of the body and line its cavities.

Epithelial tissues have the following principal functions in the body:

1. Covering or lining surfaces: skin, intestinal epithelial cells, endothelium of vasculature
2. Absorption of material: intestinal epithelial cells, renal tubule cells
3. Secretion: simple or multicellular glands
4. Reception of sensation: neuroepithelium
5. Contractility: myoepithelium

Epithelial tissues are derived from all three embryonic germ layers. Those that are situated on the outer surface of the body are derived from **ectoderm**. Those lining the digestive tract and structures derived from it originate from the **endodermal** layer. The linings of body cavities, blood vessels, urinary tract, and reproductive systems are derived from the **mesodermal** germ layer of the embryo.

General characteristics of epithelial tissues

The shapes of the epithelial cells are largely determined by the space into which they must fit. Therefore, most of the cells surface. The profile of the cells (seen from the side) will vary according to the functional requirements of the specific region and will range from very flattened cells or squamous to cells that are about as tall as they are wide (cuboidal), to those whose height is greater than the width (columnar). The nucleus of the epithelial cell tends to be elliptical and is usually placed in the central portion of the cell. Since the cell boundaries often are not clearly demarcated in light microscopic examination because of interdigitation between cells, the position of the nuclei can be useful in determining the morphological characteristics of the tissue. This is especially important in determining the numbers of layers of cells, which range from 1 to 20 layers, in the epithelial membrane.

Basal lamina

The basal lamina is found at the interface between the epithelial tissues and the related connective tissues that support them. The basal lamina is evident in electron microscopic sections, where a portion of it appears as a 20- to 100-nm layer of delicate interlacing fibrils (Fig. 1-2). This layer is known as the **lamina densa**. Between the lamina densa and the basal epithelial cells is situated an electron-lucent layer known as the **lamina lucida** or the **lamina rara**. A similar layer (lamina lucida) is sometimes seen on the opposite side of the lamina densa as well. The major constituents of the basal lamina are type IV collagen, a glycoprotein called laminin, and the proteoglycan heparan sulfate. These substances have been shown to be secreted by the epithelial tissues. Small reticular fibrils of connective tissue origin often are found to be embedded in the connective tissue side of the basal lamina and thus create a third layer, the **lamina reticularis**. These reticular fibers help in anchoring the epithelial layer to the underlying connective tissues. It should be noted that basal lamina material is also produced by muscle, adipose tissue, and Schwann's cells and is found in association with them. The basal lamina provides a selective barrier between the connective tissues and other cells. The basal lamina also influences the activity of the cells related to it, such as the control of epithelial cell location and movement.

The term **basement membrane** is used to denote the combination of basal lamina reticularis. The staining characteristics are related primarily to the properties of the reticular fibers.

Connections between cells

Epithelial cells exhibit very strong cohesive properties. These properties are partially related to glycoproteins that are some of the integral membrane proteins and a small amount of intercellular proteoglycans. The cohesive properties are partially dependent on the presence of calcium ions in the microenvironment. The cohesion between adjacent cells is strengthened by intercellular junctions that are present on the lateral boundaries of the cells. These junctions not only serve as sites of adhesion between cells to maintain the integrity of the layer but also serve as seals to prevent the movement of materials through the intercellular (paracellular) space. Some forms of junctions also allow for intercellular communication (Fig. 1-3).

Junctional complexes are most evident in the epithelial layers that serve as absorptive surfaces, such as the intestinal epithelium. The portion of the complex that is situated nearest to the lumen is the tight junction or **zonula occludens**. In these junctions, the outer laminae of the plasmalemmae of adjacent cells are fused together. Thus in these band-like or collar-like junctions the paracellular space is obliterated and the fused plasmalemmae appear to form a five-layered structure.

Situated near but on the side away from the lumen of the zonula occludens is the second element of the junctional complex, the **zonula adherens**. The adjacent plasmalemmae are not fused in this band-like junction but maintain their three-layered appearance. The intercellular space is usually wider than the usual 20 nm. The cytoplasmic surface of the junctional membranes demonstrates plaques composed of myosin, tropomyosin, alpha-actinin, and vinculin. Numerous actin-containing microfilaments insert into the plaques. The two zonular forms of junctions relate to the microfilamentous terminal web area of the apical cytoplasm and form the terminal bars of light microscopy.

The third element of the junctional complex is the **macula adherens** or desmosome. These junctions are also found elsewhere on the lateral cell walls, as well as on cells that do not demonstrate the complexes. The desmosome is a spot or plaque attachment. In many desmosomes, a dense line of material is found in the intercellular space. The cytoplasmic surface of the membranes is related to a plaque to which many of the tonofilaments of the cytoskeleton connect. Extending

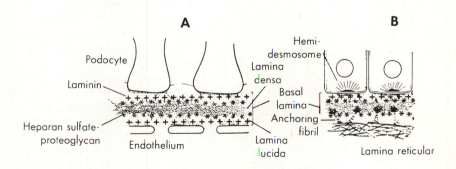

Figure 1-2.   Types of basement membranes. (*A*) The type of basement membrane that consists of only a basal lamina. The basal lamina is divided into a central **lamina densa** with a **lamina lucida** (**lamina rara**) on either side. (*B*) The more complex basement membrane underlying most epithelia.

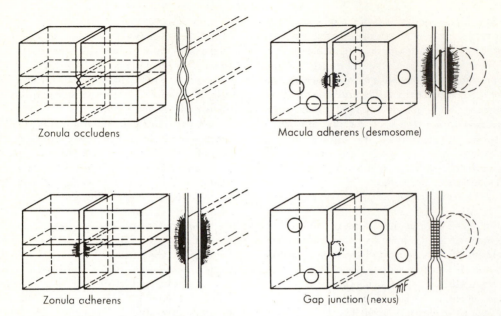

Zonula occludens

Macula adherens (desmosome)

Zonula adherens

Gap junction (nexus)

Figure 1-3. Different types of cell junctions. Note that the zonula occludens not only holds adjacent cells together but provides an effective barrier to the passage of fluids between the cells.

between the plaques to two adjacent cells are transmembrane linker filaments that bridge through the intercellular cleft and connect the two cells. These filaments are most likely responsible for the dense line found in the intercellular space. The desmosome is created by portions of two adjacent cells; one cell's contribution, a hemidesmosome, is found in regions where the basal cell membrane relates to the basal lamina.

A fourth type of junction is the nexus or **gap junction**. These junctions provide for intercellular communications and most likely do not assist in strengthening the cell-to-cell adhesion. In the nexus, integral membrane proteins form six-membered connexons. Connexons of adjacent cells align to form hydrophilic channels between the cells. Cytoplasmic ions and small molecules may pass from cell to cell through these channels.

Apical specializations

The apical aspect of many epithelial cells is modified to provide for specific functions. These specializations include microvilli, stereocilia, and cilia.

Classification of epithelia

Epithelial tissues are classified according to their structure and function. One level of classification considers the **covering epithelia** and the **glandular epithelia**. Covering epithelia are the forms of epithelia that cover or line structures. Glandular epithelia are epithelial forms that secrete substances onto a surface of the body or into the tissue fluid surrounding the cell. Glandular epithelium consists of specialized cells that secrete a fluid that is different from blood or tissue fluid. This usually involves synthesis of the macromolecules. Many of the cells will demonstrate membrane-bound storage vesicles containing the macromolecules until the gland is stimulated to release them in the production of the secretory product.

The glands that represent aggregations of glandular epithelium can be classified in a number of ways (Table 1-1).

Protein-secreting cells demonstrate all of the types of organelles necessary for the synthesis, condensation, storage, and ultimately the release of the secretory product. Secretion is usually by the process of exocytosis.

Polypeptide-secreting cells (APUD—amine precursor uptake and decarboxylation) produce and/or store epinephrine, norepinephrine, serotonin, etc. In an epithelial layer, some of the APUD cells will be in contact with the luminal surface while others will not be. When in an epithelial layer, the cells usually affect the immediately surrounding cells by means of a paracrine type of control. When in a glandular structure, the APUD cells usually function as endocrine cells by releasing their product into the circulatory system for distribution throughout the body.

Steroid-secreting cells are exceptionally rich in sER. The mitochondria have tubular cristae rather then the more common shelf-like cristae. The mitochondrial cristae and the sER contain the enzymes necessary to cleave cholesterol side chains to produce pregnenolone, and they assist in further reactions to produce steroid hormones. There is very little to no storage of steroid hormones in the steroid-producing cells; the hormone is synthesized on demand. There is, however, some intracellular storage of hormone precursors.

Stratification

The tissue layers can be further classified as being a layer of cells that is one cell in thickness (**simple**) or being composed of multiple layers of cells (**stratified**). The stratified epithelial layers are named according to the morphological configuration of the cells on the free surface of the membrane—that is, that farthest away from the basement membrane. Thus a layer that is composed of several layers of cells with the free surface cells being flattened or squamous in morphology would be classified as a stratified squamous epithelium, even though the cells in the deeper layers of the membrane might be cuboidal or even columnar in shape.

Table 1-1. Ways of Classifying Glandular Epithelium

Area into which the secretion is released

1. *Exocrine:* Secretion is released onto the surface of an epithelial layer or into a duct system that ultimately terminates on the surface. The duct system usually indicates the pattern of ingrowth of the gland during development and often indicates the point of origin from the surface epithelium.
2. *Endocrine:* Secretory elements have lost connection with the surface of the body. The secretory products are released into the interstitial space and usually are quickly taken into an immediately adjacent capillary or sinusoid (large capillary). The secretion then circulates throughout the body to affect cells that are far removed from the secreting cell.
3. *Paracrine:* Secretory cells release their secretory product into the interstitial space, but the secretion is not taken into the circulatory system. Instead, it remains in the immediate vicinity and affects the surrounding cells.
4. *Neurocrine:* Secretory cells release secretions that immediately affect adjacent cells. A specialized intercellular relationship usually exists between the cells, such as a synapse.

Pattern of duct branching

1. *Simple:* One unbranched duct (a tube of epithelial cells) leads from the surface to the secretory unit (collection of secretory cells).
2. *Compound:* The duct system branches as it proceeds from the surface orifice to the secretory units.

Mode of secretion

1. *Merocrine:* Secretory material is released from cells with no loss of cell cytoplasm. This is the predominant mode of secretion. An example: pancreatic acinar cell.
2. *Holocrine:* An entire cell, which may be highly modified, is released as a portion of the secretory material. An example: sebacous glands.
3. *Apocrine:* A small portion of the cell cytoplasm is budded off with the secretory product. This mode of secretion is almost entirely limited to the lactating mammary gland.

Type of secretion

1. *Serous:* Secretory product is rather watery. It usually is high in proteinaceous material. The cells will demonstrate abundant organelles necessary for protein secretion, such as RER, Golgi, etc.
2. *Mucous:* Secretory product is viscous. The product will contain more glycoprotein moities than serous secretions. The product is stored in large vesicles, which occupy the majority of the cell cytoplasm. The product is often dissolved during routine histological processing, giving the cell a lighter, more frothy appearance in comparison with the serous secreting cell.

Shape of the secretory unit

1. *Alveolar or acinar:* Secretory cell groups are arranged in somewhat circular or flask-shaped collections.
2. *Tubular:* Secretory cells are arranged in a tubular or cylindrical array.

The term **pseudostratified** is used to describe a simple (one cell thick) epithelium that is composed of cells of several heights. In this type, all of the cells are in contact with the basal lamina, but because of the differences in height all of the cells do not reach the surface. The nuclei are located at about the middle of the height of the cells. When the cells are viewed, the nuclei give the appearance of a stratified epithelium.

Transitional epithelium is a term that can be applied to two types of stratified cuboidal epithelium. The term is usually used to describe the epithelium that lines the lumen of the ureter and urinary bladder. The cells of the epithelium here are able to change their dimensions in such a way as to accommodate for the ever changing state of distension of the hollow viscera. When the organ is empty (collapsed), the epithelium is rather thick and the surface cells are markedly bulging; when distended, the layer is much thinner and all of the cells are flattened. The term is sometimes also used to designate that stratified cuboidal epithelium that is found in the transition from a simple columnar epithelium to a stratified squamous type.

CONNECTIVE TISSUES

Connective tissues serve to provide and maintain the form of the body. Noncellular material that is incorporated into the formation of this tissue binds the cells and tissues together. These noncellular materials consist of an amorphous ground substance, protein fibers, and the ubiquitous tissue fluid that is found primarily in the form of bound water of hydration in these tissues. The noncellular matrix (ground substance, fibers, and tissue fluid) surrounds the connective tissue cells and is produced and maintained by them.

Connective tissues not only provide for the obvious structural integrity of the body but also serve as the medium for exchange of nutrients and waste products between the blood and cells of the body. The connective tissues are also the medium in which the immunologically competent cells and the phagocytic cells of the body function.

The amorphous ground substance is colorless, transparent, and homogeneous. It fills the spaces between the fibers and cells of connective tissue. It is composed primarily of glycosaminoglycans and glycoproteins. An older term for glycosaminoglycans is acid mucopolysaccharides. These materials are composed primarily of glucosamine, galactosamine, gluconic acid, or iduronic acid. These usually bind with a protein to create a proteoglycan molecule. In the proteoglycan molecules, the carbohydrate portions account for 80 to 90% of the weight. Because of ionic characteristics, the proteoglycans can bind large numbers of cations (usually sodium) and are intensely hydrated.

Hyaluronic acid (the only nonsulfated compound), dermatan sulfate, chondroitin sulfate, keratan sulfate, and heparan sulfate are the major proteoglycans of connective tissue. Dermatan sulfate is usually found in conjunction with type I collagen fibers in the tendons, ligaments, and dermis. Chondroitin sulfate is found in conjunction with type II collagen in cartilage. Heparan sulfate is associated with type III collagen or reticular fibers.

Structural glycoproteins have importance in cellular interactions related to connective tissue. Fibronectin serves to help attach cells to the basal lamina and to each other. (Cancer cells do not produce fibronectin.) Laminin, found in the basal lamina, assists in the adhesion of cells to the type IV collagen found there. Chondronectin assists in chondrocyte adhesion to type II collagen in cartilage.

The fibroblastic connective tissue cells produce not only the substance of the matrix but also the fibrous component. Three types of proteinaceous fibers are recognized in connective tissue: collagenous, reticular (a form of collagenous), and elastic. These fibers are not distributed equally in all connective tissues. The predominant fiber type determines the nature of the connective tissue in many respects. Collagen is the protein from which collagenous and reticular fibers are formed. The principal amino acids are glycine, proline, and hydroxyproline. Hydroxyproline and hydroxylysine are characteristic of collagen. Five forms of collagen have been demonstrated. Some of the forms are produced not only by the recognized connective tissue cells but also by muscle cells, Schwann's cells, and hepatocytes. Each tropocollagen molecule (building unit of collagen) is composed of three subunits (alpha-peptide chains) that form a helix. The variations in combinations of the alpha peptides determine the different characteristics of the collagen types.

The common locations of the types of collagen are as follows:

Collagen type I: tendons, ligaments, dermis, bone
Collagen type II: cartilage
Collagen type III: reticular fibers
Collagen type IV: basal laminae
Collagen type V: embryonic tissues

Collagen is formed in the following manner:

1. Polypeptide alpha chains are assembled on polyribosomes of rER and injected into the endoplasmic reticulum.
2. Hydroxylation of proline and lysine occurs in the endoplasmic reticulum.
3. Hydroxylysine undergoes glycosylation.
4. The alpha chains with attached registration peptides forming procollagen are secreted from the cell.
5. Procollagen molecules are stripped of registration peptides and are altered into insoluble tropocollagen.
6. Tropocollagen molecules polymerize with others to produce collagen fibrils, probably with the interaction of surrounding proteoglycans.
7. Fibrillar structure is locked by the formation of covalent cross-linkages between adjacent tropocollagen molecules.

The tropocollagen molecules are 280 nm in length, and when overlapped with adjacent molecules a pattern of striation is produced that repeats each 64 nm when viewed with the electron microscope after appropriate staining. The synthesis and polymerization of collagen are dependent on several factors. Several of the factors are genetically determined and represent defects in enzyme activity or improper translation actions. Vitamin C, ascorbic acid, is important in the hydroxylation of proline. The effect of vitamin C was historically recognized through the prevention of scurvy (collagen disease) by adding citrus fruits to the diets of sailors.

Collagen fibrils are united to produce larger and larger bundles, which then are known as fibers. Collagen fibers are inelastic but flexible.

Reticular fibers are a form of collagen fiber (type III) that range in diameter from 0.5 to 2 μm. Reticular fibers are important in providing the stroma (supporting latticework of fibers) for many of the glandular organs and hematopoietic organs, as well as surrounding muscle and nerve fibers.

Elastic fibers and lamina are composed of the amorphous protein elastin. When synthesized and released into connective tissue spaces, the protein tends to form laminae, or layers. However, when it is formed in association with microfibrils into an encircling sheath, the elastin and microfibrils are organized into elastic fibers. The elastic tissue is able to stretch 150% and return to its original length. Elastic tissue is produced not only by connective tissue cells but also by muscle cells.

Cells

The cells of connective tissue include mesenchymal cells, fibroblasts and fibrocytes, chondroblasts and chondrocytes, osteoblasts and osteocytes, macrophages, leukocytes, plasma cells, mast cells, adipose cells, endothelial cells, and mesothelial cells.

Fibroblasts are the most common type of connective tissue cell. They are responsible for the production and maintenance of the ordinary connective tissue matrix (ground substance and fibers). After it has produced the matrix, which will vary according to the function and location in the body, the fibroblast becomes somewhat smaller and is sometimes referred to as a fibrocyte, in keeping with the terminology of cartilage and bone.

Connective tissue **macrophages** (10 to 30 μm in diameter) are one form of phagocytic cell derived from a precursor marrow cell that produces monocytes. The monocytes migrate into the respective tissues and organs (connective tissue in this case) and become a rather stable population of tissue phagocytes. The phagocytes serve to ingest material (usually foreign in origin) and to digest it. They participate in the immune responses of the body (antigen-antibody) and in the cell-mediated responses to infection.

Mast cells are located in the dermis, digestive tract, and respiratory tract, among other sites. These 20- to 30-μm-diameter cells possess many basophilic granules in the cytoplasm. These secretory granules are 0.3 to 0.5 μm in diameter and are heterogeneous in consistency. It has been shown that there are two populations of cells, one containing heparin in the granules, the other containing chondroitin sulfate. Although mast cells are found almost entirely in connective tissue, it has been shown that they originate in the bone marrow.

The surface of the plasmalemma contains specific receptors for IgE. When the immunoglobulin is affected by appropriate antigens, the cell degranulates, releasing histamine, heparin, leukotrienes, and ECF-A. These pharmacologically active materials affect the cells in the immediate microenvironment (paracrine effect).

Types of connective tissues

The cells, ground substance, and fibers of connective tissue are organized into classes or types of tissue (Table 1-2).

Connective tissue proper.   **Loose (areolar) connective tissue** is abundant within the body, as it supports epithelial membranes, fills spaces between organs, and surrounds blood vessels, to name several functions. It contains all elements of connective tissue (i.e., cells, matrix, bound tissue water), but

Table 1-2. Types of Connective Tissues

Connective tissue proper
1. Loose (areolar)
2. Dense
   a. Regular (e.g., tendons)
   b. Irregular (e.g., dermis)

Supporting connective tissues
1. Cartilage
2. Bone

Connective tissues with special properties
1. Mucous tissue: embryonic
2. Elastic
3. Reticular
4. Adipose tissue
5. Hematopoietic tissue
   a. Lymphoid
   b. Myeloid

the amorphous ground substance predominates. The ground substance serves as the medium in which most of the interstitial fluids of the body are situated and as such is important in the diffusion of materials from the vasculature to cells and vice versa. The presence of the ground substance serves as a physical barrier to microorganisms and to injected materials.

Dense connective tissues (proper) have a high proportion of fibers in comparison with ground substance. The designations of regular versus irregular are determined by the major orientation of the fiber bundles within the tissue. In dense regular tissue, the bundles of fibers are rather precisely arranged, usually in line with the forces playing on the tissue (e.g., tendons, ligaments). The dense irregular tissues (dermis of skin, organ capsules) demonstrate a felt-work or mat-like appearance of fibers passing in a variety of directions and are thus able to respond to stresses from more than one dimension.

Supporting connective tissues. **Supporting connective tissues** consist of cartilage and bone. The intracellular matrix of cartilage has a firm consistency and is also resilient. Cartilaginous tissue serves as support for soft tissues and as self-lubricating surfaces in joints. It plays a very important role in the development and growth of many of the bones of the body. As connective tissues, the various types of cartilage consist of cells, matrix (ground substance and fibers), and bound water or tissue fluid. The three forms of cartilage are **hyaline cartilage** (the most prevalent), **fibrocartilage**, and **elastic cartilage**. All three forms are avascular, thus the cells within the cartilage masses must be nourished by means of fluid diffusion through the matrix. The cartilage masses may grow (increase in size) by both interstitial growth, which is the production of cells and matrix within the mass, and by appositional growth, in which the mass is enlarged by accretion of cells and matrix on the surface of the mass. Mature cartilage usually possesses a tissue layer, the perichondrium, that contains the vascular supply of the cartilage, reserve cells to form more cartilage on the surface, and connective tissue fibers to connect the cartilage to surrounding tissues.

The most common type of cartilage in humans is hyaline cartilage. Elastic cartilage is similar in composition to hyaline cartilage, with the exception that the elastic cartilage has many elastic fibers embedded in the matrix in addition to the collagenous fibers found in both types of cartilage. Fibrocartilage tremendously emphasizes the fibrous component of the tissue and serves as an intermediate tissue between dense regular connective tissue and the supporting connective tissues such as bone.

The matrix of hyaline cartilage contains abundant collagen type II fibrils embedded in a ground substance consisting primarily of the proteoglycans—chondroitin sulfates and keratan sulfate—and hyaluronic acid.

The cells of cartilage, chondroblasts, and the more mature chondrocytes synthesize, release, and maintain the components of the cartilage matrix. Although the cells are active in the synthesis, they tend to be larger and more basophilic. The matrix secreted by the chondroblasts forms around them so that they are ultimately entrapped within it. The cell-containing spaces are known as lacunae. While the cartilage mass is small or growing, mitotic division of chondroblasts occurs within the lacunae. The subsequent cells are able to produce additional matrix between themselves and to move apart (interstitial growth). However, as the bulk of the mass increases, the cells produced by mitotic divisions are no longer able to form separate lacunae. Thus it is not uncommon to find several chondrocytes situated within the same lacuna in mature cartilage.

The matrix immediately surrounding the lacuna is the matrix that has been most recently secreted. Because cross-linkages between the proteoglycan molecules and in the collagen fibrils have not formed and the proteoglycans are in a greater proportion than the collagen, the matrix stains more basophilic than the cosinophilic staining matrix located farther away from the lacunae. The more eosinophilic staining matrix is older and demonstrates a higher degree of bonding between its constituents. The basophilic ring around the lacuna is often called the capsular or territorial matrix, while the older matrix located between the lacunae is known as the interterritorial matrix.

While cartilage is young or is in a thin sheet, it may grow by both interstitial and appositional growth. However, as the mass increases and cross-linking reactions increase in the matrix, the ability to grow interstitially decreases. Chondroblasts in the perichondrium are able to continue producing matrix and to add to the surface of the mass by appositional growth. As the cartilage ages, the chondrocytes often are unable to properly maintain the surrounding matrix. As this process progresses or if the chondrocytes die, the matrix tends to accumulate calcium salts and is said to calcify. If calcification takes place in the cartilage mass, the cells separated from the nutrient source by the calcified matrix are isolated from appropriate nutrition and die.

Bone is one of the hardest tissues of the body because of the deposition of calcium compounds in the fibrous matrix. As the major constituent of the skeletal system, it serves to support softer tissues, protects vital organs in the cranium and the thoracoabdominal cavities, surrounds the blood-producing bone marrow, and acts as a very important reservoir for calcium, phosphates, and other ions.

Like cartilage and all of the other connective tissues, bone incorporates cells (osteoblasts and osteocytes), a matrix of ground substance and collagen fibers, and a small amount of tissue fluid. In addition to the bone-forming and bone-maintaining cells, a population of cells normally exists in bone that participates in its destruction. These large, multinucleated cells known as osteoclasts are of a different immediate origin (derived from hematopoietic tissue) than the bone-forming cells.

As with cartilage, the formative cells, osteoblasts, synthesize and secrete the intercellular matrix. As they do so, they eventually allow themselves to be surrounded by the matrix and come to lie within lacunae. In contrast to cartilage, however, the osteoblasts preserve long cellular processes (filopodia) that extend into the matrix as it is surrounding the cells and allow for intercellular connections between adjacent cells. Through these connections and the small amount of space that surrounds the filopodia in the form of canaliculi, all living osteocytes are ultimately in contact with a surface of the bone that will provide a vascular supply. The canaliculi are necessary because there can be no tissue fluid exchange through the matrix once the calcium salts are deposited in the ossification process.

The vascularized surfaces of bone are usually associated with a layer of osteoblastic cells. The cells are not constantly producing new matrix. The surfaces of bone adjacent to a vascular supply include (1) the external surface covered with the periosteum, (2) the internal surface delineating the marrow cavity, which is covered by a cell layer known as the endosteum, and (3) the surface of numerous small canals that extend into the bone substance from either the periosteal or endosteal surface. The canals, haversian and Volkmann's canals, contain small blood vessels that are able to ramify throughout the osseous tissue as they follow the canals. The major orientation of the haversian canals is longitudinal or parallel to the long axis of a gross long bone. The haversian canals are lined with osteoblastic cells. The location of the free or vascularized surfaces of bone is important to understand not only in terms of the vascularization of the bone, but also for how it influences bone development, growth, and remodeling. Osseous tissue can be altered almost exclusively at these surfaces and can be added to only at these surfaces by the process of appositional growth.

The formative and maintaining cells of bone, osteoblasts and osteocytes, respectively, are derived from a stem cell line known as the osteoprogenitor cell. The osteoprogenitor cells are in turn derived from mesenchymal cells. Bone-degrading cells, or osteoclasts, are derived from the monocyte line of blood cells. The osteoclastic cells migrate into the bone from blood-forming tissues via the circulatory system and transform into large multinucleated cells. The resorption or breakdown of osseous tissue is an integral part of bone growth and remodeling. The osteoclastic activity assists in the regulation of the appropriate amount of bone substance related to the functional demands placed on it.

The intercellular substance of osseous tissue is composed of an inorganic component of minerals that are predominantly calcium phosphate salts and other ions, which account for approximately 50% of its dry weight. It also includes an organic matrix (ground substance and collagen fibers), which accounts for the other half. The organic matrix consists predominantly

(95%) of collagen type I fibers. These collagen fibers are embedded in the ground substance that contains chondroitin sulfates and keratan sulfate. Two unique components have been recognized: bone sialoprotein and osteocalcin. These two components may assist in the control of the calcification of the matrix.

The process by which osseous tissue is formed is as follows:

1. Osteoblasts, derived from osteoprogenitor cells, synthesize and secrete the ground substance and collagen of the connective tissue matrix. In the case of bone, this matrix is known as osteoid.

2. Osteoblasts also extrude matrix vesicles, which are membrane-bound vesicles that are about 100 nm in diameter. The vesicles contain several enzymes and possess a membrane that allows for the accumulation of calcium phosphate within the vesicle. After vesicle rupture, the contained calcium phosphates most likely serve as nucleation sites, resulting in the formation of hydroxyapatite crystal that form in the matrix. (These vesicles are also found in other calcifying tissues such as cartilage and predentin.) The hydroxyapatite crystals are oriented so that the long axes of the crystals are parallel to the collagen fibers.

3. Osteoid, as it is produced by the osteoblasts, is usually applied to a surface (appositional growth). The osteoblasts gradually surround themselves with the osteoid, which is rapidly mineralized. Once the osteoblast is surrounded, it soon ceases to secrete larger amounts of matrix components and changes to a less active cell, the osteocyte. Each osteocyte is active in maintaining the integrity of the bone substance that is adjacent to it.

4. If the bone is remodeled, the degradation or breakdown of osseous tissue is done primarily through the action of large multinucleated monocyte-derived osteoclasts. These cells are also found on the free surfaces of bone and release enzymes that cause a decalcification and digestion of the matrix in the immediate area of the cell. The indentation created by the osteoclast is often known as a Howship's lacuna.

5. The osteocytes that are liberated from their lacunae by the breakdown of the osseous tissue may be activated to an osteoblastic type of cell or they may undergo necrosis.

Connective tissues with special properties. Connective tissues with special properties form a separate category because the major fiber type is not collagen type I as found in the regular connective tissues.

Mucous tissue is an embryonic or immature form of connective tissue in which the ground substance predominates. The ground substance often changes its nature, and the proportion of fibers is increased as the tissue matures.

Elastic connective tissue, as a separate entity, is found in the ligamenta flava and the ligamentum nuchae. These ligamentous structures, related to the posterior aspect of the vertebral column, are in a position where they must be able to stretch in order for the column to flex anteriorly but at the same time must give structural integrity to the column.

Reticular tissue is most important as the scaffolding or stroma that supports the parenchyma (secretory cells) of the various organs such as the liver or supports the cells in bone marrow and lymphatic organs. The reticular fibers are a form of collagen (type III) and are synthesized by fibroblasts in the region.

Adipose tissue is a form of loose connective tissue in which many of the cells are specialized adipocytes. These cells store lipids, primarily in the form of triglycerides, which serve as an energy source for the body. The adipose tissue also serves as a physical insulating layer as the subcutaneous fascia, a shock absorber in the plantar aspect of the foot, and as "packing material" between many organs.

Adipose tissue exists in two forms: the more common yellow unilocular form of adipose tissue and the less prevalent brown multilocular form. The adipocytes of unilocular fat store the lipid contents in one droplet within the cell. As the droplet enlarges, the nucleus and organelles are pushed aside to the periphery of the cell. After routine histological preparations that dissolve the lipid, the cell has the appearance of a signet ring. The adipocytes release lipoprotein lipase, which is transferred to the endothelial cells in the region. The lipoprotein lipase hydrolyzes chylomicrons and very-low-density lipoproteins into fatty acids, which ultimately move from the capillary to the adipocyte. There they are used to synthesize triglycerides, which are then stored in the adipocyte.

Multilocular, or brown, adipose tissue is not distributed as uniformly in the body as is the unilocular form. The stored lipids are contained within the cell in multiple small droplets. The cells also contain many mitochondria. Additionally, the adipocytes are closely associated with the capillaries of the tissue. When appropriately stimulated, the metabolic activity of the individual cell related to the hydrolysis of triglycerides to fatty acids and glycerol is increased. The mitochondria alter their metabolic pathways so that very little ATP is produced and all of the energy produced is transformed into heat. This results in the production of heat in the tissue, which warms the blood passing through the tissue, ultimately distributing the warmth to the rest of the body.

Blood belongs to the group of connective tissues that have special purposes. Blood contains elements that are associated with the four basic components of all connective tissues: cells, tissue fluid, a form of ground substance, and the precursor molecules for fibers. The blood serves many functions in the body. It conveys nutrients and oxygen to cells, carries carbon dioxide and waste materials away from the cells, contains cellular and humoral agents that participate in the defense of the body, contains agents (hormones) that regulate glandular tissue and other connective tissues, assists in the regulation of body temperature, and assists in maintaining a consistent state of equilibrium (homeostasis) within the body.

The blood is composed of cells or portions of cells and a liquid intercellular portion, the plasma. The cells and/or portions of cells include red cells, erythrocytes; white cells, leukocytes; and platelets, portions of larger cells, megakaryocytes (Table 1-3). If a sample of whole blood is anticoagulated and then centrifuged, the cells are driven to the bottom of the centrifuge tube and the relative proportions can then be easily measured, with the cells forming about 45% and the plasma composing the remaining 55%. The cells are separated into two major regions, the heavier erythrocytes being moved to the bottom and the buffy coat, a layer composed of leukocytes and platelets, lying on the surface of red cell mass.

Some of the cells of the blood, erythrocytes, perform their

Table 1-3. Types of Blood Cells and Their Amounts

Type of cell	Amount
Erythrocytes	4 to 5 million/mm³
Leukocytes	6,000 to 9,000/mm³
Granular leukocytes	
Neutrophils	55 to 60% of leukocytes
Eosinophils	2 to 5% of leukocytes
Basophils	0 to 1% of leukocytes
Agranular leukocytes	
Lymphocytes	30 to 35% of leukocytes
Monocytes	3 to 7% of leukocytes
Platelets (thrombocytes)	200,000 to 400,000/mm³

function within the confines of the circulatory system. The leukocytes use the blood as a transport tissue to move them from the point of origin to the capillary bed and postcapillary venules of the tissue, at which point they will move out of the circulation and into the surrounding connective tissues. They function in the realm of the connective tissues.

Red blood cells, erythrocytes, account for the largest number of cells of the blood. Normally circulating erythrocytes are different from most cells of the body in that they do not contain nuclei in the mature stage. The nucleus is lost, exuded, during development. The erythrocytes are deformable, biconcave disks that are filled with proteins. The proteins include a variety of enzymes and, most importantly, an iron-containing protein, hemoglobin. Hemoglobin consists of four iron-containing polypeptide chains.

Leukocytes, white blood cells, are often found in the connective tissues because this is the location where they are able to be active and conduct their functions in the defense mechanisms of the body. The leukocytes circulate from the tissue in which they arise to the capillary beds and postcapillary venules of the connective tissues, where the cells pass through the vessel wall by amoeboid activity (diapedesis). Once in the connective tissue, most of the leukocytes will survive for several days and then die. Most of the leukocytes, with lymphocytes being the possible exception, remain in the connective tissues once they enter it.

The **leukocytic series** includes a granulocytic series (i.e., neutrophils, eosinophils, and basophils) and an agranular series (i.e., lymphocytes and derivatives).

Neutrophils are the most numerous of the leukocytes, or white blood cells. They measure 12 to 15 μm in diameter. While in the blood, they tend to be spherical. When in contact with a substratum, they tend to flatten and extend pseudopods, which allow them to be highly motile. Neutrophils demonstrate highly segmented nuclei, the pattern of which is not uniformly reproduced in each cell, hence the alternative name—polymorphonuclear leukocyte. The cytoplasmic granules are classified as specific granules and azurophilic granules. The specific granules are smaller and more numerous and contain an antibacterial substance and alkaline phosphatase. They do not stain intensely with either basic or acidic stains. The specific granules are primarily spherical, but rod-shaped granules have been described. The larger, less numerous azurophilic granules are lysosomes and contain lysososmal enzymes and peroxidase. In connective tissues, neutrophils are avid phagocytes. Unfortunately, as the neutrophils die, their enzyme contents are released into the interstitial space and, if abundant enough, can cause damage to the surrounding tissues.

Polymorphonuclear neutrophils are the cells that usually participate in the first response to an injury or infection and are thus commonly found in the acute phase of an inflammatory response. A sample of the sequence of events is as follows: After the neutrophils have ingested a bacterium, the specific granules fuse with and empty their antibacterial agent into the phagosome. The azurophilic granules subsequently fuse with the phagosome and empty their hydrolytic enzymes in the phagosome (which is now called a secondary lysosome). These enzymes cause lysis of the bacterium. In the process, many neutrophils die. The accumulation of dead bacteria and leukocytes constitutes a thick, yellowish material known as pus. Other leukocytes such as monocytes and lymphocytes migrate into the inflammatory response area.

Eosinophils are so named because the specific granules (lysosomes) contained within the cytoplasm stain intensely with the eosin stain used in the histological stains. The nuclei of the eosinophils also tend to be lobed, similar to those found in basophils and young neutrophils. The granules are very large, membrane-bound vesicles. The vesicles are lysosomes and contain peroxidase, histaminase, arlysulfatase, and other hydrolytic enzymes. Histaminase neutralizes the activity of histamine; arylsulfatase, or slow-reacting substance (SRS). These hydrolytic substances are also released into the surrounding tissues and thus cause a breakdown of histamine and SRS in the tissue fluid. This tends to further limit the action of the vasoactive substances released by the mast cells and basophils. The eosinophils also are known to ingest and degrade antigen-antibody reaction complexes. Eosinophils are thus potentially capable of exerting a negative feedback control on the allergic response. Eosinophils are also often found in association with tissues containing parasites.

Basophils are the least numerous of the bloodborne leukocytes. Basophils are so named because of their prominent, basophilically staining cytoplasmic granules. The granules tend to obscure the large lobulated nucleus in which the heterochromatin tends to be peripheral and the euchromatin more central. The granules and membrane-bound vesicles contain hydrolytic enzymes, heparin, histamine, and SRS. Histamine and SRS are vasoactive materials that tend to produce a dilatation of small blood vessels. Basophils are related but not identical to mast cells of connective tissue. The specific granules stain strongly with basophilic stains. Both mast cells and basophils bind immunoglobin E to its surface plasma membrane. When an allergen binds to the immunoglobin, the vasoactive materials and other contained substances are released into the surrounding tissues. These substances may cause severe vascular disturbances associated with hypersensitivity and the anaphylactic response.

Lymphocytes (a form of agranular leukocyte) are also found free within the connective tissues. Some of them are T-lymphocytes (thymus-influenced) and are responsible for cell-mediated immune responses. These cells are usually long-lived. The other population consists of B-lymphocytes (bone marrow), which when stimulated give rise to plasma cells. Lymphocytes are the primary functional cells of lymphoid tissues. They are found in blood as they move from one lymphoid organ to another and from lymphoid tissue to regular connective tissues. Three groups of lymphocytes are described: small, medium, and large. The small and medium lymphocytes are the ones normally found in the process of migration. The lymphocytes do not contain specific granules as do the previously mentioned cells and thus are grouped among the agranular leukocytes. Ribosomes give the slight basophilia seen in stained cells. The nucleus is not lobed and tends to occupy the majority of the cell.

Monocytes are the largest of the peripherally located leukocytes. They are the precursor cells to the system of cells known as the mononuclear phagocyte system. As they are in the blood, they are in transit from bone marrow to the body tissues. Monocytes remain in the blood for approximately 3 days. The nucleus is more indented than that of the lymphocyte. The chromatin tends to be arranged in a cartwheel pattern within the nucleus. The prominent Golgi and centrioles are perinuclear in location. The monocyte also contains sER and rER, as well as numerous lysosomes. During the inflammatory response, the monocytes leave the vasculature, enter the connective tissues, and transform into tissue macrophages. They participate in phagocytosis of bacteria and other cellular debris. In other situations, the monocyte serves to concentrate antigens and present them to lymphocytes.

Platelets are small cytoplasmic fragments of megakaryocytes that are found in the bone marrow. The average life span of a circulating platelet is 10 days. Although the platelets do not contain a nucleus, they possess a very well-developed plasma membrane. Platelets are important in the process of blood clotting, clot retraction, and clot dissolution. The platelet is composed of two portions, the more intensely staining chromomere or granulomere and the lightly staining hyalomere. The granules responsible for the staining of the chromomere can be classified as granules containing lysosomal enzymes and granules containing serotonin. Some microtubules are also stained as a part of the granulomere. The hyalomere contains microfilaments and microtubules that are responsible for maintaining the shape of the platelets and serve in clot retraction.

When the endothelium of a blood vessel is disrupted, several events take place. Among them is platelet aggregation and adherence at the site of injury. The platelets release serotonin, and the injured tissues release thromboplastin. The serotonin serves to assist in the constriction of the injured blood vessels and thus reduces the flow of blood through the area. Thromboplastin released by the tissues initiates clot formation. Platelets that are trapped in the clot ultimately cause the clot to retract and, after an appropriate interval, to dissolve.

Normal **plasma** is composed of the following elements and proportions: water, 90 to 92%; proteins, 7 to 8%; and other material, which include electrolytes, nonprotein nitrogenous substances (e.g., urea, nutrients, gases, hormones, enzymes), 1 to 2%.

Plasma cells, which are derived from B-lymphocytes, are found in areas subject to penetration by bacteria and foreign protein. They synthesize many of the antibodies (globulins) found in the blood. As such, the cell is rich in rER. The Golgi is paranuclear and creates a clear area in the cytoplasm when viewed with the light microscope (nuclear hof). The chromatin pattern in the nucleus is often described as being arranged in a cartwheel configuration.

Proteins are the largest of the dissolved substances. They exist in three major groups: fibrinogens, globulins, and albumins. Fibrinogens are synthesized in the liver and function in the clotting of blood. Albumins are also synthesized in the liver; they are the small proteins and serve to create the major portion of the osmotic pressure found in the plasma as it is contained within blood vessels. Globulins, which include immunoglobulins, play a role in the immunologic defense of the body. Most of the nonprotein constituents of the plasma are small enough to pass readily through the endothelium of the capillaries and small venules. Thus the intercellular, interstitial fluid is derived from the plasma and reflects its composition. In regions where the tissue fluid does not enter a connective tissue after emerging from the vessels, the extracellular fluid has usually passed through an epithelium, other than the endothelium, that modifies the composition of the fluid that is permitted to pass across the barrier.

Hematopoiesis. Hematopoiesis occurs in three phases. The first phase is found in the blood islands of the embryonic yolk sac. In the second phase, the major amount of hematopoiesis occurs in the liver and lymphoid tissues. In the third phase, hematopoiesis takes place in the red bone marrow and lymphoid organs. It has been shown that the blood cells are derived from a single, common stem cell. The stem cell is located in the bone marrow during the marrow phase of hematopoiesis.

The process of **erythropoiesis** is influenced by a hormone produced by the kidney, erythropoietin. The first separately recognizable cell in the red blood cell line is the proerythroblast. This cell is relative large, measuring about 15 μm in diameter. The nucleus is spherical and contains one or two prominent nucleoli. The cytoplasm is lightly basophilic because of the presence of a good number of free ribosomes. The next stage of development is represented by the basophilic erythroblast. This cell is somewhat smaller than the proerythroblast. It has a smaller nucleus and a more intensely basophilic cytoplasm because of an increased population of polyribosomes. As the polyribosomes synthesize the cytoplasmic proteins, predominantly hemoglobin, the cytoplasm takes on an additional eosinophilic cast. This stage in development is called a polychromatophilic erythroblast. Although the polychromatophilic cell is approximately the same size as the basophilic erythroblast, the nucleus has continued to condense and is smaller and more basophilic in staining. The polychromatophilic erythroblast transforms into the normoblast stage, which is characterized by a very condensed, almost pyknotic nucleus and a much greater eosinophilic cast to the cytoplasm. The hemoglobin staining is almost that of the mature erythrocyte. The nucleus of the normoblast is lost as the cell migrates out of the marrow space and into the vascular compartment. The early anucleate cell is called a polychromatophilic erythrocyte because the cytoplasm still contains a few groups of polyribosomes that produce a light network of basophilic staining material in the cytoplasm. The newly formed erythrocytes are also known as reticulocytes and constitute approximately 1 to 2% of all circulating red cells. An increased number of reticulocytes is usually indicative of an increased release of erythrocytes from the marrow in response to an increased demand for peripherally circulating cells.

Erythrocytes last approximately 120 days in the peripheral circulation. At that time, they tend to become more fragile or less malleable. The macrophage system in the liver, spleen, and bone marrow plays a role in the phagocytosis of the degenerating cells. The iron that had been bound in the hemoglobin is released and made available for new hemoglobin synthesis. The remaining portions of the hemoglobin molecules are further degraded and excreted as the bilirubin of bile.

The **granulocytic** series of leukocytes is also developed within the bone marrow during the definitive phase of hematopoiesis. The first, separately recognizable cell in this series is called the **promyelocyte**. The promyelocyte has a large spherical nucleus, and the cytoplasm contains scattered azurophilic granules. The promyelocyte gives rise to the **myelocyte** stage of cell development. By the time the myelocytes can be differentiated, specific granules have begun to be formed within the cytoplasm of the respective cells. Thus they can be designated as basophilic myelocytes, eosinophilic myelocytes, and neutrophilic myelocytes. The myelocytes are somewhat smaller in diameter than the promyelocyte and possess a smaller, usually slightly indented nucleus. As maturation and differentiation progress in each of the cell types, the number of specific granules increases and the nucleus becomes more deeply indented. The deep indentation of the nucleus gives rise to the lobed appearance that is one of the ultimate characteristics of these cells. This intermediate stage is known as the **metamyelocyte** stage. With further development, the nucleus of the neutrophil becomes segmented into three to five interconnected segments. With further maturation in each line of cells, the specific granules continue to increase in number and size, producing the appearance of the mature cells when combined with the deeply indented nuclei.

Granulocytes remain in the circulation for approximately 8 to 12 hours. As they exist in the blood contained in the peripheral vessels, the leukocytes may be divided into two groups or pools of cells. The circulating pool consists of those cells that are in the central stream of blood in the vessels and are moving with it. The second or marginating pool of leukocytes is found primarily in the capillary and postcapillary venule portion of the vascular tree. The marginating cells are applied to the wall of the small vessels and are not actively circulating. Many of them will subsequently migrate through the vessel wall to enter the surrounding connective tissues.

Blood platelets are cytoplasmic fragments of large cells that are situated in the bone marrow, megakaryocytes. The cytoplasm of the megakaryocyte is compartmentalized by the formation of strings of small plasma membrane vesicles. When the vesicles coalesce they thereby create small, separate, segregated units of cytoplasm that contain the organelles characteristic of platelets. The units break free from the megakaryocyte and enter the bone marrow vascular sinuses by passing through the endothelial cell apertures. The megakaryocyte subsequently regenerates the shed cytoplasm and continues to produce more platelets.

Red bone marrow, which is actively involved in producing blood cells, is found entirely within spaces contained in bone, either the medullary cavity of long bones or within the spaces of spongy bone. The red bone marrow consists of blood vessels, specialized units of blood vessels known as sinuses, and a sponge-like network of hematopoietic cells. When viewed in tissue sections, the hematopoietic cells appear to lie in groups or cords between the sinuses. The sinuses of red bone marrow are unique vascular units. The sinus occupies the position of a capillary in the regular vascular bed, that vessel unit interposed between arteries and veins. The sinus wall consists of an endothelial lining, a basal lamina, and an outer adventitial cell covering. The outer adventitial cells are also known as reticular cells. These cells extend sheet-like processes into the substance of the hematopoietic cord and to a degree support and organize the developing blood cells. The reticular cells also produce reticular connective tissue fibers. Additionally, they may play a role in stimulating the differentiation of stem cells into blood cells. When blood cell formation and passage of mature blood cells into the sinuses is active, the adventitial cells and the basal lamina material are displaced by the blood cells as they approach the endothelium lining the sinus. In order to enter the sinus, the blood cells and platelets must pass through an aperture within the endothelial cell and not pass between adjacent endothelial cells.

When the bone marrow is actively producing blood cells, the cords of hematopoietic tissue contain primarily developing blood cells and megakaryocytes. The cords may also contain macrophages, mast cells, plasma cells, and some fat cells. The specific types of blood cells tend to develop in nests or clusters that are indicative of the presence of the precursor cell. Each cluster giving rise to erythrocytes contains a population of macrophages. The erythrocyte clusters tend to be situated near the sinuses, as are the megakaryocytes. The cell clusters developing into the leukocytes tend to be situated farther from the sinuses.

If the bone marrow is not actively producing blood cells, it tends to be populated by fat cells and is designated as yellow bone marrow. Yellow bone marrow, which is the predominant type in adults, retains its potential to be hematopoietic and may be activated when necessary.

MUSCLE TISSUE

Muscular tissue is characterized by aggregates of specialized cells whose primary function is to contract or shorten. The cells are elongate and arranged in parallel arrays that allow them to work together to produce movement. The cell is highly modified in order to conduct an excitatory impulse along the surface of the muscle cell and into the interior of the cell. The muscle cells are also highly modified by the presence of numerous cytoplasmic microfilaments, which comprise the bulk of the cell. The microfilaments, actin and myosin, are found in other cells, where they play a role in movement of microvilli, cell migration, exocytosis, and cell division. In muscle cells, however, the microfilaments are more precisely organized and used to produce mechanical work.

Muscle tissue is subclassified on the basis of appearance and the location of the contractile cells. If the cells contain long bundles of microfilaments that are oriented in repeating patterns to produce the appearance of striations, they are said to be striated. If the microfilaments are not oriented sufficiently to produce striations, the muscle cell and tissue are said to be nonstriated or **smooth**. Striated muscle is found related to the

skeletal system, in skeletal muscle, where it functions to produce movement of the bones and hence the entire body. In the heart, the striated cardiac muscle produces movement of the blood. Although the microfilaments or myofilaments are arranged in essentially the same type of pattern in both types of striated muscle cells, the morphology of the cells of the two types of striated muscles are markedly different. Smooth muscle is found predominantly in the walls of blood vessels and viscera.

Skeletal muscle

Skeletal muscle is composed of elongated, parallel, striated cells that are known as fibers. The cells are multinucleated. The fibers are surrounded and held together by connective tissue. Each muscle fiber is innervated by a branch of motor neuron. A motor neuron together with all of the muscle fibers it innervates is termed a motor unit. Motor units range in size from one nerve cell supplying three to five muscle fibers in a muscle such as one of the extrinsic ocular muscles to one neuron supplying several hundred muscle cells in the muscles of the back and lower extremities.

Skeletal muscle is associated with connective tissue that organizes the muscle tissue into three levels of organization. Endomysium is the lightest connective tissue sheath and surrounds each individual skeletal muscle fiber. It is composed of delicate, loose connective tissue and contains the capillaries that supply the muscle fiber as well as the nerve fibers passing to innervate the muscle fibers. The perimysium surrounds bundles of skeletal muscle fibers and thereby divides the larger muscle mass into smaller fascicles. It in turn is the means by which larger blood vessels and nerve bundles pass through the muscle mass. The epimysium is the outermost layer of connective tissue associated with the skeletal muscle. It surrounds the gross muscles and blends with the connective tissues surrounding and separating the muscle masses.

Skeletal muscle fibers are usually relatively long. They are formed by the fusion of many single cells (myoblasts) to become a long multinucleated cytoplasmic unit. The multinucleated cytoplasmic mass is surrounded and delimited by a common plasma membrane, known in muscle tissue as the **sarcolemma**. In the mature muscle fibers, the nuclei occupy the region immediately under the sarcolemma and thus are peripherally situated. The sarcolemma possesses an associated basal lamina. With electron microscopic studies, small cells (satellite cells) have been found lying between the sarcolemma of the muscle fiber and the basal lamina. These satellite cells represent myoblasts that did not become incorporated into the muscle fibers as they were forming and serve as potential sources of muscle tissue for regenerative purposes. Such cells are not found in smooth muscle or cardiac muscle.

Skeletal muscle has been shown to exist in two major histochemical types, with some fibers being intermediate between the extremes. The two major types are known as red muscle and white muscle. The red muscle fibers are smaller in diameter, have relatively numerous mitochondria, are rich in myoglobin, and demonstrate a strong succinic dehydrogenase reaction. Red fibers compose slow-twitch motor units found in phasic muscles, have a great resistance to fatigue because of a large oxygen-binding capacity and numerous mitochondria, but tend to be somewhat weaker than white muscle fibers. The red muscle fibers are found and predominate in the postural muscles of the body. White muscle fibers, on the other hand, tend to be larger, possess fewer mitochondria, and demonstrate a weaker succinic dehydrogenase reaction. White muscle fibers predominate in the fast-twitch muscles or spurt muscles that are not used to maintain posture. White fibers are somewhat stronger than red but fatigue rather rapidly or switch to anaerobic metabolism sooner during use. The motor neuron supplying the muscle fibers is said to determine the histochemical nature of the fibers.

A major portion of the cytoplasm of skeletal muscle (sarcoplasm) is composed of contractile proteins organized into long intracellular fibrils (myofibrils) that are just visible with the light microscope. The myofibrils are, in turn, composed of myofilaments that are composed of actin and myosin. The paracrystalline orientation of the repeated subunits of the myofibrils gives the muscle fiber the cross-striation characteristic of skeletal muscle (and cardiac muscle) when the muscle fibers are viewed in longitudinal sections (parallel to the long axis of the cell or fiber).

The cross-striations of striated muscle seen with the light microscope in stained sections are the A band, the I band, the Z line, and occasionally an H band and an M line (Fig. 1-4). The A band is coexistent with myosin filaments (interdigitating with actin filaments). The I band, which is bisected by the Z line, contains actin filaments, which are attached to the Z line material. The pattern of A band, I band, Z line is repeated numerous times along the myofibril. The functional unit of the myofibril is known as the sarcomere and is defined as that portion of the myofibril lying between two successive Z lines. The myosin filaments (thick filaments) are found with the A line and are situated equidistant between the Z lines. The thin filaments (actin) are connected to the Z line. The thin actin filaments are found in the I band, where they are the only population of filaments, and extend into and interdigitate with the thick filaments in the A band. The Z line or disk serves to anchor the thin filaments of adjacent sarcomeres. If the sarcomere were viewed in a series of cross-sections, the following would be observed: Starting with the Z line and progressing to the middle of the sarcomere, (1) the Z line

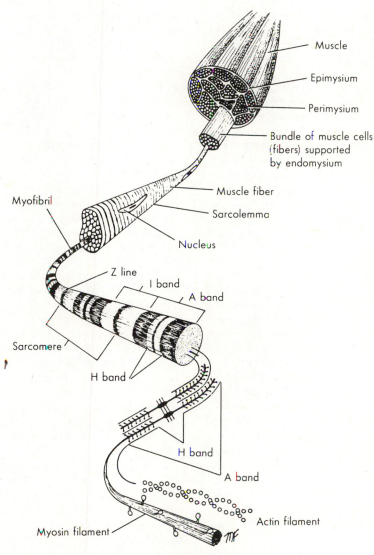

Figure 1-4. The cross-striations of striated muscle.

appears as a latticework of small filaments (alpha-actinin) onto which connect the actin filaments; (2) I band, containing actin filaments arrayed in an hexagonal pattern; (3) beginning of the A band as the thick myosin filaments are found lying within the hexagonal array of actin filaments, with each myosin filament being surrounded by six actin filaments and each actin filament relating to at least one myosin filament; (4) H zone of the A band, which demonstrates only the thick or myosin filaments; and (5) the M line, situated in the middle of the H zone, which demonstrates small transversely oriented filaments connecting adjacent myosin filaments. As the sections progress from the midregion of the sarcomere to the next Z line, the pattern is reversed—that is 4, 3, 2, and 1.

The basis of contraction of muscle lies in the interaction of the thick (myosin) and thin (actin) filaments. Several assumptions are assumed to help explain the process: (1) The thick and thin filaments can increase or decrease the extent of interdigitation in the A band region. (2) Each of the two types of filaments remains a constant length during the contraction process. (3) The two populations of filaments are separately stabilized so that the process of movement between the filaments might be effectively harnessed into useful movement. During contraction, the thin filaments are drawn toward the middle of the sarcomere, shortening the sarcomere and thus drawing the Z lines closer together. In the process, the longitudinal dimension of the I band is decreased, as is the longitudinal dimension of the H zone of the A band. The A band itself remains constant in length. As each individual sarcomere shortens, the net effect is to shorten the entire muscle. As the sarcomere shortens, it also increases slightly in diameter, thus the entire muscle will thicken during contraction. The sarcomere can contract to a maximum of less than 50% of its resting length; thus the gross muscle can contract far less that 50% of its effective resting length. The thin filaments are composed of G-actin molecules, which in aggregate form f-actin, which is organized by tropomyosin and troponin molecules. The thick filaments are composed of myosin molecules, which in turn are subdivided into a light meromyosin and a "hinged" movable head of heavy meromyosin. Then the myosin molecules are combined into the myosin filament. The heavy meromyosin heads project outwardly and are in a position to make contact with binding sites on adjacent thin filaments. In the absence of calcium, the tropomyosin and troponin of actin form a complex that prevents the cross-bridging linkage of the actin and myosin filaments. When calcium is present, the troponin-tropomyosin complex is repositioned and thus allows contact between the heavy myosin of the myosin filament and the actin filaments. During the cross-bridging linking reaction between the myosin and actin filaments, the heavy meromyosin head "swings" and draws the temporarily attached actin filament toward the middle of the sarcomere. Each swing of the myosin head accounts for a movement of approximately 100 nm, thus a series of repeated swings is necessary to produce maximal contraction. The energy required for the production of the swing of the myosin head is provided by ATP in the muscle cell. ATP is also necessary to break the bonding linkage between the myosin and actin filaments. Thus in the absence of ATP the muscle not only cannot contract but also cannot relax.

In order to produce effective contraction, the stimulus transmitted to the muscle cell by the motor neuron and transferred to it by the motor end-plate must be distributed not only along the length of the muscle fiber but also must be transmitted into the depths of the cell so that all areas of the fiber may contract simultaneously and effectively. This requirement is met by the formation of tubular invaginations of sarcolemma that extend deeply into the cell. Thus any membrane changes related to the passage of a depolarizing, excitatory potential would automatically be directed not only the length of the fiber but also into the inner aspects of the fiber by means of the tubular invaginations. Because the tubular invaginations are oriented predominantly in a radial pattern that is transverse to the longitudinal axis of the fiber, the tubular invaginations bear the name transverse tubule or T-tubule. In striated skeletal muscle the T-tubules have been shown to relate to each A band-I band junctions within the sarcomeres. Thus each sarcomere will have two T-tubules related to it. The paracrystalline organization of the sarcomeres in the adjacent myofibrils of the striated muscle cells might be a result of the T-tubules or a cause of the pattern. Another requirement for the control of contraction of striated muscle is the provision for an absence of calcium ions in the perifibrillar cytoplasm during the relaxed or noncontracting period of the muscle and, conversely, the presence of calcium ions to cause the molecular transformations necessary to allow for the cross-bridging linkages between the actin and myosin filaments in the sarcomeres during the contracting phase. This provision is accomplished by a specialization and elaboration of the sER of the muscle cell. The special term **sarcoplasmic reticulum** is given to this form of sER. The sarcoplasmic reticulum is organized as a series of tubular networks around the A band and the I band, respectively, in each sarcomere of the skeletal muscle myofibril. The individual tubules of the networks are joined to form a more regular ring-like channel around the myofibril. These ring-like channels have been named **terminal cisternae** or **terminal sacs**. Thus each network of sarcoplasmic reticulum surrounding an I band or A band will possess a terminal cisterna at either end of the region. The terminal cisternae run parallel and closely adjacent to the T-tubules. The sarcoplasmic reticulum is capable of sequestering calcium ions from the cytoplasm into the lumen of the reticulum, as well as quickly releasing the calcium into the surrounding cytoplasm. The combination of the T-tubules and contiguous terminal cisternae constitute the triad.

The sequence of events that couples a wave of excitation and contraction is as follows: (1) the depolarizing membrane potential is transmitted from the motor neuron via the motor end-plate to the sarcolemma of the muscle cell. The impulse wave is transmitted via the membrane along the length and around the circumference of the muscle fiber. As the impulse travels on the surface sarcolemma, it also travels into the interior of the fiber via the T-tubules. (2) The excitation wave causes alterations in the terminal cisternae that are relayed to the remainder of the sarcoplasmic reticulum and cause a release of calcium ions. (3) The freed calcium ions cause a reconfiguration of the tropomyosin and troponin molecules to allow the heavy meromyosin head to link with the G-actin. (4) In the presence of ATP, the myosin head swings and moves the actin filament toward the midregion of the sarcomere. In the presence of ATP, the temporary cross-linkage between the actin and myosin is broken and the myosin head returns to its original position. If calcium is still present, the events of cross-linkage formation, swing, and release are repeated. (5) When the excitatory changes in the sarcolemma revert to the resting state, the sarcoplasmic reticulum stops releasing calcium ions and begins to draw the ions back into the reticulum. (6) In the absence of the calcium ions, the tropomyosin and troponin return to the protective configuration, which inhibits cross-linkage formation. The contraction stops. In addition to the T-tubules and sarcoplasmic reticulum situated in the vicinity of the sarcomeres of the myofibrils, there are also many mito-chondria to supply ATP and glycogen granules to provide reserve energy sources.

The contact of a motor neuron with the muscle fibers is called a motor end-plate or neuromuscular junction. The myelin sheath that covers the axon terminates immediately proximal to the motor end-plate, but the nerve-muscle junction is covered by cytoplasmic extensions of Schwann cells, which are called teloglia in this situation. The axon terminals lie in small grooves in the muscle fiber, where they form neuromuscular synapses. The axon terminal contains numerous synaptic vesicles containing the neurotransmitter acetylcholine and many mitochondria. The muscle fiber cytoplasm immediately adjacent to the neuromuscular junction also contains many mitochondria. Numerous smaller grooves, (junctional folds or subneural clefts) extend from the bottoms of the major grooves containing the axon terminals. These junctional clefts increase the surface area of the sarcolemma that can be exposed to the neurotransmitters released from the axon terminals. Basal lamina material extends into the synaptic space of the junction and also covers the entire junction. When acetylcholine is released from the axon terminal, it diffuses through the synaptic cleft and interacts with receptors in the sarcolemma of the muscle. The receptors in turn initiate changes in the sarcolemma that causes an action potential to be spread from the junction to all parts of the fiber. Acetylcholin-esterase found in relation to the synaptic cleft quickly inactivates the previously released acetylcholine so that additional con-tractile activity is not generated in the muscle in response to residual neurotransmitter.

Skeletal muscle tissue contains two functional types of fibers. The vast amount of the skeletal muscle consists of fibers that are specialized to contact. A much smaller number of fibers take part in the formation or specialized neural receptors that monitor the state of contraction and the rate of contraction of the surrounding muscle fibers. The specialized receptor is called a neuromuscular spindle. The muscle fibers situated within the connective tissue capsule are known as **intrafusal fibers**. The intrafusal fibers serve as transducers for the nervous system. In comparison, the muscle fibers that produce the forceful contractions of muscle tissue are termed extrafusal fibers (fusal = spindle). The neuromuscular spindle is a receptor for the nervous system and consists of special muscle fibers and neuron terminals surrounded by a capsule. A large fluid-filled space separates the special muscle cells and the capsule. Two kinds of muscle cells are found within the spindle: nuclear bag fibers and nuclear chain fibers. A typical neuromuscular spindle may contain four nuclear bag fibers and up to twice as many nuclear chain fibers. A nuclear bag fiber demonstrates an expanded midregion to accommodate an aggregation of nuclei; the nuclear chain fiber has the nuclei arrayed in longer longitudinal groupings of nuclei. The nuclear bag fibers are contacted by primary afferent endings that spiral around it. The nuclear chain fibers receive primary afferent endings that spiral around their midregion and secondary afferent nerve endings that relate to the ends of the muscle fibers. Both types of intrafusal fibers receive motor innervation via small motor neurons known as gamma motor neurons.

Cardiac muscle

With the light microscope, cardiac muscle seems to be arranged in long fibers somewhat similar to skeletal muscle. The cardiac muscle demonstrates cross-striations that are organized in the same manner as those in skeletal muscle. However, additional transversely oriented markings are also observed. These transversely oriented marks are known as intercalated disks. The intercalated disks are the regions of cell-to-cell junctions that join individual cardiac muscle cells end to end to form the longer units of muscle. Thus cardiac muscle consists of single uninucleated cells containing centrally placed nuclei that are joined to form interlacing fibers and layers of muscle within the heart.

Cardiac muscle contains numerous large mitochondria that are frequently as long as a sarcomere. The sarcoplasmic reticulum is also well developed but not quite as well as that of skeletal muscle, especially in the regions similar to the terminal cisternae. The transverse tubules are larger than those of skeletal muscle and related to the sarcomeres of the myofibrils at the level of the Z lines. Basal lamina material also extends into the transverse tubules. The process of contraction in cardiac muscle is similar to that of skeletal muscle but is somewhat slower. The difference can partially be explained by the less numerous T-tubules and the less well organized sarcoplasmic reticulum. The less numerous, larger T-tubules may very well serve to transmit extracellular fluid into the depths of the cell, as well as to carry the action potential in the sarcolemma. The myofilaments within the cardiac muscle cells tend to branch and interlace, as do the cardiac muscle cells themselves. The cardiac muscle of the ventricles of the heart is better developed than that of the atria. The atria cells demon-strate 0.3- to 0.4-μm diameter granules (atrial granules) in the juxtanuclear region of the cell in addition to the usual cellular organelles related to any muscle cell. The atrial granules are thought to contain atrial natiuretic hormone, which may assist in the renal processing of sodium.

Smooth muscle

Smooth muscle consists of fusiform (spindle-shaped) cells that range in length from 20 μm to over 200 μm. As in striated muscle, the contractile proteins consist of actin and myosin. However, the contractile proteins are not as highly oriented in the smooth muscle cells, hence no appearance of sarcomeres or striations. The actin and myosin filaments occupy a large portion of the cytoplasm of the smooth muscle cell, and they interact with each other in a manner similar to those of striated muscle. Interspersed throughout the cell and adjacent to the plasmalemma are oval electron-dense areas. The dense areas or dense bodies are composed of alpha-actinin, the same material that composes the Z lines of striated muscle. Thus the contractile apparatus of smooth muscle is much the same as that of striated muscle. Smooth muscle does not, however, demonstrate a transverse tubule system or as elaborate a sarcoplasmic reticulum. Numerous pinocytotic vesicles called caveolae probably function in a manner similar to the transverse tubules, and the sarcoplasmic reticulum has been shown to sequester calcium.

Smooth muscle cells often contact neighboring cells and establish nexus-type junctions. These junctions allow for the easy transmission of electrical stimuli as well as intracellular substances. Smooth muscle is innervated by postganglionic neurons of the autonomic nervous system. The axons pass among the smooth muscle cells. Neurotransmitter substances are found in enlargements of the axons that are near muscle cells. In most organs, the smooth muscle cells appear to act as though they were made of functionally connected sheets or bundles. In such functional groups, each muscle cell is not individually innervated by an efferent nerve ending. However, the gap junctions that join the cells are thought to spread the contractile impulse throughout the functional group. In other organs, in which the tissue responds more rapidly, each smooth muscle cell is contacted by an efferent, motor autonomic nerve ending even though the adjacent cells are connected with nexus-type junctions.

Smooth muscle cells are surrounded by basal lamina material, except where they are joined to neighboring cells by nexus junctions. The smooth muscle cells themselves produce the basal lamina. In some situations, the smooth muscle cells are capable of synthesizing collagen fibers and elastic tissue components.

NEURAL TISSUE

Neural tissue is distributed throughout the body as an integrated communications network. Anatomically, the nervous system is divided into a central portion, often called the CNS, and a peripheral portion, often called the peripheral nervous system (PNS). The brain and spinal cord compose the central portion of the system, while nerve fibers and small aggregates of nerve cell bodies (ganglia) are found in the peripheral portion. The central and peripheral portions of the nervous system are somewhat arbitrary and are most useful for descriptive purposes because neurons whose cell bodies are situated within the spinal cord or brain stem possess cell processes that extend into and compose a portion of the peripheral part of the system. Conversely, nerve cells that possess cell bodies situated in peripheral sensory ganglia extend cell processes not only into the more peripheral portions of the system but also into the central portion.

Structurally, neural tissue consists of two classes of cell types. One type is the functional unit of the nerve system, the nerve cell or neuron (Fig. 1-5). The other class of cells is the supporting cells of the tissue. This class includes the neuroglia cells found within the central portion of the system and Schwann cells and satellite or capsular cells found in the peripheral part.

Neurons

Neurons respond to environmental changes or stimuli by altering the electrical potential differences that exist between the inner and outer surfaces of the plasmalemma (neurolemma).

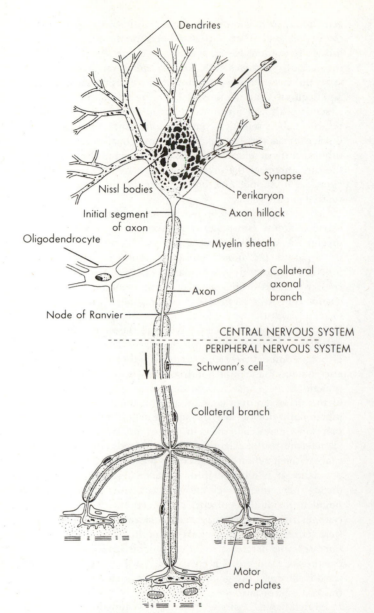

Figure 1-5.   Schematic drawing of a Nissl-stained motor neuron. The myelin sheath is produced by oligodendrocytes in the CNS and by Schwann's cells in the peripheral nervous system. The neuronal cell body has an unusually large, euchromatic nucleus with a well-developed nucleolus. The perikaryon contains Nissl bodies, which are also found in large dendrites. An axon from another neuron is shown at upper right. It has three end bulbs, one of which synapses with the neuron. Note also three motor end-plates, which transmit the nerve impulse to striated skeletal muscle fibers. Arrows show the direction of the nerve impulse.

Such cells are said to be excitable or irritable. Neuron plasmalemmae react quickly to stimuli by altering the membrane potential. The alteration may be restricted to the zone of stimulation and will lose strength as it spreads from the point of origin (generator potential) or the altered potential may be spread to adjacent plasmalemma without any loss of strength of the altered potential (action potential). The two basic functions of the nervous system are (1) to detect, integrate, analyze, and transmit all information generated by sensory stimuli affecting the body and (2) to organize and coordinate, either directly or indirectly, most of the functions of the body, including the somatic motor, visceral motor, endocrine, and mental processes.

Neurons or nerve cells are the independent anatomic and functional units of neural tissue. They possess rather complex morphological and physiological characteristics. Most neurons consist of three components: (1) A **nerve cell body** or **perikaryon** contains the nucleus and the major number of organelles involved on the metabolic and synthetic activities of the cell. It thereby is the trophic center of the cell. In some neurons, the perikaryon also serves as a portion of the receptive region of the cell. Extending from the cell body are usually found many cell processes. One of the processes is usually the axon, and the other are dendrites. (2) The **dendrites** serve to enlarge the receptive area of the neuron. The plasmalemma in the receptor zone of the neuron reacts to stimuli by the formation of generator potentials. These alterations in membrane potential are not propagated but will return to the resting state as the impulse spreads from the stimulus point. (3) The **axon** serves to transmit the neural impulse to regions that may be distant from the neuron. The plasmalemma of the axon transmits a propagated impulse or action potential that retains its strength as it passes along the axon. The axon usually terminates by branching into terminal arborizations. Each branch of the arborization terminates on a cell with the formation of end bulbs or boutons. The end bulb or bouton is thereby a portion of a synapse, most specifically the presynaptic components.

Neurons can be classified according to their shape or the number of processes. The simplest embryonic cell has one process and is said to be unipolar. With later development another process is added, making the cell bipolar. Some of the neurons associated with special senses remain bipolar throughout life. The two poles of a transitory bipolar neuron stage are said to move together and seem to fuse or emerge from the cell body at a single point to create a cell configuration known as a pseudounipolar cell. This type of cell is found in many of the sensory ganglia. The most numerous cell configuration demonstrates many processes and is thus known as a multipolar neuron and is the cell configuration for motor neurons (both somatic and visceral motor) and most internuncial cells or interneurons. Neurons may also be classified according to their function within the nervous system. Neurons that receive sensory stimuli and transmit them to the central portion of the system are said to be sensory neurons, or afferent in nature. Motor neurons or efferent cells transmit impulses away from the central portion of the system and thereby affect other tissues of the body, most notably muscle and glandular tissue. Interneurons or internuncial neurons connect the sensory and motor neurons and are resonsible for the vast complex functional chains or circuits.

The perikaryon is the part of the neuron that contains the nucleus and surrounding cytoplasm, exclusive of the cell processes. It is primarily a trophic or metabolic center but may also serve as a portion of the receptive zone of the cell as excitatory and inhibitory endings from other neurons end on it. The nucleus in most nerve cells is large, spherical, and contains a prominent nucleolus. The euchromatin is uniformly and finely dispersed. Most neuron have numerous dendrites,

which are direct extensions of the cell body and serve to greatly increase the amount of surface available to receive and integrate information from other neurons. Dendritic branches tend to become thinner as they extend away from the soma. The composition of the cytoplasm in the dendrites is very similar to that found in the perikaryon, with the exception that no Golgi complexes are found within the dendritic tree. Aggregations of polyribosomes and rER (Nissl substance) are routinely found in the dendrites of multipolar neurons, as well as in the perinuclear cytoplasm. Numerous neurofilaments and microtubules extend into the dendritic arborizations.

Most neurons have only one axon, the process that transmits a propagated impulse, although a few have no true axon. The axon is usually the longest of the cell processes and tends to be constant in diameter thoughout its length for an individual cell. All axons originate from the axon hillock, which is usually a portion of the perikaryon. This physiological region is called the initial segment. The axon hollock may be differentiated from dendrites by the absence of Nissl substance in the axon hillock and the presence of many microtubules and neurofilaments converging from the perikaryon into the axon through the hillock region. Thus the axon hillock will usually appear as a lightly stained region of the cell.

In multipolar neurons, a specialized physiological region exits in the region of the axon hillock or just distal to it. This region is known as the initial segment. It is at the initial segment that nonpropagating generator potentials of the receptive zone may raise the membrane potential to the critical threshold and initiate the formation of a propagated action potential that will then travel the length of the axon. The initial segment of the axon is characterized by the presence of a thin layer of electron-dense material immediately subjacent to the plasmalemma, the dense undercoating. In contrast to dendrites, axons retain a rather constant diameter and usually do not branch extensively until the terminal arborization is reached. Axonal cytoplasm or axoplasm contains neurofilaments and microtubules, some sER, and a few mitochondria. It does not contain large numbers of ribosomes or rough-walled endoplasmic reticulum, hence the axoplasm is dependent on the perikaryon for its maintenance.

The cytoplasm of the ends of the terminal arborizations contains numerous synaptic vesicles. The vesicles usually have a diameter within the range of 20 to 65 nm, but larger vesicles are occasionally observed. The shape and content of the synaptic vesicles have been correlated with the function of the synapse. Round, clear vesicles are associated with acetylcholine-mediated excitatory transmission at the neuromuscular junction, within the autonomic nervous system, and within the central portion of the nervous system. Flattened vesicles measuring 20 by 50 nm are often observed in the terminal boutons that are thought to be inhibitory in nature. Norepinephrine-containing vesicles usually are 40 to 60 nm in diameter and contain a dense core with a diameter of 15 to 25 nm. Neurosecretory neurons originating in the supraoptic and paraventricular nuclei demonstrate large (120 to 150 nm) vesicles that contain oxytocin and vasopressin along with their associated neurophysins. When aggregated, these large vesicles are visible with the light microscope in the form of Herring bodies.

The synaptic vesicles and their contained neurotransmitters are necessary for the transmission of an impulse from the presynaptic region of the synapse to the postsynaptic portion. The mediators are liberated at the presynaptic membrane by exocytosis and diffuse across the synaptic cleft. On reaching the postsynaptic membrane, the plasmalemma of the next cell, the transmitters act on the membrane to initiate an excitatory or inhibitory response. The synaptic vesicle membranes that have fused with the presynaptic plasmalemma undergo endocytosis and are reused to form new synaptic vesicles.

Supporting cells

Several types of cells are found in association with the nerve cells of the CNS. These cells are classified as **neuroglia** or glial cells. Neuroglia include several varieties: astrocytes, oligodendrocytes, microglia, and ependymal cells. The astrocytes and oligodendrocytes are sometimes referred to as the macroglia. Neuroglial cells do not generate action potentials and they do not form synapses with other cells. Oligodendrocytes form the myelin sheaths of the axons of the central neurons and possibly are essential for the maintenance and viability of the neurons.

Astrocytes are the largest of the glial cells and possess many long cellular processes. The nuclei are centrally placed in the cell body and tend to stain lightly with routine stains. Many of the cell processes end in association with blood capillaries. The slightly expanded pedicles are termed vascular feet and completely surround the blood vessels. Cell processes of other astrocytes participate in forming the peripheral boundary or limiting membrane of the brain and spinal cord as they lie immediately subjacent to the pia mater. Thus the neural cells do not come into contact with nonneural tissue. Astrocytes also provide structural support to the neural tissue. Protoplasmic astrocytes are most numerous in the gray matter of the nervous system. Here the glial cells support and surround the cell bodies of the nerve cells and partially insulate the synapses that occur on the perikarya and dendrites. The protoplasmic astrocytes demonstrate an abundance of granular cytoplasm and tend to posses many rather short, thick processes. Fibrous astrocytes, on the other hand, possess longer, thinner, less numerous cell processes. The fibrous astrocytes are found primarily in the white matter of the central portion of the nervous system.

Oligodendrocytes are much smaller than astrocytes, their nuclei are smaller and more intensely staining, and their processes are less numerous and shorter than the other macroglial cells. Oligodendrocytes are found in both the gray and white matter regions of the central portion of the nervous system. In the gray matter, the oligodendroglia tend to be localized near the perikarya. In the white matter, the oligodendroglia appear in rows situated among the myelinated fibers. The oligodendrocytes produce the myelin sheaths of the CNS. Each oligodendrocyte tends to provide a portion of the myelin sheaths for several adjacent nerve cell processes.

Microglia cells are small, rather densely staining, and elongated. The microglia tend to be found very near the blood vessels located within the brain and are most likely representatives of the bloodborne mononuclear phagocyte system.

Ependymal cells are found lining the ventricular system of the CNS and are derived from the neuroepithelium, as are the other true glial cells. Most ependymal cells possess motile cilia that may serve to produce movement of the cerebrospinal fluid. Ependymal cells demonstrate an abundance of mitochondria, an apical Golgi apparatus, and small amounts of rER. The lateral surfaces of many cells exhibit gap junctions and zonulae adherentes with adjacent cells. In most areas, the ependymal cells do not form an impermeable barrier to the movement of fluid and small molecules or ions from the cerebrospinal fluid to the intercellular fluid of the brain or vice versa. However, in the region of the choroid plexuses, the ependymal cells provide the barrier that determines the materials that are allowed to pass through it. Most ependymal cells demonstrate a flattened base and do not extend into the subjacent neural tissue. However, in the region of the third ventricle, especially in the hypothalamus, the ependymal cells send long processes into the subjacent neural tissue and may play a role in transferring substances from the cerebrospinal fluid to the more deeply lying neurosecretory cells.

The small amount of connective tissue that is found in the central portion of the nervous system is situated in perivascular sheaths that are present around the larger vessel. Support of the neural tissue is thus derived from cells, predominantly the astrocytes. The astrocytes not only form the supporting elements of the central portion of the nervous stem but glial cells, primarily the astrocytes, determine the nature of the endothelial cells of the capillary beds situated within the neural tissue. If the astrocytes are present and are normal, the endothelial cells will form a continuous, very selective vessel. However, if the astrocytes are abnormal or are in regions where astrocytes are not found, the capillary endothelium will be less selective and will even demonstrate fenestrations.

CARDIOVASCULAR SYSTEM

The cardiovascular system consists of the **heart, blood vessels,** and **lymphatic vessels.** The heart provides the primary force to move the blood through the vascular system. Vessels carrying blood from the heart, **arteries,** branch into many generations as they proceed to the peripheral tissues. In each generation the diameter of the individual vessels becomes smaller but the total cross-sectional area of all the vessels in that particular generation increases. The arterial vessels ultimately give rise to the smallest vessels of the system, the **capillaries.** It is at the capillary level that there is an exchange of dissolved gases and molecules of nutrient or waste material between the blood plasma and the tissue fluid. **Veins,** vessels transporting blood to the heart, are formed by the convergence of the efferents from the capillary beds.

The **lymphatic vascular system** begins as blind-ended capillaries that anastomose to form larger and larger vessels. The lymphatic system ultimately terminates in the blood vascular system. The function of the lymphatic system is to return the excess tissue fluid created at the blood vascular capillary bed to the blood. In the process, the contained tissue fluid, now known as lymph, is passed through peripheral lymphatic tissue and exposes the cellular lymphatic tissue to possible foreign material, which will cause the initiation of an immune response.

Blood not only carries dissolved gases and nutrients or metabolic waste products, but also transports substances such as hormones produced by the nervous system and the endocrine organs that assist in the integration of the physiological activities of the organism.

All structures in the circulatory system, except for some

modifications at the smallest vessel level, are constructed of three layers or **tunics**. The specific composition of the tunics is different in the various classes and subclasses of vessels and is based on the physiological demands placed on the respective vessels. The tunics, or general layers, of the vessels are (1) tunica intima, (2) tunica media, and (3) tunica adventitia.

The **tunica intima** consists of a layer of **endothelial cells** that line the vessel's interior surface. The endothelial cells lie on a basal lamina. Just peripheral to the endothelial layer and its associated basal lamina is the **subendothelial layer**. This layer consists of loose connective tissue and occasionally a few smooth muscle cells. The major orientation of the connective tissue fibers and the smooth muscle cells tends to be longitudinal in relation to the long axis of the vessel.

The **tunica media** consists primarily of concentric layers of tightly spiraled or **circularly arranged smooth muscle cells**, which are often interspersed with elastic tissue, collagen fibers (type III), and proteoglycans. The extracellular substances are produced by the smooth muscle cells of the region. In the arterial system, the tunica media is separated from the tunica intima by a prominent elastic lamina, **the internal elastic lamina**. In large arteries, the tunica media is separated from the tunica adventitia by a thinner **external elastic lamina**. These elastic lamina and those that might be found in the media of larger arteries are fenestrated to allow for the diffusion of tissue fluid to nourish the cells of the media. In capillaries and small venules, the tunica media is represented by **pericytes**.

The **tunica adventitia** is composed primarily of collagenous and elastic fibers that demonstrate a longitudinal orientation. The collagen in the adventitia is type II. The adventitia serves to unite the vessel with the surrounding connective tissue.

In larger vessels, the vessel wall is nourished by smaller vessels situated in the tunica adventitia and outer tunica media. These small vessels are known as the vasa vasorum (vessels of the vessel). The vasa vasorum of the large veins tend to penetrate further into the tunica media than they do in comparable arteries because of the lower transmural pressure and the lower oxygen tension of the blood contained within the vein. Lymphatic vessels are also found in the outer regions of the larger vessels.

The vessels of the circulatory system can be divided into two major groups according to the size or diameter of the vessel. Vessels, either arterial or venous, that posses a diameter greater than 0.1 mm are said to compose the macrovasculature while those with a diameter of under 0.1 mm compose the microvasculature. The macrovasculature consists of vessels of transit, which are primarily involved in the transportation of blood from one region of the body to another. The vessels participate in the process of exchange of substances between the blood contained within the vessels and the tissue fluid surrounding the vessels.

Capillaries are the smallest of the blood vessels and are composed of a single layer of endothelial cells and their associated basal lamina. The usual dimensions of a capillary are a diameter of 7 to 9 μm and a length of 0.25 to 1.0 mm. Capillaries can be divided into four general groups, based on the morphology of the endothelial cell and the size of the capillary. The most common type of capillary is the **somatic**, or **continuous**, capillary. This type is found in muscle tissue, nerve tissue, connective tissue, and exocrine glands. The endothelial cells do not demonstrate fenestrae. However, the endothelial cells do demonstrate numerous pinocytotic vesicles located within the cytoplasm of the cell. The spaces between adjacent endothelial cells tend to be closed by cell-to-cell junctions and/or overlapping extensions of the peripheral portions of the cells. The **visceral** or **fenestrated** capillary is found in the intestinal tract, the peritubular plexus of the kidney, and many endocrine glands. The endothelial cells of this type of capillary demonstrate many areas in which the plasmalemma of the luminal and abluminal surface of the cell is brought together to form a circular region, about 60 to 80 nm in diameter, in which there is no cytoplasm. This thinned region, a fenestra (window) is closed by a diaphragm that is thinner than the unit membrane of the plasmalemma and does not demonstrate the trilaminar structure of the cell membrane. The fenestrae allow for easier movement of macromolecules through the endothelial layer than that occurring by pinocytosis while still providing some selectivity in the materials that may pass through the layer. The third type of capillary possesses another form of **fenestrated endothelium**. Here the fenestrae are not closed by a diaphragm but are frank openings that extend through the cell cytoplasm. These capillaries are found within the renal glomerulus. The last type of capillary is the **sinusoid**. The sinusoid is much larger in diameter (30 to 40 μm) with a slower flow of blood, the periphery often is often associated with phagocytic cells, and the basal lamina is usually discontinuous. Sinusoids are primarily found in the liver and hematopoietic organs.

The capillary plexus joins the arterial and venous vessels. The vessels supplying the capillary bed, arterioles, branch into small vessels that possess a discontinuous layer of smooth muscle and are called **metarterioles**. The metarterioles serve to assist in the regulation of blood flow through the capillary bed and provide a pathway through the plexus if the plexus is not perfused. The final structure controlling the flow of blood into the capillary plexus is the **precapillary sphincter**. The density of the capillary plexus in any tissue is related to the metabolic activity of the tissue.

The function of the capillary bed of the circulatory system is related to the properties of the capillary endothelial cells themselves and consists of three major components:

1. It provides a selectively permeable barrier between the blood contained within the vascular system and the surrounding tissue by serving as the exchange site for gases such as oxygen and carbon dioxide, nutrient substrates, and metabolic wastes. The exchange mechanisms include movement of fluids and materials through the boundary of the endothelial cells and basal lamina by means of intercellular clefts between cells that are temporarily opened under appropriate conditions, the fenestrae formed within individual endothelial cells, and pinocytotic vesicles that are capable of transporting substances from one surface of the boundary cells to the other surface.

2. Metabolic functions of the endothelial cells include conversion of angiotensin I to angiotensin II. The capillary cells also serve to inactivate compounds circulating in the blood such as bradykinins, serotonin, prostaglandins, norepinephrine, etc. The cells also contain enzymes that are active in the breakdown of bloodborne lipoproteins to triglycerides and cholesterol and assist in the transportation of these molecules across the cell boundary.

3. The capillary endothelial cells also prevent the formation of platelet aggregates or platelet breakdown. If the endothelial

boundary is broken, connective tissue elements are exposed to the blood and the clotting reaction is initiated.

CHARACTERISTICS OF LARGER BLOOD VESSELS

The three major generations of arterial vessels are named from large to small: (1) **elastic arteries**, (2) **muscular arteries**, and (3) **arterioles**. Each generation of artery is accompanied by an equivalent generation of venous vessel.

Arterioles are vessels with an overall diameter of 0.5 mm or less and possess a narrow lumen. The tunica intima of arterioles usually consists of endothelial cells of the continuous or somatic type that rest on a basal lamina and a very scanty amount of subendothelial connective tissue. An internal elastic lamina is present in larger arterioles but is usually missing in smaller ones. The tunica media is composed of one to five layers of circularly arranged smooth muscle cells with a small amount of supporting connective tissue. The tunica adventitia is thin, and no external elastic lamina is present.

Muscular arteries, medium-sized arteries, compose most of the named arteries of the body. In this class of vessel the tunica intima is composed of endothelial cells of the somatic or continuous type and a thin subendothelial layer of loose connective tissue that contains an occasional smooth muscle cell. An internal elastic lamina is always present and often very well developed. The tunica media consists of 5 to 40 layers of smooth muscle with an intermingling of elastic laminae and collagen fibers. An external elastic lamina is usually present and well defined as it lies between the tunica media and tunica adventitia. The tunica adventitia consists of collagenous fibers and elastic fibers, primarily longitudinal in orientation, that serve to tie the vessels into the surrounding connective tissues. Nerves, vasa vasorum, and lymphatics are present in the tunica adventitia.

Elastic arteries such as the aorta and its major branches and the pulmonary trunk and arteries appear yellow when viewed in the fresh state. This coloration is due to the large amounts of elastic connective tissue (yellow) contained within the tunica media of the vessels. The tunica intima consists of the usual endothelial cell later and its related connective tissue. The subendothelial layer is clearly evident and contains many connective tissue fibers along with fibroblasts and smooth muscle cells. The major orientation of the fibers and smooth muscle cells is longitudinal or parallel to the major axis of the vessel. The tunica media is composed of 40 to 70 concentric laminae of elastic connective tissue. The laminae are fenestrated and intermingled with smooth muscle cells, fibroblasts, collagen fibers, and ground substances. The tunica adventitia is relatively light and consists of elastic and collagenous fibers that merge with surrounding loose connective tissue.

Elastic arteries are also known as conducting arteries. Under usual circumstances, the elastic arteries are forced to dilate by the bolus of blood delivered from the ventricles of the heart on contraction (systole). During diastole (relaxation of the heart ventricle), the elastic recoil of the elastic vessels, walls creates a smaller, secondary (diastolic) pressure on the blood within the lumen of the vessel and assists in driving the blood farther into the circulatory system. The elastic arteries thereby physically buffer the pressure changes within the system.

The muscular arteries are also known as distributing arteries. Under the control of neural and hormonal influences, they determine the flow of blood to the various organs and regions of the body. Arterioles, metarterioles, and precapillary sphincters then control the final distribution of blood within the capillary beds (plexuses) of the organs or regions.

Veins are the vessels that return blood from the capillary beds of the body to the heart. In general, veins have a thinner wall and larger lumen than the comparable companion arteries.

Venules are the smallest generation of veins. Venules are formed by the coalescence of the vessels comprising the capillary beds. The diameter of venules will range from 0.2 to 1 mm. Although thinner walled than the comparable arteries, the veins demonstrate the three-tunic configuration of the cardiovascular system. In venules, the tunica intima is composed of an endothelial layer and related basal lamina, which is associated with very little or no subendothelial layer tissue. The tunica media is also very thin and may consist of only a few circularly arranged smooth muscle cells and connective tissue. The tunica adventitia, which is the thickest lamina, is composed of longitudinally arranged connective tissue cells and fibers along with some smooth muscle cells. Small postcapillary venules are important regions of resorption of tissue fluid into the vascular system as well as a location where white blood cells are able to migrate from the circulatory system into the connective tissues. This migration is especially evident during the inflammatory response that is initiated by damage to tissues.

Small and medium-sized veins that accompany the distributing or medium-sized arteries demonstrate a thin tunica intima that rests on a thin subendothelial layer, whose connective tissue and smooth muscle elements are longitudinal in orientation. The tunica media is again composed of a thin layer of circularly arranged smooth muscle and connective tissue fibers and cells. The tunica adventitia is the thickest layer and is composed of longitudinally oriented bundles of smooth muscle, collagen bundles, and elastic fibers.

The **largest veins** demonstrate a well-developed tunica intima with an endothelial and subendothelial layering, again oriented longitudinally. The tunica media is thin and circularly arranged, while the tunica adventitia is very thick and demonstrates prominent longitudinal bundles of smooth muscle and connective tissue.

The veins of the limbs (those areas that are below the heart in a quadruped) possess valves that are semilunar in shape. These valve leaflets are arranged in pairs and serve to divide the column of blood into smaller segments. The valve leaflets are formed from folds of the endothelial and subendothelial tissue.

The heart maintains and demonstrates the typical three-layered construction of the system. The **endocardium** is internal and is homologous to the tunica intima of the vessels; the **myocardium** is the middle layer and is homologous to the tunica media, and the **epicardium** is external and similar to the tunica adventitia. The endocardium consists of the usual endothelial cells and subendothelial connective tissue and smooth muscle. Situated between the subendothelial layer and the myocardium is a transitional zone known as the subendocardium, which contains elements of the impulse-conducting system of the heart, most specifically the Purkinje fibers of the bundle branches, some nerve fibers, and small veins.

The **myocardium** consists of multiple layers of **cardiac muscle tissue**, which are arranged in spiral configurations and compose the walls of the atria and ventricles of the heart. The bundles of cardiac muscles and layers tend to interlace and intermingle. The bundles are oriented ultimately to attach to the fibrous cardiac skeleton, which surrounds the valves of the heart and separates the atrial musculature form the ventricular muscle mass.

The **epicardium** consists of a layer of mesothelial cells and their intimately related connective tissue elements that cover the external surface of the heart. This layer is the visceral pericardium of gross anatomy. Situated between the epicardium and the myocardium is a layer of connective tissue known as the **subepicardium**. The subepicardium consists of loose connective tissue, adipose tissue, and contains the major coronary arteries and cardiac veins.

The **cardiac muscle tissue** is composed of two major types of muscle cells. One group of cardiac muscle cells is specialized to contract and thus provide the propulsive force that moves the blood through the circulatory system. The other group of muscle cells composes the impulse-generating and conducting system of the heart. The cardiac cells that form the contractile elements of the heart are single cells that are usually uninucleated but occasionally demonstrate two nuclei. The cells tend to branch. The nuclei are centrally placed within the cytoplasm of the typically branched cell. The cardiac muscle operates as a functional syncytium. In order to do this, the cells are joined together by intercalated disks. The intercalated disks, which are located at the ends of the individual fibers and join adjacent cells together end to end, are composed of two regions. One region is oriented transversely to the major longitudinal axis of the joined cells and is actually a fascia adherens type of cell junction. This transverse portion of the intercalated disk serves to transmit the contractile force from one cell to another and thereby unite the cells into a contractile mass that needs very little connective tissue to harness the contractile force of the cells. The intercalated disk also demonstrates a longitudinal section. In this region of the disk, which is found at the lateral aspects of the ends of adjacent cells, are located desmosomes and gap junctions. The gap junctions serve to transmit the electrical depolarization impulse that triggers contraction of the cells from one cell to another. Thus each individual contractile cardiac muscle cell is not contacted directly by an element of the conduction system.

The **impulse-generating** and **conducting tissue** of the heart is composed of very specialized cardiac muscle tissue. Instead of being specialized to contract, the cells are altered to generate a spontaneously depolarizing membrane potential and to conduct the impulse throughout the heart. The system is composed of the sinoatrial (SA) node situated subepicardially in the right atrial wall near the superior vena cava, the atrioventricular (AV) node, located in the right atrial side of the interatrial septum, the AV bundle, and the left and right bundle branches. The SA node has the more rapidly cycling impulse-generating cells located within it and thus serves to drive the system. The SA node fibers are smaller than the usual atrial muscle cells and are oriented circularly around the nodal artery. There appears to be a series of preferred pathways within the atrial musculature to transmit the impulse to the contractile atrial muscle fibers and to the AV node. The AV node is also composed of modified muscle cells that are smaller than the atrial muscle. The AV bundle extends from the AV node through the cardiac skeleton to reach the interventricular septum, where the bundle divides into left and right bundle branches that proceed subendocardially on the septum. The modified cardiac muscle cells forming the AV bundle and its branches are known as Purkinje cells. They are larger than the contractile cardiac cells, so they can conduct the surface impulse more rapidly. The Purkinje cells demonstrate very few myofibrils within their cytoplasm. They demonstrate abundant glycogen granules within the cell. The Purkinje cells contact contractile cardiac cells by means of gap junctions. The bundle and bundle branches direct the impulse to the region of the papillary muscles and apical musculature of the ventricles, from which the impulse spreads back toward the cardiac skeleton. Thus the region of the ventricles that is situated farthest from the ventricular outflow channels (valves) contracts first and serves to milk the blood out of the chamber.

The **lymphatic portion of the circulatory system** begins as blind-ended tubules of capillary dimensions within the connective tissues of the body. The lymphatic system serves to collect the excess tissue fluid that is generated at the capillary bed and transport this fluid, now called lymph when in the lymphatic vessel, back to the deep central veins, where the lymph is placed back into the blood. Lymphatic capillaries are different from blood capillaries in that the lymph capillaries do not demonstrate a continuous basal lamina. The endothelial cells are also not united by cell-to-cell junctions. The endothelial cells of the lymphatic capillaries are attached to connective tissue fibers by means of a spot of basal lamina material. When the connective tissue is spread by the collection of an overabundance of tissue fluid, the lymphatic capillaries are pulled open and thus allow the fluid to enter the channels more easily. The lack of a continuous basal lamina and occluding junctions allows the lymphatic capillaries to receive macromolecules, particulate matter, and even microorganisms and cells that would not be able to pass into the blood capillaries. These materials that can thereby enter the lymph are free to circulate throughout the body if not stopped by lymph node tissues.

The larger lymphatic vessels demonstrate a thin-walled structure very similar to small veins. The lymphatic vessles possess abundant valves to direct the contained lymph from the periphery to the more centrally paced terminations in the lymphatic system.

INTEGUMENT—SKIN AND ITS APPENDAGES

The **skin** is the largest single organ of the body. It accounts for approximately 16% of the body weight and has a surface area of between 1.5 and 2.25 m², depending on body size.

The skin is composed of two tissue layers: (1) the **epidermis**—stratified squamous keratinizing epithelium of ectodermal origin and (2) the **dermis**—irregular fibroelastic connective tissue of mesodermal origin, which can be further subdivided into a loose irregular connective tissue stratum immediately subjacent to the epidermis (the papillary layer) and a deeper much denser layer (the reticular layer). The papillary region contains the vascular plexus that supplies the nutrients not only for the immediately surrounding connective tissue but also for the more superficially situated epithelium, the epidermis. The papillary layer also contains many encapsulated nerve endings. The deeper reticular layer provides the strength of the skin. Although the reticular layer is dense, irregularly arranged connective tissue, there is a predominant or prevailing orientation for the larger fibers that will vary according to the location within the body. This prevailing pattern gives rise to the Langer's lines, which if possible are followed in a parallel fashion when incising the skin. The resulting incision will tend to close, not open, because of the natural tensions within the connective tissues.

Deep to the dermis is a layer of subcutaneous tissue composed primarily of adipose tissue. The histological name for this region is the **hypodermis**. It will contain the secretory portions of many of the sweat glands of the skin, encapsulated nerve endings, and blood vessels, passing to and from the skin.

The **epidermis** is entirely cellular. On the palms of the hands and soles of the feet, it is much thicker than on the remaining parts of the body. These areas of the hands and feet are said to be covered with **thick skin** while the majority of the body is covered with **thin skin**. It is important to note that the designation of thick or thin skin is based solely on the structure (thickness) of the epidermis.

The epidermis demonstrates a continual progression of cells that proceed from the area of proliferation through several steps of differentiation and ultimately are cast off from the body surface. The stages of these processes are best seen in thick skin, although similar events occur in thin skin. The reserve population of cells is found in the **stratum basalis**. This layer rests on the basal lamina, and many of the cells demonstrate hemidesmosomes that strengthen the attachment to the basal lamina. The stratum basalis is also known as the **stratum germinativum** because the germinal (multiplying) cells are situated in it.

The progression of differentiation of the **keratinocytes** of the epidermis is as follows:

As the cells in the stratum germinativum undergo mitosis, one of the daughter cells remains in the germinal layer to proliferate later while the other daughter cell is moved superficially toward the surface of the body. The cells in this layer demonstrate many desmosomes joining adjacent cells. Because of the many desmosomes, the cells show many projections after artifactual cell shrinkage related to dehydration in preparation for histological study. The name **stratum spinosum** has been used to describe this layer. Cells in the stratum spinosum are capable of undergoing mitosis and do so, thus adding to the total population of cells. The term **malpighian layer** is often applied to the combined layers of the stratum germinativum and stratum spinosum. Within the stratum spinosum, the cells continue to proliferate intracellular fibrils, the formation of which was initiated in the stratum germinativum.

As the cells are forced superficially by the continued proliferation of cells in the deeper layers, the cells undergo a further change. Another proteinacous material synthesized within the cell is known as **keratohyalin**. This protein, initially appearing as granules, tends to bind to the intracellular filaments, and at this stage the protein tends to stain basophilically. Because of the granular appearance of the cytoplasm of the cells in this general layer of the epidermis, the stratum is known as the **stratum granulosum**. The cells of the stratum granulosum also demonstrate vesicles whose contents are secreted from the cell membrane-coating material. The substance is composed of glycosaminoglycans and phospholipids and serves as an intercellular cement or filler. This substance assists greatly in producing the relatively impervious barrier properties of the epidermis that are essential for life on land.

Within the next more superficial layer, the **stratum lucidum**, the epidermal cells are flattened and demonstrate no nuclei and few or no metabolic organelles. The cell is packed with filaments bound together to form a matrix. This layer stains rather lightly and acidophilically.

The stratum lucidum cells continue to be flattened and internally compacted as they are moved into the **stratum corneum**. Now these cells are in essence plates of proteinacous material, primarily keratin, that is found in the form of intracellular filaments that are joined together by keratohyalin granules.

In the outermost layers of cells of the stratum corneum, enzymatic breakdown of the intercellular substance and other cell-to-cell junctions occurs. This layer of loosened cells is often designated as the **stratum disjunctum** and is the site from which the cells are desquamated from the body.

Melanocytes compose another major component of the epidermis. These pigment-producing cells are found in the stratum basalis. Long cellular processes extend into the stratum spinosum. Melanin pigment granules are synthesized within the melanocyte and secreted into the keratinocytes surrounding the melanocyte cellular processes. The number of melanocytes varies from one region of the body to another, but for a given body region the number of cells is fairly constant regardless of race or gender. The variations in skin color among individuals are the result of different types of melanin and the rate of degradation of the melanin granules once they are within the keratinocyte.

Other cells within the epidermis include the Langerhans cells and Merkel cells. Langerhans cells are thought to be related to the mononuclear phagocyte system of the body. Merkel cells are thought to relate to nerve endings within the epidermis and thus serve as receptors for the nervous system.

The epidermal layers of epithelium also give rise to the epidermal appendages of the skin: sweat glands, hair, and nails. Sweat glands are found almost everywhere on the body surface. **Eccrine (merocrine) sweat glands**, which produce the serous fluid of perspiration, are simple tubular glands whose duct passes through the epidermis to the deeper areas of the dermis and often into the hypodermis. There the secretory portions of the tubules may be found as loosely coiled tubules surrounded by myoepithelial cells and a capillary plexus. The secretory portion contains two types of cells: (1) **clear cells** which are important in transepithelial fluid transportation and salt resorption, and (2) **dark cells**, which contain many synthetic organelles and glycoprotein-containing vesicles. The duct is usually composed of cuboidal cells and may be stratified.

A second type of sweat gland, the **apocrine sweat gland**, is present in the axillary, areolar, and the genital and circumanal regions. The glands are simple tubular glands, but the secretory portions are much larger than the merocrine glands and are situated in the hypodermis. The ducts of the apocrine glands terminate in hair follicles. The apocrine glands most likely secrete their product by the merocrine mode and not by the apocrine mode. The secretion of the apocrine glands is a rather viscous substance, which, when decomposed by bacteria, helps to produce the distinctive body odor for each individual.

A **hair follicle**, arising from the epidermis, produces an aggregation of keratinized cells known as a **hair shaft**. In humans, the size and density of hair is not sufficient to provide thermal protection as in animals but instead provides a very rich system of sensory transducers, which when moved influence the peritricheal nerve endings. Hair follicles are distributed over the entire body except for the regions of thick skin, the lips, glans penis, labia minora, and clitoris. Hair growth is influenced by genetic factors, the general state of health, and the hormonal balance of the individual.

Each hair arises from a tubular epidermal invagination, the hair follicle. During the growth phase of the follicle (producing a hair), the base (deep end) of the follicle is expanded to produce a **hair bulb**. The hair bulb caps and partially surrounds the **dermal papilla**, which contains a capillary plexus essential to the nutrition of the hair bulb and developing hair. During periods of growth, the epithelial cells that compose the hair bulb are equivalent to the stratum germinativum of the epidermis. They proliferate and produce cells that differentiate into the following cell types:

1. **Medullary cells** are found in thick hair (e.g., scalp). They are derived from the apex of the hair bulb and form the center of the hair shaft. The cells tend to be large and heavily vacuolated.
2. Cells derived from the central portions of the hair bulb produce heavily keratinized cells that form the compact hair cortex.
3. The cells from the periphery of the hair bulb produce the outer layer of cells of the hair shaft, the **cuticle**.
4. Cells of the hair follicle that are in the area of transition from the hair bulb to the follicular wall produce the **internal root sheath**. This layer of cells is found only in the areas of the follicle deep to the entrance of the sebacous glands.

The cells composing the tubular wall of the follicle are continuous with the surface epidermis and demonstrate the usual layering near the orifice of the follicle. Deeper in the follicle, the cells equivalent to the germinal layer produce the **external root sheath** layer of the follicle. The basal lamina and supporting connective tissue are continued downward around the hair follicle and become known as the **glassy membrane**. The connective tissue immediately surrounding the epithelial follicle is somewhat condensed and has been named the **mesodermal** or **connective tissue sheath**.

The **arrector pili muscle** attaches to the connective tissue sheath and to the dermis. When the muscle fascicles contract, they tend to move the hair follicle from a somewhat oblique position to a more vertically oriented position, making the hair "stand on end." That movement tends to place pressure on the **sebacous glands** associated with the neck of the hair follicle, expressing **sebum**, the product resulting from the holocrine secretion of the gland, into the follicle and ultimately to the surface of the skin.

The natural color and shape of the hair are determined by the melanocytes situated in the hair bulb and the shape of the bulb itself, respectively. The melanocytes produce melanin granules that are incorporated into the medulla and cortex of the shaft. The shape of the bulb determines the shape of the hair shaft; circular shafts produce very straight hair whereas more elliptical shafts produce varying degrees of curling.

The **nails** that are found on the distal dorsal surface of each digit are also produced by the ectodermal epithelial cells. The manner of production is somewhat similar to that of hair in that the formative region, the **nail matrix**, has been invaginated into the underlying connective tissue. The matrix is divided into **dorsal** and **vental portions** by the **nail plate**, which is formed by the accretion of cells produced by the proliferation of cells in the matrix and their subsequent keratinization. The ventral matrix often extends under the nail plate distal to the point at which the plate emerges from the **nail groove**, forming the light-colored **lunula**. The nail plate rests on the nail bed, which is composed of modified epidermis. If the nail matrix is destroyed accidentally or intentionally, no nail plate will be formed distal to the injured region; hence the surgical treatment for ingrown nails.

The keratinized products of the skin, i.e., the hair and nails, are composed of hard keratin whereas the stratum coneum of the skin is composed of soft keratin.

RESPIRATORY SYSTEM

The **respiratory system** consists of the lungs and a series of passages that join the lungs to the external environment. As such, the respiratory system can be divided into two portions, (1) the conducting portion and (2) the respiratory portion. The **conducting portion** consists of the nasal cavity, the nasopharynx and oropharynx, larynx, trachea, several generations of bronchi, and several generations of bronchioles, which end with a generation known as the terminal bronchioles. The **respiratory portion** begins as a continuation of the bronchiolar generations with the respiratory bronchiole and continues with alveolar ducts and ultimately the alveoli. The conducting portion of the system is constructed not only to conduct or carry air to and from the respiratory portion but also to condition the incoming air by warming, humidifying, and cleansing it. The terminal portion of the conducting portion also controls the flow and distribution of air to and from the respiratory areas. The respiratory portion of the system, composing the major portion of the sponge-like lungs, is constructed to provide a minimal but sufficient boundary for exchange of gases between the inspired air and the plasma of the blood. Needless to say, the lungs are very highly vascularized organs, receiving the entire output of the right ventricle of the heart.

As stated above, the **conducting portion** of the respiratory system is constructed to provide a **patent passage** of inspired and expired air. This passage can be varied in diameter and length. It is also lined with a mucosa that is responsible for conditioning the inspired air. The primary structural components maintaining patency of the conducting portion are bone and cartilage, with additional layering of muscle and other connective tissues. The skull and pharyngeal musculature provide the necessary support for the nasal cavity and naso- and oropharynx. The cartilages and musculature of the **larynx** maintain the patency of that region and lead into the trachea. The larynx not only maintains the lumen of the conducting portion of the respiratory system but also provides a zone of sensitivity and protection from entry of large amounts of foreign material into the lower respiratory system. It also provides the structural supports for the elements responsible for phonation.

The supporting elements of the **trachea** are in the form of **incomplete rings of hyaline cartilage**. The open ends of the rings are directed posteriorly, where they are united by smooth muscle fibers, the **trachealis muscle**. The cartilage rings are joined longitudinally by collagenous and elastic fibrous connective tissue.

The pattern of support of the conducting portion of the system changes from incomplete cartilage rings in the trachea and first two generations of bronchi to a pattern of **cartilaginous plates** that surround the lumen of the **intrapulmonary bronchi**. The plates demonstrate processes that tend to interdigitate to provide support between the plates. Fascicles of smooth muscle situated in the lamina propria form spirals that encircle and extend along the length of the intrapulmonary bronchi. The spiraling muscle fascicles are found predominantly within the deep lamina propria (between the mucosa and cartilage). **Elastic tissue fibers** become more and more numerous as the bronchi are followed peripherally into the smaller-diameter generations. As the tubular structures reach a diameter of about 1 mm, the cartilage plates terminate but the smooth muscle and elastic tissue continue. The tubular portions of this size and nature are known as **bronchioles**. The patency of the bronchioles is maintained primarily by the centrifugal tensions placed on the walls by the connective tissue fibers in the surrounding lung substance.

The mucosa of the conducting portion of the respiratory system is composed of a **pseudostratified columnar epithelium**. The epithelium is composed of representatives of six main cell types:

1. **Columnar ciliated cells** are the most numerous. Each cell possesses several hundred cilia on the apical surface.
2. **Mucous goblet cells** are the second most numerous cell type. These cells are unicellular mucous glands.
3. **Brush cells** are columnar cells of two forms that represent
   a. immature ciliated columnar cells or goblet cells
   b. sensory receptor cells for the nervous system
4. **Basal cells** are in contact with the basal lamina but do not extend to the free surface of the epithelial layer. They are germinal, replacing cells for the tissue.
5. **Granule cells** are short cells that contain many small granules and are thought to be related to the APUD system of diffuse endocrine-secreting cells. They probably serve to help regulate the functioning of the secretory cells in the vicinity.

The mucosa of the conducting portions of the system also demonstrates many glands, predominantly mucous in nature, situated in the lamina propria. The multicellular glands and the goblet cells are most numerous in the larger respiratory passages and become less numerous in the smaller, more peripherally situated generations of bronchi. The glands of the lamina propria are absent in the bronchioles, and the goblet cells are scattered.

Ciliated cells are especially abundant in the upper portion of the respiratory system. The cilia are organized to beat toward the pharyngeal region. Ciliated cells are found extending into the peripheral, small bronchioles and thus are located farther peripherally in the system than are the glandular elements.

The conducting portion of the system also conditions the inspired air. The **conditioning process** involves **cleansing, humidifying,** and **warming the air** being taken into the lungs. The warming is accomplished, under usual conditions, by exposing the air to a rather dense vascular plexus situated in the lamina propria, deep to the epithelium of the nasal cavity. The blood within the plexus gives up heat to the air so that by the time the air is in the nasopharynx, it is almost at body temperature. The oral cavity, pharynx, larynx, and trachea are much less efficient in warming the air.

The goblet cells of the nasal epithelium are augmented by many serous glands situated in the lamina propria. Serous and mucous glands are also found within the lamina propria of the larynx, trachea, and larger bronchi. The combined secretions of the multicellular glands and the goblet cells form a watery mucous covering layer for the epithelium. The **mucous coat** accomplishes several purposes:

1. The mucous coat **provides water** to evaporate into the inspired air, thus humidifying it. In the process, the mucous layer loses water and becomes more viscous.
2. The mucous coat **traps by adhesion or adsorption** materials or small organism that impact on its surface.
3. The mucous layer contains **immunoglobulins**, secreted by the lymphoid tissue situated in the lamina propria, that are protective against foreign materials. Thus materials trapped in the mucous coat are partially or totally "neutralized."
4. The deeper portion of the mucous coat is more watery (less viscous) than the superficial portion that has given up some of its water content. The cilia of the respiratory epithelium are situated, embedded, in the deeper layer. Ciliary action, directed toward the pharynx, gradually moves the mucous coat and its entrapped contaminants out of the nasal cavity and paranasal sinuses to the pharynx as well as out of the bronchioles, bronchi, trachea, and larynx to the pharynx.

It is important to note that the ciliated cells of the respiratory epithelium extend further peripherally within the system than do the glandular elements. It is also important to note that hereditary or environmental conditions that inhibit proper ciliary action or create a mucous layer that is too viscous or tenacious will impede the functioning of the **mucociliary ladder** or **mucociliary escalator**.

The **respiratory portion** of the system consists of the structures in the lungs in which gaseous exchange may occur between the air contained within the lumen and the blood contained within the tremendously rich capillary–small-vessel plexus situated within the walls of the air spaces (alveoli). The respiratory portion is initiated with the **respiratory bronchioles** (bronchioles that demonstrate small alveolar outpocketings from the wall but possess more wall surface than outpocketings) and continues to **alveolar ducts** (channels that have many more alveolar outpocketings than the previous generation, hence less wall surface), which in turn give rise to areas known as **atria**. The atria communicate with **alveolar sacs** or **alveoli** and represent or serve as a common or central space for the openings of the smaller alveoli, somewhat similar to an atrium and surrounding rooms in a building.

The respiratory bronchioles and alveolar duct walls are formed by strands of smooth muscle forming spirals around the lumen. Alveoli emerge between the spiral fascicles. The epithelium of the respiratory bronchioles and alveolar ducts is usually composed of a single, simple layer of columnar or cuboidal ciliated cells. No glandular elements are readily apparent.

The walls of the **alveoli** (alveolar sacs) are composed of epithelial cells of two types, type I and type II pneumocytes. Type I demonstrate an extremely attenuated but nonfenestrated squamous morphology, and type II (alveolar cells) tend to be somewhat cuboidal in shape and are often situated in the "corners" of the alveoli. Together the two cell types constitute a complete, unbroken, epithelial lining of the alveoli in that although the type I (squamous) cells demonstrate pinocytotic vesicles in the cytoplasm, there are no fenestrations and all of the epithelial cells are joined to adjacent cells by means of occluding junctions. The squamous type I cells are the primary areas of gaseous exchange. The type II cells produce the pulmonary surfactant that coats the inner aspect (next to air space) of the alveoli. The epithelial cells rest on a basal lamina, which in turn rests on the pulmonary interstitial connective tissue. The pulmonary interstitial tissue is composed of collagenous and elastic fibers (predominantly elastic) and contains the pulmonary vasculature. The connective tissue fibers prevent overdistension of the alveoli and also provides the means of elastic recoil during expiration.

The structures that are always interposed between the air and blood plasma constitute the **blood-air barrier**. At the narrowest, these include the type I pneumocyte and its related basal lamina and the capillary endothelial cell and its related basal lamina. Often the basal laminae of the two cell types of the barrier fuse into a single layer. In other areas, interstitial fibers and interstitial space may intervene between the endothelial cells and the epithelial cells with their respective basal laminae. Gases must also pass through the surfactant and other possible intra-alveolar secretions as they traverse the blood-air barrier, as well as the erythrocyte plasmalemma if the gas is transported within the red blood cell.

EMBRYOLOGY

GAMETOGENESIS (Fig. 1-6)

The formation of gametes is the first step in embryologic development. The gonads produce cells that contain one-half of each of the 23 pairs of chromosomes, the **haploid** chromosome number. These cells, the gametes, then restore the full complement of chromosomes upon union of a female and of a male gamete, forming 23 pairs or the **diploid** number. **Meiosis** is the type of cell division unique to gametogenesis.

Spermatogenesis

Within the seminiferous tubules of the testes, germ cells proliferate in very great numbers. **Spermatogonia** are diploid cells that are very active mitotically. They divide and produce more spermatogonia. Some of the spermatogonia **differentiate into primary spermatocytes**. Note that in going from a spermatogonium to a primary spermatocyte that *no cell division occurs*. Thus, one spermatogonium, which is diploid, produces one primary spermatocyte, which is also diploid.

The diploid **primary spermatocyte** has replicated DNA and proceeds into meiosis 1, which is a **reductional** cell division whereby two **haploid secondary spermatocytes** are formed. This reduction in chromosome number is achieved by the pairs of chromosomes lining up on the equatorial plate of the mitotic spindle during **metaphase**. As the cell completes metaphase and goes into **anaphase**, one of each chromosome pair migrates toward its respective pole so that when the cell divides each daughter cell (secondary spermatocyte) contains one of each pair and is thus **haploid**. The chromosomes at this stage are still replicated—that is, they contain two chromatids.

Because each replicated chromosome is intact following meiosis 1, no DNA replication occurs and thus there is no interphase between meiosis 1 and meiosis 2.

The haploid secondary spermatocyte enters meiosis 2, which is an **equational** division in that the haploid chromosome number is not further reduced. The chromosomes line up linearly on the equatorial plate of the metaphase spindle, and as anaphase begins, the two chromatids of each chromosome disjoin and migrate to opposite poles as daughter chromosomes. The cells resulting from this division are haploid **spermatids**, each chromosome existing in the unreplicated state.

To recapitulate, one spermatogonium differentiates into one primary spermacyte. The primary spermatocyte's DNA is replicated and can be quantified as 4 n. This primary spermatocyte enters meiosis 1 (a reductional division) and forms two secondary spermatocytes. Because the members of the pairs of chromosomes have been separated, the amount of DNA is now 2 n. The two secondary spermatocytes undergo meiosis 2 to produce four spermatids. Each spermatid has a quantity of DNA designated as n because each chromosome is now composed of a single chromatid.

Spermatids undergo a process of differentiation (*no cell divisions*) called **spermiogenesis**. During this process, a spermatid is transformed into a sperm, with its head, neck, middle piece, and tail. It has its chromatin substance in a very dense state located in the head of the sperm. The middle piece is a compact aggregation of mitochondria, and the tail is a motile flagellum.

Spermatogenesis (which includes spermiogenesis) takes about 64 days. Sperm leave the testes and are stored in the **ductus epididymis**, where they undergo further maturation.

Oogenesis

The ovaries produce the haploid female gametes, the ova, using the same basic mechanisms as in spermatogenesis but with some remarkable differences in the process.

Oogonia are found only prenatally. The primordial germ cells migrate to the developing ovary and differentiate into oogonia. The proliferation of the oogonia ceases in late gestation, and virtually all the primary oocytes are formed prior to birth. Widely varying estimates of the number of primary oocytes have been made, but the point is that at birth a couple of million of these cells are present in the two ovaries. By the time the menstrual cycles begin, only 30,000 to 40,000 are present, and of these only 300 to 400 are destined to undergo ovulation. The remainder undergo atresia.

The **diploid oogonia** differentiate into diploid primary oocytes. These cells enter the prophase of meiosis 1 and stop in

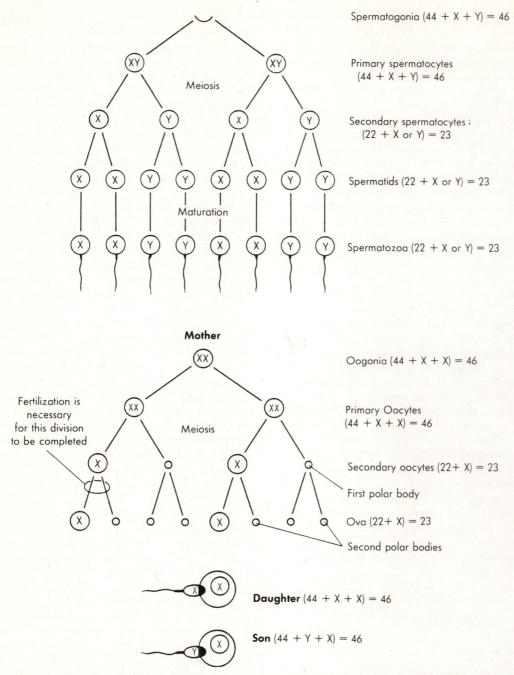

Figure 1-6.   Chromosomal changes during spermatogenesis and oogenesis, with ultimate formation of zygote.

prophase. These cells may remain in this arrested stage for decades, and thus this is called lengthy prophase. The meiosis 1 prophase has several stages, and the one in which the oocyte remains is **dictyotene.**

As a female enters puberty and menstrual cycles commence, in each cycle 12 to 15 or so of these primary oocytes and associated cells and tissues (collectively called the ovarian follicle) complete meiosis 1. Each primary oocyte produces one **haploid secondary oocyte** and one **first polar body.** Each of these has one-half of each chromosome pair, but the cell

division is unequal in that virtually all the cytoplasm goes to the secondary cell, only a scant amount to the polar body. The first polar body may go through meiosis 2, but regardless of whether it does or not it is ultimately destined to degenerate and disappear.

The secondary oocyte with its haploid complement of replicated chromosomes bypasses interphase and enters meiosis 2. Here it **stops in metaphase until fertilization** takes place. If and when fertilization occurs, meiosis 2 is completed and the second polar body is formed. The ovum contains the fertilizing sperm. The nucleus of the ovum and the sperm nucleus form female and male **pronuclei**, respectively. The DNA is replicated, the pronuclei fuse in a process called syngamy, and the zygote that is formed subsequently begins the first mitotic cell division (cleavage).

To summarize oogenesis, one diploid oogonium differentiates into one diploid primary oocyte. The primary oocyte enters prophase of meiosis 1, where it remains until it proceeds in development during a subsequent menstrual cycle. The primary oocyte completes meiosis 1 and produces a haploid secondary oocyte and the first polar body. The secondary oocyte then enters meiosis 2, in which it stops in metaphase, where it remains until fertilized. Upon fertilization, it completes meiosis 2 and forms the second polar body and an ovum, which contains the fertilizing sperm and goes on to form the zygote.

FEMALE SEXUAL CYCLE (MENSTRUAL CYCLE)

In discussing the female sexual cycle, four structures must be considered: the (1) uterus, (2) ovaries, (3) brain (hypothalamus), and (4) pituitary gland (anterior pituitary or adenohypophysis).

Uterus

This pear-shaped organ lies in the pelvis. Its lumen is lined by a mucous membrane called the **endometrium**. This is composed of an epithelium underlain by a vascular, succulent lamina propria. The endometrium is that part of the uterus that is subject to a wide range of states depending on the part of the cycle the woman is experiencing. During menstruation, it is this tissue which is partially shed. It is this layer of the uterus within which the conceptus implants following fertilization. It is this layer that is a specific "target organ" of the ovarian hormones estrogen and progesterone.

Ovaries

As the name implies, the ovaries are the female gonads— those structures that produce the ova (eggs), the female germ cells. The ovaries contain follicles that are composed of **oocytes** (those cells destined to become ova) and **follicle (granulosa) cells**, which are important in producing hormones (especially progesterone). The ovarian follicles are surrounded by ovarian stroma (a loose, cellular connective tissue), and the stroma immediately surrounding each follicle forms more or less of an envelope called the **theca**. This contains cells that are destined to secrete estradiol.

At the time of the onset of puberty, the ovaries contain 30,000 to 40,000 immature follicles (primary follicles). About 1% of these will complete the process of maturation (**oogenesis**) and undergo **ovulation**. The remaining follicles will eventually disappear in a process called **atresia**. During each cycle, approximately 12 to 15 primary follicles are somehow selected and stimulated to proceed in oogenesis. Of these, only one will complete the process and go to ovulation; the remaining follicles will undergo atresia.

Brain (hypothalamus)/pituary gland

This portion of the brain secretes hormones called releasing hormones (factors). These hormones enter a vascular structure called the hypothalamic/hypophyseal portal system, which comprises vessels starting in the hypothalamus and ending in the pituitary (hypophysis), specifically the anterior pituitary. These releasing hormones act on anterior pituitary gland cells and cause them to secrete their respective hormones. The releasing hormone relevant to this discussion is luteinizing hormone releasing hormone (LH-RH), also called gonadotropin releasing hormone (Gn-RH). As this latter name implies, it causes the anterior pituitary to secrete gonadotropic hormones (follicle-stimulating hormone [FSH] and luteinizing hormone [LH], which have their trophic effects on the gonads (ovaries).

THE MENSTRUAL CYCLE

At the onset of menstruation, part of the endometrium and some serous fluid begin to flow from the uterine lumen into the vagina and onto the body surface. This usually lasts 3 to 7 days, and normal amount of flow is 45 ml (but can range up to 90 ml in normal women). At this time the hypothalamus secretes Gn-RH (LH-RH), which travels via the portal sytem to the anterior pituitary and stimulates that gland to begin secreting FSH and LH, particularly FSH. The FSH stimulates the growth and development of the selected follicles (it is not known how the specific follicles are chosen).

For 11.5 to 12 days from the onset of menstruation, the follicles develop and begin to secrete their own hormones— estradiol and progesterone, especially estradiol. During this 11.5 to 12-day interval, the levels of FSH and LH diminish somewhat. At the end of that time, the estrogens being secreted by the ovaries have a **positive feedback effect** on the hypothalamic/pituitary axis and there is an "LH surge," during which the amount of LH secreted increases 8- to 10-fold. FSH secretions also increase several hundred percent. This LH surge brings about **ovulation**.

Ovulation is the rupture of the ovarian follicle and the shedding of the developing ovum (actually a secondary oocyte stopped at metaphase of meiosis 2), which is surrounded by a covering of granulosa cells. These granulosa cells resemble a radiating crown around the oocyte and thus have come to be referred to as the **corona radiata**. The parts of the follicle that leave the ovary at ovulation enter the oviduct and begin their 4-day passage to the uterine lumen. The portion of the follicle that remains in the ovary becomes a gland called the **corpus luteum**, which continues to secrete estradiol and progesterone.

During menstruation, the endometrium is reduced to just its basal portion. This begins to regenerate owing to the secretion of estrogen by the ovarian follicles. Thus, up to the time of ovulation this is called the **proliferative (estrogenic) phase**. The endometrium becomes 2 to 3 mm thick. Following ovulation, the corpus luteum produces large amounts of estradiol and especially progesterone. The estradiol continues to stimulate proliferation, and the progesterone stimulates the development of the endometrium's secretory capabilities. Thus, from ovulation to the next menstruation is called the **secretory (progestational) phase**.

During the period between ovulation and the onset of menstruation, the levels of estradiol and progesterone remain high except for the last 2 days. These hormones, especially progesterone, have a **negative feedback effect** on the hypothalamus and inhibit it from secreting LH-RH (Gn-RH). The anterior pituitary thus is no longer being driven to secrete FSH and LH. The diminished levels of these gonadotrophic hormones have the effect of involution of the corpus luteum, with the resultant drop in estradiol and progesterone secretion. This loss of ovarian hormones leads to vasospasms in the endometrium, resulting in transient ischemia. The ischemia brings about necrosis of part of the endometrium, and after 2 days or so the endometrium is partially shed into the uterine lumen along with some serous fluid, commencing menstruation.

The depressed levels of estrogen and progesterone at these times just mentioned means that their inhibitory effect (negative feedback) on the hypothalamus is also diminished, and thus the hypothalamus is free once again to secrete LH-RH (Gn-RH), which drives the anterior pituitary to secrete gonadotropins, which stimulate the maturation of another 15 or so ovarian follicles, and so on.

FERTILIZATION

The average ejaculate contains 200 to 500 million sperm. The average volume of ejaculate is 3.5 ml. If the sperm count is 20 million/ml or higher, the male is probably fertile. Below that, he is probably sterile.

Another factor in fertility is the number of sperm that are abnormal and/or immobile. Sperm motility is important, but most of the transport of the sperm up to the oviduct is via contractions of the female reproductive tract. Prostaglandins may stimulate this action.

Ova are usually viable for only about 12 to 24 hours following ovulation. Sperm survive longer, about 24 hours, but records indicate 3 days or more may be possible.

Sperm undergo **capacitation** (a process of activation), usually in the uterus or oviduct. This takes about **7 hours** and is a matter of removal of a glycoprotein coat and seminal plasma proteins from the cell membrane associated with the **acrosome** (modified Golgi), which forms a cap on the head or front end of the nucleus but underlies the cell membrane. Capacitation does not involve any morphological changes in sperm.

The **acrosome reaction** occurs after capacitation, as the sperm penetrates the corona radiata. The acrosome membrane fuses with the overlying cell membrane, and acrosomal enzymes are subsequently released, facilitating passage of sperm through corona radiata and zona pellucida via hyaluronidase and zona lysin (plus trypsin-like substances), respectively. **Acrosin** is the substance(s) facilitating penetration of the zona pellucida. Once a sperm penetrates the zona there is a **zona reaction,** which prevents penetration of the zona by other sperm. This is elicited by the release of cortical granules from the secondary oocyte. These granules contain lysosomal enzymes.

Following are the six steps of fertilization:
1. The sperm passes through the corona radiata.
2. The sperm penetrates the zona pellucida.
3. The sperm head attaches to the surface of the secondary oocyte.
4. The secondary oocyte completes second meiotic division, and a female pronucleus is formed.
5. A male pronucleus is formed.
6. The pronuclei fuse, and the first mitotic division (cleavage) takes place.

First week

Cleavage results in a solid ball of cells (blastomeres), which is called a **morula.** All cells in the morula seem alike, and there is no apparent differentiation. A cavity forms within this spherical mass of cells, and then the conceptus is called a **blastocyst** and the cavity the **blastocoele.** Here two cell types can be seen—the **trophoblast,** which will give rise to extraembryonic structures, and the **inner cell mass,** which will form the embryo. The journey down the oviduct from the site of fertilization takes about 4 days. As the conceptus enters the uterine cavity, it is in the blastocyst stage. The zone pellucida is lost, and on the sixth day **implantation** begins. This most frequently occurs on the posterior wall of the superior part of the uterus. Humans have **interstital implantation,** which means that the conceptus comes to lie entirely within endometrial tissues. In the first week then, there is one embryonic germ layer, which is the inner cell mass.

Second week

The inner cell mass undergoes some delamination of cells toward the blastocystic cavity. These delaminated cells are called **primitive endoderm** or **hypoblast.** This implies that another endoderm develops later. Current thought is that these hypoblast cells move to the periphery of the embryonic disk and a definitive endoderm forms later. At any rate, during the second week there are two germ layers.

Third and fourth weeks

In the third week there is a great deal of activity in the conceptus. The embryonic disk develops a primitive streak in the upper layer of its cells, and in this region cells of the **epiblast** (those cells that did not delaminate to form hypoblast) migrate through to form the definitive endoderm and the mesoderm so as to form three germ layers. The notochord forms from the cranial end of the primitive streak region called the **primitive pit and knot.** It extends cranially, and mesoderm comes to lie on either side, ectoderm dorsally, endoderm ventrally. The notochord goes through a sequence of steps of becoming hollow and flattened, transiently lying within endoderm so as to form the midline of the roof of the primitive gut for a brief time. The notochord subsequently assumes a rounded, rod-like shape and moves dorsally so that the endoderm then closes in the midline ventral to the notochord. While all this is happening, there develops a transient canal connecting the amniotic cavity with the yolk sac, and this is called the **neurenteric canal.**

Also during this time the neural plate forms as a thickened ectoderm extending in the midline from cranial to caudal ends of the embryonic disk. It develops into a groove and then a tube, which finally closes at both ends and separates from the surface ectoderm. This forming of a tube, closing both ends, and separation from surface ectoderm occurs in the fourth week. The beginning of the cardiovascular system develops, with **blood islands** forming within mesoderm in the yolk sac and within the embryo. These coalesce and form a reticulum of primitive vessels, which eventually extends throughout the embryo and yolk sac and to the other extraembryonic membranous membranes. In the region of the heart, two tubes form. These fuse into the single primitive heart tube, which by the end of the third week or early fourth becomes contractile and begins a very slow and inefficient pumping of the blood.

The so-called somite period (days 20 to 30)

As the name implies, the somite period is characterized by the appearance of somites, segmented columns of mesoderm running craniocaudally and lying on either side of the notochord. Beginning on day 20, about three pairs of these form each day, beginning in the occipital region and proceeding caudally. Although somites continue to form after day 30 (42 to 44 pairs ultimately are formed), the somite period ends on that day.

Also during this period, the rapid development of cardiovascular and nervous systems continues. The early development of musculoskeletal, gastrointestinal, and pharyngeal systems and regions begins. It is during the third and fourth weeks that the embryo is so very sensitive to teratogenic agents. If the embryo is assaulted by such substances or actions in the first couple of weeks there is no hope of survival, because so large a percentage of cells are affected and damage is so extensive that viability is nil. During the third and fourth weeks, most of the systems are beginning to differentiate, and this is the most vulnerable time.

PLACENTA AND MEMBRANES (Fig. 1-7)

The trophoblast gives rise to extraembryonic structures only. It is a group of cells of pluripotentiality from which arise various cell types. Early in development, at 6 days, when implantation begins, some of these cells specialize into a syncytium on the outer surface of the conceptus. This is the **syncytiotrophoblast** (or syntrophoblast). These cells erode the endometrium and facilitate the penetration of the conceptus into that tissue layer. The trophoblast (now called **cytotrophoblast**) remains as an undifferentiated cell layer that functions as a germinal layer and thus has much mitotic activity. In addition to forming more cells that become part of the syntrophoblast, it forms cells that come to lie on the inner surface of the cytotrophoblast and are called **extraembryonic mesoderm**. Once these three layers of the trophoblast are formed (syntrophoblast, cytotrophoblast, and extraembryonic mesoderm), they are referred to collectively as the **chorion** or **chorionic membrane**. The portion of the chorion on the side away from the uterine cavity undergoes a particularly rapid development, which results in the formation of **chorionic villi**. These persist and come to form part of the placenta. Because of the copious villi, this part of the chorion is called the **chorion frondosum**. Villi form all around the surface of the conceptus, but the portion other than the frondosum has only small, transient villi, which disappear early in development. This part of the chorion then becomes smooth and is called the **chorion laeve**.

The endometrium reacts to its invasion by the conceptus by undergoing the **decidua reaction**. This is characterized by the presence of somewhat large, ovoid cells filled with glycogen and having a rather distinctive appearance. They appear to arise from the cells of the endometrial stroma and are found in particular abundance at the interface of maternal and fetal tissues. The portion interfacing with the chorion frondosum is the **decidua basalis**, the portion forming a covering or capsule over the chorion laeve is the **decidua capsularis**, and the portion of the endometrium not in direct contact with the chorion is the **decidua parietalis**. As the fetus grows, it protrudes more and more into the uterine lumen and eventually obliterates the lumen. As this happens, the decidua capsularis thins out and finally disappears. The chorion laeve then comes into apposition with the decidua parietalis.

The chorionic villi progress through three stages:
1. **Primary villus:** An outer layer of syntrophoblast, a core of cytotrophoblast.
2. **Secondary villus:** Outer layer of syntrophoblast, next an inner layer of cytotrophoblast, and a core of extraembryonic mesoderm.
3. **Tertiary (definitive) villus:** Same as the secondary villus, except that the mesodermal core becomes vascularized.

Villi extend from the chorionic plate to the decidua basalis (anchoring or stem villi). These develop secondary and tertiary branches. The outer surface of the chorion, which interfaces with the decidua, is formed of cytotrophoblast cells and called the **cytotrophoblastic shell**. Between adjacent anchoring villi, **placental septa** form, partially partitioning some anchoring villi from adjacent villi. The villi and surrounding placental septum form a **maternal cotyledon**. Maternal blood extravasates into the intervillus spaces from arteries of the endometrium and is drained away via endometrial veins. The surfaces of the intervillus spaces are entirely formed of syntrophoblast. The portion of the villus between the maternal blood of the intervillus spaces and that in the villus capillaries constitutes the **placental membrane**. As this matures, it becomes thinner and simpler. At its most mature, it is composed of syntrophoblast and its basal lamina, plus the endothelium of the chorionic capillaries and its basal lamina.

Implantation is completed by day 11. Endocrine function of syntrophoblast begins on or about day 8. Keep in mind that this tissue is very much of an endocrine gland, secreting gonadotropins and so on.

On the inner side of the chorion, the **amnion** forms. These cells separate from the chorion and come to form a dome-like cover over the dorsal (ectodermal) side of the embryo. These cells are the amniotic ectoderm. On the side away from the embryo and toward the chorion, extraembryonic mesoderm forms the outer layer of the amnion. The space inside the chorion and outside of the amnion and embryo is the **extraembryonic coelom** or **chorionic cavity**. As the fetus grows, it comes to be contained within the amnion, which of course must grow to accommodate the fetus. The amnion grows more rapidly than does the chorion, so that eventually the chorionic activity becomes virtually obliterated.

The embryo never loses contact with the chorion. This connection is the **body stalk** (connecting stalk). Through this run the umbilical vessels, and projecting into it from the embryo is a diverticulum of hindgut called the **allantois**. This is vestigial in humans. The body stalk becomes enwrapped by the amnion as the latter grows and progressively enfolds the fetus. Also enwrapped by the amnion is the expansion ventrally of the gut called the **yolk sac**. As the embryo grows, the connection between the gut (midgut) and the yolk sac narrows and is called the **yolk stalk** (or vitelline duct). The yolk sac eventually loses this connection. The amnion enwraps the yolk stalk, allantois, body stalk, umbilical vessels (those that are related to the allantois), and vitelline vessels (those of the yolk sac). All these

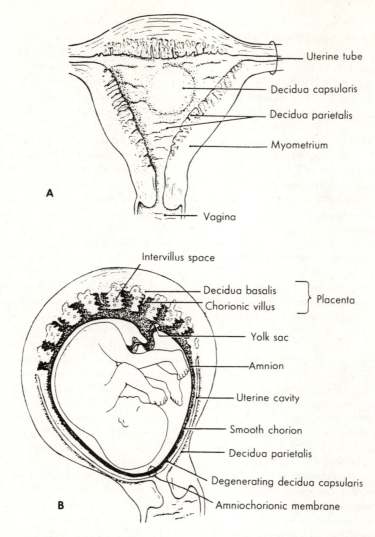

Figure 1-7. (*A*) A frontal section of the uterus showing the elevation of the decidua capsularis caused by the expanding chorionic sac of a 4-week embryo, implanted in the endometrium on the posterior wall. (*B*) Sagittal section of the gravid uterus showing the relation of the fetal membranes to the decidua.

together form the **umbilical cord.** For a time, the intra-embryonic coelom is continuous with the extraembryonic coelom through the umbilical cord. The extraembryonic coelom, allantois, and right umbilical vein disappear as development progresses. The **mucoid connective tissue** of the cord is called **Wharton's jelly.**

DIAPHRAGM

The diaphragm is formed from the septum transversum (central tendon), cervical somites (skeletal muscle), meso-esophagus, body wall, and pleuroperitoneal membranes. The most common congenital malformation is **posterolateral defect of the diaphragm** (1 in 2,000). This defect allows the herniation of abdominal viscera into the thorax, which embarrasses the breathing mechanism and is due to the pleuroperitoneal membrane's failure in formation or fusion with other parts of the diaphragm. It occurs on the left side five times more often.

BRANCHIAL APPARATUS, HEAD AND NECK

The branchial apparatus surrounds the developing pharynx. The pharynx is the most rostral portion of the foregut and is lined with endoderm. It develops a series of **pharyngeal pouches.** These pouches, also lined with endoderm, form or give rise to various structures. The first pouch forms the eustachian tube and middle ear cavity and extends into the mastoid air cells. The second becomes the tonsillar fossa, in which lie the palatine tonsils. The third gives rise to thymus and inferior (III) parathyroids; the fourth to superior (IV) parathyroids; the fifth is rudimentary, combines with fourth, and gives rise to the calcitonin-secreting cells of the thyroid (parafollicular cells).

While pharyngeal pouches are developing inside, **pharyngeal clefts** are forming on the outer surface. These are, of course, lined with ectoderm. The only one that normally remains is the first, which forms the external auditory meatus. The pouches and the clefts almost meet, but normally do not break through so as to form a communication between pouches and clefts. The tissues that lie between adjacent pouches or clefts are column-like walls of the pharynx. These are the **branchial arches** (also called pharyngeal arches or visceral arches). There are said to be six pairs, with the fifth being transient at best. The fifth can be ignored. These arches are numbered from cranial to caudal; each has a cartilage, a cranial nerve, and an aortic arch (an artery that extends from the ventrally located aortic sac to the dorsally located dorsal aorta):

I (mandibular arch): Cartilage (Meckel's), first aortic arch, trigeminal nerve

II (hyoid arch): Cartilage (Reichert's), second aortic arch, facial nerve

III: Cartilage, third aortic arch, glossopharyngeal nerve

IV: Cartilage, fourth aortic arch, vagal nerve

VI: Cartilage, sixth aortic arch, vagal nerve

Keep in mind that there is a single aortic sac from which paired aortic arches extend dorsally to open into the paired dorsal aortae.

Arch I. The face forms from its maxillary and mandibular prominences. Also associated with face development is the **frontonasal process.** The cartilage serves as a transient model for the mandibular bone, the aortic arch disappears except for a small contribution to the maxillary artery, and the trigeminal nerve accommodates the three parts of the face well—frontonasal process derivatives innervated by ophthalmic division, maxillary process derivatives by the maxillary division, and mandibular process derivatives by the mandibular division. The cartilage also forms the malleus and incus, ossicles of the middle ear.

Arch II. The cartilage is associated with formation of the **stapes, styloid process, stylohyoid ligament, lesser cornu and adjacent body of the hoid bone.** The second aortic arch disappears (forms the transient stapedial artery). The facial nerve innervates skeletal muscle derived from mesenchyme, and these are **muscles of facial expression.**

Arch III. The cartilage forms the rest of the **body of the** hyoid and *major cornua.* The third arch forms the common carotid and proximal portion of internal carotid. The **stylopharyngeus** is the only skeletal muscle developed from the mesenchyme and thus is the only skeletal muscle innervated by the glossopharyngeal nerve.

Arches IV and VI. The cartilages form the larynx. The left fourth arch forms the arch of the aorta and the right fourth arch forms the proximal part of the right subclavian artery. Pulmonary arteries arise from the sixth aortic arches. The skeletal muscles of the soft palate (except the tensor veli palatini, which is from the first arch and innervated by V_3), the pharynx (except stylopharyngeus), and the larynx and esophagus are derived from mensenchyme and innervated by cranial nerve X.

Note: Much recent research indicates that neural crest has many more derivatives than were previously attributed to this embryonic tissue. Within the branchial arches, neural crest seems to give rise to all or most of the tissues or structures there except the skeletal muscle, which arises from mesodermally derived mesenchyme.

Malformations of the branchial apparatus

Congenital auricular sinuses and cysts. Of minor importance, these are small pits or cysts around the auricle, usually anterior to it. They may be remnants of the first branchial cleft or just due to ectodermal folds that occur during the formation of the auricle.

Branchial sinus or lateral cervical sinus. Cervical sinus is the depression from which clefts two, three, and four extend. Problems are usually due to failure of the sinus or the second groove (cleft) to disappear during normal development. Such may develop from the pharyngeal pouches, but they are rare. When present, they open into the palatine tonsil region. These remnants may take the form of cysts rather than sinuses.

Branchial fistula. When the second pouch and second cleft persist, a canal extends from the side of the neck to the palatine tonsil region.

First arch syndrome. This is maldevelopment of the first arch and appears to be the result of too little neural crest migrating into the arch during the fourth week. This results in inadequate development of the zygomatic bones, causing the eyes to slant downward. Malformations of the lower lids, deformed middle and internal ears, a hyoplastic mandible, defective eyes, and cleft palate also may result.

Congenital thymic aplasia and absence of the parathyroid glands. The third and fourth pouches fail to differentiate into thymus and parathyroid glands.

Ectopic parathyroid glands. These vary considerably in number and location. They can be found in the region of the thyroid and/or thymus glands.

THYROID GLAND AND TONGUE

Thyroid gland

The thyroid gland does *not* arise from a pharyngeal pouch but rather as a ventral midline endodermal diverticulum. Some endoderm at the junction of the anterior two-thirds of the tongue and posterior one-third of the tongue proliferates and forms a column of cells that descends into the neck and forms the thyroid follicles in a shield-shaped gland that lies on the anterior surface of the upper two or so tracheal cartilages. This column of cells is the **thyroglossal duct,** and the place where this originates is marked by the presence of a small midline pit called the **foramen cecum.** This normally disappears as development progresses, but it may persist. Some remnant of this duct may remain to form the **pyramidal lobe** of the thyroid gland.

Tongue

During the fourth week, a midline swelling forms in the floor of the pharynx, the **median tongue bud** (tuberculum impar). Following this, the ventromedial portions of the first branchial arches form the two **distal tongue buds** (lateral lingual swellings) on each side and somewhat anterior to the median tongue bud. The anterior two-thirds of the tongue (oral portion) forms from the distal tongue buds. The median sulcus and median septum of the tongue form where these buds fuse.

Congenital malformations include thyroglossal duct cysts and sinuses. These may occur anywhere along the path of the duct from tongue to gland. They are in the midline of the neck, usually just inferior to the hyoid. **Lingual thyroid** occurs when the duct does not extend inferiorly. Ectopic thyroid can be seen anywhere along the normal path of the thyoglossal duct.

The posterior one-third (pharyngeal) portion of the tongue forms from two elevations posterior to the foramen cecum.

These arise from the ventromedial portions of the second branchial arches and come to form the **copula**. The ventromedial portions of the third branchial arches form the **hypobranchial eminence,** which overgrows the copula so that the latter disappears, just as did the median tongue bud.

The anterior two-thirds of the tongue forms from the first branchial arch and receives its general sensory innervation from the mandibular division of the trigeminal nerve, but its special visceral sensory innervation (taste) is supplied by the chorda tympani branch of the facial nerve. The posterior one-third develops from the third branchial arches and receives both its general sensory and special visceral sensory (taste) innervation from the glossopharyngeal nerve. The junction of anterior two-thirds and posterior one-third is marked in adults by the **sulcus terminalis.** In the tongue, the blood vessels, lymphatics, and connective tissue are derived from mesenchyme. The occipital somites form the skeletal muscles, which are innervated by cranial nerve XII.

Taste buds begin to appear in the eighth week in the vallate papillae, followed by those in the fungiform papillae. The chorda tympani branch of the facial nerve (VII) supplies the taste buds on the fungiform papillae, and those on the vallate papillae are supplied by terminal branches of the glossopharyngeal nerve (IX).

Congenital malformations of the tongue include **cysts and fistulas** that are related to the thyroglossal duct and its remnants. **Tongue-tie** (ankyloglossia) occurs frequently (1 in 300) and is due to the frenulum extending too extensively to the tip of the tongue and partially immobilizing it. It usually stretches in time and requires no active solution.

NASAL PASSAGES AND PALATE

The nasal passages and their outgrowths, the paransal sinuses, are formed from surface ectoderm and thus will have general sensory afferent, cranial nerve V innervation. Each side starts as an invagination of the thickened olfactory placodes (ectoderm). Only maxillary and ethmoidal sinuses are present at birth. At about age 2 years, the ethmoids grow into the frontal region and form frontal sinuses, into sphenoid bone and form sphenoidal sinuses.

The palate has hard parts, with the premaxilla being the more anterior, midline portion and palatal processes of the maxillary and palatine bones forming their respective sides of the rest of the hard palate. The soft palate arises from the same structures as the adjacent portions of the hard palate. The premaxilla arises from the median palatine process of the intermaxillary segment of the maxilla (frontonasal process). The remainder of the palate arises from the palatal process of the first (mandibular) branchial arch (maxillary prominences).

The premaxilla is that portion of the upper jaw that holds the incisor teeth.

Lines of fusion form between frontonasal prominence structures (philtrum, premaxilla) and the palatine processes of the maxillary prominence. Failure of fusion can and does occur anywhere along these lines. All the congenital malformations of the palate reflect some such failure and can occur to any extent.

Keep in mind that the nasal septum (from the frontonasal prominence) also plays a role in palate formation.

RESPIRATORY SYSTEM (Fig. 1-8)

At 24 weeks of gestation and fetal weight of 1000 g, the fetus may be viable should it be delivered early. Obviously, the longer the fetus can be carried past that point the better. The development of the respiratory and nervous systems is critical to the fetus's survival in case of premature birth. In the respiratory system, the constraint is the adequate development of the pulmonary vasculature, not the presence of sufficient pulmonary alveoli. It should be noted, however, that surfactant (secreted by the type II alveolar cells) is present only in very small amounts at 24 weeks and is not secreted in adequate amounts until toward the end of normal gestation. The nervous system must be developed to the degree such that the neuromuscular mechanisms for breathing movements are functional.

THE DIGESTIVE SYSTEM (Fig. 1-9)

Foregut

The pharynx has already been discussed. The esophagus is uncomplicated ordinarily, but its main problem, if there is one, is that it remains short. This results in the stomach lying at least partially within the thorax.

Caudal foregut

The caudal foregut is in the abdomen and gives rise to stomach, pancreas, liver, and upper one-fourth of the duodenum. It is supplied by the coeliac trunk. Because of the rotation, the dorsal border of the stomach comes to lie toward the left as the greater curvature, the ventral border to the right as the lesser curvature. Rotation also accounts for the right vagal trunk lying more on the posterior surface, the left vagal trunk on the anterior surface.

Midgut

The midgut gives rise to the remainder of the duodenum, all of the rest of the small intestine, the cecum, the ascending colon, and the transverse colon approximately to the left (splenic) flexure. It is supplied by the superior mesenteric artery (which is derived from the vitelline arteries). This is the part of the gut continuous with the yolk sac (connection called the yolk stalk). Parasympathetic innervation is supplied by the vagi.

This portion of the gut herniates into the umbilical cord at the end of the fifth week or early part of sixth week. This hernia is reduced on the 10th week. As the gut returns to the abdominal cavity, the first part to return is the jejunum. As the gut returns to the abdominal cavity, the gut rotation begins. The gut is returned on the 10th week, but the final movements of rotation go on for some time.

Hindgut

The hindgut forms the left colic flexure, descending colon, sigmoid colon, and rectum. It is supplied by the inferior mesenteric artery. Parasympathetic innervation is supplied by sacral spinal cord segments S2, S3, and S4.

Anus

The anus forms from the proctodeum and is lined with ectoderm. It is continuous with the hindgut.

Congenital malformations of the gastrointestinal tract are illustrated in Figures 1-8 and 1-9.

UROGENITAL SYSTEM

The urinary system is derived from the intermediate mesoderm. It begins as a ridge of tissue extending from the occipital region caudally to the cloaca. The most rostral part is the pronephros (head kidney), which never functions in humans and only contributes in that some of the tubules join to form the pronephric duct, which extends from the head region caudally into the mesonephros. Once the pronephric duct extends into the more caudally located mesonephric region, it is called the mesonephric (wolffian) duct. This duct continues caudally and eventually opens into the cloaca (lower portion of the hindgut). Opening into the mesonephric duct are numerous mesonephric tubules, which seem to form a very dilute urine for a time. As more caudal tubules are formed, those of the more cranial region of the mesonephros disappear. Those mesonephric tubules that persist are taken over in the male and become vasa efferentia in the male gonad.

Just cranial to the entrance of the mesonephric duct into the cloaca, a small diverticulum forms—the ureteric bud. This outgrowth from the mesonephric duct becomes the ureter. It grows cranially and extends into a portion of the intermediate mesoderm called the metanephric blastema, which is destined to form the nephrons of the metanephric (definitive) kidney. These nephrons formed from blastema open into the branches

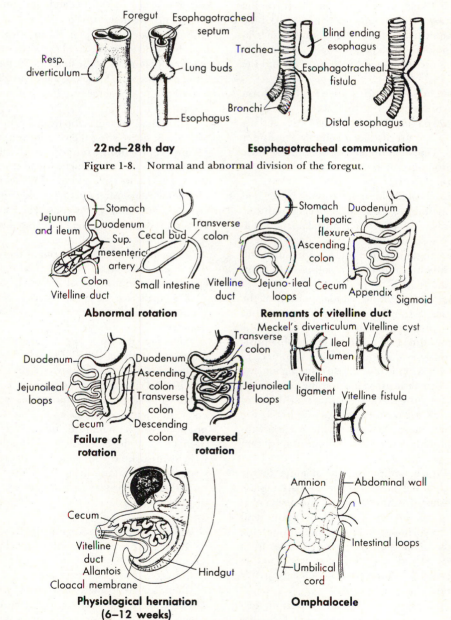

22nd–28th day   **Esophagotracheal communication**

Figure 1-8. Normal and abnormal division of the foregut.

Abnormal rotation   **Remnants of vitelline duct**

Failure of rotation   **Reversed rotation**

Physiological herniation (6–12 weeks)   **Omphalocele**

Figure 1-9. Congenital malformations of the gastrointestinal tract.

of the ureteric bud so that the distal convoluted tubule portion of the nephron opens into the arched collecting ducts of the ureteric system.

The ureteric bud forms the arched collecting ducts, calyces, ureteric pelvis, and ureter. The metanephric blastema forms the nephrons.

In the **genital system**, the **mesonephric duct** (wolffian duct) persists in the male and largely disappears in the female. Running approximately parallel to the mesonephric duct is the **paramesonephric (müllerian) duct.** This persists in the female and largely disappears in the male.

In **males**, the mesonephric tubules form the **vasa efferentia**, which open into the mesonephric duct's cranial end, which becomes the **epididymis.** The more caudal portion of the mesonephric duct becomes the **vas deferens.** Just before the vas deferens opens into the cloaca (or that part that gives rise to the prostatic urethra), it develops a diverticulum that forms the **seminal vesicle.** Note here that in females virtually all of the mesonephric duct disappears, and thus the seminal vesicle in the male has no homologue in females. Male remnants of paramesonephric ducts are the appendix of the testis and the prostatic utricle.

In **females**, the paramesonephric (müllerian) ducts form the **oviducts** (fallopian tubes or uterine tubes) from their more cranial portions. The two paramesonephric ducts fuse caudally in the midline to form the **uterus** and probably the **upper portion of the vagina.** Female remnants of the mesonephric ducts are the epoophoron (related to ovarian medulla), paroophoron, and the Gartner's duct.

The cloaca is a portion of the hindgut. It must be divided by a transverse bar of mesoderm called the **urorectal septum.** This results in the cloaca giving rise from its dorsal portion (that posterior to the urorectal septum) to the rectum and from its ventral portion to the **urogenital sinus.** From this sinus will arise the **urinary bladder** and the **urethra** and its derivatives (e.g., bulbourethral glands).

The urethra forms from the more caudal portion of the urogenital sinus. In males, the portion of the urethra continuous with the bladder is the **prostatic urethra.** Into this open the right and left **ejaculatory ducts.** These ducts are mesonephric ducts distal to the seminal vesicles and thus carry secretions of those glands plus secretions of the testes. Also opening into the prostatic urethra is the **prostatic utricle**, a midline evagination from the posterior wall of the urethra. It is a small cul-de-sac of unknown significance. Its origin is alluded to above in relation to the paramesonephric ducts. Numerous little outgrowths develop from the endoderm of the prostatic urethra, together forming the **prostate.**

The prostatic urethra extends from the bladder to the urogenital diaphragm. The urethra traversing the diaphragm is called the **membranous urethra.** Beyond the urogenital membrane, the urethra enters the bulb of the penis and extends the length of the corpus spongiosum and through the glans penis. This is the penile portion of the urethra, from which form the **bulbourethral (Cowper's glands)**, as well as the little outpocketings of the urethral mucosa called the penile urethral (Littre's) glands.

In females, the urethra is much shorter. That portion next to the bladder has endodermal outgrowths that form the **paraurethral (Skene's) glands and ducts.** These, therefore, are homologues of the prostate. Beyond the paraurethral glands, the female urethra opens into the **vestibule.** This is derived from urogenital sinus and is bordered by the labia minora. This region is comparable (homologous) to the penile urethra.

From the endoderm in this region, a pair of glands form the **major vestibular glands of Bartholin.** Between the urethral and vaginal orifices, other tiny glands form (**minor vestibular glands**). These are homologous to penile urethral (Littre's) glands.

The development of the **external genitalia** is illustrated in Figures 1-10 and 1-11. In **males**, the genital tubercle forms the **glans penis** and the **corpora cavernosa penis** and the **corpus spongiosum.** A groove that develops on the ventral aspect of the tubercle folds over and encloses the adjacent portion of the urogenital sinus, forming the **penile urethra** (Fig. 1-11).

In **females**, the genital tubercle forms the glans clitoris, corpora cavernosa clitoris, and labia minora.

The groove that forms on the ventral aspect of the tubercle is bounded laterally by folds, the **urethral folds.** In males, these folds fuse and enclose part of the urogenital sinus as the **penile urethra.** In females, these folds do not fuse but rather form the **labia minora**, which enclose that area called the vestibule. Into the vestibule open the urethra, vagina, and the vestibular glands.

The **gonads** also develop from the intermediate mesoderm. Mesothelium covering their peritoneal cavity surface is called **germinal epthelium** (a misnomer). This epithelium proliferates and forms **sex cords**, which extend inward from the surface. These cords are surrounded by the **mesenchyme** of the urogenital ridge. Migrating from the endoderm of the yolk sac are the **primordial germ cells.** These migrate from the yolk sac, up the dorsal mesentery, and into the right and left gonadal regions of the urogenital ridge.

Thus, in the developing gonads there are three sources of cells—sex cords from the germinal epithelium, the mesenchyme, and the primordial germ cells.

Sex cords give rise to the **Sertoli's cells** in the **seminiferous tubules** of males, and to the **granulosa** (follicle) cells of the ovarian follicles in females.

Mesenchyme gives rise to **interstitial (Leydig's) cells** in males and to **theca cells** (of follicles) in the female.

Primordial germ cells give rise to **spermatogonia** in males which act as virtually lifelong germinal cells in the seminiferous tubules. Some differentiate into **primary spermatocytes**, which enter the meiotic divisions and so on. In females, these form **oogonia**, which undergo all their divisions (mitotic) during the prenatal period. Thus, the cells in the primordial female follicles are **primary oocytes**, 15 to 20 of which each month will undergo maturation during the menstrual cycle.

Descent of the testes is completed about the eighth month of gestation (Fig. 1-12).

Congenital malformations of the urogenital system

In **hermaphroditism**, the external genitalia are not consistent with the gonads. True hermaphrodites (very rare) have both ovarian and testicular tissue.

Female pseudohemaphrodites have 46,XX genotype. This is most commonly caused by adrenogenital syndrome, which is a result of congenital virilizing adrenal hyperplasia. Ovaries are normal, but the suprarenal glands produce large

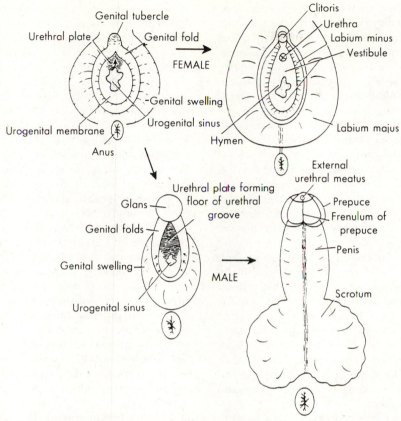

Figure 1-10.   The development of the external genitalia.

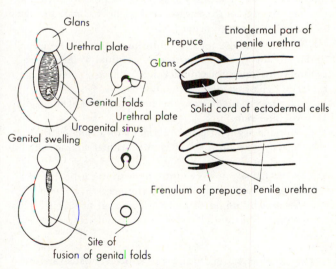

Figure 1-11.   Development of the penile portion of the male urethra.

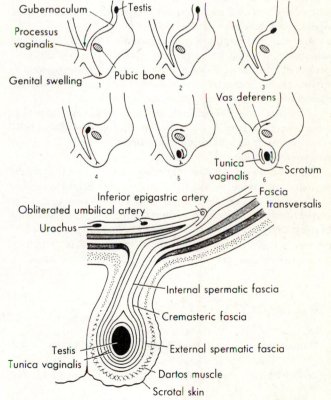

Figure 1-12.   Descent of the tests and formation of the inguinal canal.

quantities of androgens, which enlarge the external genitalia, sometimes to the extent that they appear to be nearly masculine.

Male pseudohermaphrodites have 46,XY genotype. The testes fail to produce adequate testosterone and müllerian inhibiting substances. The testes may be normal or rudimentary. The external genitalia vary widely in their development or lack of it, and remnants of the paramesonephric ducts may be larger or more persistent.

Testicular feminization is rare, transmitted by a recessive sex-linked gene. Testes are present, and the genotype is 46,XY. There may be a defect in the androgen receptor mechanism such that the labioscrotal and urogenital folds do not develop into male structures. Testes are in the abdomen or inguinal canals and may descend into the labia majora. The external genitalia are female, but the vagina is a cul-de-sac, and the uterus and uterine tubes are rudimentary or missing. Breasts develop, but menstruation does not occur.

Hypospadias occurs in 1 of every 300 males. The urethral orifice opens onto the ventral side of the glans or the shaft of the penis. The penis often has a marked ventral bend in it, called a **chordee.** Four types of hypospadias are described: (1) glandular, (2) penile, (3) penoscrotal, and (4) perineal. The perineal is rarest and occurs where scrotal folds do not fuse; the urethral orifice is between the two halves of the scrotum. In the others, the urethral folds have failed to fuse, leaving the urethral orifice located as indicated by the name. The cause is failure of the fetal testes to produce adequate androgens and/or inadequate receptor sites for the hormones.

Epispadias is much rarer than hypospadias by about 100 times. It can occur without other problems, but most frequently it occurs along with exstrophy of the bladder. The cause is unclear, but the genital tubercle may form too dorsally, and when the urogenital membrane ruptures, the urogenital sinus opens onto the dorsal side of the penis.

Uterine and vaginal malformations occur as a result of improper fusion of the paramesonephric ducts or failure of proper development of one or both ducts. The critical developmental period is around the 8th week. The uterus and even the vagina can be duplicated to varying degrees.

Cryptorchidism (undescended testes) is very common among premature males (30%) and occurs in about 3% of full-term males. It occurs unilaterally or bilaterally. The testes frequently complete descent postnatally.

Congenital inguinal hernia occurs much more frequently in males. The processus vaginalis remains patent, and intestines can herniate into the scrotum. It is frequently associated with cryptorchidism. Hydrocele forms when the abdominal opening of the processus is too small to permit herniation of viscera but allows passage of fluid into the scrotal and/or testicular portion, where it accumulates.

CIRCULATORY SYSTEM

Veins

Three pairs of veins appear in the embryo: (1) vitelline veins returning blood from the yolk sac, (2) the umbilical veins returning blood from the placenta, and (3) the cardinal veins returning blood to the heart from the fetus itself.

Vitelline veins contribute to the hepatic portal vein. An anastomotic network is formed around the gut by these veins, and by persistence of some of these anastomotic connections and loss of some parts of the veins, the normal relationship of the portal vein around the duodenum is achieved.

Umbilical veins start out paired, but the right one quickly disappears. The left one persists throughout gestation, with the exception of that portion between the liver and sinus venosus, which drops out early. In place of that segment of the left umbilical vein, a shunt from the liver to the inferior vena cava develops de novo—the **ductus venosus.**

Cardinal veins are more complicated. Cranial to the heart are the **anterior cardinal veins.** These return blood to the heart from the head, neck, pectoral girdle, and upper limbs. An anastomotic vessel develops de novo between the two anterior cardinal veins. This latter vessel facilitates the flow of venous blood from the left head, neck, and upper limb into the right anterior cardinal vein and becomes the **left brachiocephalic vein.** Caudal to the heart are the **posterior cardinal veins,** which drain the remainder of the body. Note that as the anterior and posterior cardinal veins return to the heart, they join each other on their respective sides to form right and left **common cardinal veins** (ducts of Cuvier), which flow into right and left horns of the **sinus venosus,** respectively. On the left, the remnant of the left common cardinal is the **oblique vein** (of Marshall) of the left atrium. The portion of the left anterior cardinal vein between the left brachiocephalic vein and the heart disappears. On the right side, the superior vena cava is formed by the right anterior cardinal and the right common cardinal. The only remnants of the posterior cardinal veins are the arch of the **azygos vein** (right cardinal) and the junction of the **common iliac veins.**

Cardinal veins also form the **inferior vena cava.** Posterior (caudal) to the heart are **posterior cardinal veins, supracardinal veins,** and **subcardinal veins.** Following is a summary of inferior vena cava development:

1. Hepatic segment from the proximal part of the right vitelline vein.
2. Prerenal segment from the right subcardinal vein.
3. Renal segment from the subcardinal-supracardinal anastomosis.
4. Postrenal segment from the right supracardinal vein.
5. The lowest portion of the inferior vena cava where it is formed by union of the two common iliac veins is a remnant of the right posterior cardinal vein.

Heart

The heart is formed from the **sinus venosus, atrium, ventricle, bulbus cordis,** and **truncus arteriosus.** It is first recognized as a pair of longitudinally oriented **heart tubes,** which quickly fuse. Into the caudal end of these tubes empty the various veins described above, and from the cranial end exit the arteries. The tube folds on itself whereas the caudal end comes to lie dorsal (posterior) to the more cranial end and assumes a somewhat sigmoid shape. This whole process of heart development is long, complicated, and dynamic. It is suggested that it be studied one part at a time, simply noting what embryonic structure becomes what definitive or "adult" structure.

be studied one part at a time, simply noting what embryonic structure becomes what definitive or "adult" structure.

Atrium. This is a single structure that must be septated into a right and left side. There is a **septum primum**, which extends in the midline from cranial to caudal. Because throughout gestation right and left sides of the heart must maintain an open communication, the septation of the heart must allow for this. As the septum primum is formed, there remains an opening between right and left atria as long as the septum is still incomplete. The area where the septum is incomplete is known as the **foramen primum**. However, as the septum primum approaches the **endocardial cushions** (swellings that form in the region of constriction between the atrium and ventricle and that divide this atrioventricular passage into right and left atrioventricular canals) and prepares to fuse with them, this foramen primum is steadily reduced and is destined to disappear. In order for the communication between right and left atria to be maintained, the septum primum develops another foramen near its cranial end—the **foramen secundum**. A second septum (**septum secundum**) forms to the immediate right of the septum primum. It grows from anterior to posterior and never forms a complete septum, but rather leaves an oval opening called the **foramen ovale**. The septum secundum overlaps the foramen secundum of the septum primum. Much of the septum primum degenerates, but the more caudal portion persists and serves as the **valve of the foramen ovale**. This valve functions to prevent refluxing of the blood from left atrium back into the right atrium. The foramen ovale facilitates the passage of the oxygen-rich blood from the placenta from right atrium into left atrium, thus bypassing the fetal pulmonary circulation.

At birth, the increased pressure within the left atrium effects the closure of the foramen ovale. On the right side, the interatrial septum has some landmarks of these structures. The **limbus of the fossa ovalis** is formed from the free edge of the septum secundum as it overlapped the foramen secundum. The foramen ovale is closed, and thus on the right side one sees the fossa ovalis. A probe patency of the foramen ovale is found in 20 to 25% of normal adult hearts.

The **right atrium's** smooth-walled portion, the sinus venarum, is formed by absorption of the right horn of the sinus venosus. The valve of the sinus venosus also becomes incorporated and contributes to the interatrial septum and forms the crista terminalis and the valves of the inferior vena cava and the coronary sinus.

The **left atrium's** smooth-walled portion is formed by absorption of the developing pulmonary vein and its tributaries. This vein arises de novo.

The original atrium forms the **auricular appendages** of the definitive atria.

Primitive ventricle. A muscular **interventricular septum** forms from the apex of the ventricle and extends cranially. The cranial edge is crescent shaped. Its growth at first is largely due to differential growth on each side. This also causes the formation of the **interventricular sulcus** or **groove**. Between the free edge of this septum and the endocardial cushions is an opening called the **interventricular foramen**. This allows communication between the ventricles until the end of the seventh week. The closure is effected by fusion of the **right bulbar ridge, left bulbar ridge,** and the fused **endocardial cushions**. The **membranous portion** of the interventricular septum is formed from endocardial cushion tissue extensions that fuse with the **bulbar septum** and muscular portion of the interventricular septum.

Bulbus cordis, truncus arteriosus, and aortic sac. The aortic sac is septated (**aorticopulmonary septum**) so that the portion of the sac that opens into the sixth aortic arches is separated from that portion that opens into the third and fourth aortic arches. Thus, the aorta will be continuous with the derivatives of third and fourth aortic arches and the portion of the aortic sac associated with them, and the pulmonary trunk with the sixth aortic arches and the associated portion of the aortic sac. The aorticopulmonary septum is continuous with the septum formed by the truncal ridges. The trunca septum is in turn continuous with the bulbar ridges, which fuse to form a septum also. Thus, the aorticopulmonary, truncal, and bulbar septa all are continuous and form a spiral septum that divides the outflow tract into the aorta and pulmonary trunk. The bulbar ridges (septum) divides the bulbus into the **infundibulum** of the right ventricle and the **aortic vestibule** of the left ventricle. The truncus forms the semilunar valves and the portion of the aorta and pulmonary trunk associated with those valves. The aorticopulmonary septum of the aortic sac forms the remainder of these vessels.

Valves. The **semilunar valves** of the aorta and pulmonary trunk form from ridges or swellings. Two cusps of each valve (those that form right and left adjacent cusps of the two valves) form from swellings on the truncal ridges. The ventral valve swelling forms the anterior cusp of the pulmonary semilunar valve, and the dorsal valve swelling forms the posterior cusp of the aortic semilunar valve.

Bicuspid and tricuspid valves form from swellings of subendocardial tissue in the region of the atrioventricular canals.

Arteries (Fig. 1-13)

The **truncus arteriosus** opens into the **aortic sac**. It is from this that the aortic arches arise. Remember that the flow of blood is in the order of the following structures, and that should make understanding their derivatives easier.

Truncus arteriosus: Proximal portions of pulmonary trunk and aorta

Aortic sac: First part of aortic arch (left horn) and brachiocephalic artery (right horn)

Sixth aortic arch: (Distal pulmonary trunk from aortic sac), proximal portion of each pulmonary artery; distal portion of left sixth arch forms ductus arteriosus (ligamentum arteriosum)

Fourth aortic arch: Right forms first part of right subclavian artery, left contributes to aortic arch (that portion between left horn of aortic sac and left dorsal aorta)

Third aortic arch: Forms common carotid and proximal portion of internal carotid

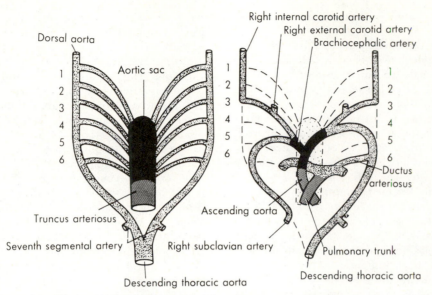

Figure 1-13.   Formation and fate of the aortic arch arteries.

Dorsal aortae: Right remains only as part of the subclavian artery, left becomes distal portion of aortic arch and descending aorta

The persistence of the left sixth's distal portion (as **ductus arteriosus/ligamentum arteriosum**) accounts for the recurrent laryngeal branch of the left vagus following its course caudal to the arch of the aorta and lateral to the ligamentum arteriosum.

Changes in circulation after birth are as follows:
1. The foramen ovale closes and becomes the fossa ovalis.
2. The ductus arteriosus becomes the ligamentum arteriosum.
3. The ductus venosus becomes the ligamentum venosum.
4. The umbilical vein from the umbilicus to the liver becomes the ligamentum teres hepati (which runs within the caudal border of the falciform ligament).
5. At birth, the right ventricular wall is thicker than that of the left ventricle, but by the end of the first month this situation is reversed.
6. The umbilical arteries, distal to the origin of the superior vesicle artery, become the medial umbilical ligaments (seen on the inner surface of the lower anterior abdominal wall and extending to the umbilicus).

Congenital anomalies of the cardiovascular system

Dextrocardia.   Should the heart tube bend to the right instead of to the left, the heart itself and the great vessels are reversed. This may occur with **situs inversus,** in which the viscera are transposed also. That often is the only defect, and the heart and its great vessels function normally. When the dextrocardia occurs alone, heart defects are more common.

Ectopic cordis.   This is very uncommon. The sternum may be split, and the pericardium may be open. The lateral folds fail to fuse so that the sternum and pericardium are defective.

Atrial septal defects (ASD).   These can range from a probe-patent foramen ovale to more serious anomalies.

1. **Secundum-type ASD.** This very common type of defect involves both the septum primum and the septum secundum. There may be excessive resorption of the septum primum and the foramen ovale will not close. The septum secundum may be defective, and the foramen ovale will be too large to be closed by the septum primum.
2. **Endocardial cushion defect with primum-type ASD.** The endocardial cushion is defective, and the septum primum does not fuse with it, leaving a patent foramen primum. This may also cause a cleft in the mitral valve's anterior cusp. A worse problem occurs when the endocardial cushions do not fuse. This large defect in the central part of the heart results in atrioventricularis communis (common atrioventricular canal). This is relatively uncommon, but it is seen in 20% of those with Down's syndrome.
3. **Sinus venosus-type ASD.** This very rare defect occurs in the superior portion of the interatrial septum and is due to incomplete absorption of the sinus venosus into the right atrium and/or a defective septum secundum.
4. **Common atrium.** The septa fail to develop.

Persistent truncus arteriosus.   Truncal ridges fail to form a complete septum. The bulbar ridges may also fail to fuse. The septum may form but have a defect in it called the "aortic window." This affords communication between the pulmonary trunk and the aorta.

Transposition of the great arteries.   The aorta arises from the right ventricle, the pulmonary trunk from the left. Venous drainage into the atria is often normal. The conus arteriosus apparently develops abnormally, so that when it is incorporated into the ventricles it is not properly septated.

Unequal division of the truncus arteriosus.   This is best seen in the tetralogy of Fallot: (1) pulmonary stenosis, (2) overriding aorta, (3) interventricular septal defect, and (4) hypertrophy of the right ventricle. The truncus must be divided equally to properly form the pulmonary trunk and the aorta. Should one be favored, it must be at the expense of the other, with the defects that follow.

Aortic stenosis and atresia. The semilunar valve cusps fuse at their edges, leaving a small opening in the case of stenosis, no opening in the case of atresia.

Coarctation of the aorta. This usually develops just before or just after junction of ductus arteriosus (preductal and postductal, respectively). The incidence in males is twice that in females, and this defect is often concomitant with patent ductus arteriosus.

Aortic arch anomalies. These include right retroesophageal subclavian, right arch of aorta, and double aortic arch.

NERVOUS SYSTEM

The nervous system begins in the middle of the third week as a thickening of the ectoderm in the midline called the **neural plate.** This develops a **neural groove,** which runs longitudinally, and on either side of the groove develop **neural folds.** The folds become more marked, grow toward the midline, and begin to fuse in the future occipital region. This results in the beginning of the formation of the **neural tube** with an opening on the cranial end and one on the caudal end, the **anterior** and **posterior neuropores,** respectively. This fusion of the neural folds extends cranially and caudally. On days 24 to 25 the anterior neuropore closes, and on day 26 to 27 the posterior closes. The neural tube thus comes to be closed at both ends and completely separated from the surface ectoderm, which simply closes over the dorsal surface where the neural plate and so on originally formed.

Cells form from the region of the neural folds, and these cells lie as a sheet wedged in between the neural tube and the surface ectoderm. These are the **neural crest** cells.

The cells that line the neural tube are the germinal cells in that they are mitotically active. The proliferation of cells results in some cells migrating away from the lining cells, coming to form an **intermediate zone** or **mantle layer,** which consists of cells that have begun their differentiation. Some are **neuroblasts** (immature neurons) and some are **glioblasts.** As differentiation continues, the developing neurons begin forming axons that extend toward the surface of the neural tube. These processes come to form an outer, relatively nonnucleated layer called the **marginal zone.** When the mitotic activity ceases, the cells lining the ventricular cavities become the **ependymal layer.** The marginal layer is the **white matter,** the mantle layer the **gray matter.**

Neuroblasts are postmitotic once they migrate away from the ventricular (proliferative) zone and form the mantle layer. These cells are incapable of further mitotic activity and enter into the process of differentiation and maturation. Glioblasts are mitotically active, as are glia throughout life. They give rise to astrocytes and oligodendrocytes. Microglial cells are traditionally described as histiocytes of the CNS and of mesenchymal origin.

The neural tube quickly develops some identifiable organization. The proliferation of the cells is such that the mantle layer (gray matter), when viewed in cross section, has on each side of the tube a dorsal (posterior) region called the **alar plate** and a ventral (anterior) region called the **basal plate.** A sulcus extending longitudinally in the lateral wall of the ven-

tricular cavity soon forms between the alar and basal plates, and this is the **sulcus limitans.** This is seen from the rostral midbrain down throughout the remainder of the brain stem and the entire spinal cord. It is not seen in the forebrain. The alar plate develops sensory/associative (integrative) function, and the basal plate develops motor function.

Neural crest derivatives seem to increase in diversity and number almost daily. They include the following:

1. Neurons whose cell bodies are found in the peripheral nervous system (e.g., dorsal root ganglion cells, autonomic ganglia cells, cranial nerve sensory ganglia cells).
2. Some books claim that leptomeninges (pia and arachnoid) form from neural crest, others that they are formed from mesoderm.
3. Dentin (teeth).
4. Adrenal medulla (adrenal cortex from mesoderm).
5. Neurilemma cells (Schwann cells).
6. Satellite (capsule) cells (those enveloping cell bodies of neurons of the peripheral nervous system).
7. Melanocytes.
8. Most structures from branchial arches *except* skeletal muscle.
9. Aorticopulmonary septum.
10. Walls of the great vessels.

Myelin is formed in the CNS by the oligodendrocytes, in the peripheral nervous system by Schwann (neurilemma) cells. Myelination occurs about the time a given tract or nerve becomes functional. Phylogenetically older tracts myelinate first. Myelination begins about the 20th week and continues into the postnatal period.

The spinal cord development is as described above. It is the simplest and is virtually the same throughout the extent of the cord.

The cranial end of the neural tube undergoes much more rapid and remarkable development. Three dilatations form in the cranial end of the neural tube—the three **primary brain vesicles.** These are the **prosencephalon (forebrain), mesencephalon (midbrain),** and the **rhombencephalon (hindbrain)** (Fig. 1-14).

The prosencephalon develops into the telencephalon (cerebral hemispheres) and **diencephalon** (the thalami).

The mesencephalon does not further divide and thus remains simply mesencephalon.

The rhombencephalon forms the **metencephalon** (pons and cerebellum) and the **myelencephalon** (medulla oblongata).

The alar and basal plates form in the brain stem (midbrain, pons, medulla). The general rule applies here. Derivatives of the basal plates include all cranial nerve motor nuclei for both skeletal muscle and autonomic innervation. All others are from alar plate. These latter nuclei include the obvious sensory nuclei (e.g., solitarius, spinal nucleus of V) and also nuclei such as the inferior olivary, pontine, cerebellar, red, etc. The cerebellum is an alar plate derivative.

The diencephalon and telencephalon are apparently derived from alar plate.

The **pituitary** has a dual origin. A diverticulum of the oral ectoderm develops in the midline and extends posteriorly toward the base of the diencephalon. This diverticulum is called **Rathke's pouch.** From this the anterior pituitary

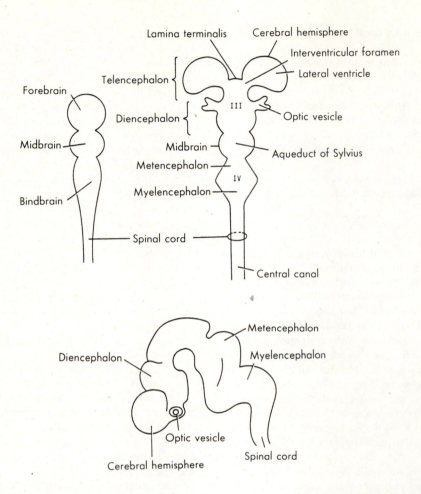

Figure 1-14.   The forebrain vesicle divides into the telencephalon and the diencephalon, and the hindbrain vesicle into the metencephalon and myelencephalon. The cerebral hemisphere on each side is seen to develop as a diverticulum from the telencephalon.

develops. Specifically, the parts of pituitary derived from Rathke's pouch are the partes distalis, tuberalis, and intermedia. The neurohypophysis develops from the ventral aspect of the hypothalamus (diencephalon) and includes the pars nervosa, infundibular stem, and median eminence. The connection of Rathke's pouch with the oral ectoderm is normally lost. However, occasionally remnants of this connection remain and are the source of craniopharyngiomas.

In the brain, the neural tube becomes very irregular in its conformation. Some areas develop extensively and form thick walls, and other areas remain very thin. In those places where only ependymal cells remain, vascularized tufts of pia form and come to lie enfolded in this ependymal layer. These are the **choroid plexuses.** Each ventricle has one. The medial walls of the two cerebral hemispheres develop in this way. These are called the **choroid fissures** where the choroid plexuses push into, as it were, the lateral ventricles.

THE EAR

External.   The pinna develops from tubercles that surround the first pharyngeal cleft. The meatus arises from the first pharyngeal cleft. The tympanic membrane develops from the membrane between the first pharyngeal cleft and pouch with endoderm forming the inner layer, mesoderm the middle layer (stroma), and ectoderm the outer layer.

Middle.   The cavity (including the eustachian tube) develops from the first pharyngeal pouch (endodermally lined). The malleus and incus arise from cartilage of the first branchial arch. The stapes develops from cartilage of the second branchial arch.

Inner.   The membranous labyrinth (semicircular ducts and their cristae; utriculus and saccule with their maculae; cochlear duct with its organ of Corti) develop from the **otic placode,** osseous labyrinth from petrous bone (part of chondrocranium).

THE EYE

The anterior epithelium of the cornea arises from ectoderm. The stroma and endothelium develop from mesenchyme. The sclera and choroid coat arise from mesenchyme. In the iris, the stroma arises from mesenchyme, the posterior epithelial layers develop from the optic cup (neural ectoderm), and the sphincter and dilator muscles are derived from the optic cup. The retina arises from the optic cup (a diverticulum of the diencephalon). The lens develops from surface ectoderm.

Congenital malformations of the nervous system

The incidence of congenital malformations of the nervous system is about 0.3%. Defects fall into three categories: (1) structural, (2) disturbances in organizaiton of the cells, and (3) metabolic errors. Of these, a large majority are due to failure of the neural tube to close, as in spina bifida cystica and meroanencephaly. These may involve only the neural tube, but sometimes the defects also involve the overlying skeletal structures.

Metabolic errors frequently lead to severe mental retardation. They are often inherited. Problems include accumulation of toxic substances, such as in phenylketonuria, and deficiencies of substances, as in congenital hypothyroidism.

Malformations of the ventricular system of the brain can be serious. These result in **hydrocephalus.** One type of hydrocephalus is internal or obstructive, in which there is blockage somewhere within the ventricles that prevents normal CSF flow. The other type is external or communicating hydrocephalus, in which the flow of CSF in the subarachnoid space is blocked. In a majority of cases, hydrocephalus is associated with spina bifida with meningomyelocele.

Chromosomal abnormalities can arise during gametogenesis, as in trisomy 21 (Down syndrome).

Infections that occur prenatally and postnatally can result in mental retardation.

Development of the vertebrae

The vertebrae develop from sclerotomes. In order for the segmental vessels and spinal nerves (which are segmented) to properly access the vertebral canal, each vertebra is formed of parts of two adjacent sclerotomes. The vertebral column has two primary curvatures, thoracic and sacral. As the infant learns to sit and eventually to stand, the secondary cervical and lumbar curvatures appear. Congenital anomalies include **Klippel-Feil syndrome** (brevicollis) and **spina bifida.** The latter was described in nervous system malformations. Klippel-Feil features a short neck and low hairline. The number of cervical vertebrae is often less than normal, and often several are fused (not segmented). The number of cervical nerve roots may be normal. The nerve roots tend to be small, as are the intervertebral foramina. Patients are often otherwise normal, but this malformation may be found along with others.

GROSS ANATOMY

UPPER LIMB

Dermatomes of the upper limbs are illustrated in Figure 1-15.

Cutaneous innervation includes the supraclavicular nerves (medial, middle, lateral; C3, C4), upper lateral brachial cutaneous (branch of axillary nerve), lower lateral brachial cutaneous (radial), posterior brachial cutaneous (radial), medial brachial cutaneous (medial cord of brachial plexus), medial antebrachial cutaneous (medial cord of brachial plexus), lateral antebrachial cutaneous (terminal branch of musculocutaneous),

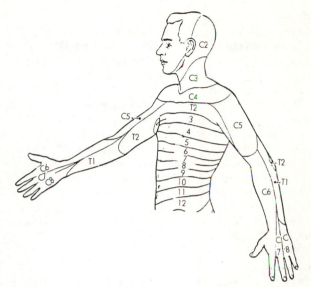

Figure 1-15.   Dermatomes of the upper limbs.

posterior antebrachial cutaneous (radial), medial (ulnar) portion of the hand—dorsal and palmar sides including the hypothenar eminence and the little finger and half of the ring finger supplied by the ulnar nerve, the radial portion of the hand on the palmar side by the median nerve (all that on the palmar surface not innervated by the ulnar), and the dorsum of the hand not innervated by the ulnar, served by the radial nerve **except** for the distal phalanges of the lateral three and one-half digits (served by the median nerve).

Visible cutaneous veins include the following: the **dorsal venous arch on the hand,** the **cephalic vein** (courses up the lateral [radial] side of the antebrachium and brachium, along the deltopectoral groove [between the deltoid and pectoralis major muscles] and is a tributary of the axillary vein), and the **basilic vein** (courses up medial [ulnar] side of antebrachium and brachium and in the proximal end of the brachium joins with the venae comitantes of the brachial artery to form the axillary vein).

Muscle groups

Pectoral muscles include the pectoralis major and minor muscles, which serve in adduction and medial rotation of the upper limbs. They are innervated by the lateral and medial pectoral nerves (from respective cords of the brachial plexus). **Scapular** muscles include the **rhomboids** (C5, root of brachial plexus), which adduct and rotate the scapula; the **rotator cuff muscles** (**subscapularis** [subscapular nerves] to the lesser tuberosity of the humerus; the **supraspinatus** and **infraspinatus** [suprascapular nerve], and the **teres minor** [axillary nerve], all three to the greater tuberosity of the humerus); the **latissimus dorsi** (thoracodorsal or middle subscapular nerve), to the floor of the bicipital groove, which extends the shoulder, medially rotates and adducts the upper limb; the **serratus anterior** (long thoracic nerve), which draws the scapula ventrally and rotates it (denervation results in "winging" of the scapula); the **trapezius** (**XI** innervation), to the clavicle and spine of the scapula (rotation, elevation, depression, adduction of the scapula); the **levator scapulae** (C3, C4, and dorsal scapular nerve [C5]), to the superior angle of the scapula (elevates scapula); and the **teres major** (lower subscapular nerve), to the medial lip of bicipital groove (extends the shoulder, adducts and medially rotates the upper limb).

Brachial flexors (musculocutaneous nerve) include the **coracobrachialis**, the coracoid process of the scapula to the medial side of the middle of the humerus shaft (flexion and adduction of the arm); the **biceps brachii**, the short head from the coracoid process of the scapula, the long head from the supraglenoid tuberosity of the scapula, to the radial tuberosity and deep fascia of antebrachium (flexion of the arm and forearm, supination of the hand); and the **brachialis**, from the distal half of the humerus to the coronoid process of the ulna (flexion of the forearm).

Brachial extensors (radial nerve) include the **triceps brachii**, three heads with the long head from the infraglenoid tuberosity of the scapula, the medial and lateral from the humerus, which inserts on the olecranon process of the ulna (extends the forearm [elbow] and long head extends and adducts the brachium at the shoulder joint).

Antebrachial flexors (median nerve except flexor carpi ulnaris and medial half of flexor digitorum profundus, which are by ulnar nerve) have a common origin from the medial epicondyle of the humerus: the pronator teres (median nerve passes between its two heads), flexor carpi radialis, palmaris longus, flexor carpi ulnaris, flexor digitorum superficialis (inserts on middle phalanges), flexor digitorum profundus (inserts on distal phalanges), flexor pollicis longus, and pronator quadratus.

Antebrachial extensors (all by radial nerve) have a common origin from the lateral epicondyle of the humerus: the brachioradialis (actually a flexor of the elbow joint), extensor carpi radialis longus and brevis, extensor digitorum communis, extensor digiti minimi, extensor indicis proprius, extensor pollicis longus and brevis, abductor pollicis longus, supinator, anconeus, and extensor carpi ulnaris.

Thenar muscles (median nerve except the deep head of the flexor pollicis brevis, which is by the ulnar nerve) include the flexor pollicis brevis, opponens pollicis, and abductor pollicis brevis.

Hypothenar muscles (ulnar nerve) consist of the flexor digiti minimi, opponens digiti minimi, and abductor digiti minimi.

Other hand muscles are the lumbricales (associated with the tendons of the flexor digitorum profundus), the medial two of which are innervated by the ulnar nerve, lateral two by the median nerve; and the interossei (ulnar nerve), three palmar and four dorsal. Note: PAD and DAB—palmar interossei abduct, dorsal abduct.

Articulations of the upper limbs are as follows: interphalangeal—hinge (ginglymal), metacarpophalangeal—condyloid; metacarpal-carpal—gliding except for first with trapezium (saddle); intercarpal—gliding (arthrodial); radius-carpal—gliding (note that the ulna does not articulate with the carpals); proximal and distal radius-ulnar—pivot (trochoid); humerus-ulna—hinge; humerus-radius—gliding; glenohumeral (shoulder) —enarthrodial (ball and socket); acromioclavicular—gliding; and sternoclavicular—gliding.

Arteries

The upper limb is supplied via the **axillary artery**. As the subclavian artery passes over the first rib and enters the axilla, its name is changed to axillary artery. It is described as having three portions indicated by the artery's relationship to the pectoralis minor. The first part lies above the pectoralis minor and has one branch, the highest or **supreme thoracic**, which supplies the first intercostal space. The second part of the artery lies behind the pectoralis minor and has two branches, the **thoracoacromial trunk** and the lateral thoracic. The thoracoacromial trunk has four branches, which describe its distribution—acromial, deltoid, clavicular, and pectoral. The lateral thoracic extends along the lateral thoracic wall. The third part of the axillary artery lies lateral to the pectoralis minor and has three branches—**anterior** and **posterior humeral circumflex arteries** and the **subscapular artery**. The circumflexes encircle the proximal end of the shaft of the humerus. The posterior is consistently much larger and accompanies the axillary artery through the axilla and out through the quadrangular space. The subscapular artery has a large branch called the **circumflex scapular** artery, which passes through the triangular space and into the infraspinatous fossa of the scapula. After the circumflex scapular branch is given off, the subscapular continues as the **thoracodorsal** artery, which courses with the thoracodorsal nerve, which supplies the latissimus dorsi muscle.

The axillary artery passes out of the axilla, past the tendon of the teres major, and is renamed the **brachial artery**. The brachial gives rise to the **deep brachial** (profunda brachii) artery, which courses distally and laterally as it passes posterior to the humerus in the **spiral groove**, where it joins the **radial nerve**. The deep brachial has muscular branches to the posterior compartment muscles and gives rise to the **radial collateral** and **middle collateral** arteries for anastomoses around the elbow. The brachial artery itself passes distally through the brachium as it supplies anterior compartment muscles, and it gives rise to the **superior** and **inferior ulnar collateral** branches. These latter two vessels also participate in the elbow anastomosis. The brachial artery passes over the cubital fossa into the antebrachium and branches into **radial** and **ulnar arteries**.

The **radial artery** extends distally along the radius and deep to the brachioradialis muscle. Near its origin, the radial artery gives rise to the **radial recurrent** artery to the elbow anastomosis. The radial artery continues into the hand, makes a minor contribution to the **superficial palmar arch**, and continues to be the main source of the **deep palmar arch**.

The **ulnar artery** gives rise to anterior and posterior ulnar recurrent branches and to the **common interosseous artery**, which branches into **anterior interosseous** and **posterior interosseous** arteries. The posterior interosseous has a branch called the **interosseous recurrent** artery, which contributes to the elbow anastomosis. The ulnar artery courses distally deep to the flexor carpi ulnaris muscle, continues across the wrist, and provides the main source of supply to the superficial palmar artery and perhaps a minor contribution to the deep palmar arch.

Veins

The venous return approximately parallels the arteries. The large cutaneous veins were described above as visible cutaneous veins. The **axillary vein** is formed by the merging of the basilic vein with the venae comitantes of the brachial artery. This occurs approximately at the level of the tendon of the teres major muscle as these vessels enter the axilla.

Innervation

The cutaneous innervation has been described above, and the innervation of major muscle groups is included in the description of the muscles. The innervation of the upper limb is via the brachial plexus.

Upper limb neural lesions

Upper lesions of the brachial plexus (Erb-Duchenne palsy) result from depression of the shoulder ipsilaterally and extreme displacement of the head to the opposite side. C5 and C6 roots suffer excessive traction or tearing. The nerves most drastically affected are the nerve to the subclavius, the supra-scapular nerve, and the axillary nerve. Muscles involved include the subclavius, supraspinatus, infraspinatus, deltoid, teres minor, biceps brachii, brachialis, and coracobrachialis. The limb will be limp and hanging at the side and medially rotated because of the pectoralis major's unopposed action. The forearm will be pronated because of loss of the biceps brachii (supinator of the forearm and flexor of elbow). This is called "waiter's tip." Sensation will be lost down the lateral side of the brachium.

Lower lesions of the brachial plexus (Klumpke's palsy) result from excessive abduction of the upper limb, and the major loss is spinal nerve T1. This segment is carried in the median and ulnar nerves and is important in the innervation of the intrinsic hand muscles. This results in claw hand because the metacarpophalangeal (MP) joints are hyperextended and the interphalangeal (IP) joints are flexed. The MP joints are extended by the extensor digitorum communis because this muscle is unopposed by the now paralyzed interossei and lumbricales. The IP joints are flexed because the long flexors of the digits are unopposed by these same paralyzed muscles. Sensation will be lost along the medial side of the limb.

Long thoracic nerve lesion results in "winged scapula" because the serratus anterior is paralyzed. In abduction of the brachium above the head, the serratus anterior aids in rotating the scapula; thus, patients cannot raise their arm above their head. Injuries can occur as the result of pressure on the posterior cervical triangle, of accidents during surgery, stabbing, etc.

Axillary nerve injuries can occur when prolonged pressure is applied to the axilla—for example, from using a poorly adjusted crutch, in extreme downward pressure of the head of the humerus as in a shoulder dislocation, or from a fracture of surgical neck of the humerus. Lesion of this nerve results in loss of innervation to the teres minor and deltoid muscles and to the skin of the upper lateral brachial area.

Axillary branches of the **radial nerve** are the (1) posterior brachial cutaneous, (2) nerve to the long head of the triceps, and (3) nerve to the medial head of the triceps. **Spiral groove branches** are the (1) lower lateral brachial cutaneous, (2) posterior antebrachial cutaneous, (3) nerve to the lateral head of the triceps, (4) nerve to the medial head of the triceps and the anconeus. In the **anterior compartment** proximal to the elbow are the (1) nerve to brachialis, (2) nerve to the brachioradialis,

and (3) nerve to the extensor carpi radialis longus. In the **cubital fossa** are the deep branch and superficial branch of the radial. The superficial branch is sensory and extends to the dorsum of the hand to innervate the skin of the lateral three and one-half fingers proximal to the nail bed. The deep branch supplies the supinator and extensor carpi radialis brevis and all the posterior compartment muscles of the antebrachium.

The most common sites of injury are in the axilla and in the spiral groove. The injuries that occur in the axilla are due to shoulder dislocation with the humerus pushing into the axilla, a poorly adjusted crutch, and generally any condition that causes excessive pressure in the axilla. Injuries in the axilla can result in paralysis of the triceps, anconeus, and long extensors of the wrist. With the extensors of the wrist paralyzed, the result is wristdrop. With the wrist in the flexed position, the strength of finger flexion is greatly compromised, as is the grip. Brachioradialis and supinator are also paralyzed, but the biceps brachii can still effect supination.

Injuries of the radial nerve in the spiral groove can occur when the shaft is fractured or when prolonged pressure is exerted on the posterior side of the brachium (e.g., prolonged use of a tourniquet). The injury usually occurs in the distal part of the groove after the branches to the triceps, anconeus, and some of the cutaneous nerves have formed. Motor loss includes inability to extend the wrist (wristdrop), and sensory loss is seen on the proximal end of the thumb. Injury to the deep branch of the radial results in loss of the long extensors of the digits. The supinator and extensor carpi radialis longus are usually preserved, and thus no wristdrop occurs.

Because it is so well protected, the **musculocutaneous nerve** is infrequently injured. The coracobrachialis, biceps brachii, and most of the brachialis are paralyzed. Radially innervated muscles assist in elbow flexion. The lateral ante-brachial cutaneous nerve is compromised, and anesthesia can result.

Injuries at the elbow result in paralysis of the long flexors of the digits (except those innervated by ulnar) and the pronators. The hand is supine, wrist flexion is weak, and there is some wrist adduction. The index and middle fingers cannot flex at the MP joints, and little flexion occurs at the MP joints of these fingers. Thenar eminence muscles atrophy. The ring finger and little finger are flexed because of intact ulnar innervation.

Injuries at the wrist also result in loss of the thenar muscles. The thumb is laterally rotated and adducted. The thumb cannot be apposed, and this makes the injury serious because this diminishes function so drastically. Loss of the median nerve distribution to skin of the hand also occurs.

In **carpal tunnel syndrome,** burning or prickling pain is felt along the median distribution. Unattended, it can result in motor losses described for injuries at the wrist. Skin over the thenar eminence is still innervated because the palmar cutaneous branch of the median nerve passes superficial to the transverse carpal ligament.

Injuries at the elbow deprive innervation to the flexor carpi ulnaris and the ulnar half of the flexor digitorum profundus. The **ulnar nerve** distribution within the hand will be lost. Because of the loss of the interossei, the fingers cannot be adducted or abducted. Grip is impaired, as demonstrated by patients trying to hold onto a piece of paper. They will do so by relying on the flexor pollicis longus, which strongly flexes the

IP joint of the thumb (Froment's paper sign). The MP joints become hyperextended as a result of loss of two lumbricales and all of the interossei. The ulnar two lumbricales are lost, and thus these two fingers become more markedly hyperextended and the IP joints flexed because the long extensors are not being opposed by muscles inserting upon extensor expansion—the "claw" deformity (main en griffe). Sensory loss is to the skin of the hand supplied by the ulnar nerve.

Skeleton

The following is a list of the bones of the upper limb and their salient features: **clavicle, scapula**—spine, acromion, coracoid process, supra- and infraspinatus fossae, glenoid cavity, supra- and infraglenoid tuberosities; **humerus**—head, neck, greater and lesser tubercles, bicipital groove, medial and lateral epicondyles, olecranon fossa, coronoid fossa, trochlea, radial fossa, capitulum; **radius**—head, neck, tuberosity, styloid process; **ulna**—olecranon process, coronoid process, trochlear notch, radial notch, styloid process; **carpal bones**—trapezium, trapezoid, capitate, hamate, scaphoid, lunate, triquetral, pisiform; **metacarpals** (5); and **phalanges** (14).

LOWER LIMB

Dermatomes of the lower limbs are illustrated in Figure 1-16.

Cutaneous innervation includes the following: cluneal nerves (cluneal and gluteal are interchangeable terms)—superior (L1–3), middle (S1–3), and inferior (from posterior femoral cutaneous); lateral femoral cutaneous—from lumbar plexus L2, L3; lumboinguinal—patch of skin just distal to inguinal ligament, from the genitofemoral nerve; ilioinguinal—to the scrotum and adjacent thigh; anterior and medial femoral cutaneous—from the femoral; posterior femoral cutaneous—from the sacral plexus (S1–3); saphenous nerve—from the femoral; to the medial leg and ankle (L3, L4); cutaneous branch common peroneal—lateral side of the proximal leg (L5, S1, S2); superficial peroneal cutaneous—anterolateral leg and dorsum of the foot (L4, L5, S1); deep peroneal cutaneous—between the great and second toe (L4, L5); sural cutaneous—posterior leg and lateral foot (S1, S2); plantar side of foot—saphenous on the medial side, tibial on the heel, medial plantar on plantar foot and medial three and one-half digits, lateral plantar on plantar foot and lateral one and one-half toes, and sural on the lateral side.

The **superificial veins** of the lower limb of particular note are the **great saphenous vein**, which begins on the medial side of the foot and ankle and courses cranially on the medial side of the limb and empties into the femoral vein through the saphenous hiatus (foramen ovale) in the region of the femoral triangle (just below inguinal ligament); and the **small saphenous vein**, which begins on lateral ankle/foot and courses cranially up the posterior surface of the leg and is a tributary of the popliteal vein.

Muscle groups

Gluteal muscles. The piriformis is the "key" to the gluteal region. It extends from the anterior surface of the sacrum through the greater sciatic notch to the femur. The tensor fasciae latae, gluteus minimus, and gluteus medius all are

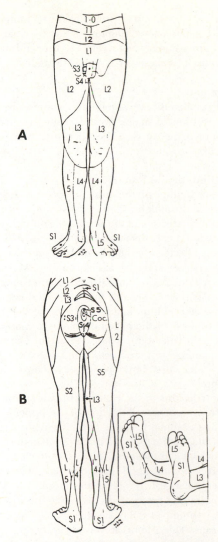

Figure 1-16. Dermatomes of the lower limbs: *A*, anterior and *B*, posterior views.

innervated by the superior gluteal nerve. As a group, they function to medially rotate and abduct the thigh. The gluteus maximus (extends and laterally rotates thigh; inferior gluteal nerve), the obturator internus (nerve to obturator internus), the superior and inferior gemelli, the quadratus femoris (nerve to the quadratus femoris), the obturator externus (obturator nerve), the iliopsoas (lumbar nerves; flexes the pelvis over the thigh), and the pectineus (obturator nerve; flexes, adducts the thigh) all laterally rotate the thigh.

Thigh muscles. **Anterior compartment** muscles all are innervated by the femoral nerve: the sartorius (flexes and laterally rotates the thigh; flexes the knee), quadriceps femoris (rectus femoris portion that crosses both hip and knee joints; vasti lateralis, intermedius, medialis—flexes hip, extends knee). The **medial compartment** is innervated by the obturator nerve except where noted; this muscle group adducts and flexes the thigh: gracilis, adductors longus, brevis, and magnus. The magnus also gets innervation from the tibial division of the sciatic nerve, and its actions also include extension and rotation of the thigh. The **posterior compartment** innervation is via the tibial portion of the sciatic, except the peroneal division to the short head of the biceps (extend the hip, flex the knee). The muscles are the biceps femoris, semimembranosus, and semitendinosus.

Leg muscles. The **posterior compartment** muscles are all innervated by the tibial nerve (flexor compartment): the triceps surae—soleus (which crosses only the ankle joint) and gastro-cnemius (crosses both the knee and ankle joints); the plantaris; the popliteus—flexes the knee, rotates the leg medially, "unlocks" the knee; the flexor hallucis longus; the flexor digitorum longus, and the tibialis posterior—plantar flexor and foot inverter. **Anterior compartment** muscles all are innervated by the deep peroneal nerve and are extensors; the tibialis anterior, extensor hallucis longus, extensor digitorum longus, and peroneus tertius. **Peroneal compartment** muscles all are innervated by the superficial peroneal nerve and plantar flex and evert the foot.

Foot muscles. **Dorsal foot muscles** are extensors of the toes (except little toe) and are served by the deep peroneal nerve. **Plantar foot muscles** are as follows: first layer—abductor hallucis, flexor digitorum brevis, abductor digiti minimi; second layer—flexor hallucis longus, flexor digitorum longus, quadratus plantae, lumbricales (four) associated with the tendons of the flexor digitorum longus; third layer—flexor hallucis brevis, adductor hallucis, and flexor digiti minimi brevis; fourth layer—four dorsal and three plantar interossei. Innervation is via the medial plantar nerve for the abductor hallucis, flexor hallucis brevis, first lumbrical, and flexor digitorum brevis. All others are served by the lateral plantar nerve.

Articulations of lower limb

Articulations of the lower limb are as follows: inter-phalangeal (hinge); metatarsal-phalangeal (condyloid); meta-tarsal-tarsal (gliding); and intertarsal (gliding). The **ankle** (talocrural) joint is mainly a hinge joint: the tibia and its malleolus, fibula's malleolus, and the talus. Of the tibiofibular joints, the proximal one is gliding, distal is syndesmosis. **Knee** articulations are the tibial condyles and femoral condyles. Major ligaments include the capsule, lateral and medial menisci, medial (tibial) and lateral (fibular) collaterals, anterior and posterior cruciates, and the transverse. The **hip** articulation is the head of the femur in the acetabular fossa. Major ligaments include the capsule (iliofemoral, ischiofemoral, pubofemoral), the ligament of the head of the femur (round ligament), the acetabular labrum, and the transverse articular.

Arteries and veins

Three major arterial stems supply the lower limb—**superior** and **inferior gluteal arteries** and the **femoral artery**. The gluteals pass through the greater sciatic foramen and distribute mainly to the gluteal region. The femoral artery is the continuation of the external iliac artery, which changes its name as it passes under the inguinal ligament. Within a short distance into the thigh, the femoral gives rise to the large **deep femoral artery** (**profunda femoris**), which supplies much of the medial and the posterior compartments of the thigh. The femoral continues on into the adductor (Hunter's) canal

(bounded by the vastus medialis muscle, the sartorius muscle, and the adductor longus and magnus muscles), along with the femoral vein. These vessels and the femoral branches of nerve to the vastus medialis and saphenous nerve also enter the adductor canal. The vessels extend through the canal and pass through the adductor hiatus (in the tendon of the adductor magnus) to enter the popliteal fossa. Here the femoral vessels become the **popliteal vessels**. Just distal to the knee, the artery ends by dividing the **anterior and posterior tibial arteries**. The anterior tibial passes between the tibia and fibula and extends down through the anterior compartment of the leg and onto the dorsum of the foot as the **dorsalis pedis artery**. This artery passes between the first and second metatarsals and is the main contributor to the **deep plantar arch**. The posterior **tibial artery** gives off a branch called the **peroneal artery,** which supplies the peroneal compartment. The posterior tibial continues down the leg between superficial and deep muscle groups and passes around the posteromedial side of the ankle and onto the superficial structures of the plantar side of the foot.

Venous return approximately parallels the arteries. The large cutaneous veins were described previously.

Skeleton

The **hip bone** (innominate bone) comprises the ilium, pubic bone, and ischium: the iliac crest; iliac tubercle; anterior superior, posterior superior, anterior inferior, and posterior inferior spines; ischial spine; ischial tuberosity; pubic tubercle, crest; pectineal line (crest); iliopectineal line; superior ramus of the pubic bone; ischiopubic ramus; obturator foramen, groove; arcuate line of the ilium; greater sciatic notch; lesser sciatic notch; pubic symphysis; body of the pubic bone; body of the ischium; body of the ilium; iliopectineal eminence; and acetabulum—notch, fossa, and lunate surface. The **femur** comprises the head, fovea capitis; neck; greater and lesser trochanters; trochanteric fossa; intertrochanteric line, crest; shaft; linea aspera; popliteal surface; medial and lateral condyles, epicondyles; intercondylar fossa; and the patellar surface. The **tibia** consists of the condyles, intercondylar eminence, tuberosity, shaft, and medial malleolus. The **patella** is situated at the front of the knee. The **fibula** is composed of a head, neck, and lateral malleolus. **Tarsal bones** include the talus; calcaneus; navicular; cuboid; and first, second, and third cuneiform bones. There are five **metatarsal bones** and 14 **phalanges**.

Lower limb neural lesions

Femoral nerve. This nerve arises from L2–4. It enters the thigh under the inguinal ligament in the lacuna musculorum at a point midway between the anterior superior iliac spine and the pubic tubercle. It lies about 1 cm lateral to the femoral pulse. Within an inch or less of the inguinal ligament it forms its terminal branches. Injuries that result in complete severance of the nerve are rare. Stab wounds in the region of the femoral triangle might effect such an injury. Should the femoral nerve be severed, the knee cannot be extended. The adductor muscles can be used to compensate somewhat in walking. Cutaneous innervation over the anterior and medial thigh might be lost. Loss of the saphenous branch of the nerve would mean loss of sensation on the medial side of the leg, ankle, and foot.

Sciatic nerve (L4—S3).   The peroneal and tibial divisions enter the gluteal region through the greater sciatic notch inferior to the piriformis muscle. The peroneal division will occasionally penetrate the piriformis and thus be separated from the tibial division. The two divisions may or may not become joined as they course distally. The sciatic nerve courses through the gluteal region midway between the posterior superior iliac spine and the ischial tuberosity and descends in the midline within the posterior compartment of the thigh. At a variable distance above the popliteal fossa, it splits into its two divisions.

The sciatic nerve is subject to injury in cases of penetrating wounds, dislocations of the hip joint, and pelvic fractures. Injudicious injections in the gluteal region can also injure the nerve. Injury much more frequently involves the peroneal division. Should the sciatic nerve be completely involved in a lesion, flexion of the knee is weak but still possible via sartorius and gracilis muscles, innervated by the femoral nerve and obturator nerve, respectively. All muscles below the knee would be paralyzed and footdrop manifested.

Common peroneal nerve (division of sciatic nerve; L4—S2). Because it is subcutaneous as it winds around the neck of the fibula, it is particularly vulnerable. Lesion would result in paralysis of the anterior and lateral compartment muscles. In such a situation, the foot is plantarflexed (footdrop) and inverted (equinovarus). Cutaneous sensations on the antero-lateral sides of the leg and the dorsum of the foot would be lost.

Tibial nerve (division of sciatic nerve; L4—S3).   This nerve courses through the popliteal fossa and then passes deep to the gastrocnemius and soleus muscles. On those rare occasions when it is seriously injured, the leg muscles of the posterior compartment and the plantar muscles of the foot are paralyzed. The unopposed muscles of the other two compartments dorsiflex and evert the foot (calcaneovalgus). The cutaneous sensations of the sole of the foot would be lost.

Obturator nerve (L2—4).   This nerve forms anterior and posterior divisions and passes into the thigh through the obturator foramen. The posterior division is distributed to the adductor magnus (which is also innervated by the tibial division of the sciatic), the obturator externus, and possibly the adductor brevis; the anterior division supplies the other muscles of the adductor compartment. The nerve is only infrequently damaged by hip dislocations, penetrating wounds, etc. It is sometimes damaged during vaginal delivery. Lesion of the nerve results in loss of the adductors of the thigh and cutaneous innervation of the medial thigh.

HEAD

Skull

The **calvaria** consists of frontal, parietal (2), occipital, and temporal (squamous portion) bones.

The **anterior cranial fossa** comprises the ethmoid (crista galli, cribriform plate), frontal (orbital plates), and sphenoid (body and lesser wing) bones and the foramina— the cribriform plate of the ethmoid for central processes of olfactory nerve (I) and anterior and posterior ethmoidal foramina (for vessels and nerves of the same name).

The **middle cranial fossa** includes the sphenoid (body, sella turcica, sphenoid tubercle, dorsum sellae, clinoid pro-

cesses, greater wing), temporal bones (petrous and squamous portions), and the foramina—the superior orbital fissure (III, IV, ophthalmic of V, VI, superior ophthalmic vein) lies between lesser and greater wings of sphenoid; the foramen rotundum (for V_2) in the sphenoid bone; the foramen spinosum (for the middle meningeal artery) in the sphenoid bone; the foramen ovale (for V_3) in the sphenoid bone; the foramen lacerum (internal carotid), formed by the temporal, sphenoid, and a small part of the occipital bones; and the optic canal (II, ophthalmic artery, sympathetics).

The **posterior cranial fossa** comprises the following structures: the occipital bone, petrous portion of the temporal bone, the parietal bone (minor contribution), and foramina— the foramen magnum (spinal cord/medulla junction, vertebral arteries, anterior and posterior spinal arteries, cranial nerve XI) in the occipital; the internal auditory meatus (VII [including nervus intermedius], VIII, labyrinthine artery) in the temporal bone; the jugular foramen (IX, X, XI) formed by the petrous and occipital bones; the hypoglossal canal (XII) in the occipital bone; and the condylar canal (emissary vein) in the occipital bone.

The **orbit** consists of frontal, ethmoid, sphenoid, zygomatic, lacrimal, palatine, and maxillary bones.

The bones of the face are the frontal, maxillary, zygomatic, nasal, and the mandible. The foramina include the supraorbital (notch or foramen) (supraorbital vessels, terminal branches of the ophthalmic division of V) in the frontal bone; the infra-orbital vessels (terminal branches of V_2) in the maxillary bone; zygomaticofacial (branches of V_2) in the zygomatic bone; and the mental (mental branches of V_3)—mandible.

The **nasal cavity** consists of the perpendicular and cribriform plates of the ethmoid; the superior and middle conchal bones (processes of ethmoid); the vomer; the palatine processes of the maxillary bone; the horizontal processes of the palatine bones; the inferior conchal bone; and the septal cartilage. Nasal spaces include the sphenoethmoidal recess—the sphenoidal sinus opens here, cribriform plate for central processes of I (olfactory cranial nerve); superior meatus—between the superior and middle conchal bones—the posterior ethmoidal sinus opens here; middle meatus, between the middle and inferior conchal bones—the frontal, maxillary, anterior and middle ethmoidal sinuses open here; the inferior meatus, below the inferior conchal bone—the nasolacrimal duct opens here; the vestibule— the entrance to the nasal passages, where hair can be seen; the atrium, or area in the nasal passages anterior to the meati; and the choanae, the anterior and posterior openings of the nasal passages.

The **hard palate** consists of the premaxilla (holds the incisors and is part of the maxilla), the palatine processes of the maxilla, the horizontal processes of the palatine bones, the nasal septum, which fuses in the midline on the superior side, and the foramina—incisive for the passage of the terminal branches of the greater palatine vessels from the oral cavity into the nasal cavity, and the greater and lesser palatine foramina for vessels and nerves of the same name as they pass from the pterygopalatine fossa onto the inferior surface of hard and soft palates, respectively.

The **mandible** consists of the body; ramus; coronoid process (temporalis muscle inserts here); condylar process (articulates with temporal bone); mandibular foramen, on inner side of ramus—transmits inferior alveolar nerve and vessels; and the chin region, whose anterior surface is the **mentis** (thus terms such as symphysis menti, mentalis muscle, mental foramen) and whose posterior side is the **genio** (thus such names as genial tubercle, genioglossus muscle, geniohyoid muscle).

The **articulations of skull bones** include the temporomandibular joint (TMJ) which comprises the condylar process of the mandible articulating with the mandibular fossa of temporal bone and is a synovial joint (hinge–sliding); the sutures; the articulation of the teeth with the alveolar processes of the maxilla and the mandible—immovable joints known specifically as gomphoses; and the ossicles (of the middle ear), which articulate with each other via synovial joints.

In the **fetal skull**, cranial sutures form postnatally. Frontal bones fuse to form the frontal suture. The anterior fontanel is situated midline at the junction of the frontal and parietal bones. The posterior fontanel is located in the midline at the junction of the parietal and occipital bones. In the midline, the parietal suture extends from the anterior to the posterior fontanel and between the parietal bones. The coronal suture extends transversely between the frontal and parietal bones. The lambdoidal suture extends transversely between the parietal and occipital bones. At the sphenoid fontanel, the pterion will form (at the junction of the frontal, sphenoid, temporal, and parietal bones). The mastoid fontanel is superior to the forming mastoid process.

Muscles

The muscles of facial expression are innervated by cranial nerve VII. Attachments include many on the facial skin. Prominent ones include the orbicularis oculi, orbicularis oris, buccinator, depressor and levator anguli oris muscles, and the zygomaticus (major and minor). The stylohyoid and posterior belly of the digastric muscles are not involved in facial expression but are innervated by cranial nerve VII.

The muscles of mastication, innervated by cranial nerve V_3, are as follows: masseter, lateral and medial pterygoids, temporalis, tensor veli palatini, mylohyoid, and anterior belly digastric. (The tensor tympani is innervated by this nerve but is involved in hearing, not mastication or swallowing.)

The intrinsic tongue muscles lie in all three planes and are innervated by cranial nerve XII. The extrinsics are all "glossus" muscles and are innervated by XII except the palatoglossus muscle (supplied by X). The genioglossus protrudes the tongue from the mouth and is peculiar in receiving motor innervation via only the contralateral cerebral cortex. The other tongue muscles benefit from bilateral corticobulbar involvement. A neural lesion of cranial nerve XII results in the protruded tongue deviating toward the side of the weakened muscles.

All of the **soft palate muscles** are innervated by cranial nerve X except the tensor veli palatini, which is supplied by V.

Of the **pharyngeal muscles**, the stylopharyngeus is innervated by cranial nerve IX, the three constrictors by X.

The orbit

The sclera and cornea comprise the outer coat of the **eyeball**. The choroid is the middle coat—choriocapillaris, ciliary body, and iris stroma. The retina is the inner coat. The neural portion is light sensitive; the nonneural portion is the ciliary epithelium and the epithelium on the posterior side of the iris. The lens is an epithelial structure with basement membrane on its surface, which forms the lens capsule; it is suspended by the suspensory ligament, which extends from the equator of the lens to the processes of the ciliary body. Contraction of the ciliary muscle reduces tension on the ligament and allows the lens to assume a more spherical shape (thickens in anterior/posterior dimension), increasing its refractive power. The intrinsic muscles are smooth muscle and include the parasympathetically innervated ciliary muscle (of the ciliary body), the iridial sphincter, and the sympathetically innervated iridial dilator muscle. The vitreous chamber is the space bounded by the lens, suspensory ligament, and ciliary body anteriorly and by the neural retina laterally and posteriorly. It is filled with vitreous humor. The anterior chamber lies anterior to the iris and posterior to the cornea. The posterior chamber lies posterior to the iris and anterior to the peripheral part of the lens and its suspensory ligament. Aqueous humor fills the anterior and posterior chambers, which communicate via the pupil. Aqueous humor is continuously formed by the ciliary body and its epithelium, flows into posterior chamber, through the pupil into the anterior chamber, to the angle, and ultimately drains into the venous system.

Extrinsic ocular muscles are all skeletal muscles. Cranial nerve VI (abducens) innervates the lateral rectus for lateral gaze. Cranial nerve IV (trochlear) innervates the superior oblique for intorsion when the eye is turned laterally and depression of eye when turned nasally. Nerve and muscle are tested by having the patient look nasally and down. Cranial nerve III (oculomotor) supplies all the rest of the muscles. Superior and inferior recti are pure elevators/depressors, respectively, when the eye is turned laterally. The inferior oblique elevates the eye when turned nasally, extorts it when turned laterally. The medial and lateral recti turn the eye medially and laterally, respectively. The levator palpebrae superioris elevates the eyelid.

The lacrimal gland lies in the upper lateral part of the orbit. Its ducts open through both superior and inferior fornices of the conjunctiva into the conjunctival sac. It is parasympathetically innervated by a complicated course beginning in the superior salivatory nucleus (in the pons) and traveling via various branches of cranial nerves VII and V.

The blood supply is mostly via the ophthalmic artery (a branch of the internal carotid).

Cranial nerve V_1 (ophthalmic division of V) provides sensory supply to the eyeball and orbit. Sympathetic innervation is from intermediolateral nucleus of the T1 segment of the spinal cord and superior cervical sympathetic ganglion. The latter sends postganglionic fibers into the orbit via the internal carotid and its branches, but some of these fibers may "hitch" a ride with cranial nerves entering the orbit also. Parasympathetic innervation is via the Edinger-Westphal nucleus of the oculomotor nerve and involves the ciliary ganglion, which contains the second-order neurons.

The ear

The **external ear** includes the pinna (auricle) and external auditory meatus. Numerous nerves provide sensory innervation, but the predominant ones are cranial nerves V_3 and X. Also contributing are VII, IX, and cervical spinal nerves 2 and

3. The external meatus extends anteriorly, medially, and inferiorly and ends at the tympanic membrane.

The **middle ear** includes the cavity that connects with the nasopharynx via the eustachian tube (auditory canal) and with the mastoid antrum and air cells. Sensory innervation is via cranial nerve IX. Significant structures are the three ossicles— malleus, incus, stapes. These articulate with one another via synovial joints. The malleus is attached to the tympanic membrane and picks up vibrations due to sound waves and transmits them to the incus, which transmits them to the stapes, which transmits them into the inner ear through the oval window. Because the tympanic membrane is much larger than the oval window, this mechanism amplifies the sound. The tensor tympani muscle (V_3) attaches to the malleus, and the stapedius muscle (VII) attaches to the stapes. Their functions are not entirely clear, but it seems that they are capable of adjusting the mechanism so as to increase efficacy. They may also serve a protective mechanism.

The **inner ear** is a labyrinthine structure contained within the petrous portion of the temporal bone. The **osseous labyrinth** has three **semicircular canals** (superior or anterior, lateral, posterior), all of which open into the **vestibule.** The vestibule is continuous with the **vestibular aqueduct,** which opens into the posterior cranial fossa. Also continuous with the vestibule is the **cochlea,** a spiral structure of about two and one-quarter turns. Within the osseous labyrinth is the **membraneous labyrinth,** which contains specialized sensory epithelia capable of serving as end organs for vestibular and auditory function. Within the osseous semicircular canals lie the membranous **semicircular ducts,** which have patches of specialized sensory epithelia called **cristae** that detect angular acceleration/deceleration. The semicircular ducts open into the membranous **utricle,** which lies within the vestibule. The utricle's sensory epithelium is a **macula,** which responds to gravitational stimuli and aids in orientation of the head to gravity. The utricle is continuous with the **endolymphatic duct** and **sac,** which lie within the vestibular aqueduct and posterior cranial fossa, respectively. Also continuous with the endolymphatic duct and lying within the vestibule is the **saccule,** which has a **macula** too. The function of the saccule is not so clear, but it seems to respond to vibratory stimuli and functions to work in the vestibular system. The saccule is also continuous with the membranous **cochlear duct,** which lies within the cochlea. The sensory epithelium of the cochlear duct is the **organ of Corti.** The membranous labyrinth is filled with **endolymph,** the osseous with **perilymph.** The osseous labyrinth opens into the subarachnoid space via the **cochlear aqueduct,** and perilymph is quite similar to CSF. The membranous labyrinth's endolymph is secreted continuously and is resorbed into the vascular system, apparently from the endolymphatic duct and sac.

The scalp

The following mnemonic device describes the scalp structures: **S** = skin; **C** = connective tissue (subcutaneous); **A** = aponeurosis (gallea aponeurotica within which the frontalis and occipitalis muscles are embedded); **L** = loose areolar connective tissue (danger space because it is a tightly bound space that can harbor infections, communicate with the cranial cavity); and **P** = periosteum.

The mouth

Tongue muscles were discussed previously. The anterior two-thirds of the tongue is innervated by V_3 for general sensations, by VII for taste. The posterior third is innervated by IX for both general **and** gustatory sensations. The floor of mouth underlies the tongue. The frenulum of the tongue extends from the underside of the tongue to the floor. On either side of it are sublingual papillae through which the ducts of the submandibular glands open (Wharton's ducts). Sublingual folds extend posterolaterally along the floor of mouth, starting at the frenulum. These are underlain by the sublingual glands. The lingual artery is a branch of the external carotid. It approaches the tongue from the underside and courses close to the midline. Cranial nerve XII (the hypoglossal nerve) courses approximately parallel to the lingual artery.

The **teeth** articulate with the alveolar arches of the mandible and maxilla via immovable joints (gomphoses). The adult dental formula is 2-1-2-3 for both jaws. The **buccal cavity** is between the teeth and cheeks/lips. The parotid duct opens by the upper second molar. The **fauces** is the general site of continuity of the oral cavity and the oropharynx. The palatoglossal and palatopharyngeal folds are the faucial pillars, and the palatine tonsil lies between the pillars in the tonsillar fossa.

Arteries

The **external carotid** supplies the face/mouth region. It typically has superior thyroid, facial, occipital, lingual, ascending pharyngeal, maxillary, transverse facial, and superficial temporal branches. The maxillary artery is perhaps the most complicated in that it has several named branches, which include the inferior alveolar, deep temporal, middle meningeal, numerous muscular branches, posterior superior alveolar, infraorbital, and the terminal branch named the sphenopalatine artery, which passes through the pterygopalatine fossa and into the nasal passage.

The **internal carotid** has no branches of significance outside of the cranial cavity. This artery enters the carotid canal and passes into the foramen lacerum to gain entry into the cranial cavity. It has branches to the pituitary. It forms an S-shaped vessel as it courses from the foramen lacerum and through the cavernous sinus. This portion is called the carotid siphon. Its named major branches are the ophthalmic (which accompanies the optic nerve through the optic canal and into orbit), anterior cerebral, anterior choroidal, and posterior communicating. It terminates as the middle cerebral artery.

Vertebral arteries arise from the subclavian artery. They course through the transverse foramina of the upper six cervical vertebrae, giving off small segmental branches to supply the spinal cord and vertebrae of the region. They enter the cranial cavity through the foramen magnum and run anterior to the medulla, where they give off the anterior spinal arteries (which fuse to form a single vessel that extends down the length of the spinal cord), posterior inferior cerebellar arteries, and posterior spinal arteries (which may arise from the posterior inferior cerebellars). The vertebral arteries fuse in the midline to form the basilar artery, which lies on the basal surface of the pons (in the basilar sulcus). The basilar artery's branches include the anterior inferior cerebellar, labyrinthine or internal auditory (which in a majority of cases arises from the anterior inferior cerebullar), numerous pontine branches, superior cerebellar. The basilar terminates by dividing into posterior cerebral arteries. The **circle of Willis**, an arterial circle at the base of the brain, is composed of the following vessels: left internal carotid, left posterior communicating, left posterior cerebral, right posterior cerebral, right posterior communicating, right internal carotid, right anterior cerebral, anterior communcating, left anterior cerebral, and back to the left internal carotid.

Cranial nerves

I (olfactory). The neurons lie in the olfactory mucosa, which is in the sphenoethmoidal recess of the nasal passages. The central processes of these neurons extend into the cranial cavity by passing through the cribriform plate of the ethmoid bone. These central processes attach to the olfactory bulb of the telencephalon. This serves olfaction and is a special visceral afferent (SVA).

II (optic). Neurons of the retina (ganglion cells) extend their axons from the eye to the diencephalon and mesencephalon as the optic nerve, chiasm, and tract. Their function is vision, as a special somatic afferent (SSA).

III (oculomotor). Nuclei lie within the mesencephalon. The oculomotor nucleus is general somatic efferent (GSE) and innervates extrinsic eye muscles (see above). The accessory oculomotor nucleus (nucleus of Edinger-Westphal) is general visceral efferent (GVE) and provides parasympathetic innervation to the ciliary muscle and iridial constrictor muscle, which function in light and accommodation reflexes. The nerve attaches to the midbrain in the interpeduncular fossa. It passes from the cranial cavity through the superior oribital fissure and into the orbit.

IV (trochlear). The trochlear nucleus lies within the midbrain and provides motor (GSE) innervation to the superior oblique muscle of the eye. It is unique in that it attaches to the dorsum of the brain stem and arises from the contralateral nucleus. The nerve leaves the cranial cavity by passing through the superior orbital fissure into the orbit.

V₁ (ophthalmic division of V). This division is sensory only, and the cell bodies lie in the semilunar (trigeminal) ganglion. The ophthalmic supplies the dorsum of the nose, the orbital contents, the upper lid skin, the conjunctiva, and the skin and scalp of the frontal region back to the vertex. It exits via the superior orbital fissure into the orbit and is general somatic afferent (GSA).

V₂ (maxillary division of V). This too is sensory only, and the neurons lie in the semilunar (trigeminal) ganglion. It supplies the maxillary region of the face, including the skin of the lower lid, the nasal passages and paranasal sinuses, and the upper jaw (teeth and palate). It exits via the foramen rotundum into the pterygopalatine fossa (GSA).

V₃ (mandibular division of V). This division is both motor (SVE) and sensory (GSA). The sensory neurons lie in the semilunar (trigeminal) ganglion. Sensory distribution is to the mandibular region, including the floor of the mouth, the tongue, and the lower teeth. The motor portion neurons form the motor nucleus of V and innervate the muscles of mastication and others (lateral and medial pterygoids, temporalis, masseter, mylohyoid, anterior belly of the digastric, tensor veli palatini, and tensor tympani). It exits the cranial cavity via the foramen ovale and passes into the infratemporal fossa.

The trigeminal nerve attaches to the brain in the middle of the middle cerebellar peduncle.

VI (abducens nerve). This nerve is motor only. It supplies the lateral rectus muscle. Its nucleus lies in the pons, and the nerve attaches to the brain at the pontomedullary junction. It exits the cranial cavity via the superior orbital fissure and passes into the orbit (GSE).

VII (facial nerve). This nerve is both motor and sensory. The portion arising from facial motor nucleus (SVE) in the pons contains those axons only and is called the facial nerve. The parasympathetic fibers (GVE) that arise from the superior salivatory nucleus join sensory fibers for taste (SVA) and fibers for general sensations (GSA) and extend from the brain as the nervus intermedius. The seventh nerve attaches to the brain at the cerebellopontine angle (along with VIII). Both the facial and intermedius leave the cranial cavity via the internal auditory meatus along with VIII. Its branches include the greater petrosal, the nerve to the stapedius, the chordae tympani, and the branches of the facial nerve after it exits via the facial canal through the stylomastoid foramen. These branches are named for the area of face/neck they supply— temporal, zygomatic, buccal, mandibular, and cervical. Note that all those branches radiating across the face are motor to skeletal muscles (of facial expression) and have no sensory distribution. Parasympathetic function of VII is to supply all the glands of the head **except** the parotid.

VIII (vestibulocochlear nerve). This nerve is sensory only (SSA). It has two parts—auditory and vestibular. The **auditory portion** carries impulses from the organ of Corti (auditory function), has cell bodies in the spiral ganglion, and attaches to the brain at the cerebellopontine angle and terminates in the dorsal and ventral cochlear nuclei. The **vestibular portion** of VIII carries impulses from the cristae of the semicircular ducts and the maculae of the utricle and saccule for vestibular function. The ganglion is the vestibular ganglion. This portion of VIII attaches to the brain at the cerebellopontine angle also. Cranial nerve VIII exits the cranial cavity via the internal auditory meatus.

IX (glossopharyngeal nerve). This nerve is both motor and sensory. Two motor functions are performed by IX—skeletal muscle (SVE) (stylopharyngeus only) and parasympathetic (GVE). The SVE fibers arise from the nucleus ambiguus, and the GVE fibers from the inferior salivatory nucleus. The only parasympathetic function is to supply the parotid gland. The sensory functions include taste (SVA) and general visceral sensations (general visceral afferent, or GVA). Both the taste and general sensory fibers are distributed to the posterior third of the tongue. IX has a small distribution of general somatic sensory (GSA) to the skin of the external ear. IX exits the cranial cavity via the jugular foramen.

X (vagus nerve). This nerve is both motor and sensory. It has the same two motor functions as IX—skeletal muscle (SVE) of the soft palate (except tensor veli palatini by V), pharynx (except stylopharyngeus by IX), all laryngeal muscles and skeletal muscle of esophagus; parasympathetic (GVE) to autonomically innervated structures beginning in the neck and continuing to the left colic flexure. SVE fibers arise from the nucleus ambiguus, and parasympathetic (GVE) fibers from the dorsal motor nucleus of vagus. Sensory function includes a small GSA distribution to the external ear, a small SVA distribution to the taste buds associated with the epiglottis, and a large GVA distribution that parallels the parasympathetic fibers. X exits the cranial cavity via the jugular foramen.

Both IX and X attach to the brain as a series of rootlets arranged in a line posterior to the olive.

XI (spinal accessory nerve). This nerve is motor only (SVE). Its cell bodies lie in the ventral horn gray matter of the upper five spinal cord segments. Fibers exit the cord laterally between the dorsal and ventral roots, turn cranially, and ascend posterior to the denticulate ligament. They pass through the foramen magnum and exit the cranial cavity via the jugular foramen. XI supplies the sternocleidomastoid and trapezius muscles.

XII (hypoglossal nerve). This nerve is motor only (GSE). The cell bodies form the hypoglossal nucleus in the medulla. It supplies the tongue muscles. XII attaches to the brain as a series of rootlets ventral to the olive along the anterolateral sulcus of the medulla. The hypoglossal nerve leaves the cranial cavity via the hypoglossal canal (foramen).

Veins

The venous drainage of the head is very largely effected by the internal, external, and anterior jugular veins. The internal jugular drains much of the cranial cavity. The external drains the face and anterior scalp. The anterior jugular is a variable vein that connects with the internal jugular and brachiocephalic veins. The external jugular is a tributary of the subclavian, and the internal jugular joins with the subclavian and forms the brachiocephalic vein. The facial veins somewhat parallel the external carotid branches. The main tributaries of the internal jugular veins are the venous dural sinuses plus some superficial facial veins.

NECK

The anterior cervical triangle is formed by midline of the neck, the anterior border of the sternomastoid muscle, and the lower border of the body of the mandible. The posterior cervical triangle is formed by the posterior border of the sternomastoid, the anterior border of the trapezius, and the clavicle.

Parts of the **cervical fascia** named here are of the **deep cervical fascia.** The **superficial investing fascia** (remember that this is still deep fascia) starts at the spines of the cervical vertebrae and extends so as to invest the trapezius, sternomastoid, and strap muscles. The **prevertebral fascia** invests the deep neck muscles closely associated with the cervical vertebrae. Anterior to the bodies of the vertebrae this splits so as to have an **alar component** and thus forms a "danger" space. The **visceral compartment fascia** invests the larynx/trachea, esophagus, and thyroid.

Extensions of all three of these deep cervical fasciae combine to form the **carotid sheath,** which contains the carotid vessels, the internal jugular vein, and the vagus (but not the sympathetic trunk). As the brachial plexus forms and extends into the axilla it is covered in an extension of prevertebral fascia called the **axillary sheath.**

Larynx

The larynx is composed of cartilages, connective tissue, mucous membrane and skeletal muscles and acts primarily as a sphincter to protect the lower respiratory tract. It has also been adapted to function as the voice box for phonation. The major cartilages are the epiglottic at the base of the tongue, the thyroid, cricoid, and the paired arytenoid cartilages.

The larynx is divided into the **vestibule, glottis,** and **infraglottic** (or subglottic) area. The vestibule is that portion from the laryngeal aditus to the vestibular (false vocal cords) folds. The glottis includes the vocal folds (ligaments) and the space between them (rima glottidis). The infraglottic or subglottic space is that from vocal folds inferiorly to the trachea. Between the vestibular and focal folds on each side is the **ventricle,** which extends laterally and superiorly as the **saccule.**

The muscles of the larynx are the cricothyroid, thyroarytenoid, vocalis (portion of thyroarytenoid), lateral cricoarytenoid, arytenoideus, and posterior cricoarytenoid. This latter muscle is the only one that *opens* the rima glottidis; all the others close it and aid in the larynx functioning as a sphincter.

The laryngeal branch of the superior thyroid artery (from external carotid) passes into upper part of the larynx by piercing the thyrohyoid membrane to supply the supraglottic space (vestibule). It is accompanied by the internal branch of the superior laryngeal nerve (branch of X).

The inferior laryngeal artery is the terminal branch of the inferior thyroid artery (a branch of the thyrocervical trunk from the subclavian artery) and supplies the infraglottic space. It is accompanied by the inferior laryngeal (terminal) branch of the recurrent laryngeal nerve of X.

The **superior laryngeal nerve** (from X) has an internal branch that supplies the vestibule and an external branch that supplies the cricothyroid muscle. The **inferior laryngeal nerve** (from the recurrent laryngeal branch of X) innervates all the other laryngeal muscles and provides sensation to the infraglottic space.

The vocal folds are the superior borders of the **conus elasticus,** a dense connective tissue structure extending from the vocal folds to the cricoid cartilage. It is overlain by the mucosa of this area.

THORAX

Pectoral region and breast

Landmarks include the manubrium, body, and xiphoid process of the sternum; the suprasternal notch (between the medial ends of clavicles, above the manubrium); the sternal angle (between the manubrium and the body) (attachment of the costal cartilages of second pair of ribs); the infrasternal notch; the clavicle; acromion process of the scapula; the anterior axillary fold (over pectoral muscles); the posterior axillary fold (over latissimus dorsi); and the lines—midsternal, parasternal, midclavicular, anterior axillary, midaxillary, and posterior axillary.

The mammary gland extends from rib two to rib six, from the side of the sternum to the midaxillary line. It consists of the areola (with glands of Montgomery); the nipple (about the fourth intercostal space); the retinacula cutis; and the retromammary space (between the membranous layer of the superficial fascia and the deep fascia [pectoralis muscle fascia]). The blood supply includes perforating branches of the internal thoracic artery and branches of the axillary artery, especially the lateral thoracic. Venous drainage is to the axillary, internal thoracic, and intercostal veins.

Nerve supply is via the supraclavicular nerves (C3, 4) and T2-6 (nipple by the fourth intercostal).

Lymphatic drainage is from most of the glandular tissue, areola, and nipple to the anterior pectoral nodes. The medial breast can drain into retrosternal channels and communicate with lymph vessels of the opposite breast. It can also drain into the epigastric region. The skin (not including areola/nipple) drains radially into surrounding lymph glands.

The pectoral region includes the clavicle, deltoid, deltopectoral groove (in which runs the cephalic vein), and pectoralis major (clavicular, costal, and sternal heads). The **clavipectoral fascia** extends from the clavicle, enfolds the subclavius, and continues to invest the pectoralis minor muscle. Beyond the pectoralis minor, this fascia blends into the axillary fascia and forms the **suspensory ligament of the axilla**.

The **axillary artery** is the continuation of the subclavian artery as the latter passes over the first rib to enter the axilla. It has three parts—medial to the pectoralis minor, posterior to the p. minor, and lateral to the p. minor. Part one has one branch (supreme thoracic), part two has two branches (thoracoacromial [deltoid, clavicular, pectoral, and acromial branches] and lateral thoracic), and part three has three branches (subscapular [circumflex scapular and thoracodorsal branches], anterior humeral circumflex, and posterior humeral circumflex [which accompanies the axillary nerve through the axilla]).

The **serratus anterior** muscle originates from the upper eight or nine ribs and extends around the thoracic wall and inserts on the deep side of the vertebral border of the scapula. It interdigitates on the anterolateral wall of the thorax with the external abdominal oblique.

Nerves of this region include the medial and lateral pectoral nerves, which supply both pectoralis major and minor muscles. They arise from medial and lateral cords of the brachial plexus, respectively. The intercostal nerves have their basic plan of lateral and anterior branches that are cutaneous. Intercostal muscles are, of course, innervated by intercostal nerves. The lateral branch of the second intercostal nerve is quite large and extends to supply the skin of the axilla and medial portion of the proximal brachial skin, and this is the intercostobrachial nerve.

Thoracic wall, pleura, and pericardium

Ribs. The upper seven are true ribs, and lower five are false. Ribs 11 and 12 are floating. The head, neck, tubercle, angle, body, and costal groove are parts of most ribs. The first rib has *no* angle but has a scalene tubercle (for the anterior scalene muscle), anterior to which is a groove for the subclavian vein and posterior to which is a groove for the subclavian artery. It has a single articular facet on its head. Rib 10 has one articular facet on its head. Ribs 11 and 12 have one articular facet on their head, *no* necks or tubercles.

Intercostal muscles. These include the external (parallel external abdominal oblique) and the internal (parallel internal abdominal oblique). The innermost are found mainly in the lateral part of the intercostal space and can be distinguished only in that intercostal neurovascular structures course between this muscle layer and the internal intercostals. Intercostal neurovascular elements are related to the costal groove on the inferior border of the ribs (Vein, Artery, Nerve, Lymphatic—VANL). Transversus thoracis, innermost intercostal, and subcostalis muscles are comparable to the transversus abdominis.

Surface landmarks of the intrathoracic position of the heart. The **apex** is at the left fifth interspace, 3½ inches lateral to the midsternal line. The **inferior border** lies along a line drawn from the apex to the upper portion of the xiphoid process. The **clinical base** of the heart is at the level of a line drawn between two points placed in the second intercostal space an inch lateral to each side of the sternum. The **right side** is formed by the superior vena cava, the right atrium, and the right inferior vena cava and is indicated by a line drawn from the right second interspace an inch lateral to the sternum and straight down to the right fifth costal cartilage. The **left side** is formed by the left ventricle, seen as a line from a point in the left second interspace and an inch from the lateral border of the sternum and extending to the apex. The pulmonary valve is situated at the junction of the second interspace and the sternum. The aortic valve is located at the body of the sternum at the level of the attachment of the third cartilage. The mitral valve is on the left side of the body of the sternum at the level of the third interspace. The tricuspid valve is on the right side of the body of the sternum at the level of the fourth interspace.

Surface projections of the pleural reflections. The right parietal pleura extends from ½ inch above the right sternoclavicular joint to the midsternal line at the sternal angle, inferiorly to the xiphoid, along the costal margin to the 10th rib at the midaxillary line, and to the 12th rib at the paravertebral line. The left parietal pleura is a mirror image of the right except for a modest lateral deviation beginning at the fourth interspace to accommodate the heart. The lungs themselves are less extensive than the parietal pleura, and in the midaxillary line they reach the level of the 8th rib and in the paravertebral line the 10th rib (at the end of expiration).

Pleura. The visceral pleura intimately invests the lungs' surface. The costal parietal pleura attaches to the thoracic wall via the **endothoracic fascia**; the diaphragmatic pleura lies attached to the superior surface of the diaphragm; the mediastinal pleura lies in apposition to the fibrous pericardium; and the cervical pleura extends up into the root of the neck approximately an inch above the clavicle. The parietal pleura passes from costal structures onto the mediastinum near the anterior chest wall, onto the diaphragm, and onto the esophagus in such a manner as to form **pleural recesses** that are parts of the pleural cavity and into which the lung and visceral pleura do not extend completely. These recesses are named for their location—costomediastinal, costodiaphragmatic, and costoesophageal. The pleural cavity is normally a potential space.

Mediastinum. A line from the sternal notch to T1 is the upper extent; a line from the sternal angle to the disk between T4 and T5 is the lower limit. It contains the arch of the aorta; sternohyoid and sternothyroid muscles; brachiocephalic and left common carotid and left subclavian arteries; brachiocephalic veins; upper part of the superior vena cava; left highest intercostal vein; vagus, cardiac, phrenic, and recurrent laryngeal nerves; trachea; esophagus; thoracic duct; thymus; and nodes.

The **inferior mediastinum** includes the anterior, middle, and posterior mediastina. The **anterior mediastinum** contains a few lymph nodes, subserous fascia. The **middle mediastinum** contains the heart enclosed in the pericardium, the ascending aorta, proximal superior vena cava and azygous vein termination, pulmonary trunk and proximal right and left pulmonary arteries, and phrenic nerves. The **posterior mediastinum** contains the thoracic descending aorta, azygous and hemiazygous veins, right posterior intercostal arteries, vagi, thoracic splanchnic nerves, esophagus, thoracic duct, and lymph nodes.

The **pericardium** is the serous sac that encloses the heart and the proximal portions of the great vessels. Unlike the other serous sacs (e.g., pleura), it develops around an elongated tube, the heart, which subsequently folds on itself so that both ends are located on the upper portion of the heart. Thus, unlike the single, common folding of the pleura around the root of the lung, there is a folding around the arterial end of the heart and separate folding around the venous end. This results in the part of the pericardial cavity that lies between the great arteries anteriorly and the great veins posteriorly, being called the **transverse pericardial sinus**.

The common reflection of the pericardium around the veins forms a cul-de-sac of pericardial cavity on the dorsal side of the heart called the **oblique pericardial sinus**. The **visceral** layer of pericardium is also called the **epicardium**. The **parietal** layer lies in apposition to the diaphragm caudally, pleura laterally, sternum anteriorly.

Heart. Figure 1-17 illustrates the structures of the heart.

Coronary arteries. The right coronary's branches include the artery of the conus, the artery of the sinus (SA) node, the right marginal, the posterior interventricular (posterior descending), artery of the atrioventricular (AV) node, and the atrial and ventricular branches. The left coronary's branches consist of the anterior interventricular (anterior descending, LAD), left coronary circumflex, and atrial and ventricular branches.

The artery to the SA node arises from the proximal portion of the right coronary. It may arise from the left coronary, and in some cases even be double and arise from both right and left coronaries. The artery of the AV node commonly arises from the right coronary near the posterior interventricular groove, sometimes from the left coronary.

Blood supply to the anterior two-thirds of the interventricular septum is from the LAD, to the posterior third from the posterior interventricular.

Anastomoses of significance include the artery of the conus (from the right coronary) with the LAD; septal branches of the LAD and posterior descending; at the crux between terminal branches of the right and left coronaries; apex between descending arteries.

Coronary veins. These include the great cardiac vein (of Galen) (anterior interventricular), the oblique vein of the left atrium (of Marshall), the middle cardiac vein (posterior interventricular), the small (short) cardiac vein, the marginal vein of the left ventricle, the coronary sinus, the thebesian veins (venae cordis minimae—seen within heart), and the anterior cardiac veins (arise out of the anterior portion of the right ventricle, pass over the AV sulcus, pierce the anterior wall of the right atrium to open into that chamber).

Cardiac skeleton. The mitral and bicuspid valve rings, right and left fibrous trigones, aortic and pulmonary valve rings, and membranous interventricular septum compose the cardiac skeleton.

Right atrium and auricle. These include the openings of the

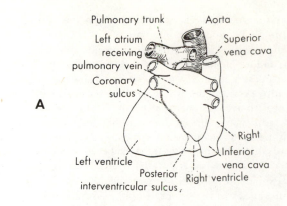

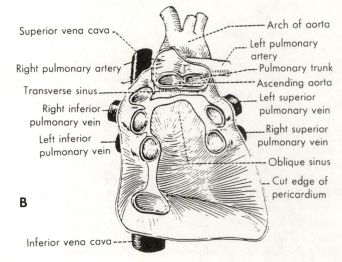

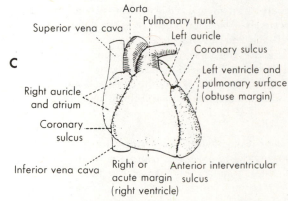

Figure 1-17. (*A*) Diagram of the heart in a posterior view; the coronary sulcus separates the base, above and to the right, from the diaphragmatic surface. (*B*) The posterior wall of the pericardial sac after removal of the heart. (*C*) Anterior view.

venae cavae, the crista terminalis (ridge between the smooth-walled main cavity called the sinus venarum and the auricle's musculi pectinati) (on the outer surface paralleling the crista is the sulcus terminalis), the valve of the inferior vena cava (eustachian), the ostium of the coronary sinus guarded by the valve of the coronary sinus, venae cordis minimae (thebesian veins), the interatrial septum, the fossa ovalis, the limbus of the fossa ovalis and the membranous portion of the interventricular septum (near the anterior portion of the base of the interatrial septum).

Right ventricle. The right ventricle comprises the tricuspid valve—anterior, posterior, septal cusps; the papillary muscles and chordae tendineae; the trabeculae carneae; the pseudo-tendons; the moderator band (septomarginal trabecula); the conus or infundibulum (smooth walled, lies immediately inferior to the pulmonary semilunar valve); the crista supra-ventricularis; the papillary muscle of the conus (may only be a chorda tendinea from conus to septal cusp), an important landmark in that the right bundle branch enters the right ventricle immediately posterior to it; and the pulmonary semilunar valve—note commissures (where two adjacent cusps are connected), lunula (free margins), and nodule (in middle of free margin).

Left atrium and auricle. These include openings for pulmonary veins (usually four), the auricle (has musculi pectinati), bicuspid (mitral) valve orifice, and the venae cordis minimae.

Left ventricle. The left ventricle comprises the bicuspid (mitral) valve; the aortic semilunar valve, with two cusps being called "coronary" because a coronary artery arises from the sinus of Valsalva related to that valve (valve cusp with which there is no associated coronary artery is called the "non-coronary" cusp); the aortic vestibule (smooth-walled area immediately inferior to the aortic semilunar valve); the trabeculae carneae; the papillary muscles and chordae tendineae; the left bundle branch; and the pseudotendons.

Cardiac conduction system. The SA node is situated at the base of the superior vena cava, between it and the right auricle. The AV node is located in muscles of the medial wall of the right atrium. Preferential conduction pathways between the SA and AV nodes are the posterior internodal tract, which follows the crista terminali; the middle internodal tract, which passes posterior to the superior vena cava down to the interatrial septum and then through the septum to AV node; and the anterior tract, which passes in front of superior vena cava to the interatrial septum and then to the AV node. The anterior tract gives off a bundle to the left atrium (Bachmann's bundle). The bundle of His (common AV bundle) leaves the AV node, passes through the central fibrous body, curves posterior to the membranous septum onto the superior margin of the muscular septum, and divides into right and left bundle branches as Purkinje fibers. Innervation of this system is to the SA node via cervical cardiac and thoracic visceral branches of the sympathetic trunk and the vagus. Sensory fibers travel back to the CNS with both sympathetic and parasympathetic fibers.

Lower respiratory tract

The trachea has cartilage rings, smooth muscle, and connective tissue. The trachea bifurcates into primary bronchi; a cartilage at the place of bifurcation is called the carina (keel). The primary bronchi at the bifurcation are enmeshed in lymphatic vessels and nodes, neural plexuses and ganglia, and bronchial arteries. Tertiary bronchi are the basic structures of the bronchopulmonary segments, which number ten in the right lung and eight in the left.

The lungs are covered in pleura. The right has three lobes (superior, middle, inferior), and the left has two lobes (superior and inferior) (Table 1-4).

Table 1-4. Divisions of the Lungs

Right bronchopulmonary segments	Left bronchopulmonary segments
Superior lobe	Superior lobe
Apical	Anterior
Posterior	Apicoposterior
Anterior	Superior lingular
	Inferior lingular
Middle lobe	
Lateral	
Medial	
Inferior lobe	Inferior lobe
Superior	Superior
Medial basal	Anteromedial basal
Anterior basal	Posterior basal
Posterior basal	Lateral basal
Lateral basal	

ABDOMEN

Anterior abdominal wall

Subdivisions are the right and left hypochondriac, right and left lateral, right and left inguinal, epigastric, umbilical, and pubic regions.

Quadrants are the right and left superior quadrants and right and left inferior quadrants.

Vertebral levels are the intertubercular plane (tubercles of the ilium) at L5; bifurcation of the aorta at the disk between L4 and L5; umbilicus at L4; and transpyloric plane at L1–2.

Palpable structures are the iliac crests, anterior superior iliac spines, pubic tubercles, pubic crest, and pubic symphysis.

Landmarks include the linea alba, lines of Langer (not a landmark per se, but are a reflection of the organization of the fibers of the dermis and are important in wound healing), linea semilunaris (lateral edge of rectus sheath), rectus sheath, external abdominal oblique muscle, inguinal ligament, and superficial inguinal ring (crura and intercrural fibers).

The superficial **fascia** has a superficial layer that is fatty and eponymously named the Camper fascia; a deeper layer is the membranous layer called Scarpa's fascia. The deep fascia lies attached to the muscles; this includes the rectus sheath and the muscular fascia on the external abdominal oblique (innominate or Gallaudet's fascia).

Muscles of wall include the rectus abdominis, external abdominal oblique, internal abdominal oblique, and transversus abdominis. The rectus sheath extends between the xiphoid process and pubis. The anterior lamina of the sheath is formed by the aponeurosis of the external abdominal oblique and half of the aponeurosis of the internal abdominal oblique passing in front of the rectus abdominis. The posterior lamina is formed by the posterior half of the internal abdominal oblique aponeurosis and the aponeurosis of the transversus abdominis. The posterior lamina changes dramatically. Superior to a semicircular line (arcuate line), which lies about halfway between the umbilicus and pubic symphysis, the lamina is more stout and formed of the typical posterior lamina. Caudal to the arcuate line, the posterior lamina is formed only by transversalis fascia.

Innervation is supplied by spinal nerves T6–12. The umbilicus is innervated by T10, the pubic region by T12.

Inguinal region

The **inguinal ligament** is the inferior border of the aponeurosis of the external abdominis muscle, and extends from the anterior superior iliac spine to the pubic tubercle. The **superficial inguinal ring** has superior and inferior crura between which, lateral to the ring, they are reinforced by the **intercrural fibers.** The spermatic cord passes through the deep ring, inguinal canal, and out through the superficial ring and on into the scrotum. The inguinal canal's boundaries are as follows: The anterior wall and floor are formed by the inguinal ligament; the posterior wall is formed by transversus abdominis aponeurosis and fascia, and the roof is formed by the internal abdominal oblique muscle and its aponeurosis.

As the testes decend, they pass through the abdominal wall and pick up layers of fascia, some skeletal muscle, etc. as they do so. The testes become vested with these layers as they pass through the wall and into the scrotum, and these layers are added in the order in which they are encountered: The tunica vaginalis (derived embryologically from an extension of the peritoneum into the developing scrotum—the processus vaginalis) is the serous sac investment that folds around the testis much as the pleura enfolds a lung. The internal spermatic fascia is derived from the transversalis fascia. The cremasteric fascia is skeletal muscle fibers and fascia that extend from the internal abdominal oblique muscle and its aponeurosis. The muscle fibers form the cremaster muscle. The external spermatic fascia is an extension of the fascia of the external abdominal oblique.

The **spermatic cord** includes the vas deferens, testicular artery, genital branch of the genitofemoral nerve (to the cremaster muscle, skin of the scrotum, and adjacent thigh), pampiniform venous plexus, artery to the vas deferens (from superior vesicular), and artery to the cremaster (from the inferior epigastric).

The **round ligament** is a remnant of the gubernaculum. It extends from the uterus through the deep inguinal ring, through the inguinal canal, out through the superficial inguinal ring, and into the labium majus, where it fans out to attach to the connective tissue there.

The **deep inguinal ring** lies lateral to the superficial ring, and the inferior epigastric vessels extend cranially from the external iliacs about halfway between the two rings. The inguinal (Hesselbach's) triangle is bound by the lateral edge of the rectus sheath, the inguinal ligament, and the inferior epigastric vessels. **Direct inguinal hernias** pass through this triangle as they push through the abdominal wall and out through the superficial inguinal ring. **Indirect inguinal hernias** pass through the abdominal wall lateral to the inferior epigastric vessels, through the deep inguinal ring, down the inguinal canal, and out the superficial ring.

The inferior portion of the external abdominal oblique aponeurosis known as the **inguinal ligament** (Poupart's ligament) extends from the anterior superior iliac spine to the pubic tubercle and crest. Beneath this ligament and the superior pubic ramus and adjacent portion of the ilium is a space that is divided into a medial area called the **lacuna vasculorum** and a lateral space called the **lacuna musculorum.** In the vascular portion, from medial to lateral, are the femoral ring within which is a large lymph node (of Cloquet), the femoral vein, and the femoral artery. The boundaries of the femoral ring (which leads into the femoral canal, which extends into the proximal thigh region as a cul-de-sac a few centimeters long) are medially the transversalis fascia over the lacunar ligament, laterally the femoral vein, inferiorly the pectineal ligament, and superiorly the inguinal ligament. The muscular space is filled with the iliopsoas muscle and the femoral nerve. A **femoral hernia** passes through the femoral ring and into the femoral canal.

As the inguinal ligament approaches the pubic tubercle, some of its fibers curve inferiorly and laterally as the lacunar (Gimbernat's) ligament. These fibers then continue laterally on the pectineal line of the pubic bone as the pectineal (Cooper's) ligament.

Peritoneal cavity

Diaphragm. This fibromuscular sheet originates from the inferior edge of the thoracic cage, vertebra T12, and the xiphoid process. It has a large tendinous central portion called the central tendon, which is considered its insertion. Its skeletal muscle fibers are innervated by the phrenic nerves, which are composed of fibers from cervical spinal nerves 3, 4, and 5. It has three major openings in it. The inferior vena cava hiatus is at vertebral level T8; the esophageal hiatus lies at the vertebral level T10, and the aortic hiatus is at T12.

Posterior surface of the anterior abdominal wall. The urachus extends from the apex of the urinary bladder to the umbilicus as the **median umbilical fold** (ligament). The umbilical arteries extend from the internal iliac arteries. Their last patent branches are the superior vesicle arteries. Beyond that point they are no longer patent but continue onto the abdominal wall, and their course takes them to the umbilicus. They form the **medial umbilical folds** (ligaments). The inferior epigastric vessels (from the external iliac vessels) extend onto the abdominal wall and enter the rectus sheath. These form **lateral umbilical folds** (ligaments).

The **supravesicular fossae** lie between the median umbilical ligament and the medial umbilical ligaments; the **medial inguinal fossae** lie between the medial and lateral inguinal ligaments; and the **lateral inguinal fossae** are lateral to the lateral umbilical ligaments.

Peritoneum. The parietal layer lines the abdominal cavity. Reflections occur that form mesenteries, ligaments, etc. Underlying the parietal peritoneum is some subserous connective tissue. A fascia lies next to the subserous tissue and covers the anterolateral wall, continuing over the caudal side of the diaphragm and the anterior surface of the quadratus lumborum and psoas muscles. This is usually referred to as the **transversalis fascia** but may change its name in specific regions to reflect that region (e.g., over the iliacus it is the iliac fascia).

As the liver develops, it bulges caudally out of the substance of the septum transversum (diaphragm), and as it does so it pushes the peritoneum ahead of it. Extending from the umbilicus to the liver is the umbilical vein, and this vessel also displaces peritoneum and comes to be enfolded within it. Thus the **falciform ligament** is formed. Extending posteriorly from the liver to the caudal foregut (stomach and upper duodenum) are the biliary ducts (common hepatic and common bile ducts), which are accompanied by the hepatic arteries and the hepatic portal vein. These too carry peritoneum with them as the liver grows and pushes caudally, and this portion of the peritoneum becomes the lesser omentum.

The falciform ligament extends from the posterior surface of the anterior abdominal wall to the liver. When it reaches the liver, its two sheets diverge as they extend over the surface of the liver and so enfold it and become the visceral peritoneum of the liver. This peritoneal tissue continues around the liver and extends from its posterior side as the lesser omentum, which extends from the liver to the lesser curvature of the stomach (gastroheptic ligament) and the upper portion of the duodenum (hepatoduodenal ligament). As the visceral peritoneum passes over the liver, an area of the cranial surface of the liver is in direct apposition with the diaphragm, and thus the peritoneum passes around that. The area of the liver not covered with visceral peritoneum is the **bare area** of the liver. The reflection of the peritoneum around this area is called the **coronary ligament**, whose right and left lateral extents are called **right** and **left triangular ligaments**. All these reflections of the peritoneum are from the **ventral mesentery**. Because of the way these peritoneal reflections form and of the rotation of the gut during development, the peritoneal cavity comes to be divided into a lesser sac (which lies largely posterior to the lesser omentum and stomach) and a greater sac (the remainder of the peritoneal cavity). The communication of the greater sac and the lesser sac (also called the omental bursa) is the epiploic foramen (of Winslow), which is bound by the duodenum, the inferior vena cava, the hepatoduodenal ligament, and the liver.

The dorsal mesentery suspends the GI tract from the dorsal body wall. The portion that extends from the dorsal wall to the greater curvature of the stomach is highly modified (exaggerated) and forms the **greater omentum**. This extends from the greater curvature of the stomach and drapes caudally over the anterior surface of the other viscera to varying lengths (but often well toward the level of the pubic symphysis) and turns back up cranially posterior to the descending layer to fuse onto the anterior surface of the transverse colon and back to the dorsal body wall fused with the transverse mesocolon.

The remainder of the dorsal mesentery has a less complicated arrangement. Because the gut is so long and goes through developmental umbilical herniation and remarkable rotation, some parts remain suspended from the body wall by a mesentery and others come to lie in direct contact with the body wall and thus have no mesenteries. If one follows the GI tract through the abdominal and pelvic regions one finds an alternation of intra- and retroperitoneal conditions. In the following sequence of viscera, those with a mesentery are underscored: stomach and upper duodenum, distal duodenum, remaining small intestine (jejunum and ilium), cecum/ascending colon, transverse colon, descending colon, sigmoid colon, rectum. The most extensive portion of the mesentery, which suspends the jejunum and ilium, attaches to the posterior abdominal wall in a structure called the **radix**. Other mesenteries are specifically named (e.g., mesogastrium, mesocolon,

etc.). The arrangement of the peritoneum of the pelvic viscera is discussed in that section.

Gastrointestinal tract

Stomach.   The stomach is made up of the greater and lesser curvatures, angular incisure; fundus; body; pylorus (antrum, canal, sphincter); and internal modifications known as rugae (longitudinal mucosal folds).

Duodenum.   The first part (next to stomach) has a mesentery and receives the common bile duct and the main and accessory pancreatic ducts. The common bile duct and main pancreatic duct join to form the hepatopancreatic duct, which passes through the duodenal wall and opens into the lumen via the duodenal papilla. This papilla is due to the dilated portion of the hepatopancreatic duct, which is known eponymously as the ampulla of Vater. The hepatoduodenal duct is encircled by smooth muscle (the sphincter of Oddi), which controls the flow of bile and pancreatic exocrine secretions.

The second part descends, the third courses horizontally toward the left, and the fourth part ascends somewhat and extends to the duodenal-jejunal junction. Some connective tissue and smooth muscle extend from the right crus of the diaphragm to this junction, called the suspensory muscle of the duodenum or the ligament of Treitz. The last three parts are retroperitoneal (no mesentery). The duodenum is about 10 to 12 inches long.

Jejunum.   This portion of the small intestine is about 8 feet long. It has a mesentery that is relatively less fat laden than that associated with the ileum. Its arteries are arranged in a single rank of arcades with long vasa rectae. Its mucosal lining is remarkable in that the plicae circulares (Kerckring's valves) are the most developed of the small intestine.

Ileum.   This is the longest portion of the small bowel, about 12 feet. Its mesentery contains much fat, and the arteries form several ranks of arcades and short vasa rectae. It is remarkable also for the large lymphatic nodules within its mucosa, Peyer's patches. It ends at the ileocolic junction, where there is a sphincter.

Cecum.   This is the beginning of the ascending colon. It extends caudally as a cul-de-sac from the ileocolic junction. The **vermiform appendix** extends from its caudal end.

Large intestine.   This is subdivided into the ascending, transverse, descending, and sigmoid colon. The latter is continuous with the rectum. The large bowel is characterized by modifications of the muscularis externis that form three longitudinal ribbons of muscle, the **teniae coli**. The colon has **sacculations** (haustra). On the external surface are fat-filled redundancies of the peritoneum called **appendices epiploicae**.

Blood supply.   The **celiac trunk** arises from the abdominal aorta and has three branches—left gastric, splenic, and common heptic. This trunk supplies the caudal foregut derivatives—stomach, upper duodenum, pancreas, and biliary system—plus the spleen.

The **superior mesenteric artery** supplies the derivatives of the midgut—lower duodenum, jejunum, ileum, ascending, and transverse colon.

The **inferior mesenteric artery** supplies the derivatives of the hindgut—descending colon, sigmoid colon, and rectum.

Nerve supply.   **Parasympathetic** supply is by the vagus as far as the left colic flexure. Beyond that point, the parasympathetic innervation is by sacral nerves 2, 3, and 4. **Sympathetic** innervation is by the thoracic and lumbar splanchnic branches of the sympathetic trunk. Sensory fibers run with both the parasympathetics and the sympathetics. Pain sensations are usually carried by fibers coursing with the sympathetics. The spinal cord segmental distribution is as follows: caudal foregut T6–9, midgut T8–12, hindgut T10–L2. Pelvic visceral sensations travel with sacral nerves 2, 3, and 4.

Liver. This organ has right, left, quadrate, and caudate lobes. The remnant of the umbilical vein is the ligamentum teres hepati, which lies between the quadrate and left lobes. The gallbladder lies between quadrate and right lobes. The ductus venosus (carries blood from the umbilical vein to the inferior vena cava in the fetus) becomes the ligamentum venosum and lies between left and caudate lobes. The inferior vena cava passes between the right and caudate lobes. That area of the liver where the hepatic ducts, hepatic portal vein, and hepatic arteries enter or leave the liver is called the **porta hepatis.**

A line drawn from the bed of the gallbladder to the ligamentum venosum approximates the boundary between functional right and left lobes of the liver—the distribution of the blood carried by right and left hepatic arteries. This means that the quadrate and part of the caudate lobes are part of the functional left lobe.

Gallbladder. The gallbladder stores and concentrates bile. Upon stimulation (e.g., cholecystokinin), its smooth muscle contracts and bile is expressed from its lumen, down the cystic duct, and into the common bile duct. The cystic duct has a spiral ridge of mucosa called the **spiral valve** (of Heister). It probably acts to maintain patency of the cystic duct rather than as a valve. The gallbladder fills retrogradely as bile flows through the hepatic ducts and into the common bile duct and then back up through the cystic duct into the gallbladder. The right and left hepatic ducts join to form the common hepatic duct. This joins with the cystic duct to make the common bile duct. The latter extends to the duodenum to fuse with the main pancreatic duct (see above).

Spleen. This lymphoid organ lies in the upper left quadrant. It is supplied by the splenic artery from the celiac trunk. The large splenic vein joins with the superior mesenteric vein to form the hepatic portal vein. The inferior mesenteric artery is frequently a tributary of the splenic vein but may be a tributary of the superior mesenteric vein, or it may open into the junction of splenic and superior mesenteric veins.

Kidneys. These lie attached to the cranial portion of the posterior abdominal wall. **Renal fascia** invests the kidneys cranially and down to the caudal pole but does not close around the caudal end of the kidneys. Within the renal fascia and outside the renal capsule is **perirenal fat.** This is most abundant on the posterior side of the kidney. Between the renal fascia and the posterior abdominal wall is **pararenal fat.** The parietal peritoneum passes anterior to the kidneys and the renal fascia.

The kidneys are concave medially, forming the renal **hilum.** The space within this concavity of the kidney is the renal **sinus.** Within the sinus are the renal vessels, the minor and major calyces, the renal pelvis, some lymphatics, and connective tissue.

The kidney parenchyma is organized into cortex and medulla. The collecting system opens into minor calyces, which coalesce to form major calyces. These in turn open into the renal pelvis. The renal pelvis leaves the renal sinus and narrows into the ureter. The cortex is the outer part of the parenchyma and contains the renal corpuscles and the associated portions of the nephrons. The medulla contains parts of the nephrons and the collecting ducts. The human kidney has an average of about 12 lobes.

The blood supply is by the renal arteries. These may be single large vessels from the aorta, but it is not uncommon to see in addition some aberrant renal arteries. The blood is drained away via the renal vein and its tributaries. The renal vein opens into the inferior vena cava. The right renal vein differs from the left in that the left has two significant tributaries—the left gonadal vein and the left inferior phrenic (or left suprarenal) vein. These vessels on the right side are direct tributaries of the inferior vena cava. This is a reflection of the development of the inferior vena cava.

Arteries of the abdomen

Inferior phrenic arteries. These paired arteries arise from the abdominal aorta or from the celiac trunk. They supply the diaphragm and give rise to the **superior suprarenal arteries.**

Celiac (coeliac) trunk. The **left gastric** branch passes along the lesser curvature of the stomach; 20 to 25% of the time it has an **aberrant left hepatic** branch. It has several esophageal branches also.

The **splenic** branch provides several arteries to the pancreas, and near the spleen it has several **short gastric** branches. Other branches include the **left gastroepiploic artery,** which courses in the greater omentum along the greater curvature of the stomach. Near the spleen, the splenic artery breaks up into smaller splenic branches that enter the substance of the spleen.

The **common hepatic** artery extends from the celiac trunk and branches into **gastroduodenal** and **proper hepatic** arteries. The gastroduodenal has **superior pancreaticoduodenal** branches and terminates as the **right gastroepiploic** artery. This passes along the greater curvature of the stomach within the greater omentum and anastomoses with the left gastroepiploic. The proper hepatic has a **right gastric** branch, which extends to the lesser curvature and anastomoses with the left gastric. The proper hepatic branches into **right** and **left hepatic** branches, which serve their respective functional lobes of the liver. The right hepatic also gives rise to the **cystic artery** to supply the gallbladder.

Superior mesenteric artery. This has small branches called the **inferior pancreaticoduodenal** arteries, which supply those structures and form the only significant anastomosis with the superior vessels from the celiac trunk. Numerous and large **jejunal** and **ileal** branches extend to the small intestine. Other named branches include the **ileocolic,** which has an **appendicular** branch that passes posterior to the distal ileum and supplies the appendix. The **right** and **middle colic** branches supply the ascending and transverse colon, respectively. The middle colic anastomoses with the left colic of the inferior mesenteric artery. The various colic arteries form an arterial continuity that parallels the inner side of the large intestine. This is called the **marginal artery of Drummond.** This artery affords a very effective anastomosis between superior and inferior mesenteric arteries.

Inferior mesenteric artery. This has a **left colic** branch (see above), several **sigmoid** branches, and a terminal branch called the **superior rectal artery.** Via the rectal branch the inferior mesenteric forms anastomoses with the internal iliac artery.

Renal arteries. These paired vessels arise from the abdominal aorta. They supply the kidneys and have **inferior suprarenal** branches.

Lumbar segmental arteries. These are four paired branches of the aorta. They supply the posterior abdominal wall.

Middle suprarenal arteries. This is a paired branch of the aorta. Note that other suprarenals are superior (from inferior phrenics) and inferior (from the renals).

Middle sacral artery. This single, midline branch of the aorta descends caudally on the anterior surface of the sacrum. It is the remnant of the caudal portion of the dorsal aorta. It may give rise to the paired fifth lumbar segmental arteries.

Veins of the GI tract

Inferior vena cava. This great vein is formed by the union of the two **common iliac veins.** Its tributaries include the **lumbar segmental veins,** the **right gonadal vein,** the **renal veins,** and the **hepatic veins.** It leaves the abdomen by passing through the hiatus of the inferior vena cava of the diaphragm and opens into the right atrium.

Hepatic portal system. The **inferior mesenteric vein** drains the same structures supplied by the inferior mesenteric artery. It is most frequently a tributary of the **splenic vein,** but it may open into the **superior mesenteric vein** or the junction of that vein with the splenic vein that forms the **hepatic portal vein.**

The **superior mesenteric vein** drains the area supplied by the artery. It, along with the artery, passes anterior to the left renal vessels and the third part of the duodenum. The uncinate process of the pancreas curves posterior to these two vessels. It joins with the splenic vein to form the hepatic portal vein.

The **splenic vein** drains those structures supplied by the artery and joins the superior mesenteric vein to form the hepatic portal vein. The inferior mesenteric vein is frequently a tributary.

The **hepatic portal vein** passes anterior to the third part of the duodenum and posterior to the neck of the pancreas. It has **gastric veins** as tributaries. The right and left gastric veins may form a loop-like structure related to the lesser curvature of the stomach and the lesser omentum; this is called the **coronary vein.** The hepatic portal delivers blood to the liver. It passes within the hepatoduodenal ligament posterior to the bile ducts and the hepatic artery. The blood of the hepatic portal vein passes into the hepatic sinusoids, where it is joined by the blood carried to the liver via the hepatic arteries. The blood is drained from the liver via the **hepatic veins,** which are tributaries of the inferior vena cava.

Venous anastomoses. The **left gastric vein** anastomoses with the **esophageal veins, which are tributaries of the azygous veins. These are involved in esophageal varices.**

The **paraumbilical veins** extend between the hepatic portal system and veins of the anterior abdominal wall around the umbilicus. These paraumbilical veins (of Sappey) course along the round ligament of the liver within the falciform ligament. The veins around the umbilicus can become engorged and form the **caput medusae.** These abdominal wall veins are continuous with the axillary and the femoral veins via the **thoracoepigastric vein.**

The **inferior mesenteric vein** via its superior rectal tributary anastomoses with the middle rectal veins, which are tributaries of the internal iliac veins.

The **retroperitoneal (Retzius's) veins** of the retroperitoneal viscera drain blood from the viscera into the body wall veins (e.g., lumbar segmental veins), which open into the inferior vena cava system.

All these anastomoses are significant in shunting blood from the hepatic portal venous system so as to bypass the liver circulation.

Posterior abdominal wall. Two pairs of large muscles form the posterior abdominal wall. The **psoas major** attaches to the bodies and the transverse processes of the lumbar vertebrae, extends across the iliac fossa, joins with the tendon of the iliacus muscle to form the iliopsoas muscle, passes under the inguinal ligament, and inserts on the lesser trochanter of the femur. It is a powerful flexor of the hip. It is the "tenderloin" muscle. There may be a **psoas minor** muscle, which lies on the anterior surface of the major and has a long tendon that inserts on the pubic bone. The other large muscle is the **quadratus lumborum,** which attaches cranially to the lower border of the 12th rib, medially to the transverse processes of the lumbar vertebrae, and caudally to the iliac crest. Both of these muscles are innervated by the lumbar spinal nerves that pass through them.

The lumbar plexus of spinal nerves is formed by nerves L1 through L4, with some possible contribution from T12. These nerves pass through the substance of the psoas major muscle. Nerves of this plexus are these as follows:

Iliohypogastric—T12 and L1. It distributes to the muscles of the anterolateral abdominal wall and the skin over the pubic region.

Ilioinguinal—L1. It has a similar course to the iliohypogastric but distributes more caudally. It passes into the inguinal canal, through the superficial ring, and supplies the skin of the scrotum, thigh, and proximal penis/clitoris.

Genitofemoral—L1, L2. This nerve passes through the substance of the psoas major and courses on its anterior surface. The genital (external spermatic nerve) branch passes through the deep inguinal ring, goes along the inguinal canal, and emerges through the superficial inguinal ring. In males it supplies the cremaster muscle, the skin of the scrotum, and adjacent skin of the thigh. In females it accompanies the round ligament of the uterus. The femoral branch (lumboinguinal nerve) follows the psoas major to the inguinal ligament, where it joins with the external iliac artery and both pass under the ligament. The nerve supplies skin on the proximal part of the anterior thigh.

Lateral femoral cutaneous nerve—L2, L3. This nerve emerges from the lateral side of the psoas major and passes across the iliac fossa toward the anterior superior iliac spine. It passes under the inguinal ligament and over the sartorius muscle to supply the skin on the lateral side of the thigh.

Obturator nerve—L2-4. This emerges on the medial side of the psoas major as the latter turns somewhat laterally to extend across the iliac fossa. The obturator nerve passes across the pelvic brim and toward the obturator foramen, through which it passes along with an artery and a vein of the same name. It supplies the adductor compartment of the thigh and the hip and knee joints. It has a posterior division that supplies the obturator externus and the adductor magnus. The anterior division supplies the adductor longus, adductor brevis, and adductor minimus (if present) and may give some fibers to the pectineus. It may have a small cutaneous distribution to the medial thigh.

Accessory obturator nerve—L3, L4.   This is present in 29% of cases. It passes over the pubic ramus and into the thigh to supply the pectineus and the hip joint.

Femoral nerve—L2-4.   The femoral passes through the psoas major muscle and extends across the iliac fossa along the lateral edge of the psoas major, which lies on the surface of the iliacus muscle. It passes under the inguinal ligament with the iliopsoas muscle and is distributed to anterior and medial thigh skin and to the extensor compartment muscles. In addition to the anterior and medial femoral cutaneous branches, it has a long branch called the saphenous nerve, whch supplies skin on the medial side of the knee, leg, ankle, and foot.

PELVIS AND PERINEUM

Female perneal structures consist of the mons pubis (mons veneris); labis majora; pudendal cleft, also called the vestibular cleft, which is bounded by the labia majora; posterior labial commissure (midline meeting of labia majora just anterior to the anus); labia minora; labial frenulum, or fourchette, the posterior junction of the labia minora; fossa navicularis (depression between the fourchette and the hymen); clitoris, with prepuce, glans, and frenulum; vestibule, which is bounded by the labia minora, into which open the urethra, vagina (introitus), major vestibular glands (of Bartholin), minor vestibular glands (tiny glands with ducts that open onto the surface between the vaginal and urethral orifices); and the hymen (carunculae hymenales).

Male perineal structures consist of the penis, with glans, prepuce, and frenulum; scrotum, with dartos tunic, septum, and raphe; and the urethral orifice.

Perineal boundaries are the pubic symphysis (with pubic arcuate ligament) anteriorly, the ischiopubic rami, ischial tuberosities, and sacrotuberous ligaments laterally, and the coccyx posteriorly. A line drawn between the ischial tuberosities divides the perinerum into urogenital and anal triangles. The perineal body (central point of the perinerum) is a fibrous body in the midline between the anus and scrotum/labial commissure.

Anal triangle.   The anus lies more or less in the center of this triangle. The ischiorectal fossa (on either side of anus) is bounded laterally by the obturator internus muscle, medially by the levator ani, posteriorly by the sacrotuberous ligament and gluteus maximus, and inferiorly by skin. It has an anterior recess that extends over the urogenital diaphragm and a posterior recess that extends posteriorly and cranially deep to the sacrotuberous ligament and gluteus maximus. It is filled with fat and connective tissue. In its lateral wall, a space within the fascia of the obturator internus forms the pudendal (Alcock's) canal, within which course the pudendal nerve and internal pudendal vessels. As these neurovascular elements pass through this fossa, they give rise to inferior rectal branches. The external anal sphincter is a ring of skeletal muscle that encircles the anus.

Urogenital triangle.   The **scrotum** lies in this triangle. It has a modified superficial fascia called the **dartos tunic,** which is formed of both the Camper and Scarpa's portions of superficial fascia of the anterior abdominal wall, which fuse into a single connective tissue structure within which are enmeshed smooth muscle fibers.

The **fundiform ligament** of the penis/clitoris is a modification of the membranous superficial fascia, which extends from the rectus sheath to the dorsum and sides of the penis.

The **suspensory ligament** of the penis/clitoris is a modification of the deep fascia and extends from the linea alba, symphysis pubis, and arcuate pubic ligament to the dorsum of the root of the penis/clitoris.

The **round ligament** extends into the superficial fascia of the labia majora.

The **fascia of Camper** continues from the anterior abdominal wall into the urogenital triangle and retains its name.

Scarpa's fascia of the anterior abdominal wall extends into the urogenital triangle but is renamed **Colles' fascia.**

The **penis** has a **glans** (covered by **prepuce** in uncircumsized males). The shaft has a single **corpus spongiosum,** within which is the penile portion of the **urethra,** and paired **corpora cavernosa penis.** At the proximal end of the penis, the corpus spongiosum becomes the **bulb,** which attaches to the urogenital diaphragm and is partially invested by skeletal **bulbospongiosus muscle.**

The two corpora cavernosa penis diverge from one another as the **crura** of the penis, and each crus becomes attached to the ischiopubic ramus of its respective side. Each crus is partially invested by skeletal **ischiocavernosus muscle.**

The clitoris also has a **glans.** The shaft has paired **corpora cavernosa clitoris,** which mimic the male structure by forming **crura** that attach to the ischiopubic rami also. The crura are partially covered by skeletal **ischiocavernosus muscle.** The vestibular bulbs are erectile tissue that lie immediately lateral to the vaginal orifice. On each side, the bulb is covered by skeletal **bulbospongiosus muscle.**

The fascia and spaces of the urogenital triangle are as follows, starting at the skin of the urogenital triangle and moving cranially:

1. Skin
2. Fascia of Camper (fatty portion of superficial fascia)
3. Colles' fascia (membranous layer of superficial fascia)
4. Superficial perineal cleft (potential space)
5. External perineal fascia (deep fascia, continuous with Buck's fascia of the penis)
6. Superficial perineal compartment, which in males contains the bulb and crura of the penis, which are covered with skeletal muscle called bulbospongiosus and ischiocavernosus, respectively, and the superificial transverse perineal muscles. In females, this compartment contains the crura of the clitoris, each covered with ischiocavernosus muscle, the vestibular bulbs which are covered by bulbospongiosus muscle, the vestibular glands (of Bartholin), and the superficial transverse perineal muscles. The floor (inferior boundary) of this compartment is the external perineal fascia, and the roof is the perineal membrane.
7. The perineal membrane is the deep fascia of the inferior side of the urogenital diaphragm and forms the roof of the superficial perineal compartment and floor of the deep pouch (deep perineal compartment).

8. The deep perineal pouch (compartment) contains the female urethra and membranous portion of the male urethra, the external urethral sphincter, the deep transverse perineal muscle, the pudendal nerve, the internal pudendal vessels, and, in males, the bubourethral (Cowper's) glands.

9. The superior fascia of the urogenital diaphragm is the deep fascia on the cranial side of the urogenital diaphragm.

The pudendal nerve arises from spinal nerves S2–4 and carries all the possible components. It gives rise to the inferior rectal nerve, as stated above, and then the perineal branch, which has a superficial branch to the skin of the scrotum/labia majora and its deep branch to muscles of the superficial compartment and urogenital diaphragm, and finally the dorsal nerve of the penis/clitoris.

The **internal pudendal artery** is a branch of the internal iliac artery. Its branches are the **inferior rectal artery**, the **perineal artery** (supply to superficial compartment and skin of scrotum/labia), the **artery to the bulb**, the **urethral artery**, the **deep artery of the crus**, and the **dorsal artery of the penis/clitoris**.

The **penis** has superficial fascia that some consider to be more of the dartos. Its deep fascia is called **Buck's fascia**. In the superficial fascia are the superficial veins of the penis, which drain into the femoral veins. Deep to Buck's fascia is the deep dorsal vein of the penis, which drains into the prostatic plexus by passing anterior to the anterior edge of the urogenital diaphragm (called the transverse perineal ligament) and posterior to the arcuate pubic ligament.

The **uterus** has the following parts: fundus (rounded, cranial portion of the uterus), body, isthmus, and cervix. The ligaments are the uterosacral, which encircle the rectum, and the cardinal (Mackenrodt's) ligaments, which provide the most significant support. The blood supply is via the uterine and vaginal arteries, which arise from the internal iliac and course in association with the cardinal ligament and inferior to which pass the ureters.

The **broad ligament** is a reflection of the peritoneum, which extends over the reproductive tract in the female pelvis. It is subdivided according to the structures to which it is attached. The part that attaches to the ovary is the **mesovarium**, and that to the uterine tube is the **mesosalpinx**. Finally, that portion of the broad ligament that lies lateral to the body of the uterus is called the **mesometrium**. The **parametrium** is the connective tissue between the leaves of the mesometrium.

Oviducts extend laterally from their attachment to the uterus. Their most lateral portion is the **infundibulum**, which has finger-like processes extending from its edge, and these are the **fimbria**. The portion medial to the infundibulum is the **ampulla**, which extends almost to the uterus. Here the oviduct narrows to a portion called the **isthmus**, which continues on to the uterine wall and is continuous with the **intramural** portion of the oviduct, so named because it passes through the uterine wall and opens into the uterine lumen.

The **ovary** is attached via the mesovarium of the broad ligament. Its blood supply is by the ovarian artery, which arises from the abdominal aorta, and the uterine artery, which is a branch of the internal iliac artery. The ovarian arteries and veins approach the ovary by coursing from the pelvic brim anteromedially and somewhat caudally. They traverse some connective tissue called the **infundibulopelvic ligament** or the suspensory ligament of the ovary. The latter is a misnomer in that it offers no support to the ovary. The **ovarian ligament** (proper ligament of the ovary) is a cord-like structure that extends from the medial end of the ovary to the uterus to attach very close to the attachment of the round ligament of the uterus. The ovarian ligament and the round ligament are remnants of the gubernaculum.

The **urinary bladder** lies posterior to the pubic symphysis, from which it is separated by Retzius's space. It is only partially covered with peritoneum. It is lined with transitional epithelium, and its walls contain much smooth muscle arranged so that upon contraction the bladder's contents are expressed into the urethra. This muscle is called the **detrusor muscle**, and it is parasympathetically innervated. Within the bladder are the ureteral orifices, between which extends the **interureteric bar** or crest, which forms the base of the **trigone**. The apex of the trigone is the urethral orifice.

The rectum lies anterior to the sacrum and coccyx. It is retroperitoneal. Its blood supply is by the superior rectal artery, a branch of the inferior mesenteric, by the middle rectal from the internal iliac, and by the inferior rectal, which branches from the internal pudendal artery. Inside it has three transverse folds called **rectal** (Houston's) **valves**, vertical folds called **rectal** (anal) **columns**, and anal valves. It ends at the anus.

The **pelvic diaphragm** is composed of **levator ani** and **coccygeal muscles**.

The **vagina** has the **introitus** as its orifice in the vestibule of the urogenital triangle. Its upper end receives the cervix of uterus, on which is the external os. The reflections from the vagina onto cervix are called **fornices**—an anterior fornix, posterior fornix, and two lateral fornices. The posterior fornix is particularly important because it is adjacent to the rectouterine pouch (of Douglas). Between the bladder and uterus is the **vesicouterine pouch**. Between the uterus and rectum is the much larger and more significant **rectouterine pouch** of Douglas. The latter extends between these two structures and ends caudally so as to be separated from the posterior fornix of the vagina by only the relatively thin vaginal wall.

The **female urethra** is short and unremarkable. It extends from the bladder through the urogenital diaphragm, within which it is surrounded by the external urethral sphincter. It opens into the vestibule. It is surrounded by the **paraurethral glands** and Skene's ducts. These are homologues of the prostate gland.

The **vas deferens** courses from the ductus epididymis as part of the spermatic cord. It enters the abdomen via the internal inguinal ring and courses from there to the base of the bladder. The ureter loops caudal to it (below it). The vas deferens dilates as it approaches the bladder to form the **ampulla**. The ampulla opens into the **ejaculatory duct**, which also receives the duct of the seminal vesicle. The ejaculatory duct passes through the prostate but does not communicate with it. Each ejaculatory duct opens into the prostatic urethra on either side of the prostatic utricle. The prostate gland surrounds the proximal portion of the urethra, and thus this portion is called the prostatic urethra. The numerous ducts of the prostate open into the prostatic urethra on either side of the seminal colliculus into the prostatic sinus.

Within the **prostatic portion of the urethra** is a ridge on its posterior wall, the **urethral crest**. This extends from the urethral orifice of the bladder throughout this part of the urethra. About midway along the urethral crest is an enlarged portion called the **seminal colliculus**. In the midline a tiny diverticulum opens onto the surface, and this is the **prostatic utricle**, a remnant of the paramesonephric ducts (müllerian ducts). The utricle is homologous to the uterus and part of the vagina.

The portion of the male urethra that passes through the urogenital diaphragm is the **membranous urethra**. It is surrounded by the external urethral sphincter. Also, the **bulbourethral glands** lie within the deep perineal pouch beside the membranous urethra. The ducts of these glands extend out of the deep pouch and open into the urethra within the bulb of the penis.

NEUROANATOMY

CEREBRUM

The cerebrum includes the telencephalon (cerebral hemispheres) and the diencephalon. These two portions of the brain are referred to developmentally and sometimes later as the **forebrain** (prosencephalon). The cerebral hemispheres are the overwhelmingly large part of the brain, and the diencephalon is almost completely enveloped by the hemispheres. In the intact, whole brain, the only part of the diencephalon that can be observed is the ventral portion, the **hypothalamus.** Of this, only the tuber cinereum, median eminence, infundibulum, pituitary stalk, and mammillary bodies are identifiable.

The cerebral hemispheres are characterized by having a layer of gray matter on the surface (**cortex**), which is arranged in folds (**gyri**) and grooves (**sulci**).

The cerebral hemispheres are organized into lobes—**frontal, parietal, temporal, occipital,** and **insula.** The insula lies at the bottom of the lateral fissure.

The lobes of the cerebral hemispheres roughly underly the cranial bones of the same names. The boundary between frontal and parietal lobes is a dependable landmark called the **central sulcus** (fissure of Rolando). The anterior boundary on the dorsolateral brain surface of the occipital lobe is a line drawn between two notch-like structures. The superior one is the **parieto-occipital sulcus**, which is a slight continuation of that sulcus onto the dorsolateral surface from the medial surface of the hemisphere. The inferior landmark is the **preoccipital notch**. A line drawn between two landmarks is the anterior boundary of the occipital lobe and the posterior boundaries of the parietal and temporal lobes.

The large, deep **lateral fissure** (of Sylvius) lies superior to the temporal lobe and inferior to the parietal and frontal lobes. At the bottom of this fissure lies the **insula** (insular lobe or isle of Reil). An imaginary line drawn from the posterior part of the lateral fissure and perpendicular to the anterior occipital boundary serves as the boundary between the parietal and temporal lobes. The terms **fissure** and **sulcus** are often used interchangeably, although a fissure is usually a much deeper and more remarkable groove or separation of structures.

The **brain stem** includes **mesencephalon** (midbrain), **pons,** and **medulla oblongata.** Overlying much of the brain stem is the **cerebellum** ("little cerebrum").

FRONTAL LOBE

This portion of the hemisphere lies anterior to the **central sulcus.** It has three horizontally oriented **gyri**—superior, **middle,** and **inferior.** The **superior** and **inferior frontal sulci** separate these gyri. The **inferior frontal gyrus** is subdivided by the anterior ramus and ascending ramus of the lateral fissure into three parts—**pars opercularis** (meaning a lid or covering), **pars triangularis,** and **pars orbitalis.** In the left hemisphere, these structure contain the **motor speech area** (of Broca, Brodmann's areas 44 and 45). Lying anterior and running parallel to the central sulcus is the **precentral gyrus.** Anterior to the gyrus is the **precentral sulcus.** The precentral gyrus has special significance in that it contains, along with the central sulcus, the primary motor cortex (Brodmann's area 4).

On the basal surface, the medial gyrus (next to the longitudinal fissure in the midline) is straight and thus called the **gyrus rectus** (straight gyrus). Lateral to the gyrus is the **olfactory sulcus,** upon which lies the **olfactory bulb and tract.** Lateral to the olfactory sulcus are several gyri and sulci, which are lumped together and referred to as **orbital gyri and sulci.** They lie on the roof of the orbit.

PARIETAL LOBE

The parietal lobe lies posterior to the central sulcus, superior to the lateral fissure, and anterior to a line dropped vertically from parieto-occipital sulcus to the preoccipital notch. Posterior to the central sulcus is the **postcentral gyrus,** which in turn is limited posteriorly by the **postcentral sulcus.** The postcentral gyrus, along with the central sulcus, contains the primary sensory cortex (areas 3, 1, 2). Extending horizontally and posteriorly from the postcentral sulcus is the **intraparietal sulcus.** Superior to this sulcus lies the **superior parietal lobule;** inferior to this sulcus lies the **inferior parietal lobule.** The superior parietal lobule is an important sensory association area. Primary sensory cortices project into this area, which in turn interprets the information, coordinates it with other sensory input, etc. The inferior parietal lobule has two parts—the **supramarginal gyrus** and **angular gyrus.** The supramarginal gyrus "caps" the posterior end of the lateral fissure. The angular gyrus encompasses the posterior end of the superior temporal sulcus. These gyri of the infratemporal lobule are included in the **sensory speech area** of the cortex, in the majority of cases in the left hemisphere (Brodmann's areas 39, 40).

OCCIPITAL LOBE

The dorsolateral surface of the occipital lobe has few distinguishing physical characteristics. This area can be referred to simply as the dorsolateral surface of the occipital lobe with occipital gyri and sulci.

TEMPORAL LOBE

From the lateral view, the temporal lobe presents a straightforward, consistent configuration. From superior to inferior, the three gyri are seen—**superior, middle,** and **inferior.** Between the middle and superior gyri is the **superior temporal sulcus.** Between the middle and inferior gyri is the middle temporal sulcus. On the posterior part of the superior surface of the superior temporal gyrus are the small, transversely oriented **transverse temporal (Heschl's) gyri**. These represent the **primary auditory cortex** (Brodmann's areas 41, 42).

On the basal surface, the temporal lobe has additional gyri and sulci. The inferior temporal gyrus continues from the lateral surface onto the basal surface. Medial to this gyrus is the **occipitotemporal sulcus** (or inferior temporal sulcus). Medial to this sulcus is the **medial occipitotemporal gyrus** (or simply occipitotemporal gyrus if the lateral gyrus is called the inferior temporal). Medial to this gyrus is the **collateral sulcus**, and, finally, medial to that sulcus is the **parahippocampal gyrus**. On the anterior end of this gyrus is a little hook-shaped bulge of the cortex, the **uncus**. The small sulcus lateral to the uncus is the **rhinal sulcus**. Along the medial edge of the parahippocampal gyrus is a crevice between it and the brain stem, and this is named the **hippocampal sulcus**.

MEDIAL SURFACE OF THE CEREBRAL HEMISPHERES

The **corpus callosum** is a massive bundle of axons connecting the two hemispheres. Such an arrangement of fibers is called a **commissure**. A commissure is a bundle of axons that connects two sides of the same level of the CNS. The sulcus next to the corpus callosum is the **callosal sulcus**, and lying next to this sulcus is the **cingulate gyrus**. In turn, the outer (more superficial) boundary of the cingulate gyrus is the **cingulate sulcus**. Note that this sulcus's posterior end swings superiorly to form the **marginal ramus** (or marginal sulcus). The dorsomedial end of the central sulcus can be identified immediately anterior to the marginal ramus. The cortex lying around this part of the central sulcus is called the **paracentral lobule**, in which pre- and postcentral gyri become continuous. Rostral to the paracentral lobule there is a small, vertical extension of the cingulate gyrus that forms the boundary between the paracentral lobule and the **medial frontal gyrus** (or the superior frontal gyrus).

Posterior to the marginal ramus of the cingulate sulcus and anterior to the **parieto-occipital sulcus** is a region of the parietal lobe called the **precuneus**. The parieto-occipital sulcus meets the **calcarine sulcus** of the occipital lobe. The wedge-shaped region bound by these two sulci is the **cuneus**. Below the calcarine sulcus is the **lingual gyrus** of the occipital lobe. The cortex in the region of the calcarine sulcus is the **primary visual cortex** (Brodmann's area 17).

The cingulate gyrus passes posteriorly and then inferior to the corpus callosum to become continuous with the parahippocampal gyrus by a thin connection called the **isthmus of the cingulate gyrus**. The lingual and parahippocampal gyri are continuous with each other also in this region.

INSULA (Isle of Reil)

This part of the cortex forms the floor of the lateral fissure. It has long and short gyri, a circular sulcus, and a little portion on its anteroinferior edge called the **limen** (threshold), over which passes the middle cerebral artery as it continues from the basal surface of the brain onto the insula.

BRAIN STEM AND CEREBELLUM

Cerebellum

The cerebellum lies on the dorsal (posterior) side of the brain stem. It is characterized by having many transverse, parallel grooves that are separated by thin folds of cerebellar cortex called **folia**. The midline portion of the cerebellum (running in the longitudinal axis) is a somewhat depressed portion called the **vermis**. The much larger, bulging, lateral portions on each side of the vermis are the **hemispheres**. The cerebellum has an **anterior lobe**, a **posterior lobe**, and a **flocculonodular lobe**. The anterior and posterior lobes are separated by the **primary fissure**. The posterior and flocculonodular lobes are separated by the **posterolateral fissure**.

Mesencephalon

Ventrally, the two very large column-like structures on the basal surface are the **cerebral peduncles** (crura cerebri). Between these peduncles is the **interpeduncular fossa**. Dorsally, the four little hillocks are the paired **superior and inferior colliculi**. They are visual and auditory reflex centers, respectively. The two pairs of colliculi form the **tectum**.

Pons

The pons is seen from the ventral and lateral aspects as a massive number of fibers extending from the basal side of the pons up into the cerebellum as the **middle cerebellar peduncle**. In the midline, on the basal surface, is the **basilar sulcus**, on which lies the basilar artery (formed by the union of the two vertebral arteries).

Medulla

On the ventral side is a midline sulcus called the **anterior median sulcus**. On either side of this sulcus are the two longitudinally oriented **medullary pyramids**. These are descending tracts called the pyramidal or corticospinal tracts. They are important in motor function, and when diseased or lesioned a salient symptom is loss of the fine digital movements.

Laterally, a sulcus extending on the dorsolateral border of the pyramid from the rostral end of the medulla down to the spinal cord is the **anterolateral sulcus**, in which are attached the fibers of the hypoglossal nerve (cranial nerve XII). Immediately dorsal to the anterolateral sulcus is an olive-shaped bulge called the **olive**. This surface landmark is the outward manifestation of the presence of the underlying **inferior olivary nucleus** of the medulla.

Dorsally, the midline sulcus is the **dorsomedian sulcus**. Rostrally, it ends at the most caudal extent of the fourth ventricle at a point called the **obex**. On either side of this sulcus lie the **dorsal columns**. The more medial of these is the **fasciculus gracilis**, which terminates in the **nucleus gracilis**, which causes a bulge called the **tuberculum gracilis**. Lateral to the fasciculus gracilis and parallel to the dorsomedian sulcus is the **dorsal intermediate sulcus**. Lateral to this sulcus and parallel to the fasciculus gracilis is the **fasciculus cuneatus**, which terminates in the **nucleus cuneatus**, which causes a surface eminence, the **tuberculum cuneatus**.

SPINAL CORD

The spinal cord is 45 cm long in males, 42 cm in females. It weighs about 30 g. At birth, it extends as low as the second or third lumbar vertebra, and in adults it extends to the level of the first or second lumbar vertebra. Its caudal end tapers into a cone-shaped **conus medullaris.** From the conus medullaris caudally, extending down the vertebral canal within the lower lumbar and sacral vertebrae, are the dorsal and ventral roots of the spinal nerves of those levels of the cord plus a small cord-like extension of the pia mater called the **filum terminale interna.** This pia and the spinal nerve roots form the **cauda equina.**

The spinal cord has two enlargements—cervical (C4 to T1) and lumbosacral (L4 to S3). These spinal cord segments provide the innervation of the limbs.

The surface of the spinal cord is marked with the **ventral median fissure, dorsal median sulcus** (and septum), and **dorsolateral** and **ventrolateral sulci** for attachment of dorsal and ventral spinal nerve roots, respectively. Above spinal cord segment T6 there is an additional sulcus, the **dorsal intermediate sulcus.**

DEVELOPMENT

The nervous system is the first system per se to make an appearance in the embryo. During the third week of gestation, the three definitive germ layers and the notochord are formed, and as these are forming the **neural plate** is formed. This is a midline thickening of the ectoderm extending from the cephalic to the caudal end of the embryonic disk. During this third week, a midline sulcus (**neural groove**) develops along the middle of the neural plate and **neural folds** develop along the lateral margins of the plate. As the end of the third week approaches, the neural folds increase in their height and approach each other in the midline. As this folding progresses, the neural folds fuse in the midline, converting the neural plate to a **neural tube.** This fusion of the lateral folds begins in the occipital region of the neural plate and simultaneously progresses cephalically and caudally. While this fusion is occurring, the forming neural tube's lumen has an opening anteriorly and posteriorly so as to communicate with the amniotic cavity. These are the **anterior** and **posterior neuropores,** respectively. During the fourth week the neural tube formation proceeds such that the anterior neuropore closes on about the 24th or 25th day, the posterior on the 26th or 27th day. Following the closure of the neuropores, the neural tube is completely separated from the surface ectoderm and does not communicate with any of the extraembryonic cavities.

As the neural folds form and grow medially to fuse in the midline, some of the cells at the junction of the neural plate cells and the surface ectoderm separate from the tube and the surface ectoderm and, bilaterally, form a flattened column of cells along the dorsolateral aspect of the neural tube. These cells are the **neural crest cells.** Some of these are destined to develop into the neurons of the dorsal root ganglia of the spinal nerves, the sensory ganglia of the cranial nerves (except those of cranial nerve I which arise from the olfactory placode, the autonomic ganglia, the adrenal medulla (and other parts of the chromaffin system), neurilemma (Schwann) cells, and the satellite (capsule) cells. Neurilemma cells ensheath all peripheral nervous system axons, both myelinated and unmyelinated. The satellite or capsule cells invest the cell bodies of the ganglion cells. These derivatives of the neural crest cells are predictable because they all are neural structures.

However, in addition to these derivatives there are several others. The neural crest cells migrate more widely from their site of formation than was previously described, and now their derivatives include melanoblasts, all the structural elements of the branchial arches (only the skeletal muscle myotubes arise from mesodermally derived mesenchyme), the aorticopulmonary septum, and the tunica media of the great vessels (in the thorax and neck).

The neural crest cells obviously must migrate extensively, as indicated by the varied derivatives and their broadly dispersed location within the body. The neural crest cells migrate into the developing structures with which they are associated and to which they contribute structurally. Those cells destined to give rise to neurons begin differentiation very early and have progressed along that process quite far by the time they reach their respective destinations. The other derivatives seem to do much of their differentiation in situ after their migration.

The neurilemma (Schwann) cells form the myelin found in the peripheral nervous system. The process of myelination occurs over a long time developmentally, and it seems to precede functional awakening of the specific neural tissue. Phylogenetically older systems myelinate earlier than do the newer systems. Unlike the CNS, the peripheral nervous system (PNS) axons all are ensheathed whether myelinated or not. Those that are myelinated have each internodal segment of mylein formed by one neurilemma cell. Each neurilemma cell can form only one internodal segment. As the individual grows, the axon must in many cases grow in length. The internodal segments increase in length so as to maintain myelin ensheathment. The process of PNS myelination is accomplished by the neurilemma cell wrapping around the axon, forming a jellyroll-like covering composed largely of neurilemma cell membranes fusing to form this lipid-rich covering. Those axons that are not myelinated are still ensheathed by neurilemma cells, with each neurilemma cell accommodating several (15 to 20 or so) axons along that particular stretch of those axons. This is repeated by one neurilemma cell after another, so that the axons are ensheathed up to their terminal portions, where they become associated with receptors of some kind.

Within the neural tube, the cells lining the lumen become the germinal layer. It is these cells that are mitotically active and from which both neuronal and glial derivatives will arise. The daughter cells that arise from the mitoses of the germinal cells migrate away from the neural tube lumen. As these cells migrate, they are destined to be neuroblasts (progenitors of neurons) and glioblasts (progenitors of glial cells). The neuroblasts differentiate rapidly, quickly assuming the shape of a primitive neuron. The cell body takes on the appearance of neurons rather quickly so that as differentiation proceeds the amount of euchromatin increases, the Nissl substance forms, etc. The axon appears just prior to the dendrites. As the axon extends from the cell body, it has on its tip a slightly bulbous expansion that contains some smooth-walled vesicles. This is the growth cone. The role of the vesicles is uncertain, but it has been suggested that the vesicles provide a ready supply of cell membrane that is needed for the growth of the axon. Once the neuroblast leaves the germinal layer cells, it has differentiated to the degree that it has lost its mitotic capabilities. The glioblasts and mature glia never lose the ability to undergo mitosis. As the cells leave the germinal epithelium of the neural tube, they move into the middle region of the neural tube's wall and there form a nucleated zone called the **mantle layer.** As the neuroblasts continue to differentiate, their axons grow toward the outer surface of the neural tube, resulting in an outer, relatively nuclear-free zone called the **marginal layer.** These changes all appear late in the third week of gestation and become marked in the fourth week. The mantle layer is the forerunner of the **gray matter,** and the marginal layer that of the **white matter.**

As the migration of the neuroblasts and glioblasts occurs, the mantle layer begins to undergo some internal organizaiton into a dorsal **alar plate** and a ventral **basal plate.** The lateral walls of the neural tube lumen come to have a longitudinally coursing groove on each side, the **sulcus limitans,** which is the boundary between alar and basal plate. This sulcus extends from the cranial end of the mesencephalon caudally throughout the remainder of the neural tube. The most cranial portion of the neural tube forms the prosencephalon or forebrain (which gives rise to the telencephalon and the diencephalon) and is apparently composed of only alar plates.

The alar plates of the neural tube give rise to nuclei that are destined to be sensory/association in function. The neurons derived from alar plate are distinguished in that they extend no part of themselves outside the CNS. It should not be inferred from the first statement of this paragraph that alar plate derivatives do not have anything to do with motor function because they do, as indicated by the fact that motor portions of the cerebral cortex arise from alar plate as does the cerebellum, the so-called head ganglion of the motor system.

The basal plates provide neurons of motor function, and many of these neurons are those that extend their axons out of the CNS into the PNS. Such neurons provide the nervous system with the "final common path" and form the links of the CNS with effectors (muscles and glands). Some cells that arise from the basal plate are interneurons and do not become contributors to the PNS.

The glioblasts of the CNS differentiate into the astrocytes and the oligodendrocytes. What the microglia really are, what they do, and from what they arise are the objects of controversy. Typically they are described as the potential macrophages of the CNS that become active when stimulated by trauma, invasion by microbes, etc. Such function has resulted in their being referred to as **reactive microglia.** Agreement about these cells is restricted to their description as small cells with a scant amount of rough endoplasmic reticulum (rER) and a number of lysosomes. Normally (in the resting state) they do not divide and have little indication of motility or phagocytosis. When stimulated, they become mitotically active and phagocytic. Two schools of thought exist as to the origin of these cells. One is that they arise from the neural ectoderm, and the other that they arise from monocytes that come into the CNS as vascularization occurs during development. It seems at present that microglia continue to be included with the neuroglia through convention.

The other glia are relatively simple to deal with. The glioblasts differentiate into astroblasts and oligodendroblasts. Some astroblasts become **fibrous astrocytes,** which are found to be associated with the fibers (axons) and thus in the white matter. Other astroblasts become **protoplasmic astrocytes,** which are found in the gray matter. Where gray and white matter interface, the astrocytes there are intermediate between the fibrous and protoplasmic forms. Astrocytes have processes that come to have an intimate association with the blood vessels within the CNS. Although not a part of the blood-brain barrier, these processes do cover a good bit of the outer surface of the CNS capillaries.

The oligodendroblasts differentiate into the oligodendrocytes. These are found in both white and gray matter. These cells develop processes that selectively enwrap axons and by coiling around these axons form internodal segments of myelin. Unlike neurilemma cells, one oligodendrocyte has numerous such processes and can form internodal segments of myelin around several different axons. Those axons of the CNS that are not myelinated are not ensheathed as are the unmyelinated axons of the PNS.

The axons of the various neurons grow toward predetermined tissues and structures in order to come into synaptic contact with them. Various theories exist about how the neurons know what to do and where to go. It is assumed that there is some sort of chemotaxis involved, but the specifics of the mechanisms involved have not been determined. It has been shown many times that many more neurons develop than are needed. For example, once the receptors on the skeletal muscle cells have come into a synaptic relationship with axon terminals, the axons extending to the muscle that do not make such a synapse atrophy and the neuron dies. This same process occurs within the CNS also, and some have termed this normal process of development morphogenetic necrosis. The generic term of *cell death* covers the entire situation, and the process is seen throughout nervous system development. Where it can be seen easily and dramatically is in the development of the spinal cord. There are the cervical and lumbosacral enlargements of the spinal cord that occur in those regions because it is they that are involved in innervation of the limbs. It is not that more neurons are initially formed in these regions of the cord, but rather that more neurons survived (i.e., did not undergo cell death), because there is much more tissue to be innervated and more receptor sites upon which synaptic formation occurs.

Experimental data related to synaptic development have had to be gathered from various experimental animals, and there seem to be no general rules that can be applied. Problems with gaining specific information about the sequence of developmental events and correlation of form and function are legion. There is a sampling problem, a problem with the heterogeneity of the cell populations studied, and the fact that a specific synapse may undergo much of its development in a matter of hours. In amphibians, researchers have tested for acetylcholine (ACh) sensitivity and its appearance as related to function of the myoneural junction. ACh sensitivity precedes function by 30 minutes to 2 hours. From 30 minutes to 2 hours after this appearance of functional ACh receptors, end-plate potentials can be recorded. Such data provide some means of correlation between developing structure and function.

Synaptogenesis begins before neurogenesis has been completed. Synapse formation, however, may be delayed for days while cells destined to form synaptic relationships lie juxtaposed and inactive. The reasons for this are unknown. No rule exists as to the sequence of development of pre- and postsynaptic structures, since in different areas of the nervous system and in the same areas but in different species presynaptic structure formations sometimes precedes postsynaptic development and vice versa. In a given area in a given species, however, the sequence is invariant.

In the development of myoneural junctions, there seems to be a restricted number of receptor sites that develop. The maturing neurons' axons grow to these sites and establish synaptic relationships. During this process, more than one axon becomes involved at a single receptor site, and by some yet undetermined mechanism only one of the axons survives and maintains the synaptic relationship. In the neuron-to-neuron synapses, this situation does not obtain, but more axons synapse on a given neuron (its cell body, dendrites, axon) during development than survive in the mature state. This is not, as it were, carved in stone, however; and considerable plasticity is achieved by synapses disappearing and new ones reforming, especially in cases of trauma or disease. Neurons sometimes die, and their axons, of course, disappear along with the synapses they have made. Other neurons' axons collateralize and form new and additional synaptic relations. Evidence points now to the differentiation of the cell in the periphery (e.g., a skeletal muscle cell), which presents receptor sites to which the differentiating axons grow and attempt to establish a synapse at these sites. This is probably due to some kind of chemotactic mechanism being involved, but none of the specifics has been determined.

Although neurons lose their mitotic capability very early in development and are not replaced by new neurons forming, the connections among neurons are not rigidly established. As indicated above, new connections can often be made in response to new demands on the nervous system (e.g., learning and memory) or to meet the established demands following trauma or disease. Once the mitotic activity of the germinal epithelium of the neural tube (those cells lining the lumen of the CNS) ceases because development has proceeded beyond that point where more cells are needed, the cells forming the lining of the neural tube become the **ependymal cells.**

The neural tube begins its development as a structure that has immediate variations from one part to another. The cephalic end undergoes rapid and dramatic developmental events very early. The most obvious sign of early differentiation is the appearance of swellings called **primary brain vesicles:** prosencephalon (forebrain), mesencephalon, and rhombencephalon (hind brain). These go on to form the **secondary brain vesicles:** telencephalon (cerebral hemispheres), diencephalon (thalami), mesencephalon (midbrain), metencephalon (pons and cerebellum), and myelencephalon (medulla oblongata).

The remainder of the neural tube forms the spinal cord. Within the spinal cord, the arrangement of the developing gray matter stays relatively simple and has some uniformity throughout. The basal and alar plates of the spinal cord gray matter develop into groups of functionally similar nuclei, with the various groups maintaining a constant physical relationship. Starting most ventrally and medially in the basal plate, the nuclei are those that provide motor innervation of skeletal muscle (all of which in this case are derived from somites). These nuclei therefore are labeled general somatic efferent (GSE). The nuclei that lie dorsolateral to the GSE nuclei provide preganglionic autonomic neurons for innervation of smooth muscle, cardiac muscle, and glands. These then are labeled general visceral efferent (GVE). Both GSE and GVE nuclei are motor and both are derived from basal plate. Dorsal to the GVE nuclei, and on the other side of the sulcus limitans, are nuclei that are associated with sensations from splanchnopleuric structures (the viscera) and are thus labeled general visceral afferent (GVA). Finally, dorsal to the GVA nuclei are neurons associated with somatopleuric structures that provide general somatic afferent (GSA) innervation. Both of the sensory nuclear groups are derived from alar plate. The GSA and GSE nuclei are found throughout the spinal cord gray matter, but the GVA and GVE nuclei are restricted to those segments of the spinal cord related to autonomic function—T1–L2 or L3 (sympathetic) and S2–4 (parasympathetic).

Passing cranially, the spinal cord merges with the medulla oblongata (hereafter referred to simply as the medulla). This most caudal portion of the brain stem consists of the mesencephalon, the pons, and the medulla.

The sulcus limitans extends throughout the brain stem, and thus there are alar and basal plates here also with the same developmental and functional significance described in the spinal cord.

The thin dorsal portion of the neural tube (**roof plate**) becomes even thinner and stretches out to become the extensive roof of the fourth ventricle associated with the hindbrain. As this broad roof plate is forming, the lateral walls move from a vertical orientation to one approaching the horizontal. The sulcus limitans is still present in the medulla and pons and persists even in adults. Thus alar and basal plates are readily identifiable. The cerebullum forms the roof of the fourth ventricle, and the pons and medulla the floor.

The floor of the fourth ventricle is called the **rhomboid fossa** because of its diamond shape. Extending in the midline the length of this fossa is the **median sulcus.** On either side of that is the **medial eminence,** the lateral boundary of which is the **sulcus limitans.** The various GSE and GVE motor nuclei are found within the medial eminence (basal plate), and the various sensory nuclei are found lateral to the sulcus limitans (alar plate).

Keeping the basic organization of the gray matter of the spinal cord in mind, the same basic pattern is seen in the brain stem. Thus, those nuclei that provide motor innervation to somitically derived skeletal muscles (GSE) will be found in the most ventromedial position of basal plate gray matter. In the brain stem, these nuclei are found in the tegmentum on either side of the midline and next to the ventricular system (including the cerebral aqueduct in the mesencephalon). It should be recalled that the brain-stem tegmentum is that portion lying ventral to the cerebral aqueduct and fourth ventricle. Thus, because cranial nerves III, IV, VI, and XII all provide motor innervation to somitically derived muscles (GSE), these nuclei can be seen to form a discontinuous column from upper midbrain to lower medulla, all lying in the position described above.

The same general rule applies to another basal plate

derivative, the GVE nuclei (parasympathetic). Cranial nerves that have such nuclei are III, VII, IX, and X. Thus, from upper mesencephalon (**Edinger-Westphal nucleus** for III), into the pons (**superior salivatory nucleus** for VII), and on to the medulla (**inferior salivatory nucleus** for IX and **dorsal motor nucleus of the vagus** for X) there is another discontinuous column of GVE nuclei lying just lateral to the GSE nuclei.

In considering the sensory nuclei, the basic plan of the GVA and GSA nuclei of the spinal cord is also maintained in the brain stem. Because the sensory nuclei are alar plate derivatives, in the brain stem these are found lateral to the sulcus limitans. The GVA function is combined with the special sense of taste (special visceral afferent [SVA]) into a single nucleus, the **nucleus solitarius**. This nucleus lies in the medulla immediately lateral to the dorsal motor nucleus of the vagus.

The other sensory nuclei of the brain stem all are GSA or special somatic afferent (SSA) for auditory and vestibular function. They are all, like the nucleus solitarius, alar plate derivatives. They all lie lateral to this GVA/SVA nucleus. GSA function for the cranial nerves is channeled entirely through the various trigeminal sensory nuclei. Although the trigeminal nerve is the largest single contributor of afferent fibers to these nuclei, VII, IX, and X also provide afferent fibers. The GSA distribution of last three nerves is confined to the skin of the external ear. There are three trigeminal sensory nuclei that extend from the midbrain down through the brain stem and into the upper two or three segments of the spinal cord. The **mesencephalic nucleus of V** extends from the upper mesencephalon to the middle of the pons. It is related to proprioception of the joints and muscles innervated by cranial nerves. The **principal** (also called chief or main) **sensory nucleus of V** lies in the middle of the rostrocaudal dimension of the pons, at the level of attachment of the trigeminal nerve to the brain stem. The function of this nucleus is related to fine, discriminative touch. Finally, the **spinal nucleus of V** extends from midpons caudally through the medulla and into the upper cervical spinal cord segments. Its function has to do with pain, temperature, and crude touch. Here again is a column of nuclei of like function lying within the brain stem.

The SSA nuclei of the eighth cranial nerve are in the upper portion of the medulla and lower portion of the pons. There are the **dorsal** and **ventral cochlear nuclei** for auditory function and the four **vestibular nuclei** (superior, medial, lateral, and inferior). These lie dorsal and lateral to the GSA nuclei.

In the development of head and neck there are two sources of skeletal muscle fibers. The one that has been described is somites. Such muscles are those that move the eyes and the tongue (III, IV, VI, XII). The other source is mesodermal mesenchyme of the branchial (pharyngeal) arches. Such muscles are histologically and functionally indistinguishable from somatically derived muscle. However, a different origin seems to require a different provision for motor innervation. Those muscles derived from the branchial arches receive motor innervation by special visceral efferent (SVE) nuclei. These nuclei are associated with cranial nerves V (**trigeminal motor nucleus** for derivatives of branchial arch I), VII (**facial motor nucleus** for derivatives of branchial arch II), IX (**nucleus ambiguus** for derivatives of branchial arch III), and X (**nucleus ambiguus** for derivatives of branchial arches IV and VI).

The SVE nuclei begin their development within the basal plate wedged in between the GSE nuclei medially and the GVE nuclei laterally. However, the SVE nuclei soon migrate ventrolaterally and come to lie within the middle of the tegmentum, but within approximately the same rostrocaudal levels as they began their development. Thus, a discontinuous column of SVE nuclei is formed, starting with the motor nucleus of the trigeminal in the midpons level, going down to the lower pons to the facial motor nucleus and into the medulla to the nucleus ambiguus. In line with these SVE nuclei is the SVE nucleus of the spinal accessory nerve (XI), which is within the gray matter of cervical spinal cord segments two through five.

The brain-stem nuclei that project largely to the cerebellum (e.g., the pontine and the inferior olivary nuclei) are derived from alar plate. The red nucleus and the substantia nigra are derived from the basal plate. The cerebellum and the entire forebrain are derived from the alar plate.

The hypophysis (pituitary gland) has a dual origin. The hypothalamus (of the diencephalon) has a downward growth called the infundibulum, which goes on to form the posterior pituitary. A diverticulum of the oral ectoderm called Rathke's pouch extends from the oral cavity to the infundibulum and partially enwraps it. Rathke's pouch forms the anterior pituitary.

The prosencephalon (forebrain) apparently arises entirely from the alar plates. The diencephalon is composed of the various thalami—epithalamus, (dorsal) thalamus, hypothalamus, subthalamus, and metathalamus (medial and lateral geniculate bodies). The telencephalon is made up of the olfactory bulbs and tracts and the cerebral hemispheres, including the extensive cerebral cortex and the basal nuclei (ganglia).

Associated with each cerebral hemisphere is a lateral ventricle. These are continuous with the third ventricle through the right and left interventricular foramina (of Monro). The third ventricle opens posteriorly into the cerebral aqueduct (of Sylvius), which runs through the midbrain. The aqueduct opens into the fourth ventricle, which is within the hindbrain. The fourth ventricle is continuous with the central canal of the spinal cord. The latter is more or less vestigial and has very little volume and contains virtually no CSF. Each ventricle has its choroid plexus. This is a combination of highly vascularized pia mater and ependymal cells. The choroid plexuses are found where the neural tube wall consists of only a single cell layer (ependyma) called the choroid fissure. These plexuses form about 70% of the CSF and secrete it into the ventricles. The roof of the fourth ventricle has three openings. In the midline at its caudal end is one called the foramen of Magendie. In each lateral recess is a foramen of Luschka. All these foramina afford communication between the ventricles and the subarachnoid space.

NEURONS

Neurons fall into three morphological groups—bipolar, unipolar (pseudounipolar), and multipolar, based on the number of axons and dendrites that extend from the cell body. The **bipolar neurons** are confined to the olfactory mucosa, the retina, and cranial nerve VIII. The **unipolar** (also called pseudounipolar) **neurons** are found in the dorsal root ganglia of spinal nerves and the sensory ganglia of cranial nerves V, VII, IX, and X. Unipolar neurons are also found in the mesencephalic nucleus of V. **Multipolar neurons** make up the remainder of this cell type and are by far the most numerous. They occur in the peripheral nervous system in the autonomic ganglia, and in the CNS they are the predominant neuron with only a very few exceptions.

Neurons typically have a **cell body,** which contains the **nucleus** and the many organelles such as **mitochondria, free ribosomes, Golgi, rER** (which is organized into regular cisternae and referred to as **Nissl substance**), **microtubules** (which serve as structural support for the cell), **neurofilaments** (intermediate filaments), and **lysosomes.** A common inclusion of neurons is **pigment. Lipofuscin** is the "wear-and-tear" pigment that is seen to accumulate with age within many neurons. **Melanin** is seen in abundance in the substantia nigra. The nucleus lies more or less centrally within the cell body, but it characteristically is eccentric in autonomic ganglia and in the nucleus dorsalis (of Clarke). The nucleus has very little heterochromatin, but it characteristically has a prominent centrally placed nucleolus.

Each neuron has a single **axon.** It is usually the largest process of the neuron, and as it extends away from the cell body it maintains a constant diameter that ranges from 0.2 to 20μm. Branches of axons are called **collaterals.** The place on the cell body where an axon attaches is called the **axon hillock,** which is usually free of ribosomes and rER, and thus it has a lighter staining appearance. This area does contain many microtubules and filaments, however. The cell membrane of an axon is called the **axolemma,** and its cytoplasm is the **axoplasm.** The proximal portion of the axon (that attached to the cell body) is called the **initial segment,** which is not myelinated and has a slightly smaller diameter than the rest of the axon. Organelles include mitochondria, smooth endoplasmic reticulum (sER), microtubules, and neurofilaments. The proteins, glycoproteins, mitochondria, and axoplasmic vesicles are manufactured in the cell body and are transported along the axon in **axoplasmic transport.**

Axoplasmic transport has three speeds—slow, intermediate, and fast. The slow is called **axoplasmic flow,** which is unidirectional and anterograde (away from the cell body) and has a speed of 1 to 4 mm/day. Such substances as cytosolic enzymes, actin, myosin, and clathrin are transported by this means. Microtubular and neurofilament proteins move in this stream also. This axoplasmic flow is required for axon growth and general maintenance of the axoplasm.

Fast axoplasmic transport travels anterogradely at a rate of 50 to 400 mm/day. Neurotransmitter-filled vesicles and membrane-associated and membrane-bound constituents that are involved in synaptic transmission move by this mechanism.

Intermediate axoplasmic transport moves mitochondria. This transport is seen to be fast anterograde transport with intermittent stops or retrograde flow.

Microtubules apparently play a key role in axoplasmic transport in that colchicine and vinblastine inhibit the process.

Dendrites are branched, tapering extensions of the cell body. Some few cells have no dendrites, but there may be many of them on a single cell. These contain most of the various organelles described for the cell. The presence of Nissl substance in them readily distinguishes them from axons.

As described in the development discussion, myelin forms around most of the axons in the CNS and PNS. The small axons are not myelinated. The general rule is that the greater the diameter of the axon, the faster the conduction of an impulse. Also, the larger the diameter of the axon, the thicker the myelin. The areas along an axon where one myelin segment abuts another is a **node of Ranvier.** At this node there is no myelin. The physical properties of the axons and the myelin are such that the depolarization (action potential) of the axolemma in myelinated axons jumps from node to node. This is called **saltatory conduction,** and it greatly increases the speed of impulse conduction.

Synapses are those places of special attachment of a neuron to another neuron or to an effector (muscle or gland). Most synapses are **chemical synapses** in which a chemical (neurotransmitter) is utilized in the mechanism to transmit an action potential from one cell to another. Another synapse type is the **electrical synapse,** which is basically a gap junction or nexus through which ions can pass readily and with virtually no loss of speed. In some cases the two are combined in **conjoint synapses.**

The neuron part that delivers the impulse to the synapse is the presynaptic terminal, and the part receiving the impulse is the **postsynaptic terminal.** The presynaptic terminal is usually an axon terminal that is somewhat expanded and called an **end bulb.** The cell membranes of pre- and postsynaptic elements that are directly involved in the synapse are modified and show thickenings. The space between the pre- and postsynaptic membranes is the **synaptic cleft,** which is 20 to 30 nm wide.

Synapses can be classified on the basis of their position on the postsynaptic neuron. The major ones are **axodendritic, axosomatic,** and **axoaxonic.** The axon terminal of the presynaptic neuron typically has numerous mitochondria and synaptic vesicles. The **synaptic vesicles** are typically spherical and have a diameter of 40 to 50 nm. Following fixation, some vesicles become flattened and others come to have a dense core. It was thought for some time that the flattened ones contain inhibitory transmitters and that the dense core ones contain catecholamines. However, these criteria seem not to be reliable enough to make these assumptions.

Synapses may have **symmetrical** or **asymmetric** appearances. Asymmetric are found in the axodendritic synapses. The synaptic cleft is 30 nm across. The asymmetry is due to the fact that the thickening of the postsynaptic membrane is thicker than that of the presynaptic membrane. The symmetrical synapse has a narrow synaptic cleft (20 nm), and the pre- and postsynaptic membranes are about equal in their densities.

Numerous neurotransmitters have been identified. Some are excitatory and some inhibitory. When an action potential reaches the end bulb of the presynaptic axon, the sodium channels in the membrane open and there is an influx of Na^+ from outside to inside the end bulb. This is immediately followed by opening of the potassium channels in the presynaptic membrane so that K^+ can pass from within the end bulb to the extracellular space. The presynaptic membrane also has calcium channels, which open briefly so that there is an influx of Ca^{2+}. Negative charges on the inner surface of the presynaptic membrane prevent the synaptic vesicles from fusing with the membrane, thus preventing the passage of neurotransmitter into the synaptic cleft. The Ca^{2+} reduces these negative charges, and the vesicles fuse with the membrane and by exocytosis release the neurotransmitter into the cleft.

The neurotransmitter released into the synaptic cleft reacts with neurotransmitter receptors in the postsynaptic membrane and elicits electrical responses. Excitatory neurotransmitters depolarize the postsynaptic membrane, and inhibitory neurotransmitters hyperpolarize this membrane. Whether the postsynaptic cell generates impulses depends on the summation of all the excitatory and inhibitory input it receives.

The fusion of synaptic vesicles with the presynaptic membrane obviously adds a great deal of membrane to the end bulb. This is accommodated by a recycling mechanism that utilizes endocytosis and involves what are called coated vesicles. Norepinephrine is also taken up in this process so that it can be used again. Other transmitters such as ACh are manufactured within the end bulb from precursors made in the cell body and transported along the axon.

Shortly after birth, all the neurons that are going to form have done so. Thus, injury to neurons can have only two possible results—regeneration of the injured neuron or death of that cell with no replacement. Regeneration of neurons in the PNS is common and enjoys a good rate of success. This is not true within the CNS. If a peripheral nerve is cut, it can be sutured together again with afferents and efferents going to appropriate tissues. The further away from the neuron cell bodies (the CNS) that the lesion occurs, the better the regeneration and return of function. Within the CNS, regeneration is limited and generally ineffective. An exception is the hypothalamohypophyseal tracts of neurosecretory fibers. A factor that makes regeneration within the PNS much better than in the CNS is that the former has endoneurial sheaths lined with Schwann cells and their basement membranes, and collectively these greatly enhance regeneration. There is nothing comparable in the CNS. Where regeneration does not occur, some compensation is achieved by collateral sprouting of surviving axons. These new collaterals form in response to the injury and seek out the receptor sites on the denervated cells.

SPINAL CORD ORGANIZATION

The spinal cord has a generally uniform organization throughout. The gray matter lies within a covering of white matter and is divided into dorsal horn gray (also called dorsal gray columns) and ventral horn gray (ventral gray columns). The dorsal gray is functionally related to sensory and association pathways; the ventral gray is related to motor function. At the junction of the dorsal and ventral gray is an area called lateral gray or intermediate gray or intermediolateral gray matter.

The gray matter of the spinal cord contains specific aggregations of neurons that comprise nuclei. In the past, some of these have been named and their identity understood. Examples of these nuclei are the nucleus dorsalis (Clarke's nucleus or Clarke's column), the substantia gelatinosa, and the nucleus proprius cornu dorsalis. Another system for identifying parts of the spinal cord gray matter identifies ten layers. After the individual who developed this system, Bror Rexed, they are now known as **Rexed laminae**. These laminae are based on the cytoarchitecture of the gray matter and appear to be consistent throughout the spinal cord. These laminae are designated by Roman numerals.

Lamina I. (This corresponds to the posteromarginal nucleus.) This is a thin layer of gray matter forming the most dorsal part of the dorsal horn gray. The thin fibers of the dorsal root terminate here and in the adjacent part of lamina II. Lamina II fibers also terminate in lamina I. The primary sensory fibers end axodendritically; those from lamina II end axosomatically. Lamina I is related to nociceptive and thermal stimuli. Whether lamina I neurons contribute a small number of fibers to the spinothalamic tract is controversial. That tract arises very largely from lamina V.

Lamina II. (This corresponds to the substantia gelatinosa of Rolando.) This lies ventral to lamina I, which covers it dorsally and dorsolaterally. The lamina is bordered medially by the dorsal funiculus. It is especially large in the enlargements of the cord. Fibers that terminate in lamina II travel in the dorsolateral fasciculus (Lissauer's tract), dorsal funiculus, and lateral funiculus. They include very small fibers, both myelinated and unmyelinated. Functional descriptions of the fibers terminating here indicate nociceptive, thermal, and mechanoreceptors. Projections from this lamina include those into the dorsolateral fasciculus, commissural fibers to the contralateral lamina II, to the lateral fasciculus proprius. Fibers from this lamina do not contribute to the long tracts. The function seems to be to modulate synaptic transmission from primary sensory neurons to secondary sensory systems. Lamina II neurons exert their synaptic influences on cells in lamina III and IV. Opiate receptors are highly concentrated in laminae I and II. There are high concentrations of substance P in these laminae, and this is typically found in areas receiving sensory afferents. Substance P has an excitatory role in central transmission of impulses associated with pain, and its release is presynaptically inhibited by enkephalin.

Lamina III. This lies parallel to lamina II. Dendritic arborizations extend into lamina I, II, IV, V. Axons form dense plexuses in laminae III and IV. These are interneurons that transmit incoming impulses to laminae that contain cells of origin of sensory tracts. Primary afferent fibers are intermediate to thick myelinated fibers.

Lamina IV. (Lamina III and IV correspond to the nucleus proprius dorsalis cornu.) Dendrites radiate up into lamina II and also receive many primary afferents. This lamina may contribute a few fibers to the spinothalamic tract, but most neurons seem to function as interneurons. Note: Laminae I, II, III, and IV in the rostral end of the cervical spinal cord merge with the spinal nucleus of the trigeminal.

Lamina V. This lamina has many large cells from which a majority of the fibers of the anterolateral system (e.g., spinothalamic tract) arise. Dendrites radiate into lamina II. Primary sensory fibers, other laminae neurons' axons, and the long descending tracts, especially the lateral corticospinal and the rubrospinal tracts, all synapse on these neurons. These long descending tracts also terminate in several other laminae.

Lamina VI. This is present only in the cord enlargements. It seems to be related to sensory data that originate in deep structures such as muscles.

Lamina VII. This is distinctive in that it is the largest of all the laminae. It occupies the intermediate zone between the dorsal and ventral horns and most of the ventral horn. The neurons present function as interneurons, but many have long axons that extend to other cord segments. Long descending tracts terminate here. Four specific nuclear groups are part of this lamina—(1) intermediolateral cell column (preganglionic sympathetics in segments T1–L2 or L3); (2) intermediomedial cell column (exists through the cord, receives primary afferents, and is related to visceral reflexes); (3) nucleus dorsalis (Clarke's column) (present from C8 through L3 and gives rise to the dorsal spinocerebellar tract); and (4) the sacral autonomic nucleus (parasympathetic preganglionic neurons in segments S2–4).

Lamina VIII. Many descending fibers terminate here, especially those of the vestibulospinal and reticulospinal tracts. Axons of neurons here project bilaterally to the same or nearby segmental levels to laminae VII and IX.

Lamina IX. These neurons lie within laminae VII or VIII. The neurons here include alpha and gamma motor neurons plus many small neurons that project up and down the cord for some distance in the fasciculus proprius.

Lamina X. This surrounds the central canal and consists of decussating axons, glia, and small interneurons. Some dorsal root fibers synapse here.

The white matter of the spinal cord lies in three **funiculi** on each side. Dorsally, between the midline and the dorsolateral sulcus (where the dorsal root fibers attach), is the **dorsal funiculus**. Laterally, between dorsolateral and ventrolateral (where the ventral roots attach) sulci, is the **lateral funiculus**. Ventrally, between the anterior median fissure and the ventrolateral sulcus, is the **ventral funiculus**. A funiculus is a large bundle of fibers that may be composed of relatively discrete groups of fibers that have specific origin, course, termination, and function (e.g., the lateral corticospinal tract).

The dorsal funiculus is rather homogeneous in its makeup. It consists largely of the ascending fibers that function in proprioception, fine touch, stereognosis, etc. Below the level of the sixth thoracic spinal cord segment, the dorsal funiculus is a single, large bundle of axons whose cell bodies lie in the ipsilateral dorsal root ganglia. These fibers form most of the dorsal funiculus below T6, and they are referred to as the **fasciculus gracilis**. They are destined to synapse in the **nucleus gracilis**, which lies in the caudal portion of the medulla oblongata. The fibers of the fasciculus gracilis are somatotopically organized such that those of the most caudal segments are the most medial within the fasciculus, and as additional fibers enter the cord from the more cranial dorsal root ganglia, they build up laterally as the fasciculus is observed extending to the medulla. Above segment T6, this same rule applies; but the fibers entering from dorsal root ganglia above this level are separated from the fasciculus gracilis by the dorsal intermediate sulcus and septum. The fibers of segments above T6 then form a separate fasciculus, the **fasciculus cuneatus**. These fibers ascend to the medulla, where they synapse in the **nucleus cuneatus**, which lies lateral and a little rostral to the nucleus gracilis. These two fasciculi are called the **dorsal columns**, and the two nuclei are the **dorsal column nuclei**.

The lateral funiculus contains numerous discrete fiber bundles, some of which are ascending (sensory) tracts and others descending (motor) tracts. In the dorsal portion of the lateral funiculus, adjacent to the dorsal horn gray matter, are two tracts that overlap considerably—the lateral corticospinal and the rubrospinal tracts. These are motor tracts, and their name indicates where they start and where they terminate. In the lateral portion of the lateral funiculus, underlying the surface of the cord, are the **dorsal spinocerebellar tract** and the **ventral spinocerebellar tract**. The dorsal tract originates in the ipsilateral nucleus dorsalis (Clarke's nucleus or column), ascends the length of the cord to the medulla, and then extends into the cerebellum via the inferior cerebellar peduncle. This tract is not seen below segment L3 because Clarke's nucleus extends from C8 to L3.

In the more ventral portion of the lateral funiculus are tracts that in some cases also lie somewhat in the ventral funiculus. The ascending tracts include the spino-olivary, spinotectal, spinothalamic, and spinoreticular. Taking some liberties, these can all be lumped together in the **anterolateral system** of ascending pathways. Those that are destined to reach consciousness must go to the thalamus, but along the way many axons terminate or collateralize into the olivary nuclei, the reticular formation, and the tectum (of mesencephalon). The descending tracts include the **medial longitudinal fasciculus, ventral corticospinal, tectospinal, interstitiospinal, solitariospinal, pontine reticulospinal, medullary reticulospinal,** and (lateral) **vestibulospinal**. The names indicate origin and termination. The specifics of these will be covered later. Tables 1-5 and 1-6 summarize the long tracts of the spinal cord.

BRAIN-STEM ORGANIZATION

Understanding the organization of the spinal cord is basic to understanding the remainder of the CNS. Think of the brain stem (the mesencephalon, pons, and medulla oblongata) as a rostral continuation of the spinal cord with the same organization upon which have been superimposed additional structures. This helps to understand the brain stem more readily. Here a review of the development can be particularly useful.

Medulla oblongata

In the caudal portion lie the dorsal column nuclei, the **nucleus gracilis** and **nucleus cuneatus** (see above). The fasciculi gracilis and cuneatus terminate in these nuclei. From these nuclei, axons form an arc-shaped bundle of fibers (on each side) that course ventrally and are called the **internal arcuate fibers**. The internal arcuate fibers decussate (**decussation of the medial lemniscus**) and turn rostrally as the **medial lemnicus**. These fibers are destined to terminate in the **ventral posterolateral nucleus** of the thalamus. The impulses project from the thalamus to the primary sensory cortex. Lateral and somewhat rostral to the nucleus cuneatus is the **accessory cuneate nucleus**. This receives input from the ipsilateral upper limb and then projects to the cerebellum via the inferior cerebellar peduncle.

Immediately ventral and rostral to the dorsal column nuclei are the **hypoglossal nucleus, dorsal motor nucleus of the vagus, nucleus solitarius, vestibular and cochlear nuclei,** and the **spinal nucleus of the trigeminal**. The physical relationships of these nuclei have been described in the section on development (see above). Lying deeper, within the tegmentum, is the **nucleus ambiguus**. Although difficult to identify without special techniques and efforts, the **inferior salivatory nucleus** (IX) extends rostrally from the dorsal motor nucleus of cranial nerve X; and the inferior salivatory nucleus blends into the **superior salivatory nucleus** (VII) as the pons is approached. Other nuclei include the distinctive inferior olivary nucleus and the accessory olivary nuclei. Numerous

Table 1-5. Major Long Ascending Tracts in the Spinal Cord

Tract	Primary neuron	Secondary neuron	Tertiary neuron	Function
Dorsal column/medial lemniscus Fasciculus gracilis	DRG, below T6; axons ascend ipsilaterally as fasciculus gracilis	Nucleus gracilis; axons form interior arcuate, which decussate and ascend contralateral as medial lemniscus	VPL nucleus of thalamus; axons project through internal capsule to cortical areas 3, 1, 2	Proprioception, fine touch for lower trunk, pelvis, lower limb
Fasciculus cuneatus	DRGs above T6; axons ascend ipsilaterally as fasciculus cuneatus	Nucleus cuneatus; axons same as for gracilis	Same as above	Proprioception, fine touch for upper trunk, pectoral girdle, upper limb, neck
Anterolateral system Spinothalamic Spinotectal Spinoreticular Spino-olivary	DRGs of all spinal nerves; axons enter via dorsal roots, synapse within dorsal gray of adjacent segments of cord	Dorsal horn gray; axons arise from Rexed laminae I and V, cross in anterior white commissure and ascend contralateral as anterolateral system, which contains all these tracts	In nuclei indicated by second portion of name. Spinothalamic goes to VPL nucleus of thalamus, which projects to cortical areas 3, 1, 2	Pain/temperature, crude touch
Dorsal spinocerebellar	DRGs of thoracic, lumbar, sacral nerves; axons ascend ipsilaterally whatever distance necessary to reach nucleus dorsalis (C8–L3)	Nucleus dorsalis (Clarke's); projects ipsilaterally as dorsal spinocerebellar tract up cord, into medulla, and through inferior cerebellar peduncle into cerebellum	Cerebellar nuclei and cortex	Unconscious proprioception to cerebellum for trunk and lower limb
Ventral spinocerebellar	DRGs of lumbar and sacral nerves; axons synapse in gray matter Rexed laminae V, VI, VII	Rexed laminae V, VI, VII; axons cross in anterior white commissure to ascend as dorsal spinocerebellar to level of superior cerebellar peduncle, into cerebellum, within which fibers cross again	Cerebellar nuclei and cortex	Unconscious proprioception to cerebellum for lower limb
Cuneocerebellar	DRGs of cervical nerves; axons ascend ipsilaterally in dorsal funiculus into medulla to accessory cuneate nucleus	Accessory cuneate nucleus, which projects via inferior cerebellar peduncle into cerebellum	Cerebellar nuclei and cortex	Unconscious proprioception to cerebellum for pectoral girdle, upper limb, neck

DRGs, dorsal root ganglia; VPL, ventral posterolateral.

Table 1-6. Major Long Descending Tracts in the Spinal Cord

Tract	Origin	Decussation	Termination	Function
Lateral corticospinal	Cortical areas 6, 4, 3-1-2	Pyramidal decussation at medulla/spinal cord junction	Rexed laminae IV, V, VI, VII, IX	All skeletal muscle groups, but most importantly on distal limb musculature; fine digital movements
Anterior corticospinal	Same as for lateral	Ipsilateral to cord segment of termination where some fibers cross	Medial portion of ventral horn gray	Axial musculature
Rubrospinal	Red nucleus	Ventral tegmental decussation	Clinically this is now unimportant and may not extend more than into cranial end of cervical cord	Dorsolateral motor system; some allege it innervates girdle and proximal limb musculature
Pontine reticulospinal	Nuclei reticularis pontine oralis and caudalis	Uncrossed; descends in MLF	Ventromedial part of ventral horn gray (Rexed laminae VII, VIII)	Movements not related to dexterity or maintenance of balance
Medullary reticulospinal	Nucleus reticularis gigantocellularis	Bilateral	Rexed laminae VII, IX	Same as pontine
Tectospinal	Superior colliculus	Dorsal tegmental decussation; descends in MLF	Ventral horn gray of cervical cord	Head movements for fixation of gaze
Medial vestibulospinal	Medial vestibular nucleus	Bilateral (more ipsilaterally); descends in MLF through cervical spinal cord	Cervical cord ventral horn gray	Head movements related to equilibrium
Lateral vestibulospinal	Lateral vestibular nucleus	Uncrossed; descends in anterior funiculus through entire length of spinal cord	Rexed laminae VII, VIII, IX throughout cord	Maintenance of upright posture

MLF, medial longitudinal fasciculus.

reticular formation nuclei lie within the reticular formation, which is a mixture of white and gray matter that forms the core of the tegmentum of all the brain stem. These nuclei are important in many functions of the CNS, including maintenance of consciousness, sleep, motor function, cerebellar function, sensory function, etc.

Organized fibers in the medulla include the following:

Medial lemniscus. (See above.)

Medial longitudinal fasciculus. This extends from the rostral end of the mesencephalon into the spinal cord at least as far as the thoracic segments. It is a composite of ascending and descending fibers. The ascending fibers are those that arise in the vestibular nuclei and course rostrally to nuclei of cranial nerves III, IV, and VI to coordinate eye movements in response to vestibular input. The descending fibers include pontine reticulospinal, tectospinal, medial vestibulospinal, and interstitiospinal tracts.

Spinal tract of V. This begins halfway up the pons and

descends down through the medulla and into the upper few segments of the spinal cord. Throughout its extent the **spinal nucleus of V** lies medial to it, and it is in this nucleus that the fibers of the tract synapse. The tract's axons arise from the sensory ganglia of V, VII, IX, and X. The last three provide some cutaneous innervation to the external ear. The axons arising from neurons in the nucleus cross the midline and ascend contralaterally as the **ventral trigeminothalamic tract** to synapse in the **ventral posteromedial nucleus** of the thalamus, which in turn projects to primary sensory cortex. The spinal tract and nucleus of V convey pain, temperature, and crude touch impulses.

Ventral trigeminothalamic tract. (See above.)

Inferior cerebellar peduncle. This massive bundle of fibers extends from the medulla into the cerebellum. Most of these fibers are afferents of the cerebellum, but some cerebellar efferents are also in this structure. Fibers that make up this peduncle include the dorsal spinocerebellar tract, cuneocerebellar tract (from the accessory cuneate nucleus), olivo-cerebellar tract (the largest single component, arising from the contralateral inferior olivary nucleus), vestibulocerebellar fibers, and reticulocerebellar. Efferents in this peduncle include flocculonodular efferents and fastigial nucleus projection fibers.

Central tegmental tract. This descriptive name indicates that these fibers lie within the central tegmentum from the upper mesencephalon to the inferior olivary nucleus. This is a discrete bundle that contains descending and ascending fibers. The descending arise from the midbrain periaqueductal gray, the midbrain reticular formation, and the red nucleus. These fibers terminate ipsilaterally in the inferior olivary nucleus. The ascending fibers originate in the reticular formation nuclei and ascend to the thalamus and hypothalamus. The ascending fibers carry a great volume of sensory information to the diencephalon, which is utilized somewhat in limbic function but whose main function has to do with sleep and consciousness. Should this tract be lesioned bilaterally, the individual would be comatose. It is this system upon which general anesthetics act. These fibers provide for wakefulness and alertness.

Spinothalamic tract. This tract is the portion of the anterolateral system that remains discrete and can be followed all the way to the ventral posterolateral nucleus of the thalamus. It carries the impulses for pain, temperature, and crude touch from the contralateral side of the body.

Dorsal spinocerebellar tract. This is an ipsilateral pathway that arises from Clarke's nucleus in the spinal cord and conveys sensory input to the cerebellum from the lower trunk and limb by passing through the inferior cerebellar peduncle.

Ventral spinocerebellar tract. This is a smaller tract that proceeds up through the brain stem to the level where it can pass into the superior cerebellar peduncle.

Pons

Two levels of the pons, a portion of the brain stem, contain the significant, landmark structures. The caudal portion of the pons contains the **abducens nucleus** and the **facial motor nucleus.** The abducens lies in the typical GSE location—that is, in the floor of the rhomboid fossa immediately lateral to the median sulcus. Its location is seen readily in the rhomboid fossa because the axons projecting from the facial motor nucleus course dorsally and medially and loop over the abducens nucleus. This causes a bulge in the floor of the rhomboid fossa, and this is the **facial colliculus**—the abducens nucleus over which pass fibers of cranial nerve VII. This loop or bend of the facial fibers is labeled the internal genu of the facial nerve. The facial motor nucleus, being SVE, lies in the center of the pontine tegmentum at this level.

The other landmark level of the pons is in the middle of its rostrocaudal dimension. It is here that the trigeminal nerve attaches to the brain stem at the middle of the middle cerebellar peduncle, which overlies the lateral side of the pons. At this level, the trigeminal fibers pass into (or out of) the pons, and lying lateral to these fibers is the **chief** (principal, main) **sensory nucleus of V.** Medial to the fibers is the **motor nucleus of V.** The main sensory nucleus serves for fine touch (two-point discrimination, etc.) for the ipsilateral face. The motor nucleus of V supplies skeletal muscles of mastication (medial and lateral pterygoids, temporalis, and masseter) plus the anterior digastric, mylohyoid, tensor veli palatini, and the tensor tympani. From this level, the **mesencephalic nucleus of V** extends cranially through the pons and well into the mesencephalon. This nucleus is GSA (proprioception for skeletal muscles and joints supplied by cranial nerves). From this level, the **spinal nucleus of V** courses caudally through the lower half of the pons, all through the medulla, and into the upper several segments of the cervical spinal cord. This nucleus (GSA) serves the sensory modalities of pain, temperature, and crude touch for ipsilateral face structures derived from ectoderm and innervated by cranial nerves V, VII, IX, and X.

Other nuclei of the pons include the various reticular formation nuclei. These are involved in descending pathways (pontine reticulospinal tract) and the ascending fibers of the central tegmental tract. The most remarkable group of nuclei are those found in the basis pontis— the pontine gray (nuclei). This large amount of gray matter is broken up into a multitude of nuclei by the great number of fibers passing longitudinally (corticopontine, corticobular, and corticospinal) and transversely (pontocerebellar) within the pons. The corticobulbar and corticospinal tracts are motor tracts that supply cortical input to the cranial nerve motor nuclei and spinal cord, respectively. The pontocerebellar fibers arise from the pontine gray, cross to the contralateral side, and pass into the cerebellum, forming the middle cerebellar peduncle. All the major lobes of the cerebral cortex project ipsilaterally to the pontine nuclei via the crura cerebri. Thus, the corticopontocerebellar pathway is formed. This facilitates a massive cerebral cortex input to the cerebellum. Other fiber bundles seen in the pons are the medial longitudinal fasciculus, medial lemniscus, spinothalamic tract, ventral trigeminothalamic tract, and lateral lemniscus. The latter is the auditory pathway. The cochlear nuclei (of the medulla) and various auditory pathway-associated nuclei form the lateral lemniscus, which courses up through the pons and terminates in the inferior colliculus of the mesencephalon.

Mesencephalon

This portion of the brain stem has two readily apparent levels. The dorsum of the midbrain is formed by the **tectum,** which is composed of the paired **superior** and **inferior colliculi.** Over the **cerebral aqueduct,** these form a roof that passes through the midbrain and connects the third ventricle with the fourth ventricle. The superior colliculi function as a visual reflex center, the inferior as an auditory reflex center. The **tegmentum** of the midbrain at the inferior colliculus level contains the **trochlear nuclei,** which lie ventromedial to the aqueduct. Also at this level is the **decussation of the superior cerebellar peduncles.** The lateral lemniscus terminates in the inferior colliculus. At the superior colliculus level are the **oculomotor nuclei** and the **red nuclei.** The oculomotor nucleus has two parts— the GSE main oculomotor nucleus for innervation of five extraocular muscles (all but the lateral rectus and superior oblique) and the GVE accessory oculomotor nucleus (of Edinger-Westphal), which supplies the smooth muscle of the ciliary body and the iridial sphincter muscle. The Edinger-Westphal nucleus does not follow the general rule of lying dorsolateral to the GSE nucleus, but rather lies dorsomedial to it. The red nucleus receives a large amount of input from the nucleus interpositus of the cerebellum via the superior cerebellar peduncle and in turn projects contralaterally to the spinal cord as the **rubrospinal tract**. This tract is not well defined in humans, and some deny its importance if not indeed its existence. The red nucleus also projects ipsilaterally in the central tegmental tract to the inferior olivary nucleus.

Other prominent structures are found in both superior and inferior collicular levels. These are the central tegmental tract, substantia nigra, reticular formation, crura cerebri, medial longitudinal fasciculus, ventral trigeminothalamic tract, and spinothalamic tract.

Table 1-7 summarizes the brain-stem nuclei and their connections.

Cerebellum

The three lobes of the cerebellum are the flocculonodular, posterior, and anterior. The cerebellum has two fissures: the primary fissure is located between the anterior and posterior lobes, and the posterolateral (dorsolateral) is between the posterior and flocculonodular lobes.

Cortex. The cortex contains molecular, Purkinje, and granule cell layers. The afferent fibers are mossy (all except those arising from the olivary nuclei) and climbing (the latter from the olivary nuclear group). The locus ceruleus sends unmyelinated aminergic fibers via the superior cerebellar peduncles into the molecular layer and uses norepinephrine as the neurotransmitter. The raphe nuclei of the reticular formation project to the cortex and use serotonergic neurotransmitters. Norepinephrine and serotonin may have opposing actions to modulate excitatory action of glutamate on Purkinje cells, with norepinephrine-enhancing and serotonin-reducing excitatory action of glutamate on Purkinje cells.

Granule cells. These cells have short dendrites with claw-like endings that synapse with mossy fibers and unmyelinated axons that extend into the molecular layer, bifurcate, and course along parallel to the folium (**parallel fibers**) to synapse with 450 Purkinje cells' dendrites (as well as stellate, basket [250], and Golgi cells). Mossy fibers branch within the white matter, extend into one or more folia, lose their myelin, branch more, and end in swellings called **rosettes,** with which several granule cells' dendrites make synaptic contact.

Glomeruli are formed in this layer, and they are synaptic complexes involving rosettes of mossy fibers, the claw-like terminals of granule cells' dendrites, and axon terminals of Golgi cells.

Purkinje cells. There are approximately 15,000,000 of these cells. They have remarkably branched dendritic trees that are oriented transversely to the folia. Primary and secondary branches are smooth, but the others have spines. Many granule cells' axons make synaptic contact with a single Purkinje cell. Purkinje cell axons are the only ones that leave the cortex, and they terminate mainly in deep cerebellar nuclei (some exceptions are those in the flocculonodular lobe). Axon collaterals synapse on other Purkinje cells, but even more on the Golgi cells. Climbing fibers (from the olivary nuclear group) extend to dendritic branches of Purkinje cells to synapse on smooth surfaces.

Basket cells. These lie within the molecular layer. The dendrites are arranged transversely within the folium, with numerous synapses with parallel fibers. Axons extend across the folium and synapse with about 250 Purkinje cells in a basket-like arrangement around the cell bodies, making synapses on axon hillocks.

Stellate cells. Parallel fibers synapse on their dendrites, and axons synapse mainly on Purkinje cell dendrites, but some synapse on granule cells.

Golgi cells. The dendrites extend into the molecular layer and synapse on parallel fibers. Purkinje axon collaterals synapse on these cells. Golgi cell axons enter the rosettes to synapse on granule cell dendrites.

Mossy and climbing fibers all are excitatory. Granule cells are the only cortical cells that are excitatory; all other cortical cells are inhibitory, including the Purkinje cells. That means that all cerebellar cortical output is inhibitory. Glutamate is probably the common neurotransmitter.

Central nuclei. Four nuclei are described: fastigial, globose, emboliform, and dentate. In humans, the globose and emboliform are considered as a single nucleus, the nucleus interpositus.

Afferents consist of Purkinje axons (gaba [−]), mossy fibers, climbing fibers (from olivary nuclear complex), pontocerebellar, reticulocerebellar, spinocerebellar, rubrocerebellar (to interpositus), and vestibulocerebellar (to fastigial) fibers. **Efferents** extend from the fastigial nuclei via the inferior cerebellar peduncle, and from the other nuclei via the superior cerebellar peduncle.

Inferior cerebellar peduncle. **Afferents** consist of the olivocerebellar, dorsal spinocerebellar, cuneocerebellar, primary and secondary vestibulocerebellar, trigeminocerebellar, arcuatocerebellar, and reticulocerebellar fibers. **Efferents** extend from the flocculonodular lobe and fastigial nuclei.

Middle cerebellar peduncle. This structure is composed entirely of pontocerebellar fibers.

Superior cerebellar peduncle. **Afferents** are the ventral spinocerebellar tract, locus ceruleus, red nucleus, and mesencephalic nucleus of V. **Efferents** are from all the deep nuclei **other** than fastigial.

Cerebellar subdivisions

Subdivisions of the cerebellum are as follows: **archicerebellum** = flocculonodular lobe + uvula of the vermis; **paleocerebellum** = vermis in anterior lobe + part of the vermis in the posterior lobe; **neocerebellum** = cerebellar hemispheres + the superior vermis of the posterior lobe; **vestibulocerebellum** = archicerebellum; **spinocerebellum** = paleocerebellum + medial parts of the hemispheres (receives spino- and cuneocerebellar fibers); **pontocerebellum** = lateral parts of the hemispheres + the superior vermis of the posterior lobe.

Vestibulocerebellum

Afferents are from the ipsilateral vestibular ganglion and nuclei and the accessory olivary nuclei via the inferior peduncle to the fastigial nuclei and cortex. **Efferents** include fibers of Purkinje cells that project to the brain stem, others to the fastigial nuclei; fibers to the vestibular nuclei and central group of reticular nuclei from the uncinate fasciculus (of Russell)—fibers leave one fastigial nucleus, cross the midline, pass through other fastigial nucleus, curve over the root of superior peduncle, and join other efferent fibers. Efferents influence motor neurons via the vestibulospinal tracts, the medial longitudinal fasciculus, and the reticulospinal tracts.

Table 1-7. Brain-Stem Nuclei and Their Connections

Nucleus	Principal afferents	Efferents and termination	Function	Deficit
Superior colliculus	Brachium of superior colliculus (primary retinal fibers and corticotectal fibers from visual cortices) Inferior colliculus Anterolateral system fibers	Tectospinal tract to cross and synapse in cervical cord gray Tectobulbar tract to motor nuclei of cranial nerves	For light reflexes, auditory reflexes to effect changes in head position Reflex actions of head structures in response to threatening movements of objects toward eye and to loud or unpleasant sound	Loss of indicated reflexes
		To pretectum and III nuclear complex	Involved in light and accommodation reflexes	
			Somatic input (via anterolateral system) is very large. This nucleus functions in some of the reflexes that are involved in reactions to pain, etc.	
Oculomotor nuclei	Bilateral corticobulbar fibers Bilateral pretectal and superior colliculus input (using the posterior commissure)	III GSE	Extrinsic eye muscles except superior oblique, lateral rectus, orbicularis oculi	Eye is abducted, slightly depressed position
		III GVE (Edinger-Westphal)	Ciliary body muscle and iridial sphincter	Mydriasis Loss of light and accommodation reflexes
Red	Superior cerebellar peduncle 1. Dentatorubro-thalamic 2. Interpositusrubro	VL, VA thalamic nucleus Rubrospinal (crossed) tract (also rubrobulbar) CTT (ipsilaterally) to inferior olivary nucleus	Part of cerebellorubro projection to thalamus to motor and premotor cerebral cortex Rubrospinal tract in humans represents most of dorsolateral portion of motor system and accompanies lateral corticospinal and excites flexors Input to inferior olivary nucleus is important feedback into cerebellum	Cerebellar signs Seldom an isolated lesion, but would contribute to signs of corticospinal loss

Table 1-7. Brain-Stem Nuclei and Their Connections (continued)

Nucleus	Principal afferents	Efferents and termination	Function	Deficit
				Cerebellar signs (however, if CTTs involved, the problems other than this tract would be of much greater import than cerebellar dysfunction)
Substantia nigra	Striatonigral	Nigrostriatal and projection to VA, VL nuclei	Basal ganglion function	Motor dysfunction— paralysis agitans (parkinsonism) and chorea
Medial geniculate body	Brachium of inferior colliculus, cortico-fugal fibers from association auditory cortex	Auditory thalamo-cortico tract (infralenticular portion of internal capsule) to areas 41, 42 (Heschl's gyri or transverse temporal gyri)	Audition	Bilateral hearing loss
Inferior colliculus	Lateral lemniscus, contralateral inferior colliculus, descending fibers via brachium of inferior colliculus	Brachium to MGB To superior colliculus	Audition Auditory reflexes Determination of direction from which sound is coming	Hearing loss, depressed reflexes
Trochlear (IV)	Bilateral corticobulbar	Contralateral IV nerve	Superior oblique muscle	Intorsion of eye, vertical diplopia, inability to depress adducted eye
Mesencephalic of V	These are primary neurons and thus have no PNS afferents	To various motor nuclei of cranial nerves, e.g., V for jaw jerk Rostrally to thalamus via unidentified pathway for ultimate projection of impulses to cortex	Proprioception of head structures supplied by cranial nerves	Presumably depressed proprioception function of head structures
Pontine nuclei	Corticopontine (ipsilateral)	Pontocerebellar fibers cross to form contralateral middle cerebellar peduncle	Part of pathway for enormous cortical input to cerebellum	Cerebellar dysfunction
Chief sensory nucleus of V	Trigeminal ganglion (plus GSA fibers from ganglia of VII, IX, X)	Dorsal trigemino-thalamic tract ipsilaterally Ventral trigemino-thalamic tract contralaterally	Discriminative touch of ipsilateral face	Loss of discriminative touch as indicated

Table 1-7. Brain-Stem Nuclei and Their Connections (continued)

Nucleus	Principal afferents	Efferents and termination	Function	Deficit
		Ascending fibers end in VPM, impulses projected to primary sensory cortex		
Spinal nucleus of V	Spinal tract of V (from neurons in trigeminal ganglion (plus GSA from ganglia of VII, IX, X)	Contralateral ventral trigeminothalamic tract to VPM thalamic nucleus	Pain and temperature for ipsilateral head	Ipsilateral loss of pain and temperature to head
Vestibular	Primary vestibular fibers Cerebellum	Ascend bilaterally in MLF to III, IV, VI Juxtarestiform body to cerebellum— flocculonodular lobe	Vestibular coordination of eye movements Cerebellar/vestibular equilibrium function	Loss of equilibrium, visual coordination
		Medial vestibulospinal tract to cervical cord in MLF (mostly ipsilaterally)	Head position	
		Lateral vestibulospinal tract (ipsilateral) throughout cord	Excite extensors of body (the antigravity muscles)	
Abducens (VI)	Bilateral corticobulbar	Cranial nerve VI	Lateral rectus muscle of the eye; turns eye laterally	Eye becomes adducted and cannot be moved
Facial motor (VII)	Bilateral corticobulbar to portion supplying orbicularis oculi muscle and above Only contralateral corticobulbar to the portion supplying muscles below the eye	Cranial nerve VII	Muscles of facial expression	Facial paralysis
Cochlear (dorsal and ventral)	Primary cochlear fibers	Contralateral inferior colliculus and the several intervening nuclei of the auditory pathway	Audition	Ipsilateral deafness
Inferior olivary	Ipsilateral CTT (from red nucleus and periaqueductal gray) Spino-olivary Cortico-olivary ipsilaterally Vestibular nuclei ipsilaterally Contralateral dorsal column nuclei Ipsilateral solitary nucleus	Most to the contra- lateral cerebellum via inferior peduncle	Provide climbing fibers to cerebellum as a relay from most major divisions of the neuraxis	Cerebellar (motor) dysfunctions

Table 1-7. Brain-Stem Nuclei and Their Connections (continued)

Nucleus	Principal afferents	Efferents and termination	Function	Deficit
	Contralateral cerebellum			
Solitarius	GVA and SVA fibers of VII, IX, X and their respective ganglia	To reticular formation for various visceral reflexes (e.g., licking movements, lip movements in response to taste) To ipsilateral VPM for projection to cortex	General visceral and taste sensory	Loss of sensory function ipsilaterally indicated
Hypoglossal (XII)	Bilateral corticobulbar to all parts except that supplying genioglossus receives only from the contralateral cortex	XII peripheral nerve to skeletal tongue muscles ipsilateral	Tongue movement	Paralysis or paresis of tongue movement ipsilaterally Tongue will deviate toward side of affected muscle
Dorsal motor of X	Visceral motor pathways via reticular formation from hypothalamus and probably other areas	Cranial nerve X	Parasympathetic to thoracic and most of abdominal viscera	Depressed parasympathetic function
Ambiguus	Bilateral corticobulbar	Cranial nerves IX, X	Skeletal muscles of soft palate, pharynx, larynx, esophagus	Paralysis of muscles indicated
Cuneatus	Fasciculus cuneatus, which arises from ipsilateral DRGs of spinal nerves for pectoral girdle, upper limb, and neck	Internal arcuate ipsilaterally and then the contralateral medial lemniscus to VPL thalamic nucleus	Proprioception and discriminative touch for ipsilateral pectoral girdle, upper limb, neck	Loss of proprioceptive function described
Gracilis	Fasciculus gracilis, which arises from the ipsilateral DRGs of spinal nerves for lower part of trunk, pelvic girdle, lower limb	Same as cuneatus	Same as cuneatus except for ipsilateral lower limb and pelvic girdle	Loss same as seen for cuneatus

CTT, central tegmental tract; DRG, dorsal root ganglion; GSA, general somatic afferent; GSE, general somatic efferent; GVE, general visceral efferent; MGB, medial geniculate body; MLF, medial longitudinal fasciculus; PNS, peripheral nervous system; SVA, special visceral afferent; VA, ventral anterior; VL, ventrolateral; VPM, ventral posteromedial.

Spinocerebellum

Afferents of the dorsal spinocerebellar tract are from the ipsilateral trunk and leg, those of the ventral spinocerebellar tract are from the contralateral leg, and those of the cuneocerebellar tract are from the ipsilateral arm and neck. Reticular nuclei transmit cutaneous input and information from primary motor and sensory cortical areas to the cerebellum; the reticulotegmental nucleus relays information from the cerebral cortex and vestibular nuclei. All three trigeminal sensory nuclei and accessory olivary nuclei are also afferents. All these may collateralize to the nucleus interpositus. Limbs are represented along the vermis in the anterior lobe and in the medial part of the hemispheres on the inferior surface of the posterior lobe. The head area is in the superior vermis and adjacent cortex in the posterior lobe. **Efferents** are as follows: the spinocerebellar cortex projects to the fastigial nucleus (vermis) and to the interpositus (medial hemispheres). Fastigial nuclei project to the vestibular nuclei and reticular formation. The nucleus interpositus projects to the central group of reticular nuclei, some to the red nuclei, some to the ventrolateral thalamic nuclei.

Pontocerebellum

Pontocerebellar fibers project to all of the cortex except the flocculonodular lobe. Efferents project to the dentate nucleus. Dentate efferents project mainly to the ventral lateral thalamic nucleus but also to the ventral anterior thalamic nucleus. Collaterals from the dentate nucleus project to the red nucleus, and collaterals of both the dentate and interpositus nuclei synapse in the inferior olivary nuclear complex.

Additional cerebellar connections. Inferior and accessory olivary nuclei fibers project contralaterally to all parts of cortex and to the nuclei. Inferior olivary nucleus fibers project to the pontocerebellum and dentate nucleus. Accessory olivary nuclei fibers project to the spino- and vestibulocerebellum and to the other three nuclei. **Afferents** to the inferior olivary are the spino-olivary, red nucleus, and cortico-olivary fibers (from ipsilateral sensorimotor cortex). Climbing fibers carry information to the cerebellum about movements not yet performed (involved in learning?). Mossy fibers mediate execution and coordination of learned movements. Dentate nucleus neurons are active several milliseconds before those in the primary motor cortex when a movement is planned.

Visual and acoustic impulses reach the superior vermis of the posterior lobe via relays in pontine nuclei—tectopontine from the superior colliculus and corticopontine from visual and auditory cortices.

Visceral functions. Stimulation of the cerebellar cortex produces respiratory, cardiovascular, pupillary, and urinary bladder responses. These responses are sympathetic in nature when the anterior lobe is stimulated, and parasympathetic in response when the tonsils are stimulated. Impulses are probably relayed to the hypothalamus via the reticular formation.

Signs of cerebellar lesions

Signs of cerebellar lesions include ataxia, dysmetria, past-pointing, adiadochokinesia, asynergy, hypotonia, intention tremor, and nystagmus.

Summary of cerebellar connections and functions

Input to the cerebellum is either via an ipsilateral pathway or a pathway that crosses the midline twice. Lesions of the cerebellum result in ipsilateral deficits.

Spinal cord input is mainly by three tracts:

Dorsal spinocerebellar. This serves the lower limbs and most of the trunk. The first-order neurons are in the dorsal root ganglia of the thoracic, lumbar, and sacral nerves. Their central processes extend into the spinal cord and synapse in the nucleus dorsalis (Clarke's nucleus). For lower lumbar and sacral nerves, this means that the entering fibers must ascend in the dorsal funiculus to reach the segmental levels where Clarke's nucleus is present (C8 to L3). Clarke's nucleus cells project axons ipsilaterally as the dorsal spinocerebellar tract, which lies on the surface of the dorsal portion of the lateral funiculus. This pathway extends up through the spinal cord, into the medulla, and into the cerebellum via the inferior cerebellar peduncle.

Cuneocerebellar tract. The first-order neurons lie in the cervical and uppermost thoracic dorsal root ganglia. These neurons' axons enter the spinal cord, travel in the dorsal funiculus, and ascend into the medulla to synapse in the accessory cuneate nucleus. This nucleus then projects into the cerebellum via the inferior peduncle. This serves the upper limb, pectoral girdle, and neck muscles.

Ventral spinocerebellar tract. This tract is quite small in humans. It serves the lower limb. The primary cells lie in the lumbar and sacral dorsal root ganglia, and their axons synapse in laminae V, VI, and VII of these segments. The secondary axons cross the midline in the anterior white commissure and ascend contralaterally through the spinal cord, medulla, and upper pons where the fibers enter the superior cerebellar peduncle and pass into the cerebellum, within which they apparently cross the midline so as to terminate on the same side of the CNS as their cell bodies.

Brain-stem input is as follows:

Inferior olivary nucleus. This has a very large input to the cerebellum. It projects axons contralaterally to enter the cerebellum via the inferior cerebellar peduncle. Afferents of the inferior olivary nucleus are multiple, but mainly they are from fibers ascending from the spinal cord (e.g., spino-olivary and collaterals from other parts of the anterolateral system), from the midbrain (via the central tegmental tract from the red nucleus, reticular formation, and periaqueductal gray), and from the cerebral cortex (cortico-olivary fibers). This nucleus has much to do with cutaneous input, cerebellar reverberating circuits, and probably learning movements and skeletal motor function.

Pontine nuclei. These project contralaterally as the middle cerebellar peduncle. Their afferents are the millions of corticopontine fibers that arise from all four lobes of the cerebral hemispheres.

Vestibular primary and secondary fibers. Some vestibular ganglion axons pass directly into the cerebellum in the inferior peduncle. A majority of primary vestibular fibers synapse in the vestibular nuclei. These, especially the inferior vestibular nucleus, then also project to the cerebellum in the inferior peduncle.

There are numerous other smaller afferents into the cerebellum. This arrangement points up the fact that all parts of the CNS projects directly or indirectly into the cerebellum.

The **efferents** of the cerebellum include the following:

1. Flocculonodular lobe Purkinje cells project directly into the brain stem to the vestibular nuclei and some of the reticular formation gray matter. These are the exception to the rule that Purkinje cells project to the deep cerebellar nuclei.

2. Flocculonodular lobe Purkinje cells project to the fastigial nucleus. This nucleus in turn projects bilaterally into the vestibular and reticular formation nuclei via the inferior peduncle.

3. The nucleus interpositus projects via the superior peduncle to the ipsilateral red nucleus, which in turn projects ipsilaterally to the inferior olivary nucleus (central tegmental tract and contralaterally to the spinal cord—rubrospinal tract).

4. The dentate nucleus projects via the superior cerebellar peduncle to the contralateral, ventrolateral, and somewhat to the ventral anterior thalamic nuclei. These in turn project to the motor and premotor cortex.

CEREBRAL CORTEX

The cerebral cortex varies in different regions. The variations reflect developmental and functional differences. All cortical areas are referred to by Brodmann's numbers (Fig. 1-18).

The **allocortex (heterogenetic cortex)** consists of the paleopallium (olfactory) and archipallium (hippocampal).

The **neocortex (neopallium, isocortex, homogenetic)** varies from one area to another, but there is a basic six-layered plan. The neuron population is estimated to be 2.6 to 14 billion. Neuron types include pyramidal and fusiform (principal cells), stellate (granule), cells of Martinotti, and horizontal cells of Cajal (interneurons). Pyramidal cells have a range in size but included are the giant cells of Betz (area 4). Fusiform cells lie in the deepest layer. Stellate cells are the most numerous interneurons. Martinotti cells have axons perpendicular to the surface. Horizontal cells of Cajal are in the most superficial layer. Projection, commissural, and associations neurons all are found in the cortex.

Layers of cortex

Thickness ranges from 4.5 mm (area 4) to 1.5 mm (area 17). The cortex is thicker over the gyrus crest than in the sulcus. Six layers are recognizable at about 7 months gestation.

1. **Molecular layer.** This is mostly neuronal processes; dendrites (mostly of pyramidal cells) and axons are from numerous sources including the cells of Martinotti. Some horizontal cells of Cajal and a few stellate cells also populate this layer.
2. **External granular layer.** Many small pyramidal and stellate cells are found in this layer; dendrites project into the molecular layer; axons extend into the deeper cortical layer, some on into the white matter. The neurons of this layer are involved in intracortical circuitry.
3. **External pyramidal layer.** The pyramidal cells in this layer increase in size from superficial to deep; dendrites project into the molecular layer; axons extend into the

white matter as association, commissural, and projection fibers.

4. **Internal granular layer.** Here are found closely arranged stellate cells. Many axons from the thalamus terminate here; axons of the local cells synapse with dendrites passing through from layer V and VI, with other stellate cells, and with cells of Martinotti.
5. **Internal pyramidal layer.** Pyramidal cells, some stellate cells, and cells of Martinotti lie within this layer, including the giant pyramidal cells of Betz (in area 4 only).
6. **Multiform layer.** The fusiform cells predominate; axons are projection, commissural, and association fibers.

Axons within the cortex lie in **radial bands** (projection, association, commissural) coming to and from the cortex and in **tangenital bands,** which are largely afferents. Heavy layers of fibers oriented parallel to the surface form outer (layer IV) and inner (layer V) **lines of Baillarger.** Afferents from the thalamus contribute to these, especially the outer. Thus, these lines are especially prominent in sensory cortex (e.g., the line of Gennari in area 17).

Most neocortex has the described six layers (homotypical cortex), but some areas do not have all six layers and are called heterotypical cortex (e.g., visual, auditory, general sensory cortices) in which layer IV stellate cells overflow into adjacent areas and layers II through V fuse into a single layer of small cells (koniocortex or **granular cortex**). The other extreme is in area IV, where II through V fuse into a layer consisting of mainly efferent pyramidal cells (**agranular cortex**).

Ventral thalamic nuclei project into the outer line of Baillarger. Other thalamic nuclei project into layers I through III.

Functional localization in cerebral cortex

Primary somesthetic area: 3, 1, 2. Area 3 is in the posterior wall of the central sulcus; it is granular heterotypical cortex. Areas 1 and 2 are in homotypical cortex. Stimulation of these areas elicits sensory (tingling) and some motor responses. The same is true of area 4 and thus the term **sensorimotor strip.** The ventral posterior thalamic nucleus is the main source of afferents; cutaneous sensations project onto the anterior part of the area, deep sensibility projects onto the posterior part. Destruction of areas 3, 1, 2 leaves crude awareness of nociceptive stimuli, and localization is poor. Thus, there is the loss of discriminative sensory function.

Second somesthetic area. This is found in the dorsal wall of the lateral fissure and may extend onto the insula. The body is represented bilaterally, but the contralateral side predominates. The afferent fibers arise from the intralaminar (to which afferents come from the reticular formation) and posterior thalamic nuclei. No clinical disorder is described for a selective lesion here.

Somesthetic association cortex. This is mainly in the superior parietal lobule and precuneus (areas 5, 7). The afferents arise from the primary somesthetic area. This cortex integrates sensory data (e.g., identifying an object held in the hand when denied visual cues). A lesion results in loss of appreciation of the significance of sensory data—**agnosia** (tactile, astereognosis, cortical neglect [right parietal lobe]).

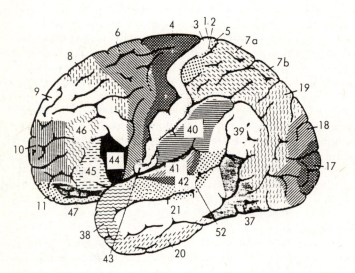

Figure 1-18. Brodmann's map.

Vision.   The primary visual cortex is area 17, which lies in the walls of the calcarine cortex. Lesion here, if complete, results in blindness. It is a thin, granular type (striate area) of cortex characterized by the lines of Gennari, which are mostly afferents from the lateral geniculate body. The association cortex is areas 18 and 19, which receive afferents from area 17. Also, there are reciprocal relationships with other areas of the cortex and with the pulvinar of the thalamus. Lesions in areas 18 and 19 result in visual agnosia. Bilateral lesion of area 19 results in visual disorientation, loss of coordination of eye movements, and inability to carry out visually guided movements of the hands.

The inferolateral surface of the temporal lobe (inferior temporal gyrus and lateral part of occipitotemporal gyrus) is also visual association cortex. It serves for storage or recall of visual memories; stimulation elicits hallucinations of scenes past; bilateral destruction of inferior portions of the temporal and occipital lobes results in **prosopagnosia,** which is impaired recognition of previously known familiar faces.

Corticotectal fibers arise from the visual cortices and project to the superior colliculus and facilitate pursuit eye movements, saccadic movements, and accommodation convergence.

Hearing.   The primary cortex lies in the ventral wall of the lateral fissure (the transverse temporal gyri of Heschl). This is areas 41 (granular heterotypical) and 42 (granular homotypical) cortex. The medial geniculate body is the main source of afferents to area 41. The association cortex lies in the floor of the lateral fissure just posterior to areas 41 and 42 (planum temporale) and area 22 (superior temporal gyrus) (**Wernicke's area**).

Taste.   This modality reaches the inferior parietal lobule posterior to the general sensory area for the mouth. The path extends from the nucleus solitarius to the parabrachial nucleus of the midbrain reticular formation and on to the ventral medial basal nucleus of thalamus to the cortex, apparently all ipsilaterally.

Vestibular cortex.   There is uncertainty as to the cortical location for this sensory function. It may be anterior and/or posterior to the primary auditory cortex.

Association cortex.   Some is specifically described as lying adjacent to the primary sensory areas in the parietal lobe and posterior temporal lobe. The anterior part of the temporal lobe seems to function for thought and memory.

Frontal cortex

The frontal cortex is responsible for motor activities, judgment and foresight, mood, and emotional tone.

The **primary motor** (area 4) is thick, agranular, and contains the giant Betz cells, which provide 30,000 (3%) of the corticospinal tract fibers. It receives input from cortical areas 6, 3, 1, and 2 and from the ventrolateral nucleus of the thalamus. It is from area 4 that 30% of the corticospinal/corticobular fibers arise. It bilaterally supplies the axial and head muscles, contralaterally the more lateral muscles, especially those of the limbs. It functions for the execution of movements.

The **secondary motor** area is ventral to the sensory motor strip in the dorsal wall of the lateral fissure (note that it overlaps with the secondary somesthetic area).

The **supplementary motor** region (part of area 6) lies on the medial surface of the hemisphere. Lesions result in paralysis and mutism.

The **premotor area** (area 6) contains no Betz cells and receives afferents from other cortical areas and the ventral anterior nucleus of the thalamus. It is programmed for skilled motor activity and directs the primary motor cortex in execution of movements.

Apraxia is the impairment of performance of learned movement in the absence of paralysis. **Agraphia** is a defect in the ability to write.

The **frontal eye field** is in the lower portion of area 8. Its loss means voluntary movement disorders, but involuntary movements (saccades, convergence) are preserved.

The **prefrontal cortex** includes association areas 9, 10, 11, and 12. This cortex has extensive connections with the other three lobes and reciprocal connections with the dorsomedial nucleus of the thalamus. The function of this cortex is related to affective reactions to the present situations on the basis of past experience. It monitors behavior and exercises control based on judgment and foresight. Stimulation of this part of the cortex elicits no motor response.

Language areas are found in the left hemisphere in the vast majority of people. The sensory language area is Wernicke's area plus the inferior parietal lobule (areas 39 and 40). The motor language center is Broca's area (areas 44 and 45). It is here that normal speech is served, but normal speech also requires the supplementary motor area. These two areas communicate via the superior longitudinal fasciculus and the arcuate fasciculus.

Aphasia is a general term for speech deficits. **Receptive aphasia** (Wernicke's) involves auditory and visual comprehension of language. Victims have trouble naming objects or repeating sentences spoken to them. **Jargon aphasia** involves Wernicke's area and the association fibers to Broca's area. The individual is fluent but unintelligible. **Conduction aphasia** results from a lesion of the arcuate fasciculus. Victims lose the ability to repeat sentences but retain relatively good comprehension and spontaneous speech. **Anomic aphasia** (isolation syndrome) occurs when the sensory language area is separated from the surrounding parietal and temporal cortex. The person is fluent, but circumlocutory speech results from word-finding difficulty. **Expressive aphasia** (Broca's aphasia) is hesitant and distorted speech with retention of relatively good comprehension. **Global aphasia** is the complete loss of ability to communicate. This results from destruction of the cortex on both sides of the lateral fissure. There is some recovery as a result of assumption of linguistic functions by the contralateral hemisphere.

Alexia is the loss of the ability to read. This may occur with or without aphasia. A lesion of the white matter of the occipital lobe of the dominant hemisphere and of the splenium affects visual cortices and the language area. **Dyslexia** is incomplete alexia.

Hemispheric dominance.   The left hemisphere is dominant in most people. Seventy percent of left-handed people still have language in the left hemisphere. The right hemisphere is involved in three-dimensional spatial perception, in singing, and in playing musical instruments.

Diencephalon

Epithalamus.   This includes the pineal body, the two habenular nuclei and the habenular commissure, and the striae medullaris thalami. The function of the pineal is still not entirely certain, but current evidence indicates that it has an antigonadotropic function. A tumor derived from parenchymatous cells can cause delayed puberty. If the tumor is such that it destroys parenchymatous cells, the result is precocious puberty.

The stria medullaris thalami (on each side) originates mostly from cells in the septal area of the telencephalon, but some contribution is made by hypothalamic neurons and the globus pallidus. These axons terminate in the habenular nuclei, and from these nuclei the habenulointerpeduncular fasciculus (fasciculus retroflexus of Meynert) arises and projects to the interpeduncular nuclei lying in the roof of the interpeduncular fossa. Via relays in the reticular formation, the interpeduncular nuclei influence neurons in the hypothalamus and preganglionic autonomic neurons.

Thalamus. Numerous nuclei are found in the thalamus, and their connections and functions are multiple (Table 1-8).

Hypothalamus. This portion of the diencephalon lies at the base of the brain. Its importance is much greater than its size, which is all of about 4 g. It lies ventral to the hypothalamic sulcus, and it has many named nuclei and myriad connections.

It is the center of the neuroendocrine axis. It is the head ganglion of the autonomic nervous system and is a major and vital component of the limbic system. In addition to its many neuronal connections, the hypothalamus responds to properties of blood that passes through it—temperature, osmotic pressure, and hormone levels. It also has hunger and satiety centers.

Hypothalamic nuclei. These can be divided into medial and lateral, with the columns of the fornix and the mamillothalamic tract serving to separate the two. The medial zone contains the **preoptic nucleus, paraventricular nucleus, dorsomedial nucleus, ventromedial nucleus, infundibular nucleus,** and **posterior nucleus.** In the lateral zone are **supraoptic, lateral nucleus, tuberomammillary,** and **lateral tuberal nuclei.**

Afferent connections. The hypothalamus is a central figure in the limbic system and as such receives afferents from the olfactory mucosa, viscera, somatic structures, cerebral cortex, and the limbic system. Major afferents are the following:

1. Visceral and somatic afferents. These arrive via collaterals of the lemniscal system and the reticular formation, and they traverse the thalamus.

Table 1-8. Thalamic Nuclei

Nuclei	Afferents	Efferents
Reticular (function uncertain)	Thalamocortical	To all other thalamic nuclei and all areas of cerebral cortex
Intralaminar nuclei (centromedian and parafascicular) (consciousness, alertness; vague awareness of painful stimuli; without discrimination but rather with emotional response)	Central nuclei of reticular formation and locus ceruleus	To extensive areas of frontal and parietal lobes To neostriatum (may have something to do with control of movements or it may be that the neostriatum has something to do with consciousness and arousal)
VPL and VPM thalamic nuclei, respectively	Spinothalamic and ventral trigeminothalamic	To cortical areas 3, 1, 2
Ventral nuclear group		
Medial geniculate body (MGB)	Inferior brachium	Auditory radiations to cortex (areas 41, 42)
Lateral geniculate body (LGB)	Optic tract	Optic radiations to cortex (area 17)
Ventral posterolateral (VPL)	Spinothalamic fibers (pain/temperature) Median lemniscus (discriminative touch)	Cortical areas 3, 1, 2
Ventral posteromedial (VPM)	Ventral and dorsal trigeminothalamic tracts (pain/temperature and discriminative touch)	Cortical areas 3, 1, 2
Ventral posteromedial (VPM) (in or near this nucleus?)	Vestibulothalamic fibers	Cortex posterior to the transverse gyri of Heschl
Ventrolateral (VL)	Dentatothalamic fibers Globus pallidus via thalamic fasciculus	To cortical area 4
Ventral anterior (VA)	Globus pallidus via thalamic fasciculus Dentatothalamic	To cortical area 6
Ventral mediobasal	Ascending taste pathway (nucleus solitarius to parabrachial nucleus of midbrain reticular formation)	To primary somesthetic cortex in cortical area for taste

2. Olfactory pathway fibers. These travel via the medial forebrain bundle.
3. Corticohypothalamic fibers are a direct projection to the hypothalamus from the frontal lobe.
4. Hippocampohypothalamic fibers travel via the fornix, which has afferents for the anterior thalamic nucleus, preoptic area, septal area, and mainly the mammillary bodies of the hypothalamus.
5. Amygdalohypothalamic fibers follow two courses—stria terminalis and a direct projection that passes ventral to the lenticular nucleus.
6. Thalamohypothalamic fibers project from dorsomedial and midline thalamic nuclei.
7. The midbrain tegmentum projects to the hypothalamus.

Efferent connections.   The major efferents are as follows:
1. The mamillothalamic tract (of Vicq d'Azyr) is a projection from the mammillary body to the anterior thalamic nucleus, which in turn projects to the cingulate gyrus.
2. The mamillotegemental tract extends from the mammillary body to the midbrain tegmentum.
3. Efferents that descend to the brain stem and the spinal cord are of mainly autonomic function, which includes connections to the GVE nuclei of III, VII, IX, and X via the reticular formation; likewise, projections down the cord end on the sympathetic and sacral parasympathetic neurons there.
4. The hypothalamohypophyseal tract extends from the supraoptic and paraventricular nuclei to the posterior pituitary (neurohypophysis). These fibers are secretory and release their substances (oxytocin and vasopressin) into the bloodstream. Vasopressin (secreted by the supraoptic nucleus) acts to cause vasoconstriction and is also known as antidiuretic hormone (ADH) (increases resorption from the distal convoluted tubules of the nephrons). The supraoptic nucleus acts as an osmo-receptor; if circulating blood should have a high osmotic pressure, more ADH is secreted and more water is resorbed and the osmotic pressure is reduced. The paraventricular nucleus secretes the oxytocin that causes contraction of uterine smooth muscle and of the myoepithelial cells of the mammary glands.
5. Hypothalamohypophyseal portal system. Capillaries

Table 1-8. Thalamic Nuclei (continued)

Nuclei	Afferents	Efferents
Posterior nuclear group (part of pulvinar, part of MGB, suprageniculate and limitans nuclei) (perception of pain)	Spinothalamic and ventral trigeminothalamic tracts	To insula and secondary somesthetic cortex
Lateral nuclear group		
Lateral dorsal (limbic system)	Hippocampus	To cinculate gyrus
Lateral posterior	?	Somatosensory association cortex (areas 5, 7)
Pulvinar	Retina, superior colliculus, pretectal area	Occipital cortex
Medial nuclear group		
Dorsomedial (limbic system—moods, emotional tone) (emotional aspects of pain) (something to do with memory, e.g., Korsakoff's syndrome)	Olfactory cortex, amygdaloid body, prefrontal cortex, orbital cortex, hypothalamus	Prefrontal cortex Orbital cortex Hypothalamus
Ventromedial (connections with hippocampus and parahippocampal gyrus suggest limbic system function)		
Anterior nuclear group		
Anterior nuclei	Mamillothalamic tract (of Vicq d'Azyr)	Cinculate gyrus
Subthalamic nucleus (motor system function; lesion produces hemiballismus)	Globus pallidus	globus pallidus

within the median eminence portion of the hypothalamus drain into veins that empty into the anterior pituitary and break up into sinusoids, which course among the parenchymal cells there. The hypothalamus secretes releasing hormones and release-inhibiting hormones. The releasing hormones stimulate production and release of adrenocorticotropic hormones (ACTH), follicle-stimulating hormone (FSH), luteinizing hormone (LH), thyroid-stimulating hormone (TSH), and growth hormone (GH). The inhibiting hormones inhibit release of melanocyte-stimulating hormone (MSH) and luteo-tropic hormone (or lactogenic hormone or prolactin) (LTH). The cells that secrete these hormones are influenced by both hypothalamic afferents and by hormone levels in the blood.

Functions of the hypothalamus

1. Control of the autonomic nervous system (ANS). The anterior hypothalamus and the preoptic area influence the parasympathetic portion of the ANS responses such as constriction of pupils, increase in GI motility, decreasing heart rate and blood pressure, etc. The posterior and lateral nuclei control sympathetic responses.
2. Endocrine control is effected through the portal system and the releasing and release-inhibiting secretions (see above).
3. Temperature regulation. Stimulation of the anterior portion of the hypothalamus puts into action those mechanisms that facilitate heat loss (e.g., sweating, dilation of cutaneous vessels). Stimulation of the posterior hypothalamus activates mechanisms that conserve heat (e.g., vasoconstriction of cutaneous vessels, inhibition of sweating). Shivering may be induced also as a mechanism for increasing heat production.
4. Food and water intake. Stimulation of the lateral hypothalamus increases food intake (the hunger center). The medial hypothalamus is the satiety center, and stimulation reduces food intake. The thirst center is in the lateral hypothalamus. This is stimulated by the osmolarity of the blood, which is also related to ADH secretion.
5. Emotion and behavior (limbic function).
6. Circadian rhythms. These rhythms are seen in body temperature, adrenal cortex activity, eosinophil count, renal secretion, and sleep/wakefulness. Rhythms of sleeping and waking are influenced in the anterior hypothalamus. The suprachiasmatic nucleus is a major center for controlling biologic rhythms. It receives numerous afferents, and among these are those from the retina. The suprachiasmatic nucleus projects to many other hypothalamic nuclei.

RETICULAR FORMATION AND THE LIMBIC SYSTEM

Reticular formation

The reticular formation consists of a reticulum of neurons and nerve fibers that extends from the spinal cord through the medulla, pons, mesencephalon, subthalamus, thalamus, and hypothalamus. It is now appreciated that this is not simply a homogeneous network of gray and white matter; rather, there is internal organization both anatomically and physiologically, albeit poorly defined. The reticular formation can be sub-

divided bilaterally into three longitudinal columns—median, medial, and lateral. Morphological differences include neuron cell size, which is intermediate, large, and small, respectively. The neurons are Golgi I—that is, they have long axons that project at length from the cell bodies. Pathways within the formation are multisynaptic, crossed and uncrossed, and ascending and descending. Both somatic and visceral functions are served. Fibers from the reticular formation extend into the cord and are continuous with interneurons of the spinal cord gray matter. Impulses from the reticular formation are also relayed to the cerebellum and to all parts of the cerebral cortex.

Afferents of the reticular formation include fibers from almost all of the CNS. These include direct pathways such as spinoreticular and collateralization into the reticular formation such as via the spinothalamic tract and the medial lemniscus. The cranial nerve nuclei also project into the reticular formation, including vestibular, auditory, trigeminal, and visual pathways. The cerebellum projects into the reticular formation, as do the hypothalamus, thalamus, subthalamus, corpus striatum (basal ganglia), motor, and somesthetic cerebral cortex.

Efferents of the reticular formation include reticulobulbar and reticulospinal (pontine and medullary), which pass to neurons of the motor nuclei of cranial nerves and the anterior horn of spinal cord gray matter, respectively. Autonomic pathways descend to cranial parasympathetic nuclei and on into the spinal cord to the thoracolumbar sympathetic and sacral parasympathetic preganglionic neurons. The cerebellum, cerebral cortex, substantia nigra, red nucleus, tectum, corpus striatum, thalamus, subthalamus, and hypothalamus all receive fibers from the reticular formation.

Nearly all of the other parts of the CNS are reciprocally connected with the reticular formation. Thus, those functions attributable to those parts are influenced in some way by reticular formation activity. The functions of the reticular formation are many, but the following are the principal ones:

1. Skeletal muscle control. Muscle tone, reflex activity, and reciprocal inhibition all are modulated by reticular formation.
2. Visceral and somatic sensations. All ascending pathways are influenced by the reticular formation, and this influence can be excitatory or inhibitory. This may well be involved in the so-called gating mechanism in controlling pain perception.
3. Autonomic nervous system. As stated above, the pathways to the various autonomic motor nuclei are relayed through the reticular formation.
4. Endocrine system. The reticular formation can influence the synthesis or release of releasing or inhibiting factors.
5. Biologic rhythms control.
6. Reticular activating system. As stated above, multiple ascending systems pass through the reticular formation carrying sensory information. This information is projected to the various parts of the cerebral cortex. Via these connections the individual's state of consciousness (alertness or sleep) is controlled by the reticular formation.

Limbic system

The limbic system functions to deal with our more primitive functions. It functions in control of emotional tone, rage, fear, feeding, reproducing, etc. Being more primitive in function, it is understandable that the limbic system is made up of phylogenetically older parts of the brain.

The **limbic lobe** is an old term that includes structures that form a nearly complete circle on the medial brain surface. It is made up of subcallosal, cingulate, and parahippocampal gyri.

Hippocampal formation is composed of the hippocampus, dentate gyrus, and parahippocampal gyrus. The **hippocampus** is very primitive cerebral cortex lying in the bottom of the hippocampal sulcus and forming the floor of the inferior horn of the lateral ventricle. It has only three layers, and its efferent fibers leave the hippocampus all along its medial border and form the **fimbria of the fornix**. These fibers pass posteriorly, but at the posterior end of the hippocampus they turn medially and dorsally to pass anterior to the splenium of the corpus callosum as the **crus of the fornix**. As the crus courses anterior to the splenium, it approaches the midline to run in juxtaposition with its contralateral counterpart. As the two crura approach each other, fibers from each crus cross the midline to join the contralateral crus. These crossing fibers, the **commissure of the fornix**, pass from one hippocampus to the other. The fornix continues anteriorly, the two crura coursing parallel to each other, going somewhat ventrally as they gradually separate farther from the underside of the body of the corpus callosum. This portion of the fornix takes on the name of **body of the fornix**. At the level of the interventricular foramen, the fornix makes a sharp ventral turn and becomes the **column of the fornix**, which forms the superoanterior boundary of the interventricular foramen. At the hypothalamic sulcus, the column diverges somewhat laterally and enters the substance of the hypothalamus and descends to end at the lateral side of the mammillary body.

The **dentate gyrus** lies wedged in between the hippocampus and parahippocampal gyrus. It has a "toothed" appearance due to the numerous small blood vessels that penetrate it. This gyrus accompanies the fimbria back toward the splenium, but unlike the fornix, it passes posterior to the splenium and onto the superior surface of the corpus callosum, where it becomes a thin layer of gray matter called the **indusium griseum**. The white matter fibers running in the indusium are the medial and lateral longitudinal striae. Anteriorly the dentate gyrus passes into the **uncus**.

The parahippocampal gyrus lies between the hippocampal sulcus and the collateral sulcus.

The almond-shaped **amygdaloid nucleus** is related to the tip of the inferior horn of the lateral ventricle and the anterior tip of the caudate nucleus. The **stria terminalis** (efferent fibers) exits from the posterior part of the nucleus, passes along on the surface of the tail of the caudate nucleus, follows the caudate nucleus around, and terminates in the septal area and anterior hypothalamus.

The **mamillothalamic tract** is a projection of the mammillary body to the anterior thalamic nucleus. The anterior thalamic nucleus projects to the **cingulate gyrus**. The white matter of the cingulate gyrus, the **cingulum**, projects to the hippocampus, which projects via the fornix back to the mammillary body etc. This is the **Papez circuit**.

The limbic system is difficult to confine to a limited number of structures because there are so many connections and so much reverberating circuitry. Figure 1-19 summarizes many of these connections. The central figures in this system are the hippocampus and the hypothalamus. **Afferents** of the hippocampus are as follows: (1) the cingulum (from cingulate gyrus); (2) fibers from the septal area (in midline and in the cerebrum near the anterior commissure) via the fornix; (3) the commissure of the fornix, which connects the two hippocampi; (4) the indusium griseum, which projects via medial and lateral longitudinal striae (of Lancisi); the (5) fibers from the olfactory-associated cortex; and (6) fibers from the dentate and parahippocampal gyri. **Efferents** of the hippocampus (fornix) are as follows: (1) to the mammillary body; (2) to the anterior thalamic nucleus; (3) to the midbrain tegmentum; (4) to the septal nuclei, preoptic area, and anterior hypothalamus; and (5) to the habenular nuclei via the striae medullares thalami. Along with various emotional functions, the hippocampus is involved in recent memory.

Lesions. Lesions of the reticular formation can cause loss of consciousness. Limbic system lesions result in dysfunction of the emotions and the visceral responses that accompany them. Lesions of the amygdaloid complex unilaterally or bilaterally can result in decreased aggressiveness, emotional instability, and restlessness; increased interest in food; and hypersexuality (**Kluver-Bucy syndrome**). There is no loss of memory. The temporal lobe is sometimes the focus of epilepsy seizures that are preceded by an olfactory or acoustic aura.

Basal ganglia

The basal ganglia should be called nuclei, but convention is such that this misnomer is accepted. The components of this group are the **corpus striatum** (caudate nucleus + putamen + globus pallidus), **subthalamic nucleus**, and **substantia nigra**. The caudate and putamen are histologically, developmentally, and functionally a single entity that becomes divided by the development of the internal capsule's anterior limb. Taken together, they are referred to as the **striatum** or **neostriatum**.

The striatum receives afferents from the entire neocortex, the intralaminar nuclei (of the thalamus), and the substantia nigra. It projects to the globus pallidus, which in turn relays these impulses to the motor and premotor cortex through the ventral anterior and somewhat the ventrolateral thalamic nuclei. The neostriatum (caudate and putamen) have a reciprocal relationship with the substant nigra, and the paleostriatum (globus pallidus) has such a relationship with the subthalamic nucleus. These connections function to modulate the activity of the corpus striatum.

The basal ganglia transfer and modify information coming from the entire cortex and then forward it to the motor and premotor areas.

Internal capsule

This very large structure is composed of many millions of the afferent and efferent fibers of the cerebral cortex. The cortex itself has billions of neurons, and many of these give rise to projection fibers that go to all other parts of the CNS. The afferent fibers are also very numerous and extend to all parts of the cortex.

In a horizontal section of the cerebrum, the internal capsule has a V-shaped configuration with the concave side facing laterally. This shape has facilitated designating parts as **anterior limb, genu,** and **posterior limb**. Filling the concavity is the **lenticular nucleus** (putamen + globus pallidus). Medial

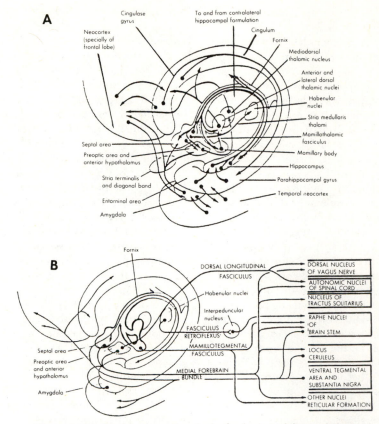

Figure 1-19. Limbic connections in the forebrain and diencephalon.

to the anterior limb is the **caudate nucleus,** and medial to the posterior limb is the **thalamus.** Within the capsule there is functional localization.

Olfactory pathway

The olfactory pathway is unique in a number of ways, but what is most significant is that it is the only sensory pathway that is a part of and feeds directly into the telencephalon.

The **olfactory mucosa** lies in the sphenoethmoidal recess of the nasal passages. The bipolar neurons that form the **olfactory nerve** lie within this mucosa. Their peripheral processes project toward the surface. The central processes are very small and unmyelinated; they pass through the cribriform plate of the ethmoid bone and synapse with **mitral cells** in the **olfactory bulb.** Tufted and granular cells also synapse on the mitral cells. The input to the olfactory bulb is bilateral in that each olfactory bulb projects to the other via the medial olfactory stria, which crosses in the anterior commissure.

The **olfactory tract** courses back to the anterior perforated substance and divides into **medial** and **lateral olfactory striae.** The medial has been described above. The lateral stria passes to the olfactory area of the cortex (in the region of the uncus).

Visual pathway

Because of the presence of the lens in the eye, the image projected onto the retina is upside down and backward. Thus, the visual and retinal fields are not the same. Once the image is projected onto the retina, the projection back through the visual pathway is such that those impulses arising from the right side of each retina project to the right visual cortex, the left side to the left cortex. Also, those impulses arising from the upper portions of the retina remain upper in the optic radiations and visual cortex.

The pathways are quite straightforward. The ganglion cells of the retina project as **optic nerves** that extend posteromedially to the **optic chiasm,** in which the fibers from the medial half of each retina cross. A lesion of the optic nerve would result in the loss of vision of that eye. The fibers from the right half of each retina then pass into the **right optic tract,** those from the left half into the **left optic tract.** Lesions of the optic chiasm result in loss of vision related to the fibers damaged by the lesion. For example, a midline lesion of the chiasm that cuts the crossing fibers damages those fibers carrying impulses from the medial half of each retina. The visual field loss, therefore, would be bilateral temporal hemianopia. A lesion of an optic tract would result in the visual field deficit of right (or left) homonymous hemianopia. The optic tract extends to the **lateral geniculate body** of the thalamus, where about 90% of the fibers synapse. The neurons of the lateral geniculate body project as the retrolenticular portion of the internal capsule and form the **optic radiation.** The radiation fibers sweep back through the white matter of the cerebral hemisphere, and the inferior fibers pass anteriorly and inferiorly toward the tip of the temporal lobe and swing around the lateral ventricle and then sweep posteriorly to the visual cortex. These inferior fibers form **Meyer's loop.** Because of their course they may be involved in discrete lesions, and when this happens the impulses arising from the lower left (or right) quadrant of each retina are denied ultimate delivery to the visual cortex. For example, if the lower left retinal quadrant fails to project to the cortex, then the visual deficit would be the opposite—upper right quadrantanopia.

The visual cortex is that of the calcarine sulcus, the cuneus, and the lingual gyrus, all on the medial side of the occipital lobe. This is area 17. The most posterior portion receives impulses from the retinal fovea. The cuneus receives fibers from the upper portion of the retina, the lingual gyrus from the lower portion. Lesions of these specific cortical areas result in the predictable visual field deficits.

Visual reflexes

Oculocephalic (doll's eye) reflex.   This is elicited by rapidly rotating the head from side to side. If the brain stem is **intact,** the eyes will move conjugately in the direction opposite to that of the movement of the head. If the brain stem is **not intact,** eyes do not move at all or movement is not conjugate.

Oculovestibular (caloric) reflexes.   Cold water in the external auditory canal results in inhibition of the lateral semicircular canal of that side. That leaves the contralateral lateral semicircular canal unopposed. The result is that the **slow** movement of the eyes will be **toward the treated side** and the **fast** movement will be **away from the treated side.** Warm water will have the opposite effect. The mnemonic used here reflects the **fast** movement: COWS—cold opposite, warm same (in relation to stimulated side).

Position of eyes at rest
1. Eyes turned **toward** the side of paralyzed limbs indicate brain-stem involvement.
2. Eyes turned **away from** the side of paralyzed limbs indicate cerebral hemisphere involvement.
3. Roving eye movements indicate an intact brain stem.
4. The eyes are vertically dysconjugate in some brain-stem lesions (skew deviation).

Pupils
1. Brain-stem areas controlling consciousness are close to pathways subserving pupillary reactions.
2. Midbrain damage—pupils in midposition, fixed to light.
3. Pontine lesions—pinpoint pupils.
4. Unilateral pupillary dilatation may indicate uncal herniation (through the tentorial notch).

Pupillary pathways are resistant to metabolic insult and thus can be valuable in distinguishing metabolic coma from structural disease.

Occipital corticotectal projections.   These fibers originate from pyramidal cells of layer V of Brodmann's areas 17, 18, and 19 of the cerebral cortex. They project via the brachium of the superior colliculus to the tectum (superior colliculus). The specific projections from the tectum and pretectal area are not well defined. This pathway is used in reflex eye movements (e.g., tracking a moving object). If these areas of cortex are stimulated, the eyes will turn **away** from the side stimulated.

Frontal eye field (Brodmann's area 8) projections.   These neurons also project via the superior brachium to the superior colliculus and the pretectal area. From the tectal area fibers project in a poorly defined path to the peripeduncular pontine reticular formation (PPRF) (also called the "lateral gaze center"), which lies lateral to the abducens nucleus. Stimulation of area 8 of the cortex results in the eyes moving horizontally **away** from the side stimulated. This pathway is related to volitional eye movements. Stimulation of the lateral gaze center results in the eyes turning horizontally **toward** the side stimulated.

The light reflex.   This reflex is the constriction of the pupil when an eye is exposed to an increase in light intensity.

Afferent limb
1. Axons of the retinal ganglion cells (optic fiber layer) exit the retina at the optic disk to become optic nerve fibers.
2. Optic nerve fibers extend posteriorly to the optic chiasm, where those arising from the medial half of the retina cross to enter the contralateral optic tract and those from lateral half of the retina pass into the ipsilateral optic tract.
3. Optic tract fibers project toward the lateral geniculate body, but those involved in this reflex bypass that nucleus and enter the brachium of the superior colliculus.
4. Fibers of the superior brachium terminate in the superior colliculus and adjacent pretectal area, the latter apparently being of much more direct significance for this reflex.

Efferent limb
1. Pretectal area neurons project bilaterally to the Edinger-Westphal (accessory oculomotor) nuclei.
2. Each Edinger-Westphal nucleus projects ipsilaterally to ciliary ganglion and synapses.
3. Postganglionic ciliary ganglion neurons innervate the iridial sphincter muscle (and muscle of the ciliary body), and the pupil constricts.

The light reflex involves the **direct response** (the pupil of the stimulated eye constricts) and the **consensual response** (the pupil of the other eye also constricts). The bilateral connection from the pretectum to the Edinger-Westphal nuclei facilitates this bilateral response. Absence of either a direct or a consensual reaction indicates lesion somewhere in the pathway. This reflex does *not* involve the cerebral cortex.

If an optic nerve were severed, the ipsilateral eye would obviously have no vision and no direct responses. In such a case, however, light stimulation of the contralateral eye would still elicit a consensual response. Were the third nerve severed unilaterally, then the efferent limb of the reflex arc would be disrupted and there could be no direct response in the side denervated or consensual response if the other eye were stimulated. Light shone into the eye to which the third nerve had been cut would still elicit a consensual response.

Fixation reflex.   This is the reflex direction of the eye toward an object attracting attention, as in optokinetic nystagmus. This is usually a cortical reflex, in that it involves the visual cortical areas. This reflex is seen in an individual riding in a car and fixing on figures in the passing landscape (e.g., telephone poles). The individual will focus on and follow an object until it passes beyond the edge of the visual field and then very rapidly move the eyes to fix on another object, etc. This is the so-called railway nystagmus. Optokinetic nystagmus requires the attention of the individual and thus the attribution to the cortex. Suffice it to say, there are subcortical structures that are and can be involved, but for purposes of this discussion it will be considered cortical. The **afferent limb** consists of visual pathways to the cortex. The **efferent limb** consists of corticofugal connections to the superior colliculus and pretectum, and from these somehow to the nuclei of cranial nerves III, IV, and VI. Normally, it is necessary for the optic impulses to be consciously perceived if they are to elicit the fixation reflex.

Accommodation reflex.   This involves the adjustment of the system for near vision.

1. Convergence of the eyes (medial recti muscles, innervated by the GSE component of III).
2. Contraction of ciliary muscle (GVE of III) to reduce tension on the suspensory ligament of the lens so that the lens can assume a more spherical configuration and increase refractive power.
3. Constriction of pupil (GVE of III).

Normally, this reflex occurs only when a near object is looked at and thus, if both eyes are used, is accompanied by fixation. Therefore, a person's attention and a desire to see the object clearly are involved in this reflex. This may require some volitional effort, especially if the individual is fatigued. Occipital eye fields are probably those that are involved, not the frontal eye fields. The **afferent link** is the visual pathway to the occipital cortex. The **efferent link** is the corticofugal fibers to pretectum, from which the appropriate parts of the oculomotor nuclei are stimulated.

Argyll Robertson sign.   The pupil will accommodate but will not react. The light reflex is impaired (pupil does not constrict), but on accommodation the pupil does constrict. The explanation for this has never been entirely satisfactory. It has been suggested by the findings of some investigators that the Edinger-Westphal nucleus has different cells for accommodation and for the light reflex. It has also been suggested that the neurons effecting pupillary constriction in the light reflex are different from those effecting pupillary constriction in the accommodation reflex. In damage to the oculomotor nerve, pupillary reflex constriction to light and accommodation and convergence are often affected to a corresponding degree. In postdiphtheritic paralysis of accommodation, the light reflex is retained.

The Argyll Robertson sign is found first and foremost in patients with syphilis of the CNS, and particularly in tabes dorsalis (90%). It is also found in other diseases (encephalitis, disseminated sclerosis, syringobulbia, tumors of the pineal, superior colliculus, or third ventricle).

The explanation of the Argyll Robertson sign is made especially difficult in that the sign can occur unilaterally. The pupil often has an irregular outline. It has been suggested that the stroma of the iris is damaged and/or that the nerves coursing through the stoma are affected. Credence is gained for this explanation by the preservation of the irregularity of the pupil after death. The problem with this explanation is that it does not do away with the questions arising from the preservation of the light reflex. No satisfactory CNS pathology has been offered either.

Adie's pupil (myotonic pupil).   The reaction to light is absent if tested in the customary manner, although the size of the pupil will change slowly on prolonged exposure to a bright light or if the individual remains in the dark for a considerable time. The reaction on convergence is slowed, sometimes requiring 5 seconds or more for completion, and the widening of the pupil on gaze into the distance is prolonged over a similar period of time. In the majority of cases, only one pupil is affected. Such a pupil will react promptly to mydriatic and miotic drugs. This pupil will react dramatically to a 2.5% solution of mecholyl instilled into the conjunctival sac. The normal pupil is not affected by this drug. This pupil appears in the third and fourth decades and is commonly associated with absence of or a decrease in the muscle-stretch reflex.

Meninges

Pia mater.   This is a delicate, vascular layer of connective tissue that is intimately attached to the surface of the CNS. There is no space, real or potential, between the pia mater and the CNS surface.

Arachnoid mater.   This is a thin, delicate layer of connective tissue with collagen fibers that extend from the arachnoid to the pia. Thus, the pia mater and the arachnoid can be considered as a single unit—the leptomeninges. The slender connective tissue fibers that extend between the pia and arachnoid are called **trabeculae**. These trabeculae traverse the space between the pia and the arachnoid that is called the **subarachnoid space**, which is filled with **CSF**. The arachnoid, unlike the pia, does not closely follow the surface of the CNS, and thus in some places the subarachnoid space is much larger than in others. Those areas where this space is exaggerated are called **cisterna**. There are several of these, but the of the more significant ones are the following:

1. Lumbar cistern—in the lower lumbar region of the vertebral column and through which course the spinal nerve roots of the cauda equina.
2. Cisterna magna (cerebellomedullary cistern)—lies in the space formed where the cerebellum overhangs the caudal pons and the medulla.
3. Lateral cistern—related to the lateral cerebral fissure.
4. Interpeduncular cistern—between the cerebral peduncles.

Dura mater.   This is a thick, dense, irregular connective tissue sheet that encases the CNS and the other two meninges. Between the dura and the arachnoid is a potential space called the **subdural space**. This is only a potential space, and thus normally there is nothing within it. The dura found in the vertebral canal is separated from the vertebrae by the **epidural space**. This is occupied by a plexus of veins (Batson's veins), fat, and other connective tissues.

In the cranial cavity, the dura mater fuses with the periosteum lining the inner surface of the bones that form the cranial vault. In some places, the inner layer of the dura (true dura) is separated from the periosteal dura so that a space is formed. Such spaces are lined with endothelium and are called **dural venous sinuses**. For all practical purposes, all these sinuses are connected and drain most of the blood from the brain and into the internal jugular veins.

Reflections of the inner layer of dura mater in the cranial cavity form large structures that separate parts of the brain and offer some support. One of the largest is the **falx cerebri**, which is a sickle-shaped structure oriented longitudinally and extending down the midline so as to separate the two cerebral hemispheres. In its superior border courses the **superior sagittal sinus**, and in its free, inferior border one finds the **inferior sagittal sinus**. Toward its posterior end the falx fuses with another dural reflection that is transversely oriented and lies under the occipital lobe and overlies the cerebellum—the **tentorium cerebelli.** This is attached on each side to the clinoid processes of the sphenoid bone (related to the cavernous sinus), the petrous ridge of the temporal bone, and along the inner surface of the occipital bone. The falx cerebri's posterior portion is continuous with the tentorium's dorsal surface. Where these two reflections meet there is the **straight dural venous sinus,** into which empty the great cerebral vein (of Galen) and the inferior sagittal sinus. The tentorium cerebelli has a gap in it called the **tentorial notch,** which accommodates the mesencephalon.

In the midline, the unpaired dural sinuses include superior and inferior sagittal, straight, and occipital. At the internal occipital protuberance of the occipital bone, there is the **confluence of the sinuses** (torcular Herophili). This confluence is that point where the straight sinus, the superior sagittal sinus, the occipital sinus, and the two lateral sinuses all are continuous. A majority of the time, the superior sagittal sinus blood turns into the right lateral sinus and that of the straight sinus into the left. Paired sinuses include the transverse sinus (along the lateral attachment of the tentorium cerebelli to the occipital bone), superior petrosal (along the tentorium cerebelli's attachment to the petrous ridge of the temporal bone), inferior petrosal (along the inferior portion of the posterior border of the petrous bone, temporal), cavernous sinus (on either side of the sella turcica, the sphenoid body), and sphenoparietal (along the lesser wing of the sphenoid and opens into cavernous). The lateral and the superior petrosal sinuses meet at the lateral end of the petrous ridge to empty into the sigmoid sinus, which follows an S-shaped course to the jugular foramen to empty into the beginning of the internal jugular vein. The other tributary of the internal jugular vein is the inferior petrosal sinus. It should be kept in mind that all the venous dural sinuses have walls composed of dura mater.

Blood supply to the CNS

Spinal cord. Two anterior spinal arteries arise from the intracranial portions of the vertebral arteries. They fuse while passing over the anterior surface of the medulla and form a single vessel that courses in the anterior median fissure of the spinal cord. This continues for the full length of the cord. It supplies midline structures of the medulla, and in the spinal cord it gives off branches to the right and to the left alternately. The anterior spinal artery supplies blood to the anterior two-thirds of the spinal cord substance. The two posterior spinal arteries also arise from the intracranial portion of the vertebral arteries (or from the posterior inferior cerebellar arteries, which arise from the vertebrals). These do not fuse, but proceed independently down the dorsolateral aspect of the spinal cord in relation to the dorsal roots and the posterolateral sulcus. The posterior spinal arteries are very small and are discontinuous.

The spinal cord does not rely entirely on these spinal arteries. Segmental branches are supplied all along the way. In the cervical region of the cord, the vertebral arteries give off small radicular branches that follow along the nerve roots, supplying them, and onto the cord itself to augment the blood supply. In addition, other cervical arteries such as the profunda cervicalis and ascending cervical send small branches. In the thoracic region of the spinal cord, the posterior intercostal arteries have radicular branches. In the lumbar area there are also segmental arteries, which arise from the lumbar segmental branches of the abdominal aorta. Certain segments of the spinal cord are especially vulnerable to vascular problems. The upper segments of the thoracic region are more dependent on the radicular augmentation, which if diminished or lost can cause damage that is extensive and very serious. In the lumbar enlargement area there is a particularly remarkable anterior radicular branch, the **arteria radicularis magna (of Adamkiewicz),** which usually arises on the left side from an intersegmental branch of the aorta from a lower thoracic or upper lumbar vessel. This vessel is a major source of blood for the lower two-thirds of the spinal cord. For unspecified reasons, the cervical cord's radicular arteries arise bilaterally, but below that level, these arteries are much more prominent on the left side. The spinal cord ends at about the level of the first or second lumbar vertebra.

The brain. The internal carotids brings about 80% of the blood supply to the brain, the vertebral arteries the remaining 20%. At the base of the brain, both of these pairs of arteries enter into the formation of an anastomotic circle of arteries, the **circle of Willis.** Cerebral vessels anastomose rather extensively on the surface of the brain, but once branches penetrate into the substance of the brain they become essentially end arteries.

Arteries commonly involved in vascular problems include the **lenticulostriate arteries,** which arise from the proximal portion of the middle cerebral on the base of the brain. The name indicates the distribution. These are so frequently involved in cerebrovascular accidents that they have been named the **arteries of cerebral hemorrhage (of Charcot).** Another significant branch is one that arises from the anterior cerebral just before it reaches the anterior communicating artery. This branch is the **medial striate artery (recurrent artery of Heubner).** It supplies the ventral part of the head of the caudate nucleus, the adjacent portion of the putamen, the genu and anterior limb of the internal capsule.

The veins from the CNS drain into the dural venous sinuses. Only a few are named and need to be mentioned. There are cerebral veins over the dorsolateral surface of the hemispheres. Of these are perhaps three that should be pointed out. The first is the **superficial middle cerebral vein,** which courses in the lateral fissure. Extending dorsally and somewhat posteriorly from that vein and opening into the superior sagittal sinus is the **superior anastomotic vein of Trolard.** Another vein extends from the superificial middle cerebral vein to the transverse sinus, the **anastomotic vein of Labbé.** The internal cerebral veins fuse to form the **great cerebral vein (of Galen),** which along with the inferior sagittal sinus opens into the straight sinus. Because veins have so many anastomoses, there is seldom a problem with venous drainage.

Cerebrospinal fluid and ventricles

The CNS is hollow in that it contains spaces, all of which are continuous. Each cerebral hemisphere contains a **lateral ventricle,** and each opens independently through the **interventricular foramen (of Monro)** into the **third ventricle,** which is contained largely within the diencephalon. The third ventricle is continuous caudally with the **cerebral aqueduct (of Sylvius),** which runs through the midbrain and connects the third ventricle with the **fourth ventricle,** which lies over the pons and medulla and under the cerebellum. The fourth ventricle narrows sharply and is continuous with the vestigial **central canal** of the spinal cord. The caudal portion of the roof of the fourth ventricle has a midline and two lateral openings that allow the ventricle to communicate with the subarachnoid space, specifically the cerebellomedullary cistern (cisterna magna). The midline opening is the **foramen of Magendie,** and the lateral openings are the **foramina of Luschka.** It is via these openings that the CSF passes from the fourth ventricle into the subarachnoid space. The subarachnoid space envelops the entire CNS, but numerous communicating devices open into the superior sagittal sinus, the **arachnoid villi** or **granulations** (pachionian bodies).

The CSF is formed continuously and is drained away in equal amount. The **choroid plexuses** (highly vascular modifications of the pia mater and ependyma which are found to be associated with each ventricle) produce about 70% of the CSF. Approximately 18% is made as capillary ultrafiltrate, and the remaining 12% is metabolic water. At any given time, there is about 140 ml of CSF; 23 ml is in the ventricles, the remainder in the subarachnoid space. This is manufactured at a rate of about 0.35 ml/minute, or about 500 ml/day.

The brain floats in the CSF, and thus a brain weighing 1500 g in air weighs about 50 g in CSF. CSF does more than serve as a liquid cushion or container. It is involved in endocrine functions, and it has various electrolytes within it. Releasing and inhibiting substances are secreted into it, and the CSF contributes to the creation and maintainence of the neurons' microenvironment. CSF pressure is low. In the recumbent position, the lumbar cistern pressure is 100 to 150 mm H_2O. In the sitting position, this pressure doubles.

BIBLIOGRAPHY

Barr ML, Kiernan JA: The Human Nervous System, 5th ed. JB Lippincott, Philadelphia, 1988.

Carpenter MB, Sutin J: Human Neuroanatomy, 8th ed. Williams & Wilkins, Baltimore, 1983.

Clementi CD (ed.): Gray's Anatomy, 30th ed. Lea & Febiger, Philadelphia, 1985.

Cormack DH: Ham's Histology, 9th ed. JB Lippincott, Philadelphia, 1987.

Fawcett DW: A Textbook of Histology, 11th ed. WB Saunders, Philadelphia, 1986.

Ger R, Abrahams P: Essentials of Clinical Anatomy. Pitman Books, Turnbridge Wells, England, 1986.

Heimer L: The Human Brain and Spinal Cord. Springer-Verlag, New York, 1983.

Hollinshead WH: Anatomy for Surgeons, 3rd ed. Harper & Row, New York, 1981.

Junqueira LC, Carneiro J, Long JA: Basic Histology, 5th ed. Appleton & Lange, East Norwalk, 1986.

Kandel E, Schwartz JH: Principles of Neuroscience, 2nd ed. Elsevier, New York, 1985.

Moore KL: Clinically Oriented Anatomy, 2nd ed. Williams & Wilkins, Baltimore, 1985.

Moore KL: The Developing Human, 4th ed. WB Saunders, Philadelphia, 1988.

Peele TL: The Neuroanatomical Basis for Clinical Neurology, 3rd ed. McGraw-Hill, New York, 1977.

Sadler TW: Langman's Medical Embryology, 5th ed. Williams & Wilkins, Baltimore, 1985.

Snell RS: Clinical Embryology for Medical Students, 3rd ed. Little, Brown & Co., Boston, 1983.

Snell RS: Clinical and Functional Histology for Medical Students. Little, Brown & Co., Boston, 1984.

Snell RS: Clinical Anatomy for Medical Students, 3rd ed. Little, Brown & Co., Boston, 1986.

Snell RS: Clinical Neuroanatomy for Medical Students, 2nd ed. Little, Brown & Co., 1987.

SAMPLE QUESTIONS

DIRECTIONS: Each question below contains four suggested answers of which **one** or **more** is correct. Choose the answer:

A if **1, 2, and 3** are correct
B if **1 and 3** are correct
C if **2 and 4** are correct
D if only **4** is correct
E if **all** are correct

1. Which of the following appear during the third week of gestation?

   1. Somites
   2. Primitive streak
   3. First indication of cardiovascular system
   4. Neurenteric canal

2. Which of the following occur during the fourth week of gestation?

   1. Both neuropores close
   2. Many somites form
   3. The heart develops rapidly and achieves effective contractions
   4. The hypoblast differentiates markedly

3. Which of the following occur as the umbilicus forms?

   1. The outer covering is chorion
   2. The body stalk is incorporated into it
   3. The right umbilical artery normally disappears
   4. The amnion becomes its outer layer

4. Which of the following contribute to the formation of the diaphragm?

1. Septum transversum
2. Pleuroperitoneal membranes
3. Mesoesophagus
4. Body wall mesoderm

5. The muscles of facial expression are correctly described as

1. derived from the third pharyngeal arch
2. innervated by the facial nerve
3. derived from somites
4. typical skeletal muscle

6. At birth, which of the following sinuses are present?

1. Sphenoidal
2. Ethmoidal
3. Frontal
4. Maxillary

7. Derivatives of the caudal portion of the foregut include the

1. pancreas
2. esophagus
3. stomach
4. distal half of duodenum

8. The paramesonephric ducts (müllerian ducts) form the

1. oviducts
2. ovaries
3. uterus
4. vestibular glands

9. The interventricular foramen is closed by fusion of the

1. endocardial cushions
2. right bulbar ridge
3. left bulbar ridge
4. septum secundum

10. The bulbus cordis gives rise to the

1. muscular interventricular septum
2. aortic vestibule
3. valve of the inferior vena cava
4. conus arteriosus

11. The sixth aortic arch is related to the

1. pulmonary arteries
2. ductus arteriosus
3. ligamentum arteriosum
4. brachiocephalic artery

12. Neural tube derivatives that are correctly matched include

1. metencephalon = pons and cerebellum
2. mesencephalon = mesencephalon
3. myelencephalon = medulla
4. telencephalon = cerebral hemispheres

13. Dermatomes found in the hand include

1. cervical 6
2. cervical 5
3. cervical 7
4. thoracic 1

14. The formation of the axillary vein involves

1. venae comitantes of the brachial artery
2. cephalic vein
3. basilic vein
4. median cubital vein

15. Innervation of the pectoralis major and minor muscles involves

1. contribution from the medial cord of the brachial plexus
2. contribution from the lateral cord of the brachial plexus
3. the medial pectoral nerve
4. the lateral pectoral nerve

16. The rotator cuff muscles include the

1. deltoid muscle
2. teres minor muscle
3. pectoralis minor muscle
4. subscapularis muscle

17. The ulna articulates with the

1. humerus
2. proximal row of carpal bones
3. radius
4. triquetral carpal

18. Lesion of the radial nerve would

1. have a negative effect on flexion of the elbow
2. result in wristdrop
3. possibly leave the skin on the posterior side of the antebrachium (forearm) anesthetic
4. result in claw hand

19. Innervation of the anterior compartment of the thigh facilitates

1. flexion of the hip joint
2. extension of the knee joint
3. cutaneous innervation of anterior and medial thigh
4. lateral rotation of the hip joint

20. Lesion of the common peroneal division of the sciatic nerve would

1. paralyze the muscles of the anterior compartment of the leg
2. diminish the victim's ability to plantar flex the foot
3. diminish the victim's ability to evert the foot
4. leave the skin of the medial side of the leg anesthetic

21. The hard palate is formed by the

1. inferior conchal bones
2. palatine processes of the maxilla
3. vomer
4. horizontal processes of the palatine bones

22. The middle ear cavity is correctly described as

1. communicating with the nasopharynx via the eustachian tube
2. containing ossicles
3. opening into the mastoid antrum
4. lying medial to the primary tympanic membrane and lateral to the secondary tympanic membrane

23. Ciliary muscle (of the ciliary body of the eye) is accurately described as

1. smooth muscle parasympathetically innervated
2. important in the light reflex
3. involved in the accommodation reflex
4. increasing tension on the lens' suspensory ligament by its contraction

24. Regarding the heart, it may be said that the

1. apex is related to the left fifth intercostal space
2. obtuse margin is formed by the left ventricle
3. right margin is formed by the venae cavae and the right atrium
4. acute margin is formed by the right ventricle

25. The anterior interventricular artery of the heart is known to

1. be paralleled by the great cardiac vein (of Galen)
2. be a branch of the left coronary artery
3. supply the anterior two-thirds of the muscular portion of the interventricular septum
4. anastomose around the apex of the heart with the posterior interventricular artery

26. Which of the following are true of the lungs?

1. The right has ten bronchopulmonary segments, the left eight
2. They are contained within right and left pleura, the cavities of which are in continuity
3. The right has three lobes, the left two
4. Most of the blood flowing through their capillaries is carried to the lungs by the bronchial arteries

27. The jejunum and ileum are known to

1. be a total of at least 20 feet in length
2. be supplied virtually entirely by the superior mesenteric artery
3. have a mesentery that attaches to the dorsal body wall via the radix
4. have a large anastomotic artery running along their inner margin, called the artery of Drummond

28. The rectouterine pouch is known to

1. lie anterior to the uterus
2. extend caudally to be only thinly separated from the anterior fornix of the vagina
3. be a known eponymously as the pouch of Retzius
4. lined with peritoneum

29. The uterine tubes are correctly described as

1. associated with mesosalpinx
2. having at their distal ends the only opening into the peritoneal cavity
3. having lumina that open into the uterine cavity
4. homologues of the gubernaculum

30. Of nervous system development, one can say that

1. the first indication of a nervous system appears in the third week
2. neural tube formation first appears in the occipital region
3. the anterior neuropore closes before the posterior neuropore
4. the neural tube is entirely separated from the surface ectoderm by the end of the fourth week

31. If a cord were hemisected in a traumatic lesion (Brown-Séquard syndrome), which of the following would be true?

1. There would be loss of pain and temperature sensations below the level of the lesion and on the contralateral side
2. There would be loss of proprioception and two-point discrimination on the contralateral side and below the level of the lesion
3. There would be paralysis/paresis ipsilaterally below the lesion
4. There would be loss of pain and temperature sensations above and contralateral to the lesions

32. The spinal nucleus of the trigeminal is known to

1. be found in the pons, medulla, and upper spinal cord
2. receive impulses of pain and temperature from ectodermally derived structures of the ipsilateral face
3. receive input from cranial nerves V, VII, IX, and X
4. project mainly ipsilaterally to the VPM thalamic nucleus

33. The medial lemniscus is correctly described as

1. part of the pain and temperature pathway for impulses carried by spinal nerves
2. a second-order neuron in a sensory pathway
3. beginning in the lower (caudal) pons
4. containing fibers destined to synapse in the VPL thalamic nucleus

34. The anterolateral system is correctly described as

1. a sensory system
2. including tracts that do not deal with conscious sensations

3. containing fibers many of which arise in Rexed lamina V

4. composed of axons that cross in the anterior white commissure of the spinal cord

35. Concerning the Rexed laminae, it may be said that they

1. are subdivisions of the spinal cord funiculi
2. all (10) are present in all spinal cord segments
3. are based on a strictly functional basis
4. divide the spinal cord gray into ten parts, six of which are in the dorsal horn

36. The supplementary motor area of the cerebral cortex is known to

1. lie on the superior border of the lateral fissure
2. be part of Brodmann area 6, on the medial surface of the hemisphere
3. be related to fine digital movements
4. be related to mutism if lesioned

37. The middle cerebellar peduncle is correctly described as

1. the largest of these peduncles
2. entirely afferent (to the cerebellum)
3. composed of axons whose nuclei lie in the contralateral pontine gray
4. providing a pathway for spinal cord input to the cerebellum

38. The inferior cerebellar peduncle is known to

1. contain axons whose cell bodies are in the contralateral inferior olivary nucleus
2. carry both cuneocerebellar and dorsal spinocerebellar fibers
3. carry both primary and secondary vestibular fibers
4. carry fibers arising from the fastigial nuclei

39. The tegmentum of the midbrain at the inferior collicular level is correctly desribed as

1. containing the red nucleus
2. the location of the decussation of the medial lemniscus
3. the level of the Edinger-Westphal nucleus
4. containing the decussation of the superior cerebellar peduncle, trochlear nucleus, and substantia nigra

40. Of the hypothalamus, one can say that

1. stimulation of its anterior portion will produce sympathetic autonomic responses
2. the medial portion is the satiety center
3. it secretes trophic hormones for the thyroid and adrenal cortex
4. it makes hormones that are secreted in response to increased osmolarity of the blood

41. Light falling on the photoreceptors of the upper nasal quadrant of the right eye will result in impulses

1. traveling through the optic chiasm

2. reaching the left medial geniculate body
3. eventually reaching the cuneus of the left occipital lobe
4. that will eventually travel in the left Meyer's loop

42. The axon hillock is correctly described as

1. the site of attachment of an axon on the cell body
2. void of Nissl substance
3. containing many microtubules and neurofilaments
4. the same thing as the initial segment of the axon

43. It may be said of the various ion channels present in the presynaptic membrane that

1. the one that opens first is the Na^+ channel
2. the one that allows the movement of an ion from within the axon terminal out to the extracellular space is that for the K^+
3. the one that changes the electrical charges so that synaptic vesicles can fuse with the presynaptic membrane is related to Ca^{2+}
4. only one is really essential for synaptic transmission

44. The cerebellar cortex is known to

1. vary in its architecture in different parts
2. have only one neuron whose axons form efferent fibers—Purkinje cells
3. have from three to six layers
4. have an output that is entirely inhibitory

45. Concerning pupillary light reflexes, it may be said that they

1. do not require cortical involvement
2. are produced directly and consensually
3. involve cranial nerves II and III
4. require skeletal muscle action

ANSWERS

1. E (all)	16. C (2, 4)	31. B (1, 3)
2. A (1, 2, 3)	17. B (1, 3)	32. A (1, 2, 3)
3. C (2, 4)	18. A (1, 2, 3)	33. C (2, 4)
4. E (all)	19. A (1, 2, 3)	34. E (all)
5. C (2, 4)	20. A (1, 2, 3)	35. D (4)
6. C (2, 4)	21. C (2, 4)	36. C (2, 4)
7. B (1, 3)	22. E (all)	37. A (1, 2, 3)
8. B (1, 3)	23. B (1, 3)	38. E (all)
9. A (1, 2, 3)	24. E (all)	39. D (4)
10. C (2, 4)	25. E (all)	40. C (2, 4)
11. A (1, 2, 3)	26. B (1, 3)	41. B (1, 3)
12. E (all)	27. A (1, 2, 3)	42. A (1, 2, 3)
13. B (1, 3)	28. D (4)	43. A (1, 2, 3)
14. B (1, 3)	29. A (1, 2, 3)	44. C (2, 4)
15. E (all)	30. E (all)	45. A (1, 2, 3)

2

PHYSIOLOGY

Michael B. Wang

The basic principle underlying all of physiology is **homeostasis**—the maintenance of a constant internal environment. A vast variety of cells, organized as tissues, organs, or systems, work together not only to maintain a constant environment but to ensure that it is optimal for the performance of body functions. Body temperature must be kept close to 37°C, blood pressure must average 100 mm Hg, oxygen content must be 20 ml/100 ml of blood, carbon dioxide tension must be 40 mm Hg, pH must be 7.4, extracellular potassium must be between 4 and 5 mEq/L, osmolarity must be 285 mOsm, blood glucose must be between 80 and 120 mg/100 ml, and so on. The mechanisms by which these values are maintained and body functions are carried out form the subject of physiology. The information necessary to understand these processes will be reviewed in the sections that follow.

FUNDAMENTAL PHYSIOLOGICAL PROCESSES

This section deals with the most fundamental physiological processes—the transport of material across cell membranes, the generation of membrane potentials, the synaptic transfer of information between cells, and the performance of mechanical work by striated and smooth muscle.

THE CELL MEMBRANE

Every cell is organized in essentially the same way. It is surrounded by a cell membrane that separates the intracellular contents from the extracellular environment. Inside the cell, the nucleus is separated from the cytoplasm by a nuclear membrane. The cytoplasm contains a number of important organelles: the ribosomes, endoplasmic reticulum, and Golgi apparatus for the synthesis and excretion of proteins; the mitochondria for the production of ATP by aerobic metabolism; and lysosomes for the digestion of intracellular debris. The cell membrane is a thin (<10 nm), compliant structure composed primarily of lipids and proteins. It is responsible for regulating the passage of material between the intracellular and extracellular fluids, for establishing and maintaining a constant intracellular environment, and for activating intracellular metabolic processes in response to signals it receives from a

variety of extracellular messengers—for example, hormones, neurotransmitters, and drugs.

The backbone of the cell membrane is a bilayer of lipid into which are inserted numerous proteins (Fig. 2-1). Most of the lipids in the membrane are phospholipids of one kind or another and cholesterol. These lipids are polarized; one end is water soluble, the other is lipid soluble. Thus they tend to line up in an orderly array with their lipid-soluble ends facing each other in the interior of the membrane and the water-soluble ends facing the exterior of the membrane. The lipids forming the interior of the cell membrane are different from those forming the exterior. The most obvious difference is the preponderance of glycolipids on the exterior of the membrane. These are probably responsible for orchestrating reactions that depend on cellular recognition, such as those involved in immunologic responses. The lipid bilayer forms a natural barrier to the passage of inorganic ions and other nonlipid-soluble materials such as glucose. However, lipid-soluble material such as gases, alcohols, and urea can easily pass through the bilayer. Some membrane proteins span the entire length of the lipid bilayer. These are called **integral** or **transmembrane** proteins. Others, called **peripheral proteins**, do not penetrate the membrane and are found either on the external or internal face of the membrane. Some of these proteins form aqueous channels or pores through which small water-soluble materials can flow. Others act as carriers, transporting materials that are either not lipid soluble or too large to fit through the pores across the membrane. Still others perform enzymatic or receptor functions. The outer surface of the cell membrane appears to be covered with a coat of

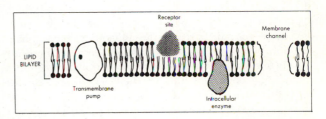

Figure 2-1. A diagrammatic view of the lipid bilayer forming the backbone of a cell membrane. Proteins, inserted into the cell membrane, serve a variety of functions such as receptors, channels, enzymes, and pumps.

carbohydrates called a **glycocalyx**. These sugars originate either as side chains of membrane glycolipids and glycoproteins or as glycolipids and glycoproteins that have been excreted by the cell and then attached to the cell membrane.

TRANSLOCATION ACROSS CELL MEMBRANES

Materials can cross cell membranes in a variety of ways. Those that can dissolve in the lipid bilayer or in the water filling the membrane pores can diffuse across the membrane. Others must be assisted across the membrane by a carrier-transport system. In some cases, the material is carried through the membrane down its electrochemical gradient. This process is called **facilitated diffusion**. In other cases, the material is carried across the membrane against its electrochemical gradient. In this case, it is called **active transport**. Water moves across membranes by a unique process called **osmosis**. Finally, the material can be enveloped by a membrane-formed vesicle, which transports the substance into or out of the cell. This type of transport is called **exocytosis** (out of the cell) or **endocytosis** (into the cell). These processes will be discussed in turn.

Simple diffusion

Simple diffusion refers to the process by which particles dissolved in a solvent (water or lipids) are kept in constant motion. The movement is driven by the heat of solution and is entirely random. That is, there is no way of predicting which way any particular particle will move. However, over time, the particles spread themselves out so their concentration is the same everywhere in the solution. The rate of diffusion depends on the size of the particle, the temperature of the solution, and the diffusibility or ease with which the particle can flow through the solvent. These characteristics are combined into a single constant called the **diffusion constant** or **coefficient** (D). When the concentration of particles in two regions of space is different, the process of diffusion leads to a net flux from the region of higher concentration to the region of lower concentration. The amount of flux is given by Fick's law of diffusion,

$$\text{Flux} = \frac{DA}{x}(C_{HIGH} - C_{LOW})$$

where A is the cross-sectional area of the boundary between the two regions, x is thickness of the boundary, and C is the concentration in each region. Molecules such as water, urea, carbon dioxide, and oxygen, which can penetrate the lipid bilayer, diffuse rapidly through cell membranes because the surface area of the lipid bilayer is so large. Ions such as sodium and potassium, which are not lipid soluble and therefore must cross the membrane through the aqueous channels, have much lower rates of diffusion. This is because there are relatively few channels in the membrane through which they can flow. In general, the diffusion coefficient of lipid-soluble materials is determined more by their lipid solubility than by their size. However, in the case of water-soluble materials, size is the most important determinant of the diffusion coefficient. Often when dealing with biologic membranes, the thickness is either not known or is assumed to be constant. Hence the flux is not normalized for thickness and Fick's law becomes

$$\text{Flux} = PA(C_{HIGH} - C_{LOW})$$

where P = the permeability constant or coefficient. D and P are related by the expression

$$P = \frac{D}{x}$$

Facilitated diffusion

Facilitated diffusion is a carrier-mediated diffusional process. Materials such as glucose and amino acids, which are not lipid soluble and are too large to fit through aqueous pores, are shuttled across the membrane by one of the integral proteins spanning the membrane. Presumably, the molecule binds to the carrier with equal affinity on the inside or outside of the membrane while the carrier goes through spontaneous reversible conformational changes. The conformational changes expose first one side and then the other side of the carrier to the inside of the cell. Net flux of material will occur if a concentration gradient exists between the inside and outside of the cell simply because there is a greater probability that the particle will bind to the carrier on the side where it is more concentrated and be released from the carrier on the side where it is less concentrated. The curvilinear line describing the relationship between the concentration gradient and flux is called **saturation** or **first-order kinetics** and is analogous to an enzyme-catalyzed reaction in which the rate of binding to the enzyme determines the rate of a chemical reaction. Of course, in carrier-mediated transport, no change in the structure of the transported molecule occurs.

Active transport processes

There are a great variety of active transport processes occurring on the cell membrane. In these processes, energy must be utilized to move materials against their electrochemical gradients. The most common of these is the sodium-potassium (Na-K) ATPase-driven pump. This enzyme pump system exists on virtually every cell and is responsible for establishing and maintaining the ionic concentration differences that exist between the inside and outside of the cell. That is, in all cells the intracellular sodium concentration is approximately 10 times lower than the extracellular sodium concentration while the intracellular potassium concentration is approximately 30 times larger than the extracellular concentration. These concentration gradients are necessary for the production of the cell's resting and action potentials. Moreover, the energy stored in the concentration gradient for sodium is used by the cell in the active transport of many other substances. This type of transport, called **indirect energy-utilizing** or **secondary active transport**, will be discussed below.

Na-K ATPase, like other carrier proteins, is an integral membrane protein. It couples the hydrolysis of one ATP molecule to the transport of three sodium ions out of the cell and two potassium ions into the cell. Although all the details are not known, it appears that the first step in the transport process is the transfer of a phosphate group from ATP to the carrier. This reaction only occurs after (or while) three sodium ions are bound to the carrier. The carrier then undergoes its first conformational change, in which sodium is transferred to the outside of the cell. In the next step, sodium detaches from the carrier, two potassium ions bind to the carrier, and the carrier undergoes a second conformation change in which the potassium ions are transported into the cell and the carrier is dephosphorylated. The carrier is now poised to begin a new cycle. Both sodium and potassium are necessary for the process to continue. Without potassium on the outside of the cell, the second conformation change could not occur. Without sodium on the inside of the cell, ATP hydrolysis could not occur. The cardiac glycoside **ouabain** and analogous drugs produce their pharmacologic effects by blocking the binding of potassium to Na-K ATPase and thus inhibiting the pump's activity.

The electrochemical gradient for sodium established by the Na-K pump can by used to transport other materials through the cell membrane against their electrochemical gradients. For example, glucose and amino acids are pumped against their concentration gradients from the lumen into the epithelial cells lining the nephron (in the kidney) and the intestinal wall (in the GI tract) by a sodium-dependent, secondary active transport system. The mechanisms underlying the behavior of this carrier are less well understood than for the Na-K ATPase pump but are thought to be based on a principle similar to that discussed earlier for facilitated diffusion. Because the electrochemical gradient for sodium is higher on the outside of the cell, it can bind to and be transported across the membrane by a membrane-bound carrier protein. There is, however, a major difference between this protein and the one used for facilitated diffusion. This protein will not undergo a conformational change unless glucose is also attached to it. As a result, both molecules cross the membrane together. The energy required for the carrier to undergo the conformational change and transport glucose into the cell is derived from the sodium electrochemical gradient. If the energy in that gradient were less than the energy required to move glucose into the cell (e.g., if the glucose concentration gradient were too high) transport would cease. Many other types of cotransport systems exist in the cell membrane, but all work in a similar way. They use the energy in the sodium electrochemical gradient established by the Na-K ATPase pump to actively transport other materials across the cell membrane.

Osmosis

Osmosis is a process in which water is driven across a membrane by a pressure gradient that is created by the presence of particles dissolved in the water. This pressure, called osmotic pressure, is a colligative property of particles. That is, like the freezing or boiling point of water, the osmotic pressure developed across a membrane depends only on the number of particles dissolved in the water and not on their charge, molecular weight, shape, etc. The osmotic pressure produced by a solute dissolved in water can be calculated using the van't Hoff equation:

$$\text{Osmotic pressure } (\pi) = c\,R\,T$$

where c = the concentration of particles, R = the natural gas constant (equal to 64 L/mOsm/°K), and T = the temperature in degrees kelvin. A simple calculation will demonstrate that osmotic pressures can be very large. For example, the concentration of plasma proteins is approximately 1.2 mOsm/L. (Note: Milliosmoles are used rather than millimoles to indicate that the number of individual particles and not molecules is being considered. Thus for example, 1 mmol of glucose = 1

mOsm; 1 mmol of sodium chloride = 2 mOsm; 1 mmol of calcium chloride = 3 mOsm, etc.) Using the van't Hoff formula,

$$\text{Osmotic pressure} = 1.2\,(64)\,(310) = 24 \text{ mm Hg}$$

Thus the plasma proteins produce an osmotic pressure approximately equal to the hydrostatic pressure within the capillaries. This pressure (called the **plasma oncotic pressure**) will become very important when considering fluid exchange across the capillaries and the filtration of fluid within the glomerulus of the kidney.

Although an osmotic pressure can be calculated for any solution, it only has meaning when two solutions are separated by a membrane that is not permeable to the solute for which the osmotic pressure is calculated. Thus, if a red blood cell (having an osmotic concentration of 285 mOsm) is placed in a sodium chloride solution having a higher osmolarity, an osmotic pressure difference across the membrane will be created and water will flow out of the cell until the two osmolarities are equal. As will be discussed below, the cell membrane is actually permeable to sodium, but because of the Na-K pump, the concentration gradient for sodium does not change and thus sodium behaves as if it were not permeable to the membrane. On the other hand, if the osmolarity of sodium were the same as that inside the red blood cell and urea were added to the extracellular fluid, the calculated osmotic pressure on the outside of the cell would be higher than on the inside. However, in this case there is no net flow of water because the cell membrane is permeable to urea. Thus the effective osmolarity is equal to the osmotic concentration of sodium chloride, which behaves as a nonpermeable solute. Urea exerts no osmotic pressure because it is permeable to the membrane. For the same reason, the osmotic pressure difference across the capillary wall is based only on the concentration of the nonpermeable plasma proteins. The other solutes within the plasma are ignored because they are permeable to the capillary.

The term **tonicity** is used instead of osmolarity when referring to just the nonpermeable particles in solution. A solution having a greater concentration of nonpermeable particles than a red blood cell is referred to as **hypertonic**; one having a lower concentration is called **hypotonic**; and one having an equal concentration is called **isotonic**. The terms hyperosmotic, hypoosmotic, and isosmotic are applied in an analogous way when the total number of particles (irrespective of their permeability) is counted. However, water will flow into or out of a cell or across a capillary membrane only when the tonicities of the two solutions are different. The volume of a cell placed in a solution having a different tonicity can be calculated using the equation

$$\pi_{INITIAL}\,V_{INITIAL} = \pi_{FINAL}\,V_{FINAL}$$

where π refers to the tonicity of the cell before and after it is placed in solution and V refers to the volume of the cell before and after it is placed in solution. Note that the volume of the cell is considered to change until it becomes isotonic with the solution. The solution is considered so large (compared with the cell) that its volume does not change.

THE RESTING MEMBRANE POTENTIAL

All cells have resting membrane potentials. These derive from two properties shared by all cells: (1) There is a difference in the concentration of ions between the inside and outside of the cell and (2) the membrane is permeable to some of these ions. As indicated previously, the Na-K ATPase pump causes sodium concentration inside the cell to be much lower than outside the cell and potassium concentration inside the cell to be much higher than outside the cell. Energy is required to establish these concentration gradients, and they in turn contain a certain amount of potential energy. As discussed above, this energy can be used to transport other substances across the cell membrane. It can also be used to create a membrane potential. To understand how this is accomplished, it is necessary to introduce a number of additional principles.

The energy contained in the concentration gradient of a substance is equal to

$$RT \ln \frac{C_{IN}}{C_{OUT}}$$

or

$$RT \ln \frac{C_1}{C_2}$$

where $\ln$ = the natural (base e) logarithm and C = the concentration of the substance inside and outside of the membrane. When the substance is an ion, any electrical field must also be considered when calculating the energy in the concentration gradient. The electrical term is equal to

$$z F E$$

where z = valance of the ion, F = the faraday, a constant (96,500) that is used to convert moles to coulombs, and E = the electrical potential energy in volts. If the two terms are equal and opposite to each other—that is, they just balance each other—then no potential energy difference exists. For example, in a normal muscle or nerve cell, the concentration of potassium inside the cell is 135 mEq/L and the concentration outside the cell is 4.5 m Eq/L. The energy in the concentration gradient is then

$$8.3 \times 310 \times \ln \frac{135}{4.5}$$

or 8750 J. The electrical potential with the same energy would be

$$\frac{8,750}{1 \times 96,500} = 0.091 \text{ V or } 91 \text{ mV}$$

The calculations are not as important as the conclusion, which is that a concentration gradient of 135 mEq/L inside the cell and 4.5 mEq/L outside the cell has the same energy as a membrane potential of 91 mV. Intuitively, it can be reasoned that the membrane potential must be negative inside the cell to balance the tendency of potassium to diffuse out of the cell

down its concentration gradient. If such a membrane potential were to exist, it would produce an equilibrium state between the concentration and electrical gradients. Such a potential is thus called an **equilibrium potential** and can be calculated, as above, by setting the two potential terms equal and opposite to each other and solving for E. When this is done, it yields

$$E = \frac{RT}{zF} \ln \frac{C_{IN}}{C_{OUT}}$$

Replacing the constants and converting from natural logs to common logs (base 10) yields

$$E = \frac{61}{z} \log \frac{C_{IN}}{C_{OUT}}$$

This is the Nernst equation. Although the value of the equilibrium potential calculated with it has many interpretations, perhaps the most useful is to equate E with the number of volts necessary to balance the energy in the concentration gradient or more simply the voltage equal to the concentration gradient.

The next concept to introduce is that of **driving force**. If the equilibrium potential calculated with the Nernst potential is equal and opposite in sign to the membrane potential actually measured across a cell membrane, no net movement of charge will occur. That is, the two energies will balance each other. However, if there is a difference, the two will be out of balance and a net flow of charge will be driven across the membrane. Since flow of charge is measured as current, the current across the membrane can be calculated using Ohm's law:

$$I = g E$$

where I = current, g = conductance (Note: this term is the reciprocal of resistance but is used in this equation because it makes the calculations easier and because it is analogous, although not identical, to membrane permeability), and E = the electrical voltage driving the current across the membrane.

The value of E, called the driving force, is the difference between the measured membrane potential and the calculated equilibrium potential. Substituting the driving force yields

$$I = g (E_{MEMBRANE} - E_{EQUILIBRIUM})$$

Table 2-1 lists the equilibrium potentials and driving forces for a number of ions of importance for nerve and muscle physiology. Notice that the driving force for sodium is much higher than the driving force for potassium. This occurs, even though the concentration gradient is not as high, because both the concentration gradient and the membrane potential are driving sodium into the cell, whereas in the case of potassium, the membrane potential is acting to oppose the diffusion of potassium out of the cell. The driving force is also called the **electrochemical gradient,** the membrane potential providing the electrical portion and the concentration gradient (whose energy is calculated using the Nernst equation) providing the chemical portion. The high electrochemical gradient of sodium allows it to be used as an energy source for the indirect active transport systems discussed earlier.

Table 2-1.
Equilibrium and Driving Forces of Ions

Ion	Conc$_{\text{INTRACELLULAR}}$ (mmol/L)	Conc$_{\text{EXTRACELLULAR}}$ (mmol/L)	Equilibrium (mV)	Driving force (mV)	Transference
Na$^+$	15	142	60	-145	0.05
K$^+$	135	4	-93	$+8$	0.95
Ca^{++}	10^{-4}	2	$+129$	—	$<<0.1$
Cl$^-$	4	120	-90	—	$<<0.1$

In a typical cell, the potassium current out of the cell is approximately equal to the sodium current into the cell. Actually, the ratio is three sodium ions out for every two potassium ions in, but the difference will be ignored to make the calculations simpler. The potassium current is

$$G_K \ (E_M - E_K)$$

and the sodium current is

$$G_{Na} \ (E_M - E_{Na})$$

Setting these two currents equal and solving for E yields

$$E_M = \frac{G_K}{G_K + G_{Na}} \ E_K \ + \ \frac{G_{Na}}{G_K + G_{Na}} \ E_{Na}$$

The terms

$$\frac{G_{Na}}{G_K + G_{Na}} \quad \text{and} \quad \frac{G_K}{G_K + G_{Na}}$$

are called the transferences for potassium and sodium. They indicate how much of the membrane conductance is due to potassium and how much is due to sodium. Thus, to calculate the membrane potential the absolute values of the conductances do not have to be known, only their ratios. Substituting the transferences in the above equation for calculating the membrane potential yields a very useful equation:

$$E_M \ = \ T_K \ E_K \ + \ E_M \ E_K$$

From this equation, it can be seen that the membrane potential for any cell depends on two factors: (1) the relative conductance of the membrane for the various ions that can travel through it and (2) the concentration gradients for those ions. An intuitive understanding of this principle can be obtained by considering what happens before there is a membrane potential. Sodium flows into the cell at a rate dependent on its concentration gradient and permeability. But as sodium flows into the cell, it makes the cell positive and thus reduces the rate of sodium flow. Similarly, potassium flows out of the cell and, as it does so, it makes the cell negative, reducing its rate of flow. Thus, as the ions flow through the membrane, they change the membrane potential. The membrane potential continues to change until it reaches a potential at which the inward flow of sodium ions equals the outward flow of

potassium ions. This is the potential calculated using the transference equation.

For example, the resting membrane potential for a typical nerve cell can be calculated using the transference equation and the values for transference and equilibrium potentials given in Table 2-1.

$$E_M = 0.95 \times -93 + 60 + 0.05 \times -85 = -85 \text{ mV}$$

The membrane potential can be changed in two ways: (1) Either the equilibrium potentials for one of the ions can be changed or (2) the transference for one of the ions can be changed. If the extracellular potassium concentration were to rise (e.g., as a result of renal failure or metabolic acidosis) to 7.5 mEq/L, the potassium equilibrium potential would become

$$-61 \log 135/7.5 = -77 \text{ mV}$$

The resting membrane potential would become

$$0.95 \times -77 + .05 \times 60 = -70 \text{ mV}$$

On the other hand, if the potassium concentration were to fall (e.g., as a consequence of diuretic therapy) to 2.5 mV, the equilibrium potential would become 104 mV and the membrane potential would become -95 mV. A decrease in the magnitude of the membrane potential is called a **depolarization,** and an increase in the magnitude is called a **hyperpolarization.** Thus, increasing extracellular potassium causes the membrane to depolarize whereas decreasing extracellular potassium causes the membrane to hyperpolarize. The same sort of changes would occur if extracellular sodium or chloride were to change, but from a physiological point of view they are not as important because (1) the transferences for sodium and chloride are so low that even large changes in their equilibrium potentials would have only a small effect on the membrane potential and (2) since their outside concentrations are so high, it is unlikely that they could ever change enough to cause a large change in the equilibrium potential.

THE ACTION POTENTIAL

The membrane potential can also be changed by changing the transference for one or more of the ions present in the intracellular or extracellular fluids. This is the basis for the action potential. Figure 2-2 illustrates the various components of the action potential. When a nerve or muscle cell is depolarized to threshold by a stimulus, it undergoes a stereotypic alteration in its membrane potential. The upstroke

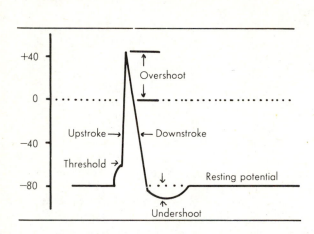

Figure 2-2. When a stimulus depolarizes a nerve membrane to threshold, an action potential is initiated. The upstroke of the action potential is produced by the inward flow of sodium, the downstroke by the outward flow of potassium. The overshoot is the period of time during which the inside of the membrane is positive with respect to the outside. The undershoot, during which the membrane is more negative than when it is at rest, is caused by a high membrane conductance to potassium.

of the action potential is caused by the inward flow of sodium ions, whereas the downstroke is caused by the outward flow of potassium ions. The ability of nerve and muscle cells to produce an action potential is derived from the special characteristics of the aqueous channels through which sodium and potassium are able to flow through the membrane (Fig. 2-3).

First, these channels are ion selective; one allows only sodium to pass through it, the other allows only potassium to pass through it. Second, the channels are gated. The sodium channels have two gates; an "h" gate on the inside of the cell and an "m" gate on the outside of the cell. The potassium channel has a single gate—an "n" gate located on the outside of the cell. Third, the gates on the channels are voltage sensitive. The m and n gates are closed when the cell is polarized and open when the cell is depolarized. The h gate behaves in the

opposite manner. It is open when the cell is polarized and closed when the cell is depolarized. Fourth, the gates are time dependent. Although they all change their positions when the membrane potential changes, they do so at different rates. The m gates on the sodium channels respond first to a voltage change, followed by the h gates and finally by the n gates.

A square micron of a nerve cell membrane may contain many hundreds of sodium and potassium ions. At rest, when the cell is polarized, most of these channels are unable to conduct current because the m and n gates are closed. However, some are open, and of those open there are approximately nine times more open potassium channels than there are open sodium channels. Thus at rest, the potassium transference is 0.95 and the sodium transference is 0.05. (Note: The chloride conductance, which does not change during the action potential, is being ignored for simplicity.) Using the transference equation and the equilibrium potentials in Table 2-2, the resting membrane potential is calculated to be −85 mV.

When the membrane is depolarized to threshold, some of the m gates open, allowing sodium ions to flow into the cell down their electrochemical gradient. The flow of positive ions into the cell causes the cell to depolarize even further. The increased depolarization causes more m gates to open, and this allows more sodium to enter the cell, causing even more depolarization. This cycle, called a **positive feedback cycle** or regenerative response, continues until almost all of the m gates are open and the cell depolarizes to approximately +40 mV. The cell does not remain at +40 mV, however, because of the subsequent change in the position of the h and n gates. As indicated above, the h gates close when the cell is depolarized, preventing any further flow of sodium into the cell, and the n gates open, allowing potassium to flow out of the cell. The flow of positive potassium ions out of the cell causes the membrane to repolarize.

The time dependency of the gates is important to the development of the action potential. If the m and h gates responded at the same time to the depolarizing stimulus, sodium would not be able to flow into the cell, because as the m gates opened the h gates would be closing. The time dependency of the gates explains several other properties of the action potential as well.

First, the hyperpolarization phase at the end of the action

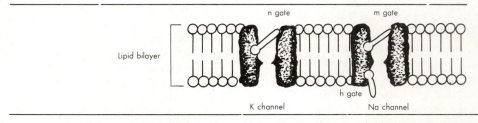

Figure 2-3.   Two voltage and time-dependent channels are responsible for the sequence of conductance changes that produce the action potential. The sodium channel is covered by an activation gate (the m gate) on its extracellular side and an inactivation gate (the h gate) on its intracellular side. The potassium channel is covered by just one gate, the n gate, located on its extracellular side. During an action potential, the m gates open first, allowing sodium to flow into the cell. This is followed by the closing of the h gate, stopping the inward flow of sodium, and the opening of the n gate, allowing potassium to flow out of the cell.

Table 2-2.
Ionic Composition of the Body Water Compartments

Ion	Plasma (mEq/L)	Plasma water (mEq/L)	Interstitial fluid (mEq/L)
Cations			
Na^+	142.0	152.7	145.1
K^+	4.3	4.6	4.4
Ca^{2+} (ionized)	2.5	2.7	2.4
Mg^{2+} (ionized)	1.1	1.2	1.1
Total	149.9	161.2	153.0
Anions			
Cl^-	104.0	111.9	117.4
HCO_3^-	24.0	25.8	27.1
$HPO_4^{2-}, H_2PO_4^-$	2.0	2.2	2.3
Proteins	14.0	15.0	0.0
Other	5.9	6.3	6.2
Total	149.9	161.2	153.0

potential results from a delay in closing of the potassium channels. The n gates, which respond last to membrane depolarization, also respond last when the membrane is repolarized. Consequently, there are more potassium channels open at the end of the action potential than there were when the cell was in its resting state, making the potassium conductance equal to 0.98. Applying the transference equation yields a membrane potential of −89 mV.

Second, the time dependency of the gates explains the altered excitability or refractory periods that occur during the action potential. During the upstroke and for most of the downstroke, applying a second stimulus will not produce a second action potential. This period of time is called the **absolute refractory period.** A stimulus applied during the upstroke has no effect, because the regenerative sodium cycle produces the same depolarization regardless of the magnitude or duration of the stimulus. This is referred to as an all-or-none response. During the initial portion of the downstroke, the stimulus is ineffective because the h gates are still closed. Stimulating the membrane will have no effect, because depolarization will cause even more of the h gates to close. When sodium is unable to pass through the sodium channels because the h gates are closed, the sodium channels are said to be inactivated.

During the latter phase of the downstroke and the hyperpolarization at the end of the action potential, enough h gates have opened to permit the generation of a second action potential. However, the strength of the stimulus must be greater than normal. This period of time is called the **relative refractory period.** It results both because many of the sodium channels are still inactivated and because the membrane is further from threshold because of the large number of potassium channels still open.

Thus far, the discussion of the Na-K pump in the generation of the membrane potential and action potential has been limited to its role in establishing the concentration gradients for sodium and potassium. Because the resistance of the membrane

at rest is fairly large, very few sodium and potassium ions leak through the membrane and the pump consumes little energy in maintaining the ionic gradients. Even during an action potential, only a few ions need to cross the membrane to produce the observed change in membrane potential. Thus only a small increase in pump activity is required to restore the steady state. Of course, if the axon fires at a high rate for a considerable duration of time, such as in a seizure, a significant amount of metabolic energy will be consumed. If the metabolic demands are too great, ionic homeostasis could be disturbed, resulting in damage or death of the neuron.

The pump also plays a small role in determining the magnitude of the resting potential. Because the pump transports three sodium ions out of the cell for every two potassium ions it transports into the cell, the pump is electrogenic. That is, each time it cycles it adds to the intracellular negativity of the cell. For example, if as a result of a large number of action potentials the intracellular sodium concentration were to rise, the pump's activity would increase. This increase could be sufficient to cause the membrane to hyperpolarize by a few millivolts. However, under most circumstances the amount of pump activity is so small that it contributes little to the resting potential. As a result, its contribution is usually ignored when discussing the factors responsible for the magnitude of the resting potential. This is a reasonable omission because, even after the pump is poisoned, it takes several hours before significant changes in ionic concentrations are observed and many hundreds of normal action potentials can be initiated.

The major function of an action potential is the transfer of information along a nerve or muscle membrane. This transfer is accomplished by the process of propagation. During propagation, the original action potential acts as a stimulus for the generation of a second action potential on a neighboring patch of membrane. The newly generated action potential then produces another action potential on the next patch of membrane and so on. Thus information is spread along an axon by the generation of new action potentials at successive patches of membrane.

Thus the action potential reaching the end of the axon has the same magnitude as the one elicited by the stimulus. When the action potential reaches the end of the axon, it does not propagate in the opposite direction because the patch of membrane just behind it is still in its refractory period. Thus, even though the action potential can propagate in any direction along the axon, propagation normally occurs in only one direction.

The speed of propagation depends on the diameter of the axon and its degree of myelinization. The axoplasm of the larger axons has a lower electrical resistance to the flow of current than the smaller axons. As a result, more current will flow to the next patch of membrane in the larger axons and threshold will be reached sooner. Because a new action potential is generated more rapidly in the larger axons, propagation proceeds more rapidly. Myelination adds resistance to the flow of current through the plasma membrane of the axon. In fact, the amount of resistance is so great that current can flow only through the small patches of membrane exposed to the extracellular fluid between the individual Schwann's cells that make up the myelin sheath. The patches of membrane, called nodes of Ranvier, occur at intervals of 0.5 to

2 mm along the axon. Thus action potentials are generated at intervals approximately 1 mm apart instead of on contiguous patches of membrane as they are in unmyelinated fibers. Because the action potentials jump from node to node, propagation in myelinated axons is called saltatory (meaning to jump or dance) conduction. In demyelinating diseases such as multiple sclerosis or after nerve injuries, the Schwann's cell sheaths produce less membrane resistance and the nodes become closer together. As a result, action potential propagation is slowed or prevented, resulting in severe deficits of sensory and motor behavior.

SYNAPTIC TRANSMISSION

Communication between neurons and other cells is essential for the production of all activity, from the simplest reflex to the most complex of our social interactions. Although a small part of this communication occurs electrically, almost all of it occurs chemically. The junction between nerve cells or between nerve and muscle or gland cells is called a **synapse,** and the process by which information passes between the two cells is called synaptic transmission. In some cases, such as the neuromuscular junction between the alpha motoneuron and a skeletal muscle fiber, only one synapse occurs. In other cases, such as on an alpha motoneuron, many thousands of synapses occur. In each case, however, the process of synaptic transmission is essentially the same. An action potential propagating along the nerve axon reaches the axon terminal, where it causes the release of a synaptic transmitter agent. The synaptic transmitter agent then diffuses across the extracellular space between the nerve terminal and the target cell, binds to a receptor on the target cell, and causes some sort of response. The process ends when the synaptic transmitter substance is inactivated. This process will be described first for the skeletal muscle neuromuscular junction and then for the more complex synaptic junctions within the CNS.

Neuromuscular synaptic transmission

The morphology of the neuromuscular synapse is illustrated in Figure 2-4. The axon from the alpha mononeuron diverges as it approaches the muscle bundle. Large axons can form several hundred branches, whereas smaller axons form just a few branches. Each branch innervates just one muscle fiber, and each muscle fiber receives a branch from only one alpha motoneuron. All the fibers innervated by a single alpha motoneuron are called a motor unit. The axon terminal loses its myelin sheath as it nears the skeletal muscle fiber and terminates in a synaptic groove or trough formed by an invagination of the muscle membrane. A 50-nm-wide space, called the **synaptic cleft,** separates the presynaptic nerve membrane from the postsynaptic muscle membrane. A connective tissue mass called the basal lamina is located within the synaptic cleft. Acetylcholinesterase, an enzyme that destroys acetylcholine (ACh), is attached to the basal lamina. The basal lamina quite possibly plays a role in maintaining the structural integrity of the synaptic region or in guiding the growth of synapses during development. However, its exact function is not known. The postsynaptic membrane, called the end-plate membrane, is approximately 0.5 mm long and forms a series of junctional folds that contain binding sites for the neurotransmitter released from the presynaptic nerve terminal.

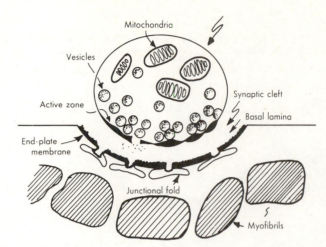

Figure 2-4. A diagrammatic view of the neuromuscular synapse. The presynaptic terminal contains transmitter-filled synaptic vesicles. When these vesicles bind to special attachment sites, they release their transmitter by exocytosis. Binding is activated by calcium, which enters the presynaptic terminal through calcium channels located close to the attachment sites. Receptors for the transmitter are located on the postsynaptic membrane. Acetylcholinesterase, a hydrolytic enzyme that terminates the synaptic response, is located in the synaptic gap between the pre- and postsynaptic membranes.

The axon terminal is specialized for the release of chemical transmitter agents. It contains numerous vesicles and mitochondria. The vesicles store the neurotransmitter, and the mitochondria provide the energy required for the synthesis of the transmitter. The inner surface of the membrane facing the junctional folds is covered with a series of structures that are **called dense bars** because they are seen as dark stripes in electron micrographs of the presynaptic nerve terminal. Synaptic vesicles collect in rows opposite the dense bars and release their stored synaptic transmitter at membrane sites associated with the dense bars. Finally, calcium-selective membrane channels appear to be lined up on both sides of the dense bars. The entire region—the dense bars and their associated vesicles, the calcium channels, and the vesicular release sites—is called the **active zone.**

Synaptic vesicles are formed from invaginations of the presynaptic membrane. The transmitter at the neuromuscular junction, ACh, is actively pumped across the vesicular membrane and becomes highly concentrated within the vesicle. The number of ACh molecules in a vesicle has been estimated to be between 5 and 10 thousand. The biosynthetic pathways involves the enzyme choline acetyl transferase (CAT), which catalyses the production of ACh from choline and acetyl coenzyme A (acetyl CoA). Choline is not synthesized in the nerve terminal and must be obtained from the extracellular fluid. It is pumped into the cell by a sodium-dependent indirect active transport system similar to the ones discussed previously. Acetyl CoA is readily available as a by-product of the citric acid cycle. Although failure to synthesize ACh at the neuromuscular junctions has not been associated with any disease processes, loss of the CAT enzyme within the hippocampus has been implicated as one of the causes of Alzheimer's disease, and some therapeutic regimens have been directed toward increasing the supply of ACh available for the affected neurons.

Release of synaptic transmitter occurs by exocytosis. The process is initiated by calcium entering the cell through the calcium channels that line the dense bars. These channels are voltage sensitive. That is, like the sodium and potassium channels discussed in connection with the action potential, they open in response to membrane depolarization. Thus, when the action potential propagates into the nerve terminal, it causes the calcium channels to open. Calcium then flows into the cell down its electrochemical gradient. Once inside the cell, calcium promotes the fusion of synaptic vesicles with release sites in the active zone. Although the mechanism by which calcium initiates exocytosis is not known, it is clear that the number of vesicles released is highly sensitive to the amount of calcium entering the cell. Thus, as will be described later when considering synaptic transmission in the CNS, small alterations in intracellular calcium accumulation can have profound effects on the synaptic transmission process.

Once the vesicles have merged with the presynaptic membrane, their interiors are exposed to the extracellular fluid and the transmitter substance diffuses out of the vesicle and into the synaptic cleft. The empty vesicle then fully merges with the presynaptic membrane. Within a minute or two after synaptic release has occurred, invaginations form on the presynaptic membrane. These invaginations, called coated pits, are covered with a fibrous protein called **clathrin**. The coated pits eventually bud off from the membrane, lose their clathrin covering, reaccumulate ACh, and once again become available for the release of neurotransmitter. The recycling of vesicles operates rapidly enough to maintain a sufficient supply of neurotransmitter for all but the highest rates of stimulation.

After being released from the presynaptic vesicle, the transmitter diffuses across the synaptic cleft and attaches to binding sites on the postsynaptic receptor. These receptors, located on the membrane of the subsynaptic folds, are a highly complex membrane protein consisting of two binding sites and a channel through which both sodium and potassium (and possibly calcium) can flow. These channels, in contrast to those that are necessary to produce an action potential, are not voltage sensitive—that is, they do not open or close in response to changes in membrane potential. Instead, they are chemically sensitive, opening only when ACh is bound to them.

The channels activated by ACh are equally permeable to sodium and potassium. However, when they are opened the amount of sodium entering the cell exceeds the amount of potassium leaving because the driving force for sodium is greater. Consequently, the opening of a single channel causes approximately 0.3 mV of depolarization. As indicated above, a single vesicle contains approximately 5,000 ACh molecules. Even when not stimulated, vesicles spontaneously fuse with the presynaptic membrane and release their contents into the synaptic cleft. Not all of the ACh reaches the postsynaptic receptors, because some diffuses out of the synaptic region and some is hydrolyzed by the acetylcholinesterase (AChase) in the cleft. However, enough ACh reaches the postsynaptic membrane to cause a depolarization of 1/2 to 1 mV. This depolarization is called a miniature end-plate potential because (1) it is small and (2) it occurs on the end-plate region of the muscle.

When an action potential invades the presynaptic nerve terminal, the calcium entering the cell causes between 200 and 300 vesicles to release their contents into the synaptic cleft. This causes a membrane depolarization of 75 mV—that is, the end-plate region of the membrane depolarizes from −90 to −15 mV. This neurally evoked depolarization is called an **end-plate potential** (EPP). The EPP cannot propagate along the end-plate region because no voltage-sensitive channels are present. Under normal circumstances, the depolarization is sufficient to reach threshold and an action potential is generated. However, this may not always happen. For example, the drug curare, used as a muscle relaxer during surgery, blocks the ACh receptors on the end-plate. This reduces the size of the EPP and interferes with neuromuscular transmission. Myasthenia gravis, an autoimmune disease in which the body produces antibodies to the ACh receptors, also causes muscle weakness by blocking neuromuscular transmission.

Inactivation of the neurotransmitter must occur soon after the receptor is activated to prevent prolonged depolarization. The enzyme AChase, attached to the basal lamina within the synaptic cleft, hydrolyzes the ACh. Acetate escapes into the extracellular fluid, and the choline is transported back into the presynaptic terminal and reused in the synthesis of new ACh. Anticholinesterases that prolong the action of ACh have been used to treat the acute effects of myasthenia gravis and other disorders in which the number of ACh receptors are diminished. Most of the pathological effects of anticholinesterase nerve gases are caused by the increased activity of the autonomic nervous system, which also uses ACh as a neurotransmitter.

CNS synaptic transmission

Synapses within the CNS have a much more diverse and complicated morphology than those in the periphery. The synapses forming on the alpha motoneuron (Fig. 2-5) serve as a model for other CNS synapses. Many thousands of synaptic terminals are located on a typical alpha motoneuron. These terminals come from hundreds of different neurons, some of which, such as Ia afferent neurons from muscle spindles or corticospinal tract neurons from the motor cortex, are located far from the alpha motoneuron. Others, called interneurons,

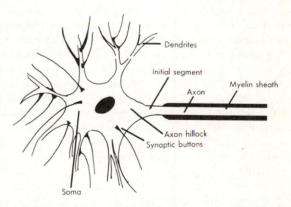

Figure 2-5. Most of the proximal dendrites and cell body of alpha motoneurons are covered with synaptic terminals. If the membrane at the axon hillock is depolarized to threshold, an action potential will be initiated. However, when the depolarization produced by a single presynaptic terminal is not sufficient to bring the axon hillock to threshold, summation of many excitatory responses is necessary. Action potential generation can be inhibited by the action of the inhibitory synapses, which keep the axon hillock from depolarizing to threshold.

are located close by and serve to relay information from a multitude of inputs. They differ from the neuromuscular synapse in a number of significant ways. First, they are smaller. Most of the synaptic terminals on alpha motoneurons and other neurons within the CNS are only a few microns in diameter. As a result, they have fewer vesicles within them and cause less of a postsynaptic effect when they discharge an action potential. Second, they contain a large variety of neurotransmitter agents that, depending on the type of receptor located on the postsynaptic membrane, can cause either excitation or inhibition. Third, their excitability can be altered by axoaxonic synapses, which cause a reduction (or sometimes an increase) in the amount of transmitter released from them.

The small size of the synaptic terminal allows only a small number of active zones to line up along the presynaptic membrane. As a result, only a few vesicles release their content into the synaptic cleft when the terminal is depolarized by an action potential. This in turn results in only a small postsynaptic effect. If the transmitter causes a depolarization of the postsynaptic membrane, the response is called an **excitatory postsynaptic potential** (EPSP). If the transmitter causes a hyperpolarization or in other ways decreases the excitability of the postsynaptic membrane, the response is called an **inhibitory postsynaptic potential** (IPSP). In either case, the magnitude of the response is too small to cause any significant change in the excitability of the alpha motoneuron. However, if the efferent fiber discharges repetitively at a high frequency, it can release enough transmitter to cause an action potential to be elicited on the alpha motoneuron (if it is an excitatory synapse) or prevent one from being elicited (if it is an inhibitory synapse). This type of summation is called **temporal summation** because the transmitter effect is summed over time. Alternatively, several excitatory or inhibitory synapses can summate by discharging at the same time. This is called **spatial summation** because the transmitter is spread out over a wide area of the cell body.

Alpha motoneurons and most other neurons within the CNS have a spike-generating region or trigger zone on their axon hillock. This is the transitional zone between the cell body and axon. A large number of voltage-sensitive channels are inserted into this region, so even a small depolarization will lead to an action potential. Phrased another way, the threshold for excitation is much lower in the axon hillock than on the cell body. The EPSPs and IPSPs produced on the cell body do not propagate (there are few voltage-sensitive channels on the cell body). However, the local depolarizations or hyperpolarizations produced by them all summate on the axon hillock. If the summed effect is sufficient to reach threshold, an action potential is generated. If, on the other hand, the IPSPs predominate, no action potential will be produced.

The ability of the presynaptic terminal to release transmitter can be altered in a number of ways. One important mechanism is called **presynaptic inhibition**. As indicated above, presynaptic inhibition is produced by the actions of an axoaxonic synapse. The transmitter released at the axoaxonic synapse causes an increase in conductance to chloride ions. As a consequence, there is a reduction in the depolarization caused by an action potential invading the nerve terminal. This can be understood by referring back to the transference equation. Recall that changing the proportion of open channels for any

ion will change the magnitude of the membrane potential. Under normal circumstances, sodium transference during the height of the action potential is 0.9 and potassium transference is 0.1. Thus the peak of the action potention is +45 mV. Chloride conductance was ignored because it was very small and did not change during the action potential. However, when the axoaxonic synapse causes chloride conductance to increase, it must be included in the transference equation. Suppose that the increase in chloride conductance caused its transference to become 0.1. Sodium transference would be reduced to 0.81 and potassium (still one-ninth of sodium) would be 0.09. Inserting these numbers into the transference equation (and again using the equilibrium potentials from Table 2-1) yields

$$0.1 \times -90 + 0.81 \times + 60 + 0.09 \times -93 = +31 \text{ mV}$$

Even this change (from 45 to 31 mV) in depolarization will have a large effect on the number of calcium channels opened. The reduction in calcium entering the presynaptic terminal will reduce the number of vesicles fusing to their release sites and thus reduce the size of the EPSP. The concentration of calcium within the cell can also be altered by the previous activity of the nerve terminal. For example, many interneurons discharge action potentials at extraordinarily high rates, called **tetanic firing**. There is insufficient time for calcium to be removed from the presynaptic nerve terminal in between action potentials, and, as a result, calcium accumulates in the terminal. Later, sometimes for more than an hour, each action potential fired by the axon terminal causes the release of an increased amount of transmitter. This process, called **posttetanic potentiation**, may serve as a model for how neuronal networks can store information for brief periods of time.

CNS receptors can operate in a variety of ways. Many receptors are analogous to the ACh receptors on the muscle end-plate. When the transmitter binds to the receptor, it causes a channel to open. The current flowing through the channel determines the change in potential produced by the transmitter-receptor complex. In most cases, within the CNS EPSPs are produced by channels that allow sodium and potassium (and possibly calcium) to pass through them. These channels differ little from those on the end-plate. The inhibitory channels most often operate by opening channels through which chloride can flow. Since in most cases the equilibrium potential for chloride is more negative than the resting potential of the neuron, chloride will flow into the cell, causing a hyperpolarization. However, even in those cases where the chloride potential is positive to the membrane potential, it still decreases the size of the EPSP (just as it decreased the magnitude of the action potential in the case of presynaptic inhibition described above) and thus acts to reduce the excitability of the neuron.

Another class of CNS receptors acts not by changing membrane conductances but by affecting the metabolic processes within the cell. This type of synaptic process is described as a second-messenger system. One of the major classes of second messengers is cyclic AMP (cAMP). In this system, the neurotransmitter binds to a receptor, called a *beta* receptor. The transmitter-receptor complex, instead of opening a channel, activates another membrane-bound protein called the G-protein. Once activated, the G-protein binds guanosine triphosphate (GTP) and then, after diffusing through the cytoplasm, associates with and activates adenylate cyclase. The adenylate cyclase then catalyzes the conversion of ATP to cAMP. The newly formed cAMP then activates a number of protein kinases, which in turn alter the activity of a large number of metabolic reactions. The duration of the effect brought about by the receptor is regulated by a number of enzymatic reactions. For example, the G-protein continues to activate the adenylate cyclase until the GTP attached to it is dephosphorylated to guanosine diphosphate (GDP) and the cAMP continues to activate protein kinases until it is hydrolyzed by a phosphodiesterase. Because these reactions occur for some time after the initial binding of the transmitter to the receptor, the effect of even a small number of transmitter molecules can be amplified many times.

Other intracellular second messengers can also be activated by transmitter-receptor binding. For example, phosphatidylinositol, a lipid common to many membranes, can be hydrolyzed by membrane-bound enzymes that are activated when a transmitter binds to its receptor. The products of the phosphatidylinositol hydrolysis, diacylglycerol and inositol triphosphate (IP_3), both can act as second messengers. Calcium also acts as a second messenger, activating calmodulin and other intracellular enzymes. Although the details of these reactions are not all completely known, it is clear that neuronal (and, as will be discussed later, muscle) activity is not regulated solely by changes in its membrane potential. In fact, it may turn out that the membrane potential changes, although easier to measure and first to be studied, may not be the most important mechanism by which synaptic transmitters communicate with their postsynaptic cells.

The identities of the synaptic transmitters within the CNS have not been easily established. To date, over two dozen transmitter candidates have been proposed. Although most of these have not met all the requirements for proof of their transmitter status, many of them are accepted as neurotransmitters. They are divided into two categories: small, low-molecular-weight amines and polypeptides.

The low-molecular-weight amines are all synthesized by cytosolic enzymes found in the nerve terminals from readily available substrates. All except ACh are derived from or are themselves amino acids. The biosynthesis of ACh has been discussed above. ACh is the most common of the transmitters in the peripheral nervous system. It is, as indicated above, the transmitter at the alpha motoneuron-skeletal muscle synapse. It is also the transmitter within all of the autonomic ganglia and for the synapses formed by the postganglionic fibers of the parasympathetic nervous system. In addition, it acts as the transmitter in a number of areas within the CNS, including the hippocampus, the thalamus, and the axons of the corticospinal tract. The catecholamines (norepinephrine, epinephrine, and dopamine) all are derived from the amino acid tyrosine. Peripherally, norepinephrine is released by the postganglionic axons of the sympathetic nervous system. Centrally it is released by cells located in many areas including the hypothalamus and the locus ceruleus of the brain. Dopamine is predominantly found in the substantia nigra, one of the basal ganglia. Destruction of these neurons is one of the causes of Parkinson's disease. Serotonin, or 5-hydroxytryptamine, is an indoleamine derived from the amino acid tryptophan. It is

found in many locations within the CNS where it is used by pathways responsible for maintaining mood and consciousness. Histamine is an imidazole, derived from the amino acid histidine. It is a ubiquitous substance involved in a variety of physiological reactions, such as inflammation, which are not related to synaptic transmission. However, it acts as one of the major transmitters in the hypothalamus and in the intrinsic nervous system of the GI tract. Cimetidine, a heavily prescribed drug used in ulcer therapy, is a histamine antagonist that prevents the histamine-induced release of hydrochloric acid from the stomach.

The major amino acid neurotransmitters are glycine and gamma aminobutyric acid (GABA), which are inhibitory, and glutamate and aspartate, which are excitatory. These amino acids are found in high concentrations in almost all neurons. However, those neurons making use of them as neurotransmitters must have the ability to sequester them in synaptic vesicles. Thus, although nerve terminals contain glutamate and GABA (which is synthesized from glutamate) in roughly the same concentrations. vesicles in inhibitory neurons only store GABA whereas those in excitatory neurons only store glutamate.

Peptide neurotransmitters differ from other transmitters in a number of significant ways. Unlike the low-molecular-weight transmitters, which are synthesized in the nerve terminal, polypeptides are synthesized in the cell body on ribosomes and transported to the nerve terminal by axoplasmic transport. Second, the polypeptides are often released from nerve terminals far from their postsynaptic cells. Their action in these cases is more to modulate the excitability of the postsynaptic cell rather than to directly affect its activity. However, polypeptides can also be released directly onto receptors of postsynaptic cells and play important roles in many cortical functions related to behavior. For example, substance P is proposed as the neurotransmitter involved in pain-reduction and pleasure-enhancing pathways, and adrenocorticotropin (ACTH) has been implicated as a mediator of the body's response to stress. Finally, polypeptides are inactivated much more slowly than the low-molecular-weight transmitters. No specific neuronal pump systems or degradative enzymes for the polypeptides have been identified. Thus, their activity is terminated only after they have diffused away from the postsynaptic cell. The slow inactivation causes the cellular responses elicited by polypeptides to continue long after the neuron releasing them has stopped firing.

SKELETAL MUSCLE

Muscle fibers are designed to convert chemical energy into mechanical energy. Two types of muscle fibers exist—**striated** muscle, which consists of skeletal and cardiac muscle, and **smooth** muscle. Although the basic principles of muscle contraction apply to all three groups of muscle fibers, there are major differences between them. The general characteristics of skeletal muscle will be discussed first, followed by a description of those aspects of contraction that are peculiar to cardiac and smooth muscle.

Skeletal muscles, as their name implies, are responsible for holding the skeleton together and moving it about. Each muscle is composed of individual muscle fibers approximately

10 to 100 μm in diameter and one to several hundred millimeters long. Individual fibers are covered with a **sarcolemma**, which consists of the cell membrane and a basement membrane containing a loose collection of polysaccharides and collagen fibers. The sarcolemma attaches to a connective tissue sheath called the **endomysium**, which surrounds each fiber. Approximately 20 to 30 muscle fibers are bundled together into fascicles held together by another connective tissue sheath called the **perimysium**. All of these connective tissue sheaths eventually merge to form the tendon, through which mechanical force produced by the muscle is transmitted to the bone.

The muscle fibers are divided longitudinally into function units called **myofibrils**. The myofibrils are approximately 1 μm in diameter and contain the thick and thin filaments that provide the force-generating capability of the muscle fibers. Myofibrils are separated from each other by the **sarcoplasmic reticulum** (SR), a diffuse network of tubules responsible for storing calcium within the fiber. In longitudinal sections, the muscle fibers are divided into dark and light bands, called **A bands** and **I bands**, respectively, which give skeletal (and cardiac) muscle fibers their striated appearance (Fig. 2-6). The thin filaments (which make up the I band) are kept in register across the muscle fiber by a dark band of protein called the **Z line**, which extends through the muscle fiber in the center of each I band. The portion of the muscle fiber between two Z lines is called the **sarcomere**. The thin filaments are attached to both sides of the Z line and extend into the middle of the sarcomere, where they interdigitate with the thick filaments. The thick filaments and the portion of the thin filaments interdigitating with them in the center of the sarcomere are responsible for the dark appearance of the A band. Thick filaments are kept in register with each other by a thin strand of protein called the **M line**, which extends through the muscle fiber in the center of the A band. The region of muscle without thick filaments, consisting of the Z line and the thin filaments attached to both sides of them, make up the I band. The central region of the A band not containing thin filaments is somewhat lighter than the rest of the A band and is called the **H band**.

The thick filaments are about 1.6 μm long and 10 nm in diameter. They are formed almost entirely by the protein myosin (Fig. 2-7). Myosin is a large molecule divided into two parts, a tail region called light meromyosin and a heavy region called heavy meromyosin. The light meromyosin is embedded in the thick filament while the heavy meromyosin projects out of the thick filament toward the thin filament. Finally, the heavy meromyosin is divided into two portions called the S_1 and S_2 fractions. The S_2 fraction forms a link between the light meromyosin and the S_1 fragment of the heavy meromyosin. The S_1 (also called the cross-bridge) is oriented perpendicularly to the thin filament. It attaches to the thin filament during muscle contraction. This will be discussed in more detail below.

The thin filaments are about 1 μm long and 7 nm in diameter. They are formed from three proteins: actin, tropomyosin, and troponin (Fig. 2-8). Actin, a globular protein, is formed into two long intertwined chains to form the backbone of the thin filaments. It combines with the myosin cross-bridge during muscle contraction. Tropomyosin is a rod-shaped molecule that is wrapped around the actin chain. It prevents actin from interacting with myosin. Troponin is a globular protein consisting of three subunits. One (Tn-T) binds to tropomyosin, another (Tn-I) controls the inhibitory activity of tropomyosin, and the third (Tn-C) contains a calcium-binding site. When calcium binds to troponin, troponin moves tropomyosin to a new position. With tropomyosin no longer blocking the interaction between actin and myosin, muscle contraction begins.

Force generation and shortening are brought about by the interaction of the thick and thin filaments. This interaction is initiated by series of events grouped together under the heading of excitation-contraction coupling. Excitation-contraction coupling begins with the generation of an action potential. The action potential propagates along the muscle fiber potential and the T tubule system. Depolarization of the T tubules causes the release of calcium from its storage sites within the TC of the SR. Calcium binds to Tn-C, causing Tn-I to undergo a conformational change during which tropomyosin moves away from its position covering the attachment sites on actin. Once the actin attachment sites are revealed, myosin cross-bridges attach to them and go through a reptitive cross-bridge cycle during which the thick and thin filaments slide across each other. The period of time during which calcium is bound to troponin and cross-bridge cycling is occurring is called the active state. The active state is terminated when the calcium is removed from the myoplasm by the calcium pumps on the SR. The mechanism of cross-bridge cycling and its relationship to force development and muscle shortening will be described below.

When the muscle is at rest, the S_2 subfragment of heavy meromyosin is lined up parallel to the thick filament and the S_1 globular subfragment is oriented perpendicularly to the thick filament facing the thin filament. When the actin attachment sites are revealed, the S_2 subfragment moves toward the thin filament and the globular head rotates so that it retains its perpendicular orientation when it binds to the actin molecule on the thin filament. Once the cross-bridge binds to the actin, it bends toward the center of the sarcomere, pulling the thin filament and the Z lines closer together. Upon reaching the end of its travel (when it forms a 45° angle with the thick filament),

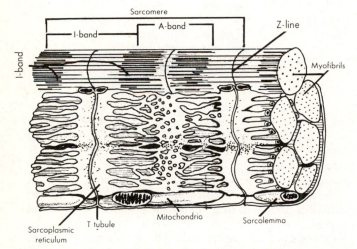

Figure 2-6. The functional unit of striated muscle is the sarcomere. Calcium is stored within the sarcoplasmic reticulum and released into the sarcoplasm when the T tubule is depolarized.

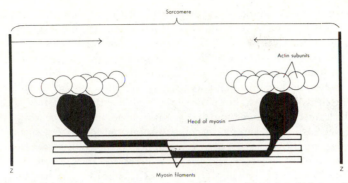

Figure 2-7. A diagrammatic view of the arrangement of myosin within the thick myofilament. The light meromyosin tails line up end to end within the thick filament while the heavy meromyosin cross-bridges are oriented perpendicular to the thick and thin filaments.

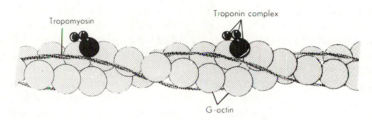

Figure 2-8. A diagrammatic view of the arrangement of the three proteins making up the thin filament. The tropomyosin covers the cross-bridge binding sites on the actin molecules, preventing cross-bridge interaction from occurring.

the cross-bridge detaches from actin, returns to its perpendicular orientation, and, if the actin sites are still uncovered, repeats the cycle. The cycling and the sliding of the thin filaments and Z line to the center of the sarcomere continues, until the calcium released from the SR is removed from the myoplasm.

ATP provides the energy for the cross-bridge cycle. As indicated above, the ATPase enzyme that hydrolyzes ATP is contained within one of the light chains on the globular head of the cross-bridge. The globular head also contains a binding site for an ATP molecule. Complete hydrolysis does not occur when the muscle is at rest because the ATPase is not fully activated until the cross-bridge combines with actin. Once binding occurs, however, the ATPase is activated and the energy required for the generation of force is liberated. The energy is used to bend the cross-bridge from its 90° to its 45° orientation. Detachment of the cross-bridge does not occur until a new molecule of ATP becomes bound to the cross-bridge. Thus, in the absence of ATP, as in rigor mortis, the thick and thin filaments remain attached to each other and the muscles become stiff and inflexible. The actual biochemical steps underlying the cross-bridge cycle are not fully understood. However, it appears that as soon as ATP binds to the cross-bridge it is hydrolyzed to ADP and Pi (inorganic phosphate). However, the ADP, phosphate, and myosin remain associated as a high-energy complex. When the cross-bridge attaches to actin, the products of hydrolysis are released, work is done, and heat is liberated.

The molecular events described above can be used to explain the mechanical features of muscle contraction. When muscle is at rest, the length of its sarcomeres is between 2 and 2.2 μm. The length is determined by the mechanical arrangement of the thick and thin filaments and the physical properties of the muscle tissue itself. The thick filaments are 1.6 μm in length and 10 nm in diameter. The thin filaments are 1.0 μm long and 7 nm in diameter. When no external tension is placed on the muscle, the thin filaments tend to come together at the center of the sarcomere, making the length of the sarcomere approximately twice the length of a thin filament. If external tension is placed on the muscle fiber, the thin filaments will be pulled apart from each other. The anatomic structure that offers resistance to the stretching of the sarcomere is not completely known but probably includes the sarcolemma and the connective tissue sheaths surrounding the muscle. These elements are referred to as the **parallel elastic component (PEC)** of the muscle because they resist extension of the muscle in parallel with the force-generating components of the muscle (i.e., the thick and thin filaments).

The force that can be generated by the muscle varies with its length prior to contraction. This can be demonstrated by an experiment in which the muscle is attached on one end to a rigid platform and at the other end to a force-measuring device called a transducer. The initial length of the muscle is set by pulling the platform and force transducer apart. The graph illustrates that force is required to increase the length of the muscle. This force is called the **passive tension** or the **preload**. The length to which the muscle is stretched is called the **initial length** or the **preload**. Note that both the initial length and the force required to set it are referred to as the preload.

Once the preload is set, the muscle is stimulated and force is produced. The contraction is called an **isometric contraction** because the total length of the muscle does not change. As shown in the graph in Figure 2-9, the amount of force produced by the muscle varies with the preload. At an initial length of 2.0 to 2.2 μm, the amount of force produced by the muscle is maximum. This is because every cross-bridge on the thick filament is able to bind to an actin molecule on the thin filament—that is, overlap between the thick and thin filaments is optimal. However, if the muscle is stretched, both the amount of overlap between the thick and thin filaments and the force developed by the muscle decrease. For example, at a preload of 2.8 μm, the cross-bridges on the central 0.8 μm of the thick filament are not opposite any actin molecules and do not participate in force generation. Thus, roughly half of the cross-bridges are unused and the force developed is half of what it was when the preload was 2.2 μm.

If the muscle is shortened below 2.0 μm, its force-generating capabilities also decrease but for another reason. In order for the muscle to shorten below 2.0 μm, the actin filaments must come in contact with each other. This produces a physical impediment to force development and thus reduces the amount of force that can be exerted on the force transducer. Shortening the muscle much beyond 1.6 μm is extremely difficult because the Z lines come in contact with the thick filaments. The relationship illustrated by the graph in Figure 2-9 is called the **length-tension relationship** and is one of the fundamental properties of muscle. The ability of the sliding filament theory of muscle contraction to explain the length-tension relationship was a major reason for its early acceptance.

In the experiment described above, the muscle was stimulated with a single action potential producing a muscle twitch. If the muscle is stimulated again, before it relaxes completely, a second contraction is produced. This is illustrated in Figure 2-10. Notice that the force of the second contraction exceeds the force of the first contraction. If the muscle is stimulated repetitively, the force continues to increase. At some frequency of stimulation, the force rises smoothly to a maximum and remains there as long as the muscle is stimulated (or until the muscle fatigues). The increase in contractile force produced by the second stimulus is called **summation**. When the stimulus frequency is high enough to produce a contraction of maximal strength, it is called a **tetanic stimulation** and the muscle is said to be tetanized or in tetanus. Repetitive

stimulation of the muscle is possible because the contractile event is much longer than the refractory period of the nerve or muscle fiber membrane. The explanation of summation and tetanus requires a closer look at the molecular mechanism underlying contraction.

The muscle fiber is a mechanically complex structure containing three different mechanical elements (Fig. 2-11). Two have already been discussed: a contractile component responsible for generating force and a parallel elastic component responsible for resisting deformation when the preload is increased. The third element is the **series elastic component** (SEC). The SEC, as its name implies, is connected in series with the contractile component. Its behavior modifies the force-generating capability of the muscle. When the muscle is stimulated and calcium binds to troponin, cross-bridge cycling begins. Each time the cross-bridges cycle, they shorten half of the sarcomere by approximately 10 nm (0.01 μm). In order for the sarcomere to shorten from a preload of 2.2 to 2.0 μm, each half sarcomere would have to shorten by 0.1 μm. This would require 10 cross-bridge cycles. Because the SEC is in series with the muscle, it is stretched by the same amount that the contractile component shortened. The force transmitted to the force transducer (or bone) depends on the stiffness of the SEC. If it is very stiff, a small number of cycles will cause a large amount of force to be generated. If it is fairly compliant, a relatively large number of cycles will be required. In other words, the force generated by the muscle depends not only on how many cross-bridges attach to the thin filaments, but also on the number of cycles that the cross-bridges go through and the elastic properties of the SEC.

Normally, the amount of calcium released from the SR of skeletal muscle is sufficient to remove the tropomyosin from all of the binding sites on actin. Typically, the SEC can stretch to about 10% of the resting muscle length. Thus, to stretch the SEC out completely (0.22 μm), the cross-bridges would have to go through 11 cycles. If each cycle required 5 msec, 55 msec would be required for the muscle to stretch the SEC all the way out and develop the maximum amount of force. Obviously, if the calcium pump on the longitudinal SR removes the calcium from the myoplasm in less than 55 msec, the muscle will not develop all the force it is capable of producing. However, if a

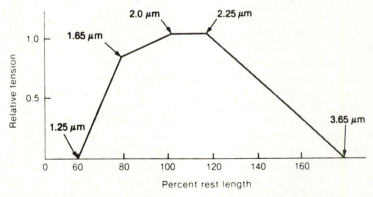

Figure 2-9.   The maximum amount of force that a muscle can produce depends on its length. Developed force is maximum at a sarcomere length of 2.2 μm because every myosin cross-bridge is opposite an actin binding site at this length.

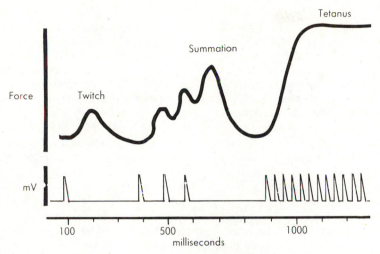

Figure 2-10.   The amount of force generated by a skeletal muscle can be varied by varying the frequency of stimulation. If a second stimulus is applied before the muscle relaxes completely, the second contraction will summate with the first, producing a larger force. Maximum force is generated when the frequency of stimulation is high enough to prevent relaxation between stimuli. The frequency producing a maximum contraction is called a tetanic stimulation.

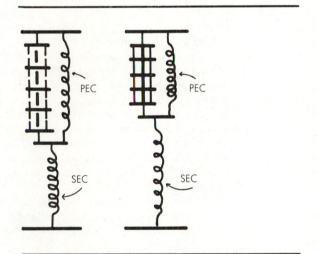

Figure 2-11. The mechanical model used to represent a skeletal muscle can be used to explain some of the muscle's properties. For example, the parallel elastic component (PEC) of the muscle must be stretched when the preload is increased. If the PEC is stiff, then more force must be applied to stretch the muscle. The series elastic component (SEC) is stretched when the muscle contracts. The force generated by the cross-bridges is transmitted to the bones (or force transducer) through the SEC. Repetitive cycling of cross-bridges is required to stretch the SEC. The amount of force generated by the muscle is proportional to the stretch of the SEC.

second stimulus is applied before all the calcium is resequestered by the SR, cross-bridge cycling will continue longer and more force will be produced. This is what occurs during summation and tetanus. Repetitive stimulation of the muscle keeps the calcium in the myoplasm, allows cross-bridge cycling to continue longer, causes the SEC to be stretched further, and

results in more force being generated. In other words, the increased force produced by a tetanic stimulus results not from more calcium being supplied to the muscle but from a longer active state.

If instead of tying the muscle to a rigid platform, as was done in the experiments described above, the muscle is attached to a weight, the weight will rise when the muscle is stimulated. This type of contraction is referred to as an **isotonic contraction** because the muscle shortens against a constant load. The load against which the muscle must shorten is called the **afterload**. The velocity of shortening is inversely related to the afterload. Also, the force generated by the muscle increases to meet the afterload and the amount of shortening the muscle is capable of producing goes down as the afterload increases. Each of these observations can be explained in terms of cross-bridge cycling. As the load increases, the time for each cross-bridge cycle is increased. As a result, shortening takes longer or velocity of shortening decreases. In order for a muscle to shorten, the force produced by the muscle must equal (or be slightly greater than) the afterload. This can be accomplished before all of the cross-bridges capable of binding to the thin filament actually do so. As soon as enough cross-bridges bind, they all cycle together, causing the muscle to shorten with a force just large enough to lift the load. As the muscle shortens to lengths shorter than 2.0 μm, its force-generating potential decreases (see Fig. 2-9). At some length, the muscle will require all of its cross-bridges just to produce a force equal to the afterload. This will be the shortest length to which the muscle can shorten. If the load is reduced, the muscle will be able to shorten further before it reaches this point.

CARDIAC MUSCLE

Cardiac muscle, like skeletal muscle, is a striated muscle. However, cardiac muscle fibers differ anatomically from skeletal muscle in a number of ways. (1) They are smaller. Cardiac muscles are rectangularly shaped and are 10 to 20 μm wide, 5 to 10 μm thick, and 75 to 150 μm long. (2) Cardiac cells are connected to each other by intercalated disks that serve to hold the cells together and contain gap junctions through which electrical activity passes from one cell to another. (3) The T tubules in cardiac muscle are larger than those in skeletal muscle and are located at the Z line rather than at the A-I junction. Also, the TC of the SR in cardiac muscle makes direct contact with the cell membrane in addition to those made with the T tubule. (4) There are many more mitochondria in cardiac muscle than in skeletal muscle. These additional mitochondria are necessary to supply the ATP required for muscle activity, which is almost entirely aerobic in cardiac muscle.

Excitation-contraction coupling also has unique features in cardiac muscle that are absent in skeletal muscle. The cardiac action potential (which will be discussed in detail in the section on the cardiovascular system) is more complex than the one produced by skeletal muscle and nerve. The upstroke of the action potential is followed by a prolonged plateau phase lasting 200 to 300 msec. The plateau is caused by the flow of calcium into the cell through voltage-sensitive calcium channels. Some of the calcium flowing into the cell during the action potential binds to troponin and contributes to the activation of cross-bridge cycling. Some of the calcium entering the cell during the action potential also binds to the TC of the SR and causes the release of calcium. This mechanism is referred to as **calcium-induced calcium release**. Calcium is also released from the TC in response to membrane depolarization just as it is in skeletal muscle.

Relaxation of cardiac muscle occurs when the calcium is removed from the myoplasm. However, cardiac muscle employs more methods than skeletal muscle to accomplish this task. In addition to calcium pumps on the SR (as there are in skeletal muscle), there are also calcium pumps on the cardiac muscle cell membrane. Thus calcium can be resequestered by the SR or pumped entirely out of the cell. More important, calcium can be removed from the cell by a **Na-CA exchange system**. The operation of this system is similar to the indirect active transport systems discussed earlier in that the energy stored in the sodium gradient is used to pump calcium out of the cell against its concentration gradient. When the cell is in its resting state, three sodium ions enter the cell down their electrochemical gradient for each calcium ion leaving the cell against its electrochemical gradient. When the cell depolarizes, the electrochemical gradient for sodium is reduced and may not be sufficient to remove calcium from the cell at the same rate (or may in fact become so small that the exchange system works backward, adding calcium to the cell in exchange for sodium leaving the cell). As a result, both voltage-sensitive channels and the Na-Ca exchange system contribute to the net amount of calcium entering the cell during the plateau of the action potential. Thus the Na-Ca exchange system plays an important role, not only in removing calcium from the cell during relaxation but in causing the entry of calcium during excitation-contraction coupling.

Another important difference between cardiac and skeletal muscle is that the amount of calcium entering the cell (across the membrane or from the SR) is not as great as in skeletal muscle and is not sufficient to saturate the troponin molecules.

Consequently, cardiac muscle is never fully activated and the force it develops is always less than that predicted by the overlap of thick and thin filaments. This condition provides cardiac muscle with a unique method of varying the force of its contraction. Cardiac muscle cannot increase its force of contraction by summation (because the action potential duration and muscle twitch are of approximately the same duration), nor can it recruit more muscle fibers (because coordinated pumping of blood by the heart requires all of its fibers to be simultaneously activated each time it beats). Cardiac muscle can alter its force by varying preload, but, as will be discussed in the section on the cardiovascular system, this is inefficient from an energetic point of view. Thus the ability to vary its force by varying intracellular calcium concentration becomes very important. Increasing contractile force by increasing calcium concentration is referred to as increasing the heart's **inotropic** or **contractile state**.

Finally, the length-tension relationship in cardiac muscle differs from that in skeletal muscle. Recall that resting skeletal muscle fibers have sarcomere lengths of 2.0 to 2.2 μm and that they can be stretched by an external force to 3.5 μm. Resting cardiac muscle fibers have sarcomere lengths of 1.6 to 2.0 μm and cannot be easily stretched beyond 2.2 μm. That is, their parallel elastic components are much stiffer than those in skeletal muscle. This too is an advantage for cardiac muscle. The preload in skeletal muscle is set by the position of the limbs or other skeletal structures. In the heart, the preload is set by the amount of blood entering the heart between beats. If the blood entering the heart were sufficient to increase the preload beyond 2.2 μm, the force developed by the heart would begin to decrease. Clearly, it is not appropriate to return more blood to the heart and then have less force available to pump it out. Thus, the stiff parallel elastic component limits the amount of blood entering the heart and prevents the sarcomeres from being stretched beyond 2.2 μm. This keeps the preload on the ascending limb of the length-tension relationship where increases in blood entering the heart result in increases in the force developed to pump it out.

These two mechanisms of increasing force development—increasing preload and increasing contractility—will be discussed more fully in the section on the cardiovascular system.

SMOOTH MUSCLE

Anatomically, smooth muscles are quite different from striated muscles. They are composed of thin and elongated (usually less than 10 μm in diameter and between 100 and 500 μm long) cells that lack the internal organization that myofibrils and sarcomeres provide to striated muscles. However, thick and thin filaments are present in smooth muscle and force development is produced by the sliding of these filaments across each other. Instead of being attached to Z lines, the thin filaments are anchored to dense bodies that are interspersed throughout the cell. The dense bodies are mechanically joined to each other and to the cell membrane by a network of very thin filaments. The force developed by the cross-bridges is ultimately transmitted through the dense bodies to the cell membrane via these very thin filaments. Although smooth muscle cells contain a SR, it is not as well developed as that appearing in striated muscle. Also, because there is no T tubule system in smooth muscle, any junctions formed by the SR must be made directly with the smooth muscle membrane.

Excitation-contraction coupling differs markedly from that occurring in striated muscle, both in terms of how calcium enters the cell and how it initiates contraction. Smooth muscles are divided into two broad categories: **multiunit** and **unitary** smooth muscles. They are differentiated primarily by how they are connected and how they are stimulated. Multiunit smooth muscles such as those controlling the diameter of the pupil are composed of individual cells isolated from each other by a basement membrane. They contract only when stimulated by the nerve fibers innervating them. In contrast, unitary muscles, such as those forming the GI tract, are connected to each other by gap junctions. Thus any electrical activity occurring in one cell is transferred to all of its neighboring cells. Unitary smooth muscle cells are normally spontaneously active. The nerve fibers innervating them are involved mostly in controlling the strength of their contractions rather than in determining whether or not they will contract. At one time, it was thought that the mechanism underlying excitation-contraction coupling would be different in multiunit and unitary smooth muscles. However, it now appears that these differences are less categorical, and the method of excitation-contraction coupling used by an individual muscle must be determined on a case-by-case basis.

Smooth muscle action potentials are primarily caused by calcium-selective voltage-sensitive channels. In some cells, such as in those in the intestine or the vas deferens, the action potential is spike-like, having an upstroke and downstroke similar to that in nerve and skeletal muscle. However, it is much slower. In nerve and skeletal muscle, the action potential duration is several milliseconds. In smooth muscle, the duration of the action potentials is 50 to 100 msecs. In other cells, such as those in the antrum of the stomach, the contour of the action potential resembles cardiac muscle with its long plateau phase. However, the smooth muscle action potential is much longer, lasting for 5 to 7 seconds. In both cases, the depolarization is caused by the entry of calcium into the cell. This calcium contributes to the activation of the contractile proteins in the smooth muscle cell.

Some smooth muscle cells, such as those in the fundus of the stomach or those surrounding the large arteries and veins, do not produce action potentials. Calcium enters these cells through voltage-sensitive channels that are opened when the cell is depolarized by an external stimulus. However, the calcium entering does not cause the cell to depolarize (probably because potassium channels are opened simultaneously), and thus an action potential does not develop. The cell is usually depolarized by a neurotransmitter or by hormone-opening channels that allow sodium and potassium (and possibly calcium) to move through them. These voltage-operated channels are a second pathway for calcium to enter smooth muscle cells.

A third mechanism for calcium entry is the opening of chemically sensitive calcium channels. These channels, called receptor-activated channels, are opened by a neurotransmitter or hormone and allow calcium to enter the cell. Calcium can also be released from the SR when the membrane depolarizes or, as in cardiac muscle, by calcium-induced calcium release.

Perhaps the greatest difference between smooth and striated muscle lies in the mechanism by which the contractile proteins are activated. In striated muscles, actin and myosin are able to bind as soon as the tropomyosin is moved away from its position on the thin filament blocking the attachment sites. There is no troponin in smooth muscle, and an analogous system does not exist. That is, there are no inhibitory proteins on the thin filament preventing interaction. Instead, the inhibition is on the thick filaments. Smooth muscle myosin cannot bind to actin unless one of the light polypeptide chains on the globular head (the S_1 subfragment) of heavy meromyosin is phosphorylated. The particular light chain that must be phosphorylated has a molecular weight of 20,000 and is thus referred to as the LC20. Calcium entering the myoplasm by any of the mechanisms discussed above initiates a chain of chemical reactions that eventually results in the phosphorylation of the LC20.

Intracellular calcium binds to calmodulin, which then binds to and activates the light chain myosin kinase (LCMK). The LCMK then phosphorylates the LC20. Initially, a large number of cross-bridges are phosphorylated by the LCMK. This number is rapidly reduced by a phosphorylase enzyme. As a result, cross-bridge cycling goes through a period of rapid cycling proportional to the percentage of cross-bridges initially phosphorylated, followed by a prolonged slower rate of cycling due to the dephosphorylation of cross-bridges. Although the dephosphorylated bridges can no longer produce muscle shortening, they are still capable of sustaining tension. This sequence of events conserves energy. The rapid cycling of cross-bridges at the beginning of a contraction produces the force development and shortening required by the muscle. However, once the necessary force is developed, it requires little energy for its maintenance because (1) the slowly cycling cross-bridges use less ATP and (2) ATP is not required to rephosphorylate those light chains from which phosphate has been removed by the phosphorylase enzyme. Eventually, the calcium is removed from the myoplasm, the LCMK becomes inactivated, the remaining activated light chains are dephosphorylated, and the muscle relaxes.

CARDIOVASCULAR PHYSIOLOGY

The blood circulates within the cardiovascular system, providing nutrients and removing wastes from the tissues of the body. There are actually two circulations in series with each other: (1) The pulmonary circulation passes through the lungs, where carbon dioxide is removed and oxygen is added to the blood. (2) The systemic circulation delivers the oxygenated blood to the various organs of the body.

These circulations are diagrammed in Figure 2-12. The left ventricle develops enough pressure to move the blood through the entire systemic circulation. After leaving the left ventricle, the blood flows through the large distributing arteries, through the small resistance arterioles, and into the capillaries, where exchange of nutrients and wastes occurs. Blood leaving the capillaries flows through the venules and veins before returning to the right atrium of the heart.

Although these processes will be discussed in detail below, it is worthwhile to provide an overview of their function. The heart undergoes a sequence of contractions (called **systole**) and

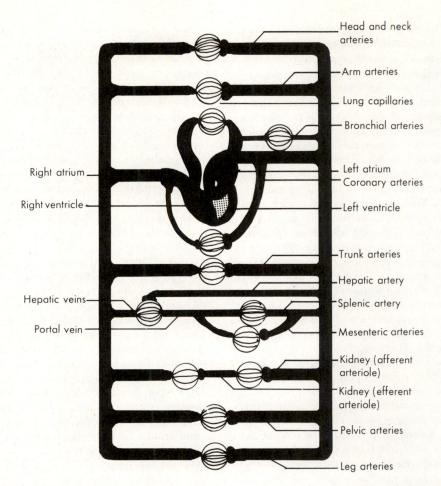

Right atrium
Right ventricle
Hepatic veins
Portal vein

Head and neck arteries
Arm arteries
Lung capillaries
Bronchial arteries
Left atrium
Coronary arteries
Left ventricle
Trunk arteries
Hepatic artery
Splenic artery
Mesenteric arteries
Kidney (afferent arteriole)
Kidney (efferent arteriole)
Pelvic arteries
Leg arteries

Figure 2-12.　A schematic diagram of the circulation. All of the organ systems are perfused in parallel, which means that blood flow to any one organ can be altered independently of all the others. However, if one vascular bed receives too much blood, another may be under-perfused. A variety of local and neural control mechanisms exist to keep the blood flow through each organ at its optimal level.

relaxations (called **diastole**) at a rate of 70 to 75 per minute. During the contraction phase, about 60% of the blood within the heart is propelled into the aorta. The volume of blood ejected with each beat is called the **stroke volume.** The volume ejected during a minute (stroke volume × rate) is called the **cardiac output.** Blood is prevented from flowing backward by a series of valves. The atrioventricular (AV) valves prevent blood from flowing into the atria during systole, and the aortic and pulmonic valves prevent blood from flowing back into the ventricle during diastole.

The distributing arteries are relatively large and elastic. Their large diameter allows the blood to pass through them without much loss of energy. Thus the pressure exerted on the blood by the left ventricle is not diminished very much in the distributing arteries. Moreover, because of the high compliance of the aorta, almost all of the stroke volume can be accommodated within it. Thus when the heart relaxes in diastole, the elastic recoil of the aorta keeps the blood moving forward.

The small arterioles offer a great deal of resistance to the flow of blood, and thus much of the hydrostatic pressure imparted to the blood by the heart is lost as the blood passes through the arterioles. The resistance vessels are very important for normal circulation. First, they are responsible for maintaining enough pressure within the distributing vessels to the head and brain for blood to flow upward against the force of gravity. Second, the distribution of blood to particular organs can be controlled by varying the resistance within the arteriole beds. For example, increasing the resistance of the splanchnic circulation and decreasing the resistance of the skeletal muscle circulation shunt blood from the gut to the muscles during exercise. Third, by reducing the pressure of the blood passing through the capillaries, arterioles prevent plasma water from being filtered across the capillary wall into the interstitial fluid.

By the time the blood reaches the capillaries, it is flowing at a slow, steady pace. This slow speed is caused by the more than 500-fold increase in cross-sectional area that occurs between the aorta and the millions of capillaries that make up the microcirculation. The slow passage through the capillaries is ideal for promoting exchange of material between the blood and interstitial fluid.

Most of the circulating blood (over two-thirds) is found within the venules and veins. As will be discussed later, this storage capacity can be used to alter the development of pressure by the heart.

ELECTRICAL ACTIVITY OF THE HEART

The heartbeat is initiated by a cardiac action potential that originates within specialized cells of the sinoatrial (SA) node of the right atrium and spreads through the atrial muscle and AV node to the His-Purkinje system, from which the ventricular muscle is activated.

CONDUCTION OF THE HEARTBEAT

Conduction from the SA node through the atrial muscle proceeds radially at a rate of less than 1 m/second. The action potentials travel for the most part through the ordinary atrial muscle fibers. Although a number of specialized conduction pathways have been identified anatomically, they do not appear to play much of a role in the normal spread of activation from the SA to the AV node.

Conduction through the AV node is very slow, less than 0.05 m/second. This slow conduction velocity accounts for the long delay (normally 120 to 200 msec) between atrial and ventricular systole, which, as will be discussed later, allows sufficient time for blood to enter the ventricle before contraction. In addition to causing a delay between atrial and ventricular contraction, the nodal cells also prevent retrograde conduction between the ventricle and atrium. The cells of the AV node have a much longer refractory period than other cells and thus are still in a refractory state when the ventricular cells depolarize. Also, because of their long refractory period, they prevent the ventricle from being driven at a rate so high that adequate amounts of blood would be unable to enter the ventricle during diastole. For example, if the atrial pacemakers were to discharge at an abnormally high rate, the long refractory period of the AV node would allow only every other or every third action potential to reach the His bundle.

The His bundle passes along the right endocardial surface of the intraventricular septum before dividing into the right and left bundle branches. The left bundle branch travels through the septum and then continues down along the endocardial surface on the left side. It eventually divides into an anterior and posterior branch. The His bundle fibers give rise to a network of Purkinje fibers, which spread out over the entire endocardial surface of both ventricles. Activation of the ventricular muscle fibers thus proceeds down along the septum and then along the free walls of both ventricles from the base of the heart to the apex and from the endocardial surface to the epicardial surface. Because the right ventricle is thinner than the left, it is activated before the left ventricle. The papillary muscles, which prevent eversion of the AV valves, are activated early in systole. The high speed of conduction through the His-Purkinje network (1 to 4 m/second) ensures that all of the ventricular muscle fibers are activated in a coordinated manner.

THE CARDIAC ACTION POTENTIALS

There are two types of action potentials in cardiac muscle cells, both different from the action potential generated in neurons and skeletal muscle cells. One is typified by the action potential produced in ventricular muscle cells. It is characterized by a rapid upstroke and a long plateau phase. The other is found in the pacemaker cells of the SA and AV nodes. It is characterized by a slowly depolarizing resting potential, a slow upstroke, and no plateau. The ionic basis for these two types of action potentials will be explained below.

The resting potential in ventricular muscle cells is usually very negative (-9 to -93 mV) because of its relatively high conductance to potassium ions. Its action potential is divided into five phases (Fig. 2-13A). The upstroke is called phase 0. This is followed by a small repolarization (phase 1), a prolonged plateau (phase 2), and a repolarization (phase 3) back to the resting potential, which is referred to as phase 4.

Phase 0, the upstroke, is analogous to the upstroke of nerve cells. When a stimulus depolarizes the membrane to threshold, sodium channels open, sodium ions flow into the cell, and the membrane potential becomes inside positive. The sodium channels then inactivate, producing the small phase 1 repolarization. However, unlike the nerve action potential, inactivation of the sodium channels does not lead to repolarization of the membrane to its resting value. Instead, the membrane remains depolarized for several hundred milliseconds before repolarization occurs.

Two unique features of cardiac muscle membranes are responsible for the plateau phase of the action potential. First, unlike the case in nerve cells, potassium conductance decreases when the cardiac cell membrane depolarizes. Second, depolarization causes the opening of calcium channels, through which a calcium current, called the slow inward current, flows into the cell. The reduced potassium conductance coupled with the increased calcium conductance is responsible for the plateau. As will be discussed below, the influx of calcium contributes to the intiation of ventricular contraction. Theoretically, the plateau could be produced by the inward flow of calcium ions without an accompanying decrease in potassium current. However, the amount of calcium flowing into the cell would have to be substantially greater if potassium conductance remained high.

The plateau phase is concluded by the outward flow of potassium ions that occurs when the potassium conductance returns to its resting value. The mechanism underlying the increase in potassium conductance is not fully understood but is assumed to result from the accumulation of calcium ions within the cell. This hypothesis is supported by the observation that the plateau phase in Purkinje action potentials is both lower and more prolonged than in ventricular muscle cells. Because the rate of calcium flowing into the Purkinje cell is less (causing less depolarization during the plateau), it presumably takes longer for enough calcium to enter the cell and initiate the repolarization phase.

The SA nodal cells from which the electrical activity of the heart originates are called **pacemaker cells**. These cells are never at rest. As illustrated in Figure 2-13B, they depolarize slowly until threshold is reached. Following the action potential, they depolarize again until another action potential is elicited. Other cells within the heart, such as those within the atria near the AV node (called junctional cells) and those within the His-Purkinje system, can also display autorhythmicity or pacemaker activity. Under normal circumstances, the heartbeat originates in the SA node because these cells depolarize toward threshold more rapidly than do the other pacemaker cells.

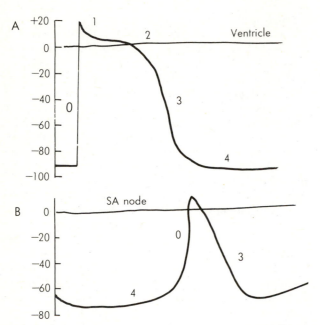

Figure 2-13. (*A*) The various phases of the ventricular muscle action potential. The upstroke (phase 0) is produced by the inward flow of sodium through fast channels. The plateau (phase 2) is produced by the inward flow of calcium ions. When the ventricular cell depolarizes, potassium conductance decreases. Repolarization (phase 3) is produced when potassium conductance returns to its resting levels. (*B*) The phases of the SA nodal action potential. Spontaneous (phase 4) depolarization is caused by the slow inward leak of sodium. Phase 0 is caused by the inward flow of calcium ions. Sodium channels do not play a role in SA nodal cell action potentials. These channels are inactivated by the low (−60 mV) resting potentials of SA nodal cells.

When the heart is controlled by SA nodal cells, the ensuing rhythm is called a **sinus rhythm.** If the SA node is damaged, the heart will be driven by an action potential originating within the AV node and is said to be under the control of a nodal pacemaker or undergoing a nodal rhythm. Pacemakers within a region of the His-Purkinje system are called **ectopic foci of activity.** These pacemakers are normally too slow ever to initiate a heartbeat. However, when they do, the sequence of ventricular activation is disturbed and the force of the heartbeat is diminished.

The action potential recorded from an SA nodal cell is illustrated in Figure 2-13*B*. The slow depolarization to threshold is called phase 4 depolarization. The upstroke of the action potential is called phase 0, and the downstroke is called phase 3. There is no plateau phase in pacemaker cells. The maximum membrane potential achieved by the SA nodal cells during diastole (the diastolic potential) is approximately −60 mV. At this potential, all of the sodium channels are inactivated and thus the upstroke is produced by the inward flow of calcium ions through calcium-specific channels. As was the case with ventricular cells, potassium conductance decreases when cardiac muscle cells depolarize and repolarization begins when the potassium conductance returns to its initial value.

The mechanism underlying phase 4 depolarization is not fully understood. The most current hypothesis suggests that the spontaneous depolarization results from the continuous

leakage of sodium and calcium into the cell. When the action potential is initiated, these channels are inactivated. This inactivation, coupled with the activation of potassium channels, then leads to the repolarization phase of the action potential. Once the cell repolarizes, the sodium and calcium channels reactivate and the whole process begins again.

THE ELECTROCARDIOGRAM

The electrocardiogram (ECG) is one of the most important clinical tools available for assessing cardiac function. It can be used to discover if there are abnormalities in the rate and rhythm of the heartbeat; if the conduction of the action potential through the heart is normal, if there is any cardiac hypertrophy or if the heart is mispositioned within the thorax; and if there is ischemic damage to the heart. However, it is important to remember that the ECG cannot be used to measure the mechanical function of the heart.

The ECG is recorded by electrodes placed on the surface of the skin. Two sets of recording leads are usually used: six limb leads (the standard limb leads, I, II, and III; and the augmented limb leads, aV_R, aV_L, and aV_F), and six precordial or chest leads referred to as V_1 to V_6. The placement of these leads and the ECG of a single heartbeat are illustrated in Figure 2-14.

The limb leads are placed on the wrists of the left and right arms and on the ankles. The standard limb leads are bipolar leads, which means that they record the difference in electrical activity between two of the limb leads. Lead I records the difference in electrical activity between the right and left arm electrodes; lead II between the right arm and left leg; and lead III between the left arm and left leg. The right leg electrode serves as a ground electrode to reduce electrical artifacts. The augmented leads are unipolar leads, which means that they record the electrical activity between them and a single reference electrode. The electrical circuit used to form the reference electrode amplifies the recording from the unipolar leads, which is why they are called augmented leads.

The deflections on the ECG recording are called the P wave, the QRS complex, and the T wave (see Fig. 2-14). The interval between the beginning of the P wave and the start of the QRS complex is called the P-R interval; that between the end of the QRS complex and the beginning of the T wave is called the ST segment.

The P wave represents the spread of electrical activity over the surface of the atria and corresponds roughly to the time of atrial systole. The pacemaker activity of the SA node is too small to cause a deflection in the ECG and so is not represented. Similarly, the electrical activity of the AV nodal cells and the His-Purkinje network is too small to cause any deflection on the ECG recording, accounting for the period of electrical silence between the end of the P wave and the beginning of ventricular muscle depolarization. The normal P-R interval is between 0.12 and 0.2 seconds. About half of this interval represents the conduction delay within the AV node. Values longer than this are referred to as a first-degree heart block and can be caused by damage to the conduction pathway between the atria and ventricles or by an increase in vagal tone to the heart. Athletes, who normally have a slow heartbeat, might also have a prolonged P-R interval, which in this case would be entirely normal.

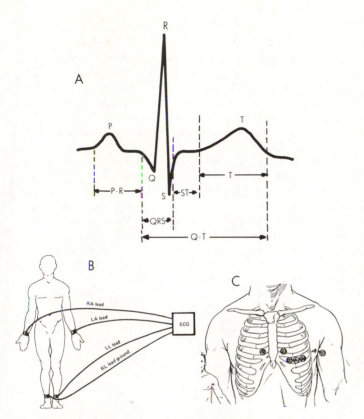

Figure 2-14. To record a standard 12-lead ECG (*A*), electrodes are placed on the limbs (*B*) and chest (*C*). The limb leads provide information about the conduction of electrical activity in the vertical plane; the chest (or precordial) leads provide information about conduction in the horizontal plane.

The QRS complex represents the depolarization of the ventricle, which is normally less than 0.1 second in duration. Values longer than this may indicate some abnormality of the conduction pathway through the ventricle. Pronounced abnormalities in the shape of the QRS complex, such as notching, may indicate a blockage of the His bundles. More bizarre shapes may indicate a beat originating within the ventricle. These are usually called premature ventricular contractions (PVCs) because they occur before the normal beat originating in the SA node is able to excite the ventricle. Their presence may be quite benign and of no clinical significance or they can represent irregularities in cardiac excitability that must be treated to prevent the possibility of ventricular fibrillation. The magnitude of the QRS complex is normally less than 1 mV. Values larger than this may indicate cardiac hypertrophy.

The steady baseline between the end of the QRS complex and the beginning of the T wave is called the ST segment. It represents the prolonged depolarization of the ventricular muscle (phase 2 of the action potential). The ST segment is generally at the same potential as the P-R interval. An ST segment that is depressed below this value or elevated above it may represent some degree of ischemic damage to the heart.

Repolarizing of the ventricular action potential is represented by the T wave of the ECG. If the T wave is inverted—that is, not in the same direction as the QRS complex—some sort of ventricular muscle disease may be present.

The deflections produced by the limb leads can be analyzed using Einthoven's triangle (see Fig. 2-15). The path of depolarization produced by the cardiac action potential as it spreads over the surface of the heart can be represented by a vector. A vector oriented from right to left and parallel to lead I is considered to have an electrical axis of 0°. A vertical vector directed downward has an electrical axis of 90°, while an upwardly directed vertical vector has an electrical axis of −90°. A vector parallel to lead II has an electrical axis of 60°, while one parallel to lead III has an electrical axis of 120°.

Although each instant in time is represented by its own unique vector, the overall shape of the deflection produced by ventricular depolarization can be understood by studying the vectors corresponding to only three moments in time: (1) the initial depolarization of the intraventricular septum (represented by a vector directed from left to right; (2) the depolarization of the left ventricular wall from endocardium to epicardium (represented by a vector directed from right to left); and (3) the final depolarization of the basal region of the heart (represented by a vector directed upward toward the head).

The magnitude of the deflection produced in any lead depends on the size and orientation of the vector representing cardiac depolarization at that time. The larger the mass of tissue depolarized, the larger the vector and the larger the

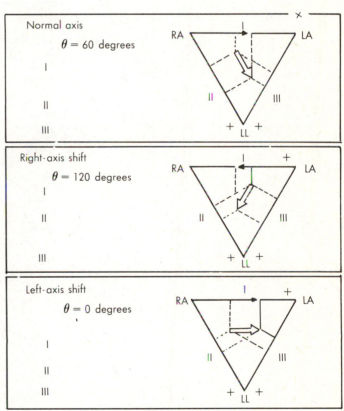

Figure 2-15. The magnitude of the ECG deflection in any given lead depends on the orientation of the vector and the limb lead. If the vector is parallel to the orientation of the limb lead, then the deflection is large; if it is perpendicular, then the deflection is small. If it is oriented in the same direction as the limb lead, then the deflection is upright; if it is in the opposite direction, then the deflection is downward.

deflection. In addition, if the vector is directed in a path parallel to the orientation of the lead, the deflection will be large and upright. If the vector is pointed in a direction opposite to the orientation of the lead, the deflection will be large and downward. If the vector is perpendicular to the lead, no deflection will be produced.

The application of this analysis to the standard limb leads is represented in Figure 2-16. The initial vector, representing the depolarization from the left endocardial surface of the septum to the right side of the heart, is oriented from left to right at an angle of −150. Because this direction is opposite to the orientation of lead I, a negative deflection is recorded. This initial downward deflection is called a Q wave. The Q wave is larger in lead I than it is in leads II or III because the orientation of the vector is almost parallel to lead I while it is close to being perpendicular to leads II and III.

The largest vector is produced by the depolarization of the left ventricular wall because this is the largest mass of tissue in the heart. The vector representing this depolarization thus produces a large upward deflection (called an R wave) in all three leads. It is largest in lead II because the orientation of the vector is most parallel to lead II. If the heart were oriented more perpendicularly, the deflection in lead I would be much smaller. Similarly, if the right ventricle were hypertrophied, the orientation of the vector would shift to a more vertical direction (closer to the right ventricle), causing the R wave to be smaller in lead I.

Finally, the depolarization of the basal portions of the left ventricle and septum produces a vector directed from left to right. This vector, like the initial vector, produces a downward deflection (called an S wave) in all three limb leads. A vector directed vertically produces a downward deflection (called an S wave) in leads II and III.

The actual shape of the ECG in any particular lead will, of course, depend on the relationship between the direction of the vector and the orientation of the lead. For example (see

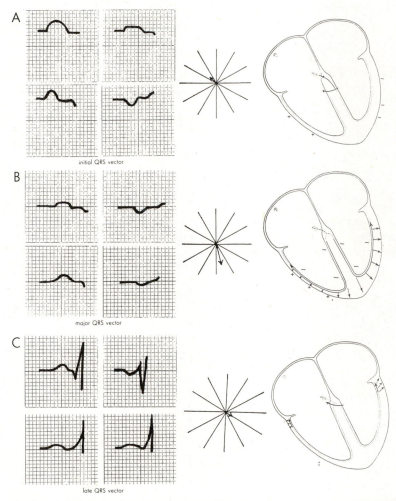

Figure 2-16. The shape of the QRS complex in any given lead depends on the changing orientation of the vector representing the spread of electrical activity through the heart. The major deflection (B) of the QRS complex is large and upright in lead II because the vector representing depolarization of the free wall of the ventricle is parallel to and in the same direction as the orientation of lead II. It is negative in lead aVr because the vector is oriented in a direction opposite to that of lead aVr.

Fig. 2-16*A*), the vector (from left to right) representing the initial depolarization of the septum produces an upward deflection (an R wave) in lead aV_R while the vector (down and to the left) representing the depolarization of the ventricular wall produces a downward deflection in aV_R (an S wave) (Fig. 2-16*B*). Recall that the Q wave is the first negative deflection of the QRS complex, the R wave is the first positive wave, and the S wave is the first negative wave following a positive wave. Thus, as illustrated by the ECG recorded from aV_R, ventricular wall depolarization is not always represented by an R wave.

The average of the deflections produced in all of the limb leads is called the mean electrical axis (MEA). For the most part, this represents the depolarization of the ventricular surface and is usually oriented from right to left along the axis of lead II. Ventricular hypertrophy, changes in the position of the heart, or conduction abnormalities that alter the normal spread of activation over the heart can change the MEA. An MEA between and 0 and 90° is considered to be normal.

The limb leads provide an analysis of the vectors directed in the frontal plane of the chest. The depolarization of the heart muscle in the anterior-posterior plane is studied using the chest leads. Because these leads are closer to the heart, the deflections produced by them are usually larger than those produced by the limb leads.

THE CARDIAC CYCLE

Figure 2-17 represents the events occurring during one cardiac cycle. The electrical events represented by the ECG have been described above. The changes in pressure and heart sounds produced during the cardiac cycle will now be described.

The heart alternates between mechanical activity when it is ejecting blood, called **systole,** and a resting state, called **diastole,** during which it is filling with blood. During diastole, blood returning to the left ventricle from the pulmonary vein causes an increase in size and pressure of the left ventricle. The initial increase in volume is quite rapid and is referred to as the **rapid filling phase.** About 70% of the blood entering the ventricle during diastole enters during this phase of filling. The rate of filling decreases toward the end of diastole because the rise of pressure within the ventricle opposes the flow of blood into it from the lungs. Near the end of diastole, the left atrium contracts, propelling a small amount of blood into the ventricle. About 10 to 15% of the ventricular volume is supplied by atrial systole.

Soon after atrial contraction, the ventricle begins to contract. The pressure in the ventricle rises rapidly, closing the AV valve. The initial phase of cardiac contraction is called the **isovolumic phase** because no change in heart volume occurs. Blood is prevented from flowing into the atrium by the closed AV valve and is prevented from flowing into the aorta because the pressure in the aorta is greater than it is in the ventricle. However, as soon as the pressure in the ventricle exceeds that in the aorta, the blood is ejected. When the heart muscle repolarizes, the ventricle begins to relax. Ejection continues until the pressure in the aorta becomes larger than that in the ventricle. The remaining phase of relaxation is called isovolumic relaxation because once again the volume of the heart cannot change. Blood is prevented from entering the ventricle from the aorta by the aortic valve. When relaxation is complete, the AV valve opens and the entire cycle is repeated.

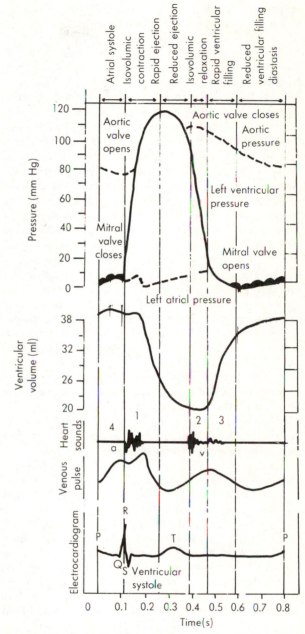

Figure 2-17. The aortic, left ventricular, and left atrial pressure pulses, cardiac volumes, phonocardiogram, venous pulses, and ECG recorded during a single cardiac cycle.

Aortic pressure rises during the ejection phase and falls during the filling phase of the ventricle. The opening of the aortic valve during ejection normally is so large that there is very little energy lost in ejecting the blood through it. Ventricular and aortic pressures thus are virtually identical. If the valve opening decreases in size, a significant loss of energy can occur and the ventricular pressure will thus have to increase to produce normal aortic pressures. As will be discussed later, this can cause cardiac hypertrophy and can lead to heart failure. The normal peak aortic pressure during ejection is 120 mm Hg. This is called the **systolic pressure.** The lowest aortic pressure is observed just before the aortic valve is opened by the next heartbeat. This pressure, normally about 80 mm Hg, is called the **diastolic pressure**. Blood pressure is reported as systolic/diastolic, and normal blood pressure is 120/80. Blood pressures above 140/90 are considered abnormally high.

A stethoscope placed over the surface of the chest can be used to listen to the heart sounds. These are represented by the phonocardiographic recordings in Figure 2-17. The mechanical events responsible for the heart sounds are not fully understood. However, their occurrence in association with particular events of the cardiac cycle provides a method of determining if any abnormalities exist. The first heart sound occurs in association with closing of the AV valve and thus represents the beginning of systole. The second heart sound occurs when the aortic valve closes and thus represents the end of systole. The third heart sound, when it can be heard, occurs during the rapid filling phase. Although it can occur in a healthy young adult or child, its presence is usually associated with heart disease. The fourth heart sound is caused by atrial systole.

The pulmonic valve of the right ventricle generally closes slightly after the aortic valve, producing a splitting of the second heart sound. The interval between the two sounds increases during inspiration and decreases during expiration. The delay in closing of the pulmonic valve results from the lower pressure in the pulmonary circulation compared with that in the systemic circulation.

Passage of blood through the valves is usually silent, so no heart sounds are heard during filling and ejection. An abnormal sound heard at these times is called **a murmur**. Diastolic murmurs can be caused by a stenotic (or narrowed) AV valve or by a leaky (insufficient) aortic valve that lets blood enter the ventricle from the aorta. Systolic murmurs can be caused by a stenotic aortic valve or by a leaky AV valve that allows blood to be forced into the atrium during ejection. In all cases, the murmurs are caused by turbulence of the blood as it passes through a partially open valve.

The pressure waves in the left atrium and the jugular vein (representing the right atrium) are also illustrated in Figure 2-17. The a wave represents atrial contraction. The large decrease in pressure following the a wave, called the x descent, is caused by the movement of the heart during systole. The x wave is sometimes interrupted by a small increase in pressure as a result of the bulging of the AV valve into the atrium. Blood begins to enter the atrium soon after the completion of atrial systole, resulting in an increase in atrial pressure called the v wave. When the pressure in the ventricle falls below that in the atrium, there is a rapid emptying of blood into the ventricle and a sudden drop in atrial pressure called the y descent.

CARDIAC MECHANICS

The basic function of the heart is to eject an amount of blood sufficient to meet the needs of the tissues. The cardiac output can be varied by varying the stoke volume and/or the rate of the heartbeat. Three factors are important in controlling the stroke volume: preload, afterload, and contractility. The influence of each of these will be reviewed in turn.

Cardiac muscle fibers behave similarly to skeletal muscle fibers in that the force of their contraction depends on the length of the individual fibers prior to contraction. However, unlike skeletal muscle, in which the initial length or preload

can be varied from 1.5 to 3.5 μm, cardiac muscle fibers cannot be stretched to more than 2.2 μm. This limitation results from the much greater stiffness of the parallel elastic component (PEC) in cardiac muscle. As will be shown below, this limitation is important to the normal function of the heart.

There is no way to determine the actual length of individual muscle fibers in an intact heart, so an indirect method must be used to determine preload. In the past the simplest method was to place a catheter in the left ventricle and measure the end-diastolic pressure—the pressure in the ventricle just before systole. Since the intraventricular pressure is proportional to ventricular volume during diastole, this is a reasonable measure. More recently, with the advent of echocardiograms that allow for the noninvasive imaging of the cardiac wall, it has been possible to measure the end-diastolic volume directly.

The relationship between end-diastolic volume or end-diastolic pressure and the stroke volume is called a Starling relationship. As indicated in Figure 2-18, an increase in preload is accompanied by an increase in stroke volume. This is predicted by the length/tension relationship discussed previously for skeletal muscle. For example, if there is a decrease in stroke volume due to some disease process or physiological perturbation, stroke volume can be increased by allowing the end-diastolic volume to increase. However, increases above the peak of the Starling curve would be counterproductive because at sarcomere lengths above 2.2 μm, increases in preload will result in a decrease in stroke volume. Thus the stiffness of the PEC in cardiac muscle ensures that the variation in preload will remain on the ascending limb of the Starling curve.

The stoke volume can also be influenced by the afterload placed on the heart. The afterload is the force that must be generated by the heart to eject its blood into the aorta. If the resistance to the flow of blood through the circulatory system increases, more pressure will have to be developed to eject the same amount of blood. A similar result will occur in aortic stenosis, when a higher than normal pressure will have to be generated by the ventricle to force the blood through the

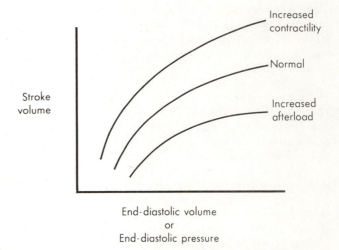

Figure 2-18. Three Starling curves illustrating the effect of increased contractility and increased afterload on the relationship between preload (measured as end-diastolic pressure or end-diastolic volume) and stroke volume.

narrowed valve orifice. Figure 2-18 illustrates the alteration in the Starling curves resulting from a variation in afterload. Note that increasing the afterload reduces the amount of blood that can be ejected at any given preload.

The force developed by a cardiac muscle cell depends on the amount of calcium entering the cytoplasm during each contraction. Recall that in the case of skeletal muscle, enough calcium entered the cell to activate all of the contractile proteins. This does not normally occur in cardiac muscle. A variety of stimuli, most notably norepinephrine released by the sympathetic nervous system or circulating epinephrine, can increase the amount of calcium available to interact with troponin. The increase in force due to an increase in calcium availability is referred to as an increase in contractility. Contractility can be decreased by diseases that affect the ability of the muscle to contract, by anesthetics such as barbiturates, or by decreases in blood supply to the heart. Drugs such as digitalis that increase the intracellular concentration of calcium can be used to increase the contractility of a diseased heart.

Regardless of its cause, an increase in contractility will produce a greater stroke volume and a decrease in contractility will produce a smaller stroke volume at any given preload (see Fig. 2-18).

From a clinical point of view, it is important to measure a decline in cardiac contractility. But as can be observed in Figure 2-18, it is difficult to separate an increase in afterload from a decrease in contractility simply by measuring the stroke volume. Both cause a decline in stroke volume. For some time, the ejection fraction—that is, the fraction of the end-diastolic volume ejected during each beat (stoke volume/end-diastolic volume)—was measured. However, this measure cannot distinguish an increase in afterload from a decrease in contractility since both will produce a decrease in ejection fraction.

Contractility can be measured independently of afterload by recording the relationship between end-systolic volume and end-systolic pressure. This relationship is actually a measure of the maximum force that the heart can produce at a given sarcomere length. To understand the rationale for this measurement, recall that during a heartbeat the heart develops pressure during its isovolumic contraction phase, shortens during its ejection phase, and then relaxes during its isovolumic relaxation phase. The contraction phase lasts longer than the ejection phase, however, so there is a period of time during which the heart is contracting but not shortening. During this time period, the heart is undergoing an isometric contraction—that is, it is generating as much force as it can at the sarcomere length it has shortened to.

Figure 2-19A illustrates the change in pressure and volume that occurs during a cardiac cycle at three different afterloads. These different afterloads were generated by varying the pressure against which the heart had to eject its blood. The lower the afterload, the smaller the heart could become before it reached the end of its shortening phase and began to contract isometrically. In Figure 2-19B the preload is varied. Notice that increasing the preload allowed more blood to be ejected but had no effect on the final volume or pressure produced by the heart at the conclusion of its ejection phase.

The heart can meet the tissue requirement for blood by adjusting its preload, contractility, or rate. However, the amount of energy expended by the heart depends on the

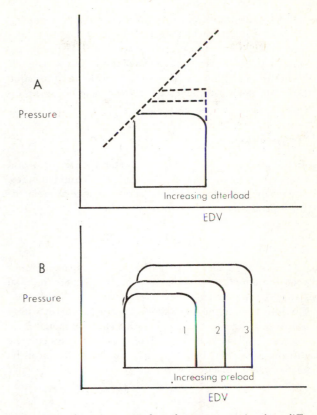

Figure 2-19. Three pressure-volume loops representing three different preloads. In this case, preload is measured by the diastolic pressure—that is, the pressure in the aorta just before the aortic valve opens. As diastolic pressure rises (from point A to B to C), the amount of blood ejected from the heart (point A to point A', point B to point B', and point C to point C') decreases. The decrease in stroke volume results from the Starling curve, which limits the end-systolic volume that can be achieved at any given afterload.

method chosen. For example, the heart can increase its stroke volume from 80 to 100 ml by increasing its preload or its contractility. However, it will require more energy to eject blood by increasing the preload than it will to eject the same amount of blood by increasing the contractility. The reason for this can be understood from the law of Laplace. This relationship can be written as

$$\text{Pressure} = \frac{\text{Stress}}{\text{Radius}}$$

where stress is the force developed by the heart wall divided by the thickness of the heart wall, or force/thickness.

To develop a given pressure thus requires more force at a higher radius than at a lower radius. Energy is used by the heart muscle to develop force. At a higher radius, more energy is required to generate the same pressure than would be the case at a lower radius. By increasing the contractility of the heart, the heart can remain at a smaller radius and thus use less energy.

When a heart begins to lose its contractility, it must increase its size to meet tissue needs for blood. When this occurs, the muscle fibers in the heart wall generally hypertrophy, increasing wall thickness. The increase in thickness reduces the force needed by each individual fiber and thus reduces the energy supply. Unfortunately, when the heart muscle hypertrophies, it is more difficult to perfuse and thus the blood supply may become inadequate even though less of it is required. Digitalis and other positive inotropic drugs can restore the contractility of the heart, making it smaller and allowing it to become more efficient.

HEMODYNAMICS

An understanding of the relationship between the heart and vascular system requires a basic knowledge of hemodynamics, the rules by which pressure, flow, and resistance are related. The most important of these relationships is

$$CO = BP \times TPR$$

where CO is the cardiac output, BP is the pressure difference between the aorta and right atria, and TPR equals the total resistance that the vascular tree offers to the flow of blood.

The resistance to the flow of blood occurs primarily within the arterioles, where the vessels are rather small and total cross-sectional area is low. In this region of the vascular system, the flow of blood is described as laminar and resistance can be calculated using Poiseuille's law:

$$R = \frac{8 \pi l}{n r^4}$$

where n = viscosity, l = length, π = density, and r = radius.

Because resistance is proportional to the fourth power of the radius, the radius of the vessel is the primary determinant of resistance. As will be described below, the radius of the arteriolar vessels can be changed by the sympathetic nervous system and so is under physiological control.

When a set of vessels is arranged in series, the total resistance offered by the vessels is simply the sum of the individual resistances. TPR is primarily related to the resistance of the arterioles because their resistance is much larger than the resistance of the distributing vessels, the capillaries, or the veins.

When the vessels are arranged in parallel, the total resistance is less than the resistance of any one vessel and is given by the formula

$$\frac{1}{R_{TOTAL}} = \frac{1}{R_1} + \frac{1}{R_2} + \ldots \frac{1}{R_n}$$

where R_{TOTAL} = the total resistance and R_1, R_2, and R_n are the resistances of the individual vessels.

All of the organs perfused by the systemic vascular system are in parallel. Changing the resistance of any one thus will affect the resistance of the whole. Equally important, the distribution of blood to each of the organs is proportional to their resistance. In contrast, the flow through organs organized in series will be the same regardless of the resistance offered by any one of them. Since the systemic and pulmonary circulations are in series with each other, the cardiac output of the left and right hearts must, on average, always be the same.

The velocity of blood through any vessel is given by the formula

$$V = Q/A$$

where V = velocity, Q = flow, and A = area. This relationship indicates that the velocity of blood decreases as the area through which it is flowing increases. This is why the blood flow through a capillary bed with a large cross-sectional area is much slower than blood flow through the aorta or any of the distributing arteries, which have a much smaller cross-sectional area.

Arterial pressure

As blood is ejected from the heart, it enters the aorta, raising the blood pressure. When ejection ceases and the heart relaxes, the blood drains out of the arteries, lowering the blood pressure. The pressure wave produced by the flow of blood through the arterial system is illustrated in Figure 2-20A. The peak of the pressure wave is called the systolic pressure; the trough is called the diastolic pressure; and the difference between the systolic and diastolic pressures is called the pulse pressure.

The magnitude of the pressure wave depends on the amount of blood ejected and the compliance (C) of the aorta. Compliance is a measure of distensibility. It is expressed as the change in volume produced by a given change in pressure, or

$$C = \frac{V}{P}$$

If this expression is solved for P to yield

$$P = \frac{V}{C}$$

the change in pressure produced during ejection can be calculated from the stoke volume and compliance if it is assumed that the entire stroke volume remains in the aorta. Actually some of the stroke volume runs off into the capillaries, so the volume increment is really the stroke volume minus the runoff. For simplicity, we will assume that the volume increment is equal to the stroke volume.

Figure 2-20B illustrates how changes in compliance can affect the pulse pressure. If the compliance is low (that is, the aorta is stiff), ejecting 80 ml of blood produces a pulse pressure of 60 mm Hg. However, if the compliance is raised (that is, the aorta becomes more distensible), the same stroke volume produces a pulse pressure of only 40 mm Hg. With age, the aorta becomes stiffer and it is normal for pulse pressure to increase. Another factor affecting pulse pressure is the diastolic pressure. This is important because (as shown in Fig. 2-20B) the compliance is not linear but decreases at higher pressures. Thus if 80 ml of blood is ejected when the diastolic pressure is 80 mm Hg, the pressure will rise only 40 mm Hg, to 120 mm Hg. However, if the diastolic pressure is 100 mm Hg, ncreasing aortic volume by the same amount will cause systolic pressure to reach 160 mm Hg, an increase of 60 mm Hg.

The mean arterial blood pressure is the average pressure

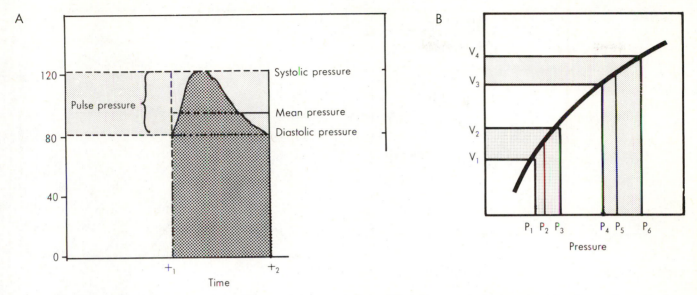

Figure 2-20. Pulse pressure is the difference between systolic and diastolic pressure. Because more time is spent in diastole, the mean pressure is closer to the diastolic pressure than to the systolic pressure. The magnitude of the pulse pressure can be calculated by dividing stroke volume by aortic compliance. (B) As mean pressure rises, pulse pressure increases because systolic pressure rises more than diastolic pressure. This occurs because of the nonlinear compliance curve of the aorta. The higher the pressure, the stiffer the aorta becomes.

within the aorta during a complete cardiac cycle. Since diastole is twice as long as systole, an estimate of the mean pressure can be obtained using the formula

$$MAP = \frac{SP + 2 \times DP}{3}$$

Mean blood pressure, as indicated above, is related to the cardiac output and the TPR by the expression

$$MAP = CO \times TPR$$

This is one of the most important relationships for understanding how blood pressure is determined and regulated by the cardiovascular system. To gain a full understanding of its significance, we must discuss how cardiac output and TPR are regulated.

Control of cardiac output

Cardiac output is the product of heart rate and stroke volume. Stroke volume in turn depends on preload, afterload, and contractility. As indicated above, the term preload refers to the sarcomere length of the muscle fibers making up the ventricular wall. This length is determined by the end-diastolic volume of the heart, which in turn depends on the total amount of blood within the circulatory system and the compliance of the vascular bed and heart.

The diagram in Figure 2-21 divides the circulatory system into four components—the veins, the arteries, the heart, and the TPR. If there is no flow in the system, the total pressure will be equal to the circulatory volume divided by the compliance.

This pressure, called the mean circulatory pressure, is normally about 7 mm Hg. If the heart begins to circulate the blood, the pressure in the veins decreases and that in the arteries increases (see Fig. 2-22). These changes in pressure occur because blood is leaving the venous system and entering the arterial system. More blood is present in the arterial system than in the venous system because when the heart starts to pump, blood is removed from the veins faster than it is able to return through the TPR. As the pressure in the arteries rises, blood is forced through the TPR at a faster rate. Blood eventually enters the veins as fast as it is removed, and a steady state is achieved.

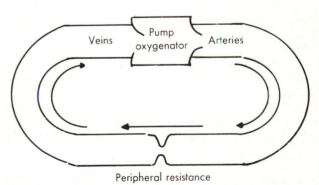

Figure 2-21. A hydraulic model to explain how changes in the characteristics of the vascular system and heart affect cardiac output (CO) and central venous pressure (CVP). The heart removes blood from the veins and pumps it through the arteries. The blood returns to the veins through the arteriolar resistance vessels.

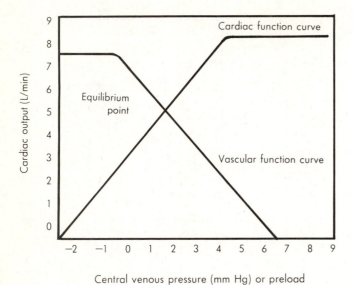

Figure 2-22. At any given time, the cardiac output and CVP are determined by the intersection of the venous and cardiac function curves.

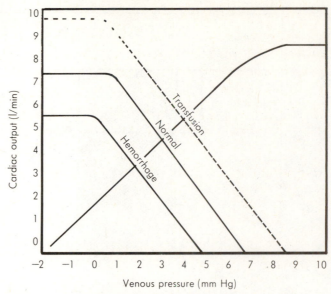

Figure 2-23. If blood volume increases (or venous capacity decreases) or decreases (or venous capacity increases), the venous function curves are shifted to the right or left.

As indicated in Figure 2-22, the larger the cardiac output, the lower the pressure in the veins. The reduction in pressure represents the reduction in total venous blood volume produced by the pumping of the heart. The blood removed from the veins is transferred to the arteries, raising the pressure within the arterial system. The increase in arterial pressure is much greater than the decrease in venous pressure because the arterial compliance is only about 1/20 of the venous compliance. Thus at a cardiac output of 5 L/minute, venous pressure decreases by 4.5 mm Hg (from 7 mm Hg to 2.5 mm Hg) while mean arterial pressure increases by 90 mm Hg, to 97 mm Hg.

The venous pressure is important because it determines the preload. Since the venous system and the heart are connected in series, the pressure within the veins will be approximately equal to that in the ventricles at the end of diastole. This pressure, the end-diastolic pressure, will determine the end-diastolic volume (recall that $P = C \times V$), which in turn determines the cardiac fiber sarcomere lengths. As shown in Figure 2-22, cardiac output increases as preload increases.

These two relationships—that between cardiac output and venous pressure and that between preload and cardiac output— are obviously intertwined since each of them is dependent on the other. In other words, if cardiac output increases, then venous pressure (and preload) decreases; if preload decreases, then cardiac output decreases. Since there can only be one cardiac output and one venous pressure, an equilibrium point is achieved by the cardiovascular system at any given blood volume, venous compliance, TPR, and myocardial contractility.

For example, if blood volume increases (as shown in Fig. 2-23), the equilibrium point will be achieved at a higher cardiac output. Conversely, if blood volume decreases, the cardiac output will decrease until a new equilibrium point is achieved. Corresponding changes will occur if TPR or contractility increases (Fig. 2-24).

An increase in contractility (or a decrease in TPR) will cause a greater stroke volume at any preload. Thus equilibrium will

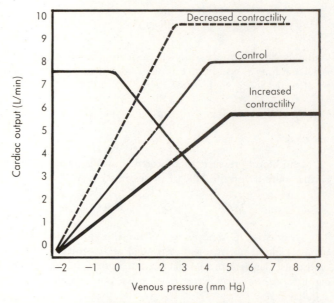

Figure 2-24. If contractility increases or decreases, the cardiac function curve is shifted to the left or right. In either case, cardiac output and CVP are determined by the intersection of the venous and cardiac function curves.

be reached at a higher cardiac output and lower venous pressure. If, on the other hand, contractility were to fall (or TPR to increase), venous pressure would increase and cardiac output would fall.

Control of blood pressure

As indicated above, the mean blood pressure depends on the cardiac output and the TPR. TPR is determined primarily by the resistance to blood flow offered by the arterioles situated between the distributing arteries and the microcirculatory beds of the various organs within the body. Their resistance, as indicated earlier, is proportional to the fourth power of their radius. Thus an understanding of how arteriolar radius is controlled is essential for an understanding of how blood pressure is controlled.

The smooth muscle fibers surrounding the blood vessels are innervated by the sympathetic nervous system. Norepinephrine, the synaptic transmitter released from sympathetic postganglionic fibers, causes contraction of the smooth muscles and constriction of the vasculature. This innervation has a significant effect on both the arterioles, where stimulation causes an increase in TPR, and on the capacitance vessels, where stimulation causes an increase in circulating blood volume. Innervation to the large distributing vessels is meager and does not have much of an effect on their diameter. Although the radius of the microcirculatory vessels can be influenced by sympathetic discharge, local factors, to be discussed below, are much more important.

The sympathetic fibers innervating the arterioles are tonically active. Decreasing their activity results in a decrease in TPR and blood pressure; increasing their activity results in an increase in TPR and blood pressure. Sympathetic discharge is controlled by a number of cardiovascular reflexes originating from a variety of peripheral receptors and CNS nuclei.

The most important of the peripheral reflexes is the **baroreceptor reflex**. Two receptors, the carotid and aortic baroreceptors, are responsible for monitoring the peripheral blood pressure. The carotid baroreceptors are located within the carotid sinus (an enlargement of the internal carotid arteries where they bifurcate from the common carotid artery) and in the aortic arch. When these regions are stretched by the blood within them, they cause an increase in the firing frequency of the nerves innervating them, the sinus nerve in the case of the carotid sinus and the vagus nerve in the case of the aortic arch baroreceptors.

Impulses from the baroreceptors eventually reach the nucleus of the tractus solitarius (NTS) in the medulla, where they form inhibitory synapses with neurons in a vasoconstrictor center. The fibers leaving the medullary vasoconstrictor area are excitatory to the sympathetic preganglionic fibers in the spinal cord. Thus when blood pressure increases, the baroreceptors are stretched, the afferent fibers are stimulated, and the discharge frequency of the fibers leaving the vasoconstrictor center is decreased. This leads to a decrease in sympathetic activity, a decrease in TPR, and a decrease in blood pressure. Conversely, if blood pressure were to fall, the discharge of the baroreceptor afferents would decrease and inhibition of the NTS fibers would decrease. This would lead to an increase in output from the vasoconstrictor centers, an increase in sympathetic discharge, and an increase in TPR.

Not every vascular bed responds equally to the change in medullary activity initiated by the baroreceptor reflexes. Most of the changes in TPR result from changes in resistance within the skin, mesentery, skeletal muscle, and kidney. The brain and coronary circulations are not affected very much at all by the baroreceptor reflexes.

Reflexes are additionally initiated by receptors on the venous side of the circulation within the vena cava, atria, and pulmonary veins. These receptors respond to changes in blood volume. If blood volume were to increase, for example, the afferents innervating these receptors would increase, causing an inhibition of the vasocontrictor centers in the medulla and a decrease in TPR. Conversely, a decrease in blood volume would result in an increase in vasoconstrictor activity. These receptors play a much more important role in the control of blood volume than they do in the control of TPR. Their ability to alter levels of aldosterone and thus affect salt and water excretion by the kidneys is discussed in the section on renal physiology.

In addition to affecting TPR, the baroreceptor reflexes also affect cardiac output. They do this in two ways. First, the medullary centers innervated by the baroreceptor afferents innervate the heart. For example, when sympathetic discharge to the resistance vessels is increased, there is a corresponding increase in sympathetic discharge to the heart. This causes an increase in heart rate and contractility, leading to an increase in cardiac output. When sympathetic discharge to the resistance vessels is decreased, not only is there a decrease in sympathetic discharge to the heart but, in addition, there is an increase in vagal activity to the atria, resulting in a decrease in heart rate.

Second, the sympathetic fibers innervate the smooth muscle surrounding the larger veins or capacitance vessels. These vessels are very sensitive to changes in sympathetic tone, displaying a significant decrease in diameter when stimulated. This decrease in diameter causes an increase in effective circulating blood volume, leading to an increase in venous pressure, preload, and thus cardiac output. In other words, constricting the capacitance vessels has the same effect on cardiac output as does an actual increase in blood volume. For this reason, constriction of the capacitance vessels is often referred to as an autotransfusion.

Cardiac output may also be affected by venous return—that is, the amount of blood returning to the heart during each cardiac cycle. For example, if an individual suddenly moves from a lying to a standing position, some of the venous blood will pool in the feet. This occurs because the weight of the blood causes an expansion in the diameter of the most dependent veins. Arterial vessels do not expand very much at all because of their rather low compliance. Similarly, if tight leg stockings are worn, the veins will not be able to expand and pooling will be less. In some cases, over 500 ml of blood can be pooled in the veins by standing. This pooling resembles the loss of blood illustrated in Figure 2-23, where cardiac output was reduced by more than 1 L. Without compensation, this can cause a fall in blood pressure of 20 to 25 mm Hg and can lead to light-headedness or syncope. This normally does not occur because of the compensatory reflexes discussed above.

The baroreceptor reflexes, sensing a decrease in blood pressure and blood volume, cause an increase in sympathetic discharge to the arteries, veins, and heart. Arteriolar diameter decreases, causing an increase in TPR. Capacitance vessel diameter decreases to produce an autotransfusion that partially replaces the blood pooled in the legs. The heart rate and contractility increase, leading to an increase in cardiac output. Taken together, these effects cause blood pressure to be maintained despite a pooling of blood in the legs. It should be noted, however, that the increase in TPR, although valuable in increasing blood pressure, also increases the afterload on the heart and thus can reduce cardiac output. A fall in cardiac output does not occur because of the concomitant increase in heart rate and contractility.

Venous valves are important in assuring that blood flows normally from the feet to the heart. The constant muscular activity associated with normal locomotion and movement periodically squeezes the veins and forces blood toward the heart. Blood is prevented from moving backward by the one-way venous valves. However, when a person is standing quietly, blood continues to enter the veins from the arterial blood, raising the pressure in the more dependent veins and forcing the valves open. Thus after a person stands motionless for a minute or so, all of the valves are opened and the entire venous system behaves as one continuous vessel.

Respiratory activity also plays a role in assuring adequate venous return. During inspiration, there is a reduction in intrathoracic pressure that causes an expansion of the very compliant veins within the thorax. The expansion of these vessels lowers their pressure, which in turn accelerates the flow of blood from the periphery to the thorax. During expiration, when intrathoracic pressure rises, the veins are partially occluded, preventing blood from entering the thorax. However, the increase in blood flow to the thorax during inspiration exceeds the decrease that occurs during expiration. Respiratory activity therefore has a positive effect overall on bringing blood into the thorax. The variation in blood flow brought about by respiration is reflected in the blood pressure. During inspiration, most of the increased blood remains pooled in the thoracic vessels so venous return to the heart actually decreases. However, during expiration, when thoracic pressure rises, this blood is forced into the heart. Thus there is a transient decrease in blood pressure during inspiration and an increase in blood pressure during expiration. A large increase in expiratory pressure such as occurs during coughing, straining at defecation, and weight lifting can cause a significant reduction of blood flow into the thorax and seriously compromise venous return.

The above discussion outlining the influence of venous return on cardiac output should not obscure the fact that in the steady state, venous return and cardiac output are the same. Thus it is as true to say that cardiac output is determined by venous return as it is to say that venous return is determined by cardiac output. It is only the transient changes in venous return such as occur when blood is pooled in the feet or in the thorax that affect cardiac output. Once a new steady state is achieved, cardiac output and venous return will be equal to each other once again. The true determinants of cardiac output are, as illustrated in Figures 2-23 and 2-24, the vascular volume, TPR, contractility, and heart rate.

The peripheral circulation

The cardiac output is divided among the various organs of the body to meet their individual metabolic needs. The adjustment of blood flow to individual organs is carried out locally by a process often called autoregulation. Strictly speaking, autoregulation refers to a process by which the flow of blood entering an organ remains constant despite variations in mean blood pressure. Without compensation, an increase in blood pressure would cause an increase in flow to each of the organs in the body. Although an increase in flow would have no obvious detrimental effect on most organs, the brain and kidney would be greatly affected. Increasing blood flow to the brain would cause an increase in intracranial pressure, while

increasing blood flow to the kidneys would cause filtration to rise. These effects do not occur, because the radius of vessels controlling the blood flow to these organs decreases in response to an increase in blood pressure, preventing flow from increasing. In a corresponding manner, a decrease in arterial pressure is accompanied by an increase in arteriolar radius, leading to an increase in blood flow.

The process of autoregulation obviously is not independent of the processes controlling cardiac output and blood pressure. For example, if a hemorrhage causes a loss in blood volume, cardiac output and blood pressure will fall. To some extent the fall in blood pressure will be ameliorated by baroreeeptor reflexes, which will increase TPR and decrease the volume of the venous capacitance vessels. To keep blood flow to an organ constant, arteriolar diameter must then increase. Thus if autoregulatory mechanisms kept blood flow to all organs constant, TPR could not increase. It consequently is impossible to maintain blood pressure and keep flow to all of the tissues constant during a hemorrhage. Those organs such as the brain and kidneys, which have a well-developed autoregulatory mechanism, are able to preserve blood flow. Those such as the skin and gut, which do not, are subjected to a reduction in blood flow.

The exact mechanism by which autoregulation is accomplished is not fully understood. However, three mechanisms have been proposed: the tissue pressure, myogenic, and metabolic hypotheses. The tissue pressure mechanism is based on the view that an increase in pressure forces fluid out of the tissue capillaries. This fluid is then thought to raise the interstitial fluid pressure enough to compress the postarteriolar vessels, preventing blood flow through the tissues. Alternatively, if arterial pressure falls, interstitial pressure falls and more blood can flow through the organ. The myogenic hypothesis is based on the observation that the smooth muscle surrounding the vessels contracts when stretched. According to this mechanism, a rise in pressure would stretch the smooth muscle around the vessels, causing them to contract and thus reducing the flow of blood through the vessel. Reducing the pressure would cause the smooth muscles to relax, thereby increasing the flow of blood through the organ. The metabolic hypothesis proposes that the buildup of metabolites by the tissues determines the caliber of the vessels. Thus when flow into the vessel is reduced, for whatever reason, metabolites would build up, causing a dilation of the blood vessels. When flow increases, these metabolites would be washed away, causing the vessel to dilate.

Microcirculation

The delivery of oxygen and nutrients to and the removal of metabolic wastes from an organ are dependent on the adequacy of blood flow through the capillary network of the organ. To a large extent, the flow of blood through the capillaries depends on the diameter of the arterioles supplying the organ. Obviously, if the sympathetic discharge to the arterioles is high, causing a narrowing of the lumen, then blood flow to the organ will be reduced. However, another important determinant of blood flow to an organ is the number of capillaries through which the blood flows.

A precapillary sphincter is present at the origin of capillaries in many tissues. The sphincter is a smooth muscle cell that envelops the capillary. When the smooth muscle cell contracts, blood is shunted away from the capillary; when it dilates, blood is allowed to flow through the capillary. The sphincter is not innervated by the sympathetic nervous system, so its contractile state depends entirely on the vasoactive metabolites surrounding it. Thus, if there is a large flow of blood through an organ, in excess of its tissue needs, most of blood will be shunted through the few open capillaries. If the metabolic needs of the tissue increase, however, such as might occur in a skeletal muscle during exercise, the consequent buildup of metabolites will result in the opening of more capillaries.

Of even more importance, if the metabolic buildup is of sufficient magnitude, it will overcome the sympathetic stimulation of the arterioles, causing even more blood to flow through the muscle. For this reason, blood flow through skeletal muscle is very high during aerobic exercise despite the large amount of sympathetic activity.

The major function of the capillary network is nutrient and waste exchange. Although some of this exchange takes place by pinocytosis and filtration, most of it occurs by diffusion.

It is not entirely certain how much if any transfer of material occurs by pinocytosis. However, pinocytotic vesicles have been observed to form on the inside of the capillary endothelium and to transfer their contents to the interstitium. It is thought that some large particles may be transported in this manner.

The amount of fluid moving across the capillaries by filtration depends on the hydrostatic and osmotic pressures of the capillary and interstitial water. The hydrostatic pressure within the capillary depends on the ratio of the pre- and postcapillary resistances and the pressure in the arteriole supplying the capillary. For example, if the arteriolar pressure is 40 mm Hg and the precapillary resistance is three times that of the postcapillary resistance, it means that three-fourths of the pressure drop will occur before the blood enters the capillary—that is, the capillary pressure will be 10 mm Hg. However, if the two resistances are equal, then only half of the pressure drop will occur over the precapillary resistance, and the capillary pressure will be 20 mm Hg. Thus any factor tending to retard the flow of blood out of the capillaries, such as an increase in right ventricular end-diastolic pressure, will cause an increase in filtration of fluid from the capillary.

The hydrostatic pressure in the interstitial fluid surrounding the capillary is most often given as zero. However, recent evidence has indicated that this value might be below atmospheric in some tissues. Certainly, the interstitial fluid pressure in the thorax is less than zero. In the kidneys, the pressure is normally near 10 mm Hg. This high interstitial pressure results from the inextensible capsule surrounding the kidney.

The osmotic pressure in the capillaries is normally 25 mm Hg and is due to the presence of plasma proteins, primarily albumin and globulins. There is little if any plasma protein in the interstitium, partly because the capillaries are essentially nonpermeable to the proteins and partly because the lymphatics are so efficient at removing whatever proteins do manage to pass across the capillary wall. Some tissues, such as the lung, have fairly leaky capillaries, so the interstitial osmotic pressure becomes significant.

These forces, the osmotic and hydrostatic pressures, are called **Starling forces** and determine the rate of fluid movement across the capillaries. The net amount of exchange is given by the expression

$$\text{Fluid flow} = k \left[(P_{CAP} + \pi_{TISSUE}) - (P_{TISSUE} + \pi_{CAP}) \right]$$

where k = the filtration constant for the capillary membrane. This constant includes both the surface area and hydraulic conductivity of the capillary. Since under most circumstances the permeability of the capillary to the movement of water does not change, an increase in k represents an increase in the number of capillaries though which the blood is flowing.

In most capillaries, only about 2% of the plasma flowing through them is filtered, and much of this occurs in the early portion of the capillaries. In the kidneys, over 20% of the plasma is filtered and filtration occurs over the entire length of the capillary. In contrast, in the intestine, capillaries absorb fluid over their entire length. The amount and direction of fluid transport in any tissue can be determined if the Starling forces and blood flow are known. Most of the filtered water moves through the spaces between the epithelial cells. Some, however, passes through the endothelial cell membrane.

Fluid filtered out of the capillaries at their arterial end may be partially reabsorbed at the venous end, where the hydrostatic pressure is less. In most tissues, however, fluid is filtered from one group of capillaries and reabsorbed by another. Only about 85% of the filtered plasma is reabsorbed by the capillaries. The remainder is returned to the circulation through the lymphatic system.

The terminal vessels of the lymphatic system consist of highly permeable closed-end capillaries. Excess water and proteins filtered out of the capillaries of the vascular system enter the lymphatic capillaries and are carried to the more central lymphatic vessels. A series of one-way valves forces the fluid to flow toward the heart. Although the net amount of water filtered from the capillaries is only a fraction of 1%, the daily lymphatic flow equals the total circulating plasma volume. In addition, protein filtered from the capillaries can only be returned to the circulation through the lymphatics. Any compromise of the lymphatic circulation thus would have profound consequences.

The largest amount of fluid and nutrient exchange across the capillaries occurs by diffusion. Although only 2% of the water flowing through the capillaries is exchanged by filtration and osmosis, almost 400 times the water flowing through the capillaries moves back and forth by diffusion.

Small water-soluble molecules and most lipid-soluble molecules pass easily through the capillary membrane by diffusion. As a result, there is seldom a concentration gradient across the capillary endothelium. If there is a large distance between the nearest capillary and a target organ, a gradient may be established, however. Similarly, if there is some limitation to free diffusion, a difference in concentration may exist between the interstitium and capillary fluid. In most cases, blood plasma reaches diffusional equilibrium with the interstitial fluid as it passes through the capillaries.

Special circulations

The control of blood flow through any organ is a function of the mean arterial blood pressure and the resistance offered by that organ to the flow of blood. We have previously discussed how blood pressure is controlled and the general factors regulating vascular resistance.

This concluding section will describe some of the peculiarities of blood flow regulation in skeletal muscle, the skin, the brain, and the heart.

Blood flow through skeletal muscle is varied both by reflexes initiated in response to changes in blood pressure and by the metabolic activity of the muscle. When skeletal muscle is at rest, blood flow is determined by the amount of sympathetic discharge. If blood pressure decreases, sympathetic discharge increases, reducing blood flow. If blood pressure rises, sympathetic tone is reduced and blood flow increases. Since skeletal muscle has a greater mass than any other organ, changes in its vascular resistance can have a significant effect on blood pressure.

However, if skeletal muscle becomes metabolically active, its blood flow increases dramatically. With maximum exercise, flow can increase by more than 20-fold. Under these conditions, it is the buildup of metabolites rather than the amount of sympathetic discharge that determines the vascular resistance. Blood flow during exercise is also influenced by the compressive forces generated by muscle contraction. When muscles contract, they increase the flow of blood through the veins by squeezing on them. The venous valves prevent retrograde flow of blood during contraction. Thus the amount of blood in the muscle is reduced when it contracts. This facilitates the entry of blood into the muscle when it relaxes. If the contractions are particularly strong and sustained, the arterial supply can be compromised and blood flow will decrease or even stop.

Skeletal muscle vasculature also autoregulates. That is, in the absence of any neural or humoral input, blood flow through skeletal muscle is constant over a fairly wide range of blood pressures. However, despite this high autoregulatory capacity, blood flow through skeletal muscle varies to meet the needs of blood pressure maintenance and metabolic demands. If the muscle is at rest or even exercises lightly, vascular resistance will depend on the amount of sympathetic stimulation. With an increase in exercise, the production of metabolites controls the resistance of the arterioles and blood flow into the muscle increases.

Blood flow through the skin is primarily determined by reflexes responsible for regulating body temperature. When temperature falls, blood flow through the skin decreases; when temperature rises, blood flow increases. This occurs most dramatically in the cutaneous vessels of the hands, the feet, the ears, the lips, and the nose. These regions are primarily perfused by arteriovenous anastomoses in which blood can flow directly from the arteries and veins without passing through a capillary bed. These anastomoses are under the exclusive control of the sympathetic nervous system and are regulated by the reflexes that control body temperature. Other vessels within these areas and other regions of the body (in which blood flows through a capillary network) are somewhat under the control of local metabolic factors. However, in all areas of the skin, the primary factor controlling blood flow is the amount of discharge produced by the sympathetic nervous system.

The coronary circulation is controlled almost exclusively by the metabolic demands of the cardiac muscle fibers. However, the rate of blood flow at any given time in the cardiac cycle is strongly influenced by the mechanical forces generated by the heart muscle and the pressure of the blood flowing into the heart.

Blood enters the myocardium through the right and left coronary arteries, which arise at the root of the aorta. The right coronary artery supplies the right atrium and ventricle, while the left coronary artery (which divides into descending and circumflex branches) supplies the left side of the heart. Most of the blood passing through the myocardial capillaries drains into the coronary sinus, from which it empties into the right atrium. Some of the blood drains directly into the left ventricle through the thebesian veins and becomes part of the anatomic shunt (to be described in the next section).

The change in right and left myocardial blood flow during the cardiac cycle is illustrated in Figure 2-25. During diastole, when the heart is relaxed, blood flow is proportional to the aortic pressure. It is thus highest at the end of systole, when the aortic and pulmonic valves close and the heart begins to relax, and it then falls during the remainder of diastole, as blood pressure falls. Blood flow reaches its lowest level during the isovolumic contraction phase, when aortic pressure is lowest and myocardial wall tension is highest. Blood flow increases somewhat during the ejection phase, following the aortic pressure wave. The variations in blood flow during the cardiac cycle are greater on the left side than on the right side because both the myocardial wall tension and blood pressure are higher on the left than they are on the right side of the heart. In fact, as shown in Figure 2-25, blood flow on the right side might actually be higher during systole than it is during diastole.

The compressive forces of the myocardium also influence the distribution of blood flow between the endocardium and epicardium. Because the endocardial surface is exposed to a higher pressure during systole, its blood flow is lower than that to the epicardium. The lower blood flow on the endocardial surface allows a buildup of metabolites to occur during systole, and thus during diastole there is a larger blood flow to the endocardium than there is to the epicardium. On average, the blood flow to these two regions is about the same.

However, the increase in blood flow to the endocardium during diastole depends on the dilation of the endocardial coronary vessels. In periods of low blood flow, such as during episodes of low blood pressure or periods of coronary occlusion, the endocardial vessels are already maximally dilated. Thus there is no means to increase blood flow during diastole, and as a result, endocardial blood flow falls below epicardial blood flow. For this reason, the endocardial surface is more likely to be damaged by coronary artery disease than the epicardial surface is.

Although the mechanism coupling myocardial blood flow to metabolism is not known, the most likely mediator is adenosine. When an adequate supply of oxygen is not available, cardiac muscle fibers generate adenosine, a potent vasodilator of coronary vessels, and coronary blood flow increases.

The sympathetic nervous system has very little, if any, direct influence on the diameter of the coronary blood vessels. However, sympathetic stimulation to the heart increases coronary blood flow because, by increasing heart rate and contractility, the sympathetics increase the metabolic requirements of the heart.

More than any other tissue, the brain is dependent on an

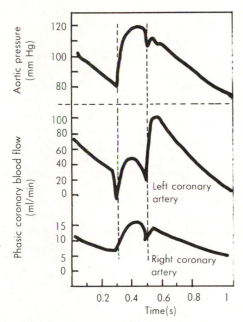

Figure 2-25. The coronary flow is dependent on the ventricular pressure (which compresses the vessels in the ventricular muscle) and the aortic pressure (which forces the blood through the coronary vessels). Coronary blood flow is lowest during isovolumic contraction, when aortic pressure is lowest and ventricular pressure is highest. Coronary flow is highest at the beginning of diastole, when aortic pressure is still high but ventricular pressure is at its lowest value. Diastole flows are not much higher on the right side of the heart because right ventricular pressures are not high enough to produce a large decrease in coronary flow.

adequate supply of oxygen and nutrients for its survival. Removal of oxygen or glucose for even a short period of time can produce global damage to brain cells. A great deal of current research is directed toward finding methods of reducing the damage caused by ischemic episodes following strokes.

Cerebral vessels have a well-developed autoregulatory mechanism and thus are able to keep blood flow to the brain fairly constant over a wide range of perfusing pressures. The distribution of blood flow to various parts of the brain is locally controlled by metabolic activity. When an individual walks, blood flow to the motor area increases; when he or she sits and listens to music, blood flow to the auditory areas increases.

These autoregulatory and metabolic control mechanisms can be overridden by changes in arterial carbon dioxide tension. If carbon dioxide levels increase, blood flow to the brain increases; if carbon dioxide decreases, then blood flow decreases. The dizziness associated with the drop in carbon dioxide tension produced by prolonged hyperventilation results from a decrease in cerebral blood flow.

If blood flow to the brain is compromised by an elevation in CSF pressure, a powerful cardiovascular reflex called the Cushing response is initiated to restore blood flow. This reflex, by producing a profound vasoconstriction to all organs of the body (except the heart), causes a large increase in mean arterial blood pressure. Although the coronary vessels are not constricted by the Cushing response, there is an increase in vagal nerve activity, which by slowing the heart reduces the metabolic

demands of the myocardium. This reflex demonstrates just how committed the circulatory reflexes are to supplying an adequate amount of blood to the brain.

RESPIRATION

The primary function of the respiratory system is to bring oxygen to the alveolar capillaries and remove carbon dioxide from them. However, the lungs also function as endocrine organs, being the major site at which angiotension II is formed by angiotensin-converting enzyme, and as a filter, removing cellular debris from the circulatory system.

The respiratory system consists of a network of airways for conducting air into the lungs and an alveolar system for exchanging gas (Fig. 2-26). Air passing through the pharynx enters the trachea. The trachea divides into left and right main bronchi. These bronchi divide again and again, forming terminal bronchioles after the 16th division. The terminal bronchioles give rise to transitional bronchioles, which continue to divide, forming smaller and smaller branches, eventually giving rise to alveolar sacs by the 23rd division. The bronchioles and associated alveoli distal to a terminal bronchiole are called primary lobules or acini.

The function of the conducting airways is to bring air into the lungs. Since no gas exchange occurs within these tubes, they are referred to as **anatomic dead space**. Typically the anatomic dead space in a 70-kg male is 150 ml (approximately 1 ml/pound).

The respiratory bronchioles, which have some alveoli

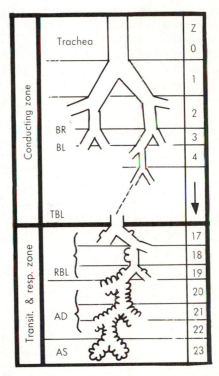

Figure 2-26. The trachea divides into two bronchi, which each divide into two bronchioles, etc. The first 16 generations are the conducting airways. The next 7 generations permit gas exchange and are referred to as the respiratory zone.

associated with them, and the alveolar ducts, which are completely lined with alveoli, are referred to as the respiratory zone. When the lung is at rest, the volume of the respiratory zone is approximately 3,000 ml. There are approximately 500 million alveoli per lung, forming a surface area of some 75 m² over which gas exchange can take place.

During inspiration, the intercostal muscles and diaphragm contract to expand the chest, drawing a tidal volume of approximately 500 ml into the airways; 150 ml of this remains in the anatomic dead space, and the remainder (the alveolar ventilation) enters the respiratory zone. When the respiratory muscles relax, the elastic properties of the lungs cause them to passively return to their resting volume.

Air flows into the airways by bulk flow along the negative pressure gradient established between the atmosphere and the alveoli when the lungs expand. However, the enormous cross-sectional area of the alveolar sacs and alveoli significantly reduces the velocity of airflow within them. Fortunately, the alveoli are small enough (approximately 300 to 400 μm in diameter) to allow equilibration between gas entering the terminal bronchioles and the alveoli to occur in less than 1 second. The remainder of this section will be divided into a discussion of ventilation (the process of moving air into the lungs) and gas exchange (the process of oxygen delivery and carbon dioxide removal).

VENTILATION

The static lung volumes.   The amount of gas in the lungs at any given time can be altered by expanding or contracting the lungs. When the lungs are reduced to their smallest volume by maximally contracting the expiratory muscles, the remaining gas volume is called the **residual volume** (RV) (Fig. 2-27). When the lungs are maximally expanded, the gas volume they contain is called the **total lung capacity** (TLC). The difference between these two values—that is, the maximum amount of air that can be drawn into the lungs during a single breath—is called the **vital capacity**. The volume of gas in the lungs when the respiratory muscles are relaxed is called the **functional residual capacity (FRC)**.

As will be described later, these volumes can change under a variety of conditions, including disease processes. Thus it is important to be able to measure them properly. The vital capacity can be measured by simple spirometry. A spirometer (see Fig. 2-27) is a device used to measure the amount of air drawn into or expelled from the lungs. It consists of a cylinder turned upside down and suspended in a tank of water by a pulley system. The cylinder acts as a reservoir for gas and moves up and down as air is added to or removed from it. A chart recorder is used to measure the movement of the cylinder. When the device is properly calibrated, the amount and rate of gas movement can be accurately recorded.

To measure the vital capacity, the subject inhales as deeply as possible and then expels as much of the gas as possible. The movement of the recording pen measures the difference between the maximum and minimum volumes of gas in the lungs—that is, the vital capacity. When the subject breathes normally, the movement of the pen records the tidal volume—the amount of air entering the lungs with each breath. The spirometer can also measure the inspiratory capacity (the amount of gas that can be inhaled starting from the FRC) and the expiratory volume (the amount of gas that can be expelled, starting from the FRC). However, the actual volumes contained in the RV, FRC, and TLC cannot be measured by simple spirometry. For these, the helium dilution technique is required.

In this technique, the spirometer is filled with a known volume of air ($V_{INITIAL}$), containing a known concentration of helium ($C_{INITIAL}$). The subject is then connected to the spirometer at a time when his or her lungs are filled with the volume to be measured (V_{LUNGS}). After several minutes, the helium concentration within the spirometer becomes reduced (from $C_{INITIAL}$ to C_{FINAL}) as it is mixed with the air inside the lungs. If the concentration of helium (C_{FINAL}) within the spirometer is measured after equilibration has occurred, the volume of air in the lungs at the time the subject was connected to the spirometer can be measured using the following equation:

$$V_{LUNGS} = \frac{V_{INITIAL}(C_{INITIAL} - C_{FINAL})}{C_{FINAL}}$$

For example, suppose a subject is connected to a spirometer containing 10 L of gas with a helium concentration of 10% when the lungs are fully expanded (TLC). The original amount of helium in the spirometer is

$$V_{INITIAL} \times C_{INITIAL} = 10 \text{ L} \times 10\% = 1 \text{ L}$$

After the gas in the spirometer equilibrates with the gas in the lungs, the concentration of helium is reduced to 6%. However, the amount of helium

$$(V_{INITIAL} + V_{LUNGS}) \times C_{FINAL} = (10 \text{ L} + \text{TLC}) \times C_{FINAL} = 1 \text{ L}$$

has not changed.

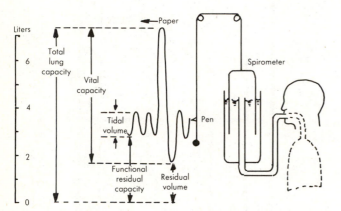

Figure 2-27. A spirometer can be used to measure vital capacity (the amount of air that can be expelled from the lungs after they are maximally inflated). It can also be used to measure the various components of the vital capacity such as tidal volume, inspiratory reserve volume, etc. However, the amount of air remaining in the lungs after a maximum expiration, the residual volume, cannot be measured with a spirometer and, as a result, neither can functional residual capacity or total lung capacity.

Setting the two expressions for the amount of helium equal to each other and solving for TLC yields

$$TLC = 10 \text{ L} (10\% - 6\%) / 6\% = 6.67 \text{ L}$$

If the subject is connected to the spirometer after making a maximum expiratory effort, then RV will be measured; if connected when the muscles of respiration are relaxed, then FRC will be measured.

Alveolar ventilation.   The amount of fresh gas reaching the lungs with each breath is called the **alveolar volume**. As indicated above, approximately 500 ml of gas enters the lung with each breath. However, 150 ml of this is dead-space gas—gas remaining in the tracheobronchial tree after the previous ventilation. Thus the alveolar volume (V_A) is the difference between the tidal volume (V_T) and the dead-space volume (V_D):

$$V_A = V_T - V_D$$

If, instead of measuring the volumes of gas moved with each breath, the volumes moved each minute are measured, the relationship becomes

$$\dot{V}_A = \dot{V}_E - \dot{V}_D$$

The dot above the volume symbol indicates volume per time. V_E is called the **minute volume** and is usually determined by measuring the amount of gas expelled from the lungs each minute. The minute volumes are simply the lung volumes multiplied by the frequency (F) in breaths per minute.

Since only alveolar ventilation is available for gas exchange, it is important to be able to measure this value. In a normal subject, alveolar ventilation can be determined by subtracting the estimated dead space within the conducting airways (1 ml/pound) from the tidal volume.

It can also be measured by Fowler's method, which is based on the difference between the composition of the gas in the conducting airways and that in the alveoli. The subject takes a single deep breath of gas containing 100% oxygen and then breathes out through a nitrogen gas analyzer. The initial portion of the expelled gas will be the pure oxygen that remained in the conducting airways and thus will contain no nitrogen (Fig. 2-28). The last portion of the expelled gas will represent the mixture of the freshly inhaled pure oxygen and the alveolar gas present in the lungs prior to the deep breath. The transition between these two gas mixtures will be partly anatomic dead-space gas and partly alveolar gas. Fowler's method assumes that approximately half of the transitional air is dead-space air (see Fig. 2-28).

Physiological dead space (the volume of gas not available for gas exchange with the blood) is composed of both alveolar and anatomic dead space. An accurate measure of the dead-space volume can be found using the Bohr equation:

$$V_D = V_T \times \frac{F_A CO_2 - F_E CO_2}{F_A CO_2}$$

The terms involving F refer to the fractional concentrations of the gases. For example, if $F_E CO_2$ equals 3%, it means that 3% of the expired air is composed of carbon dioxide.

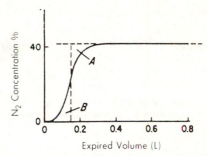

Figure 2-28. Anatomic dead space is the volume of gas in the airways that does not participate in gas exchange. In Fowler's method, the anatomic dead space is measured by taking a deep breath of 100% oxygen and then breathing out through a nitrogen gas analyzer. The first portion of gas expelled contains pure oxygen (no nitrogen). The last portion of gas expelled is alveolar air and contains a constant percentage of oxygen and nitrogen. The transitional portion, containing a varying percentage of oxygen and nitrogen, is divided into two equal volumes by a vertical line. The dead space is estimated as the volume at which the vertical line intersects the expired gas axis.

The Bohr equation is derived from the assumption that all of the carbon dioxide found in the expired air comes from the alveolar air. Thus the amount of carbon dioxide in the expired air,

$$V_T \times F_E CO_2$$

is also equal to

$$V_A \times F_A CO_2$$

Substituting $V_T - V_D$ for V_A yields

$$(V_T - V_D) \times F_A CO_2$$

Setting

$$V_T \times F_E CO_2 = (V_T - V_D) \times F_A CO_2$$

and solving for V_D yields the Bohr equation.

Respiratory muscles

The lungs are expanded by the downward movement of the diaphragm, the up and outward movement of the ribs produced by the contraction of the external intercostal muscles, and the lifting of the first two ribs by the contraction of the accessory muscles of inspiration. During normal quiet respiration, the diaphragm is responsible for two-thirds of the tidal volume, the intercostal muscles producing the remainder of the chest expansion. The accessory muscles only become involved when there is vigorous respiratory effort. The diaphragm is innervated by the phrenic nerve, which originates in the third, fourth, and fifth spinal cord segments. Should the phrenic nerve be damaged, as for example in a spinal cord injury, the intercostal muscles, which are innervated by thoracic motoneurons, would be able to sustain respiration.

Expiration is normally a passive process resulting from the elastic recoil of the expanded lungs. However, under increased respiratory effort, air is pushed from the lungs by the abdominal muscles, which push the diaphragm up, and the internal intercostals, which pull the rib cage down and inward.

The oxygen consumption associated with the work of breathing is normally fairly low, amounting to no more than 5% of the oxygen brought into the circulation by the lungs. Although this percentage rises with exercise, the oxygen cost of increased ventilation is usually not a factor in limiting physical activity.

Elastic resistance to inspiration. When the chest wall expands the thoracic cavity, it causes the lungs to expand as well. This occurs because of the adhesion between the parietal pleura surrounding the internal surface of the chest and the visceral pleura surrounding the parenchyma of the lung. The space between these two pleural membranes, called the intrapleural space, is filled with a thin film of pleural fluid. In order for the chest to expand, it must overcome the forces produced by the elastic recoil of the lungs. The amount of force exerted by the chest wall on the lungs can be determined by measuring the negative pressure that builds up within the pleural space. The pressure is created by the opposing forces of expanding chest and recoiling lungs. As long as the adhesion between the parietal and visceral pleura is maintained, the expanding chest will pull the lungs along with it.

The ratio of lung volume and intrapleural pressure (the force required to expand the lung) is referred to as **compliance**. Lung compliance is normally measured as the slope of a static pressure-volume curve (Fig. 2-29). Such a curve is produced by measuring the intrapleural pressure required to hold the lung at a given volume. Under static conditions, when air is not flowing into or out of the lung, the intra-alveolar pressure is atmospheric or zero. Actually, the pressure is 760 mm Hg (or whatever the barometric pressure is that day), but in pulmonary medicine, pressures are measured as differences from atmospheric. Thus the transpulmonary pressure (the difference between the intra-alveolar pressure and the intrapleural

pressure) expanding the lung is simply the intrapleural pressure.

Normally the lungs are very compliant, requiring a pressure of a few centimeters of water to move air in and out of the lungs. But as can be observed from Figure 2-29, the compliance (the slope of the pressure-volume curve) decreases at high lung volumes. This indicates that it is easier to expand the lungs when their volume is low than when their volume is high. Later we will discuss the differences in compliance at different regions of the lungs and the changes in compliance that occur under different physiological and pathological conditions.

The magnitude of the lungs' compliance is due to the forces resisting expansion: The greater these forces, the lower the compliance. There are two main factors controlling the compliance of the lungs. One is related to the lung tissue itself, and the other is related to the surface tension of the alveoli wall. Most of the tissue resistance to expansion is related to the elastin and collagen fibers within the lungs, although the blood vessels and bronchioles make a significant contribution. In order to expand the lungs, force must be applied to stretch these fibrous elements. As with most biologic tissues, the more they are stretched the more they resist expansion. This accounts for a portion of the nonlinearity of the pressure-volume curve.

The other force against which the respiratory muscles must work is the surface tension produced by the thin film of liquid surrounding the inner surface of the alveoli walls. Surface tension arises whenever there is an air-liquid interface and is due to the molecular forces within the liquid pulling down on the molecules at the surface. These forces act against the intrapleural pressure, making it more difficult to expand the lungs. The magnitude of these forces can be appreciated by noting the tremendous increase in compliance that occurs when a saline solution rather than air is used to inflate the lungs (Fig. 2-29).

The surface tension of the lungs is increased significantly by a coating of material, called surfactant, that is secreted by epithelial cells within the alveoli. Surfactant is composed in large part of a phospholipid (dipalmitoyl phosphatidylcholine) that is synthesized in type II alveolar epithelial cells. Synthesis of surfactant begins in the 32nd week of gestation. The inability of prematurely born infants to produce adequate amounts of surfactant causes respiratory distress syndrome in which the respiratory muscles are unable to develop the forces necessary to overcome the high surface tension of the lungs.

By reducing surface tension, surfactant greatly reduces the respiratory effort required to expand the lungs. In addition, it also acts to keep the lungs from collapsing during expiration. An appreciation of Laplace's law is required to understand the role of surfactant in maintaining the stability of alveoli at low lung volumes. According to Laplace's equation ($P = T/r$), the pressure (P) within an alveolus with a small radius (r) will be greater than the pressure within a large alveolus. Since all the alveoli in a given lobule are interconnected, this will cause small alveoli to empty their contents into larger ones. Surfactant helps to prevent this from occurring because it has a greater effect on small alveoli than on large ones. As the alveolus becomes smaller, the surfactant molecules become more tightly packed and thus produce a greater reduction in surface tension. Thus as the radius of an alveolus becomes smaller, its

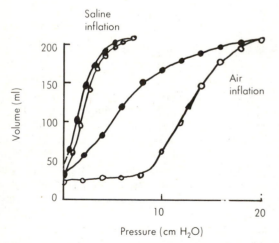

Figure 2-29. It is much more difficult to inflate an air-filled lung than a saline-filled lung because of the surface tension that develops at the interface between the air and liquid lines lung tissue. The saline-filled lung also shows less hysteresis (difference between the pressures developed during inflation and deflation) because it fills and empties more uniformly.

surface tension is proportionally reduced, and the pressure within it remains the same.

The chest wall, like the lungs, is an elastic structure. If unopposed by the recoil force of the lungs, the chest would expand to a point at which its volume would double. Thus when the lungs are at rest—that is, at FRC—the recoil force of the lungs is just balanced by the expanding force of the chest wall. As a result of these opposing forces, the expiratory muscles have to work against the elastic resistance of the chest wall to reach residual volume. On the other hand, expansion of the lungs to about 80% of TLC is made easier by the recoil force of the chest wall. Beyond this volume, the inspiratory muscles have to work against the combined recoil forces of the lungs and the chest wall.

Airway resistance. When the chest expands, the pressure within the alveoli is reduced below atmospheric pressure, drawing gas into the lungs. The rate of gas flow is proportional to the pressure gradient (P) divided by the airway resistance (R):

$$\dot{V} = P/R \quad \text{or} \quad P = \dot{V} \times R$$

Note: In the previous section V referred to velocity of blood and Q to flow of blood. In this section V refers to volume of air, $\dot{V}$ to flow of air, and v to velocity of air.

The resistance is in turn dependent on the geometry of the airways and the rate of gas flow. At low flow rates, the gas flows along the airways in a regular pattern referred to as laminar flow. Under these conditions, the rate of airflow can be calculated using the Poiseuille equation:

$$V = \frac{Pnr^4}{8\,\pi\,l}$$

in which π = viscosity, l = length, and r = radius of the airway. Under these conditions, airway resistance is equal to

$$\frac{8\,\pi\,l}{r^4}$$

As was the case for blood flow in small arterioles, the most important determinant of airway resistance is the radius of the bronchiole because a halving of the radius produces a 16-fold increase in resistance.

As flow rates increase, the regular pattern disappears and turbulence occurs. The disorganized and circular movements of the gas particles that characterize turbulent flow cause some of the energy in the pressure gradient to be dissipated, making it more difficult to move the gas forward. The loss of energy is proportional to the square of the flow rate. Thus the resistance to airflow increases as laminar flow becomes turbulent. The flow rate at which turbulence occurs can be approximated from Reynold's number, which is equal to

$$\frac{2\,rvd}{\pi}$$

where d = density and v = average velocity of the gas particles. If Reynold's number exceeds 2,000, flow is almost always

laminar. However, the highly branched structure of the tracheobronchial tree and the irregular surface of its walls cause turbulence when Reynold's number is much less than 2,000. In fact, there is some degree of turbulence in much of the airways, even at normal rates of breathing. Thus the pressure drop along the airways is a complicated function of flow rate.

$$P = K_1\dot{V} + K_2\dot{V}^2$$

Most of the resistance to airflow occurs in the upper portion of the airways. Almost one-third to one-half of the resistance is caused by the nasopharynx and trachea, and much of the rest is produced in the upper airway. There is almost no resistance to airflow in the respiratory zone of the bronchial tree despite the small diameter of the individual bronchioles. The large reduction in resistance occurs because the cross-sectional area of the bronchial tree increases dramatically within the lower airways as a result of the enormous number of branches in parallel. Because of this small contribution to the overall resistance to airflow, significant disease can develop within the lower airways without producing any clinical signs.

The resistance of the airways can be altered physiologically and pathophysiologically. During inspiration, the intrapleural pressure increases, causing the airways to expand and resistance to fall. When the lung volume is decreased during expiration, intrapleural pressure decreases, causing a decrease in airway diameter and an increase in airway resistance. These alterations in airway diameter with changes in ventilation explain why it is easier to breathe at high lung volumes than at low lung volumes.

Drugs and hormones can also change airway resistance. For example, circulating epinephrine binds to beta receptors on the airway smooth muscle, causing a reduction in tone and a decrease in resistance. Thus during exercise, when catecholamine levels increase, airway resistance is reduced and breathing becomes easier. In contrast, airway resistance is increased by irritants such as cigarette smoke and products of cell metabolism such as histamine, which is released from mast cells located within the lining of the airway walls.

Airway resistance plays an important role in determining the rate at which gas can be moved into and out of the lungs. For example, if an individual expands his or her lungs to TLC and then exhales with maximum force, the greatest flow rate is achieved at the beginning of expiration, when the airways are widest (Fig. 2-30). As the volume in the lung decreases, the intrapleural pressure and diameter of the airways decrease. The decrease in airway diameter causes an increase in airway resistance, which in turn leads to a decrease in expiratory flow rates.

The rate of gas flow achieved at TLC is effort dependent. That is, as can be seen in Figure 2-30, if the expiratory effort is reduced, there is a reduction in the maximum rate of expiration that can be achieved. However, as is also evident in Figure 2-30, the rate of expiration at low lung volumes (below about 40% of TLC) is effort independent. That is, no matter how much effort is produced, the expiratory flow rate remains the same. The effort-independent portion of the expiratory flow curves is due to compression of the airways during expiration.

Airway compression occurs when the pressure in the thorax

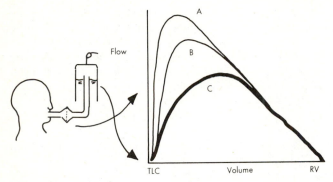

Figure 2-30. The graph shows three different inspiratory volumes (inspiration upward) followed by a forced expiration. The rate of gas flow during expiration is higher when the initial lung volume was higher. This is called the effort-dependent portion of expiration. However, as the volume of gas in the lung decreases, the rate of expiration becomes effort independent because of airway compression. At low lung volumes, as expiratory pressures increase, the intrapleural pressure also increases, increasing airway resistance.

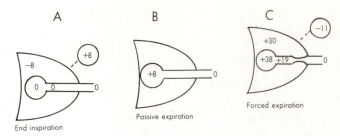

Figure 2-31. Airway compression occurs because the pressure surrounding the airways becomes greater than the pressure within the airways. Alveolar pressure is equal to the intrapleural pressure produced by the muscles of expiration plus the recoil pressure of the alveoli created during inflation. As the gas travels along the airways, its pressure decreases. If it becomes less than the intrapleural pressure, it may collapse. The airways will not collapse if there is sufficient structural (collagenous) support in their walls.

exceeds the pressure in the airways. Figure 2-31 illustrates this phenomenon. At the end of inspiration, when no gas is flowing into or out of the lung, the intra-alveolar pressure is 0 (atmospheric) and the intrapleural pressure is negative (subatmospheric) (Fig. 2-31A). As soon as the muscles of inspiration are relaxed, the elastic recoil of the alveoli causes the intra-alveolar pressure to become equal and opposite to the intrapleural pressure (Fig. 2-31B). That is, the intra-alveolar pressure becomes positive (greater than atmospheric) and begins to expel gas from the lungs. The loss of energy due to the flow of gas reduces the pressure within the airways. But because the intrapleural pressure is always negative and the airway pressure always positive, there is no compression of the airways at any point.

However, if the expiratory muscles are used to increase the rate of expiration, the intrapleural pressure becomes positive. Under these conditions the driving force for expelling the gas is increased (Fig. 2-31C) and the initial rate of expiration increases. The maximum value of expiration, however, is limited by airway compression. Again, the pressure within the airways decreases because of gas flow. But unlike the previous example, in which the airways remained opened, in this case, the intrapleural pressure becomes equal to the airway pressure at some point along its length. This point is called the **equal pressure point**. Since the intrapleural pressure exceeds the airway pressure downstream from the equal pressure point, airway compression can occur.

This model of airway compression also explains why expiratory flow rates become effort independent at low lung volumes. As the alveoli become smaller during expiration, their recoil force becomes smaller. This leads to a decrease in airway pressure and a greater amount of compression. In fact, at low lung volumes, the increase in driving force due to increased expiratory effort is nullified by an increase in airway compression. Another factor contributing to airway compression is the high flow rate itself. Recall that the pressure drop along the airways is proportional to the square of the flow rate.

Thus as flow rates increase, there is an acceleration of energy loss and a rapid drop in pressure along the airways.

Of course, airway compression will only occur if the walls of the airway are unable to withstand the inwardly directed pressures beyond the equal pressure point. Thus the structure of the airways at the equal pressure point is an important determinant of the maximum expiratory flow. For example, in emphysema, the cartilaginous support of the airways is degraded, making it easier for airway compression to occur. Moreover, the elastic recoil forces are reduced in emphysema, so the equal pressure point occurs closer to the alveoli, again increasing the amount of airway compression.

Work of breathing. The respiratory muscles supply the energy required to move air into and out of the lungs. Energy is required to overcome the elastic forces of the alveoli and the tissue and airway resistance to airflow. The work done to overcome the elastic recoil forces is determined by the pressure needed to expand the lungs to a particular volume and is represented by the area under the curve OAECD in Figure 2-32. The additional work required to overcome tissue and airway resistance is represented by the shaded area under the curve in Figure 2-32. Over 80% of this work is used to overcome airway resistance.

During expiration, the elastic energy stored in the alveoli can be used to expel the gas without involving the expiratory muscles. However, if greater rates of expiration are required, then additional energy must be expended to overcome the tissue and airway resistance.

The efficiency of breathing is the ratio of the work done in expanding the lungs to the energy used. The amount of work done in expanding the lungs depends on the combined compliance of the chest wall and lungs. Thus more work is required to expand the lungs whether the decreased compliance is due to an increase in alveolar surface tension or to an anatomic deformity of the chest wall. Diseases causing a decrease in lung compliance are referred to as **restrictive** lung diseases. More work is also required if airway resistance is increased. Diseases causing an increase in airway resistance are called **obstructive** diseases.

The pattern of respiration can be altered to minimize the

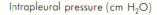

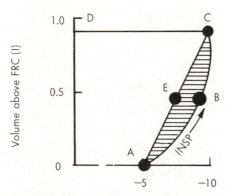

Figure 2-32. The work done by the expiratory muscles to overcome alveolar stiffness is represented by the area in the polygon OAECD; that done to overcome airway resistance is represented by the curved polygon OABCD. The work required to overcome airway resistance increases with increases in the rate of inspiration.

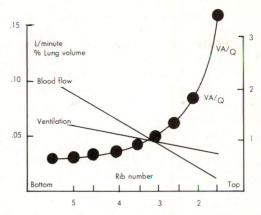

Figure 2-33. The VQ ratio is higher at the top of the lung than at the bottom. Airflow is greater to the bottom of the lung because the alveoli are smaller at the beginning of inspiration and thus can expand more. Blood flow is also greater at the bottom of the lung because the hydrostatic pressure column that must be overcome by the right ventricle is not as great at the bottom of the lung as it is at the top (in an upright person). The VQ ratio is higher at the bottom because ventilation increases 10 times while blood flow increases by only 3 times.

decrease in efficiency that occurs with respiratory disease. For example, in asthma (an obstructive disease), it is beneficial to reduce the rate of respiration and increase the tidal volume so as to limit the amount of energy dissipated in the movement of gas through the narrowed airways. In contrast, it is beneficial to increase the frequency of breathing and reduce the tidal volume in restrictive lung disease so as to reduce the expenditure of energy in overcoming the elastic recoil forces of the chest and lungs.

Regional distribution of ventilation. In the above discussion, no attention has been paid to the fact that the gas entering the lungs during respiration is not evenly distributed. Most of the inspired air is distributed to the dependent portion of the lungs. In a sitting or standing individual, this area is at the base of the lung. When one lies on one's side, the lower lung is the dependent one.

These differences are due to the mechanical effects of gravity on the lung. When in a standing position, the entire weight of the lung pulls down on the apex, expanding the alveoli at the top of the lung more than those at the bottom. Because the apical alveoli are larger, they are also stiffer and thus more difficult to expand further. Thus as the chest increases in volume, the alveoli at the base of the lung expand more than those at the apex and consequently receive a greater portion of the inspired air. Approximately three times more gas enters the base than enters the apex (Fig. 2-33). This is partly because each alveolus expands by a greater amount at the base and partly because there are more alveoli at the base.

Because of the variation in alveolar expansion, there is also a difference in intrapleural pressure. The intrapleural pressures are most negative at the apex of the lung, where the elastic recoil forces of the alveoli are greatest. This relationship is true at both high and low lung volumes. However, it has a physiological consequence at low lung volumes, when the intrapleural pressures are small. Under these conditions, the intrapleural pressure at the base of the lung may be positive and as a result compress the alveoli, preventing gas from entering

them. Under these conditions, the apical portions of the lung may actually receive a greater share of the ventilation than the base.

A similar phenomenon occurs in respiratory diseases such as emphysema, when the elastic recoil forces of the alveoli decrease. In this situation, the intrapleural pressures are reduced throughout the lung and those at the base may become greater than atmospheric even at relatively high volumes. When this occurs, the airways in the base of the lung are compressed (recall the discussion of equal pressure points above). The closure of these airways traps gas at the base of the lung, raising the volume of the FRC, and prevents fresh air from entering the base, interfering with normal gas exchange.

GAS EXCHANGE
Partial pressures. The important atmospheric gases, like all gases, obey the universal gas law:

$$PV = nRT$$

where P = pressure, V = volume, n = moles, R = the universal gas constant, and T = the temperature in degrees kelvin. In respiratory physiology, pressures are most frequently expressed as centimeters of water (1 mm Hg is equal to approximately 13 cm H_2O). More recently, the kilopascal (kP, equal to 10 cm H_2O) has been introduced. The gas law is used to calculate the volume of gas when its concentration, temperature, and partial pressure are known.

At sea level, the total atmospheric pressure is usually 760 mm Hg, or 760 torr (approximately 100 kP). The pressure contributed by each of the gases is proportional to their concentration. Thus if 20% of the gas molecules in the atmosphere are oxygen molecules, the partial pressure of oxygen will be

$$0.20 \times (760) = 152 \text{ mm Hg}$$

When the gas is inhaled, it becomes saturated with water before it reaches the lungs. At body temperature (37°C), the vapor pressure of water is 47 mm Hg. Thus the remainder of the gases in the alveoli produce a total pressure of 713 (760 − 47) mm Hg. Unless otherwise specified, the partial pressures of alveolar gases are measured when they are dried. Therefore, when calculating the partial pressure of gases from their relative concentrations, a total pressure of 713 mm Hg must be used. For example, oxygen occupies approximately 21% of dried alveolar gas, so its partial pressure is

$$0.21 \times 713 = 150 \text{ mm Hg}$$

Diffusion.   Oxygen and carbon dioxide move across the alveolar and capillary surfaces by diffusion. The amount of gas exchange can be estimated by Fick's law:

$$\text{Flow} = \frac{DA}{x} (C_1 - C_2)$$

where D = the diffusion coefficient, A = the area for exchange, x = the thickness of the diffusion barrier, and C_1 and C_2 = the concentrations on either side of the diffusing surface.

The surface area of the lung is approximately 75 m² and less than 1/2 μm in thickness, making it ideal for gas transfer by diffusion. The diffusion coefficient is determined by the properties of the gas and the alveolar membrane. Since oxygen and carbon dioxide are lipid soluble, their diffusion coefficients are proportional to their solubility in lipids. Carbon dioxide is some 20 times more soluble than oxygen, so its diffusion coefficient is 20 times greater. However, as will be discussed shortly, the concentration gradient for oxygen diffusion is approximately 10 times larger than that for carbon dioxide, and thus their rates of diffusion across the alveolar membrane are fairly similar.

The actual amount of oxygen and carbon dioxide transferred across the alveoli depends not only on the rate of diffusion but also on the rate of blood supply. For example, at resting levels of cardiac output, a red blood cell (RBC) will remain within the pulmonary capillary for about 0.75 second. This is normally enough time for the alveolar and capillary partial pressures to achieve equilibrium. A similar situation exists for carbon dioxide. Thus the volume of oxygen and carbon dioxide transferred across the alveolar epithelium is perfusion limited. The greater the blood supply, the greater the volume of gas transferred.

The situation for carbon monoxide (CO) is quite different. When molecules of carbon monoxide diffuse into the pulmonary capillaries, they combine avidly with RBCs. As a result, the partial pressure of CO in the pulmonary capillary remains near zero. Thus the only limitation of CO transfer is the amount of CO in the alveoli and the diffusion characteristics of the alveoli-capillary interface. Because diffusional equilibrium is not achieved between the alveolus and pulmonary capillary, increasing the blood flow through the capillary will not increase the transfer of CO. The transfer of CO is therefore diffusion limited.

Although oxygen also combines with hemoglobin, its affinity is much less and, as indicated above, diffusional equilibrium between the alveolus and capillary is achieved during the time a RBC is in the capillary. In fact, equilibrium is achieved by the time the RBC has traveled only one-third of the way along the path of the pulmonary capillary. Even during exercise, when the transit time of RBCs through the capillaries is much less, diffusional equilibrium normally occurs. Thus under almost all physiological conditions, the oxygen tension in the end pulmonary capillary blood is the same as that in the alveolus.

If the diffusional barrier is increased by disease, then the rate of diffusion may not be fast enough for equilibration to occur. Another situation in which diffusional equilibrium may be compromised occurs when an individual breathes a gas with a low PO_2, such as when traveling to high altitudes. Under these conditions, the RBCs are only partially saturated and can easily bind all the oxygen diffusing into the capillaries. Because of this avid absorption of oxygen, the RBCs prevent the PO_2 in the capillary from reaching that of the alveolus. Under these conditions, oxygen transfer becomes diffusion limited.

Clinically, it is important to know how much gas can diffuse from the alveolus to the capillary. This measurement, called the **diffusing capacity of the lung,** is an index of how much gas can diffuse for a given pressure difference. To perform this test, a diffusion-limited gas must be used. CO is generally chosen, although the test can be carried out using gas containing a reduced oxygen tension.

Diffusing capacity is measured by introducing a small amount of CO (less than 0.1%) into the breathing mixture and then measuring the rate of CO removal from the alveolar gas. The diffusing capacity is calculated using the following equation:

$$D_L = \frac{\dot{V}CO}{PACO}$$

This equation is derived from the Fick equation by substituting D_L for DA/x, assuming that the partial pressure of CO in the capillaries is zero, and then solving for D_L. This assumption is invalid for smokers, who may have appreciable amounts of CO in their blood. The diffusing capacity for a normal individual is typically 25 ml/minute/mm Hg.

The diffusing capacity depends on both the area and thickness of the alveolar surface available for gas exchange. A decrease in area can occur either because some parts of the lung are not properly perfused with inspired air or with an adequate supply of blood.

Pulmonary circulation.   The pulmonary circulation is in series with the systemic circulation, and thus almost all of the cardiac output passes through the lungs before it is delivered to the periphery. There are a number of notable differences between the two circulations. First, because its resistance to blood flow is so much lower than that of the systemic circulation, the pulmonary circulation can operate at much lower pressures. Second, there is much less smooth muscle surrounding the arterioles in the pulmonary circulation and a much sparser neural innervation. Thus the nervous system has very little effect on pulmonary resistance. Third, the capillaries supplying the alveoli are interconnected in such a way as to appear as a sheet of blood rather than as the tubular network characteristic of the systemic circulation.

The normal average pulmonary artery blood pressure is 15 mm Hg (systolic pressure is 25 mm Hg; diastolic pressure is 10 mm Hg). The normal left atrial pressure is between 5 and 10 mm Hg. Thus the driving force for the pulmonary circulation is less than 10 mm Hg. More importantly, gravitational forces cause the hydrostatic pressure at the top of the lungs to be less than it is at the bottom (in an erect individual). As a result, the distribution of blood flow within the lungs is influenced by the changes in intrapleural pressure that occur during breathing. These effects have caused the lung to be divided into four zones, called the zones of West.

Zone 1 is at the apex of the lung. The alveolar pressure in this region is greater than the arterial blood pressure, causing all of the blood vessels to collapse. Thus there is no blood flow in zone 1. Under normal circumstances, there are few if any alveoli in zone 1.

In zone 2, the alveolar pressure is less than the arterial pressure but greater than the venous pressure. Thus the blood flow in this region depends on the difference between the arterial pressure and the alveolar pressure, changing markedly with variations in alveolar pressure.

In zone 3, both the arterial and venous pressures are greater than the alveolar pressure and thus are not influenced by changes in alveolar pressure.

Zone 4 is at the very base of the lung. In this region, the intrapleural pressure is high enough to collapse the vessels supplying the pulmonary capillaries, causing a diminution or even cessation of blood flow. Zone 4 becomes larger at low lung volumes, when the intrapleural pressures are less negative.

Although the pressures determining blood flow are different in the four zones, the overall effect is an almost linear increase in blood flow from the top to the bottom of the lung. These differences become smaller when an individual lies down, because the effects of gravity are diminished.

Changes in lung volume alter the resistance of the pulmonary vasculature. However, lung volume affects the small vessels and capillaries close to the alveoli (called the alveolar vessels) differently from the way it affects the larger vessels within the lung parenchyma (called the extra-alveolar vessels). When the lung expands, it pulls on the alveolar vessels, causing them to lengthen and constrict somewhat. This tends to increase overall pulmonary vascular resistance. At the same time, the larger extra-alveolar vessels are pulled open by the expanding lung, decreasing their resistance. When the two effects are combined, vascular resistance is lowest at FRC and increases both when the lungs expand and when they contract.

Pulmonary vascular resistance will decrease when pulmonary blood flow increases. The decrease in resistance is primarily due to recruitment of previously closed vessels. However, because the pulmonary vessels are so compliant, they also increase in diameter when more blood is delivered to them.

Finally, the pulmonary resistance can be affected by the oxygen tension of the alveolar air. Reducing the alveolar oxygen tension (but not the pulmonary arterial oxygen tension) causes a contraction of the smooth muscles surrounding the blood vessels and an increase in vascular resistance. Although the mechanism underlying the vasoconstriction is not known, it is not due to a direct effect of oxygen. Instead, some vasoactive substance, perhaps histamine, released from epithelial cells surrounding the pulmonary vessel is responsible for the smooth muscle contraction. The response is potentiated by an increase in carbon dioxide tension and acidosis. Physiologically, it is beneficial in that it shunts blood away from poorly ventilated alveoli. However, in generalized hypoxia there can be a profound increase in pulmonary vascular resistance, leading to pulmonary hypertension and heart failure.

Fluid exchange between the capillary and interstitial spaces occurs in the lungs just as it does in the systemic circulation. However, if too much fluid enters the interstitium, the diffusion path between the alveoli and capillaries will be increased and gas exchange can become compromised. The amount and direction of fluid flow are determined by the hydrostatic and oncotic pressures (Starling forces) in the lung. Recall that

$$\text{Flow} = K[(P_C - P_I) - (\pi_c - \pi_I)]$$

The magnitude of some of the Starling forces in the lungs differs from those in the systemic circulation. For example, the average capillary hydrostatic pressure is approximately 10 mm Hg but can be twice this value at the base of the lung and can be reduced to zero at the apex. The interstitial oncotic pressure is probably between 15 and 18 mm Hg, and the interstitial hydrostatic pressure is 2 to 5 mm Hg below atmospheric. As a result of these forces,

$$\text{Flow} = K[(10 - (-4)) - (25 - 16)] = K[5]$$

there is a net flow of fluid out of the capillaries equal to approximately 20 ml/hour.

The fluid filters through the interstitial spaces to the region of the terminal bronchioles, where it is taken up by the pulmonary lymphatic system and returned to the general circulation. Pulmonary edema occurs when the rate of outward filtration exceeds the ability of the lymphatics to absorb fluid. This may occur if there is an increase in capillary permeability (K) or in capillary hydrostatic pressure. Permeability can be increased by bacterial endotoxins or by a generalized inflammation. Capillary pressure can be increased when pulmonary artery pressure is increased or when there is an increase in left atrial pressure (such as in mitral stenosis).

Excess fluid that remains in the interstitium is called interstitial edema or pleural effusion. Unless this is severe, it has little effect on gas exchange. However, if the fluid enters the alveoli, gas exchange is greatly diminished. Usually a great deal of fluid can enter the interstitium before any passes into the alveoli because of the rather high compliance of the interstitial spaces. In addition, the epithelial linings of the alveoli are connected by tight junctions and thus act as a barrier to the passage of water. However, if fluid is aspirated, it flows readily through the alveoli because of the high interstitial oncotic and low hydrostatic pressures present in the lung interstitium.

Ventilation-perfusion relationship. As indicated above, the delivery of oxygen to the capillaries is perfusion limited. That is, the amount of oxygen crossing the alveolus will depend on the amount of blood perfusing the alveolus. If the amount of blood is very low, little oxygen will be transferred from the alveoli, regardless of how much is available. On the other hand, if the blood flow is too great, the pulmonary capillaries will not receive as much oxygen as they are capable of absorbing. Thus the blood flow to each region of the lung must be matched to the ventilation of that region if oxygen transfer is to be most efficient. The mismatching of ventilation and perfusion is the most common reason for hypoxemia (a lower than normal level of arterial oxygen tension). However, it is not the only mechanism for hypoxemia. Low arterial oxygen tension (PaO_2) can also result from hypoventilation, diffusional abnormalities, and shunting of blood directly from the venous to the arterial vessels without passing through the lungs. These mechanisms are discussed briefly before ventilation-perfusion (V-Q) abnormalities will be described.

Hypoventilation is said to occur when the arterial carbon dioxide tension ($PaCO_2$) rises because the amount of ventilation is inadequate to remove all of the carbon dioxide produced by metabolism. Since there is a relatively fixed ratio (depending on diet) between carbon dioxide production and the oxygen consumed, the alveolar oxygen tension ($PACO_2$) can be calculated using the modified alveolar gas equation:

$$PAO_2 = P_IO_2 - \frac{PACO_2}{R}$$

The inspired gas oxygen tension (P_IO_2) is 150 mm Hg (recall that oxygen makes up 21% of the dry gas entering the trachea and thus oxygen tension is 0.21×713). R is the respiratory exchange quotient, which is normally 0.8. At normal body pH, the carbon dioxide tension is 40 mm Hg. Thus the alveolar oxygen tension is

$$PAO_2 = 150 - \frac{40}{0.8} = 100 \text{ mm Hg}$$

If alveolar ventilation falls, the $PACO_2$ will rise. Recall that all of the carbon dioxide produced by metabolism enters the lungs.

$$\dot{V}_A = \frac{CO_2 \text{ production}}{\% \ CO_2 \text{ in alveolus}}$$

Since $PACO_2$ is proportional to the fractional concentration of carbon dioxide,

$$\dot{V}_A \text{ is proportional to } \frac{CO_2 \text{ production}}{PACO_2}$$

And, from the alveolar gas equation, if $PACO_2$ rises, PAO_2 will fall. For example, if alveolar ventilation is reduced by half, then from the above equation, $PACO_2$ will double. This will cause PAO_2 to fall to

$$PAO_2 = 150 - \frac{80}{0.8} = 50 \text{ mm Hg}$$

If ventilation increases above that necessary to remove all of the carbon dioxide produced by metabolism, then carbon dioxide tension will fall and alveolar oxygen tension will rise. This is referred to as hyperventilation.

Note that alveolar oxygen tension can fall without a change in ventilation if the inspired oxygen tension falls. For example, the barometric pressure in Denver, Colorado (altitude of 5,000 ft), is approximately 625 mm Hg, which means that the inspired air PO_2 is $(0.21 \times [760-47])$ 121 mm Hg. Thus if there is no change in ventilation,

$$PAO_2 = 121 - \frac{40}{0.8} = 71 \text{ mm Hg}$$

Because $PACO_2$ levels are normal, the fall in PaO_2 did not result from hypoventilation. In fact, individuals exposed to significantly lower than normal oxygen tensions will usually increase their ventilation above that necessary to remove the carbon dioxide produced by metabolism. That is, they will hyperventilate, lowering their $PACO_2$ and increasing their PAO_2 toward its normal value of 100 mm Hg.

An increase in the thickness of the diffusing surface between the alveolus and capillary can also cause hypoxemia by preventing equilibration of alveolar and arterial gases. Under these conditions, PAO_2 will fall even if ventilation is adequate to remove all of the carbon dioxide produced by metabolism. The difference between the alveolar and arterial oxygen tensions is called the A-a (alveolar-arterial) gradient. As will be discussed shortly, the A-a gradient for oxygen is usually 4 to 6 mm Hg. Normally, none of this is due to diffusion limitations.

If diffusion abnormalities do occur, the A-a gradient for oxygen will be increased. However, because of the greater solubility of carbon dioxide, an A-a gradient for it is hardly ever produced, even in the presence of moderate thickening of the diffusing surface. For this reason, $PACO_2$ is a very good indicator of $PaCO_2$ and is much easier to measure.

A third abnormality resulting in hypoxemia is the shunting of blood away from the lung. Normally, a small amount of blood never flows into the lungs. For example, a portion of the bronchial circulation drains directly into the pulmonary veins without being oxygenated and the blood perfusing the heart drains directly from the thebesian veins into the left ventricle without being reoxygenated. This is called an anatomic shunt because the poor oxygenation results from a failure of the blood to enter the pulmonary circulation. Almost all of the normal A-a gradient for oxygen is due to anatomic shunts. Physiological shunts occur when the amount of blood passing through the lungs is not fully oxygenated as a result of inadequate ventilation. These and other V-Q abnormalities will be discussed next.

As indicated above, the amount of oxygen passing into the blood as it passes through a region of the lung depends on both the amount of ventilation and the amount of perfusion. This is illustrated in Figure 2-34, in which a diagram of an alveolus represents a small portion of the lung. Two extreme cases are represented. In Figure 2-34B, no blood passes by the alveolus. Thus no gas exchange occurs and the gas tensions remain equal to those in the inspired air. Because no gas exchange occurs in this portion of the lung, it is referred to as alveolar dead space. Its volume can be measured by subtracting the anatomic dead space determined using Fowler's technique from the total (or

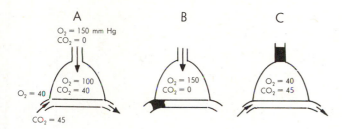

Figure 2-34. (*A*) Under normal circumstances, the average VQ ratio is 0.8. This is sufficient to increase mixed venous blood oxygen to 100 mm Hg and reduce carbon dioxide to 40 mm Hg. (*B*) If the blood flow to a region of the lung is blocked, then the alveolar gas tensions remain equal to the inspired gas. (*C*) If a region of the lung is not ventilated, then the alveolar gas tensions become equal to those of the mixed venous blood. Blood flow through regions with lower than normal VQ ratios is considered part of the physiological shunt. Regions with higher than normal VQ ratios are part of the physiological dead space and are referred to as wasted ventilation.

physiological) dead space calculated using the Bohr equation (see above).

In Figure 2-34*C*, no gas enters the alveolus. Again no gas exchange takes place and the blood in the pulmomary capillary passes through the lung without altering its oxygen or carbon dioxide tensions. This blood becomes part of the total shunt, which, as indicated above, contributes to the A-a gradient. The percentage of blood passing through the nonventilated portions of the lung can be calculated from the shunt equation:

$$\frac{Q_S}{Q_T} = \frac{C_{CAP}O_2 - C_aO_2}{C_{CAP}O_2 - C_{\bar{v}}O_2}$$

in which the Q_S is the blood flowing through the nonventilated portions of the lung, Q_T is the cardiac output, and $C_{CAP}O_2$, CaO_2, and $C_{\bar{v}}O_2$ are the oxygen contents of the end capillary blood, arterial blood, and the mixed venous blood, respectively.

The arterial and venous blood gases can be measured directly by obtaining the appropriate blood samples. The end pulmonary capillary content can be estimated from the calculated PAO_2 and the hemoglobin saturation curve (see below), assuming that no significant diffusion abnormality exists. The shunt equation assumes that the gas content of the shunted blood is the same as that of the mixed venous blood. Although this is true for blood passing through nonventilated regions of the lung or through direct right-to-left shunts, it is not true for the thebesian vein or bronchial artery shunts nor for low (but not zero) V-Q ratios (see below). Thus the shunt is a measure of the amount of blood that would have to pass directly from the venous circulation to the arterial circulation to cause the observed A-a gradient.

Most cases of V-Q abnormalities are not as dramatic as depicted in Figures 2-34*B* and *C*. More commonly there is both ventilation and perfusion but the two are not matched properly; for example, if there is too much ventilation for the amount of blood supply (i.e., the V/Q ratio is higher than normal). This large excess of gas in the alveoli prevents the $PACO_2$ from rising very much, even though a greater than normal amount of carbon dioxide is removed from the capillary blood. In the

same manner, the PAO_2 does not fall very much even though the capillary is fully saturated with oxygen. Conversely, if the V/Q ratio is lower than normal, the PAO_2 will be low and the $PACO_2$ will be high.

The V-Q ratio normally varies from the apex to the base of the lung. As indicated previously, both ventilation and blood flow are higher at the base of the lung than they are at the apex. However, whereas ventilation increases threefold from top to bottom, blood flow increases tenfold. The resulting V-Q ratios and their effect on alveolar gas tensions are illustrated in Figure 2-33. Note that the PO_2 at the apex is 132 mm Hg while that at the base is 89 mm Hg. Similarly, the PCO_2 is less than 28 mm Hg at the apex and 42 mm Hg at the base.

The regional variation in the V-Q ratio increases the A-a gradient for oxygen for two reasons. First, there is much less blood at the apex than at the base so there is more capillary blood with a lower PO_2 than there is with a higher PO_2. In contrast, the difference in ventilation at the top and bottom of the lung is not as great. Second, and more importantly, as will be discussed shortly, very little oxygen can be added to the blood by increasing tensions above 100 mm Hg because of the shape of the hemoglobin saturation curve. However, reducing oxygen tension below 100 mm Hg substantially reduces the amount of oxygen that can be added to the blood. Thus not only is there more blood with a lower oxygen tension, the amount of oxygen in the blood with a lower tension is reduced much more than the content of the blood with a higher tension is increased. When the end capillary blood from all regions of the blood combines in the pulmonary vein, the average oxygen tension in the blood is reduced below that in the alveolar air.

The effect on carbon dioxide is not as profound, because the amount of carbon dioxide removed from the blood is relatively proportional to the PCO_2. Thus the increase in carbon dioxide content occurring in blood perfusing the base of the lung is balanced by the decrease in carbon dioxide content present in blood draining from the apex of the lung.

Normally V-Q abnormalities do not cause a change in $PACO_2$ because the respiratory control system (see below) keeps the $PaCO_2$ at 40 mm Hg. Thus if $PaCO_2$ rises because of a V-Q abnormality, ventilation will increase to bring the $PaCO_2$ tension back to normal. Although the increase in ventilation will increase the arterial oxygen tension, it will not erase the deficit entirely because of the reasons discussed above.

Gas transport. Oxygen is transported from the lungs to the tissues in the blood. Although some of the transported oxygen is dissolved in the blood, well over 95% of it is combined with hemoglobin.

The amount of oxygen dissolved in the blood is a linear function of the PO_2. According to Henry's law, the amount of dissolved gas is equal to the solubility constant times the gas tension. For oxygen, the solubility constant is 0.003 ml/mm Hg/100 ml of blood. Thus the amount of dissolved oxygen in arterial blood is (0.003 × 100)/100 ml blood, or 0.3 ml/100 ml.

The bulk of oxygen is combined with hemoglobin, a complex iron-containing compound capable of binding four molecules of oxygen. Two normal types of hemoglobin exist, adult and fetal hemoglobin. Most of the fetal hemoglobin disappears during the first year of postnatal life.

The amount of oxygen binding to hemoglobin depends on the PO_2, as illustrated by the oxygen dissociation curve in

Figure 2-34. The curve is S shaped, indicating that little oxygen combines with hemoglobin at low (less than 30 mm Hg) pressures; that the amount of oxygen combining with hemoglobin rises steeply from 30 to 80 mm Hg; and that hemoglobin becomes saturated, adding little additional oxygen at tensions higher than 80 mm Hg.

When fully saturated, each gram of hemoglobin can bind to approximately 1.34 ml of oxygen. That is, the oxygen capacity of hemoglobin is 1.34 ml/g. The ratio of the actual amount of bound oxygen to the oxygen capacity is called the saturation. At a normal PaO_2 of 100 mm Hg, hemoglobin is 97.5% saturated. Typically, 100 ml of blood contains 15 g of hemoglobin. Thus the amount of oxygen bound to hemoglobin is

$$0.975 \ (1.34 \times 15) \ = \ 19.6 \ \text{ml/100 ml blood.}$$

The total oxygen content of arterial blood is then 0.3 (the amount dissolved) plus 19.6 (the amount bound), or approximately 19.9 ml of oxygen per 100 ml of blood.

It is important to distinguish the difference between the oxygen tension and the oxygen content. Oxygen tension refers to the partial pressure of the gas in solution and is an index of the amount of gas dissolved. The concentration gradient in Fick's law of diffusion refers to the gas tensions. Content, on the other hand, is a measure of how much gas is present in the blood. Although the oxygen content obviously depends on the arterial oxygen tension, the amount of oxygen delivered to the tissues is normally a function of the hemoglobin concentration. For example, if hemoglobin concentrations were to fall to half their normal values, the oxygen content would decrease to $1/2(19.6) + 0.3$, or 10.1 ml/100 ml blood, without changing the PO_2. Because the hemoglobin is almost fully saturated, doubling the PO_2 would raise the content very little. Dissolved oxygen would increase to 0.6 ml/100 ml blood while bound hemoglobin would hardly change at all.

There are several advantages to the shape of the hemoglobin saturation curve, however. Since hemoglobin can be almost fully saturated at a PaO_2 of 80 mm Hg, there can be a substantial fall in PO_2 without having very much of an effect on oxygen content. At the capillary end of the circulation, where the PO_2 is low, the steep portion of the dissociation curve promotes the release of oxygen from the hemoglobin.

Oxygen unloading from hemoglobin is also promoted by the decrease in pH and the increase in carbon dioxide and temperature found in metabolically active tissues. As illustrated in Figure 2-35, the oxygen dissociation curve shifts to the right when pH falls or temperature rises and to the left when pH rises or temperature falls. Another factor affecting oxygen unloading is 2,3-diphosphoglycerate (2,3-DPG), a by-product of RBC metabolism. The concentration of 2,3-DPG increases during periods of hypoxemia, making it easier for the RBCs to unload oxygen. The PO_2 at which hemoglobin is 50% saturated is referred to as the affinity of hemoglobin for oxygen, or the P_{50}. Increases in temperature, hydrogen ions, and 2,3-DPG all increase the P_{50}, making it more difficult for hemoglobin to hold onto oxygen at the low tensions found in the tissues but having little effect on the amount of oxygen bound to hemoglobin in the lungs, where the tensions are high.

CO affects the oxygen-binding ability of hemoglobin in two

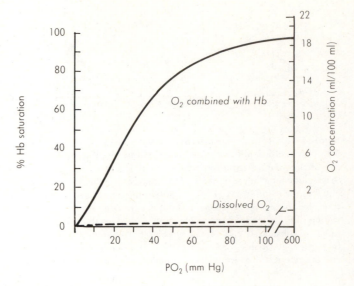

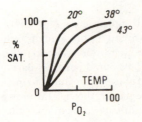

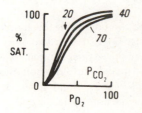

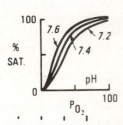

Figure 2-35. The arterial oxygen content is determined by the arterial oxygen tension and the hemoglobin concentration. Normally there are 15 g of hemoglobin per 100 ml of blood. When fully saturated, each gram contains 1.34 ml of oxygen. Thus at an arterial oxygen tension of 100 mm Hg, there are 20 ml of oxygen combined with hemoglobin in each 100 ml of blood. Relatively little oxygen is dissolved in the blood (0.3 ml/100 ml blood) at an oxygen tension of 100 mm Hg. The oxyhemoglobin saturation curve shifts to the right as temperature, PCO_2, and H^+ ion concentration increase. It shifts to the left if these variables decrease.

ways. First, its affinity for hemoglobin is some 250 times greater than that of oxygen. Whereas the P_{50} for oxygen is approximately 27 mm Hg, that of CO is less than 0.1 mm Hg. Thus even small amounts of CO can tie up a large portion of hemoglobin and reduce the oxygen-carrying capacity of the blood to dangerously low levels. Second, CO causes the affinity of hemoglobin for oxygen to increase, thus making it more difficult for oxygen to dissociate from hemoglobin when it reaches the tissues.

Carbon dioxide transit is more complicated than that of oxygen. Like oxygen, some of the carbon dioxide carried by the oxygen is in solution. But because carbon dioxide is 20 times more soluble than oxygen, the amount dissolved is a significant portion of the total. At a $PaCO_2$ of 47 mm Hg (typical of mixed venous blood), the amount of dissolved carbon dioxide is 2.8 ml/100 ml of blood. About 5% of the carbon dioxide formed by metabolism is dissolved directly in the blood.

An additional 30% of the carbon dioxide produced combines chemically with blood proteins to form carbamino compounds. Most of the carbamino groups are formed on hemoglobin. The reaction is spontaneous and occurs rapidly without enzymes. Carbamino-hemoglobin formation is favored when oxygen is not bound to the hemoglobin. Thus carbon dioxide binding increases in the tissues as oxygen is unloaded and is more easily removed from hemoglobin in the lungs as oxygen loading occurs. The reduction in carbon dioxide affinity with increased PaO_2 is called the Haldane effect. The opposite reaction also occurs. That is, the affinity of hemoglobin for oxygen decreases as $PaCO_2$ increases. This is known as the Bohr effect.

Most of the carbon dioxide carried in the blood is converted to bicarbonate by the reaction

$$CO_2 + H_2O \rightarrow H_2CO_3 \rightarrow H^+ + HCO_3^-$$

The formation of carbonic acid from carbon dioxide and water requires the presence of the enzyme carbonic anhydrase (CA). Carbon dioxide formed by tissue metabolism enters the RBCs by diffusion, where CA facilitates its conversion to bicarbonate. The hydrogen ion formed in the reaction is buffered by hemoglobin, preventing a fall in pH and allowing more bicarbonate to be formed. Bicarbonate is then transported out of the cell in exchange for chloride, maintaining electroneutrality and allowing more bicarbonate to form.

When the blood reaches the lungs, carbon dioxide diffuses from the plasma into the alveoli. This is followed by the diffusion of carbon dioxide out of the RBC, causing the above reaction to be reversed. That is, bicarbonate and hydrogen combine to form carbonic acid, which then breaks down into carbon dioxide and water. This reaction can occur rapidly because (1) hydrogen is released from hemoglobin when oxygen binds to it (the Haldane effect) and (2) RBCs contain the CA needed to catalyze the breakdown of carbonic acid.

Control of respiration

The basic respiratory rhythm is maintained by respiratory control centers in the brain stem. The medullary respiratory area is divided into a dorsal and ventral group. The dorsal group of cells controls the inspiratory drive. Although it appears that spontaneous activity in these cells can produce periodic respiratory activity, normal respiration requires some sort of excitatory input. Excitation to the dorsal group can derive from peripheral mechanical or chemical receptors or from respiratory centers higher in the brain stem. The ventral medullary center is linked to expiration rather than inspiration and only becomes involved when the respiratory effort is great enough to require an active expiration.

The apneustic center, located just below the pons, provides a tonic excitatory drive to the inspiratory center. Experimentally removing descending influences above the apneustic center produces a prolonged inspiration. The pneumotaxic center, found in the upper pons, appears to coordinate the respiratory rhythm by periodically terminating the inspiratory drive from the dorsal respiratory centers.

The cortex is not involved in the generation of the basic respiratory pattern but can be used voluntarily to increase or decrease ventilation. The range of these changes is limited, however, by the effects they produce on blood gases. Sustained hyperventilation will cause dizziness (by decreasing cerebral blood flow) and tetany (by decreasing arterial calcium concentrations). Hypoventilation causes an increase in $PaCO_2$ which will eventually lead to an automatic increase in ventilation.

The amount of alveolar ventilation is primarily controlled by the central chemoreceptors. These cells, on the ventral surface of the medulla, respond vigorously to any increase in $PaCO_2$ above 40 mm Hg or to a fall in pH below 7.4. Apparently, the central chemoreceptors respond directly to a fall in the pH of the CSF surrounding them. Thus when arterial PCO_2 rises, CO_2 diffuses into the CSF, causing a fall in pH and a rise in ventilation. Under normal circumstances, the central chemoreceptors keep arterial carbon dioxide at 40 ± 2 mm Hg.

The peripheral chemoreceptors are located at the bifurcation of the common carotid arteries and in the arch of the aorta. The carotid bodies are the more important of the two. Receptors within the carotid bodies cause an increase in ventilation when the oxygen level falls below 100 mm Hg. However, a significant response will not be produced unless there is also a rise in carbon dioxide. The peripheral chemoreceptors respond to an increase in PCO_2 more rapidly than the central chemoreceptors but do not produce as great a response. However, they alone are able to signal a change in arterial PO_2. The peripheral receptors are not sensitive to a change in arterial oxygen content unless it is profound. That is why there is no sensation of inadequate oxygen delivery during CO poisoning. Even though the oxygen content can be reduced to less than half by CO, $PaCO_2$ remains normal. Removal of the peripheral chemoreceptors does not interfere with normal respiratory control if an individual is not exposed to an environment containing a low concentration of oxygen.

A number of other peripheral receptors affect respiration. Mechoreceptors, located in the airways and the respiratory muscles, give off afferent fibers that cause a decrease in inspiration. This reflex, called the Herring-Breuer reflex, prevents very large inspirations from occurring. It is most evident in anesthetized individuals and newborns, playing a much more minor role in controlling the respiratory pattern in adults. However, pulmonary mechanoreceptors may be involved in adjusting the pattern of respiration in patients with restrictive type diseases. The increased intrapleural pressures developed during inspiration in these patients may inhibit further inspiration, helping to produce the shallow, rapid breathing patterns typical of their disease.

Irritant receptors, located in the airways and lungs, produce a rapid but shallow breathing pattern and restrict the airways in which the irritants are found. This latter response may prevent the irritating substance from penetrating deeper into the lung.

J (juxtacapillary) receptors are stimulated by the presence of pulmonary edema, causing laryngeal closing and a rapid breathing pattern. Their physiological function is not well understood but may be responsible for the sensation of shortness of breath that accompanies pulmonary edema.

GASTROINTESTINAL PHYSIOLOGY

The GI tract is responsible for providing the body with the nutrients and electrolytes it needs to sustain life. To accomplish this task food must be ingested and moved through the alimentary canal, mechanically broken down into small particles and decomposed by digestive enzymes, and finally absorbed into the bloodstream. Each of these processes will be reviewed in this section.

INGESTION

An individual ingests food to satisfy the demands of hunger and appetite. Although the composition and quantity of a meal vary among individuals, almost everyone provided with the opportunity to obtain enough food will select a diet containing adequate energy stores. Unfortunately, there is no instinctual drive to select nutritious foods, so the diets of many Americans include large quantities of food of questionable nutritional value.

Once food is placed in the mouth, it must be broken down into small particles, moistened, and swallowed. The food is broken down by the process of **chewing** (mastication). Although chewing can be accomplished voluntarily, the process is facilitated by a chewing reflex coordinated by motor centers in the reticular formation. Chewing is not essential for swallowing or later digestion. However, the process of chewing increases taste and olfactory reflexes that initiate mechanical activity of the GI tract and secretion of digestive juices. These reflexes are helpful in the digestive process. The act of swallowing begins when a portion of food is propelled from the mouth into the oropharynx by the tongue. The tip of the tongue is placed against the hard palate, preventing additional food from entering the oropharynx, and the nasopharynx is closed by the upward movement of the soft palate so food is not expelled into the nasal cavities. At this point, respiration is suspended, the glottis is closed (preventing food from entering the trachea), and the food is propelled into the esophagus by the peristaltic contraction of the pharynx and relaxation of the upper esophageal sphincter (UES).

Swallowing occurs very rapidly; less than 1 second is required to transport food from the mouth to the esophagus. Although swallowing can be initiated voluntarily, it is generally caused by the presence of food in oropharynx. Regardless of how it is begun, the act of swallowing is under the reflex control of swallowing centers in the brain stem. These centers coordinate the output of cranial nerves V, IX, X, and XII, which control the movement of the tongue and the sequential contraction and relaxation of the oropharynx and UES necessary to pass the food from the mouth to the esophagus. Destruction of these centers prevents normal swallowing from occurring, and such individuals find it very difficult or impossible to prevent aspiration of food into the trachea.

Once food enters the esophagus, it is propelled into the stomach by **peristalsis**. Esophageal peristalsis is classified as primary or secondary peristalsis depending on how it is initiated. Primary peristalsis is initiated by the act of swallowing and is essentially a continuation of the peristaltic process that began in the pharynx during swallowing. Secondary peristalsis is stimulated by the presence of food in the esophagus. Under normal circumstances, the primary peristaltic wave requires approximately 10 seconds to transport food from the UES to the stomach (liquids can move even faster under the influence of gravity). Any food remaining in the esophagus after primary peristalsis is concluded will initiate a secondary peristaltic wave. These waves will continue until all the food is removed from the esophagus.

The upper third of the esophagus is composed of skeletal muscle. Thus the sequence of activation necessary to produce a peristaltic wave through this portion of the esophagus must be coordinated by the direct action of the glossopharyngeal and vagal alpha motoneurons that innervate these muscles. The lower two-thirds of the esophagus is smooth muscle. Peristalsis in this region can be coordinated by the intrinsic (enteric) nervous system that lines the GI system throughout its length. However, it is usually controlled by vagal nerve fibers that synapse with the neurons of the intrinsic nervous system. Relaxation of the UES (the last phase of swallowing or the first phase of esophageal peristalsis) is caused by the coordinated inhibition of the efferent neurons (from the nucleus ambiguus) that innervate the cricopharyngeal muscle (the UES) and the more distal segments of the esophagus. The neural activity causes a wave of contraction (preceded by a wave of relaxation) to propagate along the esophagus. The final stage of esophageal peristalsis is the relaxation of the lower esophageal sphincter (LES). Although no anatomically distinct muscle has been identified as serving the sphincter function, the last few centimeters of the esophagus are continuously contracted. As the peristaltic wave approaches the end of the esophagus, the LES relaxes, allowing the bolus of food to enter the stomach. Like the more proximal smooth muscle portions of the esophagus, the activity of the LES can be coordinated by the intrinsic nervous system in the absence of the vagus nerve. However, it too is normally controlled by vagal efferents.

The maintained contraction of the UES reduces (or prevents) the entry of air into the esophagus. The LES acts primarily to prevent the highly acidic stomach contents from entering the esophagus. **Achlasia** is a disease of the LES in which the smooth muscle does not relax during peristalsis. As a result, food cannot easily enter the stomach. Symptomatically, patients complain of chest pain and frequent regurgitation of food. If the tone of the LES is too low, reflux of stomach acids causes esophageal injury. Similar problems can result from the failure of secondary peristalsis to remove the small amount of acid that normally enters the stomach.

MOTILITY OF THE GI TRACT

The rhythmic contraction of smooth muscle lining the walls of the GI tract is responsible for reducing the size of food particles and transporting them along the alimentary canal. The motility of the stomach can be thought of as occurring in three phases. First, the orad stomach relaxes to accommodate the food entering it during the ingestion of a meal. Second, the caudad stomach undergoes a series of contractions to break down the food particles and mix them with digestive juices. And third, the entire stomach participates in the process by which food is propelled into the small intestine. Once the food is mixed with the digestive juices of the stomach, it is called **chyme.**

The orad stomach consists of the fundus and the upper portion of the corpus. Most of the time, this region of the stomach is mechanically quiescent, exhibiting a resting tone equal to that of the abdominal cavity. Its primary mechanical function is to relax in preparation for receiving food from the esophagus. This relaxation, called receptive relaxation, allows the stomach to accept more than 1,500 ml of food with only a minimal (less than 15 cm H_2O) increase in intragastric pressure. Receptive relaxation is part of the swallowing reflex and is mediated by afferent and efferent nerve fibers traveling in the vagus nerve. The neurotransmitter responsible for receptive relaxation is not known and is referred to as a noncholinergic, nonadrenergic neurotransmitter. The tone within the orad stomach begins to increase later in the digestive process, aiding in the emptying of food from the stomach. The reflex responsible for mediating this response is not known.

The caudad stomach consists of the distal regions of the corpus and the antrum. This region undergoes periodic increases in tone during both the fasting (interdigestive) and digestive periods. During the interdigestive period, periodic bursts of phasic activity occur. These bursts, called the migrating motor complex, occur every 1 to 2 hours and last for a few minutes. They originate in the esophagus and travel all along the GI tract and are responsible for clearing the alimentary canal of any debris that remains after the digestive period. During the digestive period, the contractions occur three to five times a minute and serve to break down and mix the food with digestive juices.

The caudad stomach contractions begin in the middle corpus region and proceed in a peristaltic fashion toward the pyloric sphincter. The food is propelled in front of the contracting muscles. However, when the food reaches the terminal antrum it encounters the closed pyloric sphincter. As a result, the food is propelled back toward the orad stomach. This retropulsion of food ensures that the stomach contents are broken down into small particles before they are emptied into the small intestine. The periodic contractions of the stomach are initiated by pacemaker cells in the corpus. Pacemaker activity (rhythmic alterations in resting membrane potential) is characteristic of all smooth muscle cells in the caudad stomach. This basic electrical rhythm (BER) determines the rate of stomach contractions. The action potentials responsible for the BER are of extremely long duration (5 to 7 seconds) and resemble cardiac ventricular action potentials in waveform (Fig. 2-36). If the plateau phase reaches mechanical threshold, a contraction occurs; otherwise, it does not. The higher the

plateau, the greater the contractile force. The amount of activity in the vagal nerve fibers innervating the stomach determines the amplitude of the action potential and consequently the magnitude of the contraction. However, the frequency of the BER depends on the pacemaker activity of the smooth muscle cells and is not influenced by the vagus nerve. Nonetheless, destruction of the vagus nerve fibers interferes with the normal motility pattern of the stomach by disrupting the amplitude and peristaltic nature of muscle contractions.

Under normal circumstances, food does not empty from the stomach until it is liquefied. Thus it usually takes 2 to 3 hours to empty the stomach of food ingested during a meal. The rate of emptying is controlled by how rapidly the food is liquefied by the antral contractions, by the tone in the orad stomach and pylorus, and by the amount and type of food entering the duodenum. In general, reflexes initiated by food entering the duodenum determine the rate of gastric emptying. These reflexes involve both hormonal and neural effectors and are called, generically, enterogastric reflexes. They act to inhibit the motility of the orad and caudad stomach and to increase the tone of the pylorus and proximal duodenum. They will be considered later when regulation of gastric secretion is discussed.

Reduced gastric emptying can occur in a variety of conditions such as damage to the vagus nerve or obstruction of the gastroduodenal junction. This can result in impaired appetite, discomfort, and vomiting. Interestingly, damage to the vagus increases the rate of liquid emptying because receptive relaxation does not occur. The resulting high tone in the orad stomach causes liquids, which can easily pass through the pylorus, to empty rapidly from the stomach. Too rapid emptying can lead to diarrhea and body fluid disorders. The cause of this later effect will be discussed in more detail later.

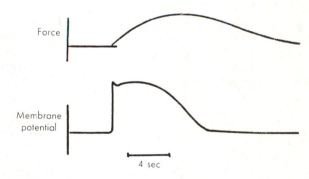

Figure 2-36. The action potential recorded from the caudad region of the stomach is 5 to 7 seconds in duration and has a prolonged plateau phase. The magnitude of the contraction produced by the slow wave is proportional to the amplitude and duration of the plateau.

The motility of the small intestine, like that of the stomach, is designed to mix the food with digestive juices and propel the food along the alimentary canal. In addition, since the intestine is the major site from which nutrients and minerals are absorbed from the GI tract, intestinal motility must also bring the food into contact with the intestinal wall. The motility of the small intestine is controlled almost entirely by the intrinsic nervous system, primarily by the myenteric plexus lying between the longitudinal and circular smooth muscle layers.

The main intestinal contractile pattern during the digestive period is called segmentation. Segmentation involves the contraction of short segments (a few centimeters) of the intestine at a time. Because these contractions are not coordinated with contractions elsewhere along the intestine, the food within the intestinal lumen can move either orad or caudad, depending on the contractile state of those regions. Over time, the food tends to move in a caudad direction because the frequency of segmentation is higher in the orad regions of the intestine than it is in the caudad regions. However, the rate of movement is very slow, allowing sufficient time for digestion and absorption of the food to occur. The migrating motor complex, described above, causes a peristalsis-like wave to occasionally sweep over the small intestine and helps to propel the residues of digestion into the large intestine.

The rate of segmentation is controlled by the BER of the intestine, which varies from approximately 12 per minute in the duodenum to less than 8 per minute in the terminal ileum. The waveform of the BER is sinusoidal with spikes (action potentials) superimposed on the slow rhythmic changes in membrane potential, called slow waves (Fig. 2-37). The amplitude of the contraction depends on the frequency of spikes appearing on the slow waves. Because the motility of the small intestine is primarily under intrinsic control, few disorders of intestinal motility achieve clinical significance. However, paralysis of the small intestine (which sometimes follows abdominal surgery) prevents normal absorption and propulsion of food. Too rapid propulsion through the intestine can also cause malabsorption by preventing the food from being adequately mixed with digestive enzymes or from remaining in contact with the intestinal wall for a sufficient period of time.

The primary function of the large intestine is to absorb water and electrolyes from its lumen and to organize the elimination of digestive wastes. The large intestine is divided into the cecum, the colon, the rectum, and the anal canal. The passage of material from the small intestine into the large intestine is regulated by variations in tone of the ileocecal junction. Analogous to the situation occurring at the pyloric sphincter, passage of food through the ileocedal junction is controlled by the amount of food present in the cecum;

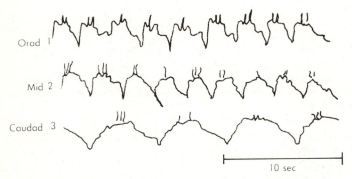

Figure 2-37. The frequency of slow waves recorded from the orad portions of the intestine is higher than that recorded from the more caudad regions. The magnitude of the contraction produced by the electrical activity of the intestine is proportional to the frequency of spikes superimposed on the slow waves.

distension of the cecum initiates reflexes that delay emptying from the ileum. Segmentation-like contractions of the colon cause the formation of **haustrations** (bag-like areas of intestine separated from each other by bands of contracting smooth muscle). These contractions, lasting 15 to 60 seconds, move the contents back and forth, allowing absorption of water and electrolytes to occur. The food slowly makes its way along the colon. Normally, it requires 10 to 15 hours to move the food from the duodenum to the rectum. During this time all but a few hundred milliliters of water is absorbed, resulting in the formation of semisolid fecal material. More rapid propulsion can occur by mass movements that sweep along the entire length of the colon, pushing the food toward the rectum. The mass movements, which occur only a few times per day, are preceded by inhibition of segmentation contractions and disappearance of the haustrations.

The rectum is usually empty of feces because its tone is normally higher than that of the sigmoid colon. However, following a mass movement or contraction of the sigmoid colon, the rectum can be filled. When this occurs, it initiates the rectosphincteric reflex, which causes the internal anal canal to open and produces the urge to defecate. Defecation can be inhibited by the voluntary closing of the external anal sphincter. If defecation does not occur, the internal anal sphincter regains its tone until more food enters the rectum. The rectum thus is able to store fecal material until defecation is convenient. Defecation is accomplished by the contraction of the distal colon and rectum and the relaxation of the internal and external anal sphincters. The movement of fecal material out of the anal canal is usually aided by contraction of the abdominal muscles and diaphragm.

The neural and hormonal control of the colon and rectum are poorly understood. However, the rectosphincteric reflex and the process of defecation are mediated in part by spinal reflexes. Thus, voluntary defecation is lost if the nerves to the anorectal area are damaged.

GASTROINTESTINAL SECRETIONS

GI secretions both moisten and dissolve food and provide the enzymes for its digestion. The mouth contains three pairs of salivary glands: the parotid, the submandibular, and the sublingual glands. Almost all of the 1 liter of saliva produced each day comes from the parotid and submandibular glands. The glands are composed of many tiny individual secretory units called **salivons**. Each salivon starts as a closed tube formed of acinar cells that secrete water, electrolytes, mucus, and enzymes. The saliva secreted by the acinar cells has a composition similar to the interstitial fluid. As it flows along the salivon, sodium and chloride are reabsorbed, making the saliva hypotonic. At the same time, potassium and bicarbonate are secreted. Thus when flow rates are low, the saliva is hypotonic to plasma and contains a higher concentration of potassium and bicarbonate than plasma. As flow rates increase, there is less time for sodium reabsorption and thus the tonicity of the saliva approaches that of plasma. The secretion of potassium and bicarbonate increases with increasing flow rates, so the concentration of these substances remains high even during copious salivation. Because of this, any fluids administered to a noneating patient with excessive salivation must contain extra potassium and bicarbonate to compensate for the salivary loss. The main organic substance in saliva is alpha-amylase. Myoepithelial cells surround the ducts of the salivon. Contraction of these cells propels the saliva into the main salivary ducts.

The main function of saliva is to moisten the food and wash it away from the taste buds and teeth. Mucin contained in the saliva helps to lubricate the food and make its passage through the esophagus easier. Although alpha-amylase can break down a significant portion of ingested starches to disaccharides, normal digestion does not require it. Saliva also performs a protective function, preventing hot foods from burning the mouth and buffering the hydrochloric acid that enters the mouth during vomiting. In addition, salivary secretions are bactericidal, destroying the bacteria that can cause dental caries and pharyngeal infections.

The parasympathetic nervous system controls the rate of salivary secretion. Efferent vagal fibers originating within the salivary nucleus in the medulla are reflexly excited by the aroma and taste of food as well as by tactile stimuli produced by the presence of food in the mouth. Stimulation of these nerve fibers directly increases the amount of saliva produced. It also increases flow rates indirectly by liberating kallikrein from the acinar cells. Kallikrein acts on a plasma protein to form bradykinin, which in turn causes an increase in blood flow. Finally, parasympathetic stimulation causes the myoepithelial cells to contract and thus increases the rate at which saliva is secreted into the mouth. Somewhat unusually, the sympathetic neurons innervating the salivary glands enhance, rather than inhibit, the actions of the parasympathetic neurons. Also, unlike in the rest of the GI tract, salivary secretion is entirely controlled by the nervous system and hormones have little or no influence.

Gastric secretions contain hydrochloric acid, pepsin, mucus, and intrinsic factor. Only the latter, necessary for the absorption of vitamin B_{12} from the ileum, is necessary for proper nutrition.

Hydrochloric acid is secreted from the parietal (or oxyntic) cells located in the mucosa covering the fundus and corpus of the stomach. The parietal cells (and the chief cells from which pepsinogen is secreted) are formed into oxyntic glands. Hydrochloric acid passes from a system of intracellular vesicles (called canaliculi) within the parietal cells into the lumen of the oxyntic glands and then into the stomach. Acid is produced in the parietal cells by a fairly complex process. First, chloride is actively pumped into the canaliculi, causing a high negative potential to develop within them. Potassium then flows passively into the canaliculi down their electrochemical gradient. Second, intracellular hydrogen is pumped into the canaliculi in exchange for potassium, producing a fluid containing a high concentration of hydrogen and chloride. Water flows into the canaliculi to preserve osmotic equilibrium with the intracellular fluid. Finally, the hydrogen secreted from the parietal cell is replaced by the following reaction:

$$H_2O + CO_2 \rightarrow H^+ + HCO_3^-$$

The bicarbonate formed by this reaction then diffuses into the blood plasma in exchange for chloride. The final result of this secretory process is the production of an isotonic fluid containing 150 mmol/L hydrogen chloride, 15 to 20 mEq/L of potassium, and no sodium.

A large luminal negative potential (-70 mV) normally exists across the stomach wall. When acid is not being secreted, the potential derives from the active reabsorption of sodium. However, when acid is secreted, the low pH inhibits sodium reabsorption. In this case, the negative potential is produced by the active secretion of chloride. The magnitude of the potential is reduced during active secretion of hydrogen because of both the active secretion of positive hydrogen ions and the inhibition of sodium transport. The final composition of gastric secretions depends on the flow rate. At low rates of flow, the gastric juice is primarily composed of nonparietal cell secretions with a composition similar to that of plasma. As flow rates increase, the electrolyte concentrations becomes similar to parietal cell secretions — that is, the concentration of hydrochloric acid increases while the concentration of sodium decreases. At very high flow rates, when the gastric juice is dominated by paritetal cell secretions, the hydrogen concentration rises to 150 mEq/L while that of potassium reaches 15 to 20 mEq/L.

Acid secretion is stimulated by gastrin (a hormone released from G cells in the antrum of the stomach), by ACh, by histamine, and perhaps by an intestinal hormone called enterooxyntin. As will be discussed below, regulation of acid secretion is accomplished by the vagus nerves (which release ACh) and by gastrin. However, the amount of acid released by these stimulants is greatly potentiated by the presence of histamine. Cimetidine, a specific blocker of the parietal cell histamine receptor (called an H_2 receptor), dramatically reduces the amount of acid secreted by the stomach without affecting other histamine receptors in the body. As a result, it has become the drug of choice for treating ulcers and other acid-produced stomach disorders.

Stimulation of acid secretion is divided into three components: the cephalic, gastric, and intestinal stages. The cephalic stage of gastric secretion is mediated by vagal nerve fibers, which are reflexly activated by the thought, aroma, or taste of food. Vagal nerve fibers entering the proximal stomach innervate ACh-containing interneurons, which directly stimulate parietal cells to secrete acid. Fibers entering the distal stomach innervate interneurons containing a gastrin-releasing peptide (thought to be bombesin). Bombesin stimulates the release of gastrin from G cells in the antrum. The gastrin then enters the circulation and, when it reaches the oxyntic glands, stimulates acid secretion.

The gastric phase of acid secretion begins when food enters the stomach. In the interdigestive period, the low pH (less than 3) of the gastric fluids inhibits the release of gastrin from the G cells. When food enters the stomach, it buffers the acid, causing the pH to rise. The increase in pH permits gastrin to be secreted from the G cells when they are stimulated.

There are two major stimulants to acid secretion during the gastric stage: distension of the stomach and protein digestive products (amino acids and polypeptides). Distension of both the proximal and distal stomach elicits reflexes that result in acid secretion. These reflexes may be mediated via long loops (vagal afferents travel to medullary centers from which vagal efferents return to the stomach) or short loops (confined to the intrinsic nervous system within the stomach wall). Efferent vagal fibers and interneurons stimulated by these reflexes synapsing within the proximal stomach stimulate parietal cells directly; those ending in the distal stomach stimulate the G cells. As indicated above, vagal stimulation of gastrin release is mediated by bombesin. Vagal stimulation also stimulates gastrin secretion by inhibiting the release of somatostatin. Somatostatin is a paracrine secretion (a hormone that reaches its target organ by diffusion rather than through the circulation) that inhibits the release of gastrin from the G cell. Thus the vagus acts on the distal stomach by both releasing a gastrin stimulant (bombesin) and inhibiting a gastrin inhibitor (somatostatin).

Protein digestion products act directly on the G cells to release gastrin. Thus vagotomy has little effect on the release of gastrin by amino acids or polypeptides. Caffeine and low concentrations of alcohol can also stimulate the parietal cells to increase acid secretion. Most of the gastric juices released during a meal occur during the gastric phase of secretion.

Only a small portion of acid secretion results from events occurring in the intestine. The primary cause of acid secretion during the intestinal phase is probably the release of gastrin from proximal duodenal cells when protein digestion products reach them. A nongastrin acid stimulus (enterooxyntin) may also be released from the intestine. Finally, amino acids absorbed into the bloodstream from the intestine act to stimulate acid secretion.

The major effect produced by the intestinal hormones is the inhibition of acid secretion. A variety of intestinal hormones, called enterogastrones, are released from the duodenum by low pH, fatty acids, and hyperosmotic fluids. The entero-gastrones inhibit acid secretion. Although both gastric inhibitory peptide and secretin can inhibit the release of acid from the parietal cells, it is not yet known whether these are the enterogastrones that act to inhibit acid secretion in response to the entry of food into the duodenum.

The other main component of gastric secretion, pepsin, is derived from pepsinogen. Pepsinogen (molecular weight 42,500) is released from the peptic (or chief) cells located within the oxyntic glands. It is converted to pepsin (molecular weight 35,000) in the gastric juices when the pH is below 5. Pepsin itself can catalyze the conversion of pepsinogen to pepsin. Pepsin initiates protein digestion by breaking apart peptide bonds. The peptic cells release pepsinogen when stimulated by ACh-containing interneurons. Thus large amounts of pepsin-ogen are released by the vagus nerve during the cephalic and gastric phases. In addition, hydrogen ion plays a significant direct and indirect role in pepsin formation. As indicated above, it directly converts pepsinogen to pepsin. Indirectly, reducing the pH initiates a local reflex, mediated by the intrinsic nervous system, that stimulates the peptic cells to release pepsinogen. Gastrin and histamine also play a role in pepsinogen release, but they are not as important here as they are in acid secretion.

Soluble mucus, a mucoprotein, is secreted from the mucus neck cells in the oxyntic glands and by pyloric glands in the distal stomach. The mucus mixes with the food and lubricates it. It is released primarily in response to vagal nerve stimulation. Another mucus secretion of the stomach is called insoluble mucus. This substance is released by epithelial cells on the surface of the stomach. It serves a protective function—first, by forming a physical barrier (approximately 1 mm thick) between the food and the stomach wall, second by preventing pepsin from digesting the stomach wall, and third by neutralizing the acidic gastric juices that come into contact with the stomach wall. When the buffering capacity of the insoluble mucus is exceeded, it precipitates into clumps that become incorporated into the gastric chyme and pass into the intestine. The barrier formed by insoluble mucus can be broken down by alcohol, aspirin, and bile salts regurgitated from the intestine. When this barrier is broken down, the potential for ulcer formation increases.

Intrinsic factor is a high-molecular-weight (55,000) muco-protein secreted by the parietal cells. Unless it is available to combine with vitamin B_{12} in the stomach, B_{12} cannot be absorbed by the ileum. Although it takes many years for the body's supply of vitamin B_{12} to be consumed, failure to secrete intrinsic factor eventually results in the development of pernicious anemia.

Pancreatic exocrine secretions are divided into two groups: a high-volume sodium bicarbonate secretion used to neutralize the acidic fluids entering the duodenum from the stomach and a low-volume enzymatic secretion that is essential for the digestion of food. The structure of the pancreatic glands resembles the salivary glands. Several acinar cells join together to form an acinus. Groups of acini merge into lobules. Epithelium-lined ductules drain the secretions from individual acini. The ductules drain into larger ducts, which in turn drain into the main pancreatic duct. The acinar cells produce the protein component of the pancreatic juices while the epithelial cells lining the ductules form the aqueous sodium bicarbonate secretion. The pancreas is innervated by both the vagus and sympathetic nerve fibers. In general, vagus nerve stimulation increases and sympathetic nerve stimulation decreases pan-creatic secretions.

At low rates of secretion, the electrolyte composition of the pancreatic juice is similar to plasma. However, as the flow rate increases, the concentration of bicarbonate rises and that of chloride falls. This change most likely comes about in a manner analogous to that occurring in the stomach. That is, at low rates of flow, the pancreatic juice is dominated by acinar cells, which produce a fluid containing digestive enzymes and a high concentration of chloride. As flow rates increase, the pancreatic juice reflects more and more the composition of the fluid produced by the ductule cells. Bicarbonate is produced in the ductule cells by the following reaction:

$$H_2O \;+\; CO_2 \;\rightarrow\; H^+ \;+\; HCO_3^-$$

However, in this case, the bicarbonate is secreted into the pancreatic juice and the hydrogen is secreted into the extra-cellular fluid. It is not certain whether bicarbonate passively diffuses or is actively secreted from the ductule cell. Normally about 1 L of pancreatic juice is formed each day and may have a bicarbonate concentration as high as 150 mEq/L.

The regulation of pancreatic secretion can be divided into cephalic, gastric, and intestinal phases. Vagal fibers stimulated by the thought or presence of food increase the rate of acinar protein secretion but have only a minimal effect on bicarbonate secretion. In addition, vagal reflexes initiated by stomach distension stimulate pancreatic secretion during the gastric phase. However, the major control over pancreatic secretions occurs during the intestinal phase of digestion.

Seventy to 80% of the pancreatic juices are secreted in response to the presence of digestion products and acid in the intestine. Hydrogen ion entering the duodenum causes the release of secretin from S cells in the mucosa. Secretin enters the circulation and acts directly on the pancreatic ductule cells to stimulate the secretion of bicarbonate and water. Although the entire intestine contains secretin-releasing S cells, the neutralization of acid in the proximal intestine prevents the more distal jejunem and ileum from releasing secretin. The amount of secretin released is proportional to both the concentration and amount of acid entering the intestine. By itself, the amount of secretin released in response to a meal cannot account for the quantity of bicarbonate and water formed by the pancreas. However, the effects of secretin are potentiated enormously by ACh and cholecystokinin (CCK).

CCK is released from intestinal cells in response to fat and protein digestion products. It stimulates the release of enzymes from the pancreatic acinar cells and, as indicated above, potentiates the effect of secretin on the ductule cells. CCK-containing cells are found over much of the small intestine.

Bile is essential for the normal absorption of lipids and the fat-soluble vitamins A, D, E, and K. Its secretion can be divided into three components: formation of bile by the liver (and bile duct epithelial cells), concentration of bile in the gallbladder, and flow of bile from the gallbladder to the intestine. Bile acids are synthesized from cholesterol in the liver. They are complex carboxylic acids resembling cholesterol in their basic structure but, unlike cholesterol, they contain several hydroxyl groups. Because of this, they are amphipathic—that is, their hydroxyl groups make them hydrophilic while their ringed nucleus and attached methyl groups make them lipophillic. The bile acids synthesized in the liver are cholic and chenodeoxycholic acid. When sufficiently concentrated, the lipophilic portions of the bile acids combine with each other to form water-soluble micelles. As will be described below, micelle formation is necessary for the absorption of lipids.

Under normal circumstances, the bile secreted by the liver is continuously reused. After traveling from the liver through the gallbladder and entering the duodenum, the bile acids are actively reabsorbed by the terminal ileum. Once absorbed, the bile acids are taken up by the portal circulation and returned to the liver. Within the liver, they are actively removed from the plasma by the hepatocytes and become available for resecretion. This cycle is referred to as the enterohepatic circulation. The total body store of bile acids (approximately 2 g) is recirculated twice during a typical meal containing the normal amount of fats. Thus the liver only has to synthesize enough bile acids to replace the small amount lost in the stool each day. In addition to the primary bile acids actually synthesized by the liver, secondary bile acids (deoxycholic and lithocholic acid) are formed by bacteria that are endogenous to the intestine. These secondary bile acids are absorbed by the terminal ileum and participate in the enterohepatic circulation. The bile acids are made more water soluble by conjugation with the amino acids taurine and glycine to form bile salts. The liver also secretes cholesterol and bilirubin into the bile for elimination in the stool.

After being secreted by the hepatocytes, the bile acids travel through the hepatic ducts to the gallbladder. The gallbladder concentrates the bile acids by reabsorbing water. Water reabsorption is secondary to the active transport of sodium across the gallbladder epithelium. Most likely, the transport process is coupled to the reabsorption of bicarbonate and/or chloride, so it is an electrically neutral process. In addition to increasing the concentration of bile acids, the reabsorption of water also increases the concentration of potassium and calcium, which are not reabsorpbed by the gallbladder. The high concentration of organic substances within the gallbladder can lead to the formation of gallstones. Precipitation of these organic compounds (primarily cholesterol) is usually prevented by the formation of bile salt micelles that incorporate cholesterol into them. Gallstones can be dissolved in some cases by feeding bile acids to patients. The increased micelles formed by the exogenously administered bile will eventually solubilize the gallstone.

During the fasting state, the bile flowing from the liver is stored in the gallbladder and does not enter the duodenum because the sphicter of Oddi keeps the terminal bile duct closed. During a meal, the smooth muscle within the wall of the gallbladder contracts to expel the stored contents into the intestine. The major stimulus for gallbladder contraction is CCK, which is released from the intestine in response to the presence of food digestion products. CCK tends to relax the sphincter of Oddi, thus allowing the bile to enter the intestine.

DIGESTION AND ABSORPTION

The fundamental purpose of the GI system is the digestion and absorption of minerals and nutrients. In addition to absorbing digestive products, the intestine must also reabsorb the large amount of water, electrolytes, and other materials (such as bile salts) that are secreted by the GI tract during the digestive process. These processes (digestion and absorption) are primarily carried out in the small intestine. The absorptive surface area of the intestine is increased greatly by folds (or villi) found in the intestinal wall and by the numerous microvilli projecting from the apical side of the epithelial cells or enterocytes. The enterocytes are responsible for carrying out the digestive, absorptive, and secretory functions of the intestine. Goblet cells, which are also present within the villi, secrete mucus. These specialized intestinal cells differentiate from stem cells found at the base of the villi. As the newly formed stem cells migrate toward the surface of the villi, they become more and more specialized. When they reach the tip of the villus, they are sloughed off and become part of the mucus lining. The entire intestinal wall is replaced in 4 to 5 days.

Approximately 9 L of fluid must be absorbed from the GI tract each day. Although part of the water and electrolyte load of the intestine derives from dietary sources, most of it results from the copius secretions of the salivary glands (1 L), the stomach (2 L), the liver and pancreas (2 L), and the intestine (3 L). Ninety-five percent of this fluid is absorbed in the small intestine (primarily in the ileum) and another 4% is absorbed in the colon. Thus, under normal circumstances, less than 100 ml of water is lost through the GI tract. The colon is unable to absorb more than 2 or 3 L of fluid each day. Thus if intestinal absorption is impaired, the amount of fluid entering the colon can overcome its absorptive capacity, resulting in diarrhea.

The primary absorptive process in the intestine is the active transport of sodium across the epithelial wall. There are three potential forms of active transport. Most of the sodium (approximately 80%) is actively absorbed in a cotransport process involving glucose or amino acids. Additional amounts of sodium are absorbed by an electrically neutral sodium-chloride pump. The remainder of the transported sodium enters the intestinal cell down its electrochemical gradient and is actively transported from the basolateral surface by a Na-K ATPase. Water moves easily across the intestinal wall to maintain osmotic equilibrium.

In the duodenum, water normally flows into the intestine from the interstitial fluid to make the chyme isotonic to plasma. As the chyme moves along the intestine, salt and other osmotically active particles are absorbed, followed by the osmotic flow of water. Thus the fluid within the intestine remains isotonic to plasma. However, its composition is quite different from that of plasma. The sodium concentration of the chyme is reduced from 140 mEq/L to approximately 125 mEq/L by the time it reaches the ileum, while the concentration of chloride is reduced to less than 60 mEq/L. In contrast, the bicarbonate concentration of the chyme is increased to over 70 mEq/L by the intestine. This reduction in chloride concentration and increase in bicarbonate concentration is brought about by a bicarbonate-chloride exchanger located on the apical surface of the epithelial cell. The concentration of potassium in the chyme rises in the intestine from 4 mEq/L to approximately 9 mEq/L.

In the colon, sodium absorption occurs primarily by one mechanism: sodium enters the apical surface down its electrochemical gradient and is pumped out of the basolateral surface by the Na-K ATPase pump. The reabsorption of sodium reduces its concentration to under 40 mEq/L. Chloride is absorbed either by the chloride-bicarbonate exchange system or by passively following sodium across the epithelial wall. However, unlike the situation in the intestine, the epithelial lining of the colon is fairly tight. This can prevent osmotic equilibrium from occurring and thus allows the excretion of a hypertonic stool. The osmolarity of the stool is normally 350 to 400 mOsm/L. Potassium is actively secreted into the colon by the epithelial cells. As a result, the potassium concentration rises to over 90 mEq/L. Because of the high concentration of potassium and bicarbonate in the colon, excessive loss of intestinal fluids through vomiting or diarrhea will cause hypokalemia and metabolic acidosis.

The absorption of electrolytes from the intestine is not precisely regulated. However, sympathetic stimulation of the intestine can increase the rate of sodium reabsorption. Also, and probably more importantly, the reabsorption of sodium by the colon is controlled to some extent by aldosterone. In the presence of aldosterone, the sodium concentration in the stool can be reduced to approximately 2 mEq/L. At the same time, aldosterone causes the potassium concentration to rise to approximately 150 mEq/L. Aldosterone increases sodium reabsorption and potassium secretion by the epithelial cells of the colon in a manner similar to that in the distal nephron of the kidney. In the presence of aldosterone, the apical membrane becomes more permeable to sodium and potassium. Thus more sodium can enter the epithelial cell down its electrochemical gradient. The excess intracellular sodium is then pumped into the interstitium, across the basolateral membrane, by the Na-K ATPase. Similarly, the high apical permeability permits the increased amount of potassium entering the cell (due to the increased pump activity) to flow into the intestinal lumen.

Any factor interfering with electrolyte or nutrient reabsorption can cause diarrhea. Thus ingesting large quantities of nonabsorbable ions (such as magnesium sulfate) increases the osmotic pressure of the chyme and result in retention of water by the intestine. Diseases that interfere with saccharide absorption or that cause excessive electrolyte secretion (such as cholera and other bacterial infections) also result in retention of fluid and diarrhea. Interestingly, choleretic diarrhea can be reduced by the administration of glucose because the proximal intestine absorbs a greater than normal amount of sodium in the process of absorbing the added glucose load.

Nutrients are absorbed from the intestine after being digested into small particles. The dietary carbohydrates (sucrose, lactose, and starches) must be decomposed into monosaccharides before they can be absorbed by the intestine. Salivary alpha-amylase (ptyalin) is capable of digesting complex starches to the disaccharide maltase. However, its action is terminated by the low pH of the stomach so less than 60% of the ingested carbohydrates are digested before the chyme empties into the intestine. Once the chyme enters the intestine, the remaining starches are digested to maltose and other small polysaccharides by pancreatic alpha-amylase. Specific intestinal enzymes secreted from the enterocytes break down the maltose, sucrose, lactose, and other small polymers of glucose into their component monosaccharides. As indicated above, the monosaccharides are then absorbed by a sodium-dependent cotransport process.

Approximately 40% of the ingested proteins are digested in the stomach by pepsin. Pepsin is particularly important for the digestion of meats because of its ability to break down collagen. The remainder of the proteins are digested by a variety of proteolytic enzymes secreted by the pancreas and epithelial lining of the small intestine. As soon as the individual amino acids are released by the digestive enzymes, they are carried across the intestinal epithelium by a sodium-dependent active transport system similar to that which transports the monosaccharides. Separate carriers are available for neutral, basic, and acidic amino acids. In addition, proline and hydroxyproline have their own specific transport carrier system.

Fats are digested almost exclusively within the small intestine by pancreatic lipase. However, digestion cannot occur until the fats are made water soluble. This is carried out by the bile salts. The lipophilic portion of the bile salts dissolves in the surface of the fat molecule, while their water-soluble ends dissolve in the digestive juices. The addition of bile salts to the fat particles causes them to break into smaller particles when agitated by the segmentation contractions of the intestine. Bile salts attach to the smaller particles, and the fragmentation process is repeated. Eventually, the fats are emulsified into particles less than 1 μm in diameter. The lipases can then digest these small particles into monoglycerides and free fatty acids.

The free fatty acids and monoglycerides are kept in solution (and prevented from reforming triglycerides) by bile salt micelles. As indicated above, when sufficiently concentrated, 20 to 40 bile salt molecules can form small globular particles, approximately 25 nm in diameter, called micelles. The lipophilic portions of the bile salts coalesce in the center of the micelle, while the hydrophilic ends dissolve in the water of the digestive fluids. When the micelles come into contact with the intestinal epithelium, the monoglycerides and free fatty acids dissolve in the epithelial cell membrane and enter the cell. Once inside the cell, the monoglycerides and free fatty acids reform as triglycerides and aggregate into small particles. The particles are coated with a beta-lipoprotein (synthesized by the endoplasmic reticulum) and then transported out of the cell by exocytosis. The extracellular fat globules, called chylomicrons, enter the lymphatic system and are carried into the thoracic duct, from which they enter the circulation. A small portion of the more water-soluble short-chain fatty acids enter the circulation directly through the portal capillaries.

RENAL PHYSIOLOGY

The primary function of the kidneys is to regulate the volume and contents of the extracellular fluid. The kidneys carry out these functions by a combination of filtration, reabsorption, and secretion. About 20% of the cardiac output (approximately 1,200 ml/minute) of blood flows through the kidneys. Of this, approximately 125 ml of ultrafiltrate is formed each minute. From this, various materials are reabsorbed and returned to the blood and other materials are added. After being processed by the kidneys, the volume of filtrate is reduced to approximately 1 ml/minute and the concentrations of the various materials dissolved in it are quite different from the original filtrate. When working normally, the kidneys (along with the GI system and the lungs) excrete any unused materials ingested or produced each day so as to maintain the constancy of the extracellular fluid bathing the body's cells. This section will review the mechanisms by which the kidneys accomplish this task.

BODY FLUIDS

Total body water is equal to approximately 60% of total body weight. Of this, two-thirds is intracellular fluid and one-third is extracellular fluid. The extracellular compartment is divided between the interstitial fluid (which makes up three-fourths of the extracellular fluid) and the blood plasma (which makes up one-fourth of the extracellular fluid). A small portion of the extracellular fluid (for example, the fluid in the digestive system, the joints, the eyes, etc.) is called the transcellular fluid because it mixes very slowly with the rest of the interstitial fluid.

The volume of each fluid compartment can be measured with the Fick dye-dilution technique. This method involves the administration of a substance that distributes in only one of the fluid compartments. For example, if a dye such as Evans blue, which does not cross the capillary epithelium (or the red blood cell membrane), is injected, it will eventually distribute evenly within the blood plasma. After allowing mixing to occur, a sample of plasma is withdrawn and its concentration of Evans blue is measured. Its volume of distribution is then calculated using the following formula:

$$\text{Volume} = \frac{\text{amount injected} - \text{amount lost from plasma}}{\text{concentration}}$$

The total blood volume can be determined from the plasma volume if the hematocrit is known. The hematocrit is the percent of blood composed of red blood cells and is normally 35 to 40% in women and 40 to 45% in men. Dividing the plasma volume by the hematocrit yields the total blood volume:

$$\text{Blood volume} = \frac{\text{plasma volume}}{\text{hematocrit}}$$

Total body water can be measured using tritiated water; extracellular space by injecting radiolabeled sulphate. Interstitial volume is measured by subtracting the value for plasma volume from that for extracellular volume.

Table 2-2 illustrates the ionic composition of the three compartments. Notice that there is a difference between the concentration of solute in the plasma and the plasma water. This difference is due to the presence of proteins in the plasma. Approximately 7% of the plasma volume is due to protein, leaving 93 ml of water for each 100 ml of plasma. As a result, the solute in each 100 ml of plasma is actually dissolved in 93 ml of water. The values for plasma water can be obtained from those for plasma by dividing by 0.93. Laboratory values are usually reported in terms of plasma volume. Thus in conditions such as hyperlipidemeia or hyperproteinemia, where the volume of water in the plasma is less than normal, the reported concentration of electrolytes may be abnormally low even though the total body content of the electrolyte is normal. For example, if the laboratory analysis of plasma sodium is lower than normal because the percent of water in plasma is less than 93, the condition is called pseudohyponatremia.

Interstitial water also differs from plasma water because of the presence of plasma proteins. Most of the proteins in plasma are negatively charged. As a result, the concentration of positive ions is higher in plasma than in the interstitium and the concentration of negative ions is lower.

A variety of units are used to describe solute concentration. For most ions, concentration is given as mEq/L—that is, the number of moles of charge per liter of water. For example, 10 mmol of sodium (Na^+) is equal to 10 mEq whereas 10 mmol of calcium (Ca^{++}) is equal to 20 mEq. Solute concentration is usually given in terms of millimolar or millimolal. The term millimolar refers to the number of mmol/L of solution, whereas millimolal refers to the number of mmol/kg water. There is very little difference in these two units when interstitial or intercellular water concentrations are compared. However, because of the presence of plasma proteins, plasma molar concentrations differ from plasma molal concentrations in the same way as plasma and plasma water concentrations differ. We will ignore the differences between these measures in this book.

Normal plasma osmolarity is 285 mOsm/L. The bulk of this osmolarity is made up of sodium (which has a concentration of 142 mEq/L) and its associated anions, chloride (110 mEq/L) and bicarbonate (24 mEq/L). The remainder is produced by potassium, blood urea, glucose, and a number of so-called lesser anions and cations. Normal glucose concentration is approximately 100 mg/100 ml, or 5.5 mmol/L). Urea is usually reported as blood urea nitrogen or BUN and is normally 15 mg/100 ml or 5 mmol/L. A reasonable estimate of plasma osmolarity can be made by doubling the sodium concentration.

The concentration of particles in solution determines the osmotic pressure of that solution. Thus plasma, having an osmolar concentration of 285 mOsm/L, has an osmotic pressure of 5,500 mm Hg. Recall that osmotic pressure can be calculated using the van't Hoff equation:

$$\text{Osmotic pressure} = RT \times \text{Conc} = 19.3 \times 285 = 5,500 \text{ mm Hg}$$

The flow of water between compartments is proportional to the osmotic pressure difference that exists between them. Notice from Table 2-2 that the osmotic pressure of plasma is some 25 mm Hg higher than that of the interstitial fluid. The difference is due to the presence of plasma proteins and is called the oncotic pressure. As explained in the discussion of capillary fluid exchange, the flow of water into the capillaries by osmosis is opposed by the capillary hydrostatic pressure. However, unless there is an opposing hydrostatic pressure difference, the osmolar concentration throughout the body will always be the same because any differences that develop will be rapidly dissipated by the osmotic flow of water. Solutions in osmotic equilibrium with each other (that is, when there is no osmotic flow of water between them) are called isotonic. In discussing body fluids, solutions that cause red blood cells to shrink are called hypertonic; those that cause red blood cells to swell are called hypotonic; and those that cause no change in red blood cells are called isotonic.

Pure water is extremely hypotonic, and any red blood cells placed into it will immediately swell and hemolyze. Thus pure water should never be administered intravenously. However, if pure water is experimentally infused into a vein, it will rapidly be incorporated into the circulation, causing the osmolarity of the plasma, interstitial fluid, and intracellular fluid all to be reduced.

For example, the following calculation illustrates the theoretical effect of infusing 1 L of pure water into a vein:

Initial osmolarity of plasma	= 285 mOsm/L	
Total volume of plasma	= 3.5 L	
Total osmotic content	= 285 × 3.5	= 997.5 particles
New volume	= 4.5 L	
New concentration	= 997.5/4.5	= 222 mmol/L

But as soon as the water enters the circulation, it will begin to flow into the extracellular fluid, causing it to be diluted as well. Thus the theoretical osmolarity of the total extracellular compartment (plasma and interstitium) will be as follows:

Initial extracellular fluid volume	=	14 L	
Total extracellular osmotic content	=	285 × 14	= 3990 particles
New volume	=	15 L	
New concentration	=	3990/15	= 266 mmol/L

However, as soon as the water enters the interstitial fluid, it will begin to flow into the intracellular fluid, making the intracellular and extracellular fluid compartments equal to each other. Thus the actual change in plasma osmolarity caused by the infusion of 1 L of pure water is as follows:

Initial body water	= 42 L	
Total body osmotic content	= 285 × 42	= 11,970 particles
New volume	= 43 L	
New concentration	= 11,970/43	= 278 mmol/L

In working through these calculations, notice that no exchange of particles between the intracellular and extracellular compartments occurred. Similarly, no exchange of particles would occur if a saline solution were infused into the extracellular fluid. Thus, if 1 L of a 570-mmol solution of sodium chloride were added to the extracellular fluid, all of the added salt would remain in the extracellular fluid. This restriction of sodium chloride is a consequence of the Na-K ATPase pump, which keeps the intracellular sodium concentration low. However, the osmolarities of all the fluid compartments eventually become equal to each other. Thus the effect of adding the hypertonic sodium chloride solution is calculated as follows:

Initial body water	=	42 L
Total osmotic particles	=	43 L
New total osmotic particles	= 11,970 + 570	= 12,540
New concentration	= 12,540/43	= 292 mmol/L

Since the added particles remained in the extracellular fluid, the new volume of the extracellular fluid is

$$\frac{3,990 \text{ (initial particles)} + 590 \text{ (added particles)}}{292 \text{ (new concentration)}} = 15.7 \text{ L}$$

and the new volume of the intracellular fluid is

$$\frac{7,980 \text{ (total particles)}}{292 \text{ (new concentration)}} = 27.3$$

In this case, the entire liter of added saline remained in the extracellular fluid. Thus, if 1 L of a 570-mOsm/L solution of sodium chloride were added to the extracellular fluid, all of the added salt would remain in the extracellular fluid. This restriction of sodium chloride is a consequence of the Na-K pump.

If 1 L of isotonic saline were infused into a vein, no osmotic gradients would be generated and thus all of the fluid would remain in the extracellular compartment. However, note that because sodium chloride diffuses freely between the plasma and interstitial fluid, only one-fourth of the isotonic fluid would stay in the plasma. The other 750 ml would end up in the interstitial fluid.

The important conclusion to be drawn from these calculations is that water added to the body distributes throughout all the fluid compartments while salt (and other osmotically active solutes that cannot cross cellular membranes) remain within the extracellular fluid. Similarly, if water is lost from the body, for example by sweating, two-thirds of it comes from the intracellular fluid and one-third comes from the extracellular fluid.

MORPHOLOGY OF THE KIDNEY

The kidneys are oblong-shaped organs (approximately 11 cm long) encased in a tough fibrous capsule (Fig. 2-38).

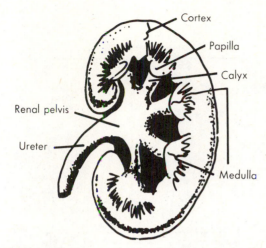

Figure 2-38. A cross-sectional view of the kidney. Urine formation begins in the glomeruli, which are located within the cortex. The filtrate flows through the renal tubules, located within both the cortex and medulla, and through the collecting ducts, located within the medulla. It empties into the calyces. The urine then flows through the renal pelvis and ureter on its way to the bladder.

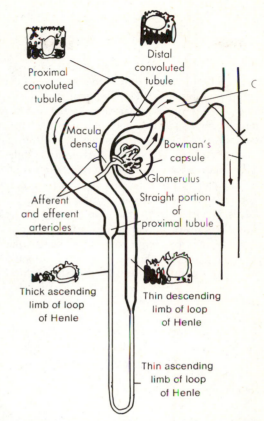

Figure 2-39. The nephron begins as a blind sac, called Bowman's capsule. It continues as the proximal tubule, loop of Henle, distal tubule, and collecting tubule before ending in the collecting duct.

Beneath the capsule is the renal cortex, and below that the renal medulla. The medulla is divided into 10 to 15 pyramid-shaped structures called the renal pyramids. The base of each pyramid lies on the border between the cortex and medulla, and its apex extends into the deeper portions of the medulla. The tips of each pyramid (called papillae) coalesce into minor and major calyces, which in turn form the renal pelvis. The ureters originate from the pelvis and carry the urine formed by the kidneys to the bladder.

The bulk of the renal mass consists of the 1.2 million nephrons that perform the reabsorptive and secretory functions of the kidney. Each nephron begins as an enlarged sac (Bowman's capsule) surrounding a capillary tuft called the glomerulus (Fig. 2-39). These two structures are often referred to as the renal capsule. The proximal tubule arises from Bowman's capsule and in turn gives rise to a loop of Henle, a distal tubule, a connecting segment, and a collecting duct. Urine formed by the nephron drains through the papillae into the minor calyces. Each of these tubular segments can be further subdivided and are lined by epithelial cells specialized for the particular function they serve. These will be described later in more detail in conjunction with the role performed by each region of the nephron.

There are two populations of nephrons. Those with glomeruli in the cortex (cortical nephrons) have short loops of Henle that either do not enter or barely enter the medulla. The other group of nephrons have glomeruli located on the cortical-medullary border and are called juxtamedullary glomeruli. These nephrons possess long loops of Henle that course deep within the renal medulla. Although they comprise less than 15% of the total number of nephrons, they provide the kidney with the ability to form a concentrated urine.

The renal artery enters, and the renal vein and ureter leave the kidney through a slit on its medial surface called the hilus. The renal artery divides into a series of smaller arteries—the interlobar, arcuate, and interlobular arteries. The afferent arterioles that branch from the interlobular arteries give rise to a capillary tuft called the glomerulus, from which the renal filtrate is formed. The glomerular capillaries join together to form the efferent arteriole, which in turn gives rise to a second set of renal capillaries called the peritubular capillaries. These capillaries surround the renal tubules and both provide material for secretion into the tubules and serve to carry reabsorbed material from the tubules into the general circulation. A special set of peritubular capillaries, called the vasa rectae, travel alongside the loops of Henle in the medulla and contribute, in a manner to be described later, to the kidney's ability to regulate water balance.

The **juxtamedullary apparatus** (JGA) is a specialized organ of the kidney and is responsible for the secretion of the hormone renin. It is composed from portions of the afferent and efferent arterioles and the distal nephron. The epithelial cells lining the distal tubular portion of the JGA are morphologically different from the other cells of distal nephron and are called the **macula densa**. The macula densa makes extensive contact with the efferent arteriole and to a lesser extent with the afferent arteriole. Modified smooth muscle cells, called myoepithelial cells, surround the afferent and efferent arteriolar portions of the JGA. These cells are responsible for synthesis and release of renin. As will be discussed in more detail later, renin release can occur when the macula densa is stimulated by excess NaCl delivery to the distal tubule, by increased pressure within the afferent arteriole, and by sympathetic stimulation of the JGA.

GLOMERULAR FILTRATION

The first step in urine formation is the filtration of plasma water from the glomerulus. The filtrate passes from the glomerular capillaries, into Bowmans's space (the extracellular fluid within the renal capsule), and then into the proximal tubule. As indicated above, approximately 125 ml/minute or 180 L/day of ultrafiltrate is formed. The filtrate is called an **ultrafiltrate** of plasma because it contains no plasma proteins. The concentration of the substances dissolved in the ultrafiltrate is essentially the same as that found in plasma water.

The forces involved in the filtration process are called Starling forces. These are the same types of forces involved in capillary exchange in the systemic and pulmonary circulations discussed earlier. However, there are important quantitative differences. Net filtration is defined by the relationship

$$GFR = K[(P_{CAP} + \pi_{BS}) - (\pi_{CAP} + P_{BS})]$$

where the hydrostatic pressure in the glomerular capillaries and in Bowman's space is P_{CAP} and P_{BS}, respectively, and π_{CAP} and π_{BS} are the corresponding oncotic pressures.

Because there are virtually no proteins in Bowman's space, the extracellular oncotic pressure is zero. In contrast, there is a significant extracellular hydrostatic pressure due to the continuous flow of filtrate into an essentially rigid kidney. This pressure is normally 10 mm Hg but can rise to much higher levels if, for example, the ureter is blocked and urine cannot flow out of the kidney. Under these conditions, the process of filtration can be reduced or stopped, leading to renal failure.

The hydrostatic pressure of blood entering the afferent arteriole is much higher than that in most systemic capillaries, averaging about 40 to 45 mm Hg. Although this pressure falls somewhat as the blood flows through the glomerulus, it is not a significant drop. The lack of change in hydrostatic pressure is in sharp contrast to what occurs with the oncotic pressure. Because of the large amount of water filtered out of the plasma, the protein concentration and hence the oncotic pressure increases markedly (Fig. 2-40), from 20 mm Hg at the afferent end of the glomerulus to 35 mm Hg at the efferent end.

Combining these Starling forces yields a net filtration pressure of

$$[(45 + 0) - (20 + 10)] = 15 \text{ mm Hg}$$

at the beginning of the capillary and

$$[(45 + 0) - (35 + 10)] = 0 \text{ mm Hg}$$

at the end of the capillary. These figures indicate that the bulk of filtration occurs in the early portion of the glomerulus and that filtration ceases before the blood leaves the glomerulus. The point along the capillary at which filtration stops is called the filtration pressure equilibrium point. The Starling forces equation can be simplified to

$$GFR = K P$$

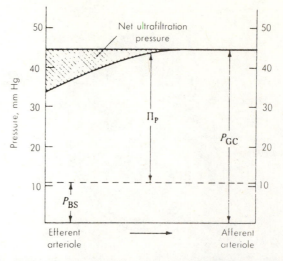

Figure 2-40. The amount of filtration from the glomerulus is dependent on the hydrostatic pressures within the glomerular capillaries, which push water out, and the hydrostatic pressure of the renal capsule and oncotic pressure of the glomerular capillaries, which oppose the outward filtration of water. The net filtration pressure decreases as blood flows through the glomerulus because of the increase in oncotic pressure that results from the filtration of water out of the capillaries. The reduction in capillary hydrostatic pressure along the capillary is small enough to be ignored.

where P = the average filtration pressure. K represents the hydraulic conductivity of the glomerular capillaries. Its value depends both on the permeability of the capillary membrane to water and on the surface area available for filtration. Hydraulic conductivity is quite a bit higher in the kidney than in other capillaries because of the unique structure of the glomerular capillary wall. Moreover, as is described below, it can be varied by the mesangial cells, which by contracting can prevent the flow of blood through portions of the glomerular capillaries.

The endothelial cells lining the capillary wall form fenestrations or holes approximately 70 nm in diameter through which all of the substances dissolved in the plasma water (e.g., electrolytes, amino acids, and glucose) can easily pass. These fenestrations are covered by thin diaphragms that do not appear to offer any significant impediment to the flow of material through them. The outer surface of the endothelial cells is covered by a basement membrane approximately 350 nm thick. The basement membrane is composed of a glycoprotein that contains a preponderance of fixed negative charges. These charges prevent the flow of the negatively charged proteins out of the glomerulus despite the large size of the fenestrations appearing within the capillary wall.

Epithelial cells (called podocytes) within the glomerulus form projections called foot processes or pedicels, which line the outer surface of the basement membrane. The individual pedicels are approximately 50 nm from each other. The space between the pedicels is called a slit pore, and a thin membrane called the filtration slit membrane extends from one pedicel to another. Thus the filtrate leaving the capillary must pass through the basement and filtration slit membranes before entering Bowman's space. The role played by the slit pore and its membrane in the filtration process is not known.

Mesangial cells are modified smooth muscle cells that are usually found between the basement membrane and the capillary endothelial cell. They perform two functions, one of which is phagocytosis. Foreign substances, cellular debris, etc., that find their way into the glomerulus are taken up by the mesangial cell and removed. In addition to this housekeeping-function, the mesangial cells are capable of contracting and thus reducing the cross-sectional area of the capillaries. As a result, they can play an important role in regulating GFR by altering the amount of capillary surface area available for filtration.

REGULATION OF RENAL BLOOD FLOW AND GFR

Under resting conditions, renal blood flow (RBF) is 20% of the cardiac output or approximately 1,200 ml/minute. Although this is far more than the kidneys need to meet their metabolic needs, the kidneys do require a significant amount of oxygen. Almost 10% of the basal oxygen used by the body is consumed by the kidneys in transporting materials across the epithelial walls of the nephrons. Flow through the outer cortex of the kidneys is greater than that through the inner cortex, which in turn is greater than that through the medulla. Since the number of glomeruli in the outer regions of the kidneys exceeds that in the inner regions, it is likely that the amount of blood per glomerulus is fairly constant throughout the kidneys. When blood flow through the kidneys is reduced, as for example during hemorrhage, blood is shunted from the cortex to the medulla, where the glomeruli with long loops of Henle are located. This presumably preserves the kidneys' ability to concentrate the urine despite a reduction in total RBF.

RBF can be autoregulated. That is, RBF remains constant in the face of large changes in arterial pressure (Fig. 2-41). When blood pressure falls, the afferent arteriole dilates to increase the percent of the cardiac output entering the kidney whereas an increase in blood pressure is met by an increase in the resistance of the afferent arteriole. Two general explanations have been offered to explain autoregulation.

The myogenic theory proposes that the smooth muscle of the afferent arteriole is sensitive to stretch. When perfusion pressures increase, the afferent arteriole responds to being stretched by contracting; when perfusion pressures decrease, the afferent arteriole relaxes. These changes in smooth muscle tone maintain blood flow at a constant level. The metabolic theory proposes that a reduction in blood flow causes the buildup or release of a vasodilatory substance and that an increase in perfusion washes these metabolites away, restoring normal blood flow. It has been difficult to identify the metabolic mediator for autoregulation; prostaglandins, adenosine, and various kinins are among the most likely candidates.

Despite the ability of the kidney to autoregulate its blood flow, blood flow through the kidney can change under a variety of physiological conditions. For example, RBF is reduced when an individual is frightened, is in pain, or is hemorrhaging. These changes are made possible by the rich innervation of the afferent and efferent arterioles by the sympathetic nervous system and the presence of angiotension II receptors on these arterioles.

Even more important than regulation of RBF is the

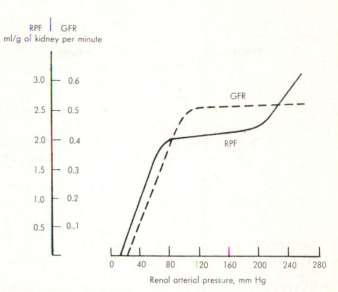

Figure 2-41. Renal blood flow is kept constant over a wide range of renal artery pressures by a variety of autoregulatory mechanisms. Glomerular filtration rate can be autoregulated over an even wider range of arterial pressures.

regulation of GFR. Under normal circumstances, GFR is 125 ml/minute. This value is maintained despite variations in RBF (Fig. 2-41). The kidney maintains its function even when presented with a reduced amount of blood. Three factors are important in determining GFR: RBF, glomerular capillary pressure, and the filtration coefficient (K) of the glomerular capillaries.

As discussed above, the removal of water from the glomerulus by filtration increases the capillary oncotic pressure and thus reduces the net outward filtration. When oncotic pressure equals net outward hydrostatic pressure, filtration equilibrium is said to occur and further filtration ceases. If the filtration fraction (GFR/renal plasma flow) reaches 33%, filtration equilibrium will occur. Under these conditions, an increase in RBF will cause a corresponding increase in GFR. However, when the filtration fraction is less than 30% (as it is in humans), filtration equilibrium does not occur and increases in RBF result in a decrease in filtration fraction. Under these conditions, increases in RBF have much less of an effect on GFR.

However, even small changes in capillary pressure have a profound effect on GFR because the net filtration pressure is very small. The magnitude of the capillary pressure depends on the perfusing pressure and the ratio of afferent and efferent arteriole resistances. If afferent arteriole resistance decreases or efferent arteriole resistance increases, capillary pressure increases. In contrast, an increase in afferent arteriole resistance or a decrease in efferent arteriole resistance causes a decrease in capillary pressure. When blood flow to the kidney is decreased or increased, capillary pressure is maintained at a normal value by the appropriate changes in afferent and efferent arteriole resistance. These changes in arteriolar resistance are mediated by a number of phenomena that still are not well understood. Tubuloglomerular feedback is one of these mechanisms. It is thought that an increase in the flow of filtrate through the macula densa region of the distal tubule causes the release of hormone, which causes a decrease in GFR by constricting the afferent arteriole or dilating the efferent arteriole or a combination of both. Although angiotensin is often cited as the mediator of tubuloglomerular feedback, recent evidence has called this into question and the identity of the mediator is not really known.

As indicated above, the filtration coefficient (K) of the glomerulus can be influenced by the actions of the mesangial cells. Angiotension II is one of the most potent stimulators of mesangial cell contraction. Renin can be released from the JGA by any of the mechanisms described above or by any cellular process involving the release of prostaglandin I_2 (PGI_2) or PGE_2. Renin activates angiotensinogen, producing angiotensin I, which is then converted to angiotensin II by a converting enzyme present within the kidney parenchyma. The angiotensin II causes the mesangial cells to contract. This results in a decrease in glomerular capillary area and a reduction in GFR. Epinephrine and antidiuretic hormone also cause mesangial cell contraction and may also play a role in the autoregulation of GFR.

MEASUREMENT OF RBF AND GFR

Renal blood flow and GFR are measured by the clearance technique. Clearance is a measure of how effectively a particular substance is removed (cleared) from the plasma as it passes through the kidney. It is measured by determining how much plasma per minute (or hour or day) is totally cleared of the substance. For example, if all of a particular substance is removed from the plasma as it passes through the kidney, the clearance of that substance is equal to the renal plasma flow (RPF). If half of it is removed, the clearance is equal to one-half of the RPF. The important point to emphasize is that the unit of clearance is flow and not volume or mass.

Para-aminohippuric acid (PAH) is almost totally removed from the plasma as it passes through the kidney, so its clearance is equal to the RPF. The formula for calculating the clearance of any substance is as follows:

$$C = \frac{U \times \dot{V}}{P}$$

where C = clearance, U = urinary concentration of the substance, $\dot{V}$ = the rate of urine formation, and P = plasma concentration of the substance. This formula is derived from the principle of mass conservation. That is, the amount of material appearing in the urine (U × V) must be equal to the amount of mass cleared from the blood (C × P). Thus if the material is synthesized or degraded by the kidney, the clearance of the material will be over- or underestimated, respectively.

The RBF can be calculated from the RPF if the hematocrit (Hct) is known using the following formula:

$$RBF = \frac{RPF}{1 - Hct}$$

For example, to measure RBF, PAH is infused until its concentration reaches a steady-state value, typically 0.05

mg/ml. If a urine sample is found to contain 20 mg/ml when the flow rate is 2 ml/minute, then

$$RPF = \frac{U_{PAH} \times \dot{V}}{P_{PAH}}$$

$$= \frac{15 \text{ mg/ml} \times 2 \text{ ml/min}}{0.05 \text{ mg/ml}}$$

$$= 600 \text{ ml/min}$$

Then, assuming a typical hematocrit of 0.45,

$$RBF = \frac{600}{1 - 0.45} = 1090 \text{ ml/min}$$

The GFR can be measured by calculating the clearance of a substance such as insulin or creatinine, which are neither reabsorbed nor secreted by the kidney. That is, the amount of the material entering the nephron by filtration is exactly equal to the amount of material that appears in the urine. Thus, from the principle of mass conservation,

$$GFR \times Pin = Uin \times \dot{V}$$

where Pin and Uin are the plasma and urine concentrations of inulin, respectively.

Solving for GFR yields

$$\frac{Uin \times \dot{V}}{P}$$

which of course is the formula for the clearance of inulin.

Inulin is a small polysaccharide and is ideal for the measurement of GFR because absolutely no reabsorption or secretion of inulin occurs, it is not bound in any way to plasma proteins, it is freely filtered through the glomerulus, and it is not metabolized at all by the kidneys. It is the substance of choice for clinical or experimental studies where accuracy is at a premium. However, inulin is expensive, difficult to measure in the laboratory, and must be continuously administered to patients intravenously to establish a steady-state plasma level. Thus for routine clinical studies, the clearance of creatinine is used. This substance is somewhat secreted by the kidneys and cannot be measured precisely. However, it is produced a constant rate by muscle metabolism and thus has a steady plasma concentration. Also because it is continuously produced, its 24-hour excretion rate can be estimated as 20 mg/kg of lean body mass. This allows the clinician to estimate whether a patient told to collect a 24-hour urine sample has followed instructions. For example, a 70-kg male should produce approximately 1.5 g of creatinine daily. If the urine contains much less than this, an incomplete urine sample should be suspected.

PROXIMAL TUBULE

The ultrafiltrate flows out of the glomerular capillary through Bowman's space and across the epithelial lining of

Bowmans's capsule to enter the proximal tubule. The first half of the proximal tubule (pars convoluta) forms a series of bends, while the latter half (pars recta) is straight. The epithelial cells lining both sections of the proximal tubule are characterized by an extensive brush border composed of microvilli. These microvilli greatly expand the surface area of the cells and contain a variety of enzymes, such as carbonic anhydrase, that are vital for normal renal function. The individual epithelial cells are connected to each other by tight junctions at the luminal surface and are separated from each other by a basolateral space at the peritubular surface. The cells along the proximal tubule are different from each other anatomically and have been divided into three sections labeled P1, P2, and P3. These sections are also different functionally. For example, most of the glucose reabsorbed by the proximal tubule occurs in the P1 segment, whereas most of the PAH is secreted into the proximal tubule in the P2 segment.

The proximal tubule actively reabsorbs many of the substances within the ultrafiltrate. Among the most important of these are sodium, glucose, amino acids, bicarbonate, potassium, phosphate, and calcium. Water is reabsorbed along with these substances in order to maintain osmotic equilibrium, while substances such as urea and chloride that are dissolved in the ultrafiltrate are reabsorbed by solvent drag.

Altogether the proximal tubules reabsorb approximately two-thirds of the salt and water presented to them. The reabsorption is termed **isosmotic** because water always follows at a rate sufficient to maintain osmotic equilibrium. The reabsorption of other substances such as glucose and bicarbonate, which have their own transport systems, is independent of salt and water reabsorption.

SODIUM REABSORPTION

Regulation of extracellular sodium content is important because the volume of the extracellular fluid is directly related to sodium content. Consequently the amount of sodium reabsorbed must be accurately controlled. This control is carried out in the distal tubule and will be covered in detail later. Reabsorption in the proximal tubules is obligatory and amounts to approximately two-thirds of the filtered sodium. Most of the sodium is reabsorbed by the sodium-potassium ATPase active transport system. Sodium flows across the luminal membrane of the epithelial cell, down its concentration gradient, and is then pumped out of the cell by Na-K ATPase transporters on the basolateral membrane of the epithelial cell. As indicated above, water follows the reabsorption of sodium by osmosis. Although the mechanism is not entirely understood, it is thought that sodium pumped out of the epithelial cells accumulates in the basolateral spaces, creating an osmotic gradient between the luminal and peritubular fluids. Most of the water flows through the cells, not because the cell membranes are extraordinarily permeable to water but because of the high surface area of the cells compared with the tight junctions between the cells. Once within the basolateral spaces, the salt and water flow into the peritubular capillaries and are returned to the general circulation.

The same Starling forces involved in forming the ultrafiltrate are involved in moving the salt and water from the basolateral spaces into the peritubular capillaries. The oncotic pressure in the peritubular fluid is much higher and the hydrostatic pressure much lower than in the glomerulus. As a result, the net pressure favors reabsorption. These forces also participate in matching the amount of salt and water reabsorbed to the amount filtered. For example, if an increase in glomerular pressure causes an increase in GFR and filtration fraction, the oncotic pressure in the peritubular capillaries would be higher and the hydrostatic pressure lower than normal. These forces would increase the reabsorption from the proximal tubule. Similarly, a decrease in GFR and filtration fraction would cause oncotic pressure to be lower and hydrostatic pressure to be higher, reducing the amount of salt and water reabsorbed from the proximal tubule. This process, called **glomerulotubular balance,** keeps proximal tubular reabsorption at two-thirds of the filtered load.

In addition to maintaining isotonicity, electroneutrality must also be preserved. In the early part of the convoluted tubule, most of the filtered bicarbonate is reabsorbed by a process coupled to the secretion of hydrogen. Since bicarbonate is negatively charged, it is coupled to sodium, and chloride is not reabsorbed. Consequently, as water leaves the proximal tubule, chloride concentration rises. In the distal portions of the proximal tubule, chloride flows through the tight junctions down its electrochemical gradient. Sodium follows passively to preserve electroneutrality. Approximately 25% of the sodium reabsorbed in the proximal tubule is reabsorbed by this process.

The tight junctions in the proximal tubule are relatively leaky. As a result, differences in sodium concentration between the luminal and peritubular fluids cannot be maintained. Normally, this is not a problem because the osmotic flow of water out of the proximal tubule keeps the luminal and peritubular sodium concentrations equal. However, if the concentration of sodium within the proximal tubule falls below that in the peritubular fluid, back-leak of sodium will occur. This situation can arise when there are nonreabsorbable solutes within the filtrate. For example, if mannitol (a nonreabsorbable sugar) is administered or if the reabsorption of bicarbonate is inhibited by a drug or the concentration of glucose in the filtrate exceeds the transport capability of the proximal tubule (see below), the amount of water reabsorbed from the proximal tubule will not be sufficient to maintain equality between luminal and peritubular fluids. As a result, luminal sodium concentration falls, back-leak occurs, and the amount of sodium reabsorbed decreases.

The rate of back-leak, for a given concentration gradient, depends on the permeability of the tight junctions to sodium. As indicated above, this is quite high in the proximal tubule so the amount of back-leak can be significant. Because the amount of sodium reabsorbed by the proximal tubule is limited by the concentration gradient that can be sustained, its transport is called **gradient limited.** If the sodium concentration within the lumen falls below 100 mmol/L net reabsorption ceases. That is, the maximum concentration that can be produced between the lumen and peritubular fluids is approximately 40 to 50 mmol/L. When nonreabsorbable solutes reduce the ability of the kidney to reabsorb water, diuresis (excess water excretion) occurs. This type of diuresis is called an osmotic diuresis because it is produced by osmotically active particles that retain water in the proximal tubule.

GLUCOSE AND AMINO ACID REABSORPTION

Almost all of the glucose and amino acids filtered into the proximal tubule are reabsorbed. The reabsorption is carried out by a sodium-dependent indirect active transport process. The carrier proteins are located on the luminal and brush border membranes. When sodium binds to the glucose carrier, the carrier's affinity for glucose increases. After both molecules bind to the carrier, the carrier undergoes a still poorly understood conformation change during which the binding sites are exposed to the interior of the cell. Sodium then detaches from the carrier, the carrier's affinity for glucose is reduced, and glucose detaches from the carrier. Glucose leaves the cell, across the peritubular membrane down its concentration gradient by facilitated diffusion. The carrier responsible for aiding the diffusion of glucose from the cell is identical to carriers on other cells, such as the red blood cell, which normally aid in the movement of glucose into the cell. A similar process is involved in the reabsorption of amino acids. Each carrier is fairly specific for only a few substances. For example, the glucose carrier will bind D-glucose and D-galactose but not mannitol, D-fructose, or L-glucose. Similarly, specific carriers for neutral, basic, and acidic amino acids have been identified.

The energy for the transport of glucose and amino acids comes from the sodium gradient established by ATP hydrolysis. In the early part of the proximal tubule, when the glucose concentration in the filtrate is still high, only one sodium ion is needed to supply the transport energy. However, at the end of the proximal tubule, when the last bit of glucose is reabsorbed, two molecules of sodium bind to the carrier. In either case, sodium reabsorption in conjunction with glucose and amino acids is significant, accounting for approximately 25% of the sodium reabsorbed by the proximal tubule.

In contrast to the active reabsorption of sodium, which was characterized as gradient limited, glucose, amino acid, and other carrier-mediated reabsorptive and secretory processes are characterized as transport limited. Figure 2-42 illustrates the effect that increasing plasma concentrations of glucose has on filtration, reabsorption, and excretion. The filtered load of glucose increases in proportion to the plasma concentration. The carrier can initially handle all of the glucose presented to it. However, as the amount of filtered glucose increases, the ability of the carriers to transport it decreases. The carriers eventually become fully saturated, and any additional glucose entering the proximal tubule is excreted in the urine. No significant reabsorption occurs after the filtrate leaves the proximal tubule.

The transport maximum (Tm) for glucose is approximately 375 mg/minute. Assuming a normal GFR of 125 ml/minute, the Tm is achieved at a plasma glucose concentration of 300 mg/100 ml. However, as can be seen in Figure 2-42, glucose appears in the urine at a plasma concentration of 200 mg/100 ml. This value, the plasma concentration at which a substance reabsorbed by a Tm-limited system first appears in the urine, is called the renal threshold for the transport process. The failure of the carrier to remove all of the glucose before its Tm is reached is called **splay**. Splay occurs for two reasons. The first is termed heterogeneity—that is, not all nephrons are alike. Some have a Tm less than 375 mg/minute and some have more. Glucose entering the nephrons with lower than average Tm appears in the urine before all of the kidneys' carriers are

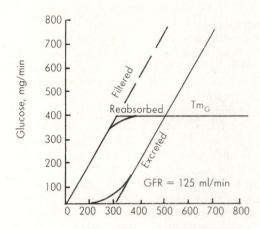

Figure 2-42. Glucose is reabsorbed by a transport maximum (Tm) limited carrier system. There are enough carriers on the proximal tubular membrane to reabsorb about 375 mg of glucose per minute. If more than this amount of glucose (the Tm) is delivered to the proximal tubule, the carriers will be saturated and the excess glucose will be excreted in the urine. Glucose actually appears in the urine before the carriers are saturated. The plasma concentration at which glucose is not totally reabsorbed (and thus appears in the urine) is called the renal threshold.

saturated. The other mechanism is based on the law of mass action. Before glucose can be transported, it must bind to the carrier. This follows first-order kinetics:

$$\text{Glu} + \text{Carrier} \rightleftharpoons \text{Glu} - \text{Carrier}$$

Regardless of the affinity of the carrier for glucose, the concentration of glucose must exceed that of the carrier before all of the carriers are saturated. Consequently, some glucose will remain in the filtrate and be excreted even though the glucose concentration is less than the Tm.

The normal plasma concentration of glucose is between 80 and 120 mg/100 ml. In diabetes mellitus, the inability to metabolize glucose causes plasma concentrations to rise significantly. If plasma glucose exceeds the renal threshold, glucose will appear in the urine. If too much glucose remains within the proximal tubule, it will cause an osmotic diuresis and compromise the kidneys' ability to regulate the extracellular fluid.

REABSORPTION OF PHOSPHATE, CALCIUM, AND MAGNESIUM

Inorganic phosphate is necessary for a large number of physiological processes including energy storage (as ATP, creatinine phosphate, etc.), acid-base balance (as a urinary buffer), and bone metabolism (as a calcium-phosphate complex). A normal diet usually contains more phosphate than required to sustain homeostatis. As a result, some 90% of the 1 g usually ingested is excreted each day.

The major site of phosphate reabsorption is the proximal tubule. Reabsorption occurs via a sodium-dependent cotransport process exhibiting a Tm. Unlike the situation with glucose, in which the Tm was far above the normal plasma concentration, the Tm for phosphate is just above the normal plasma concentration of 1.2 mmol. Thus, if phosphate concentration falls below normal all of the filtered load is reabsorbed, whereas if plasma phosphate rises above normal the excess is excreted in the urine. The difference in the renal handling of glucose and phosphate reflects the differences in their metabolism. Under normal circumstances, all of the glucose digested is either used, stored, or converted to fat. Phosphate on the other hand cannot be efficiently stored, and any excess must be excreted.

The carrier for phosphate reabsorption is localized in the brush border of the proximal tubule. At a urinary pH of 6.8, half of the phosphate exists as $HPO_4^=$ and the remainder as $H_2PO_4^-$. The carrier is only able to bind with the divalent $HPO_4^=$ and has two binding sites for sodium, both of which must be occupied for phosphate transport to occur. Once inside the cell, phosphate diffuses through the basolateral membrane down its electrochemical gradient. It is not yet known whether this is a simple diffusion through pores or a facilitated diffusion requiring a carrier. Because the percentage of phosphate in the $HPO_4^=$ form is pH dependent, a decrease in pH will decrease phosphate reabsorption by converting $HPO_4^=$ to $H_2PO_4^-$. In addition, increasing hydrogen ion concentration inhibits phosphate reabsorption because the excess hydrogen ions compete with sodium for one of the binding sites on the carrier. As will be discussed later, the pH dependence of phosphate reabsorption enhances the ability of phosphate to act as a urinary buffer.

Phosphate reabsorption is also regulated by parathyroid hormone (PTH). PTH binds to a site on the peritubular membrane of the proximal tubular cell and initiates a sequence of events that leads to a decrease in phosphate reabsorption. The PTH-receptor complex activates a regulatory protein, which in turn activates a membrane-bound adenylate cyclase, which promotes the formation of cyclic AMP. The cAMP diffuses through the cell to activate a series of kinases, which by some poorly understood manner inhibit the phosphate carrier. Calcitonin also causes a decrease in phosphate reabsorption and an increase in phosphate excretion. This effect is most likely secondary to the reduction in plasma calcium concentration caused by calcitonin. That is, the reduced calcium concentrations causes an increased secretion of PTH, which then acts to impede phosphate reabsorption. Calcitonin and hypocalcemia may both directly reduce phosphate reabsorption. However, these effects are considered to be small compared with the action of PTH. Changes in diet can influence phosphate reabsorption independently of PTH. If dietary intake of phosphate is reduced, reabsorption increases; if dietary intake is increased, reabsorption decreases. The change in phosphate handling appears to result from a change in the rate of carrier activity rather than from an increase or decrease in the number of carrier sites. However, it is not yet clear how this effect is accomplished.

Calcium homeostasis depends much more on bone metabolism than on renal function. However, the amount of calcium absorbed from the GI tract is very low, and thus almost all of the filtered calcium must be reabsorbed to maintain normal calcium stores. Most of the filtered calcium is reabsorbed in the proximal tubule in one of two ways. Either calcium passively enters the cell down its electrochemical gradient or is reabsorbed along with water by solvent drag. The calcium entering the tubular cells is pumped out on the basolateral side by a calcium-ATPase or a Na-Ca exchange system. In either case, the amount of calcium reabsorbed is dependent on the amount of sodium and water reabsorbed. Consequently, diuresis inhibits and volume contraction enhances calcium reabsorption.

PTH enhances distal tubular calcium reabsorption. Thus a decrease in plasma calcium stimulates PTH release, which in turn increases reabsorption of calcium from the distal tubule. In contrast, the reduction of PTH following a rise in plasma calcium concentration causes a decrease in calcium reabsorption. The resulting increase in calcium excretion restores the plasma calcium to normal.

Magnesium handling by the kidneys is somewhat unusual in that only about 30% of the filtered load is reabsorbed in the proximal tubules. Although reabsorption is thought to occur by solvent drag, the low permeability of magnesium to the tight junctions reduces the amount that can cross the nephron wall. The major site of magnesium reabsorption is the ascending limbs of the loops of Henle. Approximately 60% of the filtered load is reabsorbed in the loops. Although the mechanism of reabsorption is not known, it appears that whatever regulation occurs is brought about by altering the amount of magnesium reabsorbed from the loops of Henle.

SECRETION OF ORGANIC IONS

The kidneys secrete a wide variety of organic ions such as hippuric acid, bile salts, and uric acid that are produced as a by-product of metabolic activity. In addition, the plasma concentration of many drugs such as aspirin and penicillin is determined, in part, by how rapidly they are cleared from the blood by the kidney. Most, if not all, of this secretory activity takes place in the proximal tubule. The model for organic anion transport is the secretion of PAH, the substance whose clearance is an accurate reflection of renal plasma flow. Although the exact mechanism is not known, it is thought that PAH, after being actively secreted across the basolateral membrane, diffuses through the cell and is then transported across the luminal membrane by a carrier-mediated process. Endogenous cations such as acetylcholine, epinephrine, and serotonin, plus a variety of positively charged drugs, are secreted by the kidneys in a similar manner. Because these substances are secreted from the plasma by a Tm-limited transport mechanism, their clearance can be altered by changes in plasma concentration.

OTHER SUBSTANCES

The proximal tubules are also involved in the handling of other important constituents of the plasma, including urea, potassium, bicarbonate, and hydrogen. The discussion of these substances will be taken up in later sections of this chapter.

THE LOOPS OF HENLE

The loop of Henle is divided into a descending limb, a thin ascending limb, and a thick ascending limb (see Fig. 2-39). The pars recta of the juxtamedullary nephrons merges with the thin descending limb of the loop of Henle at the border of the inner and outer stripes of the outer medulla. The transition between the proximal tubule and loop of Henle in the cortical nephrons is not as clearly marked. The thin limbs of the loops of Henle are composed of small epithelial cells having a paucity of mitochondria. Although there are differences in the structure of the cells along the thin limbs, they are not sufficiently correlated with the markedly different functions of the ascending and descending limbs to warrant description. The thin ascending limb of the long loops of Henle (those arising from the juxtamedullary nephrons) give rise to the thick ascending limb at the border between the outer and inner medulla.

As was the case for the border between the proximal tubule and loop of Henle, the border between the thin and thick ascending limbs of the cortical nephrons varies with the length of the nephron, usually occurring in the region of the hairpin at the bottom of the loop. The major morphological characteristic of the epithelial cells making up the thick ascending limb is the presence of numerous mitochondria, which, as will be discussed shortly, provide the energy required for the active reabsorption of sodium chloride from the loop of Henle.

The thick ascending limb of the loop of Henle is actually the first component of the distal tubule. It begins abruptly at the outer medulla (where the thin ascending limb ends) and terminates in the cortex, where it gives rise to the macula densa. However, its function within the medulla is sufficiently different from its role in the cortex for us to consider the role of the thick ascending limb separately from that of the distal tubule.

COUNTERCURRENT MULTIPLICATION

The loop of Henle is able to perform its role in concentrating and diluting the urine because of the countercurrent arrangement of its ascending and descending limbs and because of the differences in the transport characteristics of the epithelial cells lining the two limbs. These characteristics produce a gradient in the osmolarity of the medullary interstitium that increases along its length from approximately 285 mOsm/L at its border with the cortex to 1,200 to 1,400 mOsm/L at the tip of its papilla. At the same time, the filtrate is diluted by the loop of Henle so that when it enters the distal tubule, its osmolarity is approximately 200 mOsm/L. This section describes how these two tasks are accomplished.

The filtrate entering the loop of Henle is isosmotic with the surrounding interstitium because the high water permeability of the proximal tubule epithelial cells permits complete osmotic equilibrium to occur. The descending limb is also highly permeable to water so osmotic equilibrium between it and the surrounding interstitium is also established. However, the ascending limbs (both thin and thick) are not permeable to water. Thus if sodium chloride is removed from the ascending limb, water cannot follow and the filtrate can become diluted.

Sodium chloride is actively pumped out of the thick ascending limb and enters the medullary interstitium in step 1 of the countercurrent multiplication process. Because water cannot follow, the filtrate is diluted (Fig. 2-43). Water flows out of the thin ascending limb to achieve osmotic equilibrium with the interstitium. Thus the end result of the transport process is to increase the osmolarity of the interstitium and descending limb and to decrease the osmolarity of the ascending limb. The 200 mOsm/L gradient between the interstitial and tubular osmolarity is possible because the tight junctions between the

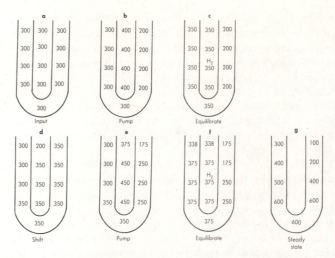

Figure 2-43. (*A*) The countercurrent multiplier in the loop of Henle is responsible for increasing the osmolarity of the medullary interstitium. (*B*) The NaCl pump on the thick ascending limb creates a gradient of 200 mOsm between the ascending limb and the interstitium. (*C*) The hyperosmotic interstitium equilibrates with the filtrate in the descending limb. (*D*) Additional filtrate enters the descending limb, and the same process repeats itself. However, because the filtrate within the deeper portions of the ascending limb is higher than before, the osmotic gradient is now higher. These steps are repeated until the salt concentration at the tip of the medulla reaches 600 mOsm. Multiplication can occur because the ascending limb is impermeable to water.

epithelial cells of the thick ascending limb do not permit much back-leak to occur. The sodium chloride transport process is more complicated than that described for the proximal tubule and will be discussed later.

This initial transport step is not sufficient to create the high osmolarity present at the tip of the medulla. In step 2 (Fig. 2-43), additional filtrate enters the loop of Henle, pushing the concentrated fluid from the deeper portions of the medulla into the thick ascending limb. The transport system again pumps sodium chloride out of the filtrate until a gradient of 200 mOsm/L is established. Again water flows out of the descending limb into the interstitium, until osmotic equilibrium is reached. Note that the interstitial osmolarity is now higher than it was in step 1. This process is repeated until a steady state is achieved. The osmolarity achieved at the tip of the medulla is a function of the length of the loops of Henle. Thus only the juxtamedullary nephrons participate in this process.

ROLE OF UREA IN URINE CONCENTRATION

Since the thin ascending limb epithelial cells do not contain mitochondria, it is assumed that they do not actively transport sodium chloride. However, the thin ascending limbs are able to participate in the countercurrent process because of the difference in urea permeability that exits in the various segments of the nephron. Urea is highly permeable to the proximal tubule epithelium and so passively follows the reabsorption of water by solvent drag. However, the concentration of urea entering the loop of Henle is higher than in the proximal tubule and may even exceed the filtered load of urea. The high urea concentration develops, in part, because the blood leaving the medulla in the vasa recta has a high urea concentration and it equilibrates with the filtrate entering the loop. Additionally, there is some evidence that urea may be actively secreted into the pars recta and that urea may flow from the urine in the pelvis, where it is highly concentrated, into the distal portions of the proximal tubule.

The descending limb is not very permeable to urea, so any changes in urea concentration are largely due to the flow of water out of the descending limb. Similarly, the ascending limb, the distal tubule, the connecting segment, and the outer collecting duct are not permeable to urea, so any urea entering the loop of Henle remains there until the distal portion of the collecting duct is reached. Here, urea permeability increases and urea flows from the nephron into the interstitium. The amoung of urea leaving the inner medullary collecting duct depends, of course, on how concentrated it is; this in turn depends on how much water has been removed from the nephron in the collecting duct. The control of water removal from the collecting duct will be discussed shortly. For now, the important point is that urea can diffuse out of the inner medullary collecting duct and maintain a high urea concentration in the medullary interstitium.

Recall that water flows out of the descending limb until osmotic equilibrium between the tubular fluid and the interstitium is reached. Because the descending limb is poorly permeable to urea, the presence of a high urea concentration in the interstitium contributes to the osmotic flow of water. As a result, the sodium chloride concentration in the filtrate rises above that in the interstitium. Now, when the filtrate enters the ascending limb, where water is not permeable, sodium chloride diffuses out of the thin ascending limb down its concentration gradient. Thus the thin ascending limb can participate in the countercurrent multiplication process despite its inability to actively transport sodium chloride.

THE VASA RECTA

The vasa recta are peritubular capillaries arising from the efferent arteriole that follow the loop of Henle into the medulla. They perform two essential functions. One is to remove all the solute and water reabsorbed from the nephrons in the medulla. The other is to preserve the high concentration of salt and urea created by the countercurrent multiplication system. The plasma entering the medulla is isosmotic with the systemic circulation. As the blood flows through the descending limb of the vasa recta, it equilibrates with the surrounding interstitium, reaching its greatest osmolarity at the tip of the loop of Henle. As the blood leaves the medulla in the ascending limb of the vasa recta, it passes through regions of lower and lower osmolarity. Water consequently enters and sodium leaves the vasa recta in an attempt to reach osmotic and diffusional equilibrium. The osmotic gradient from the outer to inner medulla is preserved because almost all of the salt that enters the vasa recta as it descends into the medulla is returned to the medulla as the blood leaves. Actually, the amount of water leaving the medulla in the vasa recta is greater than the amount that entered because the vasa recta remove the water reabsorbed from the collecting ducts. Similarly, the amount of sodium chloride leaving the medulla exceeds the amount entering, again because the vasa recta remove the salt reabsorbed from the nephron in the medulla. Since the amount of salt reabsorbed exceeds the amount of water reabsorbed, the plasma in the vasa recta leaving the medulla is hyperosmotic to the plasma entering.

EXCRETION OF A DILUTE OR CONCENTRATED URINE

The filtrate leavng the loop of Henle is hyposmotic to plasma. In the absence of antidiuretic hormone (more correctly called arginine vasopressin), the remainder of the nephron is impermeable to water. As a result, the urine excreted by the kidney is hypotonic. In the presence of antidiuretic hormone (ADH), the cortical and medullary collecting ducts become permeable to water and the filtrate can reach osmotic equilibrium with the surrounding interstitium. If maximal amounts of ADH are present, the osmolarity of the excreted urine can be as high as 1,400 mOsm, the same as the osmolarity at the tip of the medulla. Normally there is always some ADH circulating in the plasma, and so the osmolarity of the urine ranges between 200 and 1,400 mOsm. The mechanisms controlling the release of ADH and its mechanism of action will be discussed in a later section.

REABSORPTION OF SOLUTE BY THE LOOP OF HENLE

The loop of Henle reabsorbs approximately 25% of the filtered load of sodium, chloride, and potassium and, as mentioned above, about 60% of the filtered load of magnesium. Some of the sodium chloride is reabsorbed passively from the thin ascending limb. The remainder is actively reabsorbed from the thick ascending limb. The carrier on the luminal membrane is quite elaborate, containing two binding sites for chloride and one each for sodium and potassium. All four binding sites must be occupied for the carrier to operate. Once filled, the carrier undergoes a conformational change, transporting all four ions into the epithelial cell. The sodium is then removed from the cell by a Na-K ATPase on the peritubular surface, and the other ions follow down their electrochemical gradients. It is not clear whether they diffuse out of the cell through pores or are carried across by a facilitated diffusional process.

Although the transport process is electrically neutral, it results in a potential difference between the luminal fluid and the surrounding interstitial fluid. This potential creates an electrochemical gradient favorable to the flow of positive ions out of the nephron. It is assumed that magnesium and calcium reabsorption in the thick ascending limb is driven by this potential difference. The flow of these ions through the tight junctions between the epithelial cells is energetically more efficient than a transcellular route because the latter would require an active transport system to remove the ions from the cell.

THE DISTAL NEPHRON

The distal nephron consists of the distal tubule, the connecting segment, and the cortical and medullary collecting ducts. Strictly speaking, the distal tubule consists of the thick ascending limb of the loop of Henle, the macula densa, and the distal convoluted tubule. The ascending limb and macula densa have been described above. The distal convoluted tubule and connecting segment serve as a transition between the loop of Henle and the cortical collecting duct. Like the thick ascending limb, they are impermeable to water and reabsorb sodium. However, they contribute quantitatively little to the overall reabsorptive and secretory capacity of the kidney and their activity is not regulated. For example, unlike the remainder of the distal nephron, the water permeability of the distal tubule is not affected by ADH and its rate of sodium reabsorption is not influenced by aldosterone.

The collecting duct is divided into a cortical and medullary component, the medullary component being further divided into an outer and inner medullary collecting duct. Urine leaving the inner medullary collecting duct enters the ducts of Bellini, which drain into the renal pelvis. Two different cell types have been identified within the collect ducts: the principal (or light cell) and the intercalated (or dark cell). Recent evidence suggests that the principal cell is primarily responsible for the reabsorption of sodium and secretion of potassium by the collecting ducts while the intercalated cell is responsible for the secretion of hydrogen. The role played by the collecting ducts in sodium, water, and potassium balance will be discussed below. Acid secretion will be discussed in the section on acid-base balance.

SODIUM AND WATER BALANCE

Both the volume and osmolarity of the extracellular fluid must be maintained within a narrow range if normal physiological functions are to be performed. For example, adequate blood pressure and perfusion of various organs are dependent on a normal circulating volume whereas osmolarities much different from the normal 285 mOsm will cause brain cells to shrink or swell, with potentially devastating consequences. The extracellular volume is regulated indirectly by regulating the amount of sodium excreted by the kidney, while the extracellular osmolarity is regulated by adjusting the amount of water excreted. Although most of the discussion will concern the role played by the kidney in salt and water balance, the role of salt appetite and thirst in regulating ingestion should not be ignored.

As discussed previously, two-thirds of the sodium, chloride, and water filtered into the kidney is reabsorbed in the proximal tubule. An additional 25% of the salt and water is reabsorbed in the loop of Henle (water in the descending limb and salt in the ascending limb). This reabsorption is obligatory and occurs independently of the volume or osmotic state of the individual. The remaining 8 to 10% of salt and water is handled by the distal tubule and is regulated by aldosterone and ADH.

THE RENIN-ANGIOTENSIN-ALDOSTERONE SYSTEM

The alteration in aldosterone release by the adrenal cortex in response to changes in salt content is mediated by the renin-angiotensin system. Renin is a proteolytic enzyme that breaks down angiotensinogen to form angiotensin I. A converting enzyme found primarily in the lungs (but also present in the kidneys) coverts angiotensin I to angiotensin II. Angiotensin stimulates the release of aldosterone from the adrenal cortex.

Renin is synthesized and stored in specialized cells of the portions of the afferent and efferent arterioles that form the JGA. It is released directly into the blood in response to a variety of stimuli related to the circulating blood volume. For

example, changing the hydrostatic pressure within the afferent arteriole alters the amount of renin released by the JGA cells. Renin release is increased by a decrease of pressure in the afferent arteriole (reflecting a decrease in blood volume) and decreased when perfusing pressure within the afferent arteriole increases. Renal arteriole stenosis resulting in a decrease in perfusion of the kidney will cause excessive release of renin, leading to a pathological increase in circulating blood volume and pressure.

Renin can also be released by the macula densa cells in the distal tubular portion of the JGA. However, the stimulus causing macula densa activity is not fully understood. When single nephrons are studied, it appears that increased delivery of fluid or salt to the distal tubule causes the release of renin. The renin acts locally on angiotensinogen to produce angiotensin I, which is then cleaved by renal converting enzyme to form angiotensin II. The angiotensin II then acts directly on the afferent and efferent arterioles to reduce blood flow and filtrate to that particular nephron. This may be one of the mechanisms by which tubuloglomerular feedback, discussed earlier, may operate. However, both adenosine and prostaglandins have also been implicated as mediators of glomerulotubular feedback. In contrast to the observations in single nephrons, renin concentrations are found to increase when plasma sodium content or volume falls. A mechanism to explain these conflicting observations has not yet been discovered. Further complicating a full understanding of how the macula densa controls renin release is the recent finding that prostaglandins are necessary for the macula densa-mediated release of renin.

Sympathetic nerve fibers innervate both the arteriole and tubular cells of the JGA and cause increased release of renin by activating beta receptors on these cells. These fibers are presumably the efferent limb of cardiovascular reflexes originating in the arterial baroreceptors and venous and atrial stretch receptors. Thus reduction in blood volume by hemorrhage or in blood pressure by sudden changes in posture will cause sympathetic activation and release of renin by the JGA. Even when the level of sympathetic activity is below that required to cause direct release of renin, it nonetheless influences the amount of renin released by enhancing the effectiveness of the afferent arteriole pressure receptors and the macula densa.

Once released into the bloodstream, renin digests angiotensinogen (a large alpha$_2$-globulin synthesized by the liver) to form angiotensin I. Angiotensin I converting enzyme (ACE) then cleaves the two C-terminal amino acids from the decapeptide angiotensin I to form the octapeptide angiotensin II. Almost all of the ACE is found on the endothelial surface of the pulmonary microvasculature. However, significant quantities of the enzyme have also been found within other organs, including the brain and kidney. ACE inhibitors, such as captopril, are used clinically to treat the effects of elevated plasma angiotensin II such as hypertension.

Angiotensin II binds to highly specific receptor sites on a number of tissues, producing a variety of physiological effects. In addition, angiotensin II is rapidly brought into the cell by endocytosis and thus may also act by affecting the synthesis of intracellularly produced proteins. Angiotensin II antagonists such as saralasin have not found wide clinical use because they must be given parenterally and their half-life is very short.

The primary function of the renin-angiotensin system is to increase total peripheral resistance and vascular volume in response to reductions in circulating blood volume or pressure. Any reduction in blood volume, such as that occurring in hemorrhage or as a consequence of diuretic therapy or as a result of dietary salt restriction, activates the renin-angiotensin system by one or more of the mechanisms discussed above. Under normal steady-state conditions, there is little or no stimulation of the renin-angiotensin system so increases in blood volume have little effect on blood pressure or salt excretion.

Angiotensin II increases vascular resistance by causing arteriolar smooth muscles to contract. This reaction, in conjunction with sympathetic stimulation, allows blood pressure to be maintained at near normal levels even in the presence of a large hemorrhagic loss of blood. The role of angiotensin II in maintaining blood pressure is even more important when vascular volume is reduced. That is, in the euvolemic individual, blood pressure can be maintained by the sympathetic nervous system alone, whereas in a volume-depleted individual, blood pressure falls dramatically during a hemorrhage if the vasoconstrictor effects of angiotensin II are blocked. Although all vascular smooth muscles have angiotensin II receptors, those that are most prominent are in the renal and mesenteric resistance vessels.

Angiotensin II protects the body against salt and water losses by reducing blood flow through the kidneys; by directly stimulating the reabsorption of sodium by the nephron and the absorption of sodium by the GI tract; by increasing thirst and salt appetite; and perhaps most importantly, by stimulating the release of aldosterone from the adrenal gland.

Although angiotensin II receptor sites are found on both the afferent and efferent arterioles of the kidney, they are most prominent on the efferent arterioles. As a result, release of angiotensin II in response to a fall in blood volume causes a larger decrease in RBF than in GFR. The resulting increase in filtration fraction causes a rise in peritubular capillary oncotic pressure and a fall in peritubular capillary hydrostatic pressure. These effects, by increasing the Starling forces favoring reabsorption, cause an increase in salt and water reabsorption from the proximal tubule. As indicated above, there is little or no spontaneous angiotensin II stimulation of the renal vascular bed, so increases in volume do not produce corresponding increases in RBF and GFR by inhibiting renin release.

The other major effect of angiotensin II is to cause the release of aldosterone from the adrenal cortex by activating an angiotensin II receptor on the adrenal glomerulosa cells. In addition, angiotensin II stimulates the production of angiotensin II receptors, enhancing the adrenal gland's ability to respond to salt and water loss during prolonged volume depletion.

Aldosterone is a steroid hormone synthesized and stored in the adrenal cortex. Like other steroids, it produces its effect by inducing the transcription of messenger RNA within the cell's nucleus. The messenger RNA in turn enters the cytoplasm, where ribosomes use it to produce physiologically active proteins. Aldosterone produces its major effect in the principal cells of the collecting ducts, where it increases the number of sodium channels on the luminal membrane. Sodium transport by the principal cells is increased initially because the increased number of sodium channels allows more sodium to flow into the cell from the luminal fluid. Because more sodium enters the cell, more can be pumped out by the Na-K ATPase pumps on the basolateral surface of the cells. In response to the additional activity of the pump (or perhaps as a subsequent effect of aldosterone stimulation), new pump sites are synthesized by the principal cells.

In addition, the cell develops invaginations that increase the area available for sodium transport and increased mitochondrial enzyme activity to support the higher level of sodium transport. Finally, aldosterone decreases the back-leak of sodium into the collecting duct, allowing a higher sodium gradient to be maintained between the luminal and peritubular fluids. In contrast to the case for angiotensin II, aldosterone must be tonically released from the adrenal glands to preserve sodium balance. Adrenalectomized animals or patients suffering from Addison's disease (in which there is a reduction of adrenal gland activity) lose salt at an alarming and potentially life-threatening rate.

Although the renin-angiotensin-aldosterone system plays a dominant role in the regulation of extracellular volume, Starling forces are also important in determining the amount of salt and water excreted by the kidney. Earlier, the concept of glomerulotubular balance was introduced. In this mechanism, alterations in peritubular capillary oncotic and hydrostatic pressures brought about by changes in GFR keep the fractional reabsorption of salt and water by the proximal tubule at a constant value. These forces also provide the kidney with the ability to increase its excretion of salt and water in response to an isotonic expansion of the extracellular fluid. The addition of water to the plasma reduces its oncotic pressure. At the same time, the excess extracellular fluid increases the interstitial hydrostatic pressure. Both of these Starling forces act to reduce the amount of salt and water reabsorbed by the proximal tubule and lead to a saline diuresis.

The reflexes functioning to control extracellular volume have their receptors in a variety of sites including the thoracic veins, the atria, the carotid and aortic arteries, and the afferent arterioles. Each of these receptors responds to a change in circulatory pressure or volume by eliciting a reflex adjustment of renal salt and water excretion. Increases in extracellular volume lead to an increased loss of salt and water in the urine, while decreases in extracellular volume lead to a decrease in salt and water excretion by the kidneys.

The effectors responsible for these changes in renal excretion have been discussed above and are included here in summary form. Sympathetic stimulation is increased by volume depletion and decreased by volume expansion. From a cardiovascular point of view, sympathetic stimulation in response to a decrease in blood volume or pressure causes an increase in cardiac output by increasing contractility, by increasing heart rate, and by reducing venous capacitance (thus shifting blood from the venous to the arterial system). From a renal point of view, sympathetic stimulation causes the release of renin and the activation of the angiotensin-aldosterone system. In addition, the sympathetics directly enhance sodium reabsorption from the nephron and increase filtration fraction, thus increasing the percent of filtered sodium reabsorbed in the proximal tubule.

An expansion of extracellular volume causes an increase in salt and water excretion by the kidneys. Since the tonic effects of sympathetic and angiotensin stimulation are not very great, their inhibition does not have a major effect on salt and water excretion. However, reducing aldosterone secretion is an important component of the response to volume expansion. Another potentially very important effector is atrial natriuretic factor (ANF). This peptide, released from the atria in response to an increase in circulating blood volume, has a direct salt-excreting effect on the nephron. In addition, it causes a relaxation of vascular smooth muscle and thus may also be involved in reducing blood pressure.

THE ANTIDIURETIC HORMONE SYSTEM

The osmolarity of the urine is determined by the plasma concentration of ADH. As indicated earlier, the water entering the distal nephron from the loop of Henle is hypotonic to plasma, having an osmolarity of approximately 100 mOsm. In the absence of ADH, the entire distal nephron is impermeable to water. Under these conditions, a large volume (in excess of 15 L/day) of dilute urine (less than 10 mOsm) will be excreted by the kidneys. When ADH is present, the collecting duct becomes highly permeable to water and osmotic equilibrium between the filtrate and interstitial fluid will be achieved. Under these conditions, a low volume (less than 600 ml/day) of highly concentrated urine (in excess of 1,200 mOsm) will be excreted. Normally, the amount of circulating ADH is regulated to maintain an extracellular osmolarity of approximately 285 mOsm/L.

ADH increases the permeability of the collecting duct to water by increasing the number of channels through which water can flow across the cell membrane. The sequence of events leading to an increased water permeability is initiated when ADH binds to specific receptors on the peritubular membrane of the collecting duct epithelial cells. When ADH binds to the receptor, an adenyate cyclase enzyme is activated, leading to the formation of cAMP from ATP. The cAMP diffuses to the luminal surface, where it induces the opening of water channels.

ADH is a nonapeptide that is synthesized by specialized cells in the paraventricular and supraoptic nuclei of the hypothalamus. It is then transported to the axon terminals of these neurons (which form the neurohypophysis or posterior pituitary gland) for storage. When the hypothalamic neurons are stimulated, they produce an action potential, which, when it reaches the axon terminal, increases the membrane permeability to calcium. Calcium enters the nerve terminal, causing the release of ADH by exocytosis.

The release of ADH from the neurohypophysis is directly related to the osmolarity of the blood plasma. In most individuals, no ADH is released until the plasma osmolarity exceeds 275 mOsm/L. ADH release then rises rapidly, reaching a maximum at approximately 320 mOsm/L. ADH is also released in response to a decrease in blood pressure or blood volume. This effect is presumably mediated by reflexes originating in volume receptors located in the large veins, the atria, and the carotid sinus and aortic arch baroreceptors. The amount of ADH released by large decreases in blood pressure or volume is much greater than the amount released by an osmotic stimulus. However, blood volume or pressure must be decreased by more than 10% before any ADH is released, whereas an increase in osmolarity of less than 0.5% will cause a significant release of ADH. Finally ADH can be released by a number of nonosmotic nonpressure stimuli such as nausea,

hypoglycemia, and stress. The later is a particularly potent stimulus for ADH and can be the cause of the syndrome of inappropriate ADH release (SIADH) that often follows surgical or other traumas if excessive intravenous fluids are administered.

Maintenance of water balance requires that water intake match water loss. Most healthy individuals ingest about 2.5 L of water each day (this includes the small amount [350 ml] of water produced by oxidative metabolism). Of this, approximately 1,500 ml is excreted as urine, 800 ml is lost as perspiration from the skin and as respiratory gas, and the remainder is excreted in the stool. Any changes in water intake or loss (e.g., from sweating or the GI tract) will result in a rapid alteration of urine output due to the release of ADH. The ability of the osmoregulatory system to withstand osmotic challenges is enormous. For example, as indicated above, reducing the osmolarity to less than 275 mOsm/L will completely inhibit the release of ADH. Under these conditions, all of the 15 L of water reaching the distal nephron will be excreted. Thus an individual will have to go to extreme lengths to ingest enough water to reduce his or her plasma osmolarity to dangerous levels. In contrast, increases in plasma osmolarity caused by excessive water loss elicit the sensation of thirst. Plasma osmolarities above 290 mOsm/L produce a powerful drive to ingest water. Thus individuals suffering from diabetes insipidus (inability to secrete or respond to ADH), who can excrete as much as 16 L of water per day, are able to maintain their plasma osmolarities at 290 mOsm/L by matching their input to their output.

Generally, the plasma osmolarity is maintained at approximately 285 mOsm/L, in between the osmotic threshold for the release of ADH and the initiation of thirst. This permits the ADH osmotic regulatory system to respond vigorously to either an increase or decrease in plasma osmolarity. For example, if plasma osmolarity is reduced by just 1%, the amount of circulating ADH will be halved and the urine flow doubled, quickly restoring osmolarity to normal.

POTASSIUM BALANCE

Extracellular potassium concentration is normally maintained at 4 to 5 mEq/L by the kidneys. Even small deviations from this value (lowering potassium concentration below 3 mEq/L or raising it above 8 mEq/L) can cause marked changes in nerve and muscle membrane resting potentials. These resting membrane potential changes can result in skeletal muscle weakness or paralysis and potentially life-threatening alterations in cardiac muscle excitability.

Most of the total body store of potassium (50 mEq/kg) is located intracellularly. Thus even small changes in total potassium can have a significant effect on extracellular stores. For example, a normal diet contains approximately 100 mEq of potassium. If all of this were added to the extracellular fluid, the extracellular concentration of potassium would be raised by over 7 mEq/L. Thus the daily amount of potassium absorbed from the GI tract must be rapidly removed from the extracellular fluid to prevent potentially lethal increases in potassium concentration from occurring. This is accomplished by sequestering the added potassium within the intracellular fluid. Potassium is transported into cell membranes by the Na-K ATPase pump in exchange for sodium.

The action of the pump is increased by both insulin and

epinephrine. However, neither of these hormones is released in response to potassium loading. Nonetheless, under normal circumstances they are released at the appropriate time. For example, insulin is released following a meal, when potassium levels are likely to be increasing, and epinephrine is released during periods of exercise, when potassium loss from muscle cells (due to increased action potential generation) is greater than normal. The action of these hormones can be taken advantage of in a clinical setting. For example, severe acute hyperkalemia can be treated by the administration of insulin (with glucose to prevent hypoglycemia), to enhance the movement of potassium from the extracellular to the intracellular fluid.

Ultimately, however, the kidneys must eliminate the daily potassium load to maintain normal potassium balance. Since the filtered load of potassium (800 mEq/day) is far in excess of the amount excreted (100 mEq/day), the kidneys could regulate potassium by controlling the amount they reabsorb each day. Instead, the kidneys reabsorb almost all of their filtered load in the proximal tubule and collecting ducts and then regulate excretion by controlling the amount they secrete in the distal tubule.

Approximately two-thirds of the filtered potassium is reabsorbed passively from the proximal tubule. As indicated earlier, reabsorption in the proximal tubule depends ultimately on the sodium concentration gradient between the epithelial cell and the luminal filtrate. Sodium flows into the cell down its concentration gradient and is actively removed from the cell on the basolateral surface by the Na-K ATPase pump. The removal of sodium from the filtrate establishes an osmotic gradient across the cell membrane, causing water to follow sodium out of the filtrate. Materials such as potassium and urea that are dissolved in the water can then be removed by solvent drag.

Alternatively (as discussed above), potassium can flow through the tight junctions between the cells down the electrochemical gradient established by the flow of sodium across the luminal wall in the early proximal tubule and the flow of chloride through the tight junctions in the late proximal tubule. In cases of chronic hypokalemia, potassium reabsorption in the proximal tubule can exceed sodium reabsorption. This has led to the conclusion that some potassium reabsorption must be due to active transport processes on the luminal membrane capable of pumping potassium from the filtrate into the epithelial cell.

The handling of potassium by the loop of Henle is poorly understood. Potassium reabsorbed from the collecting ducts most likely enters the descending limb of the loop of Henle in the medulla and is reabsorbed from the ascending limb. The mechanism of potassium transport by a carrier that binds two chloride ions, one sodium ion, and one potassium ion has already been described. Once potassium enters the epithelial cell, it can diffuse either into the peritubular space or back into the lumen. Because the lumen is positively charged with respect to the peritubular fluid, it is more likely that potassium will be reabsorbed than that it will return to the lumen. Whatever the mechanism, however, net potassium reabsorption occurs in the loop of Henle because less than 5% of the filtered potassium appears in the early distal tubule.

The final amount of potassium excreted in the urine is regulated by events occurring in the late distal tubule and collecting ducts. In general, under normal potassium loads, potassium secretion occurs in the late distal tubule and cortical collecting duct. When potassium deficits occur, net reabsorption can result, but the amount of potassium that can be retained by the kidney is not as great as the amount of sodium it can retain. As a result, a significant amount of potassium is always lost in the urine, even when the diet contains no potassium and severe hypokalemia is present.

In contrast, increasing the amount of potassium in the extracellular fluid is met by an increased secretion of potassium. Several days of hyperkalemia are required before potassium secretion is maximized. During this time, the luminal membrane becomes more permeable to potassium and the number of Na-K ATPase pumps on the basolateral surface of the principal cells increases. These adaptations (similar to those occurring in response to low sodium levels) may be produced by aldosterone, which is released from the adrenal cortex in response to increased plasma potassium levels.

Potassium secretion is affected directly by the pH of plasma. When plasma pH rises (because of metabolic or respiratory alkalosis), potassium secretion increases. When plasma pH falls (as a result of metabolic or respiratory acidosis), potassium secretion decreases. The change in potassium secretion appears to reflect the concentration of potassium in the distal tubular cells. Decreases in plasma pH are buffered by transporting hydrogen ions into the cell (see "Acid-Base Balance"), where, to preserve electroneutrality, potassium is transported into the extracellular fluid. The reduced renal epithelial cell potassium concentration causes a reduction in potassium secretion.

On the other hand, increases in plasma pH are buffered by transporting hydrogen out of the cell. This leads to an increase in renal epithelial potassium concentration and an increase in secretion. An exception to this generality occurs when the acidosis is due to diabetes, in which case a large number of negatively charged organic ions are produced. These are poorly absorbed by the nephron and thus make the intraluminal potential of the distal tubule quite negative. The negative charge increases potassium secretion above normal, even though the intracellular potassium concentration is reduced.

SENSORY PHYSIOLOGY

The sensory system is responsible for providing the nervous system with the information it needs to carry out its function. Information transmitted by the sense organs can be used to elicit simple reflexes, to adjust various homeostatic mechanisms, to plan behavior, to produce conscious sensation, or to carry out any of many other myriad tasks performed by the brain, spinal cord, and peripheral nerve networks. This section will be concerned with the special receptors of the skin, tongue, olfactory epithelium, eye, and ear that give rise to our conscious sensations of touch, temperature, pain, taste, smell, sight, and hearing. Other receptors such as those responsible for providing the information necessary to maintain normal blood pressure, carbon dioxide tension, and postural tone are covered in the sections dealing with those functions. Regardless of the receptor's physiological function, each of them produces its sensory message in a similar way. Each has a specialized membrane receptor capable of transducing (or changing) a particular form of stimulus energy into an electrical signal. The particular energy each receptor is adapted to receive is called the **adequate** (or **appropriate**) **stimulus**. The receptor is able to detect an adequate stimulus at extremely low levels of intensity. For example, the eye can detect a single photon of light, the skin can detect deformations of less than 1 μm, and the olfactory epithelium can detect the presence of molecules at concentrations below the sensitivity of most laboratory chemical-sensing devices.

The basic conscious sensations of touch, light, sound, etc. are transmitted to the CNS through labeled lines—that is, specific neuronal pathways activated by these receptors terminate in cortical areas in which a conscious sensation is elicited. Thus the visual pathway, whether activated by light, a blow to the eye, or electrical stimulation of the visual cortex, will always elicit a sensation of light. However, complex sensations such as those used to recognize faces, identify a tune, or interpret the significance of an object being lightly passed over the surface of the skin require the integration of many different sensory signals. Although some progress has been made in understanding how this is accomplished, particularly within the visual system, much is not known. Thus the major focus of the description of each sensory system will be on how the sensory signal is generated and transmitted to the brain. How this information is integrated by the cortex will be discussed in a much more limited fashion.

The basic mechanisms underlying all sensory receptors can be described in terms of a typical mechanical receptor that transduces mechanical energy into a train of nerve action potentials. It is divided into a transducer area, where the initial conversion of mechanical energy to an electrical signal is carried out, and a spike generator, in which the electrical signal produced by the stimulus is converted into a series of action potentials.

The transducer membrane contains deformation-sensitive voltage channels. These channels are analogous to the chemical-sensitive channels, described in the section on synaptic transmission, in that they are not voltage sensitive and the number of channels opened by the stimulus is proportional to the amount of membrane deformation. Although the ionic specificity of the channel is not known, it is assumed that the flow of sodium through the channel causes the membrane to depolarize. The stimulus-produced membrane depolarization is called a **receptor potential**. The magnitude of the receptor potential can be related to the intensity of the stimulus by either of two equations:

$$(1) \quad \text{Receptor potential} \ = \ k \, I^A$$

where both k and A are constants and A is less than 1. This relationship is called the Steven's power law.

$$(2) \quad \text{Receptor potential} \ = \ k \log I$$

This equation is known as the Weber-Fechner relationship.

Both equations indicate that the relationship between the stimulus intensity and receptor potential is curvilinear. Because sensory transduction follows these types of relationships, a large range of sensory signals can be transduced. For example, using Steven's power law in which k = 1 and A = 0.5, increasing

the stimulus intensity by 10 times causes the receptor potential to increase by 3.15 times and increasing the stimulus by 100 times causes the receptor potential to increase only 10 times. If the receptor potential increased in direct proportion to the stimulus—that is, if increasing the stimulus 100 times caused a 100-times increase in the receptor potential—the receptor would soon be saturated. From a psychometrics point of view, these equations are important because they also describe the relationship between the actual magnitude of the stimulus and the intensity perceived by the person subjected to the stimulus. The correspondence between conscious sensation and the receptor potential demonstrates the important role played by receptor transduction in sensory perception.

The receptor potential does not propagate. Instead, it serves as a stimulus for the generation of action potentials on the spike-generating region of the receptor. For this reason, the receptor potential is also called the **generator potential**. The frequency of the action potentials generated by the receptor potential is proportional to the magnitude of the receptor potential. Thus the frequency of action potentials, in most cases, serves as an indicator of stimulus intensity and, because the firing frequency is proportional to an exponent (or the logarithm) of the stimulus, it is also related to the perceived intensity. In some receptors, the firing frequency remains at the same level for as long as the stimulus is applied. These are called **nonadapting, static,** or **tonic receptors**. In other receptors, the firing frequency decreases despite the continued presence of the stimulus. These receptors are called **rapidly adapting, dynamic,** or **phasic receptors**.

All the mechanisms underlying adaptation are not understood, but several have been proposed. In some cases, the linkage between the stimulus and the nerve ending is the cause of the adaptation. This is called **mechanical adaptation**. For example, in the pacinian corpuscle, described below, the mechanical stimulus is transferred to the receptor membrane on the sensory neuron by an onion-like layer of connective tissue sheaths. When the stimulus is first applied, the mechanical deformation of the outer layer of the sensory encapsulation is transmitted faithfully to the sensory membrane. However, connective tissue layers become rapidly rearranged so that the deformation is dissipated and no longer reaches the center of the capsule. Consequently, the membrane deformation disappears, the receptor membrane repolarizes, and action potential generation ceases. In other cases, the receptor membrane repolarizes even though it is still being deformed by the stimulus. This is called **neuronal adaptation**. It is thought to result from the opening of voltage- and time-dependent potassium channels. Potassium flows out of the cell through these channels, causing the membrane to repolarize despite the continued inward flow of sodium ions through the receptor channels. In some receptors, the potassium channels open rapidly, causing rapid adaptation; in others, the potassium channels open more slowly, causing correspondingly slower rates of adaptation.

The **adaptation characteristics** of a receptor determine what sort of sensory message it transmits to the CNS. For example, slowly adapting receptors are able to provide information about stimulus intensity because their firing rate remains proportional to the stimulus for as long as it is present. Rapidly adapting receptors cannot perform this task because their firing rates decrease. However, if the stimulus is applied rapidly enough it will produce a much greater firing frequency than if it is applied slowly because it will reach its full magnitude before much adaptation has occurred. Thus, the frequency of firing in rapidly adapting receptors provides the CNS with information about how rapidly a stimulus is changing. As will be detailed below, different tactile receptors have different adaptation properties, and thus each is responsible for signaling a different quality of the sensory stimulus to the CNS. It may be casually thought that sensory adaptation causes the loss of awareness of a long-standing constant stimulus, such as the hum of poorly regulated fluorescent lights, but this is not the case. In fact, the CNS has perfectly good mechanisms for preventing constant stimuli from reaching consciousness. Moreover, it would be inappropriate for it to do so by reducing the sensory input because the CNS would then lose the option of restoring the stimulus to consciousness if, because of a changing situation, the stimulus were to suddenly become important.

Two classification schemes, one based on conduction velocity and the other on axon diameter, have been used to identify sensory neurons carrying information to the CNS. Since conduction velocity is related to axon diameter, a sensory neuron classified by one criterion can be easily converted to the other. The classification schemes are important because, in some cases, the names applied to neurons conveying specific sensations correspond to their category in one of the two classification schemes. Myelinated axons are divided by diameter into type I, II, or III:

Type I:	12 to 20 μm in diameter
Type II:	6 to 12 μm in diameter
Type III:	1 to 6 μm in diameter

In the other system, myelinated axons are called A fibers and are classified by conduction velocity as alpha, beta, gamma, and delta:

Alpha:	70 to 120 m/second
Beta:	35 to 70 m/second
Gamma:	20 to 35 m/second
Delta:	1 to 20 m/second

Some of the sensory neurons named according to the above classification schemes are as follows: those originating in muscle spindles (Ia); those from Golgi tendon organs (Ib); and those from pain and temperature endings (A delta). Motor fibers are also named according to the above schemes: Alpha motoneurons have axons in the A alpha group, and gamma motoneurons have axons in the A gamma group. Unmyelinated fibers are called group IV fibers in the axon diameter system and C fibers in the conduction velocity system.

CUTANEOUS SENSATION

The skin is endowed with three major types of receptors: mechanoreceptors, thermoreceptors, and pain receptors. The mechanoreceptors are further categorized as touch, pressure, and vibratory receptors. Although there are several receptors adapted to transmit information about touch to the CNS, the major ones are called Merkel's disks and Meissner's corpuscles. Merkel's disk is a somewhat unusual cutaneous receptor because the transducer membrane is on a modified epithelial cell and not on a nerve ending. When depolarized by a mechanical stimulus, the epithelial cell releases a neurotransmitter substance that in turn depolarizes the sensory afferent neuron innervating the disk. The sensory neuron is classified as a group II or A beta fiber. The Merkel's disks are approximately 200 μm in diameter and are only activated when the stimulus is applied directly to them. They usually respond with a brief burst of activity, followed by prolonged steady discharge. Most likely they provide the CNS with information about the location of a stimulus, because of their small receptive fields, and to a lesser extent, about the magnitude of the stimulus, because of their slow rate of adaptation.

Meissner's corpuscles are encapsulated sensory nerve endings. The capsule covering the large afferent neuron (A beta or group II) containing the transducer membrane is an oblong structure approximately 30 μm wide by 150 μm long. After entering the capsule, the sensory afferent neuron forms numerous branches that make contact with the connective tissue sheaths from which the capsule is formed. These receptors are found primarily on glabrous (nonhairy) skin such as on the fingertips, where precise sensory discriminations can be made. Meissner's corpuscles are rapidly adapting and thus serve to encode the rate of stimulus application rather than its magnitude. Analogous receptors are found in association with the base of hair follicles on nonglabrous skin. These receptors are also rapidly adapting and thus can sense the movement of the hair but not determine its final position.

Ruffini's endings are long, thin (1 to 2 mm long by 150 μm wide) connective tissue structures innervated by a large (group II or A beta) afferent neuron. These receptors cover a wide area of the skin and thus are not very useful in localizing the place at which a stimulus is applied. They are extremely slow adapting neurons and thus are adapted to detect the magnitude of a stimulus. They are the receptors that transmit the information necessary to perceive the amount of pressure being applied to the skin.

The pacinian corpuscle is the fourth major encapsulated ending found within the skin. This receptor is much larger than the others, often greater than 1 mm in diameter. As indicated above, it is formed from numerous layers of connective tissue, giving it an onion-like appearance. It too is innervated by a large (A beta or group II) sensory afferent neuron. The neuron loses its myelin sheath once inside the capsule but does not branch. Because the transducer membrane on the end of the afferent fiber is surrounded by fluid, it is deformed only while the stimulus is initially applied to the capsule. The rearrangement of the lamellae after the initial application of the stimulus rapidly reduces the pressure on the receptor, causing adaptation. As a result, the neuron stops firing after producing just a few action potentials. This receptor has a large receptive field so it is not capable of detecting the location of the stimulus, and its extremely rapid adapting prevents it from detecting the magnitude and even the velocity of the stimulus. However, the receptor responds easily to a vibratory stimulus in which the pressure is repetitively applied and removed from the skin. Thus the adaptation characteristics of the pacinian corpuscle allow it to function as a vibratory receptor. It is the receptor activated when a tuning fork applied to the skin is used to test for the integrity of the sensory pathways during a neurological examination.

The sensory fibers emerging from the cutaneous receptors enter the spinal cord in the dorsal root, ascend in the dorsal columns, and synapse with secondary afferent fibers in the dorsal column nuclei, which are the gracilis and cuneate nuclei. the second-order fibers emerging from the dorsal column nuclei cross immediately and travel tot he ventrobasal nuclei of the thalamus as the medial lemniscus. Tertiary fibers exit from the thalamus, pass through the internal capsule, and eventually terminate on the somatosensory areas of the cerebral cortex. The dorsal column-medial lemniscus pathway is topographically organized—that is, those fibers coming from a particular area on the skin are segregated from those coming from other areas of the skin throughout the entire pathway. The fibers terminating on the cortex do so in an orderly fashion, with those originating on the foot ending on the medial aspects of the somatosensory cortex and those coming from the head and face ending on the most lateral aspects of the somatosensory cortex. Within the somatosensory cortex, those areas receiving the densest innervation (e.g., the fingers, lips, and tongue), have the greatest amount of cortical area devoted to them. In contrast, the back and legs, which receive sparse sensory endings, have only a small area of cortex devoted to them.

Within any area of the somatosensory cortex, the individual receptor types are represented by separate groups of neurons. Sensory receptors coming from muscles and joints are located more anteriorly, near the motor cortex, where their information is most needed. More posteriorly are located the slowly adapting neurons, and still more posteriorly, the rapidly adapting neurons. The most posterior regions of the somatosensory cortex also receive input from other sensory modalities (vision and audition) and are presumably the sites in which tactile information is integrated with vision and hearing to produce a unitary conscious awareness of the external environment.

The tactile receptors on the surface of the skin perform two major types of sensory tasks. One is to identify the type of stimulus applied: Is it for example, a slowly applied, prolonged stimulus such as might occur when the hands are placed firmly on the surface of a table, or is it a furtive, repetitively applied stimulus such as might occur when a leaf flutters on and off the face. These very different types of stimuli are recognized because of the pattern of receptor activity each one generates, the prolonged stimulus primarily affecting the Ruffini's endings and the light, repetitive stimulus affecting primarily Meissner's corpuscles. The other task of the cutaneous receptors is to identify the location and spatial extent of the stimulus. This is accomplished by receptors such as the Merkel's disks, which have small receptive fields. Thus if one Merkel's disk is stimulated, the stimulus must be within the 200 μm, forming the receptive field of the afferent neuron. However, if several Merkel's disks are activated, the sensory system must be able to distinguish two stimuli separated in space from a single stimulus applied to one area of the skin. The ability to carry out this task can be assessed by the two-point threshold test. In this test, the examiner touches the skin with a single stimulus or applies two separate stimuli to the skin and asks the subject to indicate whether a single or double stimulus has been applied.

The two-point threshold is equal to the distance at which two stimuli cannot be distinguished from a single stimulus.

The diagram in Figure 2-44 illustrates the neural basis for the ability to distinguish two neighboring stimuli from each other. If the two Merkel's disks on the ends are stimulated and the one in the middle is not, then it is a simple task for the CNS to recognize the presence of two stimuli. However, if the two stimuli each partially stimulate the disk in the middle, then the sensory information emanating from the skin is the same as when a single stimulus has been applied. However, the synaptic organization within the dorsal column nuclei accentuates the spatial separation of the two stimuli, allowing them to be distinguished from each other. As shown in Figure 2-44, neurons entering the dorsal columns send collateral branches to interneurons, which are inhibitory to the sensory fibers originating from neighboring receptors. This neuronal arrangement is called **lateral inhibition** and is the basis for the small two-point thresholds found on the surface of the skin. Because the two neurons on the end both inhibit the one in the middle, the middle neuron's activity is reduced below those at the ends. Thus it appears as if the central neuron were not stimulated, and the subject is able to recognize the presence of two stimuli. Lateral inhibition is used by other sensory systems, particularly the visual system, to provide extremely precise identification of the spatial organization of the stimulus. This will be covered in detail when vision is discussed.

Pain is a difficult stimulus to understand, in terms of both how and why it is generated. By signaling the presence of a potentially harmful stimulus, pain elicits a number of protective reflexes and behaviors that tend to eliminate the offending stimulus and reduce the damage caused by it. In this regard, pain is very useful. In fact, persons born without the ability to

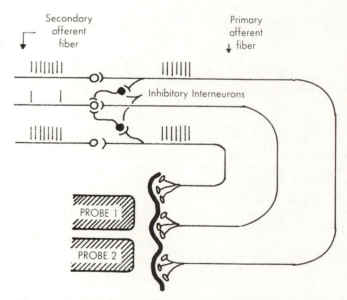

Figure 2-44. The diagram illustrates how two-point discrimination can be enhanced by lateral inhibition. In the absence of lateral inhibition, all three neurons will be stimulated equally and the nervous system will be unable to distinguish them as separate probes. With lateral inhibition, the neuron in the center will decrease its firing rate, allowing two probes to be discriminated.

perceive pain are subjected to repeated lesions resulting from the inability to avoid damaging stimuli. But pain sensations often outlast the trauma that caused them and even will occur in the absence of any obvious stimulus. Moreover, the painful stimulus exacerbates the trauma and itself results in harmful body responses. Thus a great deal of effort is being made by the research and pharmaceutical industries to develop methods for reducing or eliminating pain.

The peripheral basis for pain is fairly well understood. Free (nonencapsulated) nerve endings of unmyelinated C fibers and myelinated A delta fibers contain membranes responsive to potentially damaging stimuli. These receptor membranes, called nociceptors, respond to stimuli released from tissues provoked with high-intensity stimuli. In general, the myelinated fibers respond only to strong mechanical stimuli whereas the unmyelinated fibers respond to any noxious stimulus (e.g., heat, chemical, or mechanical stimulation). Even though the magnitude of a pain stimulus is very high, it is nonetheless an adequate stimulus for the nociceptors in that lower levels of stimuli do not activate these receptors, and although other tactile receptors may be intensely stimulated by the noxious stimulus, their activity does not give rise to a painful sensation. Although the precise stimulus required for activating the pain receptors is not known, it is thought that some chemical mediator—perhaps bradykinin, serotonin, potassium, or prostaglandin—released from the damaged tissue causes depolarization of the receptor membrane.

The pain sensation caused by activity in the myelinated nociceptor neurons is different from that caused by the activity in the nonmyelinated fibers. When the A delta fibers are stimulated, they produce a fast pain sensation. The perception is described as a sharp, prickly sensation and is easy localized on the skin. This is the type of sensation caused by piercing the skin with a sharp needle. The pain sensation elicited by the unmyelinated fibers is referred to as a slow pain. It is perceived a short time after the sharp pain sensation and is described as a dull, burning, aching type of pain that is not easily localized. Moreover, this type of pain is decidedly unpleasant and, if severe, can result in nausea, sweating, and a reduction in blood pressure. This is the type of pain that is felt after hitting the thumb a with a hammer.

These two types of pain, in addition to originating in separate neurons, also have separate pathways within the spinal cord and brain. The A delta fibers enter the cord with the dorsal root and terminate in the ipsilateral dorsal horn. Secondary fibers then cross the midline in the anterior commissure and ascend through the spinal cord as the lateral spinothalamic tract. Although most of these fibers terminate within the brain stem, many of them ascend directly to the thalamus, where they synapse on tertiary neurons that project to the cortex. This pathway is composed mostly of myelinated fibers, has few synapses, and maintains its topographical organization throughout. Consequently, it is able to provide the information needed to produce a sharp, well-localized pain sensation. The C fibers terminate in the substantia gelatinosa of the dorsal horn. A great deal of branching occurs within this region, and the pain signal travels across many neurons before being conveyed across the spinal cord to the contralateral anterolateral tract. Although these fibers ascend in parallel with those originating in the fast pain pathway, they are smaller, and almost all of them terminate within the reticular formation. Neurons activated by the slow pain pathway in the reticular formation give rise to many of the emotional aspects of the pain sensation. After passing through a number of interneurons, the pathway eventually reaches the thalamus and cortex, where it produces the dull, aching type of pain.

Acute pain, whether fast or slow, can be tolerated by most individuals and when prolonged can be treated by a variety of analgesics from aspirin to morphine. The most damaging type of pain is referred to as **chronic pain**. This is the type of pain that exists long after the initial injury has healed or, as indicated above, occurs in the absence of any identifiable stimulus. Such pain sensations are very difficult to treat and extremely debilitating to the patient. Surgical section of peripheral nerves, even of the spinothalamic tract, is often not helpful. Narcotic analgesics usually offer only temporary help and leave the patient with the additional problem of drug addiction. However, recent progress in our understanding of the pain pathways may lead to more successful treatments in the future.

Descending pathways originating in the periaqueductal gray area of the midbrain and the raphe nuclei of the pons and medulla have been found to suppress the pain pathways within the dorsal horn of the spinal cord. Although all the details are not yet known, it has been shown that serotonin and various enkephalins and endorphins act as neurotransmitters in these pathways. As indicated previously, enkephalins and endorphins are endogenous substances that act on the same receptors as morphine. Thus, these pathways may be involved in morphine's analgesic effect. A fuller understanding of the neurochemistry of these transmitters hopefully will allow the development of powerful analgesics without morphine's addictive properties and other side effects. Perhaps even more importantly, electrical stimulation of these pathways has been shown to produce a profound analgesia. This may explain some of the success attributed to acupuncture. It certainly opens the way to the development of nonpharmacologic methods of pain treatment.

In addition to their presence on the skin, pain receptors are found within the blood vessels and the viscera. The pain sensations caused by these receptors is often localized on the surface of the skin and is called **referred pain**. Most likely, referred pain occurs because the visceral pain afferents share many of the second-order neurons conveying somatic pain to the brain. The somatic location of the visceral pain can generally be used to identify the visceral organ responsible for the pain, because the both the visceral organ and somatic site will have originated from the same embryologic section. For example, cardiac pain is localized over the neck and shoulder and along the arms; esophageal pain (heartburn) is often localized over the sternum and the upper arms; and gallbladder pain can be referred to the abdomen as well as to an area on the back just beneath the scapula.

VISION

The eye is a complex optical instrument capable of focusing an image on the retina and converting it into a neuronal message. Light striking the eye must pass through the cornea, the anterior chamber, the lens, the vitreous, and all the cellular layers of the retina before reaching the light-sensitive vision receptors (Fig. 2-45). The cornea and lens act together to bring the image into focus on the retinal surface. Thus the optical system of the eye can be simplified by considering these two structures as a single refractive surface. A refractive surface can be formed from any transparent substance if the velocity of light traveling through it is different from the velocity of light in the medium just before or after it. The power of the refractive surface is related to how great the difference in velocities is and the curvature of the refractive surface. The power (in units of diopters) is calculated using the equation

$$\text{Power} = \frac{n - n'}{r}$$

where the unit of power is the diopter, n represents the refractive index (which is a measure of how much light slows down when it passes from a vacuum, or air, into another medium), and r is the radius of curvature in meters. The cornea-lens combination in the human eye has a refractive index equal to 1.4 and a radius of curvature of 0.0068 m. Since light travels from air (which has a refractive index of 1) into the cornea-lens combination, the refractive power of the eye is

$$\text{Power} = \frac{(1.4 - 1)}{0.0068} = 59 \text{ diopters}$$

Two-thirds of the refractive power comes from the cornea and one-third from the lens. However, as will be discussed below, the lens increases its power as objects are brought closer and closer to the eye in order to keep them in focus.

The power of a lens can be measured experimentally by observing where parallel rays of light shined through it come to focus. The point is called the **focal point,** and the distance from

the lens to the focal point is called the **focal distance.** Dividing the refractive index by the focal distance, measured in meters, yields the **refractive power** of the lens. The parallel rays can come from any light source, if it is far enough away. Although not strictly parallel, rays of light more than 20 feet from the eye diverge so little when they pass through the cornea that they can be considered parallel to each other from an optical point of view. If the cornea-lens combination has a refractive power of 59 D, then its focal distance is 1.4/59 = 24 mm. In the average eye, the distance from the cornea-lens combination to the retina, called the axial length of the eye, is approximately 24 mm. As a result, light coming from objects 20 feet or more from the eye are focused on the retina and can be seen clearly. (Note: Ophthalmologists often use the formula 1/power to calculate the focal distance. Applying this equation yields a focal distance of 1/59 or 17 mm. Although this is not anatomically correct, its use in optical formulas does not produce any significant errors and so it will be used in the following discussion.)

When an object is brought closer to the eye, its image is pushed farther from the cornea-lens combination. This results in a blurred image on the retina. The normal eye accommodates for the change in object position by increasing the refractive power of its lens. This is accomplished by contracting the ciliary muscles, which, by pulling on the suspensory ligaments, allow the lens capsule to retract. The refraction of the lens capsule causes the eye to bulge, which increases its curvature and thus its refractive power. The refractive power required to bring an object to focus on the retina can be calculated if the object and image distance are known using the lens formula

$$P = \frac{1}{f} = \frac{1}{o} + \frac{1}{i}$$

where f = focal distance, o = object distance, and i = image distance. Because the image is to be formed on the retina, the image distance is equal to 0.017 m.

Suppose the object is moved to a position 1 m from the eye. Then, according to the lens formula, the power of the lens will become 60 D:

$$\frac{1}{1} + \frac{1}{0.017} = 60 \text{ D}$$

The increase of 1 D in refractive power is easy for the eye to accomplish. In the young eye, the refractive power of the eye can be increased by 14 D or more, allowing an object to remain in focus even if it is brought to within 7 mm of the eye. However, with age, the ability to accommodate decreases and is usually less than 2 D at 50 years of age. The loss of accomodative power with age is called **presbyopia.** The near point, the closest an object can be from the eye and still be in focus, is a measure of how much accommodative power an individual has. The smaller the near point, the greater the power of accommodation. In the above example, with a 1-D power of accommodation, objects less than 1 m from the eye will not be in focus. This is why glasses are usually required for reading as an individual ages. The words can still be focused clearly on the retina if the print is held 1 m from the eye, but their images are too small to be distinguished from each other.

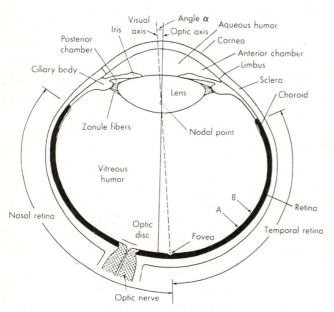

Figure 2-45. A diagrammatic view of the eye showing the path followed by two rays of light as they travel through the cornea, aqueous humor, lens, and vitreous humor on their way to the photoreceptors in the retina.

Image size can be calculated using the formula

$$\frac{O_{SIZE}}{O_{DISTANCE}} = \frac{I_{SIZE}}{I_{DISTANCE}}$$

Thus a 10-mm object placed 1 m from the eye will have an image size of

$$\frac{0.01}{1} \times 0.017 = 170\,\mu m$$

This is well within the resolving power of the eye. However, the typical letter on the page of a book is less than 1 mm wide, yielding an image size of 17 μm, which is difficult for the eye to identify. The above formula is used clinically to calculate the extent of a vision lesion. The size of the scotoma (the defect in the vision field) is mapped on a tangent screen (the object size) and then converted to an image size.

Refractive errors occur when distant objects are not focused clearly on the retina. This will occur if there is a discrepancy between the axial length of the eye and the power of the cornea-lens combination. For example, if the refractive power of the eye is 62 D, the image of a distant object will be focused in front of the eye. Such an individual is said to be **myopic**, or nearsighted. The object can be seen clearly only if it is brought closer to the eye. The person's eye functions as if it had a permanent accommodative power of 3 D. The refractive power can be corrected by placing a 3-D diverging (concave) lens in front of the eye, reducing its power to a normal value of 59 D. If the individual had an axial length of 18 mm and a refractive power of 59 D, he or she would still be myopic because the image of a distant object would still form in front of the eye. To correct the myopia, a − 3.5 D (− lens are diverging lenses) must be placed in front of the eye to reduce its refractive power to 55.5 D. The focal length of such a glasses-cornea-lens combination is 18 mm.

Hyperopia, or farsightedness, occurs when the cornea-lens combination is too small for the axial length of the eye. Thus the image of distant objects falls behind the retina. In most cases, a farsighted person can correct for the error by accommodating. However, the constant contraction of the ciliary muscle will lead to eye strain, and thus the error should be corrected by wearing glasses with a converging (convex) lens. Also, because some accommodation is used just to see distant objects, there is not enough accommodation in reserve for seeing objects brought close to the eye. The term farsightedness comes from the necessity to place objects far from the eye in order to see them clearly, not from an increased ability to see distant objects. Presbyopia can also be corrected with a converging lens.

Another common refractive error is called **astigmatism**, an uneven cornea resulting in variations in refractive power over the surface of the eye. Persons with astigmatism will therefore not be able to bring the entire image into focus. If the vertical lines are in focus, for example, the horizontal lines will not be. Fortunately, there are usually just two different refractive powers within the cornea and one of them can be changed to match the other using a cylindrical lens. Such a lens refracts light in only one plane. Hard contact lenses can also be used to correct astigmatism, because the uneven corneal surface is

replaced with the homogeneous surface of the contact lens. Soft lenses assume the contour of the cornea and so are less effective in correcting for astigmatism.

The photoreceptors for vision, the **rods** and the **cones** (Fig. 2-46), are located within the outer nuclear layer of the retina, which is closest to the pigment epithelium that lines the back of the eyeball. The rods and cones synapse with bipolar cells, which is closest to the pigment epithelium that lines the back of the eyeball. The rods and cones synapse with bipolar cells, which in turn synapse with ganglion cells. The circuitry connecting all of these cells together enables a great deal of vision processing to occur within the retina and will be discussed in detail below.

The retina contains approximately 6 million cones and 120 million rods. Most of the rods are located within a 1-mm-square area in the center of the retina called the macula. An even smaller region within the macula, called the fovea, contains only cones. This part of the eye is capable of the greatest visual acuity. Rods are dispersed throughout the retina but have their greatest density in the regions surrounding the macula. The rods are used for night vision, when the greatest amount of visual sensitivity is required. The basic structure of the rods and cones is similar (Fig. 2-46). Each has an outer segment containing the visual pigment, which detects the presence of light, an inner segment containing mitochondria to support the high metabolic rate of the photoreceptors, a nucleus, and a synaptic terminal through which the presence of

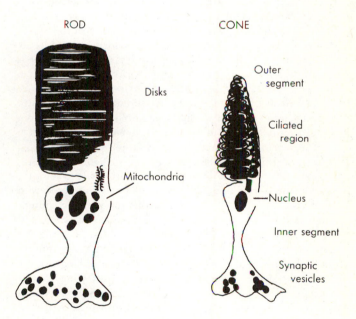

Figure 2-46. The rods and cones are the photoreceptors within the retina. The membranous disks in the outer segment of the photoreceptors contain rhodopsin. When light is absorbed by a rhodopsin molecule, it initiates a photoisomerization by which 11-*cis*-rhodopsin is changed to the all-*trans* form. During this transformation, the sodium channels within the outer segment close, the cell hyperpolarizes, and the spontaneous release of neurotransmitter decreases.

light is communicated to other cells of the retina. The average diameter of the rods, 5 μm, is twice that of the typical cone.

The photopigment is contained within membranes in the outer segment. In rods, these membranes bud off from the cell membrane to form isolated disks. There typically are some 1700 disks in each rod. These form at the base of the outer segment and migrate to the tip of the rod, where they are sloughed off and digested by phagocytotic cells in the pigment epithelium. In cones, the invaginations remain attached to the outer segment membrane.

The pigment epithelium is extremely important for the normal function and survival of the retina. As indicated above, it digests the cellular debris sloughed off the photopigments. In addition, it stores vitamin A, which it makes available to the photoreceptors for the formation of the visual pigment, and serves as a bridge between the blood vessels of the choroid and the retina, through which nutrients and wastes are exchanged. **Retinal detachment,** a not uncommon severing of the coupling of the photoreceptors and pigment epithelium, must be rapidly repaired if degeneration of the retina is not to occur.

The visual pigment is called **rhodopsin.** It consists of a chromophore (**retinal**) that alters its chemical structure when it absorbs light energy and a protein (**opsin**) that determines the particular wavelength of light striking the chromophore. Upon absorbing a photon of light, retinal is converted from its dark-adapted 11-*cis* form through a series of unstable inter-mediates to an all-*trans* form. This conformational change in the structure of retinal initiates a series of events, which will be described below, that lead to the production of a receptor potential. The photoisomerization process is referred to as **bleaching** because the dark-adapted form of rhodopsin, which is purplish, becomes transparent when the all-*trans* form of retinal is formed. Following isomerization, all-*trans* retinal and opsin dissociate from each other. Re-formation of rhodopsin occurs via two pathways. Either the all-*trans* form is immediately converted to 11-*cis* retinal by an isomerase enzyme or it is reduced to 11-*cis* retinol (vitamin A). Vitamin A is then isomerized to 11-*cis* retinol and oxidized to 11-*cis* retinal. Once 11-*cis* retinal is formed, it attaches spontaneously to opsin. Deficiencies in vitamin A lead to night blindness because not enough retinol is available for the formation of rhodopsin.

The receptor potential in the photoreceptors is unusual because the cell hyperpolarizes in response to light. In the dark, the outer segment membrane is highly permeable to sodium, causing the cell to be relatively depolarized compared with other receptor cells. When light strikes the eye, the sodium conductance of the outer segment membrane is decreased and the cell hyperpolarizes. The biochemical pathway causing this response is fairly complex. It is thought that the sodium channels are kept open by a cyclic GMP-activated kinase that is deactivated when light strikes the eye. According to this concept, the photoisomerization of retinal causes the activation of a specialized membrane protein called **transducin.** Activated transducin combines with and activates a phosphodiesterase enzyme that dephosphorylates cyclic GMP. The removal of cyclic GMP inactivates the kinase and causes the sodium channels to close.

The simplest pathway through the retina is from receptor, to bipolar, to ganglion cell. In the dark, the depolarized receptor cells continuously release an inhibitory neurotrans-mitter that keeps the bipolar cell in a hyperpolarized state. When light strikes the receptor, the rod or cone hyperpolarizes, the amount of transmitter released decreases, and the bipolar cell, freed from inhibition, depolarizes. When it is depolarized, the bipolar cell releases an excitatory transmitter, which causes a train of action potentials to be generated by the ganglion cell. The ganglion cell is the only cell in the retina that has to transmit information by generating and propagating action potentials. All the other cells in the retina are small enough for the synaptic potential elicited on one end of the cell to reach the other end without a significant reduction in size.

In the fovea, a single cone may connect to a single bipolar cell, which in turn connects to a single ganglion cell. However, there are only 1 million or so ganglion cells in the retina, half of which receive their input from 6 million or more cones. As a result, the average ganglion cell receives input from 10 to 20 cones. Even more convergence occurs in the case of rods, since more than 120 million rods must converge on less than 500,000 ganglion cells. The **receptive field** of a ganglion cell is defined as all the cones or rods making synaptic contact with the ganglion cell through bipolar cells. In general, the receptors forming the receptive field of a ganglion cell are arranged in a circular fashion. The area occupied by the receptive field can be as small as several microns in the fovea or as large as several millimeters in the periphery of the retina.

When light is shined anywhere within the receptive field, the rate of firing in the ganglion cell increases. However, if light is shined on a circular area just surrounding the receptive field, the rate of discharge is decreased. This pattern is described as **on-center, off-surround** organization to indicate that stimulation of the center of the receptive field causes excitation of the ganglion cell whereas stimulation of the surrounding area inhibits the activity of the ganglion cell. This phenomenon is called **surround inhibition** and is entirely analogous to the lateral inhibition discussed earlier in regard to two-point discrimination on the skin. The pathway mediating surround inhibition involves the horizontal cells, which, when stim-ulated by the recepts in the area surrounding the ganglion cell's receptive field, inhibit the receptors or the bipolar cells leading to the ganglion cell. The end result of this neuronal organization is the enhancement of contrast. If light entering the eye illuminates both the center and surround equally well, the ganglion cell discharge rate remains unchanged. However, if only the center is illuminated, the ganglion cell fires vigorously. On the other hand, if only the surround is illuminated, the ganglion cell's firing rate is decreased.

In addition to the on-center, off-surround organization just described, some ganglion cells have an **off-center, on-surround** organization. As their name implies, these ganglion cells fire when the surround is illuminated and are inhibited when the center is illuminated. The synaptic structure of the receptors and the position of the bipolar and ganglion cells having off-center receptive fields differs from those having on-center receptive fields. Whether these two types of ganglion cells serve different purposes or simply provide redundancy of information is not known. However, there are three different types of ganglion cells in the retina, and they do appear to serve different functions. The X type of ganglion cell has the smallest receptive field and is responsible for producing a high degree of spatial resolution. The Y type of ganglion cell has a much larger receptive field and is probably involved in generating information about the presence of a target in the visual field. Type W cells also have extensive receptive fields but project to the superior colliculus rather than to the lateral geniculate nucleus. They are involved in generating visually evoked reflexes of the eyes and head. The firing rate of amacrine cells increases markedly when an image first appears on the retina and then decreases over time. It is assumed that these cells provide ganglion cells with information about visual targets moving rapidly over the retina. Each of these cell types relays information about visual activity over the entire retina. Thus a visual image focused on the retina is analyzed simultaneously by many the neurons within the retina, and different properties of the image are conveyed to the CNS through separate pathways.

The **lateral geniculate nucleus** acts primarily as a relay station for transmitting information from the retina to the visual cortex. The lateral geniculate nucleus has six layers of cells. Layers 2, 3, and 5 receive ipsilateral input (from the temporal retina), whereas layers 1, 4, and 6 receive contralateral input (from the nasal retina). In this way, each geniculate receives the entire contralateral visual field. The type Y ganglion cells (with large receptive fields) project to layers 1 and 2 of the geniculate nucleus, whereas the other four layers receive input from the small-receptive-field type X ganglion cells. Thus the segregation of detailed information about the visual image from more global information about the presence of an object in the visual field is maintained in the lateral geniculate. Each lateral geniculate neuron receives its input from just a few ganglion cells and has the same type of on-center, off-surround receptive fields as the ganglion cells do. Although little processing of information occurs within the lateral geniculate nucleus, a great number of axons project from the visual cortex to the geniculate. These fibers may play an important role in modulating the information reaching the cortex from the retina.

The axons leaving the lateral geniculate nucleus form the optic radiations that project to the primary receiving area of the visual cortex (called **Brodmann's area 17**). The information processing that was initiated by the retina is continued in the visual cortex. The cells in area 17 are organized into large cortical columns, called **hypercolumns**. Each hypercolumn is concerned with the analysis of information from a particular spot on the retina. Each hypercolumn contains a set of smaller columns that are responsible for a particular type of analysis. For example, several geniculate cells with receptive fields on neighboring areas of the retina all project to cortical cells within a single column. The axons of these cortical cells then project to a group of other cells within the column, called **simple** and **complex cells**. The simple cells have rectangular receptive fields with an area of excitation surrounded by two areas of inhibition. Light shined anywhere in the center of the rectangle causes the simple cell to fire; light shined on the edge of the rectangle causes the cell to stop firing. The receptive field characteristics of a simple cell are derived from combining the receptive fields of several lateral geniculate cells.

The rectangular receptive field of the simple cell is usually oriented at a particular angle. A single hypercolumn will typically contain many rectangular receptive fields, each one oriented at a different angle. These cells with their rectangularly oriented receptive fields decompose an image into a series of edges.

Complex cells have much larger receptive fields. They receive their input from simple cells (with the same angular orientation) located in several adjacent hypercolumns. Because these cells have larger receptive fields, they continue to fire as the image passes rapidly over a small region of the retina. Thus the cortex does not lose track of an image when movement of the eye causes a portion of the image to move over successive hypercolumns.

The columns containing these simple and complex cortical cells receive all of their input from one side of the visual field. Separate columns within each hypercolumn receive their information from the opposite visual field. Thus each hypercolumn contains bilateral visual information that can be used for depth perception. Additional columns within each hypercolumn receive information concerned with color vision. This short description of visual information processing makes clear an important feature of the vision system—that is, visual perceptions are not obtained from a cortical projection of a retinal image. Instead, a variety of cortical cells organized into columns dissect the image into its component parts: contour, contrast, form, color, depth, and movement. This information is eventually synthesized into a unified, complex, three-dimensional image of the visual world around us. The separate analysis of different aspects of the visual image is apparent from the study of patients who have lost a particular aspect of vision perception. For example, some patients may lose the ability to perceive motion but may have perfectly adequate visual acuity and color vision. This condition is called **agnosia**—the loss of certain aspects of a sensory experience due to a deficit in information processing (as opposed to a deficit in the receptors or their projections to the cortex).

The remainder of this section will offer a neurophysiological explanation of some common perceptual qualities of the vision system.

The ability to perceive a complete image from a few lines or dots drawn on a page derives in part from the processing of information by the retinal ganglion cells. Because of their on-center, off-surround receptive fields, ganglion cell firing rates do not change when their receptive fields are evenly illuminated. Instead, their firing rates change when their receptive fields are illuminated by images with changing levels of illumination such as occur at the border between black and white lines. The CNS then uses its memory of images to create a satisfactory perception from the partial information it receives from the periphery. This is why the blind spot or even large visual field defects (scotomata) do not interfere with normal visual perceptions. Patients with visual field lesions often present with symptoms of a locomotor disorder because they are not aware that their frequent collisions with objects around them are caused by their inability to see objects. The objects are not seen because their images fall on the damaged areas of the retina. The loss of visual information does not result in a distorted visual image because the CNS creates a normal perception from the information it does receive.

Visual acuity is a measure of how well the vision system can resolve the separation between two objects placed close together. It is analogous to the two-point threshold on the skin. It is generally measured by asking a patient to read letters on a Snellen eye chart and recording the smallest line the patient can read. Acuity is reported as a fraction such as 20/30 or 20/100. The numerator indicates how far the chart is from the patient. The denominator indicates how far an average person can be from the chart and still read the letters in the smallest line the patient could read. Thus the smallest line of print an individual with 20/40 vision can read can be read by an average person standing 40 feet from the chart.

Visual acuity is greatest in the fovea for a number of reasons. First, images formed on the fovea suffer from the least distortion because they are formed by light passing through the center of the lens-cornea combination, and the blood vessels and ganglion cell axons, which cover the inner surface of the retina, do not pass over the fovea. Second, the cones in the fovea are smaller than anywhere else in the retina, and ganglion cells in the fovea have the smallest receptive fields. Third, the amount of horizontal cell inhibition is greatest in the fovea, which enhances the contrast between objects. Acuity decreases as the level of illumination decreases. This occurs partly because the opening of the pupils in dim light causes some distortion in the image, but mostly it is caused by a change in vision processing by the retina. As light levels decrease, rods become more involved in vision processing, and rods have larger receptive fields than cones. In addition, the amount of horizontal cell inhibition decreases at low light levels, decreasing the ability of the vision system to perceive the contrast between objects. The greater use of rods and decrease in surround inhibition, although decreasing acuity, increases the sensitivity of the vision system.

As the light levels decrease, the retina adapts to the dark. As discussed above, dark adaptation occurs (1) because the pupils increase in diameter, letting in more light, (2) because the size of ganglion cell receptive fields increases, and (3) because rods, which have larger receptive fields and are more sensitive to light, are more involved in vision perception at low light levels. Figure 2-47 illustrates the change in vision threshold, the lowest detectable light stimulus, that occurs when a subject enters a dark room after being subjected to a bright light. Dark adaptation is due primarily to the regeneration of rhodopsin from retinol and opsin. Regeneration of the photopigment occurs most rapidly in the cones. However, the cones cannot achieve the same sensitivity as the rods. Thus, the increase in vision sensitivity that follows after the complete adaptation of the cones is due to adaptation of the rods. At high light levels, such as in daylight, the rods are completely saturated and do not contribute to vision perceptions. This is called **photopic vision**. At low light levels, such as outdoors at night, the light intensity is below the threshold for cones. This is why astronomers do not gaze directly at dim stars. An image falling on the fovea, where there are no rods, will not be seen. Pure rod vision is called **scotopic vision**. **Mesopic vision** uses both rods and cones.

Color vision is an exclusive property of the cones. Interpretation of color is made possible by the differences in composition of the opsin contained in the photopigments of cones. These differences cause different parts of the visual spectrum to be preferentially absorbed by each of the photopigments. Three types of opsin occur—red, green, and blue.

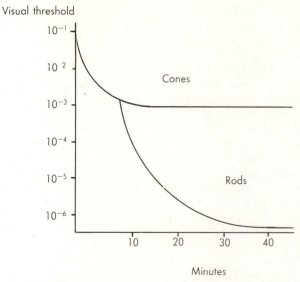

Figure 2-47. When the eyes are exposed to a bright light, the photopigments within the rods and cones are bleached, decreasing their sensitivity to light. If the person then enters a dark room, he or she is unable to detect light. Over time, the threshold for recognizing the presence of light decreases. This increased sensitivity is due to the regeneration of rhodopsin. Cones recover their sensitivity more rapidly than rods. Rods, however, are capable of detecting light at much lower intensities.

Every color causes a different combination of cones to be activated. The CNS interprets the mosaic of activity received from these receptors to assign color to the perceptions it creates. For example, yellow light causes equal amounts of activity in the red and green cones. If slightly more activity is produced in the red cones, the CNS adds a reddish hue to the yellow; if more activity is produced in the green cones, a green hue is added. Color blindness results when one or more of the opsin proteins is missing. Red-green color blindness is the most common type. This occurs when either the red or green opsin is missing. For example, if the cones that should produce red opsin produce green opsin instead, then it becomes difficult to distinguish colors in the green to red end of the spectrum because the cones respond in the same way to all of these colors. However, the person is not blind to red light (except for the far end of the red spectrum, which is not absorbed by the green photopigment. Red-green color blindness (called **protanopia** if the red photopigment is missing and **deuteranopia** if the green photopigment is missing) is caused by a sex-linked genetic defect and thus is more prevalent in males. Blue color blindness (called **tritanopia**) is far rarer and is caused by an autosomal genetic defect, so it afflicts males and females with equal frequency.

HEARING

The ear converts pressure striking the ear drum into a train of action potentials that are used by the CNS to produce the perception of sound. Sound is conducted from its point of origin to the ear as a wave. The wave consists of alternating regions of high and low pressure created by a vibrating object. For example, a tuning fork vibrating at 512 Hz (cycles per second) causes the surrounding air to vibrate at the same frequency. When the tuning fork is directed outward, it pushes the air particles together, increasing their pressure. When the tuning fork vibrates inward, the air particles move apart, decreasing their pressure. The pressure wave moves away from the tuning fork because the expanding air particles push on the air surrounding them. These in turn push on their neighbors, and so on. The maximum pressure created by the air particles is considered to be the amplitude of the sound wave. It is measured in units called decibels. The decibel scale is a ratio scale comparing the ratio of the sound being measured to some reference. In hearing, the reference is the lowest pressure detectable by the ear, 2×10^{-4} dynes/cm². Decibels are calculated as

$$\text{Decibels}_{\text{SPL}} = 20 \log \frac{P}{P_{\text{REF}}}$$

where decibels$_{\text{SPL}}$ = decibels referenced to the sound pressure of 2×10^{-4} dynes/cm², P is the pressure measured, and P_{REF} is the reference pressure.

Using this scale, a sound wave having an amplitude 100 times SPL would have an amplitude of 20 log 100 = 40. Sound waves of this amplitude are produced by quiet talking. Traffic noise is generally 80 dB, or 10,000 times larger than SPL. Sounds above 120 dB, such as those produced by rocket engines or rock bands, can be painful and damaging to the ears.

Sound waves entering the ear cause the tympanic membrane to vibrate, in turn causing the middle ear bones to vibrate. A considerable amount of sound energy is lost when the sound wave travels from air to water. This is why a person underwater cannot hear someone on shore talking. However, in order for sounds to reach the nervous system, they need to be transferred from air to the fluid environment of the cochlea. The characteristics of the middle ear bones enable them to carry out this transfer with less than the expected energy loss. The fairly complex process called impedance matching can be intuitively understood in terms of pressure amplification. Because the tympanic membrane is 17 times greater than the area of the malleus, the sound pressure is amplified by 17 times. Additional amplification occurs because of the mechanical advantage provided by the linkage of the malleus with the incus. Thus the pressure reaching the oval window from the stapes is some 22 times greater than that striking the tympanic membrane. Because the middle ear does not amplify all sound equally well, it is much more effective in the range of 1,000 to 5,000 Hz than it is at lower and higher frequencies, and hearing thresholds vary with frequency. Damage to the tympanic membrane or middle ear bones will not prevent sound from reaching the inner ear. However, the loss of amplification will cause a 25-dB loss in hearing, enough to make it difficult to hear normal conversations.

The inner ear is encased in a snail-like structure called the cochlea. Inside the cochlea are three fluid-filled canals, divided from each other by the basilar membrane and Reissner's membrane (Fig. 2-48). The scala media or cochlear duct is in the center of the cochlea, bounded above by the Reissner's membrane and below by the basilar membrane. The scala vestibuli, above the Reissner's membrane, and the scala tympani, below the basilar membrane, are connected to each

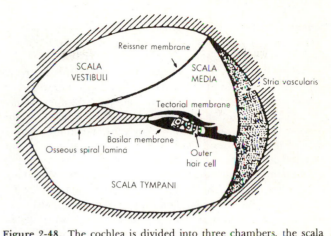

Figure 2-48. The cochlea is divided into three chambers, the scala vestibuli, the scala media, and the scala tympani. The cell bodies of the hair cells are located on top of the basilar membrane. The stereocilia projecting from the hair cells are embedded in the tectorial membrane. Sound pressure waves entering the cochlea cause the basilar membrane to vibrate up and down and the stereocilia to tilt back and forth. The movement of the stereocilia causes the hair cells to depolarize.

other through the helicotrema at the apex of the cochlea. The fluid in the scala vestibuli and scala tympani is called perilymph. Its composition is similar to that of the extracellular fluid. The scala media is filled with endolymph, a fluid having a high concentration of potassium and a low concentration of sodium. This fluid is secreted by the stria vascularis, a highly vascular tissue lining the outer wall of the cochlea. The basilar membrane is narrowest at the base of the cochlea (approximately 50 μm) and widest at the apex (almost 500 μm). Thus as the cochlea becomes smaller, the basilar membrane is becoming wider. Sounds entering the cochlea through the oval window cause the fluid in the scala vestibuli to vibrate. Although these vibrations could in theory travel through the helicotrema to the scala tympani, they actually travel directly through the scala media to the scala tympani. In doing so, they cause the basilar membrane to vibrate at the same frequency as the tympanic membrane. The vibration of the basilar membrane results in the transformation of sound energy into electrical energy by the hair cells.

The hair cells are located in the organ of Corti, which lies on the surface of the basilar membrane. The bases of the hair cells are anchored to the basilar membrane. The stereocilia on top of the hair cells extend upward toward a gelatinous structure called the tectorial membrane. There are two groups of hair cells, a single row of inner hair cells and three rows of outer hair cells. When vibration pushes the basilar and tectorial membranes down, the stereocilia between them move inward; when the basilar membrane moves up, the stereocilia move outward. Bending the stereocilia inward causes the hair cell to depolarize; bending them out causes the hair cell to hyperpolarize. Thus the up and down motion of the basilar and tectorial membrane is transformed into an outward and inward bending of the stereocilia, which in turn is transformed into an alternating hyperpolarizing and depolarizing receptor potential. The hair cells, like the touch cells in Merkel's disks, are modified epithelial cells. They communicate with their primary nerve afferents through synaptic transmission. When the hair cells depolarize, they release a synaptic transmitter, producing a train of action potentials in the auditory (eighth cranial) nerve fibers synapsing with them.

The particular hair cell activated by a sound depends on the frequency of the sound. The energy of low-frequency sounds is transmitted across the basilar membrane near the apex, where the basilar membrane is widest and most compliant. High-frequency sounds, on the other hand, are transmitted across the basilar membrane near the base, where the basilar membrane is narrowest and stiffest. Intermediate frequencies are transmitted across the basilar membrane at the point where energy transfer from the fluid in the scala vestibuli to the basilar membrane is most efficient. Only those hair cells located on the vibrating portion of the basilar membrane are activated by the sound. Thus different frequencies of sound activate different groups of hair cells. The discharge of the cochlea nerve afferents generated by the sound informs the CNS about the location of the activated hair cells and consequently about the frequency of sound entering the ear.

Although there are far fewer inner hair cells (3,500) than there are outer hair cells (13,500), almost 90% of the 30,000 auditory nerve fibers innervate the inner hair cells. That is, each inner hair cell receives 9 to 10 afferent nerve fibers. These cells are analogous to the cones within the retina in that they enable the ear to discriminate between various frequencies of sounds. Each auditory nerve fiber responds best to a particular frequency of sound, called its characteristic frequency. The characteristic frequency of an afferent neuron depends on the location of the hair cell it innervates. Neurons innervating hair cells near the base of the cochlea have high characteristic frequencies, and those at the apex have low characteristic frequencies. The correspondence between the location of the hair cell along the basilar membrane and the characteristic frequency of the afferent neuron is due primarily to the stiffness of the basilar membrane. However, the hair cells are also adapted to respond preferentially to a particular frequency. Adding the tuning characteristics of the hair cells to those of the basilar membrane enhances the frequency discrimination capabilities of the auditory system.

The auditory nerve fibers terminate within the cochlear nucleus. Fibers with high characteristic frequencies penetrate to the deeper portions of the nucleus, whereas those with low characteristic frequencies remain superficial. Thus, the tonotopic organization originating in the inner ear is maintained within the cochlear nucleus. This organization is maintained throughout the ascending auditory pathway. The auditory pathway is much more complicated than either the somatosensory or vision systems. Fibers leaving the cochlear nucleus travel bilaterally to the inferior olive. Olivary fibers from each side of the brain stem cross the midline and synapse within the inferior colliculus. Fibers leaving the colliculus join together as the lateral lemniscus and end in the ipsilateral medial geniculate nucleus. Projections from the geniculate nucleus reach the ipsilateral auditory cortex in the temporal lobe. Because of the extensive bilateral representation within the auditory pathway, lesions within the central auditory pathway do not produce major deficits in hearing.

The auditory cortex produces a perception of sound that is characterized by frequency, loudness, and direction. Frequency is primarily determined by the location of the auditory neuron in the auditory cortex. However, low-frequency sounds can also be recognized by the frequency of their action potentials. Below 500 Hz, the auditory fibers can fire at the same frequency as the sound stimulus. Between 500 and 5,000 Hz, the refractory period of the neurons prevents it from firing at the same frequency as the sound stimulus, but it can fire in phase with the sound. For example, the neuron may fire on every other cycle or every fifth cycle, etc., depending on the frequency of the sound. Thus low-frequency sounds can be discriminated on the basis of which neuron is firing as well as the frequency of its firing. However, for the most part, frequency of firing is related to the loudness of the stimulus. The more intense the stimulus, the greater the number of neurons activated and the higher the frequency of firing produced by each neuron.

The neural mechanism underlying the perception of direction illustrates just how precisely the CNS can analyze incoming information. As indicated above, cells within the superior olive receive input from both ears. Some of these neurons receive excitatory input from one ear and inhibitory input from the other. When a sound is located in front of the head, the intensity of the sound reaching one ear equals that of the sound reaching the other ear; the two inputs cancel each other out, and the olivary neuron's firing rate does not change. However, if the sound comes from one side, the intensity of the signal on that side will exceed the intensity on the other and the firing rate of the neurons within the olivary nucleus will either increase or decrease (depending on whether the excitatory or inhibitory input predominates). This mechanism works well for high-frequency sounds, because the head acts as a barrier to sounds of high frequency. However, low-frequency sounds pass around the head easily so both sides receive signals of the same magnitude regardless of where the sound is coming from. Other cells in the lateral superior olive can distinguish the location of sound because they are sensitive to when the sound reaches the two ears. Sounds located in front of the head will reach both ears simultaneously. Sounds to one side will reach the ear on that side before reaching the ear on the other side. These time differences (which can be small fractions of a millisecond) can be detected by the olivary cells. The information from these cells is transferred to the auditory cortex for processing. Lesions of the auditory cortex result in the inability to determine the direction from which a sound stimulus is coming.

TASTE

The sensation of taste derives primarily from the activity of taste receptor cells on the tongue. However, the actual perceptual experience of taste depends as much on the temperature, texture, and smell of the material bathing the tongue as it does on its taste. The appropriate selection of foods is guided to a large extent by how they taste. Carbohydrates and salts are ingested because they taste good, and alkaloids (which often are poisonous) are rejected because they taste bad. Significant nutritional and behavioral problems can develop in individuals who are unable to taste foods normally.

Taste receptor cells, like the auditory and Merkel's disk cells discussed previously, are modified epithelial cells that communicate with their primary afferent neurons through synaptic transmission. The apical surfaces of taste receptor cells are covered with microvilli. Taste receptors may be located on the microvilli or on the underlying membrane. The mechanism underlying the generation of a taste cell receptor potential is not known. However, bathing the extracellular fluid surrounding the taste cell results in a depolarizing receptor potential.

The taste cells are localized within taste buds. Each taste bud is approximately 100 μm in diameter and contains 40 to 50 taste cells. The taste cells are formed from stem cells located on the base of the taste bud. Newly formed cells migrate to the surface of the taste bud, serve as taste receptor cells for about 10 days, and then are sloughed off from the taste bud. The continuous replacement of taste cells prevents the loss of taste sensation due to mechanical, chemical (spicy foods for example), or thermal trauma. The microvilli on the surface of the taste cell protrude into the taste pore that penetrates into the center of the taste buds. Solutions bathing the surface of the tongue reach the taste receptors by dissolving in the saliva within the taste pores. The life cycle of the taste bud is dependent on the integrity of its nervous innervation. Sectioning the afferent nerves prevents the formation of new taste cells and leads to the degeneration of the taste bud. If the remaining epithelial cells are reinnervated, new taste buds will form.

Taste buds are located within papillae covering the surface of the tongue and parts of the pharynx. Several hundred fungiform papillae, each containing three to five taste buds, are located on the anterior surface of the tongue. These taste buds are innervated by the chorda tympani nerve (a branch of the facial, or seventh cranial, nerve). About a dozen circumvallate papillae are spread in a row along the back of the tongue. Each of these papillae contains more than 100 taste buds. They are innervated by the glossopharyngeal (ninth cranial) nerve.

Both the chorda tympani and glossopharyngeal taste afferents synapse within the nucleus of the tractus solitarius within the medulla. Second-order neurons then project through the medial lemniscus to the ventrobasal thalamus, and from there, third-order neurons ascend to the sensory cortex. The cortical taste area is located close to the somatosensory area on the lateral surface of the postcentral gyrus that receives projections from the tongue. This pathway is concerned primarily with the objective interpretation of taste sensations. The emotional and affective behavior elicited by taste is thought to be mediated by a pathway that ascends from the medulla and pons to the hypothalamus and amygdala.

Four primary taste sensations have been identified: sweet, salty, sour, and bitter. Sweet taste sensations are elicited by sugars and a number of other substances including amino acids, peptides, alcohols, and some lead compounds. Salty sensations are produced by common table salt (sodium chloride) and other monovalent and divalent salts. Sour tastes are derived primarily from organic and inorganic acids, and bitter-tasting substances are most often alkaloids such as quinine and caffeine. Sugars and salts must be present in fairly high concentrations (10 mmol or more) to be detected by the taste receptors, although some of the artificial sweeteners can elicit a sweet taste at much lower concentrations. Acids must also be present in high concentrations (at a pH of 3 or below) to produce a sour taste. In contrast, quinine is an effective stimulus at 10 μmol. The higher sensitivity to quinine (and other bitter-tasting poisons) makes the tongue an effective guardian against the ingestion of dangerous materials. However, the relatively high concentrations at which these substances are active makes it unlikely that they bind with a highly specific receptor site on the taste cell membrane. In fact, any given taste cell usually responds to more than one of the so-called primary taste sensations.

The inability to identify a specific taste receptor for each of the primary taste sensations makes it difficult to understand how taste sensations are interpreted by the CNS. Most likely, each taste sensation produces a unique pattern of activity in a number of afferent fibers and this pattern is then used by the cells in the cortical taste area to produce a taste sensation. Despite the seeming randomness with which taste receptors respond to one or more taste stimuli, various areas of the tongue are more responsive to some taste stimuli than others. Thus sweet-tasting stimuli are most effective when applied to the tip of the tongue; salty substances elicit the greatest response when applied to the front and sides of the tongue; and the back of the tongue produces the greatest response to sour- and bitter-tasting substances.

OLFACTION

Olfaction, like taste, provides information about the nature of chemicals that come in contact with an individual. The olfactory receptor is located on the dendrites of the bipolar nerve fibers that make up the olfactory (first cranial) nerve. There are more than 100 million olfactory nerve fibers, and they are among the thinnest in the nervous system. Their cell bodies are located within the olfactory epithelium that lies on top of the nasal cavity. The olfactory epithelium has an area of approximately 5 cm^2 and contains supporting and basal cells in addition to the olfactory cells. The basal cells continuously differentiate to form new olfactory neurons every 60 days or so. Thus the olfactory receptors are similar to taste receptors in that new cells are continuously being formed. The olfactory system is remarkable, however, because the receptors are part of the CNS, in which neurons are thought not to be capable of differentiation in the adult.

The dendrites extend for about 100 μm before enlarging into an olfactory vesicle. The olfactory vesicle is 1 to 2 μm in diameter and gives rise to 20 or 30 cilia, which extend into the mucous layer covering the olfactory epithelium. Most likely the olfactory receptor is located on these cilia. The olfactory cell axons leave the nasal cavity through the cribiform plate and enter the olfactory bulb. Second-order neurons arising from the olfactory bulb travel through the olfactory tract to the olfactory cortex on the ventral surface of the frontal lobe. This is the only sensory pathway that reaches the cortex without first synapsing within the thalamus. Fibers from the olfactory bulb also enter the hypothalamus and limbic system. These pathways presumably mediate the intense affective response that often occurs to odors. Additional fibers travel from the cortex to the olfactory bulb. These fibers may play a role in modifying the olfactory information reaching the olfactory cortex and limbic system.

Not much is understood about the mechanism by which an odorous molecule stimulates an olfactory receptor. However, olfactory stimulants must be airborne and soluble in the mucous coating of the olfactory epithelium if they are to reach the ciliary receptors. Although it has been impossible to identify any unique chemical or structural characteristics by which odorants could be classified, seven different types of smells have been suggested as odor primaries. These are camphorous (a mothball odor), musky, floral, minty, etheral (like ether), pungent (like formaldehyde), and putrid (like rotten eggs). Specific binding sites for odorous molecules are likely to be identified in the future, however, because (1) minute concentrations of the odorants (fewer than 8 molecules per olfactory neuron) are able to produce an olfactory sensation and (2) a large number of specific anosmias (the inability to recognize a particular odor) have been found.

Olfactory perceptions fade rapidly during prolonged exposure to an odorant. The adaptation is due to events within the CNS because neither the receptor potential nor the train of action potentials it generates adapts. Also, the olfactory system saturates at relatively low concentrations of odorants. Typically, a concentration of just 50 times threshold will cause a maximum firing rate in the olfactory nerve fibers. Thus it appears that the olfactory system functions primarily to identify new odors in the environment. Neither the concentration of the odorant nor its continued presence seems to be of much concern to the CNS. Perhaps this is related to the strong emotional and behavioral responses associated with olfactory sensations. For example, a great many social and sexual behaviors are elicited in animals in response to odors, called **pheromones**, released by other members of their communities. Once the behavior is triggered, no particular advantage would be derived from the continued presence of the sensation. In fact, it might be disadvantageous if the previously released odor masked the presence of a new odor entering the environment. Also, because the molecules are released in such small quantities and elicit behaviors in an all-or-none fashion, there is no need to respond over a wide concentration range. It is unclear whether humans respond strongly to the release of pheromones. However, seemingly irrational group behaviors may be due to olfactory cues. In addition, a number of psychotic reactions can be elicited by odors, and schizophrenic individuals often have increased sensitivity to, or at least awareness of, odors in their environment.

PHYSIOLOGY OF THE MOTOR CONTROL SYSTEM

Muscular activity is organized by the motor control system. The motor control system, like all control systems, is composed of receptors, integrators, and effectors. Two types of receptors are important. One group, providing information about events occurring outside the body, helps determine what motor acts are required to pursue purposeful behavior. The other group, called proprioceptors (consisting of muscle, joint, and vestibular receptors), provides information about body position and skeletal muscle activity. This information is used to plan motor activity and monitor its progress while it is being carried out. The integrators are dispersed throughout the CNS, allowing motor behavior to be controlled at the most appropriate level. The spinal cord controls simple reflexes, the brain stem controls posture, the basal ganglia controls complex patterns of movement, the cerebellum coordinates muscular activity, and the cortex plans and executes voluntary movements. A

single effector unit, the alpha motoneuron and the skeletal muscle fibers it innervates, is responsible for generating all motor activity.

This chapter will review each component of the motor control system and illustrate its role in the production of movement.

THE EFFECTORS

The alpha motoneuron is the final common pathway for all motor behavior. All movement, whether a simple reflex response to a painful stimulus or a highly complex gymnastics maneuver, is carried out by the coordinated discharge of alpha-motoneuron action potentials.

Alpha motoneurons are among the largest neurons in the CNS. Their cell bodies are 30 to 70 μm in diameter; their dendritic trees extend over several millimeters; and their axons can be longer than a meter. Over 80% of their cell bodies and dentrites are covered with synaptic terminals. They are organized into motoneuron pools both within the ventral horn of the spinal cord and the nuclei of the cranial nerves producing skeletal muscle activity. The motoneuron pools contain both the alpha motoneurons innervating a particular muscle and the gamma motoneurons, which, as will be discussed below, are responsible for controlling the activity of the muscle spindle receptors within the skeletal muscles.

The alpha motoneuron and all the skeletal muscle fibers it innervates are called a **motor unit**. This is the functional unit of the motor control system because each time an alpha moto-neuron is fired, all of its branches and consequently all of the skeletal muscle fibers it innervates are also discharged. Motor units can consist of just a few or several hundred skeletal muscle fibers. The size of the motor unit varies with the amount of control exerted over the muscle by the CNS. Thus the large postural muscles of the back have much larger motor units than those controlling the movements of the fingers.

The muscle fibers within a motor unit are separated from each other so that their force can be evenly distributed throughout the muscle. The fibers contained within a motor unit all have the same physiological and metabolic properties. Two major types of skeletal muscle fibers have been identified on the basis of several related criteria. One type is characterized by its rapid speed of contraction, its capacity for aerobic metabolism, its resistance to fatigue, and its red color. The other type is characterized by its slow contractile speed, its dependence on anaerobic metabolism, its susceptibility to fatigue, and its white color.

Table 2-3 lists several other characteristics of these two types of muscle fibers, as well as an intermediate type of fiber. The slow, aerobic, fatigue-resistant red fiber is adapted for continuous activity. It has a rich supply of capillaries to provide oxygen and a high concentration of mitochondria to utilize the oxygen for the aerobic production of ATP. In contrast, the fast, anaerobic, fatigable white fibers are adapted for sudden bursts of activity. These fibers have a sparse capillary supply and rely on their large glycogen stores and glycolytic enzymes for the anaerobic production of ATP. Slow-twitch fibers are smaller than the fast-twitch fibers and have a lower density of myofilaments within them. Thus they produce smaller forces than the fast-twitch fibers. In return for being able to generate more force, large fibers are limited in the duration of their

Table 2-3. Characteristics of Muscle Fibers

Property	Classification		
	FF(FG, IIb, white)	FR(FOG, IIa, red)	S(SO, I, red)
Speed of shortening	Fast	Fast	Slow
Resistance to fatigue	Poor	Intermediate	High
Fiber diameter	Large	Intermediate	Small
Size of motor unit	Large	Intermediate	Small
Sarcoplasmic reticulum	Large	Intermediate	Small
Vascular supply	Sparse	Intermediate	Dense
Myoglobin content	None	Little	High
Glycogen content	High	Intermediate	Low
Mitochondria	Few	Intermediate	Many
Glycolytic enzymes	High	Intermediate	Low
Oxidative enzymes	Low	Intermediate	High
Myosin ATPase	High	High	Low

activity because there is a limit to (1) how rapidly oxygen can diffuse into them and (2) how much glycogen they can store. Most muscles contain a mixture of motor unit types and are thus able to produce low levels of sustained activity as well as short bursts of high-force production.

The recruitment of motor units during the performance of a motor task is carried out in an orderly fashion. The smaller motor units containing the slow-twitch fibers are recruited before the larger motor units containing the fast-twitch fibers. This is sensible from a physiological point of view because it allows the muscle fibers to be used efficiently.

For example, there is little point in activating the easily fatigable larger motor units if the motor task requires a sustained action or a low force production. As more force is required, the larger motor units can be recruited to provide it. In this way, muscle glycogen stores can be preserved and the oxygen provided to the muscles can be used most effectively.

The synaptic organization of the motor neuron pool ensures that the orderly recruitment of motor units according to size occurs automatically. Almost all of the afferents synapsing with one neuron in a motoneuron pool will synapse with all the other neurons in the pool as well. Thus the number of channels opened, and consequently the amount of current entering the cell, will be the same in all alpha motoneurons. However, having the same amount of synaptic current does not result in the same amount of depolarization. According to Ohm's law,

$$V = IR$$

where V = the depolarization caused by the synaptic current; I = the synaptic current; and R = the resistance of the cell membrane to the passage of current.

The larger the cell, the larger its surface area and the lower its resistance. Thus the same amount of synaptic current flowing through small and large alpha motoneurons will cause a larger depolarization in the smaller cells and the larger depolarization will cause threshold to be achieved in smaller cells before it is reached in larger cells.

The type of muscle fiber in a motor unit is determined by the activity of the muscle fiber. The more active a muscle is, the more fatigue-resistant characteristics it develops. Thus exercise causes an increase in the number of capillaries supplying a muscle, in the concentration of mitochondria within a muscle fibers, and in the ability of the muscle to withstand prolonged activity without fatigue.

The mechanism by which activity produces the changes in fiber characteristics is not known. However, it is independent of how the muscle fiber activity changes. For example, electrical stimulation of the muscle at a steady rate of 10/second will produce the same changes as exercise. Similar changes can occur in a muscle if its innervation changes. This can be produced experimentally by severing the nerve to a muscle and reconnecting the peripheral stump of the nerve to the central end of a nerve that previously innervated a different muscle. If the peripheral end of a nerve going to a slow-twitch fiber is connected to the central end of a muscle that previously went to a fast-twitch fiber, the fiber will develop the characteristics of a fast-twitch fiber. Similar changes occur spontaneously after nerve injury. The growing fibers do not necessarily innervate the same fibers they innervated before they were injured. However, all the muscle fibers newly innervated by branches from the same alpha motoneuron will develop the same physiological contractile properties.

THE RECEPTORS

The CNS receives information about the muscle length and contractile force of skeletal muscles from the muscle spindles and **Golgi tendon organs** (GTOs), respectively. GTOs are large (0.5 to 1 mm in diameter) encapsulated receptors located within the tendinous insertions of skeletal muscles. They are innervated by large Ib afferent fibers. The number of GTOs in a muscle increases with the size of the muscle and the degree of control exerted over the muscle by the CNS.

Each GTO is attached to a few muscle fibers from a number of motor units. When these fibers contract, the nerve terminal within the GTO is stretched, resulting in an increase in firing rate of the IB afferents. As indicated in Figure 2-49*B*, the frequency of IB discharge increases in proportion to the amount of force generated by the muscle when it contracts. Since passive stretch of the muscle has very little effect on Ib afferent activity, the frequency of firing in the Ib afferents is a good indication of the active tension produced by the muscle.

The **muscle spindle** is much more complicated than the GTO because it contains at least two different types of afferent fibers, and more importantly its sensitivity can be altered by the CNS. Muscles over which the CNS exerts a high degree of control, such as the hand muscles, have a higher density of muscle spindles than do muscles such as those in the back, which are not under precise CNS control.

The muscle spindle (Fig. 2-50) is an encapsulated receptor containing a dozen or so modified muscle fibers within it. These muscle fibers are called intrafusal fibers to indicate that they are within the fusiform-shaped capsule. The normal skeletal muscle fibers are referred to as extrafusal muscle fibers. The intrafusal fibers' nuclei are located in the central or equatorial region of the fiber. The remainder of the fiber is composed of sarcomeres similar to those found in extrafusal muscle fibers.

The **intrafusal fibers** are classified as nuclear bag or nuclear chain, based on the arrangement of their nuclei in the center region of the fiber. The nuclei in the nuclear bag fibers are bunched up in the center of the fiber so that many nuclei can be seen in a cross-sectional view. The nuclei in the nuclear chain fibers are lined up in a single row so only one nucleus is visible in a cross-section of the muscle fiber. The nuclear bag fibers are thicker and longer than the nuclear chain fibers. Every intrafusal fiber (both nuclear bag and nuclear chain) is innervated by a branch of the single Ia afferent entering the spindle. The afferent terminals curl around the center of the intrafusal fibers and so are called **annuolospiral endings**. They are also called **primary endings** or simply Ia afferents. Smaller afferent fibers, called group II afferents, flower spray endings, or secondary endings, innervate the nuclear chain intrafusal fibers. The group II fibers terminate in the muscle region just bordering the Ia afferents. Several group II afferents may enter a single muscle spindle.

Muscle spindle afferents increase their firing rate when the muscle is stretched (Fig. 2-51*A*). Stretching the muscle causes the intrafusal muscle fibers to stretch. However, only the central nuclear region of the intrafusal fiber stretches because it is much more compliant than the sarcomere-containing polar regions of the intrafusal fibers. Stretching the central region of the intrafusal muscle fibers deforms the Ia and II afferent endings, causing them to increase their rate of firing.

The firing pattern produced by stretch is different in the Ia and II afferents. Ia afferents fire rapidly when the muscle is stretched and then level off to a slow, steady rate of discharge proportional to the amount of stretch. Thus they provide information about both the rate and amount of muscle stretch. Group II afferents produce a steady rate of discharge without going through a period of firing. Thus they provide information only about the amount of stretch. The ability of the Ia afferents to respond to the rate of muscle stretch results from their innervation of the nuclear bag fibers. The nuclear chain fibers provide the Ia and II afferents with information about the amount of muscle stretch.

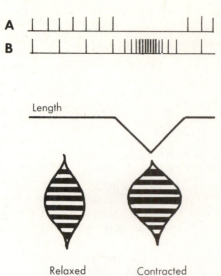

Figure 2-49. Muscle spindles are arranged in parallel with the skeletal muscle so the firing of Ia afferents decreases during muscle contraction (A). In contrast, the Golgi tendon organ is arranged in series with the skeletal muscle so the discharge rate of Ib afferents increases during a muscle contraction (B).

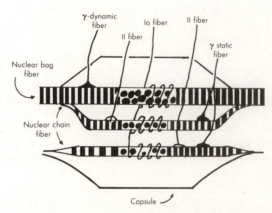

Figure 2-50. A diagram of the innervation of the intrafusal fibers within a muscle spindle. Both nuclear chain and nuclear bag intrafusal fibers are innervated by the single Ia afferent entering each muscle spindle. Group II fibers entering the spindle innervate nuclear chain fibers. Gamma motoneurons innervate both types of intrafusal fibers.

Ia and II afferent firing ceases when the muscle contracts (Fig. 2-49*A*). This is in contrast to the response of GTOs, which discharged in response to muscle contraction. The difference in the response characteristics of Ia and Ib afferents is related to their orientation with respect to the extrafusal muscle fibers. Ib afferents are in series with the muscle so they are stretched whenever tension on the extrafusal fibers increases (although as indicated above, passive increases in tension have very little effect on IB activity). Ia and II afferents are in parallel with the extrafusal muscle fibers. Thus they are stretched when the extrafusal fibers are stretched and become slack when the extrafusal muscle fibers are shortened.

The sensitivity of the muscle spindle to changes in muscle length is controlled by two types of gamma motoneurons. The

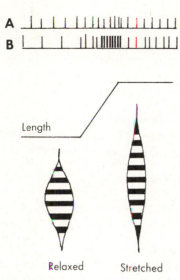

Figure 2-51. The rate of Ia discharge increases when the intrafusal fibers are stretched. If the gamma motoneurons are stimulated, the firing rate increases even more.

gamma static fibers increase the Ia afferents' responsiveness to changes in muscle length, while the gamma dynamic fibers increase the Ia afferents' response to the rate of muscle stretch. These effects are illustrated in Figure 2-51*B*, which displays the change in Ia firing rate when a muscle is stretched in the absence and presence of gamma-motoneuron activity.

When the gamma motoneurons fire, they cause the sarcomeres of the intrafusal fibers to shorten. Because the force of intrafusal contraction is so low, only the highly compliant central region of the intrafusal fibers is stretched. Gamma motoneuron discharge also prevents the cessation of Ia and II afferent discharge that occurs when the muscle contracts. As indicated above, when the muscle contracts, the central region of the intrafusal fibers becomes slack. This is referred to as unloading. Unloading can be avoided if the gamma motoneurons cause the intrafusal muscle fibers to shorten along with the extrafusal muscle fibers. Under most normal circumstances, firing of the alpha motoneurons is accompanied by firing of the gamma motoneurons so that the amount of spindle unloading during a movement is minimized. The simultaneous firing of alpha and gamma motoneurons is called **coactivation.**

SPINAL CORD REFLEXES

The Ia afferent activity initiated when a muscle is stretched elicits a reflex contraction of that muscle. A phasic stretch reflex is produced when the muscle is rapidly stretched. This can be observed as a single rapid contraction of the quadriceps muscle when the patella tendon is tapped. A static stretch reflex is produced when the muscle is stretched more slowly. This reflex provides the slight resistance to stretch generated when a normal limb is extended. It is also responsible for the steady rate of firing present in antigravity muscles that maintain an upright posture. The stretch reflex is also called the **myotatic reflex.**

The Ia afferents entering the spinal cord through the dorsal root synapse directly on alpha motoneurons innervating muscle fibers from which the afferent fibers originated. In addition, a branch of the Ia afferent synapses on inhibitory interneurons within the spinal cord that in turn synapse on alpha motoneurons innervating muscle fibers that are antagonistic to the muscle from which the Ia afferent originated. Thus the stretch reflex not only causes direct, monosynaptic contraction of the agonist muscle but at the same time causes inhibition of the antagonistic muscle. This neuronal organization, called **reciprocal innervation,** is a general feature of the motor control system. It has the obvious advantage of allowing a muscle to contract without opposition from its antagonists. Other branches of the Ia afferents cross the spinal cord to activate contralateral motoneurons, while still others ascend in the spinal cord to provide the CNS with information about changes in muscle length.

Ib afferents entering the spinal cord synapse on inhibitory interneurons that in turn synapse on alpha motoneurons innervating the muscle from which the Ib afferent originated. Thus whenever a muscle contracts, the GTOs cause a reflex inhibition of the muscle. This reflex is called the **inverse myotatic reflex** or the autogenic inhibitory reflex. It acts to limit the amount of tension a muscle can generate.

Another reflex-limiting muscle tension is mediated by Renshaw cells. These cells are located among the alpha motoneurons in the ventral horn and receive monosynaptic synapses from branches of the alpha motoneurons as they leave the spinal cord. The Renshaw cells then synapse directly on the alpha motoneurons, diminishing their activity. Renshaw cell inhibition is called recurrent inhibition. Although it might appear that the reflex inhibition of alpha motoneurons is counterproductive, it actually provides the CNS with another mechanism to control the force of muscle contraction. By changing the sensitivity of the inhibitory interneurons, the CNS can increase or decrease the amount of recurrent inhibition produced by the Renshaw cell.

The information about muscle length and tension provided to the CNS by the muscle spindles and GTOs is used in both the planning and monitoring of motor behavior. In addition, the CNS can, by altering the sensitivity of the muscle spindles and spinal interneurons, use the sensory information in the execution of motor acts. Sensitivity of the muscle spindles is increased by firing of the gamma motoneurons. The pathway by which the change in muscle spindle sensitivity alters the activity of muscle fibers is called the gamma loop. The gamma loop consists of the gamma motoneuron, the intrafusal muscle fiber, the Ia afferent, and the alpha motoneuron. The process by which the gamma loop affects muscle contraction is referred to as a **servo control** system.

In a servo system, the effector organ is activated until a predetermined condition is achieved. For example, in a servo-controlled heating system, the thermostat (the receptor) is set at a particular temperature (the set point) and the furnace (the effector) operates until the room temperature reaches the set point. In the motor control system, the servo system controls the amount of muscle shortening that occurs during a movement. Suppose, for example, that an object is to be lifted by contracting the biceps and thus flexing the arm. Instead of directly activating the alpha motoneurons innervating the biceps muscle, the servo system acts through the gamma loop.

Descending pathways from the motor cortex activate the gamma motoneurons. The gamma motoneurons in turn cause the intrafusal muscle fibers to contract, and this causes the Ia afferent fibers to discharge. (Recall that when the intrafusal fibers contract, their sarcomeres shorten and their central region lengthens.) The Ia afferents then excite the alpha motoneurons. The amount of alpha-motoneuron activity produced (and consequently, the force of biceps contraction) depends on the frequency of discharge in the Ia afferents, and this depends on how much the central regions of the intrafusal fibers have been lengthened by the gamma motoneurons. As the biceps shortens, the central region of the intrafusal fibers shortens and the Ia discharge decreases. Eventually the amount of Ia activity is too low to drive the biceps and the arm stops moving. The final position of the arm is determined by the amount of intrafusal fiber contraction produced by the gamma motoneurons.

The main advantage of a servo-guided movement over a directly produced movement is that the final position of the arm, rather than the force produced by the muscle, is specified by the CNS. If the CNS incorrectly estimated the force of contraction, the arm could overshoot the desired position (if the force was too great) or fail to achieve it (if the force was too low). Servo-guided movements occur more slowly than directly activated movements, so when speed and power are more important than final position (such as when swinging a baseball bat), the alpha motoneurons are directly activated. Regardless of whether the movement is servo guided or directly produced, the CNS coactivates the alpha and gamma motoneurons. The CNS excitation of the alpha motoneurons adds to that produced by the Ia afferents, aiding servo-guided movements, while the CNS gamma activation in a directly produced movement decreases the amount of intrafusal fiber unloading that occurs during muscle shortening.

Another, and equally important, role of the servo system is to resist movement when the load on the muscle changes or when the mechanical properties of the muscle are altered. For example, if the arm is held in a flexed position and the load on the biceps increases, the arm will extend. Extension of the biceps will cause the intrafusal fibers to lengthen, resulting in Ia discharge, alpha-motoneuron firing, and biceps contraction. Conversely, if the load is reduced, the muscle will shorten, causing Ia and alpha-motoneuron activity, and biceps contraction will be reduced.

The alteration of biceps contraction in response to length changes depends on the sensitivity of the Ia fiber to stretch, and this in turn depends on the degree of gamma-motoneuron activity. The greater the gamma-motoneuron activity at a particular extrafusal fiber muscle length, the more the muscle will resist changes in length. The GTOs also participate in maintaining muscle position. For example, if the muscle begins to fatigue, the amount of Ib activity will be reduced, causing a decrease in alpha-motoneuron inhibition. Removal of inhibition results in an increased firing frequency and thus an increase in muscle force development.

The tonic input into the spinal cord from higher centers in the brain is very important in the maintenance of normal movement. When the spinal cord is severed, total paralysis (spinal shock) occurs. Although part of the paralysis may be due to the trauma of injury, most of it is due to the loss of excitation from higher centers. Over time, reflex activity within the cord returns and, in fact, becomes hyperexcitable. Eventually, the affected limbs exhibit spasticity (abnormally high tone). The cause of the hyperexcitability is not known but appears to be axonal sprouting. That is, the degeneration of synapses on interneurons and alpha motoneurons within the spinal cord caused by the destruction of descending axons leaves room for branches of peripheral afferent fibers to form new synapses. These new synaptic connections are thought to cause the increased reflex excitability and spasticity that occur subsequent to a spinal injury.

Spinal control of posture and locomotion

When the neuroaxis above the pons is sectioned, the antigravity muscles become hyperexcitable and spastic. This condition (called decerebrate rigidity) is caused by the removal of cerebral inhibition from the brain stem. Without this inhibition, pathways from the brain stem, particularly the reticulospinal and vestibulospinal pathways, discharge at abnormally high rates. Although both the alpha- and gamma-motoneuron activity is increased, most of the decerebrate rigidity disappears if the gamma loop is severed (by cutting the dorsal roots). Consequently, the decerebrate rigidity is called gamma rigidity and is thought to result from a hyperexcitable stretch reflex. Antigravity muscles are affected more than the non-antigravity muscles, because the brainstem centers exciting them (principally in the pontine reticular formation) become more active when released from inhibition than those centers (primarily in the medullary reticular formation) exciting the non-antigravity muscles.

If, in addition to separating the cerebral pathways from the brain stem, the cerebellar pathways are also removed, the degree of spasticity is increased. If under these conditions the dorsal roots are cut, the spasticity does not disappear. Consequently, this type of condition is called **alpha rigidity**. Despite the difference in names, the two types of spasticity are caused by an increase in both alpha and gamma-motoneuron activity. However, when the removal of cerebellar inhibition is added to removal of cerebral inhibition, the amount of alpha-motoneuron discharge is so great that it can sustain the spasticity without the aid of the gamma-loop reflex.

The muscles exhibiting increased tone following a brain injury depend on the amount of cerebral damage and can be quite variable. In general, the leg extensors (antigravity muscles) almost always display increased tone. However, the arm extensors are usually hyperexcitable following a decerebrate state while the flexors are usually more excitable following a cortical or internal capsular lesion. The reasons for these differences are unclear.

Spasticity is a specific term applied to the clinical signs of cortical lesions releasing the brain stem centers from inhibition. It involves an increased reflex excitability to only one of the muscles at a joint—for example, the leg extensors or the arm flexors. Because of its reflex nature, the amount of muscle tone increases as the affected muscle is stretched. This is in contrast to the clinical sign of rigidity that occurs in Parkinson's disease. In rigidity, both muscle groups (extensors and flexors) acting at a joint display increased tone and the tone does not increase when the muscles are lengthened.

The brain stem centers help to maintain an upright posture

by increasing the sensitivity of the gamma loop in antigravity muscles. In addition, they participate in other reflex adjustments to disturbances in body position. For example, most individuals will sway back and forth during normal standing. The amplitude of the sway is decreased by a reflex contraction of the gastrocnemius muscle when the body moves forward and the reflex contraction of the tibialis when the body sways backward. However, if the gastrocnemius muscle is stretched by tilting the foot upward (so the body is pushed backward), contraction of the gastrocnemius would destabilize the posture. If this is done repeatedly, the gastrocnemius stretch reflex is inhibited. Although the pathways are not entirely known, the inhibition of the stretch reflex does not occur in patients with cerebellar lesions. Thus the cerebellum appears capable of modifying the excitability of the gamma loop to meet various postural demands.

Brain stem centers are also capable of initiating the rhythmic alterations in muscular activity required for normal locomotion. Decerebrate cats can be made to walk on a treadmill by electrically stimulating an area in the brain stem called the midbrain locomotor region. The speed and pattern of walking depend on the treadmill speed and not on the pattern of electrical stimulation. Thus as the speed of the treadmill increases, the rate of walking increases. If the speed becomes high enough, the cat will trot or gallop on the treadmill.

The pattern generators for walking are located in the spinal cord. Although each leg can be made to walk independently, under normal circumstances they are linked together so that the movement of all four limbs is coordinated. Afferent information generated during locomotion is important for normal walking to occur. For example, during normal walking, the leg acts alternately to support the weight of the body (the stance phase) and to move forward (the swing phase). As the leg is extended during the stance phase, muscular activity suddenly switches from primarily extensor to primarily flexor and the swing phase is initiated. The timing of this switch is related to the amount of leg extension. If the limb is prevented from extending, the swing phase is not initiated. The brain uses information it receives from muscle, joint, and cutaneous receptors to modify the walking behavior. It also receives information from the alpha motoneurons responsible for generating the movement. This information, called **efference copy** or **reafferance**, allows the CNS to compare its motor commands (efference copy) with the actual movements they produce (afferent feedback).

THE VESTIBULAR SYSTEM

The vestibular apparatus is a highly specialized receptor organ that detects the position of the head in space as well as any movements made by the head. It consists of a series of tubes that are continuous with the cochlea of the inner ear. It is divided into two different sensory organs—the **semicircular canals**, responsible for detecting rapid head movements, and the **utricle** and **saccule**, responsible for detecting the position of the head in relation to gravity.

Hair cells, similar to those found in the cochlea, serve as receptor cells for the vestibular apparatus. The major difference lies in the geometry of the hairs. In the vestibular apparatus, each hair cell contains one large **kinocilium** and approximately

50 smaller hairs called **stereocilia**. When the stereocilia bend toward the kinocilium, the cell depolarizes; when the stereocilia bend away from the kinocilium, the hair cell hyperpolarizes. Thus the hair cells are directionally sensitive.

The three **semicircular canals** are oriented perpendicularly to each other. Both ends of the canals are continuous with the utricle to form a structure called the ampulla. The ampulla contains a mound of tissue, called the crista, on which the hair cells are located. These hair cells are embedded in a gelatinous mass called the cupula. When the cupula moves, the hair cells bend. All of the hair cells in each semicircular canal are polarized in the same way; their kinocilia are located on the side of the hair cell closest to the utricle. When the head moves rapidly, the semicircular canals move with it but the fluid in the canals lags behind. The relative movement of the fluid drags the cupula in a direction opposite to that of the head and causes the stereocilia to bend. The amount of bending depends on how fast the head is moving. After a short time (20 to 30 seconds), the elasticity of the cupula restores the hairs to their original position and the hair cells return to their resting level of activity. Thus the hair cells are only capable of measuring changes in movement or acceleration and not movements at a constant velocity. Because the semicircular canals are organized in three planes, movements in any direction can be detected.

The horizontal canal is oriented in such a way that it is horizontal to the plane of the earth when the head is tilted slightly forward. The ampulla is located so that moving the head to the right pushes the hairs in the left semicircular canal away from the utricle (and kinocilium) while the hairs in the right semicircular canal are pushed toward the kinocilium. When the head stops moving, the canals immediately cease their motion. However, the fluid within them keeps moving, dragging the cupula along with it. Thus the hairs are bent again, although in a direction opposite to that which occurred when the movement began. Thus after ceasing a rotation of the head to the right, the fluid and cupula in the horizontal semicircular canals continue to move toward the right. This causes stimulation of the hair cells in the left semicircular canal and inhibition of the hair cells in the right semicircular canal.

The hairs of the utricle and saccule are embedded in a gelatinous mass containing a large number of calcium carbonate crystals called otoconia. For this reason, these organs are sometimes referred to as **otolith organs**. The crystals have a higher density than the fluid in which they are embedded and so "fall" downward. The hairs embedded inside the otoconia also bend. Those hair cells oriented in such a way that their hairs bend toward the kinocilium increase their rate of firing. Those in which the stereocilia bend away from the kinocilium decrease their rate of firing. Still other hair cells, in which the hairs do not bend toward or away from the kinocilium, do not change their rate of firing. In this manner, activity in a specific hair cell signals the position of the head in space. Because they are horizontally organized, the hair cells of the utricle are highly sensitive to small tilts of the head from its normal vertical position.

The vestibular apparatus gives rise to a number of reflexes that are important for maintaining balance and coordinating the movement of the head and eyes. For example, afferent neurons innervating the utricle (cranial nerve VIII) enter the vestibular nucleus, where they initiate reflexes that keep the head in an upright position. Thus if a person falls forward, the neck muscles responsible for moving the head backward will keep the head in an upright position. At the same time, leg extensors will be activated to keep the body from falling. Similar postural reflexes are elicited by the semicircular canals. When the head moves rapidly in one direction, the leg on that side is extended to act as a pivot while the leg on the other side is flexed in preparation for moving in the direction the head is turned.

One of the most important reflexes mediated by the vestibular apparatus is the **vestibulo-ocular reflex**. This reflex ensures that the eyes remain fixed on an object while the head is moving. The reflex is easily demonstrated by rotating an individual sitting on a chair. As the head moves to the right, the hair cells in the right horizontal semicircular canal are stimulated. The hair cells activate fibers of cranial nerve VIII. These fibers enter the vestibular nuclei, where they synapse with neurons whose axons travel in the medial longitudinal fasciculus to the oculomotor nuclei of the ipsilateral cranial nerve III and contralateral cranial nerve VI. Efferents from these cranial nuclei excite the medial rectus on the right and the lateral rectus on the left, causing the eye to move opposite to the direction of head movement.

At the same time as the hair cells in the right semicircular canal are stimulated, those in the left semicircular canal are inhibited. This causes relaxation of the left medial and right lateral rectus muscles, allowing the eyes to move without opposition. If the head continues to move, the eyes will eventually reach the end of their ability to rotate in the socket. This will elicit another reflex that rapidly returns the eyes to the center of the socket. These two reflexes—the slow movement of the eyes opposite to the direction of head movement and the rapid return of the eyes to the center of the socket—is referred to as **nystagmus**.

When the head stops moving, the hair cells in the horizontal semicircular canal on the opposite side will be stimulated, producing a slow movement of the eyes in the direction of previous rotation. This reflex, called **postrotary nystagmus**, lasts for 30 seconds or until the cupula returns to its original position. Destruction of the vestibular apparatus eliminates or prevents nystagmus from occurring, while irritative lesions in the vestibular system or the cerebellum can cause the presence of spontaneous nystagmus.

THE BASAL GANGLIA

The basal ganglia are a group of brain structures within the cerebrum and brain stem that are important in the generation of patterned activity. However, some aspects of parkinsonism may occur when damage to the nigrostriatal tract disinhibits a cholinergic pathway within the basal ganglia. For this reason, anticholinergic drugs used to be prescribed for parkinsonism. Currently the use of L-dopa to replace the loss of dopamine has proved to be much more effective. Its use has brought significant relief to many parkinsonian patients.

The rigidity associated with parkinsonism is different from the spasticity caused by the cortical lesions that release the reticular formation from inhibition. Unlike spasticity, which is caused by hyperactive stretch reflexes in the antigravity muscles, the rigidity of parkinsonism is caused by overactivity to both agonists and antagonists at a joint. It is often described as

"lead-pipe" or "cogwheel" rigidity. The term **lead-pipe** derives from the tendency of the limb to remain fixed at whatever position it is moved to, while the term **cog-wheel** represents the alternating rigidity and relaxation that accompany passive movement of the limb. The tremor disappears while the patient is performing a voluntary movement. Although its mechanism is not known, the resting tremor may be caused by a higher than normal discharge from those basal ganglia feedback loops that are released from inhibition. Perhaps the tremor disappears during purposeful movements because the basal ganglia are inhibited by the motor cortex or perhaps the output from the motor cortex simply overwhelms that of the basal ganglia.

The paucity of movement (akinesia) associated with parkinsonism is not caused by motor weakness or by a loss of ability to perform motor tasks. Instead it appears to be caused by a loss of the ability to initiate the motor commands, because once a task is begun it can be performed normally (within the constraints of the overlying rigidity). The general lack of ability to initiate motor activity may also account for the fixed facial expression and lack of coordinated movements that occur during the performance of a motor task (for example, the failure to swing the arms while walking).

THE CEREBELLUM

The cerebellum plays a crucial role in coordinating motor activity. When it is damaged, highly skilled movements deteriorate significantly. Interestingly, however, cerebellar disease does not cause any profound changes in muscle tone nor produce any spontaneous activity, as is the case with cortical and basal ganglia lesions. The cerebellum receives information from all cutaneous and proprioceptive receptors and thus is "aware" of the body's position at all times. Simultaneously, the cerebellum receives information from the cortex about the nature of the motor tasks being carried out. By "knowing" the goal of a motor command and how the body's musculoskeletal system responds to it, the cerebellum is able to coordinate motor activity during the execution of a movement.

The neuronal circuitry within the cerebellum is fairly simple. The cerebellum is divided into three lobes: the anterior, posterior, and flocculonodular lobes. The **flocculonodular lobe** was the earliest lobe to be developed phylogenetically and thus has been called the archicerebellum. The **anterior lobe** is more primitive (again from a phylogenetic viewpoint) than the posterior lobe and so is referred to as the **paleocerebellum**, while the anterior lobe is referred to as the **neocerebellum**.

Functionally, it is more appropriate to divide the cerebellum into longitudinally distinct areas of responsibility. Using this schema, the central regions of the cerebellum (called the vermis) and the flocculocerebellum are called the **vestibulo-cerebellum**, the intermediate regions that make extensive contact with the spinal cord are called the spinocerebellum, and the lateral regions (occupying most of the cerebellar hemispheres) are called the **cerebrocerebellum** because they have extensive feedback loops with the cerebral cortex.

The spinocerebellum receives two types of input from the spinal cord. The dorsal spinocerebellar and cuneocerebellar tracts relay information from the peripheral cutaneous and proprioceptive receptors and thus inform the cerebellum about the state of the musculoskeletal system. The ventral and rostral spinocerebellar tracts relay information from the alpha motoneurons of the spinal cord. This information is used by the cerebellum to monitor the motor commands issued by the cerebral cortex.

The cerebrocerebellum receives its information from the cortex through the corticopontocerebellar pathway. This pathway informs the cerebellum about the intention of motor commands issued by the cortex. Another important afferent pathway to the cerebellum is the olivocerebellar tract. This tract originates in the inferior olive of the brain stem and relays information from all regions of the motor control system (the spinal cord, basal ganglia, reticular formation, and the cerebral cortex) to the cerebellum.

The efferent output from the cerebellum arises from three cerebellar nuclei located beneath the cerebellar cortex. The dentate nuclei receives its input from the lateral hemispheres (cerebrocerebellum) and sends its output to the ventral anterior nucleus of the thalamus, where it is in turn relayed to the cerebral cortex. The intermediate (spinocerebellum) cerebellar cortex sends its output through the interpositus nucleus to the other centers of the motor control system. Thus both the cerebro- and spinocerebellum are part of feedback loops within the motor control system. A similar feedback loop connects the vestibular nuclei to the vermis and flocculonodular lobes of the cerebellum. Afferent fibers from the vestibular nucleus terminate within the vestibulocerebellum. Efferent information then returns to the vestibular nucleus from the cerebellar cortex through the fastigial nucleus.

The pathway traveled by fibers entering the cerebellum is the same in each region. All fibers entering the cerebellum send one branch to the cerebellar nuclei and another to the cerebellar cortex. The afferent fibers (except those originating in the olivary nucleus, which will be considered separately) are called mossy fibers. They synapse with small granule cells in the granular layer of the cerebellar cortex. Granule cell axons then ascend to the outer layers of the cerebellar cortex (the molecular layer), where they divide into two branches, called parallel fibers, that travel in opposite directions. The parallel fibers synapse with the dendrites of Purkinje cells that ascend from the Purkinje cell layer of the cerebellar cortex into the molecular layer. Purkinje cell axons project to the cerebellar nuclei to complete the internal cerebellar feedback loop.

The number of fibers involved in each individual feedback loop is staggering. Each mossy fiber synapses with several hundred granule cells, each parallel fiber synapses with over 50 Purkinje cells, and each Purkinje cell receives synapses from 100,000 to 200,000 parallel fibers.

The mossy fiber input to the cerebellum is excitatory. Thus both the cerebellar nuclei and the granule cells are activated by axons entering the cerebellum. The granule cells in turn activate the Purkinje cells. Generally a large number of granule cells must fire together to initiate a train of normal action potentials (called simple spikes) in a Purkinje cell. Interestingly, the Purkinje cell axons, which project to the same nuclear cells activated by the mossy fibers, are inhibitory. Thus afferent input to the cerebellum produces a short burst of activity in nuclear cells, followed shortly thereafter by a burst of inhibitory activity. This rapid onset and cessation of activity of the

cerebellum presumably provides the cerebellum with the timing circuits it needs to coordinate the excitation and inhibition of alpha motoneurons that is required for all sorts of motor behavior.

Three other types of inhibitory interneurons are present within the cerebellar cortex. These are the basket cells, stellate cells, and Golgi cells. The basket and stellate cells are found in the outer molecular layer of the cerebellar cortex. These cells are activated by parallel fibers and in turn inhibit the Purkinje cells adjacent to those receiving the majority of excitation from the parallel fibers. Thus they act to narrow the region of cortex excited by mossy fiber input. The Golgi cells are found in the Purkinje cell layer of the cerebellar cortex. They too are stimulated by the parallel fibers. However, unlike the basket and stellate cells, the Golgi cell axons have a feedback effect on the granule cells and inhibit them. These cells turn off the granule cells soon after they are excited by the mossy fibers. These pathways supplement the circuit described above and help the cerebellum produce a short burst of well-focused activity.

The fibers entering the cerebellum from the olivary nucleus are called **climbing fibers** because their axons wind around the dendritic tree of the Purkinje cells like a vine, making over 300 synaptic contacts. Each climbing fiber synapses with only a few Purkinje fibers, producing a short burst of activity in these cells whenever it fires. The Purkinje fiber spike train produced by the climbing fiber is called a complex spike because it consists of an exceedingly rapid burst of action potentials that diminish in size and die out within a few milliseconds. The climbing fiber input does not appear to be involved in coordinating the ongoing motor activity of the motor system but instead may participate in motor learning.

THE CEREBRAL CORTEX

The cerebral cortex is responsible for planning and executing voluntary movements. Voluntary movements can be thought of as occurring in three stages. First, the idea for the movement must be generated. Second, a plan for carrying it out must be devised. And third, the commands for the movement must be issued. Although the role played by the different regions of the cerebral cortex in each of these taks is not yet known, a consensus seems to be emerging. The motor cortex (Fig. 2-52), lying just in front of the central sulcus, is thought to contain the command neurons responsible for issuing the orders for a movement and helping to coordinate the lower motor neurons during its execution. The supplementary and premotor cortical areas, on the dorsal and medial surface of the cortex in front of the primary motor cortex, are thought to be involved in generating the motor plan. And finally, the posterior parietal cortex is thought to contain the neurons that generate the idea for a movement. This section will describe each of these motor areas and present some of the evidence supporting their proposed role in the control of voluntary movements.

The primary motor cortex is topographically organized. That is, the body is mapped onto the cortex so that activity in the most lateral portions of the cortex generate movements of the face and mouth, while those most medially generate movements of the feet (Fig. 2-53). Much more cortical area is

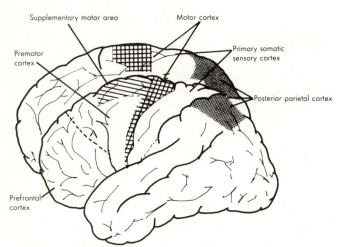

Figure 2-52. A large portion of the cerebral cortex is devoted to the control of movement. The primary motor cortex, located just in front of the central sulcus, is responsible for issuing the commands for a movement; the supplementary motor area is concerned with the planning of a movement; and the premotor and posterior parietal areas are concerned with the motivations and ideas associated with the initiation of a movement.

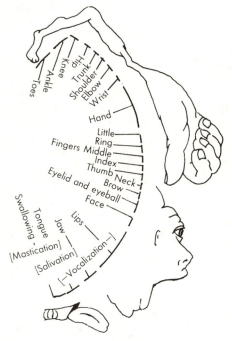

Figure 2-53. The amount of motor cortex associated with a particular muscle is related to the degree of control that must be exerted over that muscle. The homunculus maps the body parts in proportion to the area of cortex devoted to controlling them. The thumb, for example, is controlled by a cortical area as large as that required for the control of the entire trunk.

devoted to controlling muscles of the hand and mouth areas, where fine motor control is essential, than to the muscles of the trunk or legs, where coarser movements can be tolerated.

Two separate descending pathways originate within the motor cortex, the pyramidal and extrapyramidal pathways. The pyramidal pathway (consisting of the corticospinal and corticobulbar tracts) obtains its name because its axons reach the spinal cord through the pyramids found on the ventral surface of the medulla. Only about 60% of the one million or so pyramidal axons originate from neurons within the motor cortex. The remaining 40% arise from neurons within the somatosensory cortex lying just behind the central sulcus. Almost all of the pyramidal tract neurons synapse with spinal cord interneurons lying close to the alpha motoneurons controlled by the motor cortex. A small percentage (approximately 2%) of the pyramidal tract neurons arise from fairly large cortical neurons (called Betz's cells). These axons may synapse directly on alpha motoneurons and are presumably responsible for controlling movements requiring the greatest amount of precision.

The extrapyramidal system is far more diffuse. It consists of all neurons within the motor cortex that are able to control spinal motoneurons. Neurons within the extrapyramidal system synapse within the brain stem and thus relay their commands to the spinal cord through cerebral interneurons. The most important of these pathways travel through the pontine and medullary reticular formation. These neurons most likely control most of our ordinary voluntary movements. For example, if we decide to cross the room, sit down, and pick up a newspaper, the cerebral commands issued to the alpha motoneurons required to carry out these movements probably descend to the spinal cord through the extrapyramidal system. However, if we then decide to do the crossword puzzle, the hand and finger movements necessary to guide the pencil are probably controlled by the pyramidal system.

The neurons of the extrapyramidal system play another important role. They are responsible for keeping the excitatory reticulospinal tract neurons under control. These latter neurons provide a tonic excitatory input to the alpha motoneurons innervating the antigravity muscles. This is why lesions within the extrapyramidal system lead to spasticity. When the inhibitory fibers to the pontine reticular formation are destroyed, the excitatory input to antigravity muscles becomes excessive. As a result, the antigravity muscles are stimulated continuously. In contrast, lesions to the pyramidal system, although producing a deficit in fine motor control, do not lead to an increase in muscle tone and do not prevent most movements from occurring normally. Clinically, pure pyramidal tract lesions do not occur. Thus motor deficits resulting from a stroke or other traumatic brain injury are a combination of losses in both the pyramidal and extrapyramidal systems.

The neurons within the primary motor cortex are organized into columns. These columns, about 1 mm in diameter, are viewed as the basic unit through which the cortex controls movements. All of the neurons within a given cortical column appear to project to a common set of alpha motoneurons that are all concerned with a particular movement at a single joint. For example, some cells of the column might be responsible for exciting the finger muscles involved in holding a pencil while others may inhibit the extensors acting at the same joint. In other cases, where the object of the movement is joint stabilization, both the extensors and flexors would be excited by the neurons within the column. Interestingly, the cortical columns responsible for a particular movement also receive sensory information necessary to monitor the progress of the movement. For example, the columns responsible for grasping an object would receive tactile information from the palmar surface of the fingers as well as proprioceptive information from receptors within the joint and muscles involved in the movement.

The supplementary motor area is most likely responsible for translating the concept or goal of a movement into a set of neuronal firing patterns. This is the area that determines the general sequence and magnitude of muscle activity necessary to carry out a movement.

Extensive projections from the posterior parietal areas reach the supplementary motor area, which in turn sends its output to the primary motor area. In addition, the supplementary area (and the related premotor area) receive input from the basal ganglia and cerebellum. These latter projections participate in any adjustments of the motor plan that might be required during the execution of a movement.

Recent studies of motor activity during the planning and execution of a movement have provided strong evidence for the postulated role of the supplementary and premotor areas in the planning of a movement. In these studies, blood flow to the brain is measured and it is assumed that when a particular area of the brain becomes active, its blood flow is increased. When a subject is asked to carry out a simple motor task for a prolonged period, there is a large increase in blood flow to the primary motor cortex. However, when the task becomes more complex and requires alteration in muscle activity, blood flow to the supplementary and premotor areas increases as well. If the subject is asked simply to think about the movement but not to carry it out, blood flow to the supplementary and premotor areas increases without a corresponding increase of blood flow to the primary motor area.

The posterior parietal areas of the brain are assumed to be responsible for generating the idea for a movement. When these areas are lesioned, apraxias result. An **apraxia** is the inability to carry out a motor task when no deficit in the motor control system can be demonstrated. That is, there is no muscle weakness or alteration in tone, no tremors or loss of coordination, and no loss in the ability to carry out complex movements. The deficit is confined to the voluntary execution of the movement. For example, a patient may be unable to execute a military salute on command or in response to the presence of a superior officer. However, the patient will have no difficulty carrying out the same type of movement to wipe a bug away from his eyes.

BIBLIOGRAPHY

Berne RB, Leug MN: Cardiovascular Physiology, 5th ed. CV Mosby, St. Louis, 1986.

Johnson LR (ed): Gastrointestinal Physiology, 3rd ed. CV Mosby, St. Louis, 1985.

Kandel ER, Schwartz JH: Principles of Neural Science, 2nd ed. Elsevier Science Publishers, New York, 1985.

Murray JF: The Normal Lung, 2nd ed. WB Saunders, Philadelphia, 1986.

Rose BD: Clinical Physiology of Acid-Base and Electrolyte Disorders, 2nd ed. McGraw-Hill, New York, 1984.

Valtin H: Renal Function, 2nd ed. Little, Brown & Co., Boston, 1983.

Wang MB, Freeman AR: Neural Function. Little, Brown & Co., Boston, 1987.

West JB: Pulmonary Pathophysiology, 3rd ed. Williams & Wilkins, Baltimore, 1987.

West JB: Respiratory Physiology, 3rd ed. Williams & Wilkins, Baltimore, 1985.

SAMPLE QUESTIONS

DIRECTIONS: Each question below contains four suggested answers of which **one** or **more** is correct. Choose the answer:

A if **1, 2, and 3** are correct
B if **1 and 3** are correct
C if **2 and 4** are correct
D if **4** is correct
E if **1, 2, 3, and 4** are correct

1. The overshoot of a nerve action potential will decrease if the

1. extracellular potassium concentration in decreased
2. extracellular sodium concentration is decreased
3. magnitude of the stimulus eliciting the action potential is increased
4. nerve membrane is in its relative refractory period

2. The skeletal muscle end-plate potential is produced by an increase in the conductance of

1. sodium
2. calcium
3. potassium
4. chloride

3. Which of the following processes play an important role in the initiation of contraction in both smooth and striated muscle?

1. Phosphorylation of cross-bridge light chains
2. Release of calcium from the sarcoplasmic reticulum
3. Depolarization of T tubules
4. Sliding of thick and thin filaments

4. Which of the following will cause a decrease in central venous pressure?

1. Increasing cardiac output
2. Increasing venous compliance
3. Decreasing circulating blood volume
4. Decreasing contractility

5. If the mean electrical axis of the QRS complex is 0 degrees, the QRS complex will be negative in leads

1. I
2. III
3. aVf
4. aVr

6. Pulse pressure will increase if there is

1. a decrease in aortic compliance
2. a decrease in mean blood pressure
3. an increase in stroke volume
4. an increase in heart rate

7. Which of the following will increase during a hemorrhage?

1. Total peripheral resistance
2. Mean blood pressure
3. Heart rate
4. Central venous pressure

8. Keeping stroke volume constant, myocardial oxygen consumption will increase if

1. mean arterial blood pressure increases
2. aortic stenosis develops
3. total peripheral resistance increases
4. end-diastolic volume increases

9. Which of the following contribute to the alveolar-arterial gradient for oxygen?

1. Blood entering the heart from the thebesian veins
2. Areas of the lung having a low V/Q ratio
3. Blood entering the heart from the bronchial veins
4. Left-to-right intracardiac shunts

10. Which of the following lung volumes can be measured directly with a spirometer?

1. Tidal volume
2. Expiratory reserve volume
3. Vital capacity
4. Functional residual capacity

11. The work required for a single breath will increase with increases in

1. Airway resistance
2. Tidal volume
3. Respiratory rate
4. Lung compliance

12. Which of the following can occur when a normal individual hyperventilates?

1. Arterial carbon dioxide tension can be reduced significantly
2. Arterial oxygen content can be increased significantly
3. Alveolar oxygen tension can be increased significantly
4. Hemoglobin oxygen saturation can be increased significantly

13. Diarrhea can be caused by

1. a decrease in the amount of sodium absorbed by the gut
2. an increase in the quantity of bile salts present the colon
3. an increase in the quantity of fatty acids present in the colon
4. an accumulation of nonabsorbable sugars in the small intestine

14. Elimination of the enteric nervous system will

1. prevent vagus-mediated relaxation of the lower esophageal sphincter
2. prevent the release of gastrin in response to protein digestive products
3. increase the tonic activity of the small intestine
4. increase the spontaneous contractile activity of the antrum

15. Removal of the antrum is associated with an increase in

1. basal acid production
2. maximal acid production
3. the rate of gastric emptying of liquids
4. the rate of gastric emptying of solids

16. Increasing ADH secretion will decrease the

1. rate of urine formation
2. urine osmolarity
3. extracellular fluid osmolarity
4. extracellular salt content

17. Proximal tubular reabsorption accounts for almost all (greater than 95%) of the reabsorption of

1. glucose
2. bicarbonate
3. phosphate
4. sodium

18. Increasing extracellular sodium concentration will cause an increase in secretion of

1. aldosterone
2. ADH
3. renin
4. natriuretic factor

19. Glomerular filtration will tend to increase with increases in

1. renal artery pressure
2. renal afferent arterial resistance
3. renal efferent arterial resistance
4. renal artery oncotic pressure

20. Which of the conclusions below are true, given the following data?

Urinary creatinine concentration =	1.5 mg/ml
Urinary PAH concentration =	20.0 mg/ml
Plasma creatinine concentration =	1.5 mg/100 ml
Plasma PAH concentration =	5.0 mg/100 ml

Plasma glucose concentration   = 125.0 mg/100 ml
Urinary flow rate   =   1.5 ml/minute
Hematocrit   = 52

1. Filtration fraction = 0.2
2. Renal blood flow = 1,250 ml/minute
3. Filtered load of glucose = 7.5 g/minute
4. Creatinine clearance = 150 ml/minute

21. Which of the following statements concerning the function of the auditory system are correct?

1. The middle ear is responsible for amplifying the pressure of the sound waves entering the ear
2. Loss of hair cells near the base of the cochlea will affect the hearing of high-frequency sounds more than low-frequency sounds
3. The basilar membrane near the apex of the cochlea vibrates with a greater amplitude in response to low-frequency sounds than it does in response to high-frequency sounds
4. Rupture of the tympanic membrane prevents sound waves from reaching the inner ear

22. Which of the following visual abilities are greater in a darkened room than in a well-lit room?

1. Visual acuity
2. Color discrimination
3. Depth perception
4. Sensitivity to light

23. Stretch of a muscle causes a reflex response during which

1. alpha motoneurons to the stretched muscle increase their firing rate
2. alpha motoneurons to the antagonist of the stretched muscle decrease their firing rate
3. Golgi tendon organs from the stretched muscle are stimulated
4. Gamma motoneurons to the stretched muscle are inhibited

24. Increased muscle tone will develop after lesions to the

1. substantia nigra
2. posterior cerebellum
3. extrapyramidal system
4. vestibular nuclei

25. Which of the following are more likely to be observed during REM sleep than during slow-wave sleep?

1. Dreaming
2. Irregular heartbeats
3. Muscle paralysis
4. Sleep spindles

ANSWERS

1. C (2, 4)	14. B (1, 3)
2. B (1, 3)	15. C (2, 4)
3. C (2, 4)	16. B (1, 3)
4. A (1, 2, 3)	17. A (1, 2, 3)
5. C (2, 4)	18. C (2,4)
6. B (1, 3)	19. B (1, 3)
7. B (1, 3)	20. E (all)
8. A (1, 2, 3, 4) E	21. A (1, 2, 3)
9. A (1, 2, 3)	22. D (4)
10. A (1, 2, 3)	23. B (1, 3)
11. A (1, 2, 3)	24. B (1, 3)
12. B (1, 3)	25. A (1, 2, 3)
13. E (all)	

3

BIOCHEMISTRY

Ira Schwartz and Isidore Danishefsky

ACIDS, BASES, AND BUFFERS

pH AND pK

Approximately 80% of the weight of all animal cells and tissue is water. In addition, essentially all biochemical reactions take place in an aqueous milieu. Thus, it is necessary to understand the special properties of water that allow for the diversity of reactions that constitute the biochemistry of cells.

Many substances dissociate when dissolved in water to yield ions. Compounds that release protons are called acids; those that accept protons are bases. Acids that do not completely dissociate in water are referred to as weak acids. Most acids that are encountered in the cell are in the latter category. The dissociation of a weak acid can be represented by the following equation:

$$HA \rightleftharpoons H^+ + A^- \qquad \text{(equation 1)}$$

The **dissociation constant** for this reaction is given by the following:

$$K_a = \frac{[H^+][A^-]}{[HA]} \qquad \text{(equation 2)}$$

where the brackets denote the molar concentrations of the components of the reaction.

Water can be defined as a weak acid since it dissociates into protons (hydrogen ions) and hydroxyl ions.

$$H_2O \rightleftharpoons H^+ + OH^- \qquad \text{(equation 3)}$$

K_w, the ion product of water, is defined by the equation

$$K_w = [H^+][OH^-] = 1 \times 10^{-14} \qquad \text{(equation 4)}$$

Thus, in pure water the concentrations of protons and hydroxyl ions are the same and equal to 1×10^{-7}M. It is convenient to express the hydrogen ion concentration as its negative logarithm—that is, $pH = -\log[H^+]$.

Equation 2, which defines the dissociation constant of a weak acid, can be rearranged as follows so as to express it in terms of pH:

$$[H^+] = \frac{K_a[HA]}{[A^-]} \qquad \text{(equation 5)}$$

Taking the negative log of both sides of equation 5 yields

$$pH = -\log K_a - \log \frac{[HA]}{[A^-]} \qquad \text{(equation 6)}$$

or,

$$pH = pK_a + \log \frac{[A^-]}{[HA]} = pK_a + \log \frac{[salt]}{[acid]} \qquad \text{(equation 7)}$$

Equation 7, known as the Henderson-Hasselbalch equation, can be used to determine the pH of any buffer solution.

TITRATION CURVES AND BUFFERS

The addition of a strong base to a solution of a weak acid will result in an increase in the pH of the solution. A plot of the pH as a function of the amount of base added (usually in moles or equivalents) yields a titration curve. Figure 3-1 shows such a curve for the addition of sodium hydroxide (NaOH) to a solution of acetic acid. Examination of the curve reveals that there is a pH range at which even large additions of base result in a small increase in pH. This is the characteristic property of a buffer. The midpoint of the titration curve, where the pH change is smallest, corresponds to the pK_a. Thus, a buffer is a solution of a weak acid and its salt that can resist changes in pH on addition of significant quantities of base. The buffering capacity is greatest at pH values within one pH unit of the pK_a. Inspection of the Henderson-Hasselbalch equation shows that this is the case when the concentrations of the acid and its salt are equal.

The normal pH of plasma is 7.4. During metabolism, a variety of acidic products are formed. These include carbon dioxide (CO_2) (which dissolves in water to yield carbonic acid, see below), lactate, and acetoacetate. Since a pH below 7.0 or above 7.8 is incompatible with life, the plasma must contain a very effective buffering system. This is provided chiefly by the bicarbonate-carbonic acid buffer.

The components of this system are CO_2, carbonic acid (H_2CO_3), and bicarbonate (HCO_3^-):

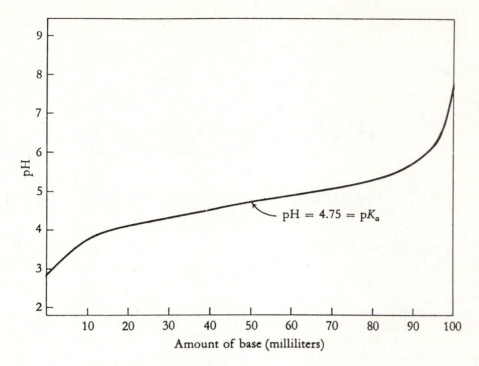

Figure 3-1. Titration curve of addition of 0.1N NaOH to a 0.1N acetic acid solution.

$$CO_2 + H_2O \rightarrow H_2CO_3 \qquad \text{(equation 8)}$$

and

$$H_2CO_3 \rightarrow H^+ + HCO_3^- \qquad \text{(equation 9)}$$

H_2CO_3 is a weak acid with a pK_a of 6.1, and the Henderson-Hasselbalch equation yields the following:

$$pH = 6.1 + \log \frac{[HCO_3^-]}{[H_2CO_3]} \qquad \text{(equation 10)}$$

The amount of dissolved CO_2 is very low as a result of the action of the enzyme carbonic anhydrase and is not easily measured. In addition, the amount of CO_2 dissolved in plasma is governed by the partial pressure of CO_2 (pCO_2) in alveoli and is given by

$$[CO_2] = 0.03 \times pCO_2 \qquad \text{(equation 11)}$$

where the concentration of CO_2 is in millimoles/liter (mmol/L) and pCO_2 is in torr (mm Hg). Combining this relationship with equation 10 generates the following expression:

$$pH = 6.1 + \log \frac{[HCO_3^-]}{0.03 \, pCO_2} \qquad \text{(equation 12)}$$

From inspection of equation 12, several important facts regarding the bicarbonate concentration and the pH of plasma can be discerned:

1. The pCO_2 in alveolar air is usually 40 mm Hg. Therefore, the concentration of CO_2 plus H_2CO_3 in plasma is approximately 1.2 mM.
2. The pH in plasma is usually 7.4. This means that the ratio $[HCO_3^-]/[H_2CO_3 + CO_2]$ is approximately 20:1.
3. Since pCO_2 is 40 mm Hg, the bicarbonate concentration is 24 mM.

ACID-BASE IMBALANCE

The efficiency of the bicarbonate buffer system in regulating plasma pH is due to the fact that PCO_2 is kept constant by the respiratory system. Thus, a decrease in plasma pH (which will result in an elevated $[CO_2]$) is compensated for by removal of excess CO_2 by the lungs. Conversely, an increase in plasma pH is corrected by readjustment of $[CO_2]$ in alveoli.

A plasma pH below 7.4 is referred to as **acidosis**, whereas a pH above 7.5 is termed **alkalosis**. These abnormalities in blood pH can be the result of either respiratory aberrations or alterations in metabolism.

Respiratory acidosis is generally the result of some pulmonary insufficiency (e.g., embolism, pneumonia, or drug overdose). This results in elevated $[CO_2]$ and a lower plasma pH. $[HCO_3^-]$ is also elevated as a result of some metabolic compensation.

Respiratory alkalosis is caused by hyperventilation. pCO_2 decreases, resulting in elevated pH. $[HCO_3^-]$ is also decreased.

Metabolic acidosis arises when high concentrations of acid are produced by cellular metabolism and are released into the bloodstream. This can be the case in ketoacidosis in diabetics and alcoholics. These acids react with bicarbonate and cause a corresponding increase in H_2CO_3 and CO_2. The excess CO_2 is removed by hyperventilation, but this may not be sufficient to correct the imbalance completely.

Metabolic alkalosis is characterized by elevated levels of plasma $[HCO_3^-]$. This causes an elevation in plasma pH. The administration of diuretics may result in this state.

PROTEINS

AMINO ACIDS

Proteins are composed of alpha-amino acids. The two structural features common to all the naturally occurring amino acids is that they possess both an amino group and a carboxyl group attached to a central (alpha) carbon as shown:

$$
\begin{array}{c}
\text{COOH} \\
| \\
\text{H}_2\text{N–C–H} \\
| \\
\text{R}
\end{array}
$$

The 20 common amino acids that are found in proteins are distinguished from one another by the composition of their side-chain R groups. Table 3-1 lists the amino acids, their structures, and the one- and three-letter designations for each.

Table 3-1. Amino Acids

Name and 3- and 1-letter abbreviations	Structure
Glycine (Gly, G)	$\begin{array}{c}NH_2\\|\\H-C-COOH\\|\\H\end{array}$
Alanine (Ala, A)	$\begin{array}{c}NH_2\\|\\H_3C-C-COOH\\|\\H\end{array}$
Valine (Val, V)	$\begin{array}{c}CH_3\ NH_2\\ \ \ |\ \ \ |\\HC-C-COOH\\|\ \ \ \ |\\CH_3\ \ H\end{array}$
Leucine (Leu, L)	$\begin{array}{c}CH_3\ \ \ \ \ NH_2\\ \ \ |\ \ \ \ \ \ \ |\\HC-CH_2-C-COOH\\|\ \ \ \ \ \ \ \ \ \ |\\CH_3\ \ \ \ \ \ H\end{array}$
Isoleucine (Ile, I)	$\begin{array}{c}CH_3-CH_2\ \ NH_2\\ \ \ \ \ \ \ \ \ |\ \ \ |\\HC-C-COOH\\|\ \ \ \ \ \ |\\CH_3\ \ \ \ H\end{array}$
Methionine (Met, M)	$\begin{array}{c}NH_2\\|\\CH_3-S-CH_2-CH_2-C-COOH\\|\\H\end{array}$
Proline (Pro, P)	$\begin{array}{c}CH_2-CH_2\ \ H\\|\ \ \ \ \ \ \ \ \ \ \diagdown COOH\\CH_2-N\\ \ \ \ \ \ |\\ \ \ \ \ \ H\end{array}$
Phenylalanine (Phe, F)	$\begin{array}{c}NH_2\\|\\\bigcirc-CH_2-C-COOH\\|\\H\end{array}$
Tryptophan (Trp, W)	$\begin{array}{c}NH_2\\|\\-CH_2-C-COOH\\|\\H\end{array}$

TABLE 3-1. (*Continued*)

Name and 3- and 1-letter abbreviations	Structure
Asparagine (Asn, N)	$\begin{array}{c}O\ \ \ \ \ \ \ \ \ \ \ NH_2\\||\ \ \ \ \ \ \ \ \ |\\H_2N-C-CH_2-C-COOH\\|\\H\end{array}$
Glutamine (Gln, Q)	$\begin{array}{c}O\ \ \ \ \ \ \ \ \ \ \ \ \ \ \ \ \ NH_2\\||\ \ \ \ \ \ \ \ \ \ \ \ \ \ \ |\\H_2N-C-CH_2-CH_2-C-COOH\\|\\H\end{array}$
Serine (Ser, S)	$\begin{array}{c}NH_2\\|\\HO-CH_2-C-COOH\\|\\H\end{array}$
Threonine (Thr, T)	$\begin{array}{c}NH_2\\|\\CH_3-CH-C-COOH\\|\ \ \ \ \ |\\OH\ \ H\end{array}$
Aspartic acid (Asp, D)	$\begin{array}{c}NH_2\\|\\HOOC-CH_2-C-COOH\\|\\H\end{array}$
Glutamic acid (Glu, E)	$\begin{array}{c}NH_2\\|\\HOOC-CH_2-CH_2-C-COOH\\|\\H\end{array}$
Lysine (Lys, K)	$\begin{array}{c}NH_2\\|\\H_2N-CH_2-CH_2-CH_2-CH_2-C-COOH\\|\\H\end{array}$
Arginine (Arg, R)	$\begin{array}{c}NH\ \ H\ \ \ \ \ \ \ \ \ \ \ \ \ \ \ NH_2\\||\ \ |\ \ \ \ \ \ \ \ \ \ \ \ \ \ \ \ |\\H_2N-C-N-CH_2-CH_2-CH_2-C-COOH\\|\\H\end{array}$
Histidine (His, H)	$\begin{array}{c}NH_2\\|\\CH_2-C-COOH\\|\\H\end{array}$
Tyrosine (Tyr, Y)	$\begin{array}{c}NH_2\\|\\HO-\bigcirc-CH_2-C-COOH\\|\\H\end{array}$
Cysteine (Cys, C)	$\begin{array}{c}NH_2\\|\\HS-CH_2-C-COOH\\|\\H\end{array}$

Amino acids can be classified in a variety of ways that depend on the composition of the side-chain R groups. Glutamic acid and aspartic acid, which contain a carboxyl group in addition to the one attached to the alpha carbon, are **acidic** amino acids; lysine, arginine, and histidine are **basic** amino acids. The remainder are referred to as **neutral** amino acids. An additional level of classification is based on other properties of the side chains. For example, phenylalanine, tyrosine, and tryptophan are **aromatic** amino acids.

All amino acids are charged at physiological pH because of the acid-base properties of the alpha-amino and alpha-carboxyl groups. Indeed, it is most appropriate to represent amino acids as the charged species. Amino acids go through several dissociations as the pH is increased:

$$
\begin{array}{ccccc}
\text{COOH} & & \text{COO}^- & & \text{COO}^- \\
| & & | & & | \\
^+_3\text{HN–C–H} & \rightleftharpoons & ^+_3\text{HN–C–H} & \rightleftharpoons & _2\text{HN–C–H} \\
| & & | & & | \\
\text{R} & & \text{R} & & \text{R}
\end{array}
$$

The constant governing the first dissociation is designated pK_1, the second is pK_2. As shown, the predominant species at neutral pH carries both a positive and a negative charge. This is referred to as a dipolar ion, or **zwitterion**. Although this species is charged, it is electrically neutral (i.e., it will not migrate in an electric field) because the net charge is zero. The pH at which this occurs varies for different amino acids and is called the isoelectric point, or pI. In the case of an amino acid that does not contain any additional ionizing groups in the side chain, the pI is the arithmetic mean of pK_1 and pK_2. If such an amino acid is titrated with base from the fully acidic form, one obtains the curve shown in Figure 3-2. This is simply the sum of the titration curves for two weak acids. At pK_1, the concentrations of the acidic and dipolar species are equal; at pK_2, the concentrations of the dipolar and basic species are equal. At any given pH, the net charge on the amino acid can be calculated from the Henderson-Hasselbalch equation.

For those amino acids that contain ionizable R groups, there is an additional pK value. Thus, for an acidic amino acid, such as aspartic acid, titration of the acidic species with base yields the following dissociations:

$$
\begin{array}{ccccccc}
\text{COOH} & & \text{COOH} & & \text{COO}^- & & \text{COO}^- \\
| & & | & & | & & | \\
\text{CH}_2 & & \text{CH}_2 & & \text{CH}_2 & & \text{CH}_2 \\
| & \rightleftharpoons & | & \rightleftharpoons & | & \rightleftharpoons & | \\
\text{HC–NH}_3^+ & & \text{HC–NH}_3^+ & & \text{HC–NH}_3^+ & & \text{HC–NH}_2 \\
| & & | & & | & & | \\
\text{COOH} & & \text{COO}^- & & \text{COO}^- & & \text{COO}^-
\end{array}
$$

The pI in this case is also the mean of pK_1 and pK_2. The isoelectric species, however, exists at an acidic pH, in contrast to the neutral amino acids.

For lysine, a basic amino acid, the following dissociations are observed:

$$
\begin{array}{ccccccc}
\text{NH}_3^+ & & \text{NH}_3^+ & & \text{NH}_3^+ & & \text{NH}_2 \\
| & & | & & | & & | \\
(\text{CH}_2)_4 & & (\text{CH}_2)_4 & & (\text{CH}_2)_4 & & (\text{CH}_2)_4 \\
| & \rightleftharpoons & | & \rightleftharpoons & | & \rightleftharpoons & | \\
\text{HC–NH}_3^+ & & \text{HC–NH}_3^+ & & \text{HC–NH}_2 & & \text{HC–NH}_2 \\
| & & | & & | & & | \\
\text{COOH} & & \text{COO}^- & & \text{COO}^- & & \text{COO}^-
\end{array}
$$

In this case, pI is the mean of pK_2 and pK_3 and occurs at a basic pH.

PROTEIN STRUCTURE

Proteins are ubiquitous in all living matter and serve a variety of functional and structural roles. Enzymes, which catalyze all cellular processes, are proteins. Some hormones (e.g., insulin, growth hormone) and antibodies are proteins. Other functional proteins include those involved in transport (e.g., hemoglobin) and muscle contraction (actin, myosin). Certain proteins, such as collagen, play important roles in maintaining cell structure.

Proteins are macromolecules built up from repeating monomer units of amino acids. The most elementary unit of protein structure is the peptide bond that links the constituent amino acids together.

$$
\begin{array}{ccccccc}
& \text{H} & \text{O} & & \text{H} & \text{O} & \\
& | & | & & | & | & \\
^+\text{H}_3\text{N–} & \text{C–} & \text{C–N–} & & \text{C–} & \text{C–O}^- & \\
& | & & \text{H} & | & & \\
& \text{R}_1 & & & \text{R}_2 & &
\end{array}
$$

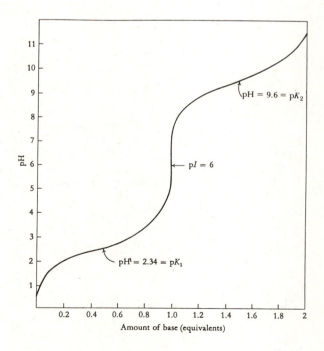

Figure 3-2. Titration curve of glycine.

A sequence of amino acids held together by peptide bonds is also referred to as a polypeptide. Since all proteins contain the same 20 amino acids and the essential covalent structure of all proteins is the same, it would appear that proteins should not differ much from one another. This is not the case, however. This is because amino acids may be repeated many times in any given protein and proteins may be composed of up to several thousand amino acid residues. This affords enough variability for almost an infinite number of proteins of unique sequence.

Protein structure is considered on several levels because proteins are large. **Primary** structure is the sequence of amino acids in a protein that are held together by peptide bonds. **Secondary** structure refers to the folding of the flexible protein protein chain as a result of hydrogen bonding between units of the protein backbone. **Tertiary** structure results from additional folding of the protein as a result of interactions between the amino acid R groups. This level of organization determines the final three-dimensional shape of the protein. Certain proteins are composed of more than one polypeptide chain. The spatial arrangement of the individual chains relative to each other is referred to as **quaternary structure**.

Primary structure

A variety of methods, both chemical and enzymatic, are employed to determine the amino acid sequence of a protein. The usual first step is determination of the amino acid composition. The peptide bonds are hydrolyzed by incubation for 24 hours in 6N hydrochloric acid at 110°C. The percent composition of each amino acid in the resultant mixture is then examined in an automated amino acid analyzer.

The most widely used procedure for determination of the N-terminal amino acid in a polypeptide is Edman's method (Fig. 3-3). Phenylisothiocyanate reacts with the free amino group to give a phenylthiohydantoin (PTH) derivative. This is followed by acid hydrolysis and chromatography to identify the PTH-amino acid. The great utility of this method is that it is nondestructive and can be employed for sequential N-terminal analysis.

C-terminal analysis is usually accomplished by treatment of the polypeptide with the enzyme carboxypeptidase. This enzyme is an exopeptidase that cleaves peptide bonds, beginning with the C-terminal amino acid.

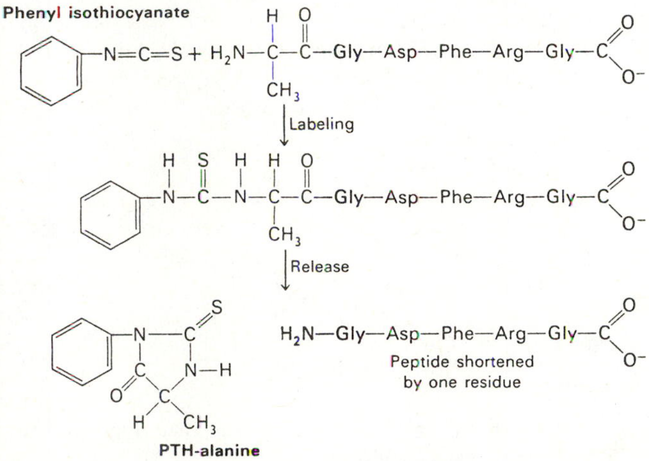

In principle, these two methods should suffice for determination of an amino acid sequence. In practice, however, the large size of most proteins makes it impractical to carry out sequence analysis on an intact polypeptide chain. Several enzymatic procedures are commonly employed to cleave the polypeptide into smaller fragments that are more amenable to complete sequence analysis by Edman degradation. **Trypsin** cleaves peptide bonds whose carboxyl function is donated by lysine and arginine, the basic amino acids. **Chymotrypsin** cleaves peptide bonds whose carboxyl function is donated by the aromatic amino acids phenylalanine, tryptophan, and tyrosine. There are additional endopeptidases that are used in sequence analysis that are not as specific as trypsin and chymotrypsin. These include pepsin and papain. Several overlapping sets of sequenced peptide fragments can be generated by the use of endopeptidases with different cleavage specificities. The entire sequence of the intact polypeptide chain can then be established by alignment of the overlapping sequences.

Secondary structure

A polypeptide chain can assume a characteristic three-dimensional shape that is the result of a number of noncovalent interactions. Hydrogen bonding between the carboxyl and amino functions of different peptide bonds within the polypeptide provides the first degree of folding, which is referred to as secondary structure.

Several types of secondary structure are possible. In the alpha helix, the protein chain is coiled so that each turn of the helix consists of 3.6 amino acid residues (Fig. 3-4). This structure is stabilized by hydrogen bonding between −C=O and −NH moieties of amino acids, which are separated from each other by three intervening residues. A polypeptide chain can also assume a more extended, zigzag shape. Two or more such chains can line up and interact via interchain hydrogen bonds. Such a structure is referred to as a beta-pleated sheet

Figure 3-3. The Edman degradation.

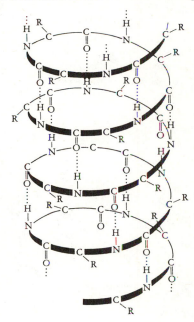

Figure 3-4. Alpha-helical structure of a polypeptide.

(Fig. 3-5). In most proteins there are regions that have no helical or sheet structure. Such stretches are known as random coils.

Tertiary structure

Every protein assumes a characteristic three-dimensional structure. The overall shape of the protein is determined by long-range interactions between the side chains of its amino acids. The most important of these are hydrophobic interactions. The driving force for this effect is the strong tendency of water molecules to hydrogen bond with each other. This results in the clustering of nonpolar amino acid side chains (e.g., valine, isoleucine, phenylalanine) so as to exclude water molecules. Further stabilization of protein structure is achieved by van der Waals interactions between the associated hydrophobic residues.

In addition to hydrophobic interactions, the amino acid side chains can interact via hydrogen bonding (e.g., asp, glu, ser, thr) and polar interactions (e.g., between the negatively charged R groups of asp or glu and the positively charged side chains of lys or arg). The tertiary structure of many proteins is also stabilized by disulfide bonds (–S–S–) between the sulfhydryl groups of two cysteine residues.

Structurally, proteins are often characterized as either fibrous or globular. Fibrous proteins are elongated and relatively insoluble in water. The structural proteins of hair (keratin) and connective tissue (collagen) are examples of fibrous proteins. These proteins generally have a uniform structure throughout. In contrast, globular proteins are not composed of repetitive structural motifs but, rather, consist of varying regions of alpha helix, beta sheet, and random coil. Such proteins are water soluble and relatively compact and spherical.

The three-dimensional structure of globular proteins can be disrupted by a variety of agents. This process is referred to as **denaturation**. High temperature or treatment with urea will result in unfolding of the polypeptide chain. In many instances, this effect is irreversible and the denatured protein is permanently inactivated.

Quaternary structure

Many proteins are composed of more than one polypeptide chain. Each of these individual chains, or subunits, has its own characteristic three-dimensional structure. The manner in which the subunits are associated with each other via noncovalent interactions is termed quaternary structure. The associated subunits behave as a single molecule in solution. Hemoglobin is an example of a protein with quaternary structure. It is composed of two copies each of two different polypeptide chains—alpha-globin and beta-globin. The individual subunits lack the oxygen-binding capabilities of hemoglobin. It is only the intact, four-subunit protein that is able to function properly.

ENZYMES

The sum of all the chemical reactions in a cell is referred to as **cellular metabolism**. These processes must proceed with both speed and accuracy. Essentially all metabolic reactions are catalyzed by a special class of globular proteins called enzymes.

THERMODYNAMICS

Free energy

In order to appreciate cellular metabolism and the interplay of individual chemical reactions in a particular pathway, it is necessary to understand the thermodynamic basis of these reactions.

For a biochemical system, the second law of thermodynamics can be represented as

$$\Delta G = \Delta E - T\Delta S$$

where T is absolute temperature, ΔS is the entropy change, and ΔE is the difference in energy between the products and reactants. ΔG is the **free-energy** change, which is defined as the energy that can be utilized to do work. ΔG is the thermodynamic value which is most important in understanding biologic reactions.

ΔG can also be defined as the free-energy change of the reaction as it proceeds to equilibrium. By convention, reactions that release energy have negative values for ΔG. Such reactions are **exergonic** and **spontaneous**. Conversely, reactions that require an input of energy have a positive value for ΔG and are said to be **endergonic** and **nonspontaneous**. By definition, at equilibrium the value of ΔG is zero.

Chemical equilibrium

Most biochemical reactions are reversible and ultimately reach a point of equilibrium at which both the forward and reverse reactions occur at equal rates. Any reaction can be characterized by an equilibrium constant. Thus, for the hypothetical reaction

$$A + B \rightleftharpoons C + D$$

the equilibrium constant is given by

$$K = \frac{[C]\,[D]}{[A]\,[B]}$$

The free-energy change of a reaction is related to its equilibrium constant by the relationship

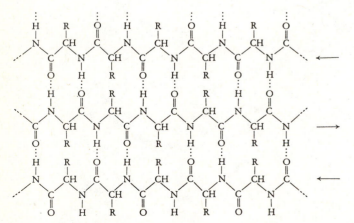

Figure 3-5.   Beta-pleated sheet structure of a protein.

$$\Delta G = \Delta G° + RT \ln K$$

where R is the gas constant (1.99 cal/mol deg), T is the absolute temperature (kelvin), and ln is the natural log (2.3 $\log_{10}$). $\Delta G°$ is the **standard free-energy change** for the standard initial conditions that all the products and reactants are present at a concentration of 1.0 M. Since at equilibrium $\Delta G = 0$, then

$$\Delta G° = -RT \ln K$$

Thus, at 25°C,

$$\Delta G° = -(1.99)\,(298)\,(2.3)\,\log K = -1363 \log K$$

Employing this relationship, it is possible to determine quickly, by inspection, whether or not a given reaction is spontaneous and will proceed with the release of free energy. If K > 1, $\Delta G°$ is negative and the reaction is exergonic. Conversely, if K < 1, $\Delta G°$ is positive and the reaction is endergonic.

In practice, few biochemical reactions begin with all the components present at 1.0 M. It is therefore necessary to consider both the **standard** free-energy change and the **initial** concentrations of the products and reactants when determining the free-energy change of a biochemical reaction at a given set of conditions.

High-energy compounds

The energy that is required for most cellular processes is derived from the oxidative metabolism of ingested nutrients. For example, the complete oxidation of 1 mol of glucose to CO_2 and water releases 686 kilocalories (kcal) of energy. Unless this energy is trapped and stored, it will be lost as heat. The predominant storage form of metabolic energy is **adenosine triphosphate** (ATP). Hydrolysis of ATP to adenosine diphosphate (ADP) and inorganic phosphate releases 7.3 kcal/mol of energy (i.e., $\Delta G° = -7.3$ kcal/mol). ATP is synthesized when energy is released during oxidative metabolism and is hydrolyzed when energy-requiring cellular processes occur.

Compounds such as ATP, which release large amounts of energy upon hydrolysis, are called **high-energy compounds**.

KINETICS

Reaction rate and catalysis

The fact that a particular reaction has a negative value for ΔG indicates only that the reaction is spontaneous in thermodynamic terms. However, it does not denote anything with regard to the rate at which the reaction will occur. This is because reactants must first be activated before they can react to form products. The amount of energy that must be provided in order for the reactants to achieve the activated state is called the **energy of activation** and is designated $\Delta G^{\ddagger}$. The rate of a chemical reaction is dependent on the value of $\Delta G^{\ddagger}$. The relationship between $\Delta G^{\ddagger}$ and ΔG is shown in Figure 3-6. Although the free energy of the products is lower than that of the reactants (and the ΔG is negative), the conversion to products can occur only after the reactants have reached the higher energy state. This activated state is sometimes referred to as the **transition state**.

Catalysts can speed up the rate of a reaction by lowering the $\Delta G^{\ddagger}$. The ΔG, however, remains unchanged. Therefore, catalysts cannot do what is impossible thermodynamically. However, if a reaction has a negative ΔG, the reaction rate can be enhanced significantly by the presence of a catalyst. The reaction rates required during normal metabolism are achieved by the action of enzymes, which are the catalysts of biochemical reactions.

Michaelis-Menten equation

The substrate in an enzymatic reaction binds to a specific site on the enzyme surface called the **active site**. The conversion of substrate to product is presumed to proceed via an

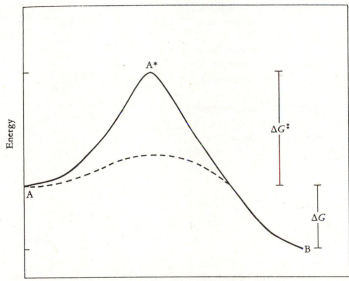

Figure 3-6.   Energy diagram for a chemical reaction. A and B are reactants and products, respectively. A* is the transition state. $\Delta G^{\ddagger}$ is the energy of activation.

intermediate enzyme-substrate (ES) complex, which is analogous to the transition state. Formation of the ES complex is the step that allows catalysis to occur. The reaction pathway is usually depicted as

$$E + S \underset{k_{-1}}{\overset{k_1}{\rightleftharpoons}} ES \overset{k_2}{\rightarrow} E + P$$

The expression that is employed for the kinetic analysis of enzymatic reactions is the **Michaelis-Menten equation**

$$v_o = \frac{V_{max}[S]}{K_M + [S]}$$

where v_o is the initial velocity of the reaction and [S] is the total substrate concentration. K_M and V_{max} are the two parameters that are used to describe the catalytic properties of an enzyme.

V_{max} is the maximal velocity at which the reaction can proceed and is attained when all the enzyme molecules have bound substrate ([E] = [ES]). If the conversion of ES to product is the rate-determining step of the overall reaction (i.e., k_2 is slow relative to k_1 and k_{-1}), then the following relationship holds:

$$V_{max} = k_2[E]$$

k_2 is sometimes referred to as k_{cat}, or the **turnover number**. This is defined as the number of substrate molecules converted to product per unit time when the enzyme is fully saturated with substrate.

K_M can be defined in several ways. It is the substrate concentration required to achieve ½ V_{max}, or the [S] at which half the active sites are filled. K_M is a collection of rate constants. If formation of ES is rapid relative to its conversion to product (k_1 and k_{-1} are much larger than k_2), then K_M is simply the dissociation constant of ES. Thus, K_M is a measure of the strength of the enzyme-substrate complex; a high value for K_M indicates weak binding, whereas a low value denotes tight binding.

An additional parameter, k_{cat}/K_M, is now being employed more frequently to define the **catalytic efficiency** of an enzyme. The larger the value for k_{cat}/K_M, the more efficient the enzyme is in achieving catalysis.

The values for K_M and V_{max} are determined experimentally by measuring the initial velocity of the reaction at several different substrate concentrations. These data are then analyzed graphically by the double-reciprocal transformation of the Michaelis-Menten equation:

$$1/v_o = K_M/V_{max}[S] + 1/V_{max}$$

A plot of $1/v_o$ versus $1/[S]$ (Fig. 3-7) yields a straight line with a slope of K_M/V_{max} and a y-intercept of $1/V_{max}$.

Inhibition of enzyme activity

Enzyme activity can be reduced or abolished by a variety of treatments or modifications. Since enzymes are proteins, any procedure that affects protein structure can inactivate an enzyme. Examples of this are denaturation by heat or extremes

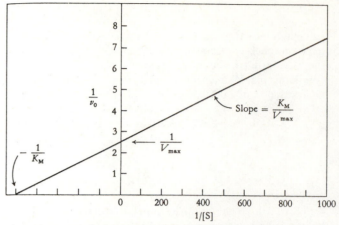

Figure 3-7. A double-reciprocal (Lineweaver-Burke) plot of an enzymatic reaction.

of pH and chemical modification of specific amino acid side chains that may be required for enzyme activity. In general, these result in *irreversible* inactivation of the enzyme.

In addition, enzymes can be *reversibly* inhibited by a variety of compounds that bind specifically to the enzyme surface. There are two major types of reversible inhibition, and these can be distinguished from each other by virtue of their different effects on the kinetic parameters K_M and V_{max}.

Competitive inhibition is characterized by the binding of an inhibitor to the active site. Since this is also the substrate binding site, there results a competition between the substrate and inhibitor for binding to the enzyme. The equation for the double-reciprocal plot in such a case is

$$1/v_o = K_M/V_{max}(1 + [I]/K_I)\,1/[S] + 1/V_{max}$$

The plot is shown in Figure 3-8. The slope is increased by a factor of $(1 + [I]/K_I)$, where [I] is the concentration of the inhibitor and K_I is the inhibitor constant (the dissociation constant of the enzyme-inhibitor complex). This means that, in the presence of a competitive inhibitor, the K_M is increased

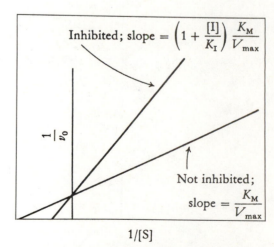

Figure 3-8. Effect of competitive inhibitor on kinetics of an enzymatic reaction.

but the V_{max} remains unchanged. An important implication of this statement is the fact that the effect of a competitive inhibitor can be overcome by addition of a huge excess of substrate.

Competitive inhibition is usually caused by compounds that are structurally related to the substrate. This has important therapeutic consequences. Many antimetabolites that are employed in the treatment of disease are competitive inhibitors of the normal enzymatic reaction. Two prominent examples are allopurinol (used in the treatment of hyperuricemia), which is a competitive inhibitor of xanthine oxidase, and methotrexate, a substrate analogue of dihydrofolate, which inhibits dihydrofolate reductase.

In contrast, **noncompetitive inhibition** is the result of the binding of an inhibitor molecule to a site on the enzyme different from the substrate binding site. Therefore, both inhibitor and substrate can be bound to the enzyme simultaneously, and even a large excess of substrate cannot reverse the effect of a noncompetitive inhibitor. The double-reciprocal equation for this type of inhibition is

$$1/v_o = K_M/V_{max}\ (1 + [I]/K_I)\ 1/[S] + 1/V_{max}\ (1 + [I]/K_I)$$

A representative plot is shown in Figure 3-9. As with competitive inhibition, in this case, as well, the slope is increased by a factor of $(1 + [I]/K_I)$. However, the K_M remains unchanged while V_{max} is decreased. Common examples of this type of inhibition are heavy metals (e.g., Cu^{2+}, Hg^{2+}, and Pb^{2+}), which react reversibly with sulfhydryl residues on the enzyme.

As mentioned above, enzymes can be irreversibly inhibited by chemical modification of amino acid residues that are required for catalysis. Such inhibitors are often useful in the elucidation of enzyme mechanisms. Two examples of compounds of this sort are iodoacetate (which reacts with the sulfhydryl moiety of cysteine) and diisopropylfluorophosphate (DFP), which reacts with the hydroxyl group of serine. The reactions of these compounds are shown in Figure 3-10.

Allosteric enzymes

Metabolic regulation of biosynthetic pathways requires that the end product of the pathway be produced only when it is

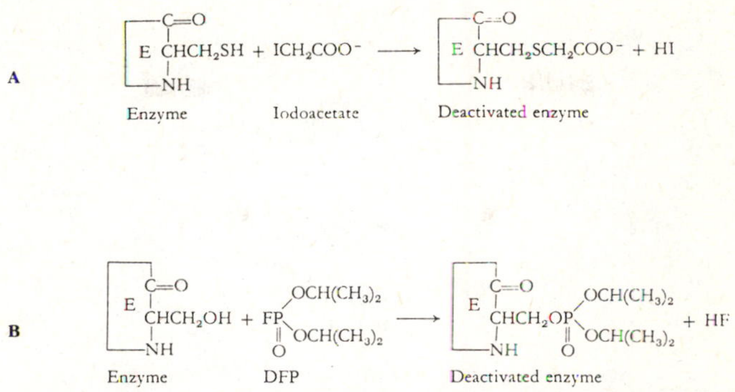

Figure 3-10. Action of irreversible inhibitors. (*A*) Reaction of iodoacetamide with cysteine residue. (*B*) Reaction of diisopropylfluorophosphate with serine residue.

needed. This control is usually accomplished by a process in which the end product inhibits the initial enzymatic reaction in the pathway. This is referred to as **end-product** or **feedback regulation**. Frequently, the enzymes catalyzing the first step are **allosteric enzymes**.

Allosteric enzymes have several properties that distinguish them from other enzymes. In addition to the active site, these enzymes have a second binding site to which allosteric **effectors** can bind (allosteric means another site). These effectors are the regulatory compounds that modulate the activity of the enzyme. Allosteric enzymes are multisubunit proteins. The active site and the regulatory, or allosteric, site are usually contained of different subunits (referred to as the catalytic and regulatory subunits, respectively).

The kinetics of allosteric enzymes also differ from other enzymes in that they do not exhibit classic Michaelis-Menten behavior. A direct plot of v_o versus [S] yields a sigmoid curve as opposed to a hyperbola. This indicates that the binding of the first substrate molecule increases the affinity of the enzyme for binding of subsequent substrate. This is thought to be the result of a conformational change in the structure of the enzyme that is induced by substrate binding.

The binding of an allosteric effector at the regulatory site also induces a conformational change, which can result in either an enhancement or inhibition of enzyme activity. The inhibition caused by a **negative** effector has characteristics that are distinct from those induced by competitive or noncompetitive inhibitors.

There are numerous examples of allosteric enzymes that play a pivotal role in metabolic regulation. These include isocitrate dehydrogenase (citric acid cycle) and aspartate transcarbamoylase (pyrimidine biosynthesis). The oxygen-binding reaction of hemoglobin also follows characteristic allosteric behavior. The properties of these enzymes will be discussed later in this chapter.

CARBOHYDRATE STRUCTURES AND METABOLIC FUNCTION

The principal carbohydrates in mammalian organisms are hexoses, pentoses, and their derivatives and polymers. The most important ones are shown in Figure 3-11. Additional ones that are generally included in the diet are presented in Figure 3-

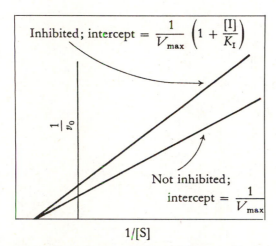

Figure 3-9. Effect of noncompetitive inhibitor on kinetics of an enzymatic reaction.

Hexoses

α-D-glucose

β-D-glucose

Designations α or β refer to configurations on carbon-1.

The above are also written as:

and

wherein the corners represent carbons unless noted otherwise.

α-D-galactose

α-D-mannose

α-D-fructose

Pentoses

α-D-ribose

2-deoxyribose

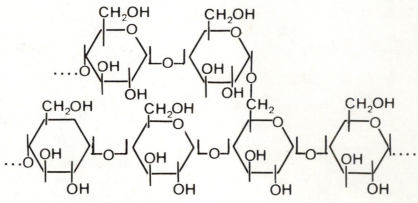

Figure 3-11. Carbohydrate structures.

12. The major carbohydrate used by cells is glucose. For other sugars to be metabolized, they must first be transformed to either glucose derivatives or related substances. When discussing the metabolism of sugars, therefore, most of the considerations involve the transformations of glucose.

The major metabolic functions of glucose are (1) utilization as a fuel for deriving energy, (2) production of intermediates for synthesis of various noncarbohydrate cellular components, (3) generation of reducing energy for biosynthetic reactions, and (4) provision of intermediates for formation of complex polymeric cellular components (e.g., nucleic acids, glycoproteins, glycosaminoglycans).

Carbohydrate digestion and absorption

Dietary carbohydrates are digested mainly in the small intestine. The enzyme **amylase**, secreted by the pancreas, catalyzes the hydrolysis of starch to the disaccharides maltose and isomaltose. These, as well as ingested disaccharides, are hydrolyzed by specific disaccharidases to their respective monosaccharides:

$$\text{Sucrose} \rightarrow \text{glucose} + \text{fructose}$$
$$\text{Maltose or isomaltose} \rightarrow 2 \text{ glucose}$$
$$\text{Lactose} \rightarrow \text{glucose} + \text{galactose}$$

The latter are absorbed from the small intestine to the portal circulation and distributed from the liver to the systemic system.

The first transformation of glucose on entry into a cell is its conversion to glucose 6-phosphate. This reaction is catalyzed

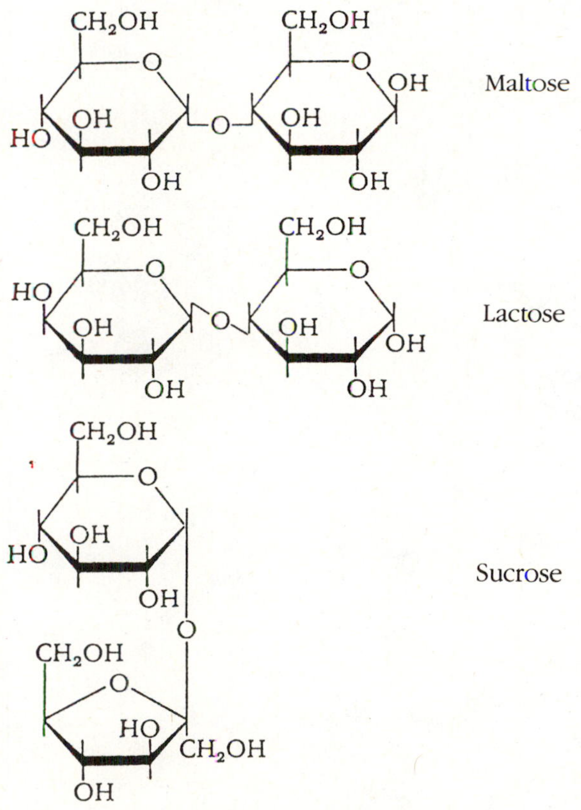

Figure 3-12. Dietary disaccharides.

by the enzyme **hexokinase**, which also requires ATP (Fig. 3-13). Glucose 6-phosphate can be metabolized by one of several pathways depending on the capabilities and immediate requirements of the specific tissue. A sequence or pathway that is common to most cells is the one termed **glycolysis**, in which the final product is pyruvic acid or lactic acid (Fig. 3-13).

Glycolysis

For glycolysis, glucose 6-phosphate is transformed to fructose 6-phosphate. The latter reacts with ATP, providing **fructose 1,6-diphosphate** and ADP. This is a critical regulatory step in glycolysis. The activity of the enzyme for the reaction, **phosphofructokinase**, is influenced by various metabolic intermediates. The mechanism for these controls will be discussed later in this section.

Frucose 1,6-diphosphate is cleaved between carbon-3 and carbon-4 to yield **dihydroxyacetone phosphate** and **glyceraldehyde** 3-phosphate. Dihydroxyacetone phosphate itself can also be converted to glyceraldehyde 3-phosphate. Thus, each molecule of fructose 1,6-diphosphate can effectively provide two molecules of glyceraldehyde 3-phosphate.

The enzyme glyceraldehyde 3-phosphate dehydrogenase catalyzes the reaction between glyceraldehyde 3-phosphate, nicotinamide-adenine dinucleotide (NAD), and inorganic phosphate to provide **1,3-diphosphoglyceric acid** and the reduced form of NAD (NADH). The former reacts with ADP to form **3-phosphoglyceric acid** and **ATP**. In the subsequent steps, 3-phosphoglyceric acid is changed to **2-phosphoglyceric acid**, which in turn is transformed to **phosphoenolpyruvic acid**. The latter reacts with ADP to yield **pyruvic acid** and ATP.

The enzyme **lactate dehydrogenase** catalyzes a reaction between pyruvic acid and NADH to yield **lactic acid** and NAD. Although lactic acid is a constant product of glycolysis in skeletal muscle, its formation is increased considerably during exercise or muscular exertion.

The steps in the glycolytic pathway, the enzymes, and the structures of the components are outlined in Figure 3-13.

It should be noted that certain steps in glycolysis require energy (in the form of ATP) and others are exergonic and release ATP. The ATP-dependent reactions are (1) the formation of glucose 6-phosphate from glucose as catalyzed by hexokinase and (2) the formation of fructose 1,6-diphosphate from fructose 6-phosphate, which utilizes the enzyme phosphofructokinase. The steps that yield ATP are (1) the conversion of 1,3-diphosphoglycerate to phosphoglycerate and (2) the formation of pyruvate from phosphoenolpyruvate. Since two molecules of the 3-carbon intermediates are formed from each fructose 1,6-diphosphate, a total of four ATP molecules are produced. The *net* yield of ATP from glycolysis is thus *two*.

Tricarboxylic acid cycle

The glycolytic reactions occur in the extramitochondrial compartment of cells. For further metabolic degradation, pyruvate is transported into the mitochondrial matrix. The overall reactions that occur at this juncture are (1) conversion of pyruvate to acetylcoenzyme A (acetyl-CoA) and CO_2 and (2) oxidation of the acetyl unit to CO_2 and water. Unlike the glycolytic steps, which can occur under anaerobic conditions, the mitochondrial processes require oxygen. Additionally, these aerobic mitochondrial reactions provide a considerable amount of ATP.

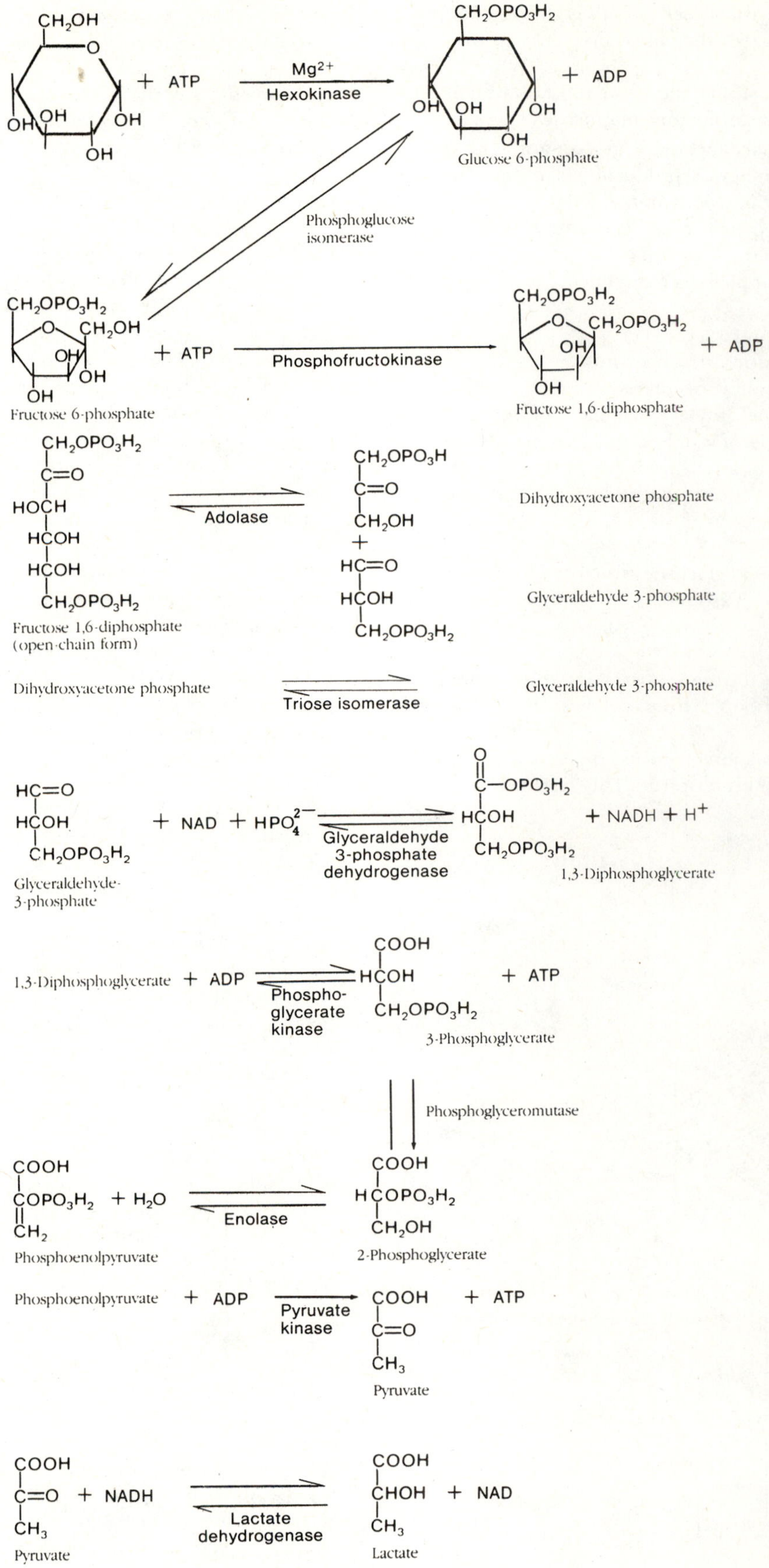

Figure 3-13. Glycolysis.

The conversion of pyruvate to acetyl-CoA is catalyzed by a multienzyme complex involving three enzymes and several cofactors. The first reaction involves decarboxylation of the pyruvate and utilizes **thiamine pyrophosphate** as a cofactor (Fig. 3-14). This step is catalyzed by a decarboxylase. In the second reaction, the two-carbon compound is transferred from the thiamine pyrophosphate to lipoate. As a result of this reaction, lipoate is reduced. The two-carbon acetyl group is then transferred from the lipoate to CoA. Both of these transfer reactions are catalyzed by the same enzyme (transacylase). The third reaction is the reoxidation of the reduced lipoate to its oxidized form. The oxidizing coenzyme in this process is NAD, which in turn is reduced to NADH.

The tricarboxylic acid cycle (citric acid cycle, Krebs cycle) is a series of reactions that effectively result in the production of CO_2 from the acetyl unit in acetyl-CoA. The steps are summarized in Figure 3-15. **Acetyl-CoA** condenses with oxalacetate to yield **citrate** and **CoA**. Citrate is transformed to **aconitate** and **isocitrate**. The latter is oxidized by an NAD-dependent enzyme, providing **alpha-ketoglutarate**, CO_2, and NADH. Alpha-ketoglutarate is degraded by a multienzyme system analogous to the one that oxidizes pyruvate. Hence, this process also requires thiamine pyrophosphate, lipoate, and NAD as cofactors. The products in the oxidation of alpha-ketoglutarate are **succinyl-CoA**, CO_2, and NADH. Succinyl-CoA, by reacting with guanosine diphosphate (GDP) and inorganic phosphate, yields **succinate** and guanosine triphosphate (GTP). Succinate is oxidized by a riboflavin-linked enzyme to produce **fumarate** and reduced flavin. Fumarate is converted to **malate**, which in turn is oxidized by an NAD-requiring enzyme to yield **oxaloacetate** and NADH. Oxaloacetate may now react with another molecule of acetyl-CoA, and the cycle is repeated.

Essentially, the overall effect of each turn of the cycle is the

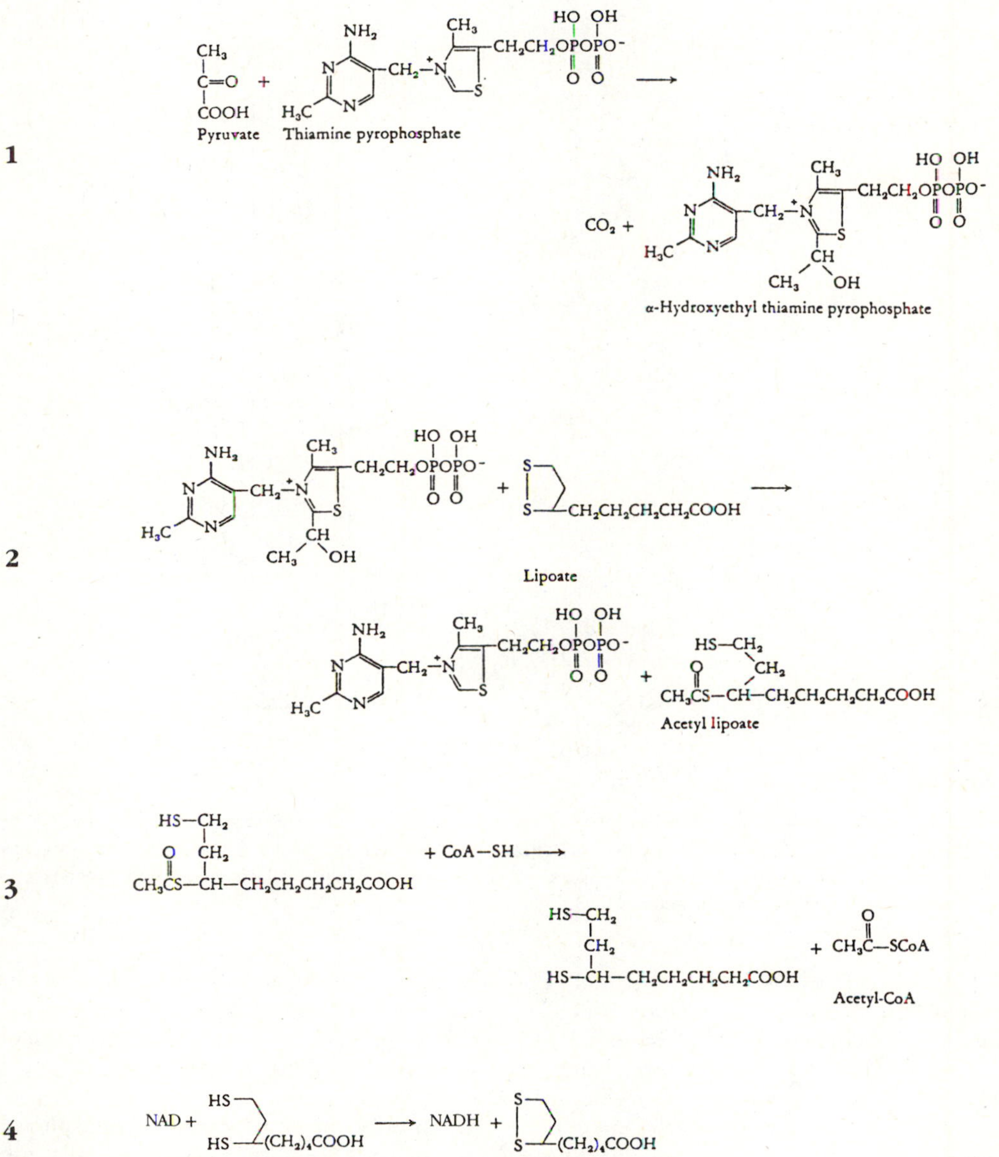

Figure 3-14. Reactions of the pyruvate dehydrogenase complex.

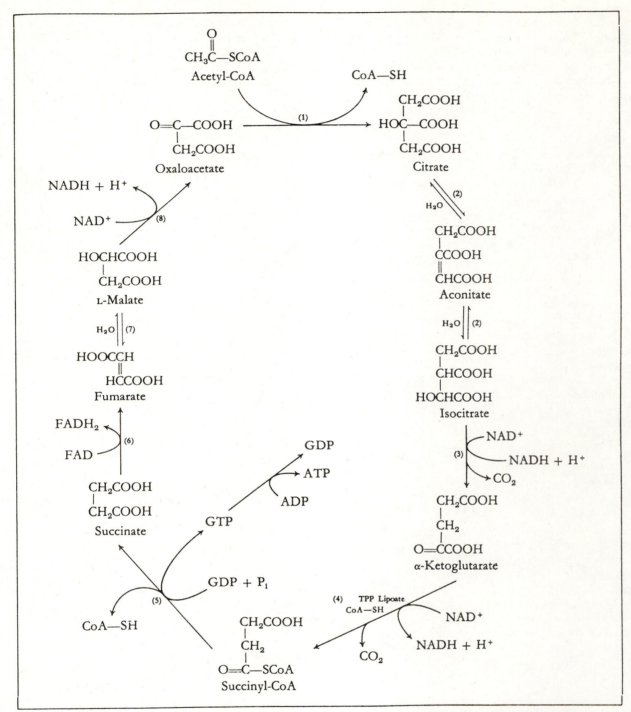

Figure 3-15. Citric acid cycle. Enzymes: (1) citrate synthase, (2) aconitase, (3) isocitrate dehydrogenase, (4) alpha-ketoglutarate dehydrogenase complex, (5) succinate thiokinase, (6) succinate dehydrogenase, (7) fumarase, and (8) malate dehydrogenase.

conversion of 1 mol of acetate, 3 mol of NAD, and 1 mol of flavoprotein to 2 mol of CO_2, 3 mol of NADH, and 1 mol of reduced flavoprotein. Additionally, a mole of GTP is produced from GDP and phosphate. Since oxaloacetate is regenerated, only small amounts of oxaloacetate are required for degrading relatively large amounts of acetate. However, since the amounts of NAD and flavoprotein are limited, the cycle cannot function unless the reduced forms of the coenzymes are reoxidized. The ultimate oxidant for these reduced coenzymes is oxygen. Thus,

the citric acid cycle can only operate under aerobic conditions—that is, when oxygen is available.

The process by which reduced coenzymes are oxidized involves a series of reactions known as the respiratory chain.

Respiratory chain and oxidative phosphorylation

The inner membrane of mitochondria contains a number of components that can exist either in a reduced or oxidized form. The former is converted to the latter on release of electrons. When the electrons are accepted by another compound, this compound is reduced. Thus, with two hypothetical materials, A and B, the following could occur:

$$A \text{ (reduced)} \rightarrow A \text{ (oxidized)} + \text{electrons}$$
$$B \text{ (oxidized)} + \text{electrons} \rightarrow B \text{ (reduced)}$$

The direction of flow of electrons (i.e., from A to B or from B to A) depends on the relative affinity or electrode potential of each system. By convention, the system with the more positive electrode potential will accept electrons from the one with a lower value. When electrons flow in this direction, the process is exergonic, or energy is released. In mitochondrial sequences, most of the energy from such oxidative reactions is utilized for the synthesis of ATP from ADP and inorganic phosphate.

Reduced NAD (i.e., NADH generated in the mitochondrial matrix) is oxidized by a membrane flavoprotein enzyme termed **NADH dehydrogenase**. In this reaction, two electrons are transferred from NADH to the flavin unit in the flavoprotein. As a result, NADH is converted to NAD and the flavin unit is reduced (Table 3-2). In an analogous manner, electrons move from the flavin via an iron system to coenzyme Q. This leaves the flavoprotein in the oxidized form, and coenzyme Q is in the reduced state. Electron transport continues from coenzyme Q through the cytochrome system. The latter consists of several iron-prophyrin-linked proteins in which the iron is 3+ in the oxidized state and 2+ in the reduced state. The electron flow from the cytochromes is

Cytochrome b $\rightarrow$ Cytochrome C$_1$ $\rightarrow$ Cytochrome C $\rightarrow$ Cytochrome a,a$_3$

The ultimate acceptor of electrons from cytochrome a is oxygen. The reduction of oxygen yields water as the product. It will be remembered that the first oxidation in the series occurred on the metabolic intermediate (e.g., isocitrate, alpha-ketoglutarate, or malate). If these are denoted as MH$_2$, the total process can be summarized as shown in Table 3-2.

Unlike the metabolic intermediates mentioned above, succinate is oxidized directly by a flavoprotein enzyme called succinate dehydrogenase. Electron transport from this flavin is to coenzyme Q, so that the step involving NADH dehydrogenase is bypassed.

As noted above, the energy released can be utilized for the synthesis of ATP. This process is termed **oxidative phosphorylation**. The transport of two electrons from a substrate to NAD through the complete respiratory chain to oxygen yields 3 mol of ATP. In contrast, a substrate that is oxidized directly by a mitochondrial flavoprotein (e.g., succinate) results in the formation of 2 mol of ATP. The explanation as to how the energy released in the oxidative steps is channeled for the synthesis of ATP is known as the **chemiosmotic theory**. It is postulated that the inner mitochondrial membrane containing the components of the respiratory chain is impermeable to protons as well as many other ions. During the oxidative processes, there is a transfer or translocation of protons to the exterior of the inner membrane. As a consequence of the impermeability of the membrane, the process results in an increased concentration of protons on the outer side, generating a proton gradient or electrochemical potential difference across the membrane. The mitochondrial membrane contains an enzyme that catalyzes the synthesis of ATP from ADP and inorganic phosphate. However, since this synthesis is an energy-requiring reaction, it will occur only when the necessary energy is supplied. The enzyme involved, **ATP synthase**, is constructed in such a manner as to be able to utilize the energy from the proton gradient for the synthetic reaction. In summary, the mechanism of oxidative phosphorylation involves (1) oxidative steps of the respiratory chain, (2) generation of a proton gradient from the energy released, and (3) utilization of the energy from this gradient for the endergonic synthesis of ATP.

It follows from this sequence that a condition that interferes with any one of the steps will inhibit the oxidation of the substrate or synthesis of ATP. For example, a limitation on the availability of oxygen will result in a decrease or inhibition of oxidation of substrates or regeneration of NAD. Any condition that inhibits oxidation will also inhibit formation of ATP. Certain substances inhibit the respiratory chain at specific sites. Thus, barbiturates are known to interfere with electron transfer from NADH to coenzyme Q. Similarly, the transfer of electrons from reduced coenzyme Q to cytochrome c (via cytochrome b and cytochrome C$_1$) is inhibited by antimycin A. The oxidation of cytochrome a by oxygen is inhibited by

Table 3-2. Reactions of the Respiratory Chain

1. $MH_2 + NAD^+ \rightleftharpoons M + NADH + H^+$

2. $NADH + H^+ + FMN \rightleftharpoons NAD^+ + FMNH_2$

3. $FMNH_2 + 2Fe^{3+}\text{S-protein} \rightleftharpoons FMN + 2Fe^{2+}\text{S-protein} + 2H^+$

4. $2H^+ + 2Fe^{2+}\text{S-protein} + \text{Coenzyme Q} \rightleftharpoons 2Fe^{3+}\text{S-protein} + \text{Coenzyme QH}_2$

5. $\text{Coenzyme QH}_2 + 2 \text{ Cytochrome b (Fe}^{3+}) \rightleftharpoons \text{Coenzyme Q} + 2 \text{ Cytochrome b (Fe}^{2+}) + 2H^+$

6. $2 \text{ Cytochrome b (Fe}^{2+}) + 2 \text{ Cytochrome c}_1 \text{ (Fe}^{3+}) \rightleftharpoons 2 \text{ Cytochrome b (Fe}^{3+}) + 2 \text{ Cytochrome c}_2 \text{ (Fe}^{2+})$

7. $2 \text{ Cytochrome c}_1 \text{ (Fe}^{2+}) + 2 \text{ Cytochrome c (Fe}^{3+}) \rightleftharpoons 2 \text{ Cytochrome c}_1 \text{ (Fe}^{3+}) + 2 \text{ Cytochrome c (Fe}^{2+})$

8. $2 \text{ Cytochrome c (Fe}^{2+}) + 2 \text{ Cytochrome a} + \text{a}_3 \text{ (Fe}^{3+})(\text{Cu}^+,\text{Cu}^{2+}) \rightleftharpoons 2 \text{ Cytochrome c (Fe}^{3+}) + 2 \text{ Cytochrome a} + \text{a}_3 \text{ (Fe}^{2+})(\text{Cu}^+,\text{Cu}^{2+})$

9. $2 \text{ Cytochrome a} + \text{a}_3 \text{ (Fe}^{2+})(\text{Cu}^+,\text{Cu}^{2+}) + \frac{1}{2}O_2 + 2H^+ \rightarrow 2 \text{ Cytochrome a} + \text{a}_3 \text{ (Fe}^{3+})(\text{Cu}^+,\text{Cu}^{2+}) + H_2O$

Net: $MH_2 + \frac{1}{2}O_2 \rightarrow M + H_2O$

carbon monoxide or cyanide. The ultimate results of the action of these inhibitors are that oxygen will not be consumed and ATP will not be produced.

Another class of substances interfere with the formation of ATP but do not inhibit the oxidative chain or oxygen utilization. Such substances are called **uncouplers**. Their action is essentially to interfere with the maintenance of the proton gradient. Examples of uncouplers are 2,4-dinitrophenol and thyroxin. A third type of inhibitor is one that interferes with ATP synthase. Such activity is exemplified by oligomycin.

Energy from total oxidation of pyruvate

The oxidation of pyruvate to acetyl-CoA as well as the reactions of the citric acid cycle result in the production of reduced coenzymes. The latter are reoxidized by the reactions of the respiratory chain, which concomitantly yield ATP. The actual amount of ATP generated can be derived from the number of molecules of reduced coenzyme that are formed. The conversion of 1 mol of pyruvate to acetylcoenzyme via the pyruvate dehydrogenase multienzyme complex leaves 1 mol of NAD in the reduced state (i.e., NADH). Oxidation of this cofactor by the mitochondrial respiratory chain generates 3 mol of ATP. The oxidation of one acetyl from acetyl-CoA by the citric acid cycle yields 3 mol of NADH and 1 mol of reduced flavoprotein-linked succinate dehydrogenase. The sources of NADH are the reactions catalyzed by (1) isocitrate dehydrogenase, (2) alpha-ketoglutarate dehydrogenase, and (3) malate dehydrogenase. Reoxidation of the NADH generated in these reactions yields a total of 9 mol of ATP. Respiratory chain reoxidation of the reduced succinate dehydrogenase flavin coenzyme yields 2 mol of ATP. Another mole of nucleoside triphosphate (i.e., GTP) is formed when succinate is formed from succinyl-CoA. This is also a potential source of ATP. A single turn of the cycle thus yields a total of 12 mol of ATP. Mitochondrial total aerobic oxidation of pyruvate thus provides 15 mol of ATP.

Aerobic oxidation of glucose

As noted above, the anaerobic degradation of glucose to pyruvate yields ATP as well as NADH. (The latter is formed in the oxidation of glyceraldehyde 3-phosphate to yield 1,3-diphosphoglycerate, Fig. 3-13). Under anaerobic conditions, NAD is regenerated from this NADH by the reaction with pyruvate as catalyzed by lactate dehydrogenase. In contrast, in the presence of oxygen, most of the pyruvate is converted in the mitrochondria to acetyl-CoA. The extramitochondrial NADH must therefore be oxidized by other mechanisms.

Although the mitochondrial inner membrane is not permeable to NADH so that the latter cannot be oxidized by the enzymes of the respiratory chain, several mechanisms exist for the effective transfer of the electrons for these NADH molecules to the mitochondria. Two principal mechanisms, known as shuttle systems, may produce this effect. One of these involves dihydroxyacetone phosphate and the enzyme glycerol phosphate dehydrogenase (Fig. 3-16). This yields glycerol phosphate and NAD. The former is then oxidized by a mitochondrial flavoprotein enzyme to produce dihydroxyacetone phosphate and a reduced flavoprotein that is oxidized via the respiratory chain. Two moles of ATP are generated by oxidative phosphory-

lation. Another shuttle system operates by the oxidation of the extramitochondrial NADH by oxaloacetate utilizing the enzyme malate dehydrogenase. The product, malate, can be transferred by a specific transport system into the mitochondrial matrix, where it is reoxidized to produce oxaloacetate and NADH. Oxidation of the latter via the oxidative chain yields 3 mol of ATP. Thus, when glucose is oxidized aerobically, the NADH produced in the glycolytic sequences can provide ATP by oxidative phosphorylation.

Energy from glucose

Metabolic degradation of glucose to pyruvate and the conversion of the latter to lactate (anaerobic glycolysis) produce a net amount of 2 mol of ATP per mole of glucose. Under aerobic conditions (i.e., when there is no limit in oxygen supply), most of the pyruvate is converted to acetyl-CoA, with the concurrent production of 3 mol of ATP by oxidative phosphorylation, or 6 mol of ATP per mole of glucose. The oxidation of each mole of acetyl-CoA to CO_2 and water by the citric acid cycle yields 12 mol of ATP, or 24 mol of ATP per mole of glucose. To the 32 mol of ATP obtained by the above reactions we can add either 4 or 6 mol of ATP from the reoxidation of extramitochondrial NADH. Thus, the aerobic metabolism of glucose yields a minimum of 36 mol of ATP.

Relatively large amounts of lactic acid are produced from glucose when the need for oxygen exceeds its supply. This occurs in muscle upon excessive exertion. Small amounts of lactate are formed in muscle, however, even when there is an ample supply of oxygen.

Pentose pathway

The pentose pathway is a sequence of reactions that utilize glucose for (1) production of reduced nicotinamide-adenine dinucleotide phosphate (NADP) (i.e., NADPH), which in turn is required for the biosynthesis of fatty acids, cholesterol, and various other tissue components and (2) synthesis of ribose nucleotides, used mainly for the synthesis of nucleic acids. The reactions of the pentose pathway occur in the **cytosol**, which is the soluble fraction of the extramitochondrial compartment.

The specific reactions and the required enzymes are described in Figure 3-17. Two of the steps are oxidations that require NADP—that is, the oxidation of glucose 6-phosphate to gluconolactone 6-phosphate and the conversion of gluconic acid 6-phosphate the ribulose 5-phosphate (a pentose) and CO_2. The subsequent steps involve interconversions of the pentose phosphates (ribose, ribulose, and xylulose) and the production of sugars with three, four, and seven carbons. It also should be noted that transketolase requires thiamine pyrophosphate for its action.

Most of the glucose metabolized in adipose tissue is degraded by the oxidative pentose pathway. The cells of this tissue actively synthesize fatty acids from acetyl-CoA, and NADPH is required for this process. Similarly, the liver consumes NADPH for synthetic reactions, and a considerable fraction of glucose is metabolized by the oxidative pathway in order to generate the reduced coenzyme. In contrast, glucose degradation in muscle cells occurs exclusively by the glycolytic pathway. These examples serve to demonstrate that the degree of utilization of specific reactions by cells of certain tissues is related to their metabolic functions and requirements.

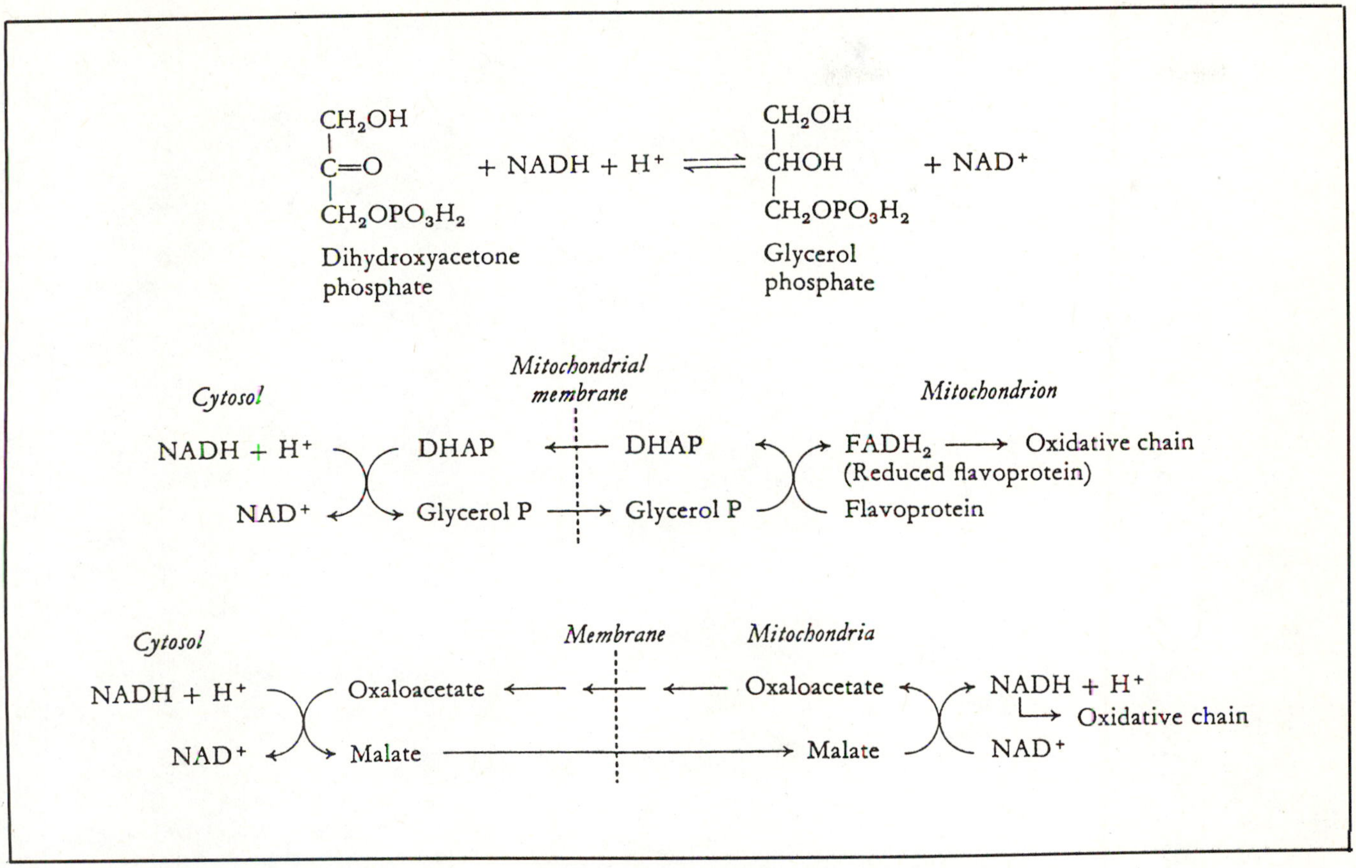

Figure 3-16. Shuttle systems for transfer of electrons into the mitochondria.

Synthesis and degradation of glycogen

Glucose is stored as glycogen in liver and muscle cells. Small amounts are also found in other tissues. The steps in the synthesis of glycogen are described in Figure 3-18. The first reaction in the synthesis involves the conversion of glucose 6-phosphate to glucose 1-phosphate. This reaction is catalyzed by the enzyme **phosphoglucomutase**. Glucose 6-phosphate then reacts with uridine triphosphate (UTP) to yield uridine diphosphate glucose. The latter functions as the donor of glucose for elongation of glycogen chains. Thus glucose from uridine diphosphate glucose is added to the end of a growing glycogen chain, forming an alpha-1,4-glycosidic bond. The enzyme for this reaction is **glycogen synthase**. Elongation of glycogen continues until about 10 glucose units are added. At this point, another enzyme catalyzes the transfer of an oligosaccharide section from the nonreducing terminus, to carbon-6 of an internal glucose residue (Fig. 3-18, step 3). This transfer results in the formation of a 1,6-linkage or a branch in the glycogen structure. New glucose units can then be added to the nonreducing ends of the chains by transfers from uridine diphosphate glucose (step 2). This addition continues to a certain point, whereupon another branching reaction occurs. The alternation of elongation and branching processes continues to yield the complex, tree-like structure characteristic of glycogen.

The first step in the degradation of glycogen is catalyzed by the enzyme **phosphorylase**. This step involves the reaction of inorganic phosphate with glycogen to yield glucose 1-phosphate and glycogen, which contains one glucose less than the original substrate (Fig. 3-19, step 1). The release of glucose 1-phosphate continues until the area of a 1,6-linkage is approached. Debranching occurs in two steps, as shown by reactions 2 and 3 in Figure 3-19. The resulting straight chain is then degraded by the action of phosphorylase until another branch point is reached. This is followed sequentially by another debranching process and further degradation by phosphorylase.

The principal product of glycogen degradation is thus glucose 1-phosphate. The latter can be converted to glucose 6-phosphate, which in turn can be processed by the glycolytic or pentose pathway. In addition to these alternatives, glucose 6-phosphate *in liver* can be hydrolyzed by the action of the enzyme **glucose 6-phosphatase** to yield glucose and inorganic phosphate. This glucose generated in liver cells is released to the bloodstream and carried to other organs for utilization. Hence, the liver is capable of contributing to blood glucose and thus regulates its concentration.

Control of glycogen metabolism

As indicated above, glycogen serves as the metabolic storage form of carbohydrates. In order to fulfill this function, it is critical that the release of glucose 1-phosphate from glycogen as well as its incorporation into glycogen should be responsive to the immediate requirements of the organism. Regulation of glycogen synthesis and degradation involve

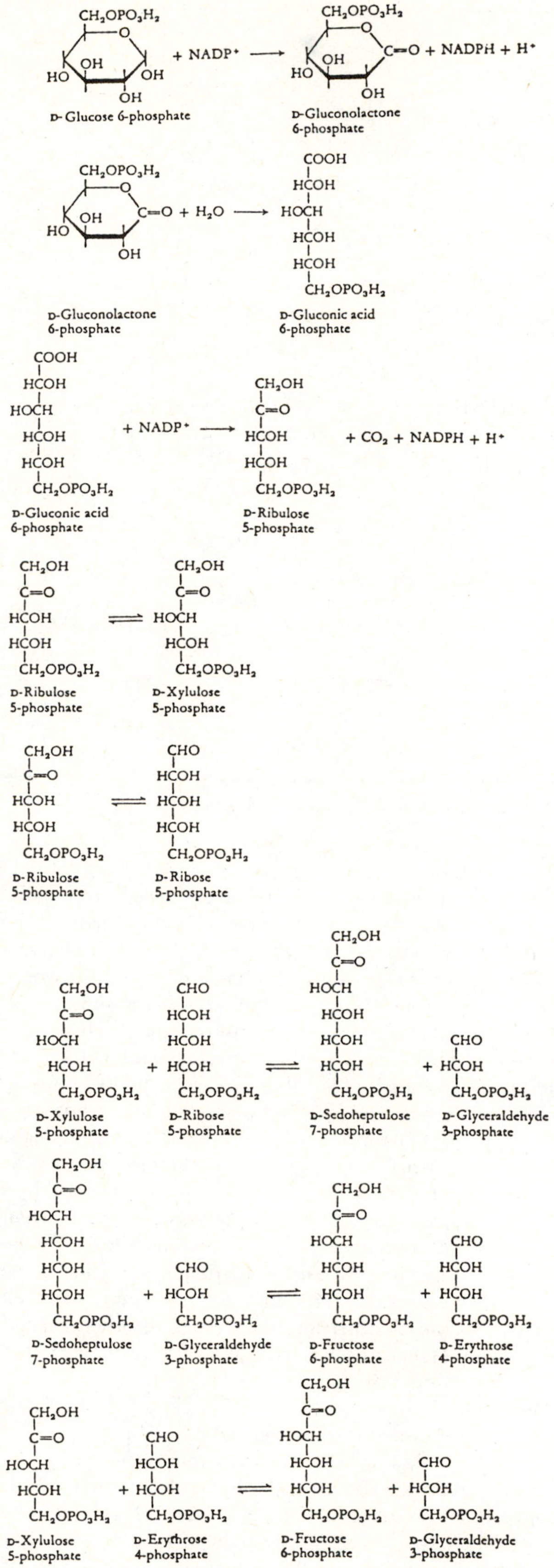

Enzyme:

$CH_2OPO_3H_2$ ... D-Glucose 6-phosphate $+ NADP^+ \longrightarrow$ D-Gluconolactone 6-phosphate $+ NADPH + H^+$ — Glucose 6-phosphate dehydrogenase

D-Gluconolactone 6-phosphate $+ H_2O \longrightarrow$ D-Gluconic acid 6-phosphate — Lactonase

D-Gluconic acid 6-phosphate $+ NADP^+ \longrightarrow$ D-Ribulose 5-phosphate $+ CO_2 + NADPH + H^+$ — Gluconic acid 6-phosphate dehydrogenase

D-Ribulose 5-phosphate $\rightleftharpoons$ D-Xylulose 5-phosphate — Pentose phosphate epimerase

D-Ribulose 5-phosphate $\rightleftharpoons$ D-Ribose 5-phosphate — Pentose phosphate isomerase

D-Xylulose 5-phosphate $+$ D-Ribose 5-phosphate $\rightleftharpoons$ D-Sedoheptulose 7-phosphate $+$ D-Glyceraldehyde 3-phosphate — Transketolase

D-Sedoheptulose 7-phosphate $+$ D-Glyceraldehyde 3-phosphate $\rightleftharpoons$ D-Fructose 6-phosphate $+$ D-Erythrose 4-phosphate — Transaldolase

D-Xylulose 5-phosphate $+$ D-Erythrose 4-phosphate $\rightleftharpoons$ D-Fructose 6-phosphate $+$ D-Glyceraldehyde 3-phosphate — Transketolase

Figure 3-17. Reactions of the pentose pathway.

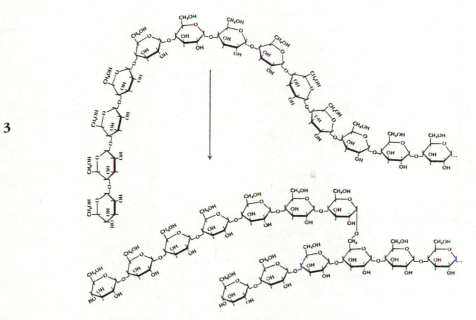

Figure 3-18. Top: Reaction catalyzed by phosphoglucomatose; 1, 2, and 3 are steps in the synthesis of glycogen.

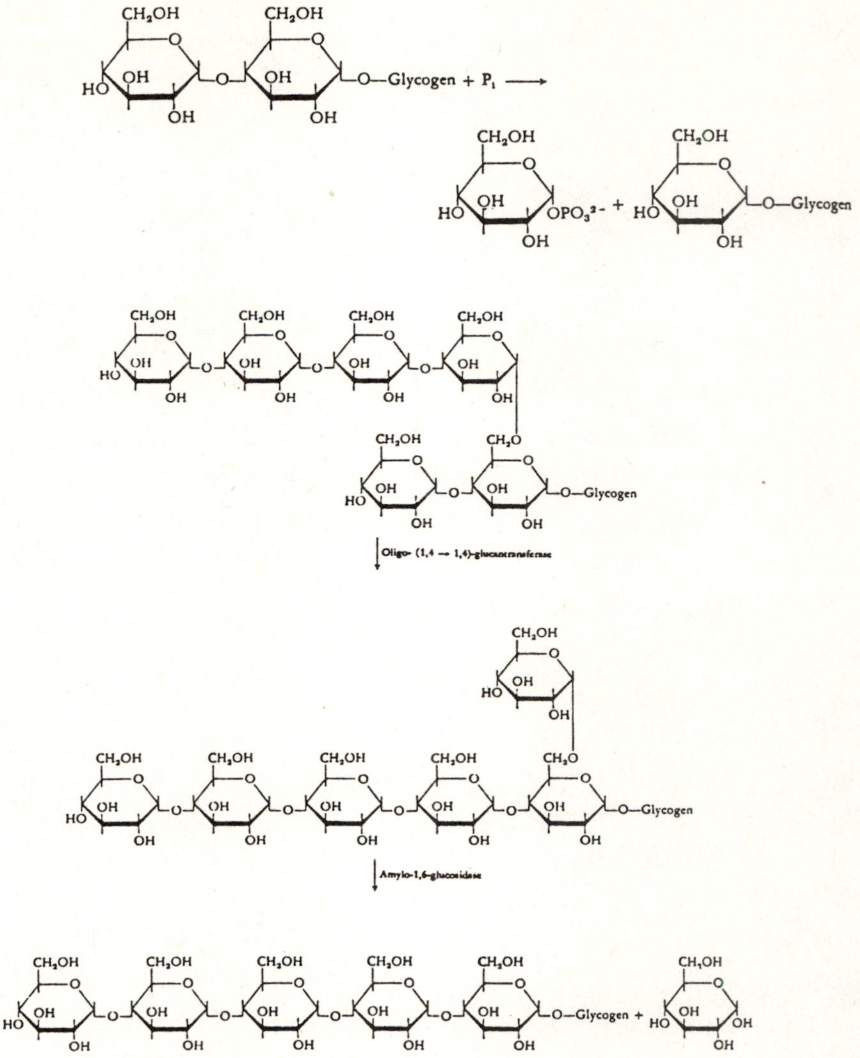

Figure 3-19. The three steps in the degradation of glycogen.

hormonal as well as enzymatic controls. Glycogen phosphorylase exists as both active and inactive forms. These are termed **phosphorylase a** and **phosphorylase b**, respectively. The inactive form is converted to the active form by the action of ATP and the enzyme **phosphorylase b kinase**. This transformation involves a conformational change in the protein and addition of phosphate to various serine residues. Also, phosphorylase a loses its characteristic activity when the phosphate is released. This reaction is catalyzed by **phosphorylase a phosphatase**. The breakdown of glycogen can thus be regulated by the activation and inactivation of phosphorylase. The hormone epinephrine is effective in enhancing the activity of phosphorylase b kinase by a sequence of reactions shown in Figure 3-20. Binding of epinephrine to muscle cells promotes the action of **adenyl cyclase**. This enzyme catalyzes the conversion of ATP to 3,6-cyclic AMP, as shown in the inset in Figure 3-20. The latter activates a **protein kinase**, which provides an active form of phosphorylase b kinase. The same protein kinase also enhances the production of inactive glycogen

synthetase (synthetase D) from the active form (synthetase I), as shown in Figure 3-20. Increased blood levels of epinephrine will therefore result in promotion of the breakdown or utilization of glycogen and minimization of glycogen synthesis or glucose storage.

Another hormone that influences glycogen metabolism in liver in a manner similar to that of epinephrine is glucagon, a protein hormone produced by alpha cells of the pancreas. Insulin effectively causes a decrease in the concentrations of cyclic AMP. It will therefore enhance glycogen synthesis and decrease the degree of glycogen degradation (Fig. 3-20).

Gluconeogenesis

Glycogen or glucose can be synthesized from various nonsugar intermediates. These include certain amino acids (e.g., glutamate, aspartate, alanine, serine) as well as lactate, pyruvate, or glycerol. The common feature among amino acids that are glucogenic is that they can be converted to either pyruvate or one of the acids of the citric acid cycle. Glycerol can

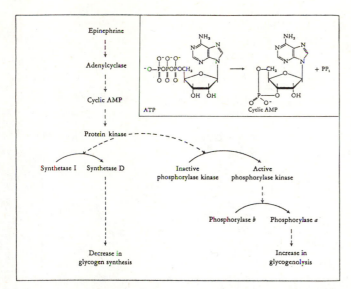

Figure 3-20. Sequence of steps in the effect of epinephrine of synthesis and degradation of glycogen.

be converted to glycerol phosphate and oxidized to dihydroxy-acetone phosphate; lactate can be oxidized to pyruvate. Most of the reactions in the glycolytic pathway are reversible. The steps that are unidirectional are the transformations of (1) phosphoenolpyruvate to pyruvate, (2) fructose 6-phosphate to fructose 1,6-diphosphate, and (3) glucose to glucose 6-phosphate. In order to produce glucose or glycogen from pyruvate, therefore, the three irreversible steps must be bypassed by alternate sequences.

Pyruvate can be converted to phosphoenolpyruvate by reactions **A** and **B** shown in Figure 3-21. The enzyme **pyruvate carboxylase** catalyzes the formation of oxaloacetate from pyruvate. This step requires energy in the form of ATP. A second enzyme, **phosphoenolpyruvate carboxykinase** causes the conversion of oxaloacetate to phosphoenolpyruvate. Energy for this step is derived from GTP. The sequence of steps by which phosphoenolpyruvate yields fructose 1,6-diphosphate is essentially the reversal of glycolysis. Fructose diphosphate is then hydrolyzed by a phosphatase as described above to yield fructose 6-phosphate. The latter is converted to glucose 6-phosphate by the action of an isomerase. Liver and kidney cells contain an enzyme, **glucose 6-phosphatase**, which yields glucose and inorganic phosphate. The glucose can be released from the liver into the bloodstream. By this mechanism, the liver can regulate the levels of glucose in the blood. Alternatively, glucose 6-phosphate can be utilized for synthesis of glycogen as shown in Figure 3-21. Many amino acids can be transformed to their respective ketoacids—for example, aspartate or glutamate could provide oxaloacetate or alpha-ketoglutarate, respectively. The ketoacids may then be converted to phosphoenolpyruvate, which yields glucose. Gluconeogenesis is an important function of the liver. In contrast, this process does not occur in muscle cells that do not contain glucose 6-phosphatase or fructose diphosphatase. The regulatory sites for glycolysis and gluconeogenesis are the reactions catalyzed by phosphofructokinase and fructose diphosphatase. Both of these enzymes are allosteric, and their activities are sensitive to concentrations of

critical intermediates. Phosphofructokinase is inhibited by ATP, NADH, and citrate. The intracellular levels of these materials are relatively high when the energy needs of the cell are satisfied. Hence, glycolysis is minimized. In contrast, when the levels of ATP are decreased, those of ADP and adenylate (AMP) are increased. ADP and AMP promote phosphofructokinase, and consequently glycolysis is enhanced.

Hormonal effects

Epinephrine and glucagon promote the breakdown of glycogen to glucose 1-phosphate, as described above. Insulin is effective in enhancing the synthesis of glycogen and in minimizing its synthesis. Insulin also facilitates the entry of circulating glucose into muscle or adipose tissue cells. Hence, insulin will cause a decrease in concentrations of blood glucose. Some steroid hormones (e.g., cortisone) increase the degree of gluconeogenesis.

Metabolism of galactose

Digestion of lactose (milk sugar) gives rise to both glucose and galactose. Galactose is metabolized in the liver and erythrocytes by the sequence shown in Figure 3-22. The enzyme **galactokinase** catalyzes the formation of galactose 1-phosphate from galactose and ATP. Galactose 1-phosphate reacts with uridine diphosphate glucose to yield uridine diphosphate galactose and glucose 1-phosphate. The enzyme for this reaction is **uridyl transferase**. Uridine diphosphate galactose is then transformed to uridine diphosphate glucose. Hence, all of the galactose is converted to glucose derivatives that can undergo further metabolic transformations.

There are two genetic disorders in which galactose cannot be metabolized. One of these is galactokinase deficiency and the other is a uridyl transferase deficiency. In both of these, the galactose that cannot undergo normal metabolism is reduced to galactitol, which deposits in the lens of the eye and causes cataracts. Additionally, in the uridyl transferase deficiency, the galactose 1-phosphate that accumulates causes mental retardation and liver damage. Children who are born with galactose disorders are treated by elimination of milk from their diet, since that is the principal source of lactose.

Other products of glucose metabolism

In addition to the pathways described above, glucose metabolism also gives rise to uridine diphosphate glucuronic acid and hexosamine derivatives. They function as building blocks for the synthesis of glycosaminoglycans, hyaluronic acid, chondroitin sulfates, heparin, and heparan sulfate. These polysaccharides are constituents of connective tissue as well as of cell membranes. Various sugars are also utilized in the synthesis of glycoproteins.

LIPIDS AND LIPID METABOLISM

Triglyceride structures and metabolic function

Triglycerides are categorized as a subgroup of **lipids**. Lipids are substances with a variety of structures whose common feature is their solubility in organic solvents and limited solubility in water. Glycerides are esters of glycerol and fatty acids (Fig. 3-23). The fatty acids that are generally found in animal triglycerides are carboxylic acids with an even number

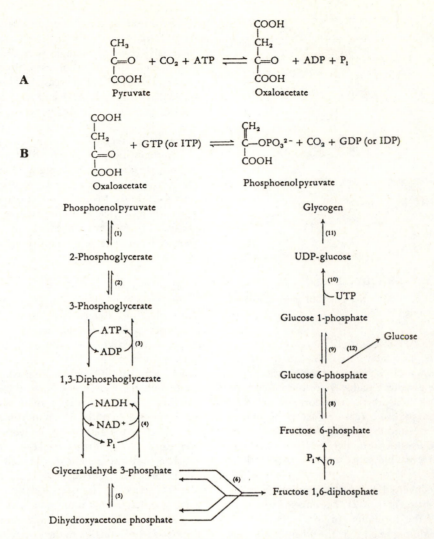

Figure 3-21. Formation of glucose and glycogen from pyruvate. The enzymes indicated by the numbers in parentheses are (1) enolase, (2) phosphoglyceromutase, (3) phosphoglycerate kinase, (4) glyceraldehyde 3-phosphate dehydrogenase, (5) triosephosphate isomerase, (6) aldolase, (7) fructose diphosphatase, (8) glucose-phosphate isomerase, (9) phosphoglucomutase, (10) UDP-glucose pyrophosphorlyase, (11) glycogen synthetase, and (12) glucose 6-phosphatase.

Galactose + ATP $\xrightleftharpoons{\text{galactokinase}}$ galactose-1-P + ADP

Galactose-1-P + UDP-glucose $\xrightleftharpoons{\text{uridyl transferase}}$ UDP-galactose + glucose-1-P

UDP-galactose $\xrightleftharpoons{\text{epimerase}}$ UDP-glucose

Figure 3-22. Metabolic transformations of galactose.

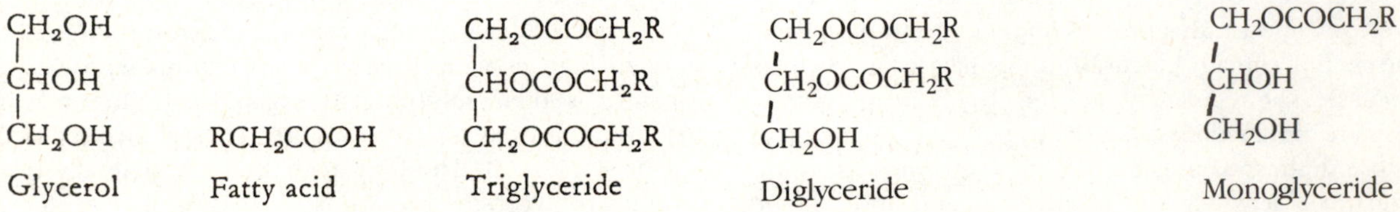

$$
\begin{array}{lllll}
CH_2OH & & CH_2OCOCH_2R & CH_2OCOCH_2R & CH_2OCOCH_2R \\
| & & | & | & | \\
CHOH & & CHOCOCH_2R & CH_2OCOCH_2R & CHOH \\
| & RCH_2COOH & | & | & | \\
CH_2OH & & CH_2OCOCH_2R & CH_2OH & CH_2OH \\
\text{Glycerol} & \text{Fatty acid} & \text{Triglyceride} & \text{Diglyceride} & \text{Monoglyceride}
\end{array}
$$

Figure 3-23. Fatty acids, glycerol, and glycerides.

of carbons. They contain long hydrocarbon chains, which may be either saturated or unsaturated. The structures of fatty acids that occur most frequently are shown in Table 3-3.

The major functions of triglycerides are to store energy and to provide a source of fuel. The free fatty acids derived from triglycerides that are stored in adipose tissue or ingested in the diet are degraded by a series of oxidation reactions, and the energy released is utilized for the requirements of the organism.

Triglyceride digestion and absorption

Triglycerides from dietary fat are digested in the small intestine by a lipase secreted by the pancreas. Bile salts derived from the gallbladder serve to emulsify the triglyceride droplets, thereby increasing the surface area available from the action of pancreatic lipase. The enzyme catalyzes the hydrolysis of the triglycerides, yielding free fatty acids, monoglycerides, and diglycerides. These products form mixed micelles with bile salts and are absorbed into intestinal mucosal cells. The glycerides and fatty acids are converted to triglycerides and combined with small amounts of specific proteins to form particles termed chylomicrons. The latter are released to the lymphatic vessels, from which they are transported to the systemic circulatory system. Since chylomicrons contain about 98% lipid and 2% protein, they have limited solubility in the blood. As a consequence, after ingestion of fats, blood has a turbid appearance. This condition is termed alimentary lipemia. Chylomicrons are normally disrupted by the action of the enzyme lipoprotein lipase, which is present on the surface of capillary endothelial cells. This enzyme catalyzes the hydrolysis of the triglycerides in chylomicrons to yield glycerol and free fatty acid. The glycerol, which is soluble, is metabolized by liver cells. The relatively insoluble fatty acids are bound to circulating albumin and transported to cells that can utilize them for energy.

Catabolism of free fatty acids

Free fatty acids are degraded by a sequence of reactions termed beta oxidation. The specific steps for stearic acid (18-carbon acid) are shown in Figure 3-24. The first step, described as activation, involves the interaction of the fatty acid with ATP and coenzyme A to yield the fatty acyl coenzyme A (acyl-CoA) (structure 2), adenosine monophosphate, and inorganic pyrophosphate. The acyl-CoA is then transferred by a specific mechanism to the mitochondria, where the subsequent reactions occur. Dehydrogenation of the fatty acyl-CoA by a flavin-adenine dinucleotide (FAD)-linked dehydrogenase yields the 2,3-unsaturated product (structure 3) and $FADH_2$. Addition of the elements of water to the latter provides fatty 3-hydroxyacyl-CoA (structure 4). Oxidation of the fatty 3-hydroxyacyl-CoA by an NAD-linked dehydrogenase yields 3-ketoacyl-CoA (structure 5) and NADH. Reaction of the 3-ketoacyl-CoA with coenzyme A results in a cleavage that results in formation of acetyl-CoA and a coenzyme A derivative of a 16-carbon fatty acid. Repetition of the reactions (except for the activation) seven more times generates eight additional moles of acetyl-CoA.

Thus, the sum total of products derived by beta oxidation of 1 mol of an 18-carbon saturated fatty acid are 9 mol of acetyl-CoA, 8 mol of reduced flavoprotein ($FADH_2$), and 8 mol of NADH. The amount of ATP obtainable from these amounts of $FADH_2$ and NADH are 16 and 24, respectively. Furthermore, oxidation of the 9 mol of acetyl-CoA to CO_2 and water via the citric acid cycle yields 108 mol of ATP. The activation step consumed the equivalent of 2 mol of ATP, since the reaction involved removal of two phosphates. Hence, the net amount of ATP obtained is 146.

Biosynthesis of fatty acids

Long-chain fatty acids can be synthesized from acetyl-CoA. This synthetic process is most prominent when there is a high intake of carbohydrates; excess acetyl-CoA is then diverted to the formation of fatty acids instead of further oxidation via the citric acid cycle. Thus, when the energy requirements are fully satisfied, adipocytes convert acetyl-CoA to fatty acids and store them in the form of triglycerides. In contrast to the degradative process, which occurs in the mitochondria, the synthetic steps take place in the extramitochondrial compartment of the cell.

The first step for the synthetic process is the reaction of

Table 3-3. Structures of Common Fatty Acids

Structure	Name	Designation*
Saturated		
$CH_3(CH_2)_{12}COOH$	Myristic	14:0
$CH_3(CH_2)_{14}COOH$	Palmitic	16:0
$CH_3(CH_2)_{16}COOH$	Stearic	18:0
$CH_3(CH_2)_{18}COOH$	Arachidic	20:0
Unsaturated		
$CH_3(CH_2)_5CH{=}CH(CH_2)_7COOH$	Palmitoleic	16:1 or Δ^9
$CH_3(CH_2)_7CH{=}CH(CH_2)_7COOH$	Oleic	18:1 or Δ^9
$CH_3(CH_2)_4CH{=}CHCH_2CH{=}CH(CH_2)_7COOH$	Linoleic	18:2 or $\Delta^{9,12}$
$CH_3CH_2CH{=}CHCH_2CH{=}CHCH_2CH{=}CH(CH_2)_7COOH$	Linolenic	18:3 or $\Delta^{9,12,15}$
$CH_3(CH_2)_4CH{=}CHCH_2CH{=}CHCH_2CH{=}CHCH_2CH{=}CH(CH_2)_3COOH$	Arachidonic	20:4 or $\Delta^{5,8,11,14}$

*The numerical designation defines the number of carbon atoms and the number of double bonds. Thus, 18:2 indicates that the acid is composed of 18 carbon atoms and contains two double bonds. The other notation, which uses the Greek letter delta (Δ) and a superscript, indicates the position of the double bond. For example, $\Delta^{9,12}$ means that there are double bonds between carbon-9 and carbon-10 and between carbon-12 and carbon-13.

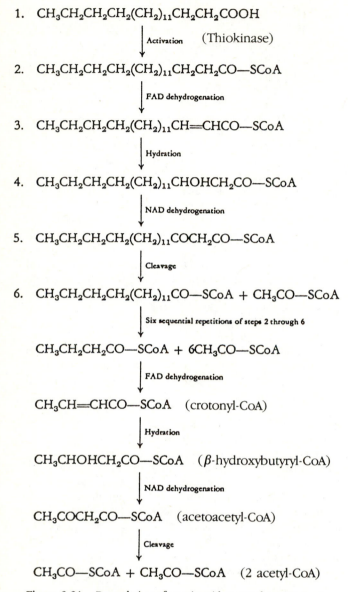

1. $CH_3CH_2CH_2CH_2(CH_2)_{11}CH_2CH_2COOH$

    ↓ Activation   (Thiokinase)

2. $CH_3CH_2CH_2CH_2(CH_2)_{11}CH_2CH_2CO{-}SCoA$

    ↓ FAD dehydrogenation

3. $CH_3CH_2CH_2CH_2(CH_2)_{11}CH{=}CHCO{-}SCoA$

    ↓ Hydration

4. $CH_3CH_2CH_2CH_2(CH_2)_{11}CHOHCH_2CO{-}SCoA$

    ↓ NAD dehydrogenation

5. $CH_3CH_2CH_2CH_2(CH_2)_{11}COCH_2CO{-}SCoA$

    ↓ Cleavage

6. $CH_3CH_2CH_2CH_2(CH_2)_{11}CO{-}SCoA + CH_3CO{-}SCoA$

    ↓ Six sequential repetitions of steps 2 through 6

$CH_3CH_2CH_2CO{-}SCoA + 6CH_3CO{-}SCoA$

    ↓ FAD dehydrogenation

$CH_3CH{=}CHCO{-}SCoA$ (crotonyl-CoA)

    ↓ Hydration

$CH_3CHOHCH_2CO{-}SCoA$ (β-hydroxybutyryl-CoA)

    ↓ NAD dehydrogenation

$CH_3COCH_2CO{-}SCoA$ (acetoacetyl-CoA)

    ↓ Cleavage

$CH_3CO{-}SCoA + CH_3CO{-}SCoA$ (2 acetyl-CoA)

Figure 3-24.   Degradation of stearic acid to acetyl coenzyme A.

acetyl-CoA with carbonate and ATP (Fig. 3-25, step 1). The enzyme that catalyzes this reaction, acetyl-CoA carboxylase, contains biotin as a prosthetic group (Fig. 3-25, structure 2). Formation of long-chain fatty acyl derivatives from acetyl units involves a multienzyme complex called the **fatty-acid synthetase** system. The enzymes of this complex are bound to each other, so that the steps that they catalyze proceed in an efficient regulated sequence.

In contrast to fatty acid catabolism, in which the intermediates are linked to coenzyme A, the biosynthetic pathway requires that the components be bound to acyl carrier protein (ACP). The latter is a small protein linked through the hydroxyl oxygen of a serine residue to phosphate, pantothenic acid, and mercaptoethanolamine (Fig. 3-25, structure 3). The carboxyl groups of the metabolites are bound as thioesters to the thiol group. Malonyl-CoA that was formed in the first step is converted to malonyl-ACP by the action of a component of the multienzyme system called **malonyl transacylase** (Fig. 3-25, reaction 1). Similarly, acetyl from acetyl-CoA is transferred to ACP (reaction 2). Malonyl-ACP then reacts with acetyl-ACP to produce acetoacetyl-ACP (reaction 3).

The subsequent step is the reduction of acetoacetyl-ACP by NADPH to yield hydroxybutyryl-ACP (reaction 4). Removal of the elements of water generates the unsaturated product, which in turn is reduced by a second NADPH to yield the four-carbon acid butyryl-ACP (reactions 5 and 6). It can be seen that this series of reactions elongates the chain by two carbons. Two more carbons can now be added by interaction of butyryl-ACP with malonyl-ACP followed by reactions analogous to reactions 3 through 6. This process is repeated until a 16-carbon fatty acid is formed. The ACP-linked fatty acid is then converted back to a coenzyme A derivative.

Fatty acids are stored in adipose tissue as triglycerides. Synthesis of the latter (Fig. 3-26, Reactions A, B, C) occurs in the endoplasmic reticulum. The fatty acyl-CoA reacts with glycerol phosphate to produce a phosphatidic acid. Hydrolysis of the latter yields a diglyceride, which then condenses with acetyl-CoA to form the triglycerides.

Synthesis of phospholipids

Diglycerides also serve as substrates for the biosynthesis of phospholipids. These include phosphatidylcholine (lecithin), phosphatidylethanolamine, phosphatidylserine, and phosphatidylinositol. The sequence for the formation of lecithin and phosphatidylethanolamine is shown in Figures 3-26 and 3-27. Choline is converted to choline phosphate, which reacts with cytidine triphosphate to yield cytidine diphosphate choline (Fig. 3-26, reactions 1 and 2). Similarly, ethanolamine is transformed to cytidine diphosphate ethanolamine (Fig. 3-26, reactions 3 and 4). Each of the cytidine diphosphate derivatives reacts with diglycerides, yielding the respective phospholipids as shown in Figure 3-27. Structures of other phospholipids, phosphatidylserine and phosphatidylinositol, are also shown in Figure 3-27.

Phospholipids are integral components of membrane structures. For example, glycerol phospholipids compose about 40% of the lipid portion of the erythrocyte cell membrane and over 95% of the lipid in mitochondrial membranes. In the circulatory system, the phospholipids occur as components of lipoproteins.

Mobilization of triglycerides

Triglycerides that are stored in adipose tissue can be hydrolyzed by **tissue lipase**. This makes free fatty acids available for export, via the bloodstream, to cells of other tissues, especially muscle. The fatty acids that are released are carried in the blood bound to albumin. The activity of tissue lipase is promoted by epinephrine. The latter stimulates adenyl cyclase in adipose tissue to convert ATP to cyclic AMP. The general mechanism for the action of cyclic AMP in this process is analogous to its action in stimulating glycogen phosphorylase. Insulin inhibits this process and thus decreases the hydrolysis of triglycerides. Moreover, insulin stimulates synthesis of triglycerides since it enhances the uptake of glucose by the cells. This action effectively decreases the requirement for fatty acids so that they will be channeled toward triglyceride formation. Additionally, glycolysis provides the intermediate (dihydroxy-

Structure 1

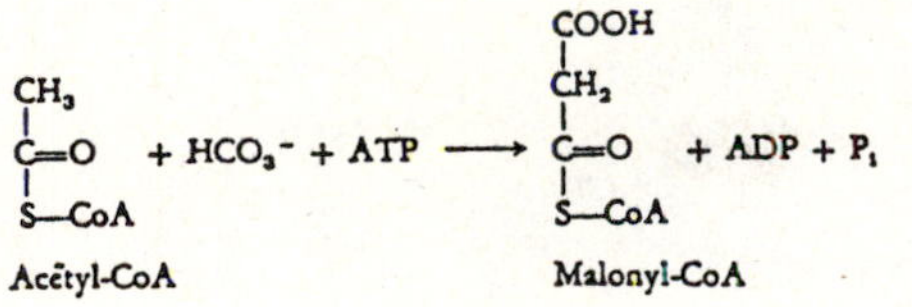

$$\underset{\text{Acetyl-CoA}}{\overset{\overset{\displaystyle CH_3}{|}}{\underset{\underset{\displaystyle S-CoA}{|}}{C=O}}} + HCO_3^- + ATP \longrightarrow \underset{\text{Malonyl-CoA}}{\overset{\overset{\displaystyle COOH}{\underset{\displaystyle CH_2}{|}}}{\underset{\underset{\displaystyle S-CoA}{|}}{C=O}}} + ADP + P_i$$

Structure 2

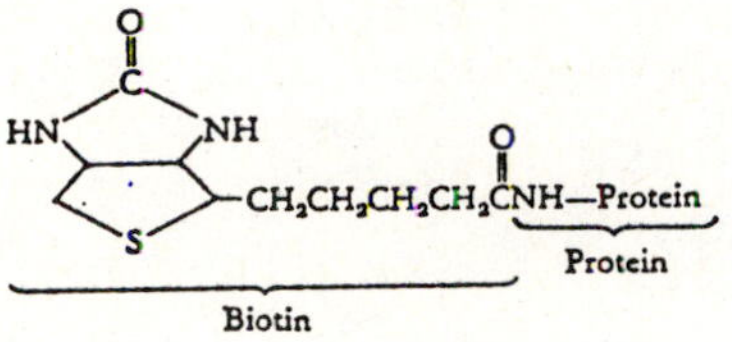

Biotin—$CH_2CH_2CH_2CH_2CNH$—Protein

Structure 3

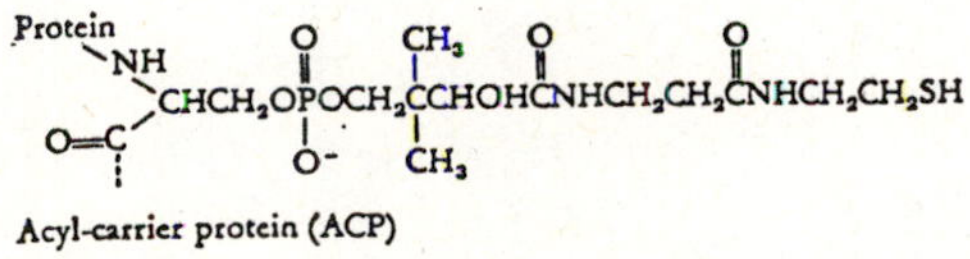

Acyl-carrier protein (ACP)

Reaction 1

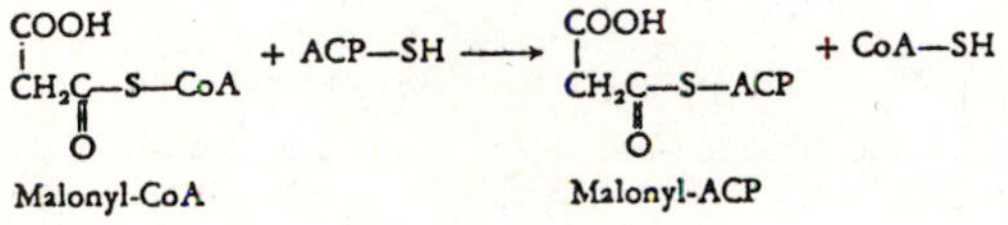

$$\underset{\text{Malonyl-CoA}}{COOH\!-\!CH_2C\!-\!S\!-\!CoA} + ACP\!-\!SH \longrightarrow \underset{\text{Malonyl-ACP}}{COOH\!-\!CH_2C\!-\!S\!-\!ACP} + CoA\!-\!SH$$

Reaction 2

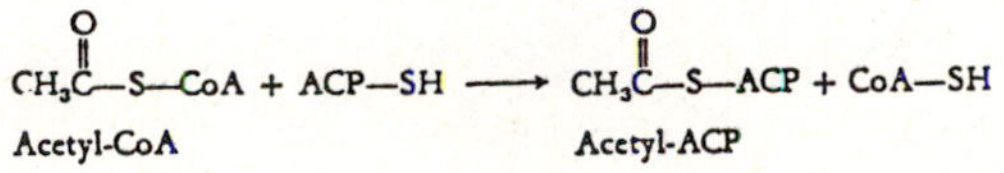

$$\underset{\text{Acetyl-CoA}}{CH_3C\!-\!S\!-\!CoA} + ACP\!-\!SH \longrightarrow \underset{\text{Acetyl-ACP}}{CH_3C\!-\!S\!-\!ACP} + CoA\!-\!SH$$

Reaction 3

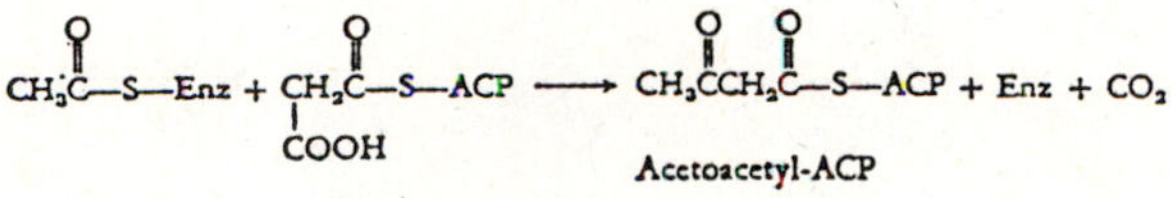

$$CH_3C\!-\!S\!-\!Enz + \underset{\underset{COOH}{|}}{CH_2C\!-\!S\!-\!ACP} \longrightarrow \underset{\text{Acetoacetyl-ACP}}{CH_3CCH_2C\!-\!S\!-\!ACP} + Enz + CO_2$$

Reaction 4

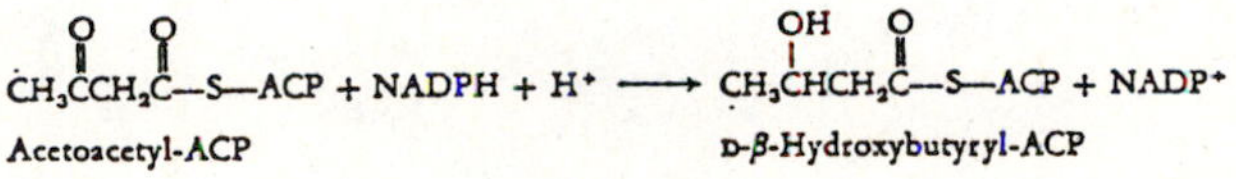

$$\underset{\text{Acetoacetyl-ACP}}{CH_3CCH_2C\!-\!S\!-\!ACP} + NADPH + H^+ \longrightarrow \underset{\text{D-}\beta\text{-Hydroxybutyryl-ACP}}{CH_3CHCH_2C\!-\!S\!-\!ACP} + NADP^+$$

Reaction 5

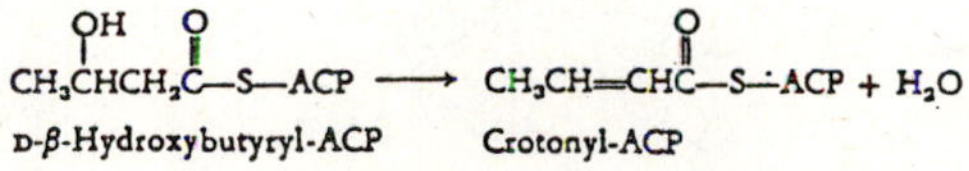

$$\underset{\text{D-}\beta\text{-Hydroxybutyryl-ACP}}{CH_3CHCH_2C\!-\!S\!-\!ACP} \longrightarrow \underset{\text{Crotonyl-ACP}}{CH_3CH=CHC\!-\!S\!-\!ACP} + H_2O$$

Reaction 6

$$\underset{\text{Crotonyl-ACP}}{CH_3CH=CHC\!-\!S\!-\!ACP} + NADPH + H^+ \longrightarrow \underset{\text{Butyryl-ACP}}{CH_3CH_2CH_2C\!-\!S\!-\!ACP} + NADP^+$$

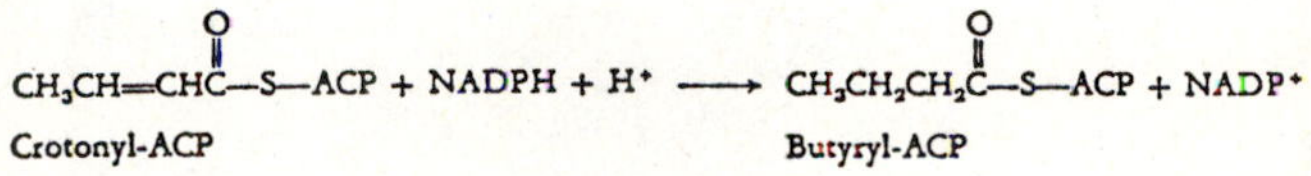

Figure 3-25. Synthesis of fatty acid from acetyl-CoA.

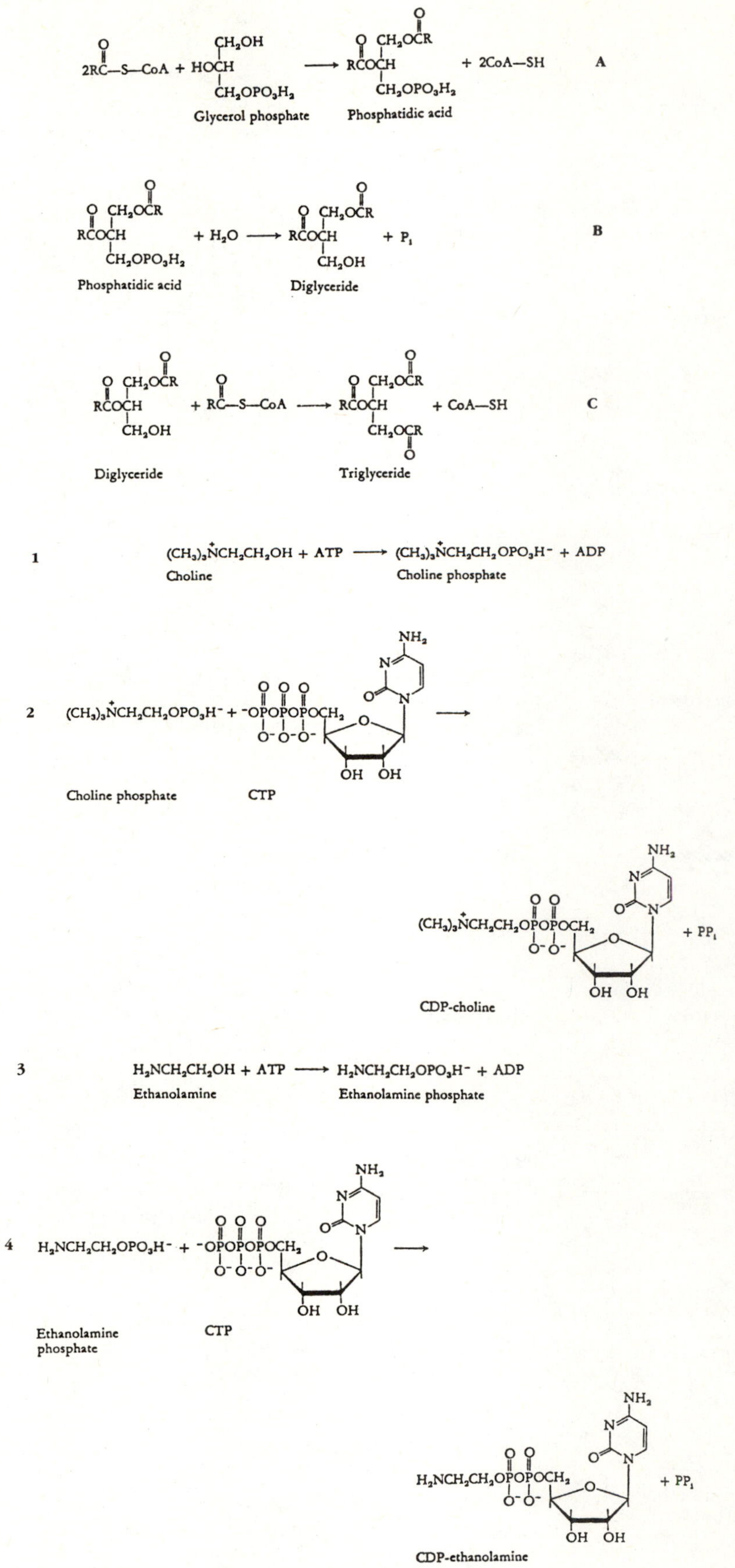

Figure 3-26. Synthesis of triglycerides and phospholipids.

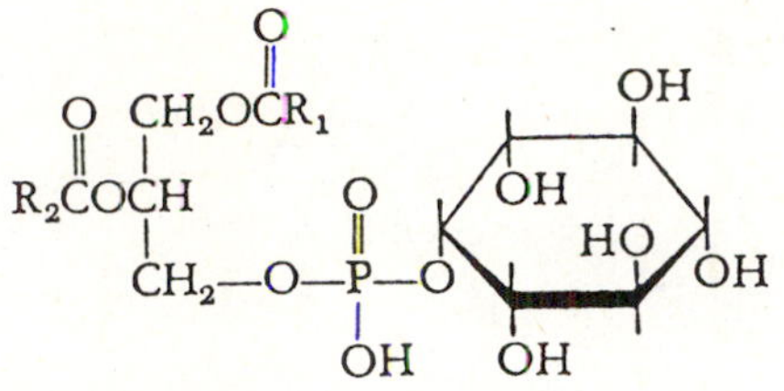

Phosphatidylinositol

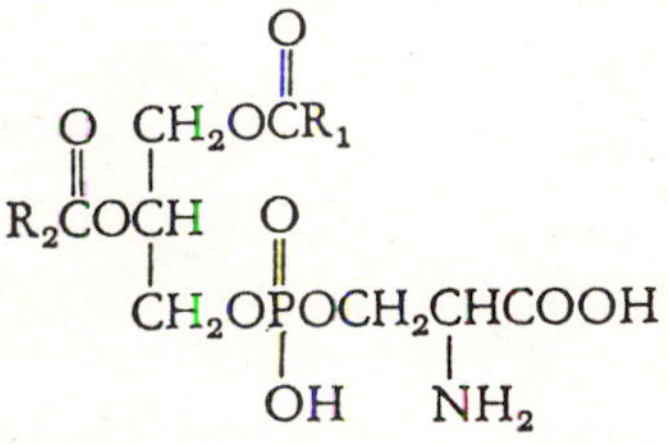

Phosphatidylserine

Figure 3-27. Structures of other phospholipids.

acetone phosphate) required for forming glycerol phosphate, which in turn is necessary for the synthesis of triglycerides.

In view of the fact that glucose can be metabolized to acetyl-CoA and that acetyl-CoA can be converted to free fatty acids, it is clear that carbohydrate can be utilized for the generation of triglycerides. Hence, ingestion of excess carbohydrate leads to the accumulation of fat. It should be noted, however, that fatty acid ingestion cannot lead to an increase in glucose or glycogen.

Ketone bodies

Degradation of fatty acid in muscle tissue yields acetyl-CoA, which can then be degraded further via the reactions of the citric acid cycle. Similar degradation occurs in the liver; however, a small but significant amount of the fatty acid metabolites is converted to free acetoacetate. This may occur either by removal of the coenzyme A from acetoacetyl-CoA or by formation of 3-hydroxy-3-methylglutaryl-CoA and its subsequent conversion to acetoacetate and coenzyme A (Fig. 3-28). Acetoacetate can be reduced to form 3-hydroxybutyrate. Some acetoacetate is decarboxylated to yield acetone (Fig. 3-28). The three products—acetoacetate, 3-hydroxybutyrate, and acetone—are called **ketone bodies**.

The liver has no mechanism for reactivating ketone bodies and therefore it cannot utilize them. They are, therefore, transferred to the bloodstream. Most of the acetone is exhaled through the lungs. Acetoacetate is taken up by muscle tissue, where it is activated—that is, it is converted to the coenzyme A derivative. The other ketone body, 3-hydroxybutyrate, is oxidized to acetoacetate and activated. The acetoacetyl-CoA can then be converted to 2 mol of acetyl-CoA by the action of thiolase and utilized for deriving energy.

As a result of the formation of ketone bodies in the liver and their transport and utilization by extrahepatic tissues, small amounts of these substances are present in the circulatory system. Normally, blood plasma contains about 0.3 to 2.0 mg of ketone bodies per 100 ml. This amount represents a steady state arising from the production of acetoacetate in the liver and its intake by muscle and other extrahepatic tissues. In certain situations, the rate of formation of acetoacetate becomes excessive. This occurs mainly during prolonged starvation or carbohydrate deprivation, as well as in persons with untreated diabetes.

When the production of acetoacetic acid and 3-hydroxybutyric acid in the liver exceeds the capacity of extrahepatic tissue for their utilization, there is an increase in the blood levels of ketone bodies. Considerable amounts of these substances are then excreted in the urine. Since the ketone bodies are acids that are ionized at the pH of blood, they are excreted as anions together with sodium ions. This loss of cations from the blood leads to a decrease in blood pH, a condition called **metabolic acidosis**. Concurrently, there is a loss of water from the system. If it is not corrected, the situation results in a comatose state and may become life threatening.

STEROID METABOLISM

CHOLESTEROL BIOSYNTHESIS AND METABOLISM

Cholesterol is an essential component of cell membranes and serves as a precursor for the biosynthesis of steroid hormones and bile salts. The body of a 70-kg adult male contains 75 to 150 g of cholesterol. Approximately 20% of this is in the metabolic pool; the remainder is contained in the tissues and is turned over slowly. The average normal adult has a serum cholesterol concentration of 150 to 250 mg/100 ml. Two sources contribute to the total cholesterol levels—diet and biosynthesis. The level of circulating cholesterol affects the amount synthesized by the tissues.

Biosynthesis

The major site of cholesterol biosynthesis is the liver. All the carbons of cholesterol ultimately derive from acetyl-CoA. The synthesis of 1 mol of cholesterol uses 18 mol of acetate, 18 mol of ATP, and 13 mol of NADPH. The committed step in cholesterol biosynthesis (Fig. 3-29) is the formation of mevalonic acid, which is catalyzed by **HMG-CoA reductase**. Fasting or ingestion of cholesterol reduces the activity of this enzyme, as well as its biosynthesis. A resumption in feeding after a fast and ingestion of carbohydrate or triglycerides (which are dietary sources of acetyl-CoA) results in increased biosynthesis of cholesterol.

About two-thirds of the cholesterol in plasma is esterified. This is accomplished by the transfer of fatty acid (usually linoleate) from the two position of lecithin to the 3-hydroxyl group of cholesterol (Fig. 3-30). This reaction is catalyzed by the enzyme **lecithin-cholesterol acyl transferase**, commonly referred to as LCAT.

Cell uptake

All cells require cholesterol for membrane biosynthesis. In general, extrahepatic cells obtain their cholesterol from the circulating pool in the plasma. Cholesterol is found in plasma primarily as low-density lipoprotein (LDL), and the mechanism for uptake involves specific LDL receptors on the surfaces of these cells.

LDL binds to the cell surface receptors, and the complex is internalized by endocytosis. The endocytotic vesicles fuse with

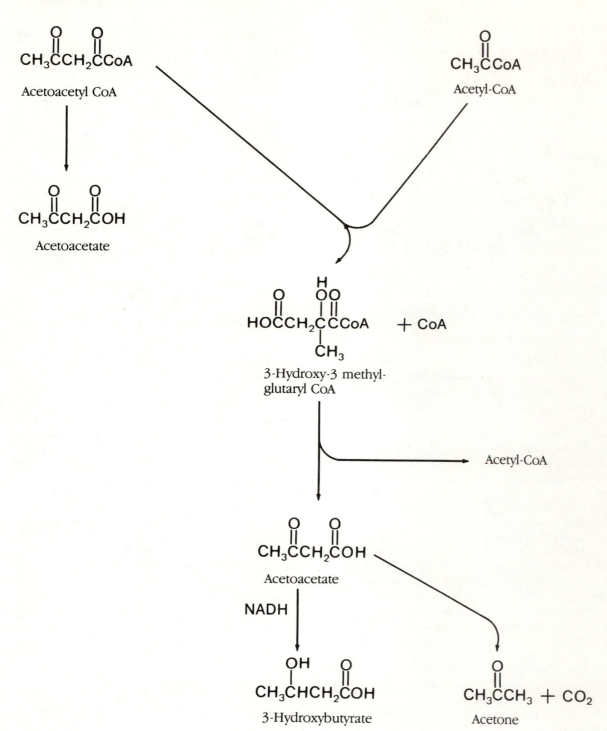

Figure 3-28.   Formation of ketone bodies.

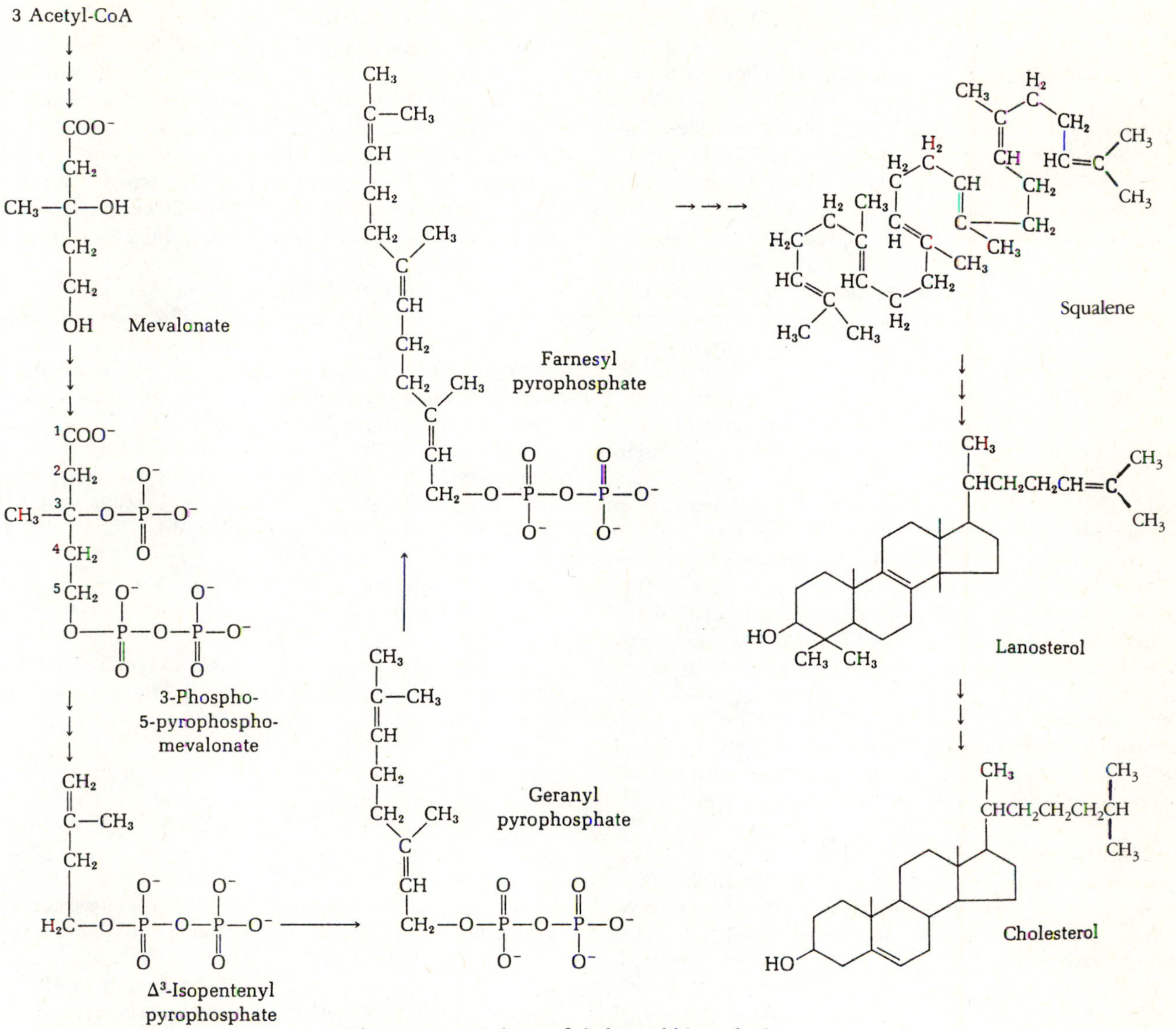

Figure 3-29.   Pathway of cholesterol biosynthesis.

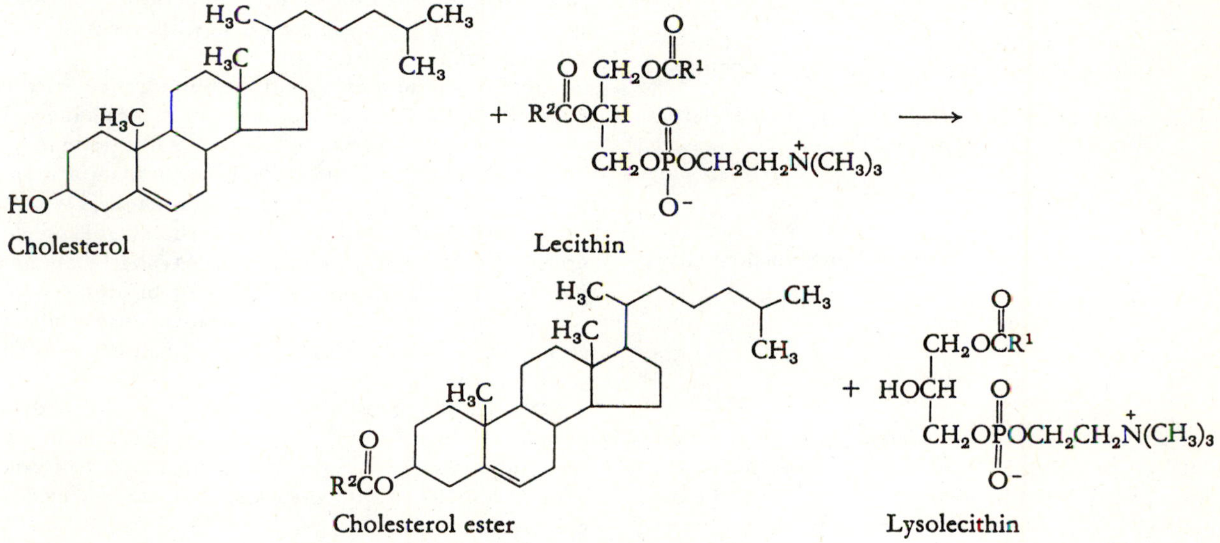

Figure 3-30.   Esterification of cholesterol.

lysosomes, and lysosomal enzymes digest the protein components and hydrolyze the cholesterol esters. The free cholesterol thus released within the cell is employed for membrane biosynthesis or reesterified for storage within the cell. In contrast to the esterification reaction in plasma described in the previous section, reesterification usually involves the transfer of oleate or palmitoleate and is catalyzed by a different enzyme, acyl-CoA cholesterol acyltransferase (ACAT).

In cells that depend on LDL uptake for their source of cholesterol, the cholesterol levels are controlled in two ways. The accumulation of free cholesterol inside the cell inhibits de novo synthesis at the level of HMG-CoA reductase, as described earlier. In addition, LDL receptor synthesis is regulated by intracellular cholesterol concentrations. When cholesterol levels inside the cell are high, new LDL receptors are not synthesized. Since the lifetime of these receptors is approximately 1 day, inhibition of receptor biosynthesis blocks further cholesterol uptake.

The importance of LDL receptors in maintenance of appropriate cellular cholesterol levels is demonstrated by a genetic disorder known as **familial hypercholesterolemia**. Patients homozygous for this disease display enormously elevated plasma cholesterol and LDL levels (plasma cholesterol normally exceeds 600 mg/100 ml). These patients generally die in childhood from coronary artery disease. Heterozygotes also have elevated plasma cholesterol levels, usually greater than 300 mg/100 ml. The latter individuals exhibit premature atherosclerosis. Homozygotes have almost no cell surface LDL receptors. The result is no cellular uptake of plasma LDL, which leads to elevation of plasma cholesterol levels.

High-density lipoprotein cholesterol

A series of studies have led to the conclusion that high-density lipoprotein (HDL) cholesterol levels in plasma are a useful predictor for risk of coronary artery disease. There is an inverse relationship between HDL levels and coronary artery disease; the higher the HDL, the lower the incidence of disease. This correlation is independent of total cholesterol or LDL levels in plasma. It appears that HDL may be responsible for the removal of arterial cholesterol.

STEROID HORMONE BIOSYNTHESIS AND ACTION

Cholesterol is the major precursor for all the steroid hormones, as shown in the following scheme:

$$Cholesterol$$
$$\downarrow$$
$$Glucocorticoids \leftarrow Progestogens \rightarrow Mineralocorticoids$$
$$\downarrow$$
$$Androgens$$
$$\downarrow$$
$$Estrogens$$

Essentially, the same biosynthetic enzymes are present in the adrenals, ovaries, testes, and placenta. Quantitative and qualitative differences in these enzymes from tissue to tissue account for the range of different products produced.

Adrenocorticol hormones

If an animal is adrenalectomized, the following are observed: (1) disturbance of electrolyte balance (increased excretion of Na^+, Cl^-, and H_2O, and K^+ retention); (2) increased blood urea due to decreased renal blood flow; (3) decrease in liver glycogen, hypoglycemia, and insulin sensitivity; (4) decreased utilization of dietary carbohydrate; (5) decreased gluconeogenesis and protein catabolism; (6) muscle weakness (probably secondary to alterations in carbohydrate metabolism); and (7) reduced ability to withstand stress.

Administration of adrenocortical extracts ameliorates all of these effects, indicating that there are substances produced in the adrenal cortex that control these processes. The variety of symptoms can be classified as two types—metabolic and mineral balance. These are regulated by glucocorticoids and mineralocorticoids, respectively.

Biosynthesis. The first step on the biosynthetic route from cholesterol to the steroid hormones is the formation of dihydroxycholesterol by hydroxylation at C-20 and C-22. These reactions occur in the mitochondria.

$$Cholesterol + 2\ O_2 + 2\ NADPH \rightarrow$$
$$dihydroxycholesterol + 2\ H_2O + 2\ NADP^+$$

A separate electron transport system is required for these reactions; it utilizes a special class of cytochromes referred to as **cytochrome P$_{450}$**. Electrons for the hydroxylation are provided by NADPH.

After hydroxylation, the C–20,22 bond is broken by the action of cholesterol desmolase, yielding Δ^5-pregnenolone. The latter compound is released into the cytosol and converted to progesterone. Progesterone is a branch point in the production of the adrenocorticoids. Its conversion to cortisol (glucocorticoid) or aldosterone (mineralocorticoid) is determined by the relative rates of reaction of two other hydroxylase enzymes, 17-alpha-hydroxylase or 21-hydroxylase (Fig. 3-31). If progesterone is first hydroxylated at C–17, then the end product will be cortisol. Prior hydroxylation at C–21 leads to the production of aldosterone.

Normal daily synthesis of adrenocorticoids is 10 to 20 mg of cortisol and only 0.3 mg of aldosterone. Glucocorticoids are not stored in the adrenal cortex, so whatever is produced is released into the bloodstream.

Steroid biosynthesis is controlled by **adrenocorticotropic hormone** (ACTH), which is synthesized in the pituitary gland. The surfaces of adrenal cells have ACTH receptors, and binding of ACTH to these receptors results in the activation of adenyl cyclase. This in turn leads to the increased synthesis of cyclic AMP, resulting in (1) increased cholesterol and glucose uptake, (2) increased production of NADPH by the pentose phosphate pathway, and (3) increased biosynthesis of the various hydroxylase enzymes. As a consequence of all of these events, pregnenolone biosynthesis is enhanced, yielding elevated levels of adrenocorticosteroids.

The half-life of circulating cortisol is 1 to 2 hours. The primary mechanism for its breakdown is the reduction of the 3-keto group and Δ^5 double bond to give tetrahydrocortisol. The latter is conjugated with glucuronic acid and excreted in the urine.

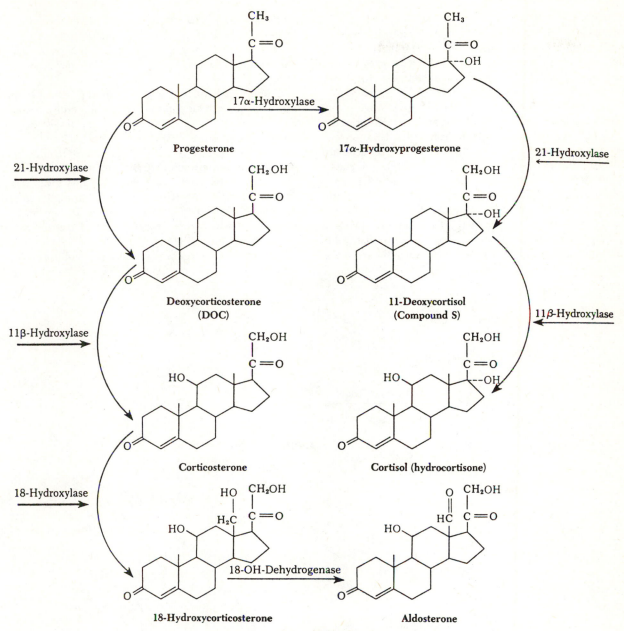

Figure 3-31. Biosynthesis of corticosteroids.

Mechanism of action. The primary metabolic action of glucocorticoids is to stimulate gluconeogenesis. The major carbon source for this process is amino acids. In muscle, this process is promoted by the stimulation of protein catabolism. In hepatocytes, amino acid transport into the cells is enhanced. Glucocorticoids also stimulate the biosynthesis of phosphoenol-pyruvate (PEP) carboxykinase, fructose 1,6-biphosphatase, pyruvate carboxylase, and glucose 6-phosphatase, all of which are gluconeogenic enzymes.

Aldosterone regulates electrolyte balance by stimulating renal sodium readsorption, which leads to sodium retention and potassium excretion. Aldosterone secretion is induced by ACTH, angiotensin II, elevated serum K^+, or low serum Na^+. Low serum Na^+ levels trigger renal synthesis of the enzyme

renin, which is involved in the production of angiotensin II. Aldosterone thus plays a major role in maintenance of normal blood pressure.

Diseases. Either hypo- or hyperfunctioning of the adrenal cortex results in a diseased state. **Addison's disease** results from hypofunction of the adrenal cortex. The result is (1) low blood pressure, (2) low basal metabolic rate, (3) subnormal temperature, (4) disturbance in electrolyte balance, and (5) hypoglycemia. This can usually be treated by administration of prednisone (Δ^1-cortisone).

Cushing's disease results from the hyperproduction of adrenocorticoids. This results in altered protein, fat, and carbohydrate metabolism and adiposity of the face, neck, and trunk.

Sex hormones

Androgens.   Androgens are synthesized chiefly in the Leydig's cells of the testes. The biosynthetic route from cholesterol to Δ^5-pregnenolone is the same as for the adrenocorticoids. The production of Δ^5-pregnenolone in the testes is stimulated by luteinizing hormone. The major pathway from Δ^5-pregnenolone to testosterone is shown in Figure 3-32.

Testosterone is the major circulating androgen. Its primary target tissues are the prostate and seminal vesicles. Testosterone enters these cells via passive diffusion and is reduced to dihyrotestosterone (DHT) by the action of 5-alpha-reductase. DHT is a more potent androgen than testosterone and cannot serve as a precursor for estrogen synthesis as is the case with testosterone.

DHT produced in the target cells complexes with a cytoplasmic receptor, enters the nucleus, and stimulates the transcription of a specific set of genes. The result is the synthesis of cell-specific proteins that are responsible for the develop-ment of male sexual characteristics. Under the influence of DHT, the testicles descend, spermatogenesis is sustained, mammary development is inhibited, and secondary male characteristics such as hair growth, muscle development, and voice mature.

Estrogens.   Estrogens are synthesized primarily in the ovaries. The biosynthetic pathway from cholesterol to testosterone is identical to that which occurs in the testes (Fig. 3-32). Specifically in ovaries, testosterone is converted in three steps to estradiol (Fig. 3-33). The three structural differences between testosterone and estradiol are (1) aromatization of the A ring, (2) a 3-hydroxyl group, and (3) no methyl group at C-19. Estradiol may be converted to estrone or estriol, but estradiol is the major circulating estrogen secreted by the ovary. The relative potencies of the estrogens estradiol to estrone to estriol are approximately 1000 to 100 to 30.

Secretion of estrogens is stimulated by follicle-stimulating hormone (FSH). Conversely, pituitary secretion of FSH is

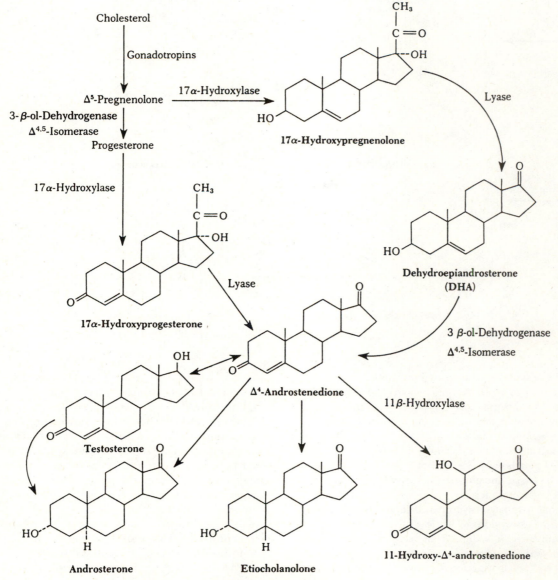

Figure 3-32.   Biosynthesis of androgens.

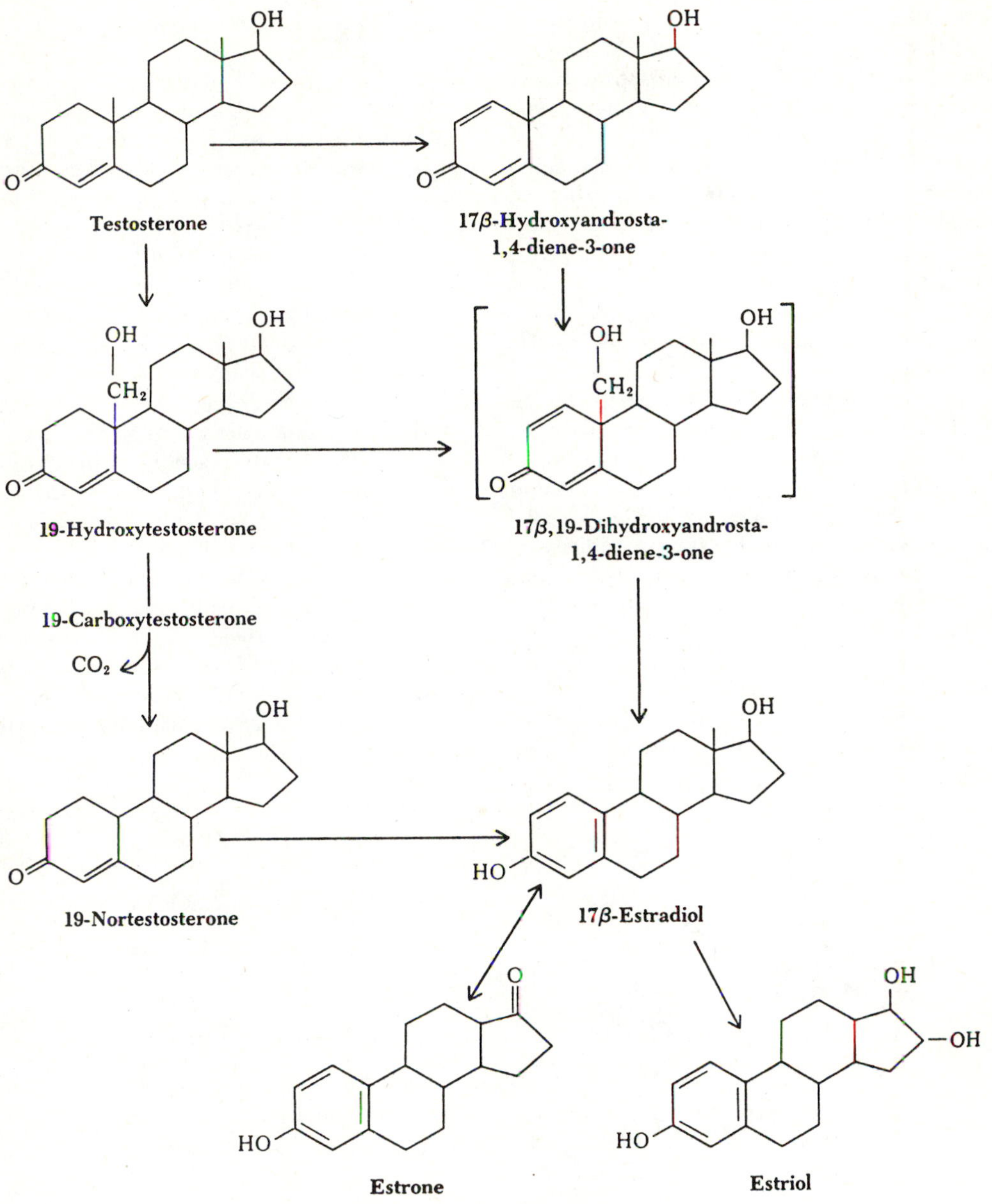

Figure 3-33. Biosynthesis of estrogens.

feedback regulated by estrogens. Serum levels of estrogen in women fluctuate, with peak levels of approximately 0.35 ng/ml of plasma occurring at 13 and 20 days of the menstrual cycle. The major target tissues are the uterus and vagina. Estrogens enter the cells and lead to increased transcription of specific genes by the cytosolic receptor mechanism described above for androgens. The major physiological effect is the development of the uterine endometrium. In addition, estrogens are required for the maintenance of the female reproductive organs.

After the release of a mature ovum, the ruptured follicle is converted to a corpus luteum by the action of luteinizing hormone. The corpus luteum secretes progesterone, which facilitates the further development and preparation of the uterine wall for implantation of a fertilized ovum. Progesterone also inhibits ovulation and stimulates mammary gland growth. Progesterone must be present for the continuation of pregnancy.

PROTEIN METABOLISM

Digestion and absorption

In order to be absorbed and utilized, dietary proteins must be hydrolyzed to their constituent amino acids. This function is performed by the proteolytic enzymes in the stomach and intestine. Gastric digestion of proteins is catalyzed by **pepsin**. This enzyme is an endopeptidase—that is, it hydrolyzes specific peptide bonds in a random manner, in the middle of the protein chains. The enzyme has a specificity for peptide bonds involving the carboxyl group of aromatic amino acids (e.g., phenylalanine, tyrosine, or tryptophan). Pepsin has a pH optimum of 2 to 3. This low pH is produced by the secretion of hydrochloric acid from the parietal cells of the stomach.

Pepsin in the stomach is produced from an inactive form, or zymogen, called pepsinogen. The latter is secreted by the chief cells of the gastric mucosa and converted to pepsin in the lumen of the stomach through the action of hydrochloric acid. Pepsin itself also catalyzes the transformation of pepsinogen to pepsin. The formation of pepsin is thus an autocatalytic process.

When the stomach contents are transferred to the small intestine, they are neutralized by the secretions of the pancreas. Pancreatic juice contains trypsinogen, chymotrypsinogen, and several zymogens in an alkaline medium. These inactive enzymes are converted to the active forms by the action of pepsin. The pancreatic enzymes catalyze further degradation of ingested proteins. Various mucosal peptidases finally convert the small peptides to amino acids.

Amino acids are absorbed from the small intestine into the portal circulation. This transport is an energy-requiring process, and different amino acids are absorbed at different rates.

The intracellular interconversions of amino acids include numerous reactions and thus present a highly complex and intricate system. One of the reasons for the multiplicity of reactions is that each amino acid has several specific pathways. However, several types of reactions are common to most amino acids. These will be considered first.

Transamination

A critical preliminary step in the catabolism of amino acids is their conversion to ketoacids. This may be accomplished by either transamination or deamination. The most general and predominant mechanism for nitrogen removal is transamination. One of the important reactions in the intermediary metabolism of amino acids is the reversible transfer of amino groups from glutamate to oxaloacetate (Fig. 3-34). The enzymes that catalyze these reactions are called **transaminases**. These enzymes are generally named according to the two amino acids involved in the transamination. Hence, the common name for the enzyme that catalyzes the reaction cited is **glutamate-aspartate transaminase**. The enzyme is also called glutamate-oxaloacetate transaminase. All the transaminases contain pyridoxal phosphate (Fig. 3-34) as a coenzyme. The latter is derived from the vitamin pyridoxine, or vitamin B_6.

All amino acids, except threonine, lysine, and proline, can undergo transamination with alpha-ketoglutarate (Fig. 3-34, equation 2). Since the reactions catalyzed by transaminases are freely reversible, they serve to form specific amino acids from the corresponding ketoacids. Liver cells have the enzymes required to synthesize all amino acids except glycine, lysine, proline, and threonine. Glutamate can function as the amino group donor in such syntheses. An example is the production of alanine from pyruvate (Fig. 3-34, equation 3). The enzyme for this reaction is **glutamate-alanine transaminase**. It may also be noted that transaminases function as a bridge between the metabolism of amino acids and glycolytic, as well as citric acid cycle, reactions.

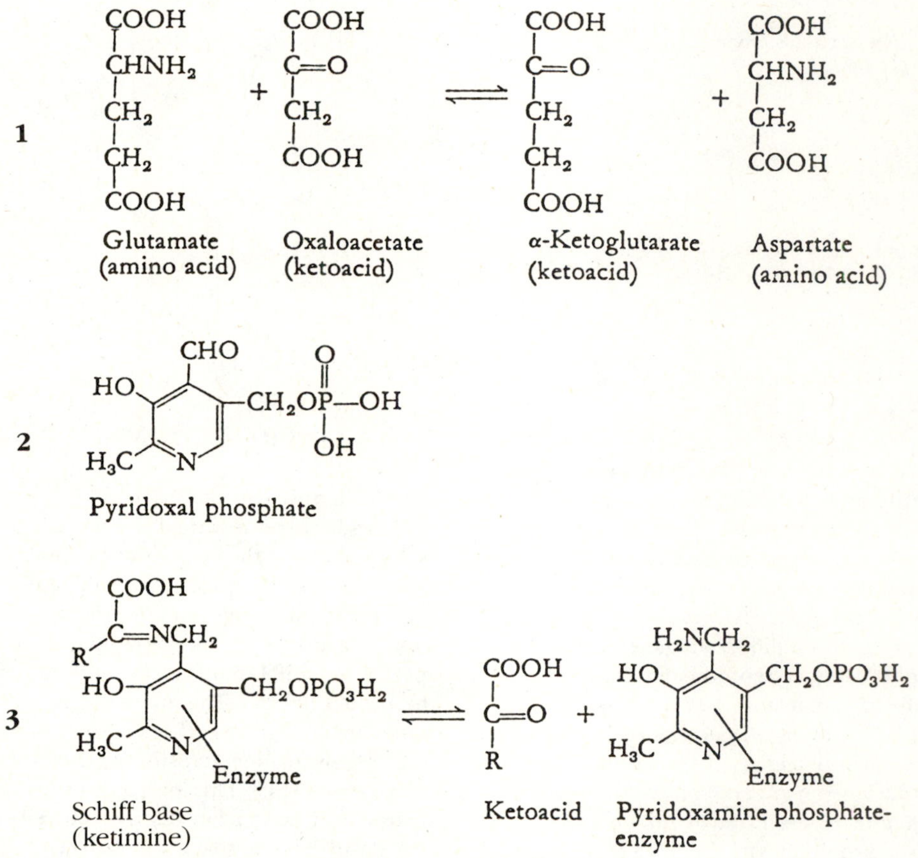

Figure 3-34. Transaminations.

Transaminases are important in clinical diagnoses because the blood levels of these enzymes are related to the functioning of cardiac muscle and liver. Glutamate-oxaloacetate transaminase and glutamate-alanine transaminase are of special clinical interest since these enzymes are lost from damaged myocardium and liver and, as a result, their concentrations in blood increases. Analyses for these enzymes thus have important diagnostic value.

Deamination

The amino group can also be removed from glutamate by oxidative deamination. This reaction is catalyzed by the NAD-linked enzyme **glutamate dehydrogenase** (Fig. 3-35, equation 1). As shown in the equation, this reaction provides a link in a process in which amino acids can be transformed to ketoacids by transamination with alpha-ketoglutarate. The glutamate that is formed in the transamination can be reoxidized by glutamate dehydrogenase to regenerate the alpha-ketoglutarate (Fig. 3-35, equation 2).

Conversely, the reverse reaction catalyzed by glutamate dehydrogenase can function to provide glutamate from alpha-ketoglutarate. The glutamate can then be utilized for synthesis of amino acids from corresponding ketoacids by transamination reactions.

Ammonia metabolism

Ammonia that is produced by the action of glutamate dehydrogenase (Fig. 3-35), as well as in various other reactions, is potentially lethal. It is removed as a result of three mechanisms. One of the reactions is the reversal of the glutamate dehydrogenase reaction. Another reaction that utilizes ammonia is the synthesis of glutamine from glutamate (Fig. 3-36, reaction 1). This involves the reaction of ammonia with glutamic acid and ATP. The enzyme for this reaction is **glutamine synthase**.

A third reaction that utilizes ammonia involves the formation of carbamoyl phosphate (Fig. 3-36, reaction 2). The latter compound is synthesized in the liver and, to a lesser extent, in other cells. Carbamoyl phosphate is an intermediate in the synthesis of urea.

Urea synthesis

Urea is the major end product of protein-nitrogen metabolism in humans. Carbamoyl phosphate reacts with ornithine to

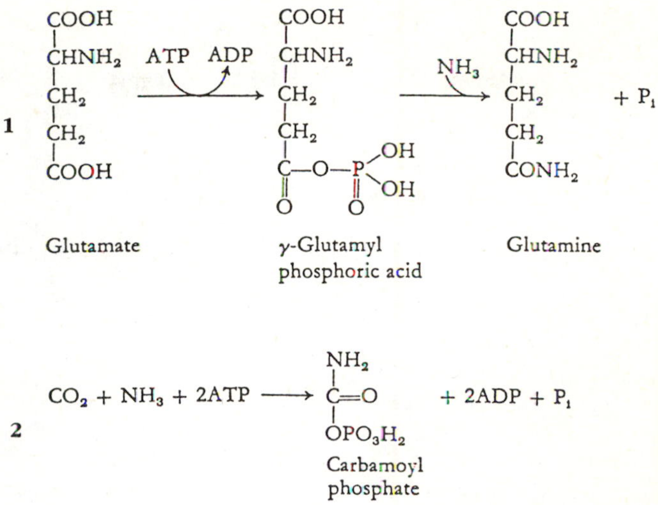

Figure 3-36. Reactions that utilize ammonia.

yield citrulline (Fig. 3-37, equation 1). Citrulline then condenses with aspartate to form argininosuccinate (Fig. 3-37, equation 2). Cleavage of argininosuccinate results in the formation of arginine and fumarate (Fig. 3-37, equation 3). Arginine is then hydrolyzed to yield urea and ornithine (Fig. 3-37, equation 4). This series of reactions constitutes a cyclic process called the **urea cycle** (Fig. 3-38).

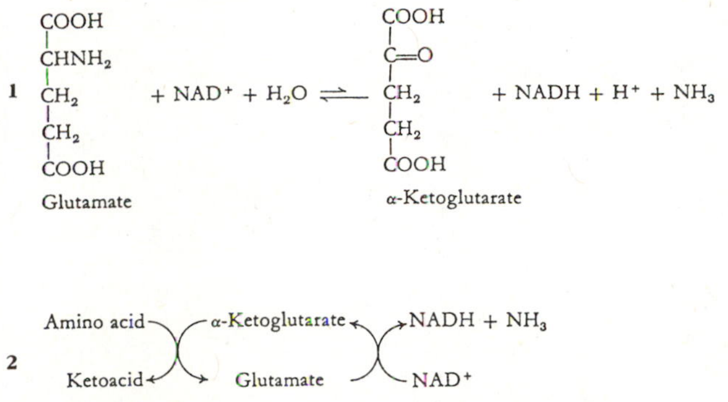

Catabolism of carbon chains from amino acids

The amino acids are convertible to either pyruvate, acetyl-CoA, or intermediates of the citric acid cycle. Thus transaminations from alanine, glutamate, and aspartate yield pyruvate, alpha-ketoglutarate, and oxaloacetate, respectively. Aspartate is converted to fumarate by the urea cycle. Only about 10% of the total human energy requirement is normally derived from proteins. When lipids or carbohydrates are restricted from the diet, greater amounts of protein are utilized for energy.

The principal degradative pathway of the carbon chains of amino acids involves their conversions to pyruvate or citric acid cycle metabolites, which can be oxidized to CO_2 and water. Additionally, these intermediates can be utilized for the synthesis of glucose or glycogen (gluconeogenesis). Such amino acids are termed **glucogenic**. Other amino acids that form acetoacetate or acetyl-CoA are called ketogenic. The specific amino acids in each category are shown in Table 3-3. The rationale for the classification may be understood by consideration of the pathways depicted in Figure 3-39.

Transmethylation

Certain amino acids can provide methyl groups for the synthesis of various intermediates. Such reactions are called **transmethylations**. The sources for the methyl groups are methionine and betaine. The latter is derived from choline as shown in Figure 3-40, reaction 1.

Methionine functions as a methyl donor by first reacting with ATP to form S-adenosylmethionine (Fig. 3-40, reaction 2). Methyl groups are transferred from S-adenosylmethionine to various acceptors (Fig. 3-41).

Figure 3-35. Activity of glutamate dehydrogenase.

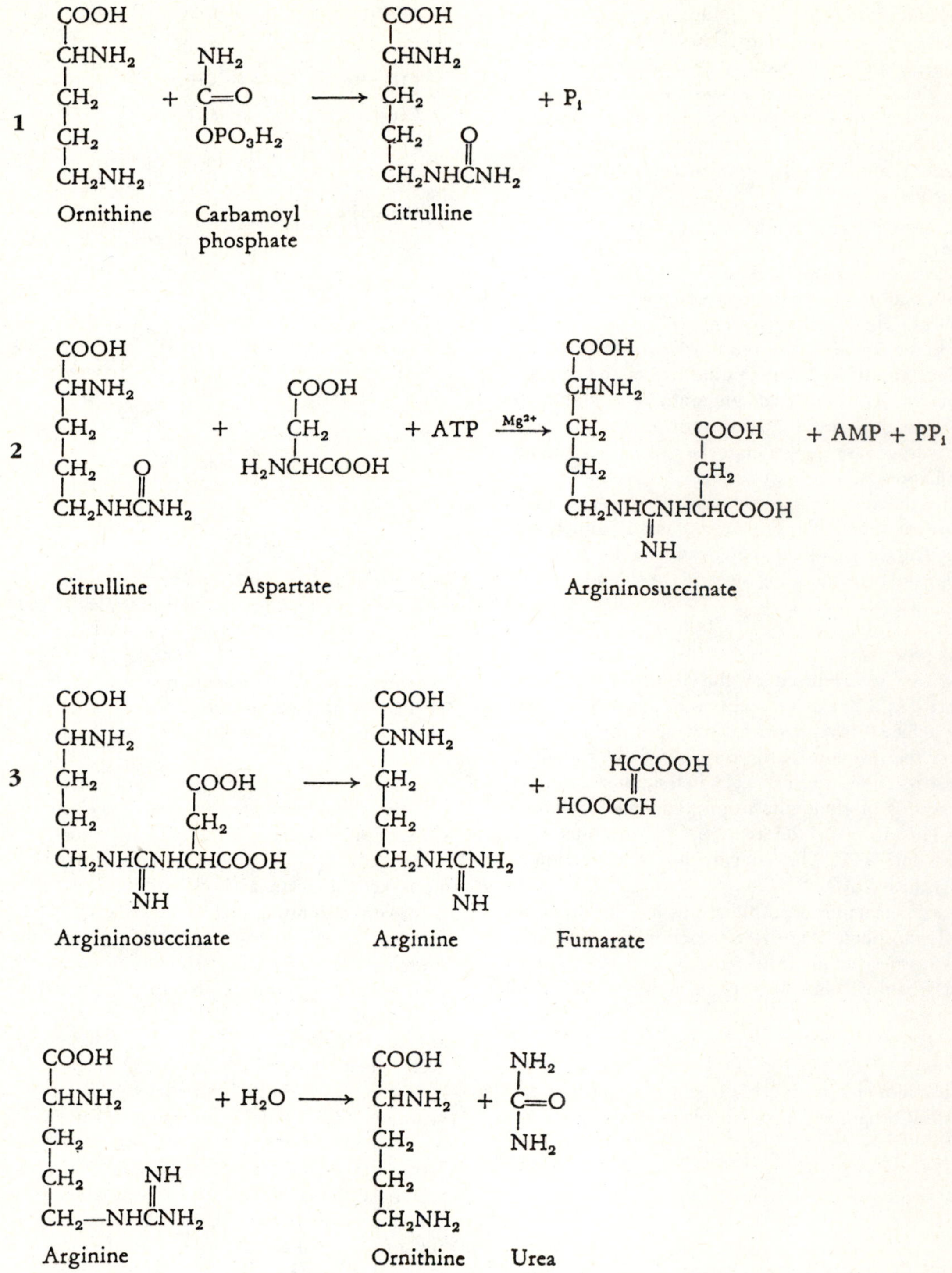

1

$$
\begin{array}{c}
\text{COOH} \\
\mid \\
\text{CHNH}_2 \\
\mid \\
\text{CH}_2 \\
\mid \\
\text{CH}_2 \\
\mid \\
\text{CH}_2\text{NH}_2
\end{array}
\quad + \quad
\begin{array}{c}
\text{NH}_2 \\
\mid \\
\text{C}=\text{O} \\
\mid \\
\text{OPO}_3\text{H}_2
\end{array}
\quad \longrightarrow \quad
\begin{array}{c}
\text{COOH} \\
\mid \\
\text{CHNH}_2 \\
\mid \\
\text{CH}_2 \\
\mid \quad\quad \text{O} \\
\text{CH}_2 \\
\mid \quad\quad \| \\
\text{CH}_2\text{NHCNH}_2
\end{array}
\quad + \text{ P}_i
$$

Ornithine   Carbamoyl   Citrulline
               phosphate

2

$$
\begin{array}{c}
\text{COOH} \\
\mid \\
\text{CHNH}_2 \\
\mid \\
\text{CH}_2 \\
\mid \\
\text{CH}_2 \quad \text{O} \\
\mid \quad\quad \| \\
\text{CH}_2\text{NHCNH}_2
\end{array}
\quad + \quad
\begin{array}{c}
\text{COOH} \\
\mid \\
\text{CH}_2 \\
\mid \\
\text{H}_2\text{NCHCOOH}
\end{array}
\quad + \text{ ATP } \xrightarrow{\text{Mg}^{2+}}
\begin{array}{c}
\text{COOH} \\
\mid \\
\text{CHNH}_2 \\
\mid \\
\text{CH}_2 \quad\quad \text{COOH} \\
\mid \quad\quad\quad \mid \\
\text{CH}_2 \quad\quad \text{CH}_2 \\
\mid \quad\quad\quad \mid \\
\text{CH}_2\text{NHCNHCHCOOH} \\
\quad\quad \| \\
\quad\quad \text{NH}
\end{array}
\quad + \text{ AMP} + \text{PP}_i
$$

Citrulline   Aspartate   Argininosuccinate

3

$$
\begin{array}{c}
\text{COOH} \\
\mid \\
\text{CHNH}_2 \\
\mid \\
\text{CH}_2 \quad\quad \text{COOH} \\
\mid \quad\quad\quad \mid \\
\text{CH}_2 \quad\quad \text{CH}_2 \\
\mid \quad\quad\quad \mid \\
\text{CH}_2\text{NHCNHCHCOOH} \\
\quad\quad \| \\
\quad\quad \text{NH}
\end{array}
\quad \longrightarrow \quad
\begin{array}{c}
\text{COOH} \\
\mid \\
\text{CNNH}_2 \\
\mid \\
\text{CH}_2 \\
\mid \\
\text{CH}_2 \\
\mid \\
\text{CH}_2\text{NHCNH}_2 \\
\quad\quad \| \\
\quad\quad \text{NH}
\end{array}
\quad + \quad
\begin{array}{c}
\text{HCCOOH} \\
\| \\
\text{HOOCCH}
\end{array}
$$

Argininosuccinate   Arginine   Fumarate

4

$$
\begin{array}{c}
\text{COOH} \\
\mid \\
\text{CHNH}_2 \\
\mid \\
\text{CH}_2 \\
\mid \quad\quad \text{NH} \\
\text{CH}_2 \quad \| \\
\mid \\
\text{CH}_2\text{—NHCNH}_2
\end{array}
\quad + \text{ H}_2\text{O} \longrightarrow
\begin{array}{c}
\text{COOH} \\
\mid \\
\text{CHNH}_2 \\
\mid \\
\text{CH}_2 \\
\mid \\
\text{CH}_2 \\
\mid \\
\text{CH}_2\text{NH}_2
\end{array}
\quad + \quad
\begin{array}{c}
\text{NH}_2 \\
\mid \\
\text{C}=\text{O} \\
\mid \\
\text{NH}_2
\end{array}
$$

Arginine   Ornithine   Urea

Figure 3-37. Reactions of the urea cycle.

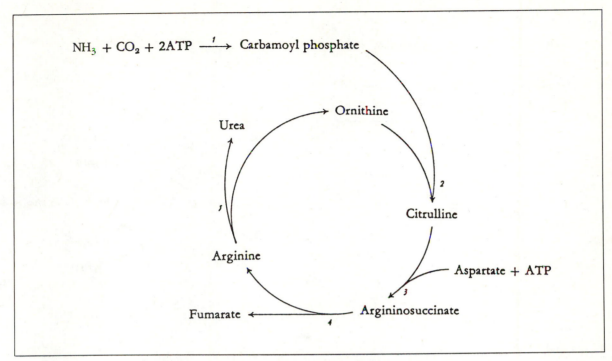

$$NH_3 + CO_2 + 2ATP \xrightarrow{\ 1\ } Carbamoyl\ phosphate$$

Figure 3-38.   Urea cycle. The enzymes for the reactions are 1, carbamoylphosphate synthetase; 2, ornithine transcarbamoylase; 3, arginosuccinate synthetase; 4, argininosuccinate lyase; 5, arginase.

Creatine

Creatine is required for muscle metabolism because it serves in the storage of energy. The first step in the synthesis of creatine is a reaction between glycine and arginine to yield ornithine and guanidinoacetic acid (Fig. 3-42, reaction 1). This reaction is common for the kidneys, liver, and pancreas. A methyl group is then transferred from methionine (via S-adenosylmethionine) to guanidinoacetic acid, providing creatine (see Fig. 3-41).

Creatine can be converted to phosphocreatine by a reaction with ATP and the enzyme **creatine kinase** (Fig. 3-42, reaction 2). Phosphocreatine is utilized for energy storage in muscle since it transfers its phosphate to ADP, forming ATP. Its availability allows for the rapid production of ATP and utilization of the latter for muscle contraction. Phosphocreatine has limited stability; it undergoes hydrolysis to form creatinine (Fig. 3-42, reaction 3). The latter compound diffuses from the muscle into the bloodstream and is excreted in the urine.

Folic acid and single carbon transfers

Certain amino acids (e.g., serine, glycine, histidine, tryptophan) provide single carbon units (other than methyl groups) for synthesis of various metabolic intermediates. The carbon carrier for such processes is tetrahydrofolic acid (Fig. 3-43), which is derived from the vitamin **folic acid**. One example in which tetrahydrofolic acid functions as an acceptor of a carbon is shown in Figure 3-44. In this reaction, serine serves as the donor of the one-carbon unit. This carbon can then be transferred from the tetrahydrofolic acid to provide for the synthesis of other products, for example, purine nucleotides.

Essential and nonessential amino acids

As seen from some of the reactions described above, many amino acids can be synthesized from intermediates of the glycolytic pathway or the citric acid cycle. Such amino acids are called **nonessential**—that is, they do not have to be included in the diet. In contrast, **essential amino acids** cannot be synthesized by the animal organism but must be included in the ingested proteins. Figure 3-45 provides a tabulation of the two categories of amino acids.

Metabolism of phenylalanine and tyrosine

Phenylalanine is converted in the liver to tyrosine by the enzyme **phenylalanine hydroxylase**. In addition, some phenylalanine undergoes transamination with alpha-ketoglutarate to yield phenylpyruvate and phenyllactate, as shown in Figure 3-45.

Normally, urine contains small amounts of phenylpyruvate and phenyllactate. In the inborn metabolic defect called **phenylketonuria**, the enzyme phenylalanine hydroxylase is missing or defective and the principal pathway for phenylalanine is blocked. In this abnormality, the serum level of phenylalanine is elevated and considerable amounts of the amino acid, as well as phenylpyruvate and phenyllactate, are excreted in the urine. Phenylketonuria is generally linked to mental retardation. The disease is so named because of the high concentrations of phenylpyruvate in the urine. Mental impairment can be prevented if the defect is recognized in early infancy and phenylalanine is restricted from the diet.

The steps in the metabolism of tyrosine are shown in Figure 3-46 (reactions 1 and 2). The p-hydroxyphenylpyruvate is then transformed by an ascorbic acid-requiring enzyme called p-

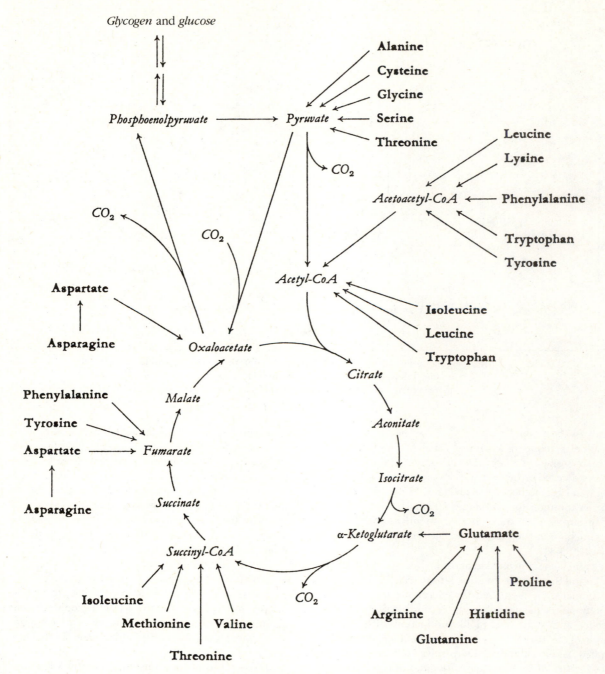

Figure 3-39. Pyruvate, acetate, and citric acid cycle components (italics) as intermediates in the metabolism of amino acids (boldface). Phosphoenolpyruvate is shown in order to indicate the pathway to glucose and glycogen (gluconeogenesis). Note that some amino acids lead into more than one site.

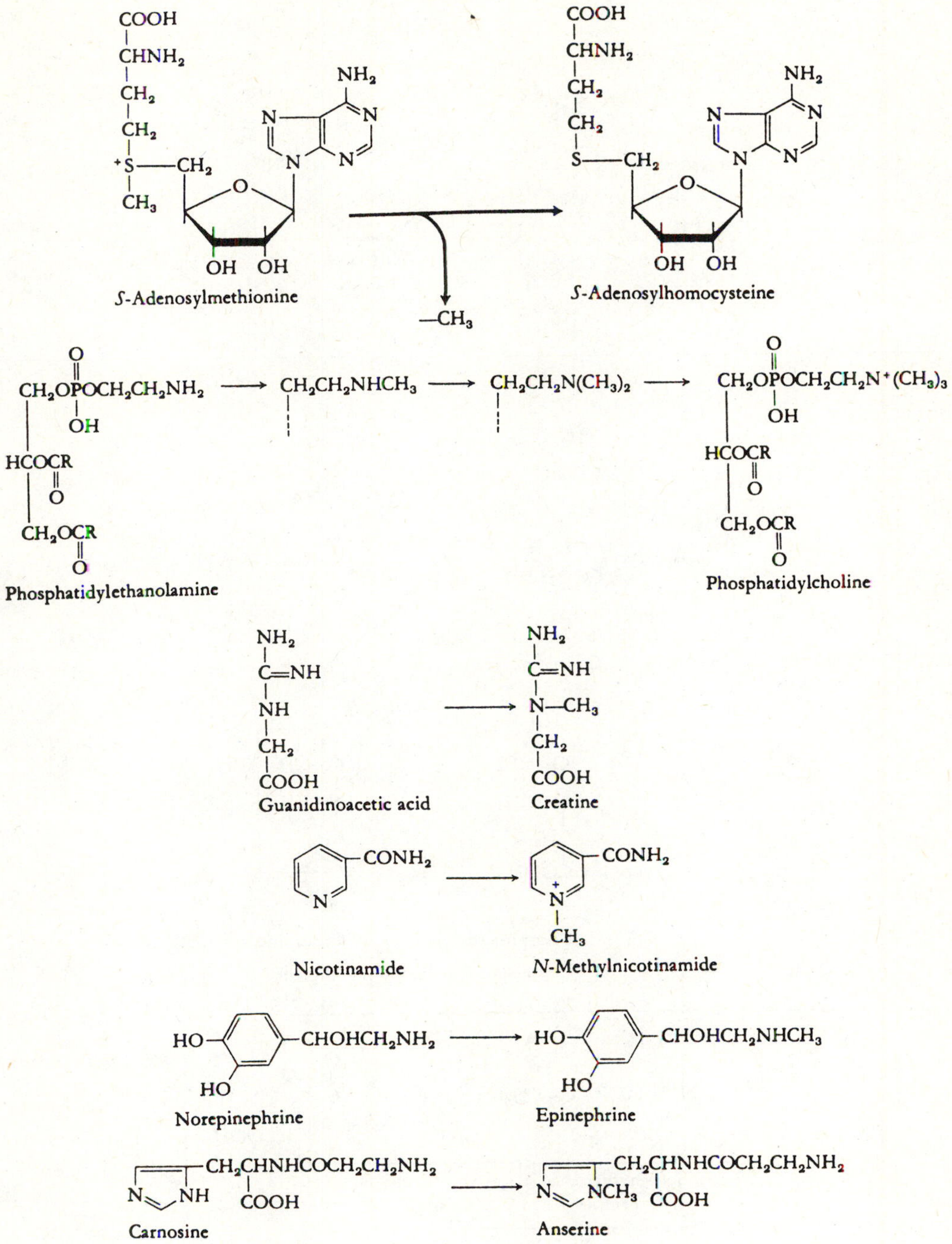

Figure 3-40. Methyl donors.

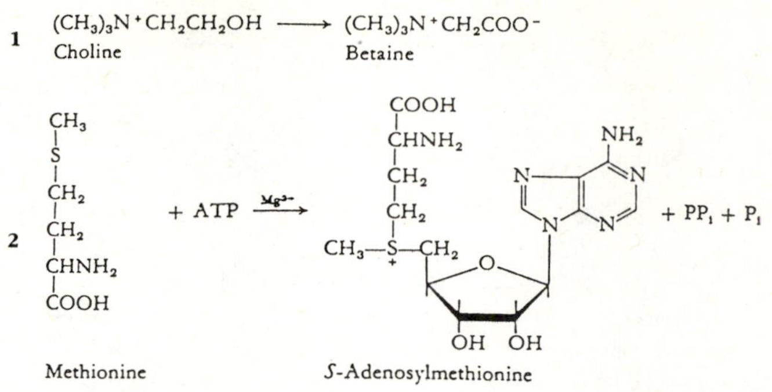

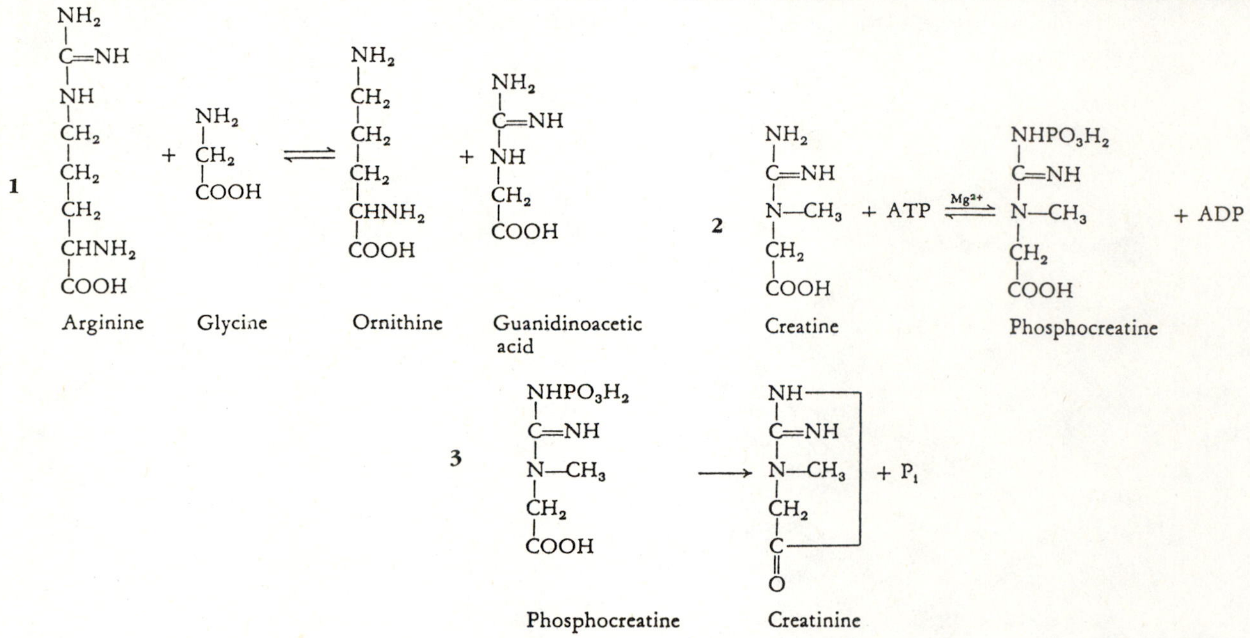

1    $(CH_3)_3N^+CH_2CH_2OH \longrightarrow (CH_3)_3N^+CH_2COO^-$
      Choline   Betaine

2   Methionine   + ATP $\xrightarrow{Mg^{2+}}$ S-Adenosylmethionine $+ PP_i + P_i$

1   Arginine   +   Glycine $\rightleftharpoons$ Ornithine   +   Guanidinoacetic
                                                                     acid

2   Creatine   + ATP $\xrightarrow{Mg^{2+}}$ Phosphocreatine   + ADP

3   Phosphocreatine $\longrightarrow$ Creatinine $+ P_i$

Figure 3-42.   Creatine metabolism.

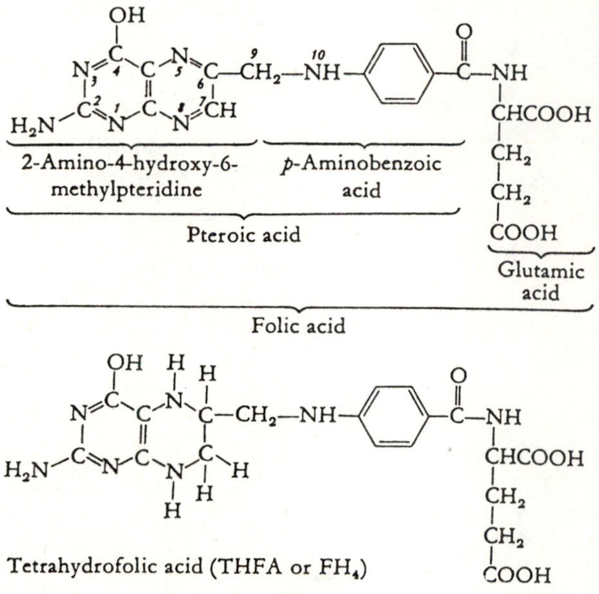

2-Amino-4-hydroxy-6-
methylpteridine   p-Aminobenzoic
                             acid
Pteroic acid   Glutamic
                                            acid
Folic acid

Tetrahydrofolic acid (THFA or FH_4)

Figure 3-43.   Structures of folate.

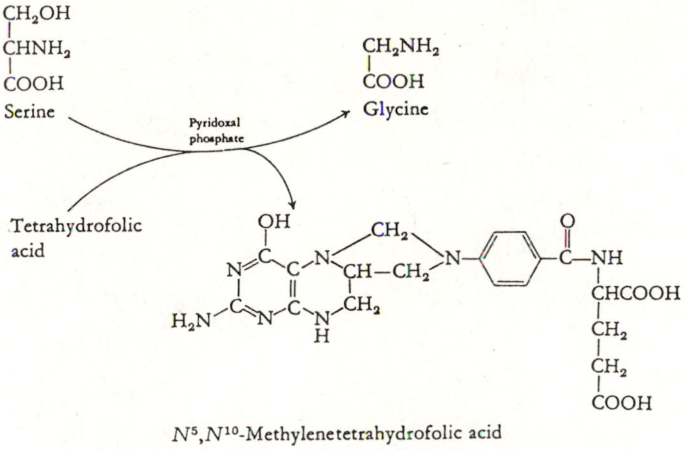

Figure 3-44. Transfer of single carbon unit to folic acid.

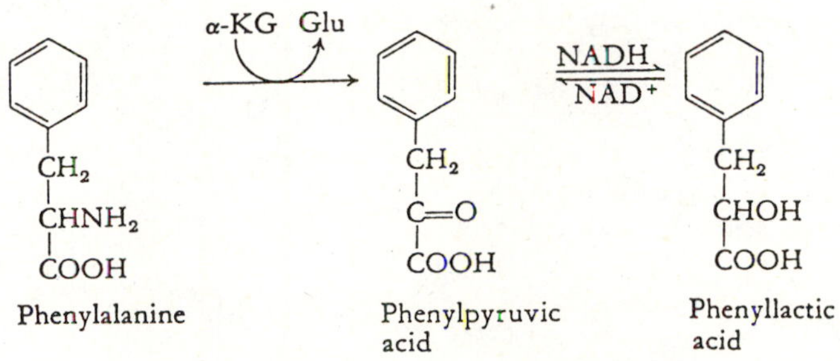

Figure 3-45. Reactions of phenylalanine.

hydroxyphenylpyruvate oxidase to p-hydroxyphenyllactate. Absence of this enzyme has been implicated as the cause of tyrosinemia I. Another enzyme defect is involved in the disease alkaptonuria. This involves the absence of the enzyme that oxidizes homogentisic acid.

Another route for tyrosine metabolism is the reaction shown in Figure 3-47. The product dopa quinone is then transformed by a series of steps to form the pigment melanin, which determines skin colorations.

In the adrenal medulla, tyrosine is converted to epinephrine as shown in Figure 3-48, equation 1. Tyrosine is also the precursor for the synthesis of triiodothyronine and thryroxine (Fig. 3-49, structures 2 and 3). Both of these thyroid hormones are stored by thyroglobulin in the thyroid gland.

Porphyrin synthesis

The central structure of a porphyrin is shown in Figure 3-49. Individual porphyrins differ from each other with respect to groups attached on the pyrrole units. Porphyrin structures occur as prosthetic groups in a number of proteins. These include cytochromes, hemoglobin, myoglobin, and various oxidase enzymes. The nitrogens in porphyrins form complexes with iron or other metals. The structure of heme, the porphyrin in hemoglobin, is shown in Figure 3-49.

Porphyrins are synthesized from glycine and succinyl-CoA (Fig. 3-50). Porphobilinogen formed in the second reaction condenses to produce the tetrapyrrole or porphyrin ring system, and they require distribution of side chains.

NUCLEOTIDE METABOLISM

PURINE BIOSYNTHESIS

Both purine and pyrimidine biosynthesis require 5'-phosphoribosyl-1-pyrophosphate (PRPP) as a key intermediate. PRPP is synthesized by the pyrophosphorylation of ribose 5-phosphate, which is derived from the pentose phosphate pathway (Fig. 3-51).

The initial step in the purine biosynthetic pathway is the condensation of PRPP with glutamine in a reaction that is catalyzed by the enzyme **PRPP aminotransferase** (Fig. 3-52). This reaction is irreversible and is the committed step in purine biosynthesis. It is under feedback regulation by any of the adenosine or guanosine phosphates that are the end products of the biosynthetic pathway.

The subsequent reactions in the pathway to inosinate (IMP) are shown in Figure 3-52. They involve the stepwise addition of carbon, oxygen, and nitrogen atoms to the purine ring from

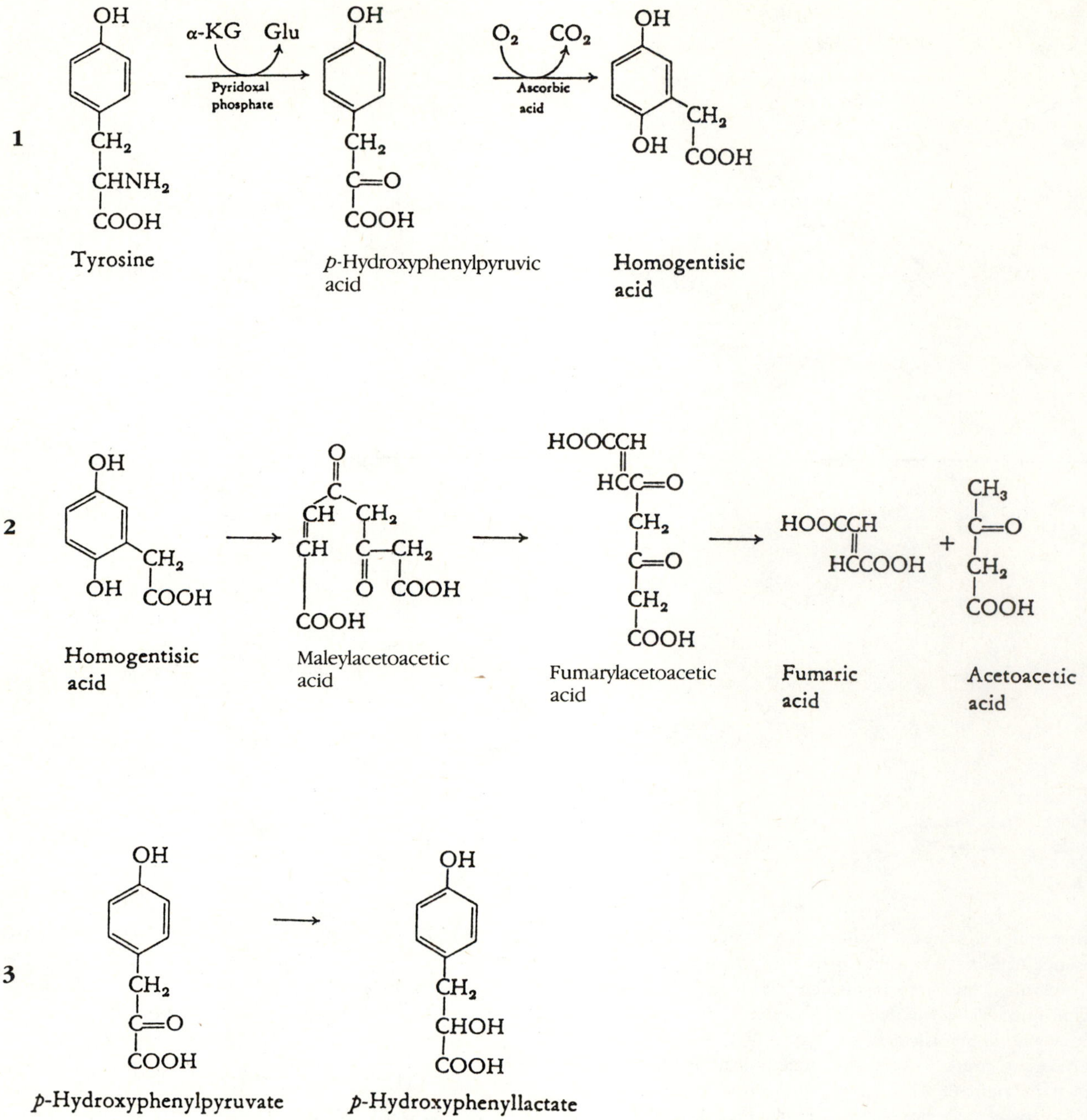

Figure 3-46.   Metabolism of tyrosine.

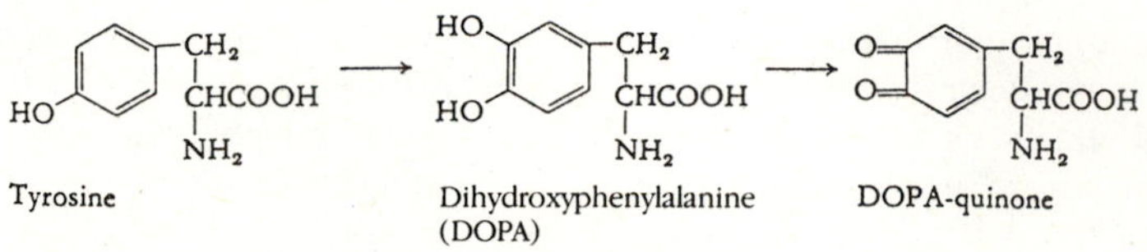

Figure 3-47.   Formation of dopa from tyrosine.

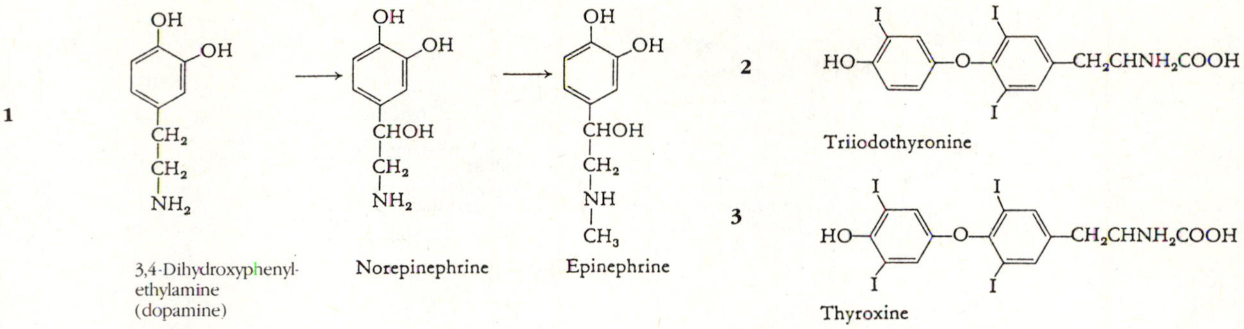

Figure 3-48. Synthesis of epinephrine and thyroxine.

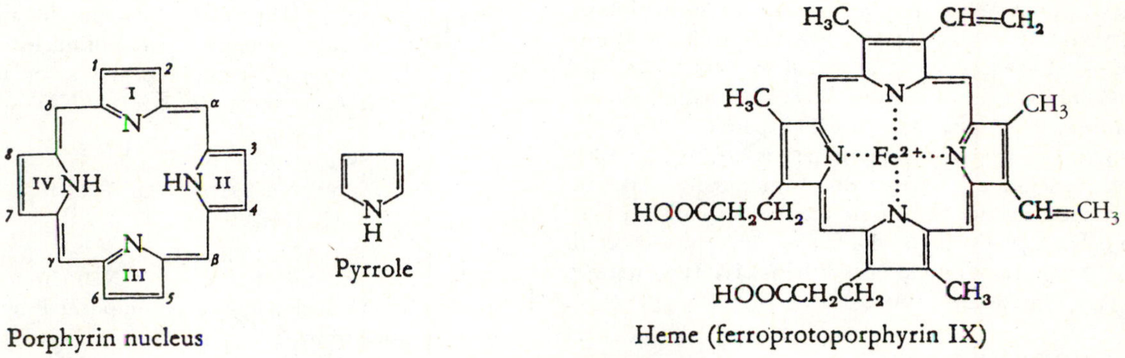

Figure 3-49. Porphyrin structures.

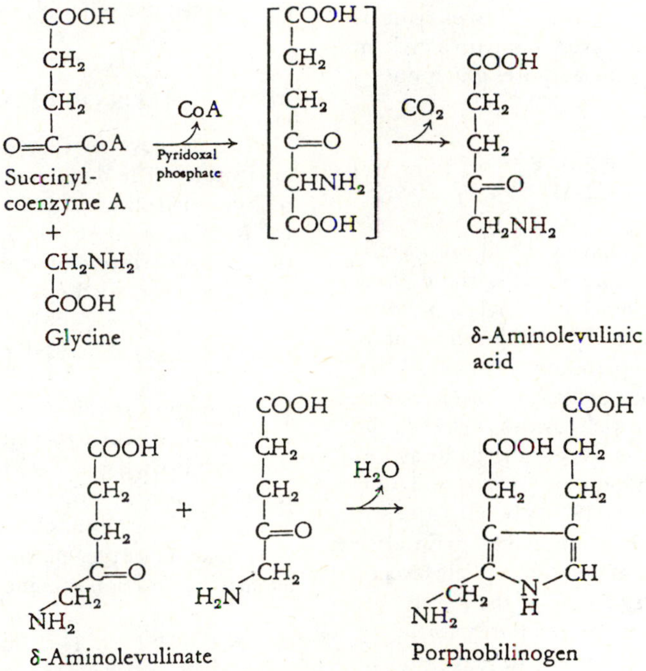

Figure 3-50. First steps in the synthesis of porphyrins.

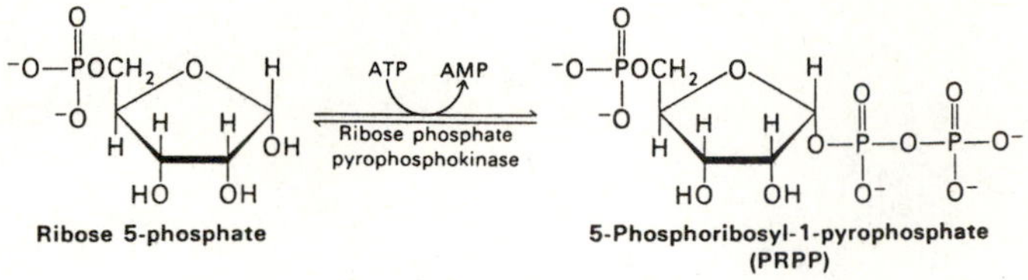

Figure 3-51. Formation of phosphoribosylpyrophosphate.

smaller precursor compounds. The intermediates formed in this process have no other role in metabolism. It is important to note the close interrelationship between amino acid and purine metabolism as exemplified by the requirements for glutamine, glycine, and aspartic acid as precursors for IMP synthesis.

IMP is not itself the end product of de novo purine biosynthesis but rather an intermediate to the formation of both AMP and GMP (Fig. 3-53). In one branch, IMP is oxidized to xanthylate (XMP), which is aminated to yield GMP. The oxidation is inhibited by the end product GMP. In the other leg of the pathway, IMP is condensed with aspartate to produce adenylosuccinate, from which fumarate is cleaved to leave AMP. The condensation step is feedback inhibited by AMP. In addition to this feedback regulation, the synthesis of GMP and AMP are balanced by virtue of the fact that the conversion of IMP to GMP requires ATP and the synthesis of AMP from IMP requires GTP (Fig. 3-53).

PYRIMIDINE BIOSYNTHESIS

The first step in pyrimidine biosynthesis is the condensation of carbamoyl phosphate with aspartate to yield carbamoyl aspartate (Fig. 3-54). This reaction is catalyzed by the enzyme aspartate transcarbamoylase (ATCase). The carbamoyl phosphate precursor is produced in a reaction catalyzed by carbamoyl phosphate synthetase (CPSase). This enzyme is distinct from a similar one that is involved in the urea cycle in that the former enzyme is cytoplasmic and uses glutamine as the amino-group donor.

$$\text{Glutamine} + \text{HCO}_3^- + 2\,\text{ATP} \rightleftharpoons$$
$$\text{glutamate} + \text{H}_2\text{N-CO-P} + 2\,\text{ADP} + 2\,\text{P}_i$$

The next step is ring closure catalyzed by dihydroorotase to produce dihydroorotic acid. In animal cells, these three enzyme activities appear to be contained in a single multifunctional enzyme. These initial reactions of pyrimidine biosynthesis are the committed steps of the pathway.

The three subsequent steps are oxidation, condensation with PRPP, and decarboxylation to yield uridylate (UMP), the initial pyrimidine nucleotide product of the pathway. In animals, UMP is a feedback inhibitor of CPSase and thus regulates the activity of the pathway. UMP may be subsequently converted to UTP (see below). The remaining pyrimidine nucleotide, cytidine, is synthesized at the triphosphate level by amination of UTP to CTP. The regulation of the pyrimidine biosynthetic pathway in bacteria is quite different from the process in animals. Bacterial ATCase is an allosteric enzyme that is subject to negative feedback regulation by CTP. Thus, in

bacteria, CTP rather than UMP is the regulatory end product of pyrimidine biosynthesis.

BIOSYNTHESIS OF NUCLEOSIDE TRIPHOSPHATES

The products of the de novo pathways are nucleoside monophosphates (NMP), but these compounds are essentially only intermediates for the production of nucleoside triphosphates (NTP), which are the precursors for nucleic acid biosynthesis. The conversion of NMP to NTP occurs in two steps:

$$\text{NMP} + \text{ATP} \rightleftharpoons \text{NDP} + \text{ADP}$$
$$\text{NDP} + \text{ATP} \rightleftharpoons \text{NTP} + \text{ADP}$$

Synthesis of nucleoside diphosphates (NDP) from their corresponding monophosphates is accomplished by phosphate group transfer from ATP. The reaction is catalyzed by base-specific kinases.

The fate of NDP is ultimately conversion to NTP in a second reaction, which is catalyzed by the enzyme **nucleoside diphosphate kinase**. This enzyme is completely nonspecific, with no preference for either the base or sugar moiety of the NDP. The phosphate donor in this case is invariably ATP, although the enzyme can use other NTPs for this purpose.

BIOSYNTHESIS OF DEOXYRIBONUCLEOTIDES

The de novo biosynthetic pathways produce only ribonucleotides. The deoxyribonucleotides are synthesized from the ribonucleotides by reduction of the hydroxyl group at the C2′ position of ribose to hydrogen. The reaction is catalyzed by the enzyme **ribonucleoside diphosphate reductase**. The conversion is carried out only at the level of NDP:

$$\text{NDP} \rightleftharpoons \text{dNDP}$$

The reduction requires an additional protein, **thioredoxin**, which is the reducing agent for this reaction. In the process, thioredoxin itself is oxidized and must be converted back to the reduced form in order for subsequent dNDP synthesis to occur. This is accomplished through the action of **thioredoxin reductase**. This latter enzyme employs NADPH as the reducing agent. The reaction scheme may be summarized as follows:

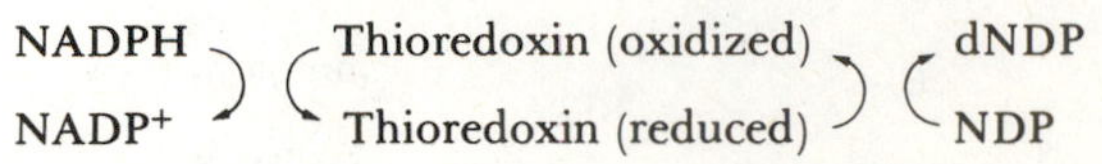

NADPH   Thioredoxin (oxidized)   dNDP

NADP⁺   Thioredoxin (reduced)   NDP

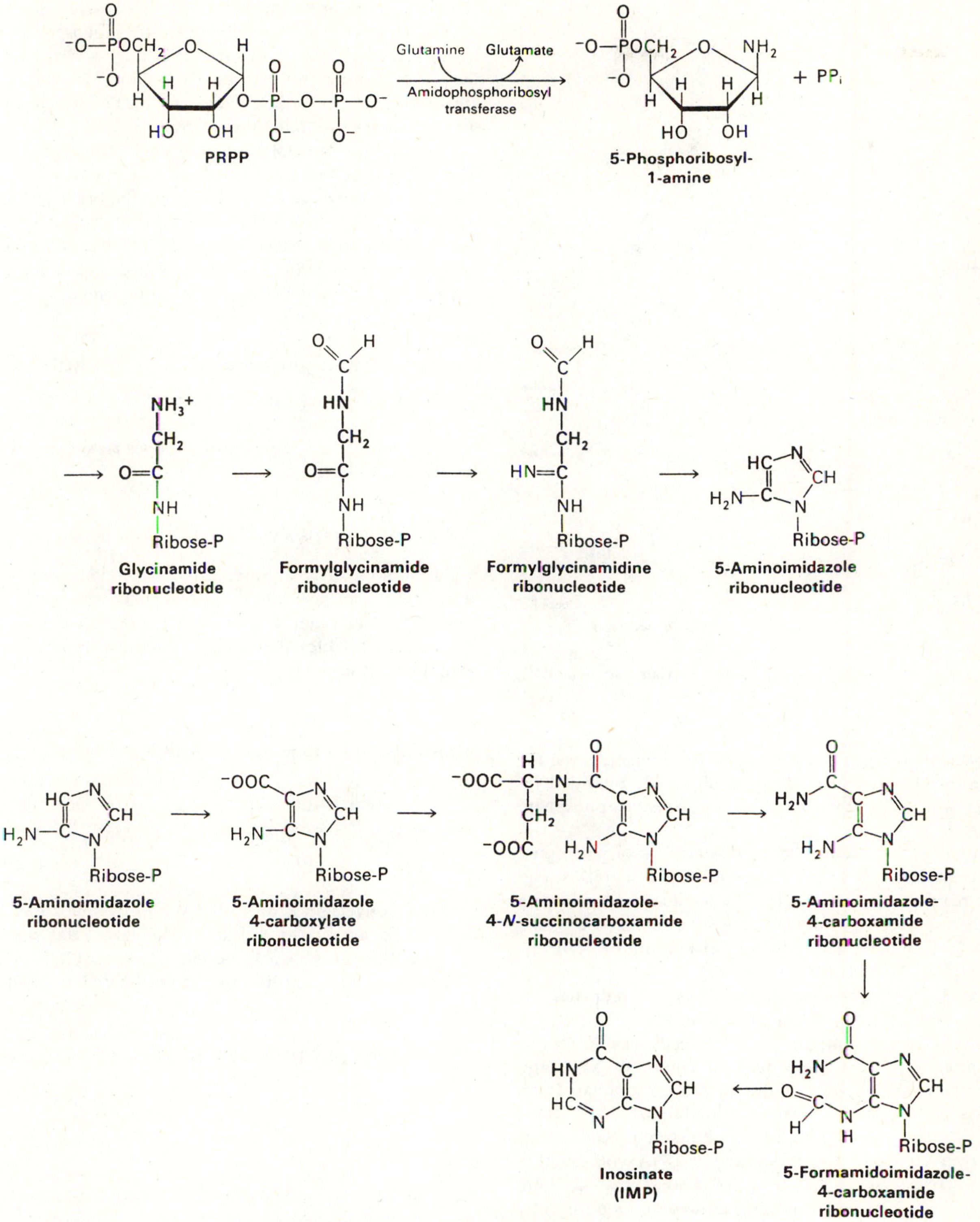

Figure 3-52.   Pathway for de novo purine biosynthesis.

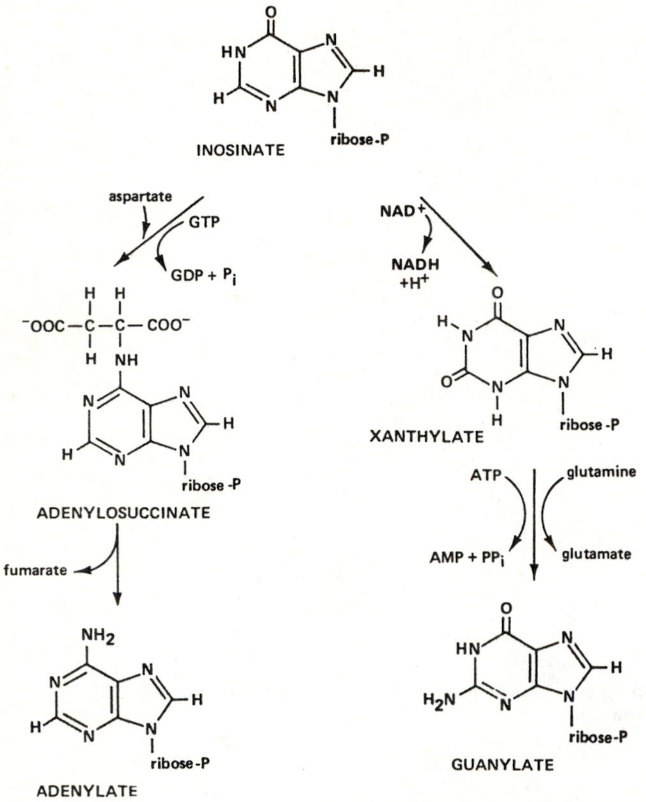

Figure 3-53. Conversion of inosinate to adenylate and guanylate.

An important point to note here is that the reducing power for deoxyribonucleotide biosynthesis is ultimately provided by NADPH, which is produced primarily in the pentose phosphate pathway.

Ribonucleoside diphosphate reductase is a very complex allosteric enzyme that catalyzes the reduction of all NDPs. The various reactions are under exquisite feedback control by its products and may be summarized as follows (Fig. 3-55):

1. ATP stimulates the reduction of pyrimidine NDPs to yield dCTP and TTP.
2. As TTP accumulates, it stimulates the reduction of purine NDPs to yield dATP and dGTP.
3. At high concentrations, dATP is a feedback inhibitor of the enzyme. Thus, when the production of dNTPs by the enzyme exceeds the requirements of cellular DNA synthesis, further reduction is inhibited.

In addition to preventing the unnecessary production of dNTPs over and above what is required for DNA synthesis, this complex regulatory mechanism also assures that all four dNTPs will be produced in roughly equivalent amounts.

THYMIDYLATE SYNTHESIS

The only de novo pathway for the synthesis of thymidylate (TMP) is by methylation of dUMP. This requires a series of steps beginning with the production of UMP by the pyrimidine biosynthetic pathway.

$$UMP \rightarrow UDP \rightarrow dUDP \rightarrow dUTP \rightarrow dUMP$$

These reactions are mediated by uridylate kinase, ribonucleoside diphosphate reductase, ribonucleoside diphosphate kinase, and dUTP diphosphohydrolase (dUTPase), respectively. The latter reaction not only provides dUMP for TMP synthesis but also prevents the accumulation of dUTP, which can be improperly incorporated into DNA.

Methylation of dUMP at C-5 to yield TMP is catalyzed by thymidylate synthetase. The reaction requires methylenetetrahydrofolate as a cofactor (methyl group donor). The resultant dihydrofolate must be reduced to tetrahydrofolate for subsequent methylation reactions to occur. This is accomplished through the action of the enzyme dihydrofolate reductase, which employs NADPH as the reducing agent. The overall scheme can be summarized as

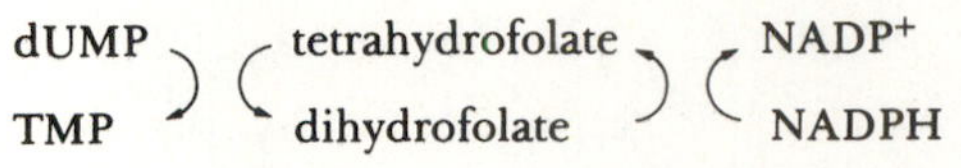

$$\begin{array}{l} dUMP \\ TMP \end{array} \Big) \Big(\begin{array}{l} tetrahydrofolate \\ dihydrofolate \end{array} \Big) \Big(\begin{array}{l} NADP^+ \\ NADPH \end{array}$$

Thymidylate can also be produced via a **salvage pathway**, as discussed below.

SALVAGE PATHWAYS

In addition to the de novo nucleotide biosynthetic pathways, most cells also have salvage pathways. These are a series of reactions that facilitate the conversion of bases and nucleosides (which are available either in the diet or by virtue of nucleic acid degradation) to nucleotides.

Conversion of a base to a nucleotide (one step)

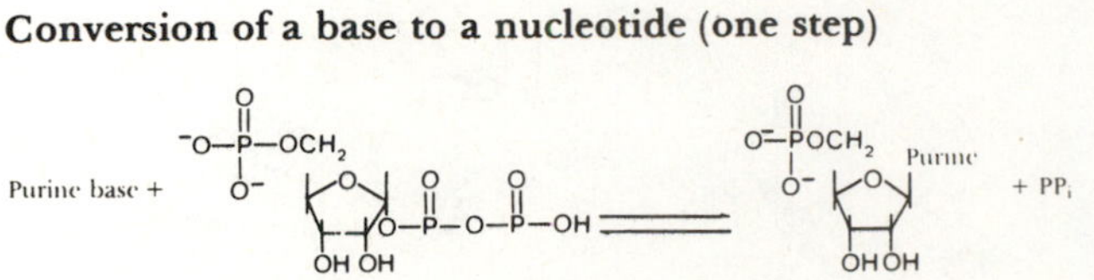

This conversion is only observed for purine bases. There are two known reactions of this type that are catalyzed by the enzymes adenine phosphoribosyltransferase (APRT) and hypoxanthine-guanine phosphoribosyltransferase (HGPRT).

Conversion of a base to a nucleoside (two steps)

$$Base + ribose\text{-}1\text{-}P \rightarrow Nucleoside\ (+\ P_i) \rightarrow Nucleotide$$

$$\overset{\displaystyle \frown}{ATP\quad ADP}$$

The first step in the conversion is catalyzed by nucleoside phosphorylase. There are three known enzymes of this class—specific for uridine, thymidine, or any purine. The second step is catalyzed by nucleoside-specific kinases.

Salvage pathways play an important role in TMP production in many cell types. They are especially prominent in rapidly proliferating cells such as intestinal mucosa and malignant tissue. Purine salvage is crucial in CNS tissue, as evidenced by the abnormalities resulting from a deficiency in HGPRT (see discussion below).

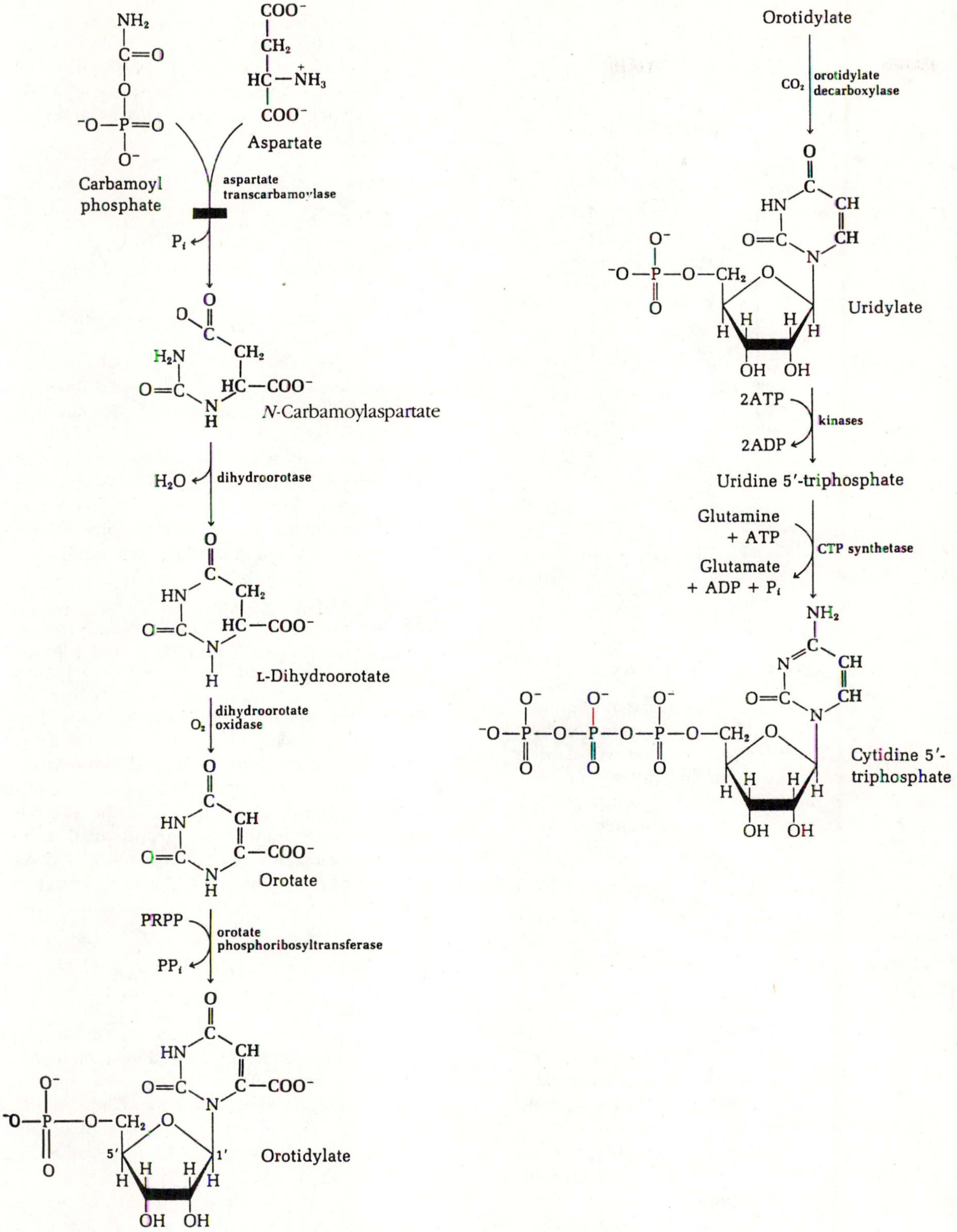

Figure 3-54. Pathway for pyrimidine biosynthesis.

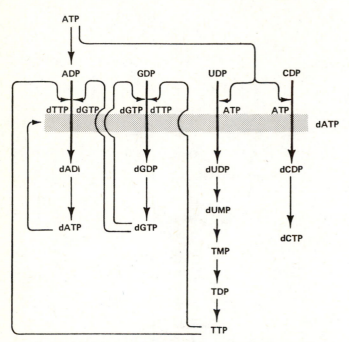

Figure 3-55. Regulation of deoxyribonucleotide biosynthesis by ribonucleotide reductase.

INHIBITORS OF NUCLEOTIDE SYNTHESIS

Since the synthesis of RNA and DNA is crucial to cellular viability, any block in the availability of precursors for these processes will result in cell death. Furthermore, there is a direct correlation between cell proliferation and the rate of DNA synthesis. This provides the opportunity to specifically block the growth of rapidly proliferating cells without affecting those that are dividing only very slowly or not at all. For these reasons, the nucleotide biosynthetic pathways have been a major target for antiproliferative and antibiotic drugs.

Several antimetabolites have their sites of action in the de novo purine biosynthetic pathway (Fig. 3-56). Any reaction that utilizes glutamine as an amino group donor (steps 1 and 4, Fig. 3-52) can be inhibited by the glutamine analogue **azaserine**. Reactions that require folic acid derivatives as carbon or methyl group donors (steps 3 and 9) will be blocked by a variety of folic acid antagonists. These include **methotrexate**, which is a structural analogue of folic acid. Folic acid is also the target of sulfa drugs, such as **sulfanilamide**. Many bacteria normally synthesize folic acid and utilize *p*-aminobenzoic acid (PABA) as a precursor in this process. Sulfanilamide, which is a structural analogue of PABA, inhibits folic acid production and thereby blocks purine biosynthesis. Sulfa drugs are thus potent antibiotics. Humans are not affected by these compounds because they depend on exogenous, preformed folic acid for their metabolism.

Methotrexate is also a potent inhibitor of dihydrofolate reductase and thus blocks the synthesis of TMP. Another drug that acts to prevent TMP production is fluorouracil. This is converted to fluorouridine monophosphate via the salvage pathway. The latter compound reacts covalently with TMP synthetase, resulting in irreversible inhibition of the enzyme and a shutdown of TMP synthesis. Both methotrexate and fluorouracil are employed in chemotherapy of a wide variety of malignancies. They will have a pronounced effect on the viability of cancerous cells because of the high DNA synthetic activity of these cells. However, they are also toxic to other normal cells that proliferate rapidly, such as bone marrow and intestinal mucosa.

CATABOLISM OF PURINES

Nucleic acids are degraded to yield purine nucleotides. The various reactions leading to the production of uric acid, the degradative end product of purine catabolism, are shown in Figure 3-57.

AMP can be deaminated to IMP by the action of adenylate deaminase, and IMP is dephosphorylated to inosine by the action of a phosphatase. Alternatively, AMP can be converted to adenosine and then deaminated by **adenosine deaminase**. The same phosphatase enzyme also transforms GMP to guanosine. Inosine and guanosine are further degraded to their component bases, hypoxanthine and guanine, in a reaction catalyzed by purine nucleoside phosphorylase. Both of these bases are converted to xanthine—guanine by deamination and hypoxanthine via oxidation. Xanthine is then oxidized to uric acid by the action of **xanthine oxidase**. It is interesting to note that the oxidation of both hypoxanthine and xanthine is catalyzed by xanthine oxidase.

Uric acid is produced primarily in liver and intestinal mucosa. Under normal circumstances, uric acid production and excretion are balanced. The average plasma uric acid level in normal males is 5 mg/100 ml, whereas that for normal females is 4.1 mg/100 ml. Approximately 500 mg of uric acid is excreted daily in the urine.

At physiological pH, uric acid is present in plasma as its sodium salt. Sodium urate has limited solubility in plasma (6.4 mg/100 ml) and tends to precipitate when the plasma levels are elevated. This often results in the deposition of sodium urate crystals in the joints. A variety of metabolic abnormalities can lead to elevated plasma urate levels, a condition referred to as **hyperuricemia**. Several of these will be discussed in the next section.

DISEASES OF NUCLEOTIDE METABOLISM

Orotic aciduria

Orotic aciduria is a rare inborn error of pyrimidine biosynthesis characterized by an accumulation of orotic acid, which is excreted in the urine. This is caused by an absence of both orotate phosphoribosyltransferase and the decarboxylase. The condition can be treated by administration of uridine, the end product of the de novo pyrimidine biosynthetic pathway.

Gout

Gout is a disease that manifests itself by hyperuricemia and severe joint pain (and possible disfigurement in extreme cases). Primary gout has a genetic component, but it can be caused by a variety of metabolic defects that result in overproduction of urate. However, any disorder that increases plasma urate levels will cause similar symptoms. Thus, patients with defects in renal excretion of urate or renal failure can also exhibit hyperuricemia. Such a situation can also arise during chemotherapy of proliferative diseases such as leukemia because of the increased levels of nucleic acid turnover.

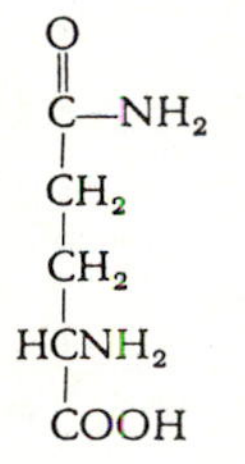

O
‖
C—NH₂
|
CH₂
|
CH₂
|
HCNH₂
|
COOH

L-Glutamine

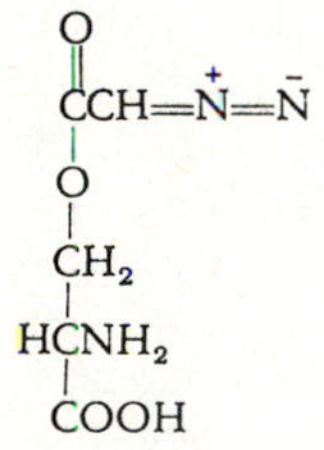

O
‖
CCH=N⁺=N̄
|
O
|
CH₂
|
HCNH₂
|
COOH

Azaserine

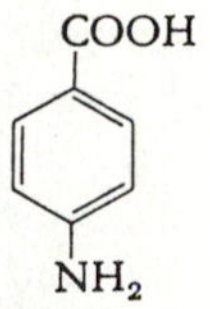

COOH

NH₂

p-Aminobenzoic acid

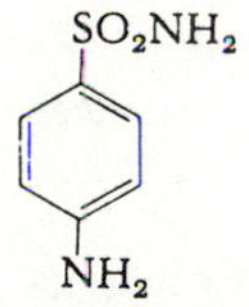

SO₂NH₂

NH₂

Sulfanilamide

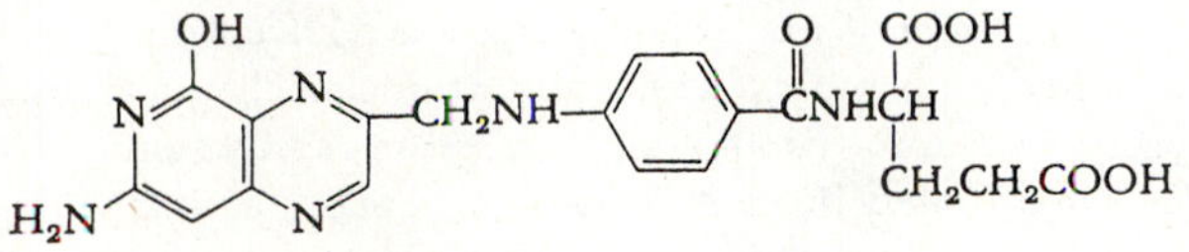

OH
|
N   N
| —CH₂NH— O COOH
| ‖ |
H₂N   N   CNHCH
                    |
              CH₂CH₂COOH

Folic acid

NH₂
|
N   N   CH₃
| —CH₂N— O COOH
| ‖ |
H₂N   N   CNHCH
                    |
              CH₂CH₂COOH

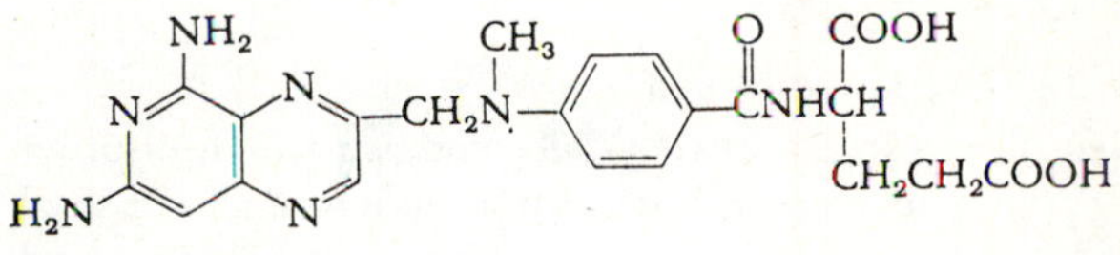

Methotrexate

Figure 3-56. Structures of several inhibitors of nucleotide biosynthesis. The structures of the corresponding natural substrates are also shown.

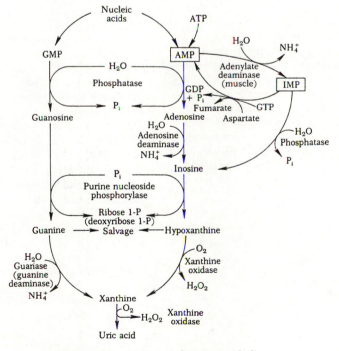

Figure 3-57. Pathways of purine catabolism.

The drug of choice for the treatment of hyperuricemia is allopurinol (Fig. 3-58), a substrate analogue of hypoxanthine. This compound is a competitive inhibitor of xanthine oxidase and thus blocks the production of uric acid. This results in accumulation of xanthine and hypoxanthine in plasma, but since these are more soluble than uric acid, the elevated levels of these compounds do not cause any clinical problems.

Lesch-Nyhan syndrome

Lesch-Nyhan syndrome is an inborn error of metabolism that is transmitted as a recessive X-linked characteristic. The clinical symptoms of the disease are developmental retardation, self-mutilation, and aggressive behavior. Patients suffering from the disease lack the salvage pathway enzyme HGPRT. As a result, they cannot convert guanine and hypoxanthine back to the respective nucleotides and these compounds are instead degraded to uric acid. These patients also manifest enhanced de novo purine synthesis due to elevated levels of PRPP.

The cause of the neurological symptoms is not clear, although it may indicate a relatively greater reliance of CNS tissue on salvage pathways for purine production than might be the case in other tissues. The hyperuricemia encountered in these patients can be treated with allopurinol, but this has no palliative effect on the neurological abnormalities.

Adenosine deaminase deficiency

Adenosine deaminase (ADA) deficiency is a genetic disorder that results in severe combined immunodeficiency. Lack of active ADA leads to an accumulation of adenosine and deoxyadenosine, which are phosphorylated to ATP and dATP. The latter compound is a potent inhibitor of ribonucleotide reductase, and its accumulation results in the inability of the cells to produce sufficient quantities of the other deoxyribonucleotides. T cells appear to most affected because they normally contain higher levels of the enzyme. The disease is fatal; the only successful treatment is bone marrow transplantation.

Purine nucleoside phosphorylase deficiency

Purine nucleoside phosphorylase (PNP) deficiency is an autosomal recessive disorder that results in immunodeficiency. In afflicted persons, T-cell function is most affected, with relatively minor effects on B cells. PNP converts inosine and guanosine to hypoxanthine and guanine, respectively. PNP deficiency results in an accumulation of guanosine and elevated levels of dGTP, which is also an inhibitor of ribonucleotide reductase. This appears to be the biochemical basis of the immunodeficiency. It is interesting to note that patients with

PNP deficiency excrete almost no uric acid because of their inability to produce the free bases.

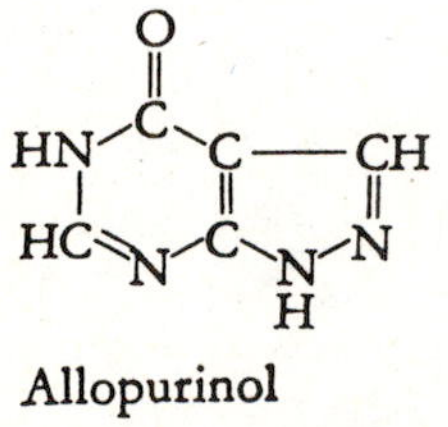

MOLECULAR BIOLOGY

The physical and metabolic characteristics of any organism are ultimately defined by its **genome**, which is composed of thousands of individual genes that contain the information for the synthesis of enzymes and other functional and structural proteins. It is the properties of these **gene products** that determine the phenotype of the individual. This genetic information is encoded as a sequence of nucleotides in DNA. The Central Dogma of Molecular Biology states that the genetic information stored in DNA is copied into RNA by a process referred to as **transcription**. This RNA in turn serves as the template for the synthesis of protein by a mechanism known as **translation**. In addition, DNA functions as a template for its own synthesis, which allows the accurate transmission of genetic information from one generation to the next. This process is referred to as **replication**.

DNA STRUCTURE

Nucleic acids are macromolecules composed of many repeating units of nucleotides. These are linked together by phosphodiester bonds. There are two major chemical differences between the two types of nucleic acids, RNA and DNA. The sugar moiety in RNA is ribose, whereas that in DNA is 2′ deoxyribose. RNA contains adenine, guanine, cytosine, and uracil as base components, and DNA contains thymine in place of uracil. The chemical structure of a small polynucleotide is presented in Figure 3-59. Note that the top nucleotide has a free (unlinked) phosphate group attached to C-5 of deoxyribose and the bottom nucleotide contains a free 3′-hydroxyl group. By convention, polynucleotides are always presented in this way—that is, they are written in the 5′-to-3′ direction. Thus, these molecules have a polarity.

The DNA of most organisms is double stranded—that is, it consists of two polynucleotide chains. These are held together by hydrogen bonding between the bases in opposite strands. Adenine is always bonded to thymine, and guanine interacts with cytosine. Each base pair (i.e., AT or GC) is said to be **complementary**, and the two opposing strands in the DNA are thus complementary to each other. The dimensions of the two types of base pairs are roughly the same, so the overall structure of DNA is not affected by the nucleotide sequence. In addition, the two strands have an opposite polarity from one another (Fig. 3-60) and are said to be **antiparallel**.

As a result of the geometry of the base pairs and their interaction by hydrogen bonding, the two strands of DNA wind around each other and form a helical structure. There are ten base pairs in every turn of the double helix. The structure shown in Figure 3-61 is that of B-DNA and is the most common structural form. Recently, a second structural form with potential biologic significance, called Z-DNA, has been discovered.

The hydrogen bonds that hold the two polynucleotide strands together can be broken by a variety of treatments, such as heating. The result is a separation of the DNA into single strands. This process is referred to as **denaturation**. Since the

Figure 3-58. Structure of allopurinol.

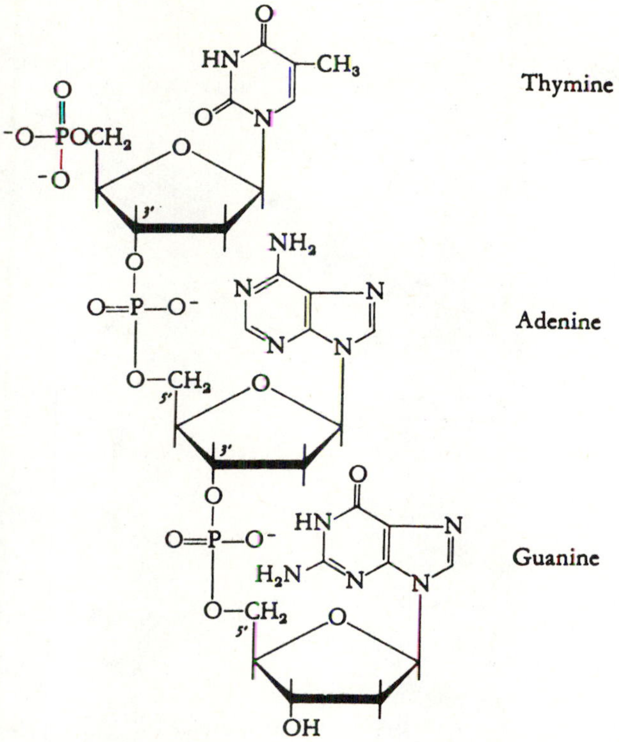

Figure 3-59.   Structure of a small polynucleotide.

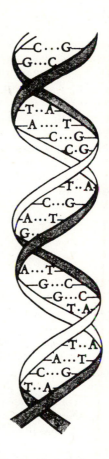

Figure 3-61.   The double-helical structure of DNA.

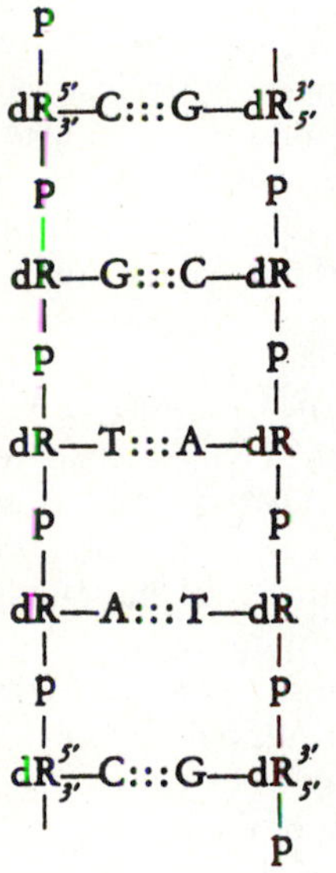

two strands are complementary to each other, the original double-helical structure can be reformed by slow cooling, which allows reestablishment of the hydrogen bonds. This is the process of **renaturation**. This property of DNA is very important for a number of procedures that are employed in recombinant DNA technology, which is discussed later in this chapter.

CHROMOSOME STRUCTURE

In eukaryotic cells, the genetic material is contained in the nucleus. DNA can be accommodated in the nucleus only because it is made very compact by virtue of complex formation with protein. Indeed, the DNA in the chromosome is compacted roughly 10,000-fold from its size as a naked DNA double helix. The major chromosomal proteins responsible for this structure are called **histones**.

Histones are small, basic proteins. In most mammalian organisms, there are five different histones—H1, H2A, H2B, H3, and H4. Twenty percent or more of the total amino acids in histones are lysine or arginine. Thus, these proteins will have a high degree of positive charge at physiological pH and will bind readily to the negatively charged DNA. In addition, histones have some affinity for each other. In particular, H3 and H4 interact with each other, as do H2A and H2B.

The chromosome also contains many other proteins. As a group, these are referred to as **nonhistone proteins** and are

Figure 3-60.   Schematic diagram depicting the opposite polarities of the two polynucleotide strands in DNA.

those that remain bound to the DNA after histone has been removed. This is a very heterogeneous class of proteins and probably comprises more than 400 individual species. The functions of these proteins include participation in DNA replication, RNA synthesis, and overall control of gene expression.

The basic, repeat unit of chromosome structure is the **nucleosome**. The structure of this particle is depicted in Figure 3-62. It is composed of a **core particle**, which contains approximately 140 base pairs of DNA and two copies each of H2A, H2B, H3, and H4. The DNA double helix is wrapped around a core of these eight histone molecules. The individual nucleosomes are connected by 20 to 50 base pairs of **linker DNA**. Histone H1 is bound to the linker. Studies have shown that essentially all the chromosomal DNA is packaged into this type of nucleosome structure.

DNA REPLICATION

The complementary base-paired structure of DNA is crucial to the mechanism of replication. During this process, the opposite strands of the DNA molecule separate and each strand serves as the **template** for the synthesis of a new, complementary strand. This mode of replication is referred to as **semiconservative**. In this manner, the sequence information contained in DNA is faithfully copied from one generation to the next.

The detailed mechanism of DNA replication is best understood for prokaryotic organisms. In most of its aspects, the mechanism appears to be the same in mammalian systems, as well. DNA synthesis is accomplished by the successive addition of nucleotides to the 3' terminus by formation of phosphodiester bonds. This reaction is mediated by **DNA polymerase**. These enzymes have been isolated from a wide variety of organisms, and they all appear to have essentially identical properties. The requirements for the reaction catalyzed by DNA polymerase include a base-paired template-primer substrate containing a 3' terminus with a free hydroxyl group and all four deoxyribonucleoside triphosphates. DNA synthesis occurs by the addition of a nucleotide to the free 3'-hydroxyl end of the primer. The choice of the appropriate nucleotide is determined by base pairing between the incoming nucleotide and the base in the template strand. This reaction is depicted schematically in Figure 3-63.

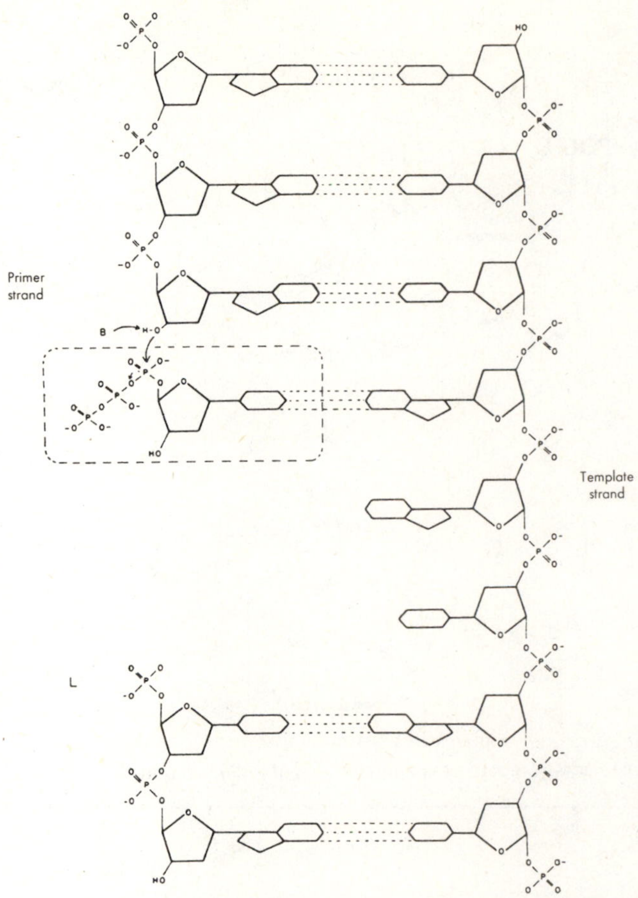

Figure 3-63. Mechanism of action of DNA polymerase.

In addition to their polymerization activity, DNA polymerases also possess an exonucleolytic activity that is involved in **proofreading**. This process is critical to the fidelity of DNA synthesis. If an incorrect nucleotide is inserted into the growing polynucleotide chain, this is detected by DNA polymerase because of the improper base pairing. The enzyme then catalyzes the cleavage of the newly formed phosphodiester bond, which reverses the error.

The properties of DNA polymerase dictate the mechanism of DNA synthesis. DNA polymerase cannot initiate synthesis of a polynucleotide de novo—that is, it can only elongate a preexisting primer strand. In contrast, RNA polymerases can direct the synthesis of the initial phosphodiester bond between two ribonucleoside triphosphates. For this reason, DNA replication begins with the synthesis of an RNA primer, which is then elongated by DNA polymerase. In most organisms, a specific type of RNA polymerase, called **DNA primase**, mediates the synthesis of the primer.

All polynucleotide chain growth occurs in a 5'-to-3' direction. Both strands of the parental DNA must unwind in order to serve as templates for the synthesis of daughter strands. These strands are antiparallel (i.e., they have opposite polarity with respect to each other). As a result, it is not possible to synthesize a continuous daughter DNA strand off both parental DNA strands simultaneously. This problem is obviated by synthesis of one of the daughter chains as short pieces. These are sometimes referred to as **Okazaki fragments**. The comple-

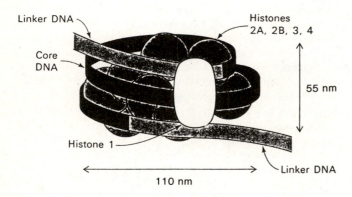

Figure 3-62. The structure of a nucleosome.

tion of the replication event requires the removal of the RNA primer and the joining of the Okazaki fragments to each other. The primer is degraded by a $5' \rightarrow 3'$ exonuclease. In *Escherichia coli*, this is a property of DNA polymerase I that also fills in the gap left by the removal of the RNA. The precise mechanism for primer excision in other organisms is not known. The newly synthesized fragments are then joined together by the action of **DNA ligase.**

The mechanism of DNA replication is thus very complex and involves the participation of a large number of enzymes. This enzymatic activity takes place at a region of the chromosome that is unwound. Such a site is referred to as a **replication fork.** A schematic diagram of a replication fork in *E. coli* is presented in Figure 3-64 and summarizes many of the aspects of DNA replication discussed in this section.

TRANSCRIPTION

The sequence of information stored in DNA is initially decoded by transcription into RNA. In addition to the chemical differences between them, RNA also differs from DNA in that it is single stranded. There are three types of RNA found in all cells, and they each serve distinct functions. Ribosomal RNA (rRNA) is a structural component of ribosomes—the site of protein synthesis. Transfer RNA (tRNA) is the molecule that shuttles amino acids to the ribosome during protein synthesis. Messenger RNA (mRNA) contains the protein coding information that determines the amino acid sequence of all proteins synthesized in the cell. rRNA and tRNA are much more abundant than mRNA and are referred to as stable RNAs because they have a much longer half-life than mRNA. RNA synthesis is catalyzed by the enzyme **RNA polymerase.** The basic mechanism of this process is essentially the same in all organisms, but the sequences in DNA that control transcription, and the enzymes themselves, vary significantly in prokaryotes and eukaryotes.

RNA synthesis

In the presence of all four ribonucleoside triphosphates and a DNA template, RNA polymerase will catalyze the formation of phosphodiester bonds. Polynucleotide chain growth occurs

in a $5' \rightarrow 3'$ direction. The sequence of the newly synthesized RNA is dictated by complementary base pairing between the DNA template strand and the incoming ribonucleoside triphosphate. Only one of the two DNA strands serves as a template for RNA synthesis. Thus, the RNA product will have a sequence complementary to that of the DNA strand that functions as the template. There are specific regions in the DNA that delineate the initiation and termination points of transcription. These sequences, as well as the RNA polymerases themselves, differ in prokaryotes and eukaryotes.

Prokaryotes.   There is a single RNA polymerase that carries out transcription of all RNA species in prokaryotes. The **core polymerase** consists of three different polypeptide subunits, one of which is present in two copies. Its structure is designated $\alpha_2\beta\beta'$. An additional subunit, referred to as sigma factor, is required for the initiation phase of transcription. Core polymerase with sigma factor attached is called RNA polymerase **holoenzyme.** Sigma cycles off the holoenzyme when elongation of the RNA chain begins and it rebinds for subsequent initiation events. Thus, only the core polymerase is necessary for the polymerization reaction once the initial phosphodiester bond has been formed.

Specific sequences in DNA, called **promoters,** are recognized by RNA polymerase holoenzyme and signal the starting points for transcription. The sequences of close to 200 promoters in *E. coli* have been analyzed, and several common features have been discerned. The promoters consist of two specific sequence elements located 10 and 35 base pairs upstream (i.e., on the $5'$ side) of the transcription start site. These are referred to as the -10 (or Pribnow) box and -35 box and contain sequences closely resembling TATAAT and TTGACA, respectively. Similarly, termination of transcription is indicated by a specific sequence in the DNA. There are two types of termination signals in *E. coli*. One is dependent on protein factor rho, which binds to RNA polymerase and recognizes a termination sequence. The other rho-independent, transcription termination site consists of a base-paired stem and loop structure followed by a short sequence rich in T residues. When RNA polymerase encounters such a sequence, its interaction with the DNA template is apparently destabilized and it is released.

Eukaryotes.   In contrast to the situation in prokaryotes, there are three RNA polymerases in eukaryotes that are responsible for the transcription of distinct classes of RNA. RNA polymerase I is the major polymerase in eukaryotes and is responsible for transcription of rRNA. The synthesis of mRNA is catalyzed by RNA polymerase II, while the production of tRNA, 5S RNA, and several other small RNAs is catalyzed by RNA polymerase III. All of these enzymes appear to be large aggregates of several polypeptide chains. The activity of RNA polymerase II can be specifically inhibited by the compound α-amanitin.

Promoters for RNA polymerase II are similar in design to those found in prokaryotes, although they differ in regard to sequence and position. These promoters most often consist of an AT-rich sequence 25 nucleotides upstream of the transcription initiation site known as the TATA box and a second region at -70 to -80 that usually contains a CAAT sequence and is referred to as the CAAT box. It is clear from many studies, however, that other sequence elements further upstream have a dramatic effect on transcription. One example of such a

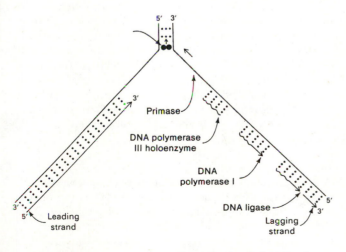

Figure 3-64.   Representation of a replication fork in *E. coli.*

sequence element is an **enhancer**. These were first discovered in viral genes but have now been found in many other organisms. Enhancers can be situated at large distances from the genes that they affect (more than several thousand base pairs) and can function in either orientation. These properties make enhancers distinctly different from promoters.

RNA polymerase III recognizes a promoter structure that is quite distinct from that of RNA polymerase II. In this case, the promoter lies within the gene that is being transcribed. The precise nature of the promoter varies from gene to gene, but in all cases the recognition site is within the sequence to be transcribed and signals the initiation of transcription at a position upstream from the promoter.

RNA processing

The initial RNA product produced by RNA polymerase action is called the **primary transcript**. In almost all cases, this RNA is further modified by nucleolytic cleavage or base modification. The only exception to this posttranscriptional processing appears to be prokaryotic mRNA. rRNA in all organisms is synthesized as a single, large primary transcript that contains the sequences of all the individual rRNA species. The primary transcript is cleaved at specific sites by a ribonuclease, which yields the mature rRNA species found in the ribosome. tRNA is also synthesized as a larger precursor molecule, which is processed to the mature form by a variety of nucleolytic cleavages. In addition, approximately 15% of the individual bases in tRNA are modified posttranscriptionally. In eukaryotes, some precursor tRNAs contain intervening sequences, or **introns,** which are not part of the final tRNA product. In these cases, the complete maturation process requires endonucleolytic cleavage on either side of the intron and **splicing** of the remaining ends to each other.

The production of mature mRNA in eukaryotes is a particularly complex process. The primary transcripts synthesized by RNA polymerase II are very large and heterogeneous and are designated hnRNA (heterogeneous nuclear RNA). hnRNA containing the sequences for a specific mRNA will also usually harbor several introns, which must be removed during maturation. The introns generally begin with a 5' GU dinucleotide and end with a 3' AG. These sequences provide a signal for the excision of the intron and the joining of the resultant RNA ends. This process is referred to as splicing. The sequences that are found in mature mRNA are known as **exons.** Most eukaryotic mRNAs are also modified at both the 5' and 3' ends. A 7-methyl G in an unusual 5'−5' linkage is located at the 5' end of the mRNA. This is known as the **cap structure** and is involved in ribosome binding. The majority of eukaryotic mRNAs have a stretch of 100 to 200 adenine residues at their 3' ends. This **poly A tail** is added posttranscriptionally by the enzyme poly A polymerase. An AAUAAA sequence is generally observed within 30 nucleotides of the poly A tail and is thought to be the signal for poly A addition.

GENETIC CODE

The sequence of nucleotides in mRNA specifies the amino acid sequence of its corresponding protein. The translation of the nucleotide sequence into the amino acid sequence is governed by the **genetic code**. This code is presented in Table

Table 3-4. The Genetic Code

First position (5' end)	Second position				Third position (3' end)
	U	C	A	G	
U	Phe	Ser	Tyr	Cys	U
	Phe	Ser	Tyr	Cys	C
	Leu	Ser	Stop	Stop	A
	Leu	Ser	Stop	Trp	G
C	Leu	Pro	His	Arg	U
	Leu	Pro	His	Arg	C
	Leu	Pro	Gln	Arg	A
	Leu	Pro	Gln	Arg	G
A	Ile	Thr	Asn	Ser	U
	Ile	Thr	Asn	Ser	C
	Ile	Thr	Lys	Arg	A
	Met	Thr	Lys	Arg	G
G	Val	Ala	Asp	Gly	U
	Val	Ala	Asp	Gly	C
	Val	Ala	Glu	Gly	A
	Val	Ala	Glu	Gly	G

3-4. Examination of the code reveals several important features which are discussed below.

Triplet code

There are 20 amino acids that commonly occur in proteins. The nucleotide sequence must be capable of unambiguously coding for each amino acid. This is accomplished by having a sequence of three nucleotides specifying a given amino acid. These triplet sequences are called **codons**.

Degeneracy of the code

It is possible to construct 64 different triplet codons from combinations of the four available nucleotides. This means that either 44 codons will not specify any amino acid or that more than one triplet can code for a specific amino acid. In fact, the latter is the case and the code is said to be **degenerate**. All amino acids except methionine and tryptophan are specified by more than one codon. In addition, degenerate codons (which specify the same amino acid) generally differ from each other by only one nucleotide, and this change usually occurs in the third position (see Table 3-4). These properties of the code minimize the lethal effects of point mutations (i.e., single base changes in DNA) because such mutations are likely to be silent (i.e., although the codon is different, it still specifies the same amino acid).

Punctuation

The only punctuation signals in the reading of an mRNA are those that specify the beginning and the end of the protein. The **initiation codon** is AUG (and in a small number of cases GUG). The first amino acid inserted into all nascent proteins is, therefore, methionine. This amino acid can be subsequently removed, so that methionine is not the N-terminal amino acid in all mature proteins. The initiation of translation at an AUG codon sets the **reading frame,** and the sequence following that AUG is deciphered three nucleotides at a time until a **termination codon** is encountered. There are three termination codons—UAA, UAG, and UGA. These three triplets do not code for any amino acid and instead signal the end of the protein sequence.

Universality of the code

With few exceptions, the genetic code is identical in all organisms, from bacteria to higher mammals. Recently, several instances of minor variations in the coding table have been discovered. The most noteworthy of these is in the mitochondria of several eukaryotic organisms, including humans. The universality of the code is extremely important in facilitating the comparisons of protein structures between related organisms by simple comparison of the nucleotide sequences of the genes. It is also critical to production of therapeutically useful human proteins in bacteria by recombinant DNA procedures. This is possible only because the code that specifies protein sequence in humans is identical to that which is operative in bacteria.

PROTEIN SYNTHESIS

As we have seen, the sequence of nucleotides in mRNA specifies the sequence of amino acids in a protein. The process by which the mRNA code is deciphered is called translation. The two major components involved in this process are tRNA and ribosomes.

tRNA

There is no inherent complementarity between nucleotides and amino acids. This means that there must exist a molecule that can bridge the gap between these two types of compounds. This is the function of tRNA. Individual species of tRNA are specific, in that a unique amino acid can be covalently attached at one part of the molecule and a second portion is capable of recognizing the cognate triplet codon that specifies that amino acid.

Structure. The sequences of several hundred tRNAs from a wide variety of organisms have been determined. They all have several properties in common. They consist of 75 to 90 nucleotides and can all be folded into a similar secondary structure, which is shown in Figure 3-65.

This structure is formed by complementary base pairing between different regions of the tRNA and is referred to as the **cloverleaf** structure. The individual stems and loops are responsible for distinct functions. The amino acid is attached to the 3' end of the tRNA via an aminoacyl ester linkage (see below). The codons in mRNA are recognized by complementary base-pairing interactions with the three central nucleotides in the **anticodon** loop. tRNAs also have a unique tertiary structure (Fig. 3-66). It is important to note that the two important functional ends of tRNA (the aminoacyl end and the anticodon) are situated at opposite ends of the molecule. tRNAs must also interact in a specific manner with ribosomes and aminoacyl-tRNA synthetases (see below). The structural elements that define these interaction sites are not presently known.

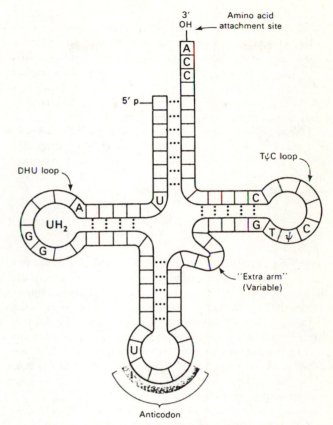

Figure 3-65.   Cloverleaf structure of tRNA.

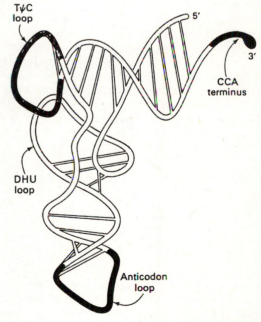

Figure 3-66.   Representation of the three-dimensional structure of tRNA.

A cell requires a minimum of 20 different tRNA species, one for each amino acid. In fact, most organisms contain 40 to 50 distinct tRNAs. Thus, individual amino acids can be carried by more than one tRNA species, which are called **isoacceptors**. In no case, however, do isoacceptors contain the identical anticodon sequence. The acceptor specificity of a tRNA is signified by a superscript—for example, tRNA^{Phe} indicates a tRNA species that can carry phenylalanine.

Aminoacylation.   For each amino acid there is an enzyme, **aminoacyl-tRNA synthetase**, which attaches the amino acid to its cognate tRNA. All isoacceptor tRNAs for a particular amino acid are handled by the same synthetase. The overall aminoacylation reaction occurs in two steps:

$$E + AA + ATP \rightarrow E{\sim}AA{\sim}AMP + PP_i \qquad (1)$$
$$E{\sim}AA{\sim}AMP + tRNA \rightarrow AA{-}tRNA + E + AMP \qquad (2)$$

In the first step, the amino acid is **activated** to an enzyme-bound, high-energy aminoacyl adenylate intermediate. In the subsequent step, the activated amino acid is **charged** onto its cognate tRNA. Thus, each aminoacylation event requires the hydrolysis of one molecule of ATP. The aminoacyl linkage in charged tRNA is a high-energy bond, and its hydrolysis provides most of the energy for peptide bond formation on the ribosome. The charged tRNA species is designated as AA-tRNA—for example, Phe-tRNA^{Phe} indicates tRNA^{Phe} amino-acylated with phenylalanine.

Peptide bond formation takes place on the ribosome. The insertion of a particular amino acid in the nascent peptide chain is determined by the interaction between the anticodon in tRNA and the complementary codon in mRNA. This means that the accuracy of protein synthesis is completely dependent on the precision with which a cognate amino acid is charged onto its tRNA. Any errors in the aminoacylation reaction will result in the insertion of an incorrect amino acid in newly synthesized proteins. For this reason, aminoacyl-tRNA synthetases have **proofreading** mechanisms that ensure that tRNAs are not charged with noncognate amino acids.

Codon-anticodon interaction.   The codon-anticodon interaction occurs by complementary, antiparallel base pairing. In most cases, the differences between degenerate codon sequences are limited to the 3′ position. It was observed that certain nucleotides in the 5′ position of the anticodon could pair with nucleotides other than the normal bases. This led to the proposal, known as the **wobble hypothesis**, that a single tRNA species could recognize more than one codon in mRNA. The wobble rules are listed below:

5′ anticodon nucleotide	3′ codon nucleotide
I	A, C, U
G	C, U
U	A, G
A	U
C	G

This means that a tRNA with G in the 5′ anticodon position can recognize not only the standard XYC codon, but also the nonstandard XYU by formation of a wobble GU base pair. For example, the major valine isoacceptor tRNA in many organisms has the anticodon sequence IAC. This single tRNA can recognize three of the four valine codons, GUU, GUC, and GUA. A second tRNA^{Val} is necessary to interact with the remaining valine-specific codon GUG. This property of codon-anticodon interactions accounts for the fact that cells do not require 61 distinct tRNAs in order to decipher the 61 sense codons in the genetic code. Indeed, the mitochondria of most mammals contain only 32 tRNAs, the minimum number required for recognition of all the codons, based on the rules of wobble pairing.

Ribosomes

Ribosomes are the organelles that serve as the site for protein synthesis. They are very complex ribonucleoprotein assemblies. Ribosome structure varies somewhat between prokaryotes and higher organisms, although the basic design of the particle is essentially identical.

Ribosomes consist of two subunits, each of which in turn is composed of RNA and protein. mRNA binds to the small subunit, whereas the site for peptide bond formation is associated with the large subunit. Ribosomes and their subunits are usually designated by sedimentation coefficient (which is a function of their size and shape). Bacterial ribosomes (e.g., those of *E. coli*) are 70S. They are composed of a 30S and a 50S subunit. The 30S subunit contains one 16S RNA molecule and 21 different proteins. The 50S subunit is composed of a 5S RNA and a 23S RNA molecule and 32 different proteins. The three-dimensional arrangement of each of these components relative to each other is highly specific and is necessary for ribosome function.

The ribosomes of eukaryotes are 80S, being composed of 40S and 60S subunits. The RNA component of the small subunit is 18S, and those of the large subunit are 5S, 5.8S, and 28S. In general, the small eukaryotic ribosomal subunit has approximately 30 proteins while the large subunit is composed of 45 to 50 proteins. Although eukaryotic ribosomes are roughly 50% larger than their prokaryotic counterparts, the functions of both particles are fundamentally the same.

Mechanism of protein synthesis

The translation of the mRNA code into protein on the ribosome occurs in three distinct phases—initiation, elongation, and termination. The only major difference in this process between prokaryotes and eukaryotes is at the level of initiation. Formation of the peptide bond takes place during the elongation phase. All the individual steps of translation require the participation of protein factors, in addition to charged tRNA, mRNA, and ribosomes.

Initiation.   The formation of the initiation complex in prokaryotes is outlined in Figure 3-67. The first step involves the binding of the 30S subunit to a specific region of mRNA that contains an appropriate initiation codon (AUG). Initiation factor IF-3 ensures that a pool of free 30S subunits is available for this step and also enhances the binding of mRNA to the ribosome. A purine-rich sequence (e.g., GGAGG) is usually situated seven to nine nucleotides upstream of the AUG codon and guides the binding of mRNA by base pairing with a complementary sequence (CCUCC) at the 3′ end of 16S RNA. The purine-rich sequence is called the **Shine-Dalgarno** region. AUG codes for methionine, and, as already pointed out, this is

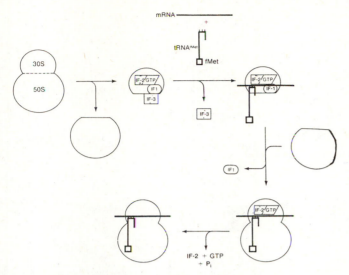

Figure 3-67. Initiation of translation in prokaryotes.

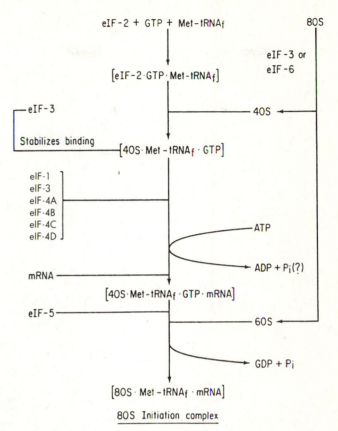

Figure 3-68. Initiation of translation in eukaryotes.

only one of two amino acids that is coded for by a single codon. The initiator AUG codon is recognized by a special initiator tRNA that has its amino terminus blocked by formylation (fMet-tRNA). Initiator tRNA binds to the 30S subunit-mRNA complex in a reaction mediated by initiation factors IF-1 and IF-2. IF-2 binds as an IF-2~GTP complex. At this point, a 50S subunit joins the complex concomitant with the release of the bound initiation factors and the hydrolysis of GTP → GDP + P$_i$. This yields a 70S ribosome with fMet-tRNA bound at the initiation site. At this point, a second tRNA can bind and the elongation phase can begin.

Eukaryotic initiation complex formation requires many more protein factors than is the case in prokaryotes. A schematic diagram of this process is presented in Figure 3-68. The special initiator tRNA is also a Met-tRNA, but in this case the amino group of methionine is not blocked by formylation. Met-tRNA$_i$ forms a ternary complex with GTP and initiation factor eIF-2. The ternary complex binds to a free 40S subunit prior to mRNA binding. eIF-6 appears to be responsible for maintaining the pool of free 40S subunits. mRNA then binds to the 40S initiation complex in a step that is stimulated by several protein factors including eIF-1, eIF-3, eIF-4A, eIF-4B, eIF-4C, and eIF-4D. eIF-3 is a very large multimeric protein with a molecular weight in excess of 500,000. This mRNA binding step also requires the hydrolysis of 1 mol of ATP. In contrast to the bacterial system, there is no specific sequence in front of the AUG initiation codon in eukaryotic mRNA that designates it as the translation initiation site. Instead, it appears that the 40S subunit binds to the 5′ end of the mRNA (which usually contains the methylated cap structure) migrates along the mRNA until the first AUG codon is encountered and thus signals the initiation of the reading frame for protein synthesis. A 60S subunit then joins the 40S "preinitiation" complex. This step is dependent on eIF-5. The 60S subunit binding step results in the hydrolysis of GTP. The resultant 80S initiation complex is now ready for the next phase of translation.

Elongation. Ribosomes have two tRNA binding sites. At the conclusion of the initiation step, initiator tRNA is bound at the ribosomal **P site**. The codon that specifies the next amino

acid is aligned in the ribosomal **A site**. Aminoacyl-tRNA forms a ternary complex with elongation factor EF-Tu and GTP, and it is the ternary complex that binds to the A site. The choice of the appropriate aminoacyl-tRNA is based solely on the codon-anticodon interaction between the mRNA in the A site and the aa-tRNA in the ternary complex. After tRNA binding, GTP is hydrolyzed and EF-Tu is released as a binary EF-Tu · GDP complex. The GDP is converted to GTP by the action of EF-Ts, thus regenerating the active ET-Tu · GTP complex, which can combine with another aminoacyl-tRNA. Once the two tRNA binding sites are occupied, formation of the peptide bond occurs by transfer of the amino acid (or nascent polypeptide chain) from the P-site-bound tRNA to the free amino end of aminoacyl-tRNA at the A site. This reaction is catalyzed by the **peptidyl transferase** center of the ribosome. This activity is an intrinsic property of the ribosome, and no additional factors are required for peptide bond formation.

After peptide bond formation, the ribosome has peptidyl-tRNA bound at the A site and uncharged tRNA at the P site. In order for translation to continue, three things must happen— deacylated tRNA must be ejected from the P site, peptidyl-tRNA must migrate from the A site to the vacant P site, and the next codon must be aligned in the A site. These events are referred to collectively as **translocation**. This process is mediated by elongation factor EF-G and requires the hydrolysis of an additional mole of GTP. The elongation phase is summarized in Figure 3-69.

The mechanism of elongation is essentially identical for all organisms. In eukaryotes, elongation factor EF-1 serves the

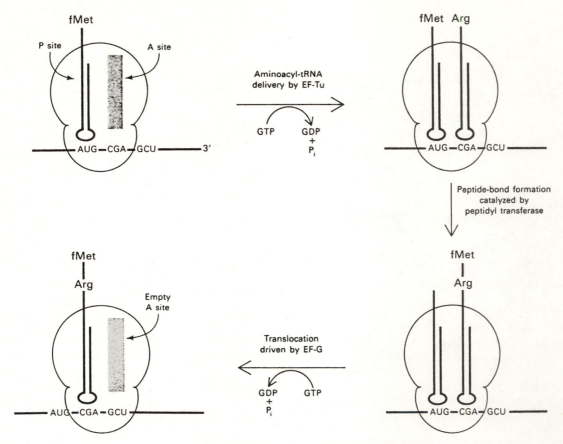

Figure 3-69. Elongation phase of protein synthesis.

functions of EF-Tu and EF-Ts, and EF-2 is the functional equivalent of EF-G.

Termination. Elongation of the polypeptide chain proceeds by successive rounds of aa-tRNA binding, peptide bond formation, and translocation. This continues until one of the three termination codons—UAA, UAG, or UGA—appears at the A site. These codons do not specify the binding of any tRNA. Instead, a **release factor** binds to the A site and stimulates the hydrolysis of the aminoacyl linkage between the nascent polypeptide and the tRNA bound at the P site. This results in release of the completed protein from the ribosome. In bacteria, there are two release factors that respond to different termination codons—RF-1 recognizes UAA and UAG, and RF-2 recognizes UAA and UGA. In eukaryotes there appears to be a single release factor that responds to all the termination codons.

Antibiotic inhibitors of protein synthesis

Many commonly used antibiotics act by inhibiting various steps of protein synthesis. Several of these antibiotics and their modes of action are listed in Table 3-5. These compounds can function as antibiotics because they act only on prokaryotic ribosomes.

Synthesis of membrane and secreted proteins

Most of the proteins synthesized in bacteria remain in the cell. In eukaryotes, however, many proteins are either secreted

Table 3-5. Antibiotics That Act by Inhibiting Protein Synthesis

Antibiotic	Mode of action

Aminoglycosides
  1. Streptomycin
  2. Gentamicin
  3. Neomycin
	Bind to 30S subunit and interfere with codon-anticodon interaction. This results in misreading of the mRNA code and causes synthesis of mutant proteins.

Tetracycline	Inhibits the binding of charged tRNA to ribosomes.
Erythromycin	Binds to 50S subunit and blocks peptidyl transferase activity.

from the cells or are inserted into the cell membrane. These latter classes of proteins are synthesized on ribosomes that are bound to the **endoplasmic reticulum**. The mechanism by which this synthesis occurs is shown schematically in Figure 3-70. The mRNAs for most of these proteins code for a special N-terminal sequence, called the **signal sequence**, which is very hydrophobic in nature. Translation begins on a free cytoplasmic ribosome, but as the hydrophobic, N-terminal **signal peptide** is formed, the translating ribosome attaches to the membrane

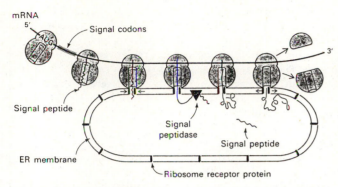

Figure 3-70. Scheme for cotranslational synthesis of membrane and secreted proteins.

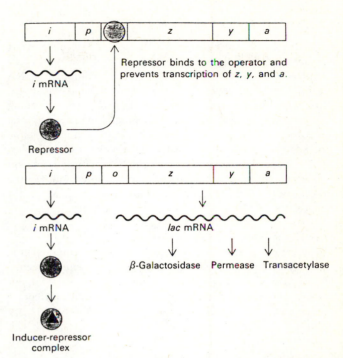

Figure 3-71.   Control of lactose operon gene expression.

of the endoplasmic reticulum. This binding is mediated by a ribonucleoprotein assembly, the **signal recognition particle**, which recognizes the nascent signal peptide and a receptor in the membrane. As translation continues, the nascent polypeptide passes through the membrane and the signal peptide is cleaved by a **signal peptidase** enzyme that resides in the membrane. Termination of translation results in a protein on the cisternal (or internal) side of the membrane.

Many membrane and secreted proteins are modified cotranslationally by the addition of carbohydrate. Proteins that contain covalently bound sugar residues are called **glycoproteins**. A variety of sugar residues, including glucose, galactose, mannose, and sialic acid, may be incorporated into the complex oligosaccharide chains of glycoproteins. The sugar residues are added to the nascent peptide chain while it is attached to the membrane of the endoplasmic reticulum or Golgi apparatus. **Glycosyl transferases** catalyze the addition of individual carbohydrate residues to the growing oligosaccharide.

CONTROL OF GENE EXPRESSION

Only a small portion of the total genetic information of an organism is expressed at any specific time. Organisms respond to different physiological and environmental requirements, as well as to a variety of developmental cues.

Genetic control in prokaryotes

In prokaryotes, genes that code for enzymes catalyzing successive steps in a biochemical pathway are often located contiguously in the genome. As a result, the expression of all the related genes can be controlled by a single molecule. Such gene clusters are called **operons**.

The best-studied example of a bacterial operon is the *lac* operon of *E. coli*. This operon consists of three genes whose products are responsible for the utilization of lactose as a nutrient. In the absence of lactose, the genes are not expressed. The introduction of lactose in the growth medium results in the transcription of the genes and the synthesis of the corresponding proteins. This type of control is called **negative regulation**, and the control circuits are presented in Figure 3-71. A specific **repressor** protein, which is coded for by a gene that is not part of the operon, normally binds to a segment of DNA, the **operator**, located adjacent to the promoter. This binding blocks transcription of the genes in the operon. The **inducer**,

lactose, forms a complex with repressor, thus inactivating it. This results in the expression of the genes. In this manner, *E. coli* will produce these gene products only if the substrate is present.

Some bacterial operons are also subject to **positive regulation**. This means that RNA polymerase is not capable of transcribing these genes by itself but, rather, requires the participation of an ancillary factor. One example of such control is the expression of **heat shock** genes. These are a group of apparently unrelated genes whose expression is induced by elevated temperature. It has been observed that these conditions induce the synthesis of a new sigma factor that allows RNA polymerase to preferentially transcribe the heat shock genes.

Active genes in eukaryotes

As described earlier, virtually all the DNA in the eukaryotic genome is organized as nucleosomes. This is true even for genes that are very actively expressed in a particular tissue. Recent studies have shown, however, that the chromatin structure at or near genes that are undergoing active transcription is different from that of bulk chromatin. **Transcriptionally active chromatin** is much more susceptible to digestion by a variety of nucleases (e.g., DNase I). Two nonhistone proteins, HMG 14 and HMG 17, appear to be specifically associated with these regions of chromatin.

Another variable appears to be the methylation state of the DNA. In mammals, 2 to 7% of the cytosine residues in total DNA are methylated at C-5. This methylation occurs almost exclusively at CG sequences. Many recent investigations have indicated that actively transcribed genes are undermethylated. Indeed, it is possible that X-chromosome inactivation in females may be the result of methylation of one of the two X chromosomes at an early stage of development.

RECOMBINANT DNA TECHNOLOGY

The past 15 years have witnessed an explosive growth in our ability to manipulate DNA at a level that was previously impossible. The enormous potential of recombinant DNA technology will impact directly on the practice of medicine, from the production of new therapeutic drugs, to the screening for rare genetic diseases, to the mapping of the entire human genome. Future physicians will therefore require a basic knowledge of recombinant DNA technology. In its simplest form, this methodology involves the identification and isolation of specific fragments of DNA and their amplification. For the production of therapeutic compounds, a mechanism for expression of the isolated DNA is also necessary.

Restriction endonucleases

Restriction enzymes are widely distributed among prokaryotic species. In these organisms, they serve the protective function of preventing transformation by the uptake of foreign DNA. These enzymes recognize a very specific nucleotide sequence in the DNA, bind to it, and cut the DNA by phosphodiester bond cleavage of both DNA strands. The recognition sequences most commonly consist of four or six base pairs and always exhibit a twofold axis of rotational symmetry (Fig. 3-72). The cleavage site is always in the same point in the sequence on each strand. This means that if the cut is asymmetric (i.e., not directly in the center of the sequence), the resulting ends will be complementary to each other. Therefore, DNAs from two distinct sources can be joined to each other if both are treated with the same restriction enzyme (Fig. 3-73). Thus, these enzymes provide two of the key ingredients for recombining DNA molecules—a method for cutting DNA into specific fragments and a means for making the ends of these fragments cohesive.

Vectors

In order to propagate a DNA fragment, it must be replicated. Only DNA fragments that contain an origin of replication, or **replicon**, have this property. A wide variety of replicon-containing DNAs that are employed for this purpose are currently in use. They are referred to as **vectors**. The most common vectors are plasmids. These are derivatives of naturally occurring extrachromosomal pieces of DNA that are commonly found in bacteria. They have two useful properties—an easily assayed phenotype (usually antibiotic resistance) and several unique restriction sites. Thus any fragment of foreign DNA that contains the same cohesive end can be joined to a vector and propagated by its replication in a host organism.

Other commonly used vectors are derivatives of bacteriophage. Plasmid and phage vectors can only be used if the host organism is a bacterium. Derivatives of several eukaryotic viruses such as SV40 and vaccinia have been employed as vectors with eukaryotic hosts.

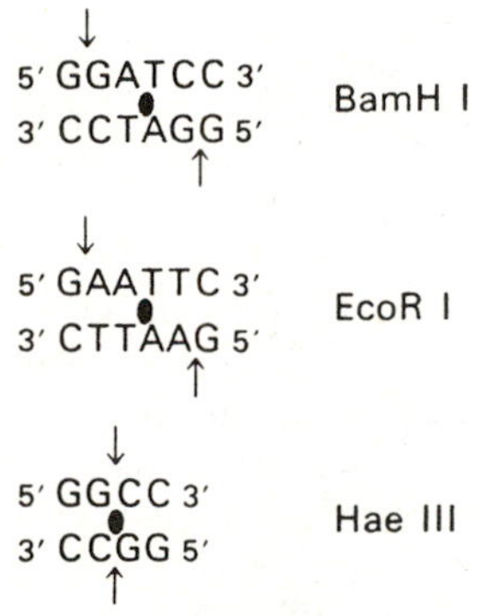

Ligation

The construction of recombinant DNA molecules requires the covalent joining of DNA fragments from different sources to each other. This is accomplished by the use of **DNA ligase**, an enzyme described earlier that functions in vivo during DNA replication. The preferred substrate for this enzyme is a base-paired DNA duplex with a nick, i.e., a 3'-hydroxyl adjacent to a 5'-phosphate. DNA ligase binds to the nick and seals it, yielding a fully covalent duplex molecule (Fig. 3-74). Under certain in vitro conditions, DNA ligase can also use DNA molecules with **blunt ends** (i.e., completely base-paired ends) as substrates.

Figure 3-75 is a schematic diagram that demonstrates the construction of a recombinant DNA molecule by the techniques described in the preceding sections.

cDNA cloning

The vast majority of the DNA in a eukaryotic genome does not code for any gene product. This makes the task of isolating the gene for a specific product from the total genome an extremely difficult task. This can be greatly simplified by first isolating the mRNA that codes for the protein of interest and synthesizing a **complementary DNA** (cDNA). The cDNA can then be cloned and analyzed. A scheme for the synthesis and cloning of cDNA is presented in Figure 3-76.

Most mRNA contains a poly A tail at the 3' end. A complementary oligonucleotide of T residues (oligo dT) can be annealed to the poly A tail by base pairing. This serves as a substrate for the enzyme **reverse transcriptase**, which can synthesize DNA from an RNA template. This results in the production of a single-stranded cDNA. After removal of the mRNA template, this cDNA can serve as the template for the synthesis of its complementary strand by elongation in the presence of deoxyribonucleoside triphosphates and DNA polymerase I. Further processing by several specific nucleases yields a double-stranded cDNA, in which one of the strands has a sequence identical to the original mRNA. The cDNA can be propagated by cloning into an appropriate vector as described earlier.

In practice, the initial isolation and sequencing of most eukaryotic genes is accomplished with cDNA.

Hybridization techniques

The complementary base-pairing properties of nucleic acids can provide an effective means for detection and analysis of genomic structure. Several widely employed techniques are based on the annealing of complementary lengths of single-stranded DNA. The identification of a specific gene among thousands of other genes is most readily accomplished by **Southern hybridization** or **blotting**. The steps in this procedure are outlined below:

Figure 3-72.   Recognition sequences of several restriction enzymes.

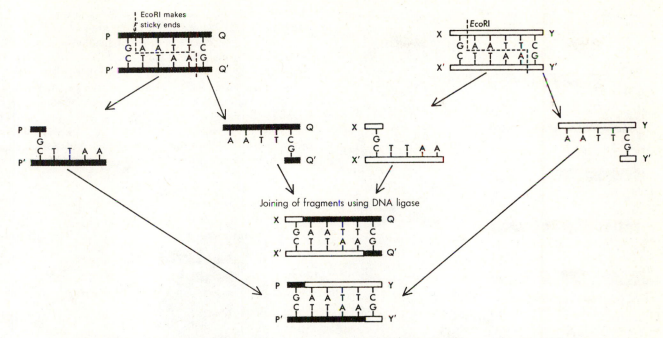

Figure 3-73. Construction of a recombinant DNA molecule by taking advantage of the complementary cohesive ends.

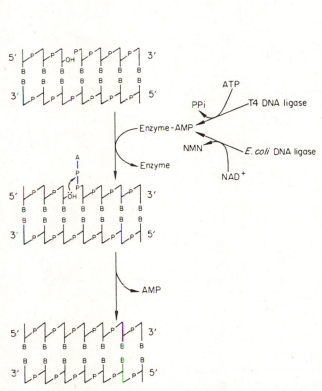

Figure 3-74. Mechanism of action of DNA ligase.

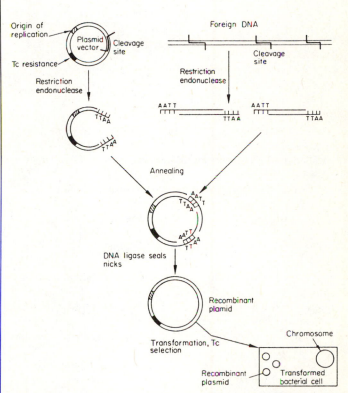

Figure 3-75. Scheme for construction and propagation of a recombinant plasmid.

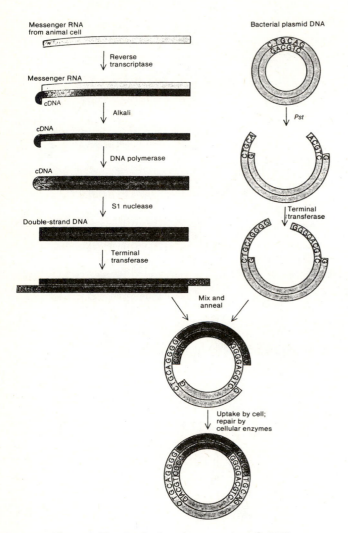

Figure 3-76.   Synthesis and propagation of cDNA.

Isolate DNA and digest with restriction enzyme
↓
Separate restriction fragments by gel electrophoresis
↓
Transfer DNA from gel to a nitrocellulose filter
↓
Incubate filter with radioactive DNA probe
↓
Analyze by autoradiography

The DNA probe is often a cDNA or synthetic oligonucleotide with a sequence complementary to a portion of the gene of interest. Since formation of hybrids depends on the existence of extensive complementarity between the two sequences, it is possible to specifically identify a single unique gene in the total genomic DNA.

One application of this procedure has been for prenatal diagnosis of genetic defects, for example sickle cell anemia. This disease is characterized by the substitution of valine for the usual glutamic acid at position six in the beta chain of hemoglobin. The corresponding alteration in the DNA sequence is a single base change, from CCTGAGG to CCTGTGG.

The normal CCTGAGG sequence is the cleavage site for the restriction enzyme *MstI*, but the mutant sequence is not. The result is that DNA isolated from an individual with the sickle mutation will contain one less *MstI* site in the beta-globin gene region than will normal DNA. If a Southern blot of *MstI*-restricted DNA is analyzed with a probe that is specific for the 5′ end of the beta-globin gene, the mutant DNA will show a larger fragment (because it is missing the restriction site). Results from this type of analysis are shown in Figure 3-77. Similar restriction site polymorphisms serve as the basis for prenatal diagnosis of other diseases.

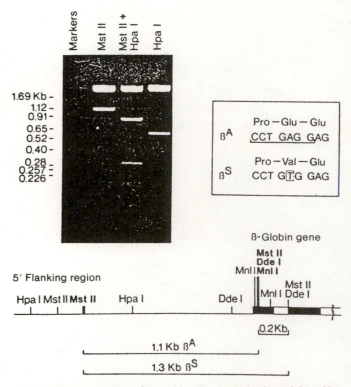

Figure 3-77.   Detection of the sickle cell mutation in beta globin (β^s) by restriction analysis, hybridization, and autoradiography (from Orkin et al: N Engl J Med 307:32–36, 1982).

BIBLIOGRAPHY

Danishefsky I: Biochemistry for Medical Sciences. Little, Brown & Co., Boston, 1980.

Lehninger AL: Principles of Biochemistry. Worth Publishers, New York, 1982.

Montgomery R, Dryer RL, Conway TW, Spector AA: Biochemistry, A Case Oriented Approach. CV Mosby, St. Louis, 1983.

Stryer L: Biochemistry, 2nd ed. WH Freeman, San Francisco, 1981.

McGilvey RL, Goldstein GW: Biochemistry: A Functional Approach, 3rd ed. WB Saunders, Philadelphia, 1983.

Schreiber WE: Medical Aspects of Biochemistry. Little, Brown & Co., 1984.

SAMPLE QUESTIONS

> **DIRECTIONS:** Each question below contains five suggested answers. Choose the **one best** response to each question.

1. In the figure below, the kinetic plots were obtained for an enzyme in the absence of an inhibitor, in the presence of a competitive inhibitor, and in the presence of a noncompetitive inhibitor. The enzyme concentration was the same in all experiments. Which point contains all the information necessary to determine the substrate concentration that will produce half maximal velocity for the competitively inhibited enzyme?

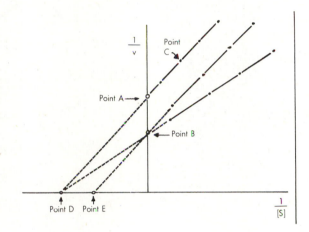

    A. Point A
    B. Point B
    C. Point C
    D. Point D
    E. Point E

2. The enzyme glyceraldehyde 3-phosphate dehydrogenase is inhibited by iodoacetamide. This suggests that one of the important amino acid residues at the active site is

    A. cysteine-SH
    B. serine-OH
    C. aspartate-COOH
    D. tyrosine-OH
    E. hydroxyproline-OH

3. If an animal were exposed to an atmosphere of the heavy isotope of oxygen (^{18}O), in which the following would the heavy oxygen most probably first appear?

    A. ATP
    B. Fatty acids
    C. Glucose
    D. Carbon dioxide
    E. Water

4. Red blood cells do not have mitochondria. As a consequence, they cannot

    A. convert glucose to pyruvate
    B. convert succinate to fumarate

    C. form ribose 5-phosphate from ribulose 5-phosphate
    D. generate ATP
    E. generate NADPH

5. The series of steps involving the conversion of

$$CH_3(CH_2)_8CH_2CH_2C{\nwarrow}^{0}_{SCoA} \quad to \quad CH_3(CH_2)_8C{\nwarrow}^{0}_{SCoA}$$

provides

    A. four ATP
    B. five ATP
    C. six ATP
    D. eight ATP
    E. twelve ATP

6. The number of moles of ATP produced by mitochondrial oxidation of 1 mol of pyruvate to carbon dioxide and water is

    A. 2
    B. 6
    C. 12
    D. 15
    E. 24

7. Free fatty acids released from adipose tissue are transported in the blood bound to

    A. chylomicrons
    B. high-density lipoproteins
    C. low-density lipoproteins
    D. albumin
    E. globulin

8. Unlike liver, muscle can utilize ketone bodies as a source of energy because muscles can convert

    A. acetone to dihydroxyacetone phosphate
    B. ketoses to aldoses
    C. acetoacetate to beta-hydroxybutyrate
    D. acetoacetate to acetoacetyl CoA
    E. acetoacetyl CoA to acetoacetate

9. Reduced NADPH generated in the oxidative pentose pathway is

    A. mostly oxidized by the mitochondrial oxidative chain and thus provides 3 mol of ATP
    B. oxidized by pyruvate, thus yielding lactate
    C. utilized as the reducing agent for the biosynthesis of fatty acids
    D. excreted in the urine
    E. oxidized directly by coenzyme Q

10. ATP is a reactant in the formation of

    A. creatine
    B. glutamine
    C. glutamate
    D. cystathionine
    E. epinephine

11. Linked to its 5' end, each Okazaki fragment is synthesized with a short stretch of

    A. protein

B. RNA
C. DNA
D. carbohydrate
E. fatty acid

12. Choose the correct statement:

A. In the activation of amino acids and formation of aminoacyl tRNA, the carboxyl group of amino acids is linked to the 3'-hydroxyl group of the ribose of the 3'-terminal adenylic acid residue of tRNA.
B. In the activation of amino acids and formation of aminoacyl tRNA, the carboxyl group of amino acids is linked to the 3'-hydroxyl group of the ribose of the 3'-terminal cytidylic acid residue of tRNA.
C. In the activation of amino acids and formation of aminoacyl tRNA, the carboxyl group of amino acids is linked to the 3'-hydroxyl group of the ribose of the 5'-terminal adenylic acid residue of tRNA.
D. In the activation of amino acids and formation of aminoacyl tRNA, the carboxyl group of amino acids is linked to the 3'-hydroxyl group of the ribose of the 5'-terminal cytidylic acid residue of tRNA.
E. None of the above.

13. Given the nucleotide sequence of the DNA template shown as 5'-T-A-C-A-G-C-A-A-A-T-T-T-C-G-A-C-A-T-3', which of the following is true?

(Use the genetic code provided. Assume no peptidase is present.)

First position (5' end)	Second position				Third position (3' end)
	U	C	A	G	
U	Phe	Ser	Tyr	Cys	U
	Phe	Ser	Tyr	Cys	C
	Leu	Ser	Term*	Term*	A
	Leu	Ser	Term*	Trp	G
C	Leu	Pro	His	Arg	U
	Leu	Pro	His	Arg	C
	Leu	Pro	Gln	Arg	A
	Leu	Pro	Gln	Arg	G
A	Ile	Thr	Asn	Ser	U
	Ile	Thr	Asn	Ser	C
	Ile	Thr	Lys	Arg	A
	Met	Thr	Lys	Arg	G
G	Val	Ala	Asp	Gly	U
	Val	Ala	Asp	Gly	C
	Val	Ala	Glu	Gly	A
	Val	Ala	Glu	Gly	G

* Chain-terminating codons.

A. The mRNA will have the sequence 5'-A-U-G-U-C-G-A-A-A-U-U-U-G-C-U-G-U-A-3' and the polypeptide formed will have the sequence N-terminal-met-ser-lys-phe-ala-val-C-terminal.

B. The mRNA will have the sequence 5'-A-U-G-U-C-G-U-U-U-A-A-A-G-C-U-G-U-A-3' and the polypeptide formed will have the sequence N-terminal-met-ser-lys-phe-ala-val-C-terminal.
C. The mRNA will have the same sequence 5'-A-U-G-U-C-G-A-A-A-U-U-U-G-C-U-G-U-A-3' and the polypeptide formed will have the sequence N-terminal-met-ser-phe-lys-ala-val-C-terminal.
D. The mRNA will have the sequence 5'-A-U-G-U-C-G-U-U-U-A-A-A-G-C-U-G-U-A-3' and the polypeptide formed will have the sequence N-terminal-met-ser-lys-phe-ser-met-C-terminal.
E. None of the above.

14. In the figure below, where is the 3' terminus of the *template* strand?

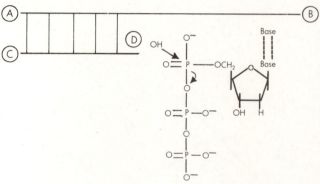

A. Point A
B. Point B
C. Point C
D. Point D
E. At none of the above points

15. All of the following statements about the repressor of the lac operon of *E. coli* are true EXCEPT that the repressor

A. is the product of a regulatory gene
B. binds to the operator region of the DNA of the lac operon
C. is a protein
D. interacts with the operator in such a way as to prevent translation of beta-galactosidase
E. can combine with lactose to form a complex that will no longer bind to the operator region

16. To elongate a nascent polypeptide chain by three amino acids, the number of GTP hydrolyzed is

A. 9
B. 6
C. 12
D. 5
E. none of the above

17. Which of the following sequences is most likely responsible for the *rho-independent* transcriptional termination in prokaryotes?

A. . . . AUUAAAGGCUCCUUUUGGAGCCUUUUUUUUUU-3'
B. . . . AUUAAAGGCUCCUUUUGGAGCCUUUAAAAAAA-3'
C. . . . AUUAAAGGCUCCUUUUGGAGCCUUUCCCCCCC-3'

D. . . . AUUAAAGGCUCCUUUUGGAGCCUUUGGGGGGG-3′
E. . . . AUUAAAGGCUCCUUUUAAAACCCUUUUGGAAA-3′

3. 1,6-diphosphoglucose
4. phosphoenolpyruvic acid

DIRECTIONS: Each question below contains four suggested answers of which **one** or **more** is correct. Choose the answer:

A if 1, 2, and 3 are correct
B if 1 and 3 are correct
C if 2 and 4 are correct
D if 4 is correct
E if 1, 2, 3, and 4 are correct

23. Cofactors in the miltienzyme complex that catalyze the conversion of pyruvate to acetyl-CoA are

1. thiamine pyrophosphate
2. pyridoxal phosphate
3. lipoic acid
4. NADP

18. Choose the correct combination of statements with respect to *E. coli* DNA replication.

1. Synthesis of the RNA primer is catalyzed by RNA polymerase or primase.
2. The $3′ \rightarrow 5′$ exonuclease activity of DNA polymerases is an error-editing mechanism during replication.
3. Of the various DNA polymerases now known, the most probable replicator of DNA in vivo is DNA polymerase III.
4. DNA ligase requires NAD^+ for its enzyme activity.

19. With respect to chromatin structure and function,

1. the nucleosome is a basic structural subunit of chromatin, consisting of a core of 8 histone molecules and 140 base pairs of DNA.
2. HMG proteins are nonhistone proteins that are important for transcriptional regulation.
3. histones are small basic proteins that are rich in lysine or arginine.
4. heterochromatin refers to chromatin regions that are transciptionally active.

20. With respect to signals that are required or that modulate transcription or translation,

1. "TATA" consensus sequence refers to a signal for in vitro synthesis of mRNA precursors.
2. "Enhancers" are promotor signals that may facilitate the entry of RNA polymerase II.
3. RNA polymerase III-directed transcription is characterized by an "intragenic" promoter.
4. A "cap" structure is required for translation of eukaryotic mRNA.

21. Ingested galactose can normally be utilized for the synthesis of glycogen. Reactions required for this purpose are

1. galactose + ATP $\rightarrow$ galactose 1-phosphate
2. galactose 1-phosphate + UDP-glucose $\rightarrow$ UDP-galactose + glucose 1-phosphate
3. UDP-galactose $\rightarrow$ UDP-glucose
4. galactose 1-phosphate $\rightarrow$ glucose 1-phosphate

22. Compounds that transfer their phosphate directly to ADP are

1. glucose 6-phosphate
2. 1,3-diphosphoglyceric acid

DIRECTIONS: The groups of questions below consist of lettered choices followed by several numbered items. For each numbered item, select the **one** lettered choice with which it is **most** closely associated. Each lettered choice may be used once, more than once, or not at all.

Questions 24–28. For each of the following descriptions, choose the associated substance. The same lettered item may be used once, more than once, or not at all.

A. Aldolase
B. Fructose diphosphate phosphatase
C. Glyceraldehyde 3-phosphate dehydrogenase
D. Gluconic acid 6-phosphate dehydrogenase
E. Glucokinase

24. Yields a pentose phosphate

25. Requires ATP

26. Requires NAD^+

27. Requires $NADP^+$

28. Yields triose phosphates

ANSWERS

1. E	11. B	21. A (1, 2, 3)
2. A	12. A	22. D (2, 4)
3. E	13. A	23. B (1, 3)
4. B	14. A	24. D
5. B	15. D	25. E
6. D	16. B	26. C
7. D	17. A	27. D
8. D	18. E (all)	28. A
9. C	19. A (1, 2, 3)	
10. B	20. E (all)	

4

MICROBIOLOGY

Joan Fung-Tomc and Richard C. Tilton

GENERAL

BACTERIAL ANATOMY

Bacteria are **prokaryotes**. They differ from higher biologic forms or eukaryotes in that bacteria lack cellular compartments and organelles. The bacterial cell (Fig. 4-1) consists of a cytoplasm bounded by a cytoplasmic or plasma membrane and usually surrounded by a rigid cell wall. Together, they are referred to as the cell envelope. In some bacteria, a capsule surrounds the entire cell. Capsules are usually composed of polysaccharides, and rarely of polypeptides. In *Bacillus*, the capsule is poly-D-glutamic acid. Capsules protect the bacterium from phagocytosis. Capsular antigens are important in serogrouping organisms. The detection of their presence free in body fluids of infected patients has been used as a rapid diagnostic test for infection.

The **cytoplasm** contains inclusion granules for temporary storage of excess metabolites and ribosomes for protein synthesis. Ribosomes exist both free in the cytoplasm and bound to the cytoplasmic membrane. Occasionally, the cytoplasmic membrane invaginates into the cytoplasm, forming mesosomes, whose function is yet unclear. The nuclear region of bacteria consists of a closed double-stranded DNA (dsDNA). This nuclear body or nucleoid is not separated from the cytoplasm by a nuclear membrane.

Flagella may be present and are responsible for the organism's motility. Flagella may be distributed around the entire cell (peritrichous) or at one or both poles of the cell. The H antigen of *Salmonella* resides on the flagella. The bacterial flagellum is an aggregate of a protein subunit called flagellin. The flagellum is attached to a basal body originating just inside the cytoplasmic membrane.

Thinner filamentous appendages known as pili are seen surrounding many gram-negative bacilli. Somatic pili serve in bacterial adherence to specific host cell receptors. The longer sex pili observed on male (F+ or Hfr) bacterial cells are necessary for conjugation and are the sites for specific bacteriophage attachment.

Under growth conditions with limited nutrients, the gram-positive *Bacillus* and anaerobic *Clostridium* strains form highly resistant spores. When growth conditions become favorable, spores germinate into vegetative cells. Sterilization by steam autoclaving and ethylene oxide gas destroys all microbial forms including spores. Disinfectants used for destroying microbial forms on inanimate objects and antiseptics used on living tissues do not destroy spores.

BACTERIAL CELL ENVELOPE

Bacteria are divided into two groups by their Gram stain characteristics (Fig. 4-2). In the Gram stain, smears are flooded with crystal violet and iodine, decolorized with alcohol, and counterstained with safranine or dilute carbol fuchsin. Gram-positive bacteria retain the crystal violet-iodine complex and are purple, whereas gram-negative bacteria stain red.

The cell walls of these organisms differ. Gram-positive bacterial envelopes contain a thick structure exterior to the

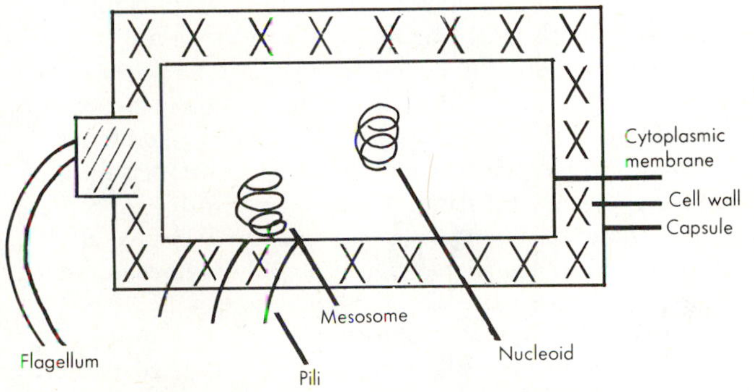

Figure 4-1. A vegetative bacterial cell.

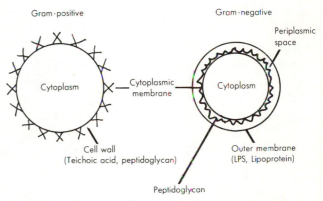

Figure 4-2. Cell envelope of gram-positive and gram-negative bacteria.

257

cytoplasmic membrane. This cell wall contains several layers of peptidoglycan, teichoic acid, and protein. Gram-negative bacterial envelopes, on the other hand, consist of a single layer of peptidoglycan exterior to the cytoplasmic membrane. An outer membrane containing protein, lipoprotein, and lipopolysaccharide (LPS) lies exterior to this layer of peptidoglycan in gram-negative bacteria. Thus, more lipid and protein are present in the cell envelope of gram-negative organisms. The space between the inner and outer membranes of gram-negative bacteria is known as the periplasmic space. Many hydrolytic enzymes including penicillinase reside in this space. In gram-positive bacteria, these enzymes are excreted extracellularly, since there is no outer membrane to retain them.

Peptidoglycan or **murein** functions in giving the bacterium its shape and its osmotic resistance. Its structure consists of a backbone with alternating *N*-acetylglucosamine and *N*-acetylmuramic acid residues, a tetrapeptide substituent, and a peptide bridge. The peptide bridge links GlcNAc-MurNAc strands of the backbone and layers of peptidoglycan, resulting in a giant macromolecular bag. The peptide cross-link of *Staphylococcus aureus* is a pentaglycine (Fig. 4-3).

The biosynthesis of murein was elucidated from the observation that a pentapeptide intermediate with an attached uridine nucleotide (Park nucleotide) accumulated in penicillin-treated bacteria (Fig. 4-4).

The uridine phosphate is cleaved and the MurNAc-pentapeptide is attached to a membrane carrier lipid (undecaprenol-P). The GlcNAc-MurNAc-pentapeptide disaccharide is synthesized and the pentaglycine cross-link introduced by glycyl-tRNA. As the peptidoglycan chain grows, the lipid carrier is removed. (This step is blocked by vancomycin and ristocetin). The terminal D-alanine is displaced during the transpeptidation or peptide cross-linking step.

Transpeptidase displaces the terminal D-alanine and acts as a receptor for the donor amino acid of the branch peptide. Penicillin binds to the transpeptidase, blocking the cross-linkage step in cell wall synthesis. Enzymes that are involved in the terminal reactions of bacterial cell wall synthesis and that bind penicillin are known as penicillin-binding proteins (PBP). PBPs can also be carboxypeptidases and endopeptidases.

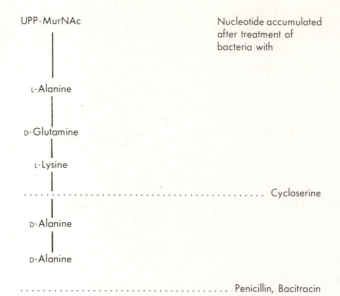

Figure 4-4. Soluble intermediates of peptidoglycan.

Penicillin blocks the transpeptidation reaction, resulting in a weakened structure and an osmotically unstable cell. Since peptidoglycan biosynthesis occurs primarily during active growth of the organism, the effect of penicillin killing is seen with actively growing cells and not with nongrowing or stationary phase cells.

The treatment of bacterial cells with penicillin can give rise to variants lacking cell wall. Unlike protoplasts and spheroplasts (see below), L-forms can grow, though slowly. In the absence of penicillin, L-forms can revert to their normal vegetative cells. Cultivation and reversion of L-forms can best be accomplished in hypertonic medium. L-forms have been suggested as a possible cause of persistent infections such as pyelonephritis and endocarditis. A class of organisms that lacks cell wall and is pathogenic is the mycoplasmas. Due to the absence of a cell wall, L-form and mycoplasmas are not killed by penicillins nor are they susceptible to other inhibitors of cell wall synthesis.

Lysozyme, an enzyme found in phagocytic lysosomal granules, hydrolyzes the peptidoglycan backbone, resulting in an osmotically unstable cell. Gram-positive bacteria are more susceptible to lysozyme than gram-negative bacteria, since lysozyme is excluded from entering the periplasmic space by the outer membrane of gram-negative bacteria. Bacteria treated with lysozyme become osmotically sensitive spheres. These spheres or protoplasts arising from the treatment of gram-positive bacteria contain a cytoplasm bounded by a cytoplasmic membrane. Gram-negative bacteria whose outer membrane is damaged prior to lysozyme treatment give rise to spheroplasts with both cytoplasmic and outer membranes.

As with all biologic membranes, both the cytoplasmic and outer membranes consist of a lipid bilayer with hydrophilic polar regions and long, hydrophobic lipid chains of the phospholipids being aligned. The lipophilic regions of membrane proteins associate with the lipid region.

The cytoplasmic membrane is involved in transport (either by facilitated diffusion or by active transport), DNA replication, and biosynthesis of cell envelope components. It also contains

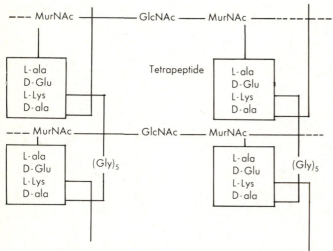

Figure 4-3. Peptidoglycan of *Staphyloccus aureus*.

the complete electron transport system and is therefore analogous to mitochondria found in eukaryotes.

The outer membrane acts as a sieve for small molecules. It also contains specific transport proteins or receptors for larger molecules. **LPS** or **endotoxin** is a molecule unique to the outer leaflet of the outer membrane (Fig. 4-5). It is composed of a lipid A portion responsible for its endotoxic properties and a polysaccharide portion responsible for its antigenicity. The somatic (O) antigen serogrouping of *Salmonella* is based on its LPS. In *Salmonella*, the LPS contains a constant core region of five sugars. O-specific side chains are added to this core. *Salmonella* strains lacking the O side chains do not agglutinate with O-specific antisera and are known as rough (R) mutants. Strains containing the O side chains contain smooth (S) LPS. The outer membrane also contains lipoprotein (Lipoprotein exists in two forms: free lipoprotein and that linking peptidoglycan to the outer membrane, known as bound lipoprotein).

As LPS is unique to gram-negative bacterial, **teichoic acid** is unique to gram-positive bacteria. Teichoic acid exists as either wall teichoic acid or membrane teichoic acid (also known as lipoteichoic acid). Teichoic acid is made up of a backbone consisting of repeating units of glycerol phosphate or ribitol phosphate. Lipoteichoic acid has been shown to be an inhibitor of the autolytic system, which is involved in cell wall biosynthesis and cell death. Monitoring antibody levels to teichoic acid has been used to differentiate between a transient versus deep-seated *S. aureus* infection (e.g., endocarditis and osteomyelitis). Teichoic acid is also the group carbohydrate of group D streptococci.

BACTERIAL CLASSIFICATION

Classification (taxonomy) is an orderly arrangement of bacteria into groups. Terminologies used in classification are as follows:

Family: A group of closely related genera. The family name usually consists of the name of its earliest genus plus the suffix acae.

Genus: A group of closely related species.

Species: A group of bacterial strains with certain dominant characteristics in common.

For example, the species *Escherichia coli* belongs to the genus *Escherichia* and to the family *Enterobacteriaceae*.

Bacteria are classified phenotypically by biochemical reactions and other characteristics. They are grouped by their DNA relatedness. This includes the genome size, the guanine-plus-cytosine (G+C) content, and DNA-DNA homology. The homology of DNA sequences between two different bacteria is determined by their degree of DNA-DNA hybridization under a variety of reassociation conditions. Double-stranded DNA is thermally denatured into single strands. The single strands of two closely related bacteria will have many similar sequences,

and complementary sequences will hybridize under a lower optimal temperature.

The phenotypic characteristics important in bacterial taxonomy include their morphology (Fig. 4-6), Gram-staining property, growth requirements, and biochemical properties.

MICROBIAL METABOLISM

The metabolic energy of bacteria needed for growth can be provided in a number of ways. Central to this is adenosine triphosphate (ATP). ATP is generated by the phosphorylation of adenosine diphosphate (ADP) through high-energy intermediates. This is accomplished by **fermentation,** when organic compounds serve as electron donors and acceptors, and by **oxidation,** when oxygen is the ultimate electron acceptor.

The major pathway of glucose fermentation is **glycolysis.** A net of two ATP molecules are generated with lactate as the end product. The overall equation for glycolysis is

$$\text{Glucose} + 2 \text{ ADP} + 2 \text{ Pi} \rightarrow 2 \text{ lactic acid} + 2 \text{ ATP} + 2 \text{ H}_2\text{O}$$

Fermentation can proceed in the absence of oxygen; it is how anaerobic organisms obtain energy. Facultative anaerobes (i.e., those that can grow either in the presence or absence of oxygen) ferment under anaerobic conditions. Glycolysis refers to conversion of glucose to lactate and the Embden-Meyerhof pathway, usually of glucose to pyruvate (Fig. 4-7). Glycolysis is homolactic fermentation. Other types of anaerobic fermentation can occur in microorganisms: heterolactic fermentation with end products of lactic acid, ethanol, and carbon dioxide; alcoholic fermentation with ethanol end products; and mixed-acid fermentation. Anaerobes can also ferment amino acids (Stickland reaction).

Respiration is the energy-yielding metabolic process in which a series of compounds serves to transport electrons to molecular oxygen. In respiration, acetyl CoA derived from oxidation of carbohydrates, fatty acids, and amino acids enters into the tricarboxylic acid (TCA or Krebs) cycle (Fig. 4-8). The resulting end product of each molecule of acetyl CoA is the reduction of three molecules of nicotinamide adenine dinucleo-

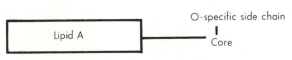

Figure 4-5. Lipopolysaccharide.

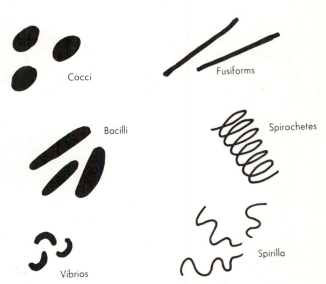

Figure 4-6. Bacterial morphologies.

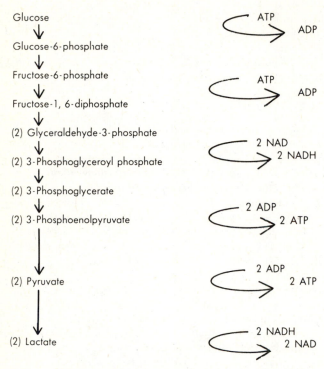

Figure 4-7. Glycolysis (Embden-Meyerhof pathway).

tide (NAD^+) and one molecule of flavin adenine dinucleotide (FAD). The NADH and $FADH_2$ (reduced forms) are fed into the electron transport chain (Fig. 4-9). Thus for each molecule of glucose, two pyruvate molecules are generated and are converted into two molecules of acetyl CoA. Respiration of one molecule of glucose results in 10 NADH, 2 $FADH_2$, 6 CO_2, and 6 H_2O. Thus an equivalent of 36 ATP molecules is generated in glucose oxidation.

The glyoxylate cycle is a modification of the TCA cycle. It converts fatty acids to carbohydrates. Two acetyl CoA residues are converted to succinate, which may be used for the synthesis of new carbohydrate.

BACTERIAL REPLICATION

Bacteria can multiply or double in cell mass quickly. The doubling time of *E. coli*, for instance, is 20 minutes. After *n* number of generations, the number of bacteria present is 2^n. The bacterial growth curve can be divided into four phases (Fig. 4-10):

1. Lag phase, when the bacteria have to adjust to their new growth conditions.
2. Log (logarithmic or exponential) phase, when the bacterial growth is maximal.
3. Stationary phase, when growth stops due to the lack of nutrients.
4. Death phase, when cells lyse.

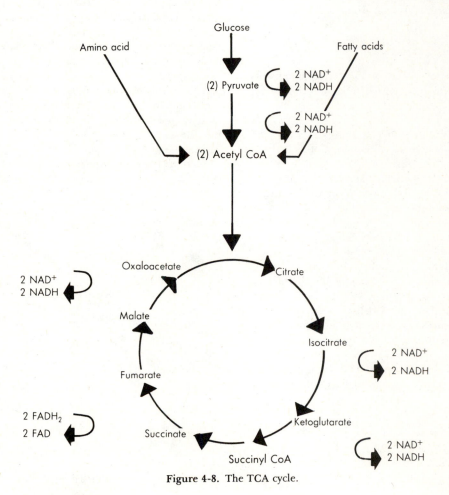

Figure 4-8. The TCA cycle.

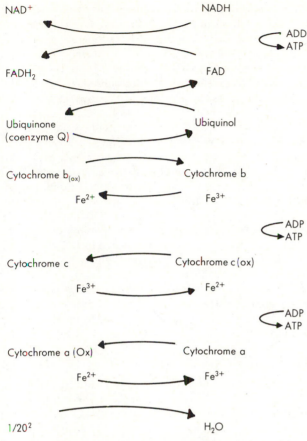

Figure 4-9. The electron transport chain.

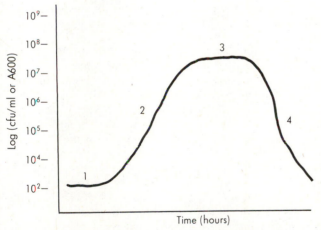

Figure 4-10. The bacterial growth curve. (1) Lag phase; (2) log phase; (3) stationary phase; (4) death phase.

DNA carries the genetic information. A DNA strand is a chain of nucleotides composed of adenine (A), guanine (G), cytosine (C), and thymine (T) bases. The two strands of DNA are complementary: A pairs with T, G with C. The sequence of nucleotides specifies the amino acid sequence of proteins. DNA is transcribed by RNA polymerase to RNA, which is complementary to one of the DNA chains. In RNA, T is replaced by uracil (U). There are three types of **RNA**: ribosomal

RNA (rRNA), transfer RNA (tRNA), and messenger RNA (mRNA). In bacteria, there is one RNA polymerase. In eukaryotes, there are three RNA polymerases, which are responsible for making the primary transcripts of rRNA (type I RNA polymerase), mRNA (type II), and tRNA (type III). RNA polymerase binds to the promoter region of DNA about 20 to 30 nucleotides upstream (in the 5' direction) of the TATAAT sequence (Pribnow box). The Pribnow box and a second consensus sequence, TGTTGACA, are critical for initiation of transcription. RNA transcription occurs in the 5' to 3' direction. At the 5' end of mRNA is a cap consisting of a methylated guanine nucleotide. Transcription terminates either by aid of a specific protein, rho factor (rho-dependent termination) or by rho-independent sites containing self-complementary regions, which form "hairpin" structures. In bacteria, **transcription and translation** (RNA-directed protein synthesis) occur simultaneously. In eukaryotes, transcription occurs in the nucleus and translation in the cytoplasm. The primary RNA transcript in the nucleus may be greater in length than the mature RNA in the cytoplasm. RNA processing occurs in the nucleus, with removal (splicing) of spacer sequences (introns) from the expressed transcript (exons). Messenger RNA transported to the cytoplasm contains poly (A) tail at its 3' end. The poly (A) tail appears to protect mRNA from enzymatic degradation in the cytoplasm. The poly (A) tail has enabled scientists to isolate eukaryotic mRNA with columns containing poly (T) sequences.

Gene expression is most often regulated at the level of transcription. Transcription may be regulated by proteins (repressors), which may inhibit it by binding at or near the promotor region, thus preventing RNA polymerase binding to the promotor region. The repressor binding site is known as the operator; the operator and promotor sequences often overlap. On the other hand, some molecules (inducers) may enhance transcription. Inducers may interact with repressors so as to detach them from the operator and thus allow RNA polymerase to bind. In some instances, a repressor may only bind to the operator in the presence of a second molecule (co-repressor). The control of gene expression may often involve both repressor and inducer regulatory effects.

Genes that encode functions in a common pathway or function are often clustered; this is especially true in bacteria. This cluster of genes (known as an **operon**) is often under the control of a common promotor. The mRNA synthesized is polycistronic (i.e., it contains the message for several functional proteins). The polycistronic mRNA, however, contains a different ribosome binding site, start codon, and stop codon for translation of each cistron.

A well-studied operon is the lactose operon, which encodes three proteins. In the repressed state, the repressor binds to the operator, preventing the transcription of Z, Y, and A genes. In the induced state, lactose interacts with the repressor, disabling its binding to the operator, and the polycistronic mRNA is transcribed (Fig. 4-11). Actually, the lactose operon also has a positive control. A catabolite activator protein (CAP) interacts with cyclic AMP (which is formed in high concentration during glucose starvation). This CAP-cyclic AMP complex binds to the DNA near the promotor region to facilitate the binding of RNA polymerase.

Translation of mRNA into proteins involves all three RNA: mRNA containing the genetic information, rRNA involved as

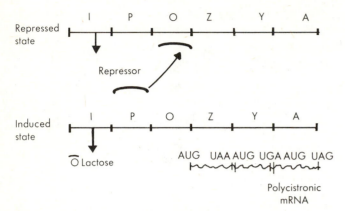

Figure 4-11. Lactose operon (Jacob-Monod). I = gene encoding repressor; P = promotor; O = operator; Y = permease gene; A = tranacetylase gene; AUG = start condon; UAA, UGA, UAG = stop condons; ⌒ repressor (binds to operator); ⌒⊙ repressor with lactose (cannot bind to operator); Z = galactosidase gene.

components of the ribosome, and tRNA for decoding mRNA via base pairing codon-anticodon interaction. There are several different (40 or more) tRNA species, each specific for one amino acid. A single amino acid may be translated by more than one codon. A codon is a nucleotide triplet on mRNA, and an anticodon is the complementary tRNA nucleotides. In addition, AUG is a start (initiation signal) codon; AUG codes for methionine, so all proteins begin with methionine. Stop (termination) codons are UAA, UGA, and UAG. As the ribosome moves down the mRNA (5' to 3'), an amino acid is added onto the growing polypeptide chain via recognition of the genetic code by aminoacyl-tRNAs.

DNA replication begins with initiation of DNA synthesis at the origin. Bacterial chromosome has one initiation site and eukaryotes, several origins of DNA synthesis. DNA synthesis moves bidirectionally as growing forks from the origin, with both strands being copied. On one of the two DNA strands, DNA replication occurs with synthesis of a leading strand, while the opposite strand consists of a lagging strand (Fig. 4-12). DNA replication is semiconservative, with a daughter DNA strand pairing with one of the parental DNA strand. The classic experiment demonstrating semiconservative DNA replication (the Meselson and Stahl experiment) used N^{15}-labeled nucleotides. The N^{15}-labeled parent strands were used as templates for synthesis of daughter strands that incorporated N^{14} (light)-deoxyribonucleotide precursors. The DNA, after one and two DNA doubling times, was banded into CsCl, and

the resulting profile showed disappearance of heavy (N^{15}-N^{15}) band with synthesis of daughter DNA strands. Thus N^{15}-N^{14} band appeared after one round of DNA replication and N^{14}-N^{14} band appeared after a second round of DNA replication.

The supercoiled DNA is unwound by **topoisomerases**, which nick DNA to relieve the coil and subsequently reseal the nick. Topoisomerase I nicks one of the two DNA strands, whereas topoisomerase II nicks dsDNA. Topoisomerase II (also known as gyrase in bacteria) consists of two subunits that can be differentially inhibited by coumermycin and quinolones. There are three DNA polymerases: In *E. coli*, they are I, II, and III; in eukaryotes they are alpha (nucleus associated), beta (nucleus and cytoplasm), and gamma (mitochondria associated). DNA polymerase I and III have 5' → 3' exonuclease activity necessary to remove RNA primers. DNA polymerases can only synthesize DNA in the presence of preexisting RNA primers. The RNA primers are synthesized by RNA primases. Deoxynucleotides are added onto the 3' end of RNA primers. DNA synthesis occurs in the 5' → 3' direction. The DNA chains with RNA are called Okazaki fragments. As the DNA polymerase approaches a second Okazaki fragment, the RNA primer on this second fragment is removed by the polymerase and the DNA segments joined by ligases.

BACTERIAL GENETICS

Bacterial genetic information may be transferred by one of three ways: transformation, conjugation, or transduction. **Transformation** is the uptake of naked DNA by competent bacteria. Transformation was first demonstrated in *Streptococcus pneumoniae* when uptake of DNA from smooth (S) cells transformed rough (R) cells to the S type. Pneumococci with the S type are encapsulated and virulent in mice, whereas the R type is not. Transformation can occur with cells exposed to $CaCl_2$, making them more permeable to DNA; this is also known as **transfection.**

Conjugation occurs between a male (F^+ or Hfr) bacterium and a female (F^-) bacterium. The F^+ cells contain a sex (F) factor, which is plasmid mediated. The F plasmid may be integrated into the bacterial chromosome, which increases the F^+ strain's ability to recombine with F^- (known as high-frequency recombination [Hfr]). The transfer of genetic material in conjugation occurs through the sex pilus of the F^+, which attaches to the F^- cell. In Hfr strains, transfer of genetic material starts at a specific locus (origin of transfer). Bacterial genes are transferred in conjugation. The proximity of these genes to the origin of transfer determines their likelihood of being transferred. The transfer may be interrupted by mechanical agitation; thus gene locations relative to the origin of transfer and to each other may be mapped with conjugation.

Transduction occurs via a bacteriophage. Transducing phages may be generalized (transfer any gene in the bacterial chromosome) or specialized (transfer specific regions of the bacterial chromosome). Thus genes that cotransduce lie close together on the chromosome. Transduction is used for mapping chromosomal genes.

RECOMBINANT TECHNOLOGY

The cloning of a specific gene involves the cleavage of DNA fragments from the chromosome or plasmid. This cleavage is

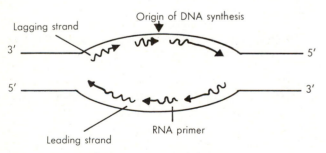

Figure 4-12. DNA replication.

achieved by either physically shearing the DNA or cleavage with restriction endonucleases. Restriction endonucleases are enzymes that cleave DNA at sequence-specific sites. Restriction enzymes may cleave DNA to give fragments with sticky ends (staggered ends with complementary sequences). These foreign DNA fragments are then attached to cloning vehicles. Cloning vehicles or vectors can replicate extrachromosomally. Vectors may be plasmid or bacteriophage. Foreign DNA fragments and vector DNA cleaved with the same restriction enzyme will have the same complementary sequences, allowing these ends to hybridize. The two DNAs are sealed and stabilized by ligase. The plasmid and bacteriophage are then introduced into a host cell such as *E. coli*. The cells that are transfected are selected, usually with antibiotic-resistance markers constructed into the plasmid. Genomic libraries can be constructed. The clone carrying a specific gene of interest may be screened for a functional activity, for antigenic properties, or with a nucleic acid probe.

HOST-PARASITE INTERACTION

The identification of the etiologic agent of disease is based on Koch's postulates. These postulates specify that

1. The agent must be present in every case of the disease.
2. The agent must be isolated from the diseased host and grown in pure culture.
3. The specific disease must be reproduced when a pure culture of the agent is inoculated into a healthy susceptible host.
4. The agent must be recoverable once again from the experimental infected host.

Disease may occur either by invasion of host cells by the microorganism or by exotoxins produced by the organisms. The ability of the microorganism to produce disease depends in part on its virulence and in part on the host's susceptibility to infection by the particular pathogen. Host factors may involve age of the host, race, and nutritional state. Microorganisms that may not produce disease in a healthy host but in one with altered immune status are known as an **opportunistic pathogens**. Host response to infection to eliminate the infecting pathogen is dependent on successful mounting of an immune response, which may be aided with antimicrobial therapy. Likewise, immunity to infection may sometimes be acquired by passive immunity or by active immunization against the specific microorganism. Passive immunity may be acquired by vertical transmission of immunoglobulins from mother to fetus, which protects the newborn during the first few months of life. Passive immunity against specific toxins or viruses can be acquired by administration of serum containing antibodies to these agents. The immunity acquired by passive immunity is short-lived (depends on the half-life of the acquired immunoglobulin in the recipient), whereas active immunity is long-lived. Active immunity may be mounted by immunization with an inactivated killed microorganism, an attenuated strain of the organism, a partially purified or purified extract of the organism, or peptides produced from cloned sequences of the microorganism.

IMMUNOLOGY OF INFECTIOUS DISEASES

IMMUNE SYSTEM

The immune system protects the host from offending microorganisms. It is composed of two arms: humoral immunity and cellular immunity. The lymphocyte class of **B cells** initiates the humoral immune response. B cells are activated by foreign antigens and transform into antibody-secreting plasma cells. **T-cell lymphocytes** mediate cellular immune response. The T-lymphocytes are dependent on the thymus for their maturation. B-lymphocytes (analogous to those derived from the bursa of Fabricius in birds) are independent of the thymus for their development; in mammals, the bursa function is replaced with liver, spleen, and bone marrow. T cells constitute 80% of peripheral lymphocytes, and B cells 20%.

An antigen can be immunogenic if it mounts an immune response, or it can be nonimmunogenic. Nonimmunogenic antigens (i.e., **haptens**) can stimulate immune response when covalently attached to a carrier molecule.

IMMUNOGLOBULINS

Antibodies are proteins belonging to one of several classes of immunoglobulins (Ig). The basic immunoglobulin structure consists of four polypeptides: two identical heavy (higher molecular weight) chains and two identical light chains. The carboxyl (C) terminus of the Ig molecule contains the constant region. The two C-terminal halves of the two heavy chains (Fc region) contain binding sites for complement and protein A. The amino (N) terminal of the heavy and light chains (Fab region) contains the variable region (the region where amino acid sequences widely vary for different antibodies) and the antigenic binding site (Fig. 4-13). There are five classes of immunoglobulins (Table 4-1), which differ in their heavy-chain constant regions. The five heavy chains, designated gamma, alpha, mu, delta, and epsilon, belong to immunoglobulin classes IgG, IgA, IgM, IgD, and IgE, respectively. Similarly, within heavy-chain classes, there are subdivisions into subclasses as IgG1, IgG2, IgG3, and IgG4. There are two types of light chains: kappa (K) and lambda (λ). The constant and variable regions of Ig are encoded by two separate genes, which are joined together for antibody synthesis. The genes for the constant and variable regions of immunoglobulin are not

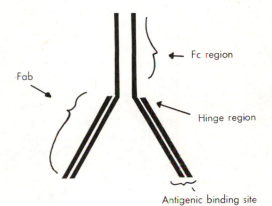

Figure 4-13. Structure of IgG molecule.

Table 4-1. Characteristics of Immunoglobulin Classes

	IgG	IgM	IgA	IgD	IgE
Sedimentation constant	7S	19S	7S (serum) 11S (mucosal sites)	7S	8S
Heavy chain	gamma	mu	alpha	delta	epsilon
Serum concentration (mg/100 ml)	1,000– 1,500	60–180	100–400	3–5	0.03
Half-life in serum (days)	23	5	6	3	2.5

contiguous. During B-lymphocyte differentiation, the two regions move closer together and form a single transcription unit (i.e., translocation). The nuclear RNA transcribed is processed to mRNA. The excised regions are introns, and the expressed regions exons. Thus a single heavy-chain variable gene can exist with a number of heavy-chain constant regions to form immunoglobulin molecules of different classes (IgM, IgG, IgA) but with the same specificity.

The rearrangement of a variable gene with constant genes of the heavy chain allows for the "heavy-chain switch" observed in B cells. This switch is observed during B-cell maturation: Bursal cells frequently contain both IgM and IgG classes, whereas individual peripheral plasma cells contain only a single major class of Ig. In addition, this switch is observed from primary (IgM) to secondary (IgG) immune response. Some specific characteristics of the different immunoglobulin classes are as follows:

1. IgG can pass through the placenta.
2. IgG and IgM can fix complement.
3. IgA has two forms. At the mucosal surfaces, IgA molecules containing a J chain and a secretory component are produced. This is known as secretory IgA.
4. IgM is a pentamer. It has five units and one J chain. It is the earliest antibody synthesized in primary response to an antigen.

LYMPHOCYTES

On its surface, each lymphocyte has specific receptors for an antigenic determinant. During lymphocyte transformation (blast transformation), the antigen binding stimulates proliferation and differentiation of the cells. Lymphocyte differentiation leads to effector cells and memory cells. Memory cells are responsible for immunologic memory of prior antigenic exposure. Subsequent exposures to an antigen result in rapid and heightened secondary response with production of specific antibodies and effector T cells. The end product of B-lymphocyte differentiation is a plasma cell. B cells have surface Ig molecules identical in specificity with those secreted when they differentiate into plasma cells. These surface Ig molecules differentiate B cells from T cells, which lack Ig on their surface. B-lymphocytes interact with antigen via these specific receptor molecules. T-lymphocytes can differentiate into

1. Cytotoxic T cells, which destroy foreign cells directly.
2. T_h, helper T cells, for B-cell differentiation and proliferation.
3. T_s, suppressor T cells for suppressing immune response.

Since T cells are antigen specific, they too have receptor molecules analogous to the membrane-bound Ig of B cells. The receptor consists of two subunits (alpha and beta); each chain contains a constant and a variable domain.

T-cell recognition of antigen also requires the presentation of this antigen on a cell with self major histocompatibility complex (MHC) proteins.

MHC proteins are involved in tissue-graft rejections. MHC proteins are either class I or class II. The class I protein is a single glycopeptide associated with $beta_2$-microglobulin. Class II molecules consist of two chains (alpha and beta). Class I molecules are involved in cytoxic T-cell antigen recognition, class II molecules with T_h and T_s recognition of antigen. T4 cells bear surface antigen OKT4, Leu3; T8 cells bear OKT8, Leu2. These specific T-cell markers are identified by monoclonal antibodies, and the nomenclatures used are adopted from those assigned by manufacturers of commercial kits.

PHAGOCYTES

Another group of cells important in host defense are phagocytes. Phagocytes represent the nonspecific element of immunity; lymphocytes are antigen-specific cells. There are two types of phagocytes: polymorphonuclear leukocytes (PMN), also known as neutrophils, and the mononuclear phagocytes (including blood monocytes and their differentiated end-stage successor, the macrophage, fixed in tissues). Neutrophils have a multilobed nucleus and cellular granules. These granules contain lytic enzymes as well as nondigestive enzymes (e.g., myeloperoxidase). The blood monocytes have an indented, kidney-shaped nucleus and granules. They have surface receptors for the Fc portion of IgG and complement component C3b. Monocytes can be differentiated into macrophages in tissues. Macrophages are like monocytes in their surface receptors for IgG and C3b. Macrophages can be activated by bacterial LPS and lymphokines released from activated T cells. Lymphokines are mediators produced by T cells, which recruit and activate macrophages to the site of T-cell interaction with antigen. These lymphokines also inhibit the departure of these cells from the site. Some lymphokines are migration inhibitory factor (MIF), macrophage activation factor (MAF), monocyte chemotactic factor (MCF), lymphotoxin, interferon, and transfer factor. Activated macrophages have increased opsonin-mediated phagocytic capabilities. Phagocyte recognition of foreign particles includes hydrophobicity, opsonin, and other factors. Microbial death can result from digestion within the phagocyte through fusion of intracellular granules with phagosome or via the production of hydrogen peroxide (H_2O_2). An intermediate of H_2O_2 production is the highly reactive free radical superoxide anion (O_2^-). H_2O_2 and O_2^- are bactericidal, but in neutrophils and monocytes, the major H_2O_2 and halide ions (I^-, Cl^-), myeloperoxidase generates strong oxidizing agents as hypochlorus acid (HOCl). The activated halide attaches to peptide bonds, leading to cleavage of these bonds. In addition, superoxides formed from H_2O_2 during phagocytosis are also toxic to bacteria.

IMMUNE RESPONSE

The immune response begins with processing (alteration) of the antigen by accessory cells (macrophages) for presentation to T- and B-lymphocytes in the lymphoid organs. Antigen-triggered lymphocytes proliferate and differentiate in the lymph node, with resulting concomitant morphological changes in the node. The lymph node can be divided into three general areas: the germinal center (outer cortical lymphoid region), the paracortial area (deep cortical area), and the medulla. B cells migrate to the germinal center and medulla, whereas T cells remain in the paracortical area. The medulla of a stimulated node contains numerous plasma cells that actively secrete antibodies. The memory and effector T cells and memory B cells eventually reenter the general circulation after antigenic stimulation.

The B-cell response to an antigen is heterogeneous, with antibodies produced being of different classes (IgM, IgG, IgA, IgD, IgE), of different affinity, and to different antigenic determinants (epitopes) on the antigen. A given plasma cell secretes only one class of antibody. IgM is the first antibody produced in response (primary immunization) to an antigen. It is a pentamer with 10 antigenic binding sites: This makes IgM effective in cross-linking antigens and in agglutination assays. IgG is produced in subsequent immune response (secondary immunization) to the antigen. It is a monomer. Both IgM and IgG fix complement. IgA can exist as a monomer, dimer, or trimer. Secretory components produced by some epithelial cells bind to the Fc portion of IgA to facilitate their secretion into the GI tract, saliva, sweat, milk, and tears. IgE exists as a monomer. It binds via its Fc portion to the surface of mast cells. Interaction of IgE with antigen activates mast cells, with resulting degranulation (exocytosis of granules containing heparin and histamine).

Antibodies eliminate foreign antigens and cells by several mechanisms:

1. Antibody binding to adhesins may prevent adherence of microbe to host cells. This could prevent microbial colonization or invasion of host cells.
2. Antibody binding to microbial toxins or other microbial products could neutralize their effect.
3. Coating of antigens or microbes with IgG and IgM stimulates their ingestion by phagocytes.

4. IgM and IgG binding to antigens can activate complement. Complement (C8 and C9) can induce cell membrane lesions, subsequent cell lysis, and cell death. Complement (C3b) binding to antigen-antibody complexes enhances phagocytosis. Other complement components (C3a, C5a, C5b-C6-C7 complex) can also initiate a localized inflammatory reaction. The complement system is composed of a group of at least 21 serum proteins, representing up to 15% of the total serum globulin. They migrate in the alpha, beta, and gamma regions on electrophoresis. These proteins interact in a sequential pathway, resulting in cleavage and biologic activation of complement components. There are two complement systems, which share much of the same pathway: The classic pathway is triggered by immune complexes, and the alternate or properdin pathway is activated by a wide range of substances (LPS, toxins, aggregated IgA). Complement components interact in precusor or proenzyme forms, the resulting cleavage yielding components with biologic activities (Table 4-2).
5. IgE antibodies bind to mast cells and basophils, causing cell degranulation and release of histamine and other mediators.

Mast cells are most numerous along the respiratory and GI tracts and under the skin, where IgE is predominantly formed. Basophils account for 0.5 to 2% of circulating white blood cells (WBCs). Mediators released by mast cells and basophils include histamine, slow-reacting substance of anaphylaxis (SRS-A), eosinophil chemotactic factor of anaphylaxis (ECF-A), serotonin, platelet aggregating factor, heparin, and bradykinin. Histamine causes smooth muscle contraction with a 10-minute duration of action. SRS-A has a longer time effect (hours) on smooth muscle contraction. ECF-A release causes an influx of eosinophils into the area of allergic inflammation, which in turn disposes of antigen-IgE antibody complexes. Bradykinin release from mast cells causes slow sustained contraction of smooth muscles, increased vascular permeability, and increased secretion by mucous glands. The physiological roles of these mediators in the defense against injury is first by causing inflammation and then by stimulating tissue repair.

Table 4-2. Biologic Activities of Complement Components

Components	Biologic Activities
C1, C3, C2	Viral neutralization
C4b, C3b	Immune adherence
C3a, C5a	Chemotatic activity for PMNs Anaphylatoxin
C3b	Immune clearance
C5	Opsonization of yeast
C2	Kinin-like substance
C5b-C9	Lysis

In intestinal parasitic nematode infections, high IgE levels are present. It is believed that the release of mediators results in leakage of serum proteins (including specific IgG and IgM antibodies against the parasite) from the intestinal blood vessels and is involved in eliminating the parasite from the intestine.

Though antibodies may be produced to antigens containing repeating, identical antigenic determinants (e.g., bacterial polysaccharides) independent of T cells, most humoral immune responses to antigens require T cells. T_h-cell response to antigen presented by macrophage results in its activation and subsequent stimulation of specific B cells. T_s cells are also generated by antigenic stimulants to suppress immune response. Lymphokines released from T cells attract and activate macrophages. The end process of cellular and humoral immunity results in removal of the antigen.

LABORATORY DIAGNOSIS

DIRECT SPECIMEN EXAMINATION

Patient specimens can be examined directly for the presence of microorganisms. This may be accomplished by microscopy of stained smears of the specimen, by detection of microbial antigen in the specimen, or by detection of microbial nucleic acid in the specimen.

The Gram stain differentiates between gram-negative (red) versus gram-positive (purple) bacteria. The size and shape of the organism may also be obtained by smear examination. In the Gram stain, the smear is first stained with crystal violet, rinsed with water, flooded with Gram's iodine, rinsed again with water, decolorized with acetone-alcohol, and then counterstained with safranine. Mycobacteria are stained with acid-fast stain. (For more detail, refer to the section on *Mycobacterium*.) *Nocardia* is partially acid fast. Treponemes from chancres can be examined by dark-field microscopy. In dark-field microscopy, a substage dark-field condenser that prevents any light rays from entering the microscope straight upward from the light source is used; thus all rays from the light source enter the objective lens only through reflections from particles (such as spirochetes) in the specimen. As a result, the spirochetes are brightly illuminated against a black field. Direct fluorescent antibody stains using fluorescein-labeled antibodies directly against specific bacteria and viruses can be useful in detecting these agents in clinical specimens.

Specific microbial antigens can be detected by a number of methods including enzyme-linked immunosorbent assay (ELISA), counterimmunoelectrophoresis (CIE), latex agglutination, and coagglutination. ELISA assays can have several formats. However, a typical ELISA assay for detecting microbial antigen may involve a solid support (e.g., microtiter plate) that has antibodies to a specific antigen absorbed on its surface. The test sample is added to the microtiter well, followed by washings to remove nonattached material in the test sample. A second antibody (either the same as the first antibody adhering to the solid support or an antibody against a different epitope on the antigen) is added. This second antibody is labeled with an enzyme. Binding of the second antibody to the antigen is detected by the addition of a substrate that generates either a visible color, fluoresces, or chemiluminesces when cleaved. In CIE, the test specimen for detection of antigen is placed in a

cathodic well and the antiserum in an anodic well. Electrophoresis drives the antigen and antibody toward each other. A precipitin line in the agarose is formed at the region containing optimum proportion of antigen and antibody. In latex agglutination, antibodies are attached to polystyrene latex particles, which agglutinate in the presence of homologous antigen. In coagglutination, protein A-containing *S. aureus* cells bind antibodies of the IgG class; the antibody-coated *S. aureus* agglutinates in the presence of homologous antigen. Microbial nucleic acids in specimens may be detected by DNA or complementary DNA (cDNA) probes. cDNA are DNA sequences synthesized from an RNA (i.e., mRNA) template with the use of reverse transcriptase. These probes contain specific sequences present in the microbe. Test sample is first treated under conditions (e.g., high temperatures) to denature dsDNA. The DNA probe is then added, and under renaturing conditions, some of the probe will hybridize with complementary DNA sequences in the test sample. Hybridization is detected by the use of radiolabeled or enzyme-labeled DNA probes.

CULTIVATION

The isolation media for bacteria and fungi can be categorized as selective or nonselective media. A selective growth medium may contain antibiotics or other agents that selectively inhibit some microorganisms and not others. An example of a selective medium is MacConkey agar, which selectively grows gram-negative bacteria. On the other hand, sheep blood agar and chocolate agar are nonselective growth media. The use of a selective medium often depends on the clinical specimen; specimens that contain normal flora often are plated onto a selective isolation medium. In contrast, specimens such as CSF or those that are normally sterile are plated onto a nonselective medium. In addition, an isolation medium can also be a differential medium. The colony morphology of a bacterium on differential medium may be a helpful clue to its identity. For example, lactose fermenters form pink colonies on MacConkey agar, but nonfermenters grow as clear colonies. Specimens that contain flora should be plated by the pure culture technique for single-colony isolation (Fig. 4-14). In most instances, a specimen is plated onto several isolation media. Depending on the pathogens anticipated from different body sites, the plates are incubated either aerobically, anaerobically, and/or in the presence of 5 to 10% carbon dioxide (microaerophilic condition). In most cases, bacteria can be isolated within 1 to 2 days; other microbes (viruses and fungi) may require longer incubation.

Anaerobes make up a large portion of the indigenous bacterial flora of the skin and of the mucosal areas of the body (colon, oral cavity, and vaginal tract). As a general rule, specimens from sites that would normally contain anaerobes

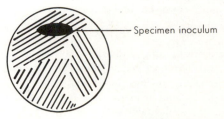

Specimen inoculum

Figure 4-14. Pure culture technique (3-part streak).

should not be cultured for anaerobic organisms. These include urine, sputum, feces, and swabs of the throat, vagina, and cervix. An exception is the culture of *C. difficile* from stools. However, *C. difficile*-associated disease is best diagnosed by the detection of *C. difficile* toxins A and/or B in feces.

CLINICAL BACTERIOLOGY

GRAM-POSITIVE COCCI

The gram-positive aerobic cocci of clinical significance are *Staphylococcus* and *Streptococcus* species. Staphylococci are gram-positive cocci in groups and are catalase positive; streptococci are gram-positive cocci in chains and are catalase negative.

Staphylococci

Staphylococci can be separated by their coagulase activity. Coagulase causes plasma to clot. Coagulase-positive staphylococci are *S. aureus*, and coagulase-negative staphylococci consist of several different species; the most common (60 to 80% of the time) is *Staphylococcus epidermidis*, and in urinary tract infections of young females, *Staphylococcus saprophyticus* has gained importance. *S. aureus* is also positive for mannitol fermentation, thermonuclease, and deoxyribonuclease (DNase).

S. aureus is involved in several types of infections, including skin infections (cellulitis, pustules, boils, impetigo, and wound infections), endocarditis, bacteremia, pneumonia, osteomyelitis, meningitis, food poisoning (via thermostable enterotoxin), and toxic shock syndrome (exotoxin C, also known as enterotoxin F). Toxic shock syndrome (TSS) predominantly afflicts menstruating females using superabsorbent tampons. A few TSS cases have been reported in males, after insect bites, or as a result of operative procedures. *S. aureus* food poisoning is the result of enterotoxins. The enterotoxins are actually neurotoxins that activate receptors of the abdominal vicera, the stimulus reaching the vomiting center via the vagus nerve. These enterotoxins are heat stable and are a heterogeneous group of single-chain globular proteins. There are six serotypes (A, B, C1, C2, D, E). The most common source of *S. aureus*-associated food poisoning is food handlers, and pork (especially ham) is the food most often implicated in the United States.

S. aureus causes nosocomial infections (e.g., nursery, cardiac surgery patients). Nasal and skin carriers of *S. aureus* spread the organisms. In recent years, nosocomial *S. aureus* strains that are methicillin resistant (minimal inhibitory concentration [MIC] > 16 μg/ml) have emerged. Methicillin resistance (also known as intrinsic resistance) of *S. aureus* has been associated with alteration in PBPs. Methicillin-susceptible strains of *S. aureus* contain four PBPs. Methicillin-resistant *S. aureus* (MRSA) possesses an additional PBP known as PBP2' or PBP2a. PBP2a has a molecular weight very close to that of PBP2. PBP2a, however, has a very low affinity for beta-lactam antibiotics. Though some strains are homogeneously methicillin resistant (i.e., the expression of resistance is uniform throughout the population of cells), most MRSA strains are heterogeneously (1 cell in 10^6) methicillin resistant. Thus conditions such as incubation at 30°C (versus 35°C), incubation for 48 hours (versus 24 hours), and test medium containing high sodium chloride are needed for enhanced expression of resistance. Vancomycin is the drug of choice for treatment of infections caused by MRSA. MRSA is usually resistant to several classes of antibiotics. Though MRSA strains are sensitive to the cephalosporin type of antibiotics in vitro, they do not respond to these antibiotics in vivo and cephalosporins should not be used. In methicillin-sensitive *S. aureus* strains that do not produce penicillinase, beta-lactam antibiotics can be used. However, in penicillinase-positive, methicillin-sensitive strains, a semisynthetic penicillin (nafcillin, oxacillin, or methicillin) is the drug of choice. Bacteriophage typing has been a useful epidemiologic marker in nosocomial outbreaks of *S. aureus* infections. (Recently, the teichoic acid antibody test has been used for the determination of deep-seated *S. aureus* infections and efficacy of anti-*S. aureus* therapy. Though it appears to be promising, additional data on its use need to be gathered.)

The coagulase-negative staphylococci, in particular *S. epidermidis*, are encountered in postoperative infections (joint prostheses), shunt infections (CSF shunts), and others. These strains often are also methicillin-resistant and should be treated with vancomycin, often in combination with rifampin or an aminoglycoside.

A screening test to distinguish *S. saprophyticus* from other coagulase-negative staphylococci, which are often skin contaminants in urine, is the novobiocin test. *S. saprophyticus* is novobiocin resistant and is clinically significant in the young sexually active female.

Streptococci

Several clinically significant streptococci are *Streptococcus pyogenes* (group A streptococci); *Streptococcus agalactiae* (group B); the enterococci *Enterococcus faecalis, Enterococcus faecium,* and *Streptococcus bovis* (previously all known as the group D streptococci); *Streptococcus pneumoniae*; and viridans streptococci. Streptococci cannot grow in the presence of 6.5% sodium chloride, whereas enterococci can. This distinguishing characteristic is important since streptococci and enterococci have different susceptibility patterns. Streptococci are penicillin susceptible, but enterococci are resistant to penicillin though sensitive to ampicillin.

Streptococci can be characterized by their hemolytic properties on blood agar plates (Table 4-3). Enterococci can be either alpha, beta, or gamma hemolytic. Beta-hemolytic strains are further differentiated by their Lancefield group antigens (i.e., group A, group B, etc.). The Lancefield group antigens are carbohydrates on the streptococcal cell wall. The group D antigen is teichoic acid. These antigens have to be extracted (either by autoclaving, enzymatic treatment, or acid treatment) and then tested with antisera against the various group antigens. Useful presumptive identification of *S. pyogenes*

Table 4-3. Hemolytic Properties of Streptococci on Blood Agar Plates

Hemolysis	Streptococcal species
Beta (complete): clearing	*S. pyogenes* *S. agalactiae*
Alpha (partial): green	Viridans streptococci *S. pneumoniae*
Gamma (none): no hemolysis	

includes its sensitivity to bacitracin (also known as Taxo A), and for *S. agalactiae*, hydrolysis of hippurate and a positive CAMP test. (In the CAMP test, streptococci are perpendicularly cross-streaked to a beta-lysin-producing *S. aureus*. If the organism is *S. agalactiae*, it will synergistically act with the beta-lysin to form a typical arrowhead hemolytic zone at the junction of the *S. aureus* and streptococci cross-streak.) Alpha-hemolytic streptococci are differentiated by optochin susceptibility or bile solubility (*S. pneumoniae* is optochin susceptible and bile soluble, whereas viridans streptococci are the reverse).

Other components of the group A streptococcal cell wall include the M, T, and R proteins. The M protein is important in virulence; it has antiphagocytic properties.

Group A streptococci are the primary cause of bacterial pharyngitis. They are the causative agents of scarlet fever, pyoderma, impetigo, cellulitis, bacteremia, endocarditis, osteomyelitis, meningitis, and pneumonia. Complications following infection with erythrogenic toxin-producing group A streptococci may be rheumatic fever and acute glomerulonephritis, which are possibly the result of immunologic response to infection: acute glomerulonephritis from immune complexes deposited in the glomeruli and rheumatic fever from antibodies made to group A streptococcal antigens, which cross-react with human heart sarcolemma. A rise in anti-streptococcal O (ASO) titer is observed after group A streptococcal pharyngitis, and antihyaluronidase after group A streptoccal skin infection. Other antibodies measured after group A streptococcal infections are anti-DNase and anti-streptokinase. Diagnosis of group A streptococcal disease includes culture, serology, and recently the detection of the group A antigen directly in throat swabs.

Group B streptococci are important pathogens in newborns. There are four serotypes: Ia, Ib, II, and III. Antibodies to these serotype polysaccharide antigens are protective. It appears that maternal antibodies to group B streptococci are vertically transmitted to the fetus and protect neonates against disease. Babies of colonized mothers acquire the streptococci during passage through the birth canal. Nosocomial passage of group B streptococci can also occur. Newborn group B streptococcal infections can be divided clinically into early-onset disease (occurring before 7 days of age, with pneumonia and sepsis) and late-onset disease (occurring after 7 days of age, with meningitis). There is a higher mortality rate (55% versus 20%) for early-onset disease. All serotypes are equal causes of early-onset disease, versus 89% of late-onset disease being serotype III. Group B streptococci can also cause a wide spectrum of diseases in adults (meningitis, bacteremia, pneumonia, postpartum infection, etc.). Diagnosis of group B streptococcal disease is made by culture and by the detection of the group B or serotype antigens directly from patient specimens.

S. pneumoniae can cause otitis media and bacteremia in children and infants, pneumonia, and other types of infection, especially in patients with Hodgkin's disease, sickle cell disease, or asplenia. There are 83 serotypes, and antibodies to these serotypes are protective. Pneumococcal vaccines are available against the common serotype. Type-specific antisera have been used in the Quellung test. In the Quellung reaction, the serotype-specific antiserum reacts with the capsular polysaccharide, giving a "capsular swelling" effect microscopically in the presence of methylene blue dye.

The antisera have also been used for the detection of capsular polysaccharide in patient specimens. The detection of these polysaccharides in sputum has correlated better than culture or Gram stain in the diagnosis of pneumococcal pneumonia. Pneumococci are lancet-shaped diplococci. The pneumococcal colony is initially dome shaped but becomes flattened from the center outward as a result of autolysis. The characteristic bile and deoxycholate solubility of pneumococci is due to lysis of the organisms in the presence of these agents. Recently, decreased penicillin-sensitive pneumococcal strains have been isolated in South Africa. This decreased sensitivity is the result of lower affinity of PBPs.

The viridans streptococci comprise 10 species of streptococci. These organisms account for 25% of cases of all infective endocarditis. They are part of the indigenous oral flora. *Streptococcus mutans* plays an important role in dental caries and plaque. Patients with valvular defects receive prophylaxis during dental manipulations.

The group D antigen is found in both *Streptococcus bovis* and the enterococci. They hydrolyze bile esculin but differ in their ability to grow on salt (*S. bovis*, no growth; enterococci, growth). The isolation of *S. bovis* has recently been associated with colonic carcinoma. Thus its isolation should be followed up with the appropriate tests to rule out any underlying GI disease. (Another organism that also has been associated with carcinoma of the bowel is *Clostridium septicum*.) Enterococci are often recovered from urine specimens. They are involved in a wide spectrum of infections. Treatment of endocarditis with enterococci requires a combined regimen of a penicillin and an aminoglycoside. Recently, clinical isolates of enterococci exhibiting high-level resistance to aminoglycosides (MIC > 2,000 μg/ml) have been reported. These strains are not killed with a penicillin-aminoglycoside combination. This resistance is plasmid mediated.

Anaerobic streptococci (peptostreptococci) and anaerobic staphylococcus-like strains (peptococci) are found associated with abscesses alone or polymicrobially.

GRAM-NEGATIVE COCCI

The gram-negative aerobic cocci of clinical importance are *Neisseria gonorrhoeae* and *Neisseria meningitidis*. *Neisseria* are kidney-shaped gram-negative diplococci. They require carbon dioxide for growth and are grown on chocolate agar. The pathogenic *Neisseria* are cold sensitive.

N. gonorrhoeae causes a wide spectrum of sexually transmitted diseases (urethritis, cervicitis, salpingitis, and pelvic inflammatory disease [PID]). Though infections can be asymptomatic, especially in females, discharge and dysuria are common symptoms. PID is noted in females a few days prior to the menstrual cycle and frequently in those using an intrauterine device (IUD). Anorectal and oropharyngeal gonorrhea in females and homosexuals may be symptomatic, presenting as proctitis or pharyngitis and tonsillitis. In rare cases, the gonococci disseminate. Disseminated gonococcal infection (DGI) occurs most frequently in females during menstruation and pregnancy. Clinically, DGI is characterized by skin lesions, arthritis, and tenosynovitis. Gonococcal strains involved in DGI are generally exquisitely sensitive to penicillin, though resistant strains have recently been reported. DGI strains are often auxotrophic for arginine, uracil, and hypoxanthine ($A^-U^-G^-$).

The laboratory diagnosis of gonorrhea includes Gram stain, culture, and recently gonococcal antigen detection. The Gram stain is highly sensitive (> 98%) and specific with urethral specimens from males, but its sensitivity drops (50 to 70%) with endocervical specimens from females. The characteristic microscopic picture of gonorrhea is gram-negative diplococci located intracellularly in PMNs. The correlation between gonococcal antigen detection and culture is also higher with urethral specimens versus endocervical specimens.

Isolation of the organism is achieved with plating onto a selective chocolate agar medium such as Thayer-Martin (TM). TM medium is then incubated under increased carbon dioxide at 37° C for 2 to 3 days. The isolate is identified as *N. gonorrhoeae* by carbohydrate assimilation test (CTA sugars: gonococci assimilate glucose and not maltose, whereas meningococci assimilate both) or by fluorescent antibodies specific for gonococci.

Treatment for gonorrhea is penicillin. Recently, strains of penicillinase-producing *N. gonorrhoeae* (PPNG) have been isolated. This beta-lactamase is encoded on a plasmid. Therapy of PPNG infections is with spectinomycin and, recently, with ceftriaxone. The B-lactamase assay should be performed on all gonococcal isolates.

Chromosomally mediated (beta-lactamase negative), penicillin-resistant strains of gonococci also exist. They have altered PBP patterns (PBP1 and PBP2). Therapy of infections with these strains can include spectinomycin, cefoxitin, or cefotaxime.

N. meningitidis meningitis is characterized by sudden onset with fever, intense headache, nausea, vomiting, stiff neck, and frequently a petechial skin rash. In fulminant infection (Waterhouse-Friderichsen syndrome), widespread intravascular coagulation results with shock and often death. *N. meningitidis* can also cause arthritis, pneumonia, and other diseases.

The meningococci are carried in the nasopharynx of approximately 5% of healthy individuals. This carriage rate is higher among homosexuals (40%) and can be as high as 70 to 80% in the general population during epidemics. Meningococcal infections occur most often in the winter and spring and are encountered in small children and adolescents. Outbreaks are the result of overcrowding, as in schools or military barracks.

N. meningitidis is classified into serogroups A, B, C, D, X, Y, Z, 29E, and W135. Serogroup A is often responsible for epidemics, whereas serogroups B and C are responsible for most sporadic cases. The group B polysaccharide is immunologically identical to the K1 capsular polysaccharide of *E. coli*.

The diagnosis of *N. meningitidis* meningitis includes CSF examination for the serogroup antigen, Gram stain for gramnegative diplococci, and isolation of the organism on chocolate agar plates. Isolation of both *N. meningitidis* and *N. gonorrhoeae* includes growth on chocolate agar at 37° C in a 3 to 10% carbon dioxide atmosphere. Both organisms are cold sensitive, thus CSF specimens for culture should never be placed in the refrigerator, since this can result in failure to isolate meningococcus.

Treatment of meningococcal disease is penicillin or ampicillin, with or without chloramphenicol. The initial therapy for meningitis in children is ampicillin with chlor-amphenicol. This is to cover for *Hemophilus influenzae* and *S. pneumoniae*, since ampicillin-resistant *H. influenzae* strains are not uncommon. Close contacts of patients with meningococcal meningitis should receive prophylaxis with sulfadiazine or rifampin. Vaccines containing groups A, C, Y, and W135 polysaccharides are available. U.S. military recruits are routinely vaccinated. There is no vaccine against group B meningococci; the group B polysaccharide is poorly immunogenic.

Moraxella (Branhamella) catarrhalis also colonizes the nasopharynx of healthy individuals. It is a gram-negative diplococcus in the family *Neisseriaceae*. It causes mainly respiratory types of infections—otitis media, pneumonia, and bronchitis. It has been reported to cause endocarditis and, rarely, a meningococcal type of meningitis. Because most strains of *M. catarrhalis* produce beta-lactamase and may be confused with meningococcus, the differentiation between these two organisms has therapeutic significance. *M. catarrhalis* does not produce acid from glucose, maltose, lactose, or sucrose. Unlike *Neisseria* strains, it does produce DNase.

GRAM-POSITIVE BACILLI

Corynebacteria

The most commonly encountered gram-positive bacilli are *Corynebacterium*. They are often irregularly shaped and have been described as resembling Chinese letters. Corynbacteria are part of the indigenous flora of the human respiratory tract, other mucous membranes, and skin. Thus isolation of corynebacteria in clinical specimens is generally insignificant. In normally sterile specimens, their isolation must be differentiated between possible specimen contamination versus an opportunistic infection. The organisms, along with their anaerobic counterparts (*Propionibacterium*), are often referred to as diphtheroids.

Toxigenic *Corynebacterium diphtheriae* strains causing diphtheria have been infected with a beta-phage containing the *tox* gene. Diphtheria is the result of the exotoxin elaborated by the bacteria, causing necrosis of the surrounding tissue. The diphtheria toxin is a heat-labile polypeptide composed of two subunits held together by disulfide bonds. The larger fragment, B, is required to transport fragment A into the cell. Fragment A contains the enzyme activity that catalyzes the transfer of adenosine diphosphate (ADP)-ribosyl from NAD to the elongation factor EF-2.

$$NAD^+ + EF\text{-}2 \rightarrow ADP\text{-ribosyl} - EF\text{-}2 + nicotinamide + H^+$$

The resulting ADP-ribosyl–EF-2 is inactive, thereby preventing peptide chain elongation.

Laryngeal diphtheria is especially serious in infants and young children, since the diphtheritic pseudomembrane formed can cause airway obstruction.

The laboratory diagnosis of diphtheria includes culture of the nasopharynx and throat. These specimens are plated onto cysteine-tellurite agar, on which *C. diphtheriae* will grow as characteristic black colonies. *C. diphtheriae* colonies appear morphologically as one of three biotypes—*gravis, intermedius,* and *mitis.* In the past, these biotypes were associated with severity of disease, however this association no longer is clear. *C. diphtheriae* is identified biochemically. Toxigenicity testing involves either the guinea pig lethality test or the in vitro Elk immunodiffusion test (Fig. 4-15).

The Schick test is a skin test used to determine whether an individual has circulating antibodies to the diphtheria toxin. A small amount of toxin is injected intradermally. A positive Schick test, characterized by swelling and tenderness at the site of injection, indicates little or no antitoxin is present in the serum.

Treatment of diphtheria is with antitoxin. Antibotics (penicillin or erythromycin) have little or no effect on the clinical course of diphtheria, but they can eliminate the carrier state. The diphtheria toxoid is given with tetanus as Td or along with pertussis and tetanus vaccines as DPT.

A *Corynebacterium* strain demonstrating multiple resistance has recently been identified in infections associated with indwelling IV catheters, in granulocytopenic patients, and in persons with previous cardiac surgery. Colonization of hospitalized patients with *Corynebacterium jeikeium* (previously group JK) strain can be high (30%). *Corynebacterium* D2 is also multiply resistant to antibiotics. Both are susceptible to vancomycin.

Listeria

Listeria monocytogenes causes meningitis and sepsis at the extremes of age, during pregnancy, or in immunocompromised patients. Outbreaks of listeriosis have been associated with infected milk or milk products. In newborns, listeriosis, like group B streptococcal disease, has two distinct clinical presentations: the early-onset septic infection occurring during the first week of life and the late-onset meningitis after the first week of life. Serotypes Ia, Ib, and IVb *L. monocytogenes* account for over 90% of all isolates. *L. monocytogenes* is characterized by its microscopic tumbling motility in a hanging drop preparation or its umbrella-type formation in motility medium at 25°C.

Bacilli

Bacillus organisms are gram-positive, spore-forming bacilli. They are generally environmental contaminants of clinical specimens, though they can rarely cause serious infections associated with immunosuppression, traumatic wounds and burns, surgical procedures, and parenteral drug abuse.

Bacillus anthracis is the etiologic agent of anthrax. Intestinal anthrax and pulmonary anthrax may occur from ingestion of infected meat or inhalation of spores. Most common is cutaneous anthrax, caused by contact with infected animals or animal products (hides, wool, etc.). Cutaneous anthrax is characterized by a lesion or boil that develops into a depressed black eschar, which may lead to septicemia, meningitis, and

death. Animal handlers are at risk and should be vaccinated against anthrax. Laboratory diagnosis of anthrax includes Gram stain examination for gram-positive rods. Colonies are nonhemolytic. *B. anthracis* is nonmotile. The capsule of *B. anthracis* is composed of poly-(D-glutamic) acid. Penicillin is the drug of choice for anthrax.

Bacillus cereus food poisoning can present as the diarrheal type, which is associated with meats, sauces, etc., or the emetic type, which is associated with rice. It is of rapid onset and persists for no longer than 24 hours. Diagnosis is based on finding at least 10^5 *B. cereus* colony-forming units (cfu) per gram of suspect food.

Clostridia

Clostridium organisms are anaerobic gram-positive, spore-forming bacilli. In humans, several clostridia species inhabit the lower GI tract. The most commonly encountered species of clostridia is *Clostridium perfringens*. *C. perfringens* may be involved in gas gangrene from a contaminated wound, postabortion septicemia, necrotizing pneumonia, and empyema. It is the third most common cause of food poisoning in the United States, followed by *Salmonella* and *S. aureus*. There are five toxin types of *C. perfringens*: A, B, C, D, and E. Type A strains are most commonly associated with food poisoning, especially with improperly cooked meats. Diagnosis is based on isolating more than 10^5 organisms per gram of suspect food. The type C strains produce a much more severe necrotizing disease of the small bowel known as enteritis necroticans. It is also known as pigbel in New Guniea. This syndrome is encountered mainly in children. Here the organism proliferates in the small intestine and produces beta-toxin.

Clostridium difficile has recently been named as the cause of antibiotic-associated pseudomembranous colitis (PMC) and diarrhea. Many broad-spectrum antibiotics including ampicillin, the cephalosporins, and especially clindamycin have been implicated. Though it is often part of the indigenous fecal flora of healthy infants, it is rarely (3%) found in healthy adults. Colonization increases (30%) in hospitalized patients without GI symptoms. The diagnosis of *C. difficile*-associated disease is based on detection of its cytotoxin in stools. The cytotoxin, or toxin B, is extracted from stool samples and inoculated into tissue culture cells. Neutralization of the cytopatic effect by *C. difficile* antitoxin is indication of toxin B activity. *C. difficile* also contains a second toxin, toxin A. This enterotoxin is often found associated with toxin B. It has poor cytotoxic activity and is detected by ELISA. *C. difficile*-associated diarrhea can often be resolved by discontinuing the antibiotic. Vancomycin is the most common antibiotic used for treatment. Bacitracin and metronidazole also have been used.

Clostridium botulinum causes three types of disease entities: infant botulism, foodborne intoxication, and wound botulism. Unlike the classic foodborne botulism, in which intoxication is the result of ingestion of preformed botulinal toxin in contaminated foods, infant botulism results from colonization of the intestine by *C. botulinum* with subsequent in vivo toxin production. The majority (94%) of infant botulism occurs in infants less than 6 months of age, and an identified source of the organism is honey. Infant botulism presents initially with constipation, followed by lethargy, poor feeding, difficulty in swallowing, and generalized weakness (the floppy baby).

Intoxication botulism, or food poisoning botulism, occurs

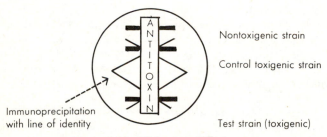

Figure 4-15. Elk immunodiffusion test.

when the toxin is absorbed through the intestine into the circulation to the neuromuscular junction and peripheral autonomic synapse. Here the toxin becomes bound to pre-synaptic terminals. The toxin blocks the exocytosis of acetyl-choline-containing vesicles, and flaccid paralysis results. There are eight serotypes of botulism neurotoxin (A, B, E, F, C, C_2, D, G). However, types A, B, E, and rarely F are associated with intoxication in humans. Type A is the most common (62% in the United States), followed by type B (28%). Type E has been associated with fish and fish products and is the cause of 10% of cases of botulism in the United States. The foods most commonly associated with botulism are vegetables (57%), followed by fish and fish products (15%), preserved fruits (12%), condiments (8%), and assorted products (9%) such as beef, pork, poultry, milk products, and soup. Type A is most often the cause of wound botulism. Wound botulism is rare and has been reported in drug users.

The botulinal toxin is like the diphtheria and tetanus toxins; it consists of two subunits. The B fragment binds to nerve cells, and the A fragment is responsible for neurotoxic effects. With some types of *C. botulinum* (e.g., A, B, and especially E), a slightly active "progenitor" toxin is produced initially and activated subsequently by a protease. Thus, portions of foods suspected to be the source of botulism should be digested with trypsin to enhance toxin activity. In addition, the laboratory diagnosis of botulism includes toxin detection in feces and serum specimens and culture for *C. botulinum* from feces and the suspected food. The toxin is not always detected in serum. This is especially true for infant botulism. Treatment of botulism is mainly supportive. If antitoxin is administered, patients must be monitored for anaphylaxis or serum sickness, since the antitoxin is of equinine origin.

Clostridium tetani exotoxin induces tetanus when the organism grows anaerobically at the site of an injury. Spores of the organism in the soil are introduced into lacerations. The tetanus toxin acts primarily on the central reflex apparatus in the spinal cord, causing excitation of the motor neurons and thus spastic paralysis. The actual mechanism of the tetanus toxin is by inhibiting release of glycine from the inhibitory snapse. Glycine is an inhibitor of neurotransmission. The tetanus toxin is synthesized as a single polypeptide that is proteolytically cleaved into two fragments. The fragment B binds to specific receptors (disialogangliosides GD_2 and GD_{16}). Treatment of tetanus is supportive. The wound is debrided to excise all devitalized tissue. Antitoxin is administered to neutralize circulating toxin, and penicillin is given to remove the source of the tetanospasmin. Prevention of tetanus is through active immunization with the tetanus toxoid in DPT or DT.

Mycobacteria

The most distinctive feature of the genus *Mycobacterium* is its staining property. It is known as an acid-fast bacillus. The acid-fast property describes its staining red with the basic dye carbol-fuchsin, but it resists subsequent decolorization with acid alcohol. Other acid-fast organisms include *Legionella micdadei*, some *Nocardia* species, ascospores of yeasts, and rhodochrous strains (a *Corynebacterium*-like organism). Acid fastness is a characteristic of the cell wall of *Mycobacterium*, but it has striking similarities to the cell wall of *Corynebacterium* and

Nocardia in that they all contain arabinose, galactose, meso-diaminopimelic acid (meso-DAP), and mycolic acid. In Gram stain, mycobacteria, corynebacteria, and nocardiae all stain positive. The mycobacterial cell wall, unlike others, contains a high lipid content (60% of its dry weight). It may also contain a cord factor (6'6-dimycolytrehalose). This lipid was once associated with virulence, since pathogenic strains appear to form cords and to have this factor. However, the cord factor has also been isolated from nonpathogenic strains.

Tuberculosis (TB) is primarily a pulmonary disease, though it can present as a skin and lymph gland infection or as intestinal TB by ingestion of milk. Intestinal tuberculosis was at one time primarily caused by *Mycobacterium bovis*. However, due to the pasteurization of milk, it has essentially been eliminated in the United States.

Humans are the sole carriers of TB in this country. Thus a history of exposure to an infected individual is important in a diagnosis of TB. *Mycobacterium tuberculosis* is spread primarily by droplet—nuclei less than 5 μm in size when the infectious material is discharged into the air by coughing.

Humans are very susceptible to TB infection but remarkably resistant to TB disease. This is probably because of our immune system. Once inhaled, the tubercle organism is ingested by the alveolar macrophage. The organism continues to multiply intracellularly and extracellularly to cause inflammation of the lung, with production of pulmonary lesions containing fibrin, PMNs, macrophages, and a few bacilli. The bacilli are drained into the regional lymph node, where they are kept in check till further dissemination via the lymphatic system and the bloodstream to the GU tract, the bone and joints, CNS, and the GI tract. By 4 to 12 weeks, dissemination, bacilli multiplication, and tissue inflammation stop as a result of sensitized T-lymphocytes, as indicated in the delayed hypersensitivity reaction seen in tuberculin testing. These lymphocytes can act directly on infected host cells by lysing macrophages combining the tubercle bacilli. Along with tubercle antigens, the sensitized T cells activate macrophages and enable them to have increased capacity to inhibit or kill the tubercle organism.

Tubercle bacilli that escape destruction are walled off from the rest of the body by macrophages, and granulomas (tubercles) are formed. This granuloma may be encapsulated with collagen and become a caseum, which may persist for years. The caseum may become hardened (tuberculoma) or may liquefy. The liquefied mass containing the tubercle bacilli drains into the surrounding lung, leaving a hollow center known as the tuberculous cavity.

In most individuals infected with tubercle bacilli, primary infection is not clinically severe. Only with subsequent reinfection or reactivation (80 to 95% of clinical tuberculosis) in these masses does the patient get clinically ill and seek medical attention. Reactivation occurs with decreased immunity, as in cancer patients, in patients on immunosuppressive therapy, in alcoholics, and in diabetics. Reactivation may occur as long as 10 years or more after primary infection.

The diagnosis of TB is based on clinical symptoms, history of exposure to individuals with TB, abnormal chest x-ray, positive tuberculin test, positive acid-fast smears, and isolation of *M. tuberculosis*. Some of the clinical symptoms of TB include a low-grade fever that increases as the disease progresses, night sweats, weakness, fatigue, and weight loss. Pulmonary TB may present with no cough when the lesions are small but may develop into chronic cough and sputum production as the lesions become more extensive. Extrapulmonary TB presents with many of the same symptoms as pulmonary TB. Unlike pulmonary TB, which is on a decline in the United States, the incidence of extrapulmonary TB has remained the same. In tuberculous meningitis, the CSF has an elevated protein, decreased glucose, and increased cell count, predominately mononuclear leukocytes.

On chest x-rays, lesions in adults are frequently observed in the upper lobes, where the oxygen tension is highest for the obligate aerobic tubercle bacilli to grow. In children, these lesions are more dispersed throughout the lung, possibly the result of a less well-developed immune system, which is unable to confine the organism.

Tuberculin purified protein derivative (PPD) comes in three strengths. The low 1-TU strength or lower is used in testing blacks and patients with TB of the skin or eyes. The skin test must be interpreted with consideration of previous exposure to atypical *Mycobacterium*. Patients with military TB (i.e., a very severe form of the disease in which the organism has disseminated and involved sites of antibody production such as the spleen or lymph node), patients on immunosuppressive therapy, patients recently receiving a viral vaccination, or patients with malignancies may exhibit anergy and thus false-negative tuberculin skin test.

The acid-fast (AFB) smear is useful in the rapid presumptive diagnosis of TB and thus permits more immediate infection control. It is also effective for monitoring the appropriateness of therapy. Besides the AFB (Ziehl-Neelsen or Kinyoun) stains, auramine O, a fluorochrome stain, can be used for tubercle bacilli detection.

Mycobacterium is usually cultured on Löwenstein-Jensen or 7H10 medium. In general, it is grown at 37°C; however, *Mycobacterium marinum*, a causative agent of skin granuloma, requires 25°C for optimal growth. *M. tuberculosis* requires at least 3 weeks to grow. BCG (Bacille of Calmette and Guérin) is an attenuated strain of *M. bovis*. In the United States, BCG vaccination is recommended only in individuals at risk of TB (e.g., household contacts of TB patients).

Mycobacterium leprae is an obligate intracellular organism. It cannot grow in vitro. Leprosy is transmitted from person to person.

The atypical or nontuberculosis mycobacteria are not transmitted from person to person. These organisms are generally found in the environment and are classified by the Runyon scheme, which is based on their colonial morphological features of pigment formation and their rates of growth (Table 4-4).

M. marinum is a common inhabitant of water. It may cause a localized skin infection at the site of injury. Sources of this organism include fish aquariums and swimming pools.

M. kansasii and *M. avium-intracellulare* are by far the most common atypical mycobacteria causing infection in humans. *M. kansasii* causes TB-like disease. It is relatively susceptible to antimycobacterial drugs, unlike most other atypical mycobacteria.

M. scrofulaceum causes cervical lymphadenitis in children. It is biochemically similar to *M. avium-intracellulare*, and the three species are sometimes grouped together and called the MAIS complex. *M. szulgai* can produce pulmonary infection. The scotochromogen *Mycobacterium gordonae* is rarely a pathogen in humans; it is frequently isolated in clinical specimens such as gastric washings. This is probably because the natural reservoir of *M. gordonae* is water and soil.

M. avium-intracellulare is commonly found as a saprophyte but can cause progressive pulmonary disease. It has been found in soil and is endemic in southeastern United States. It has been recently noted that dissemination of this infection occurs in patients with acquired immunodeficiency syndrome (AIDS). It is resistant to many antituberculosis drugs, and a combination of five to six drugs may sometimes be necessary for therapy.

Mycobacterium fortuitum has been isolated from abscesses in humans. *Mycobacterium chelonei* has been isolated from porcine heart valves used in heart valve transplants.

Antimycobacterial drugs include isoniazid (INH), rifampin, streptomycin, ethambutol, and others. INH is the most commonly used antituberculosis drug. It has the advantage that it crosses the blood-brain barrier and penetrates macrophages. It can be toxic to the liver. Streptomycin was the first drug effective in TB therapy. As a general rule, antituberculosis therapy includes at least a two-drug combination. This reduces the likelihood of development of drug resistance. A report on the susceptibility result of an antimycobacterial agent against a *Mycobacterium* species is expressed as the percent of tested bacilli

Table 4-4. Runyon Group Classifications of Mycobacteria

Runyon group	Characteristic	Potential pathogens
I. Photochromogen	Forms pigment only after exposure to light	*M. kansasii* *M. marinum*
II. Scotochromogen	Forms pigment in dark	*M. scrofulaceum* *M. szulgai*
III. Nonphotochromogen	No pigment formed	*M. avium* *M. intracellulare*
IV. Rapid growers	Grows <7 days	*M. fortuitum* *M. chelonei*

that are resistant to the drug. If more than 1% of the organism inoculum grows, the organism is considered to be resistant to this drug.

Nocardiae

Nocardia causes mycetoma but mainly pulmonary infections. The two species involved are *Nocardia asteroides* and *Nocardia brasiliensis*. They are found in the soil. Mycetoma is the result of subcutaneous implantation by contaminated thorns or splinters or, in pulmonary nocardiosis, inhalation of contaminated dust. The pulmonary infection resembles TB and may disseminate, with abscesses in subcutaneous tissues and in the CNS. *Nocardia* species stain as thin, branching gram-positive rods, which may fragment into bacilli and coccoid forms. They may be partially acid fast. Colonies can be orange, and they are speciated by their differential abilities to hydrolyze casein, tyrosine, and xanthine. Treatment of nocardiosis is with sulfonamide, with or without trimethoprim.

Actinomycetes

Actinomyces israelii is an anaerobic, gram-positive species of bacteria that produces filaments that branch and often fragment into bacilli. They are not acid fast. *Actinomyces* organisms are present in the normal oral cavity. Actinomycosis occurs as a result of injury in the oral cavity (tooth extraction, etc.), when the organism is swallowed, or by human bite. It is a chronic disease localized in the jaw, thorax, or abdomen. The suppurative to granulomatous lesions spread to the bone. Discharges from draining sinuses may contain "sulfur granule" colonies, which should be examined microscopically for filamentous branched rods and be cultured. Though other *Actinomyces* species can cause antinomycosis, *A. israelii* is the usual pathogen. Penicillin is usually effective in the treatment of actinomycosis.

GRAM-NEGATIVE BACILLI

Enterobacteriaceae by definition are aerobic gram-negative rods that ferment glucose. They are usually oxidase negative and reduce nitrate to nitrite. Some members of *Enterobacteriaceae* include *E. coli*, *Salmonella* species, *Shigella* species, *Proteus* species, *Enterobacter* species, and *Yersinia* species.

Escherichia coli

E. coli is the primary pathogen isolated from bilary tract infections (63%), from urinary tract infections (70 to 80%), and in gram-negative sepsis. *E. coli* is also a causative agent of nosocomial pneumonia and neonatal meningitis. Eighty percent of *E. coli* causing meningitis possess the K-1 antigen. *E. coli* is part of the indigenous fecal flora. Its detection in water samples, for example by the coliform count method, is an indication of fecal contamination.

There are four types of *E. coli* causing enteric disease: enteropathogenic, enterotoxigenic, enteroinvasive, and hemorrhagic. Enteropathogenic *E. coli* (EPEC) has been associated with outbreaks of acute diarrheal disease in newborn nurseries. It can also cause diarrhea in adults. EPEC strains have been limited to certain serotypes and are identified only by serological testing. The pathogenic mechanism of EPEC is unclear. The enterotoxigenic *E. coli* (ETEC) is often implicated in "traveler's diarrhea." ETEC elaborates either a large heat-

labile toxin (LT) and/or a smaller heat-stable (ST) toxin. Genes of both toxins are encoded in plasmids. The colonization factor required for ETEC to attach to the small bowel to cause disease is also plasmid mediated. The LT toxin resembles the *Vibrio cholerae* toxin (CT). Both LT and CT stimulate adenylate cyclase in the small bowel mucosal cells, leading to increased cyclic AMP levels and thus secretion of chloride by these cells. The ST toxin activates guanyl cylase. ETEC diarrhea is profuse and watery like that in cholera. The LT toxin is measured by cytoxicity in tissue culture cells, and the ST by fluid accumulation in the ligated rabbit ileal loop assay or in the suckling mice fluid accumulation assay.

The diarrhea caused by enteroinvasive *E. coli* resembles that of shigellosis, with invasion of the mucosal layer. Stools in enteroinvasive *E. coli* diarrhea contain blood, mucus, and PMNs. This enteroinvasiveness is also plasmid mediated.

The grossly bloody stool in hemorrhagic colitis is caused by *E. coli* serotype 0157:H7. This type of diarrhea has often been associated with partially cooked hamburger. It is caused by a *Shigella*-like cytotoxin to Vero and HeLa cells. The *E. coli* from hemorrhagic colitis is typically sorbitol negative. *E. coli* is identified mainly by biochemical tests. Typically, *E. coli* is indole positive, lactose positive, citrate negative, and Voges-Proskauer negative.

Salmonella

Three species of *Salmonella* causing disease are *Salmonella choleraesuis* (bacteremia), *Salmonella typhi* (typhoid fever), and *Salmonella enteritidis*. There is only one serotype of *S. chloeraesuis* and *S. typhi* but 1,500 serotypes of *S. enteriditis*. The most common serotype of *S. enteritidis* is serotype *Salmonella typhimurium*. *Salmonella paratyphi* A, *S. paratyphi* B, and *S. paratyphi* C are serotypes of *S. enteritidis*.

Salmonella is acquired from ingesting contaminated food (poultry and poultry products such as eggs, eggnog, ice cream, and dairy products) or water. Animals are the natural reservoirs of *Salmonella* except for *S. typhi*, which is transmitted from person to person.

S. chloeraesuis is highly virulent, often associated with bacteremia. *Salmonella* is second to *Campylobacter jejuni* as the leading causative agent of bacterial gastroententis in the United States. This can lead to bacteremia and even meningitis in infants or young children, especially those 2 to 4 months of age. *Salmonella* is also the primary cause of osteomyelitis in patients with sickle cell anemia.

Salmonella gastroenteritis is the result of mucosal invasion of the small and large intestines. Thus stool specimens from patients with salmonellosis may contain large numbers of neutrophils and red blood cells (RBCs). *Salmonella* gastroenteritis presents with abdominal cramps, pain, and diarrhea.

Besides gastroententis and bacteremia, the third form of *Salmonella* infection is typhoid fever. Typhoid fever is caused by *S. typhi* and in milder forms by *S. paratyphi* A and *S. paratyphi* B. The organism can be isolated from the blood early in disease and from urine and feces after the first week. *S. typhi* is a facultative intracellular microorganism, capable of intracellular multiplication within macrophages. Chronic foci of infection in typhoid carriers are in the biliary tree.

Isolation of *Salmonella* from feces includes the use of selective, differential media such as Hektoeon agar, xylose-lysine-deoxycholate (XLD), or *Salmonella-Shigella* agar. These agars differentiate lactose from nonlactose fermenters and detect the production of hydrogen sulfide (colonies with black centers). Often an enrichment broth (such as selenite broth or gram-negative broth) is added to the fecal specimen workup for enrichment for *Salmonella* (i.e., indigenous bacteria are inhibited but *Salmonella* is able to grow). *Salmonella* are motile, nonlactose-fermenting rods. With the exception of *S. typhi,* they produce gas from glucose fermentation. Hydrogen sulfide is produced, though *S. typhi* shows blackening only at the aerobic portion of the triple sugar iron (TSI) stab. *Salmonella* are biochemically identified as *S. typhi*, *S. choleraesius*, or *S. enteritidis*. They should be serogrouped for confirmation. *Salmonella* contains a number of antigens useful in its serotyping. These include the H (flagellar), O (somatic, also known as the LPS), and Vi (specialized capsular K) antigens. Ninety-eight percent of *Salmonella* infections in United States belong to one of the five somatic groups: A, B, C (C1 and C2), D, and E. The serotyping classification of *Salmonella* is known as the Kauffmann-White classification. *S. typhi* agglutinates with the Vi antiserum but not with the D grouping serum. After a suspension of *S. typhi* has been heated, the reverse is observed, with no agglutination with Vi antiserum but agglutination with the D grouping serum. A given *Salmonella* strain may form either one of two kinds of H antigen at different times. The flagellar H antigens are specified by two genes, H1 and H2. The expression of one flagellar antigen (phase) versus the other is dependent on a reversible inversion of DNA in this region.

The serological test for salmonellosis (Widal's test) is one of the febrile agglutination tests. Antibodies to the O and H antigens are measured. Interpretation of the Widal's test should consider any previous infection or vaccination with typhoid or paratyphoid vaccines and, for immigrants, the endemicity of these diseases in the foreign countries involved. Of the febrile agglutination tests (*Brucella, Francisella*, and *Ricksettia*), the Widal's test is perhaps the least useful. Salmonellosis is most often diagnosed by a positive culture.

Uncomplicated *Salmonella* gastroenteritis does not always require antibiotic treatment. In fact, antibiotics may prolong the carrier state. However, in infants less than 2 months old, in the elderly, and in persons with extraintestinal infections, antibiotics should be administered. Most *Salmonella* strains are susceptible to chloramphenicol, ampicillin, and trimethoprim-sulfamethoxazole. Plasmid-mediated resistance to these antibiotics occurs, especially in certain countries where antibiotics can be readily obtained over the counter. Thus susceptibility testing should be performed on *Salmonella* isolates. There has been some controversy in recent years about whether the incorporation of antibiotics in animal feed may promote drug resistance in *Salmonella* isolates.

Shigella

The genus *Shigella* is composed of four species: *Shigella dysenteriae* (group A), *Shigella flexneri* (group B), *Shigella boydii* (group C), and *Shigella sonnei* (group D). *S. dysenteriae* (Shiga's bacillus) is the most pathogenic, causing serious disease with fever and colitis and occasionally death. *S. sonnei* is the least pathogenic, with milder symptoms and shorter duration. The severity of the disease also is dependent on the host (increased severity in children, the elderly, and malnourished patients)

and on the infecting dose. As few as 10 organisms of *Shigella* can cause infection.

Outbreaks of shigellosis occur under conditions of overcrowding and poor sanitation, such as in day-care centers, mental institutions, and jails. Humans are the natural hosts of *Shigella*.

Shigella infection is limited to the mucosal area of the large and small intestine. Unlike in salmonellosis, systemic spread is extremely rare. The pathogenesis of *Shigella* is invasion, with bloody and purulent stools. This virulence is plasmid mediated. In addition, *S. dysenteriae* elaborates an enterotoxin (Shiga's toxin).

Shigella is isolated from stools on the same media used for isolation of *Salmonella*. It does not produce hydrogen sulfide. It does not ferment lactose, except for *S. sonnei*, which ferments lactose slowly. *Shigella* organisms differ from *Salmonella* in that they are also nonmotile. *Shigella* specifies are identified biochemically and antigenically. Shigellosis is treated with fluid and electrolyte replacement and with antibiotics such as trimethoprim-sulfamethoxazole, ampicillin, tetracycline, or chloramphenicol. Multidrug-resistant strains exist, and therapy depends on the susceptibility pattern of the isolated strain.

Yersinia species

The three clinically significant *Yersinia* species are *Yersinia enterocolitica, Yersinia pseudotuberculosis*, and *Yersinia pestis*. The first two species are responsible for yersiniosis, whereas *Y. pestis* is the etiologic agent of plague. *Y. enterocolitica* gastroenterocolitis occurs more frequently (two-thirds of cases) among children. It is transmitted via milk or water or from puppies and kittens. There appears to be an association between serotype of *Y. enterocolitica* and geographic location. *Y. pseudotuberculosis* is associated with acute mesenteric lymphadenitis in humans. Humans are incidental hosts. The reservoirs of *Y. pseudotuberculosis* are birds and mammals.

Plague is a systemic disease that can be acquired from contact with infected animals or their fleas (bubonic plague) or with aerosols from infected animals or patients (pneumonic plague). Wild rodents are the natural reservoir of plague. Plague is characterized by enlarged lymph nodes (bubo), fever, prostration, and a history of exposure to rodents or fleas. Untreated bubonic plague has a 50% fatality rate. The most effective antibiotic against *Y. pestis* is streptomycin.

Other Enterobacteriaceae

Klebsiella pneumoniae, Enterobacter species, *Serratia marcescens*, and *Proteus* species often are causes of bacteremia, pneumonia, and urinary tract infections. In many cases, these Enterobacteriaceae are nosocomially acquired. Hospitalized patients often (50%) are predisposed to oropharyngeal colonization by these organisms. *K. pneumoniae* pneumonia is most frequently community acquired. *S. marcescens* colonies can be red pigmented, though the majority are nonpigmented. The treatment of infections by these organisms is based on antibiogram patterns. Indole-negative *Proteus* (i.e., *Proteus mirabilis*) is usually more susceptible than indole-positive *Proteus*-like species (*Proteus vulgaris, Morganella morganii, Providencia stuartii*, and *Providencia rettgeri*).

Vibrio species

The *Vibrio* species of medical importance include *V. chloerae, Vibrio parahaemolyticus, Vibrio alginolyticus*, and *Vibrio vulnificus*. The first two species are associated with GI infections and the later two with extraintestinal infections. All reside in seawater. Cholera can present as a mild watery diarrhea to acute diarrhea with abdominal cramps, nausea, vomiting, dehydration, and shock. The diarrhea is watery (often described as rice-water), with no blood or mucus. Cholera occurs after the ingestion of contaminated water or raw or undercooked seafood (crab or other shellfish). Cholera outbreaks in the United States have occurred around the Gulf Coast. There are two serotypes of *V. cholerae*: serotype 01, which has historically caused epidemics of cholera, and non-01, which is often associated with sporadic cases of cholera. The *V. cholerae* 01 strain can be further subdivided immunologically into serotypes Ogawa (AB), Inaba (AC), or Hikojima (ABC). They can be biotyped into the classic strains or as El Tor strains. There is a higher ratio of asymptomatic to clinically ill cases with El Tor than with the classic strain. *V. chloera* produces an enterotoxin that is made up of two subunits. The H, heavy (or A), subunit activates adenylate cyclase, causing increased levels of cyclic AMP and hypersecretion of salt and water. The five B subunits bind to the receptor ganglioside GM_1 on the cell membrane. A killed vibrio vaccine is available today, though it is only protective for short duration (3 to 6 months). Isolation for *V. chloerae* from feces and vomitus includes culture onto thiosulfate citrate bile salt (TCBS) agar.

V. parahaemolyticus causes gastroenteritis. In Japan, it is responsible for 25 to 70% of all gastroenteritis. As with *V. cholerae*, infection is introduced by seawater or seafood. Foot wound infection with this organism has been reported.

V. parahaemolyticus produces a heat-stable hemolysin that is responsible for the Kanagawa reaction (i.e., hemolysis on Wagatsuma agar containing human or rabbit RBCs). Although 97% of diarrheal isolates exhibit a positive Kanagawa reaction, only 1% of *V. parahaemolyticus* isolated from seafood or seawater exhibits this property.

V. vulnificus infections can present as a wound infection or as septicemia. Wound infection usually follows exposure to seawater, and patients with underlying disease (diabetes, alcoholism, etc.) are at risk. In 75% of *V. vulnificus* septicemia cases, there is an underlying hepatic disease. Septicemia is associated with ingestion of raw oysters.

Campylobacter species

Campylobacter organisms are slender, curved rods, sometimes described as seagull shaped. *C. jejuni* accounts for more cases of gastroentertis than *Salmonella* or *Shigella*. It is acquired from improperly cooked food such as chicken, unpasteurized milk, or infected pets (especially puppies and kittens). Stools usually contain blood and mucus. Though the enteritis is frequently self-limiting, prolonged illness may occur. Laboratory diagnosis includes isolation of the organism from stools on selective growth medium. The medium is incubated at 42° C in an atmosphere with reduced oxygen with added carbon dioxide.

Other *Camplyobacter* species that can cause disease in humans are *Campylobacter fetus* subsp. *fetus* and *Campylobacter pylori* (previously *C. pyloridis*). *C. fetus* subsp. *fetus* is associated with septicemia and not diarrhea. Infections in animals can result in abortion in sheep and cattle. *C. pylori* has been isolated from biopsy specimens of humans with gastritis and peptic ulcers.

Other gram-negative fermentative rods that rarely cause infections include *Pasteurella multocida* and *Francisella tularensis*. *P. multocida* is part of the indigenous oral flora of many animals. The majority of infections involving this organism include animal bites or scratch wounds from dogs and cats. *F. tularensis* is the etiologic agent of tularemia, a zoonotic disease. Humans may acquire the infection via direct contact with infected animals, especially rabbit or tick bites resulting in an ulceroglandular infection, via inhalation (pneumonic disease), or ingestion (typhoidal type of infection). Diagnosis of tularemia includes isolation of the organism from lesions, sputum, or blood or by serologically demonstrating seroconversion or increase in agglutination antibody titer to *Francisella* antigen. Streptomycin or gentamicin is the antibiotic of choice for tularemia.

Pseudomonads

The best-known nonfermentative gram-negative bacillus is *Pseudomonas aeruginosa*. It is responsible for 10 to 20% of nosocomial infections. *P. aeruginosa* is an environmental organism. It has been isolated from fruits, vegetables, plants, aqueous solutions, and topical medication. Normal adults have a low incidence (< 10%) of carrying the organism in their upper respiratory or GI tract. Major predisposing factors of *P. aeruginosa* colonization include prolonged hospitalization, neutropenia, and other immunocompromised status. Infections with *P. aeruginosa* include bacteremia, pneumonia, skin infections, urinary tract infections, and pleuritis. Mucoid isolates of *P. aeruginosa* are common and unique isolates from the lungs of cystic fibrosis patients.

P. aeruginosa is oxidase positive and motile. Epidemiologic characterization of these strains has included serotyping, pyocin typing, and bacteriophage typing. Other pseudomonads of clinical significance include *Pseudomonas cepacia, Pseudomonas maltophilia, Pseudomonas mallei*, and *Pseudomonas pseudomallei*. The first two species are opportunistic pathogens of compromised patients. *P. mallei* is the etiologic agent of glanders, an infection primarily of equines. *P. pseudomallei* causes melioidosis in Southeast Asia and parts of Australia.

P. aeruginosa is one of the most antibiotic-resistant bacteria causing human infections. The mucoid strains are even more resistant. The therapy most commonly used in the treatment of *P. aeruginosa* infection is ticarcillin or carbenicillin in combination with an aminoglycoside. Strains can be resistant to gentamicin and tobramycin; most are sensitive to amikacin. Several third-generation beta-lactams (ceftazidime, piperacillin, cefoperazone, and cefotaxime) and quinolones also have antipseudomonas activity. *P. cepacia*, in contrast to other *Pseudomonas* species, is resistant to aminoglycosides and predictably susceptible to chloramphenicol and trimethoprim-sulfamethoxazole.

Legionella species

Legionellosis presents as two distinct disease entities: Legionnaires' disease and Pontiac fever. Both are characterized by malaise, myalgia, anorexia, headache, nonproductive cough, and fever. They differ in that Pontiac fever is self-limiting, not associated with pneumonia or death, and thus does not require treatment. The disease is most often caused by *Legionella pneumophila* (especially serogroup 1) and less often by other *Legionella* species, as *L. micdadei*. Diagnosis includes isolation of the organism on specialized media (as buffered charcoal yeast extract [BCYE] with or without antibiotics), direct detection of the organism in bronchopulmonary secretion by a direct immunofluorescence test, and the indirect immuno-fluorescence assay for demonstrating seroconversion or anti-body titer rise. Erythromycin is the treatment of choice for legionnaires' disease.

Brucella

Brucella is an intracellular parasite that causes abortions in animals. In humans, brucellosis presents with fever, chills, generalized aching, weight loss, arthralgia, and sweats. Trans-mission to humans occurs either by direct contact with infected animals or animals parts, unpasteurized milk or dairy products, or by inhalation. In the United States, most cases of brucellosis occur in animal handlers. Laboratory diagnosis includes isolation of the organism from blood or bone marrow after prolonged incubation of the cultures, but most often by serological demonstration of agglutinating antibodies to *Brucella*. In the serological test, antibodies to *Brucella canis* are not detectable.

Haemophilus influenzae

H. influenzae, along with *S. pneumoniae* and *N. meningitidis*, is responsible for the majority of cases of bacterial meningitis in the United States. It accounts for nearly 70% of bacterial meningitis among children younger than 5 years. The serotype b of *H. influenzae* is most commonly encountered in meningitis. Secondary cases of *H. influenzae* meningitis have occurred in day-care centers and among siblings. It can also cause pneu-monia, otitis media, epiglottitis, and conjunctivitis. In many instances, these nonmeningitis diseases are caused by non-typable *H. influenzae* strains, which may be part of the normal respiratory tract flora. The HIB vaccine composed of the capsular antigen ribosyl ribitol phosphate is currently being used in children 2 years of age. Rifampin prophylaxis has been used in household and day-care center contacts. *H. influenzae* meningitis is treated initially with an ampicillin-chloramphenicol combination. In some areas, ampicillin-resistant strains can account for as much as 40% of all *H. influenzae* isolates. In most of these instances, ampicillin resistance is the result of a plasmid-mediated beta-lactamase. Rarely, nonbeta-lactamase ampicillin-resistant isolates as well as chloramphenicol-resistant isolates can be found. The ampicillin-resistant, nonbeta-lactamase-producing *H. influenzae* appears to have altered penicillin binding proteins. Though chloramphenicol is gene-rally considered a bacteriostatic drug, it is bactericidal against *H. influenzae* and *S. pneumoniae*. Laboratory isolation of *Haemo-philus* includes growth on chocolate agar in an atmosphere of increased carbon dioxide. The detection of type b capsular polysaccharide in body fluids (e.g. CSF, urine, serum) has been useful in the early diagnosis of *H. influenzae* type b meningitis.

Bordetella species

Pertussis, or whooping cough, is caused by infection with *Bordetella pertussis*, though it may also be caused by *Bordetella parapertussis*. It is characterized by an initial catarrhal stage with mild respiratory symptoms, progressing to a paroxysmal stage with violent coughs. Fatality occurs most frequently in infected infants under 1 year of age. Prevention is through active immunization with a vaccine consisting of a suspension of killed bacteria adsorbed on aluminum salts. In rare instances, vaccinees may experience severe reactions such as convulsion, fever, or encephalopathy. These individuals should not receive further doses of the pertussis vaccine. Fears of adverse reactions to the vaccine have resulted in decreased pertussis vaccination in some countries. This, however, has lead to several lethal cases of pertussis in infants and young children. The benefit of immunization outweighs the relatively rare adverse reactions to the vaccine. Laboratory diagnosis of pertussis is based on examination of a pernasal nasopharyngeal specimen for the organism by direct fluorescent microscopy. Also, a duplicate pernasal nasopharyngeal swab and throat swab should be submitted for culture. Isolation media used are the Bordet-Gengou agar or Regan-Lowe agar. *Bordetella* grows as tiny colonies, requiring 3 to 5 days for growth. Microscopi-cally, *Bordetella* organisms are small, gram-negative rods or coccobacilli. *B. pertussis* can be differentiated from other *Bordetella* species is not producing urease.

Anaerobes

Anaerobes do not normally cause disease, unless the intact body surface is broken such as in accidental and surgical wounds. Anaerobes can be solely the causative agent, but often coinfect with aerobic bacteria in a wide variety of infections such as abscesses, oral and dental infections, chronic otitis media and sinusitis, gas gangrene, bacteremia, wound infec-tions, postoperative surgical infections, and postabortal sepsis. Clues suggesting anaerobic infection include foul-smelling specimens, proximity of the infection to a mucosal surface, gas in the tissue or discharge, and characteristic morphology on Gram stain. Some characteristic microscopic morphology of anaerobes are as follows: spindle-shaped gram-negative bacilli with tapered ends, *Fusobacterium*; gram-positive bacilli with Chinese letter arrangement, *Propionibacterium*; thin filamentous, long branching, gram-positive bacilli, *Actinomyces*.

The anaerobes most frequently isolated from clinical specimens include *Propionibacterium acnes*, *Peptococcus*, *Peptostrepto-coccus*, *C. perfringens*, *Bacteroides fragilis* group, *Bacteroides melanino-genicus*, and *Fusobacterium nucleatum*. The *B. fragilis* group is the most commonly encountered, and their clinical importance is accentuated by the occurrence of their resistance to penicillin and other antimicrobial agents. The *B. fragilis* group consists of *B. fragilis*, *Bacteroides thetaiotamicron*, *Bacteroides distasonis*, *Bacteroides vulgatus*, *Bacteroides ovatus*, and *Bacteroides uniformis*. *B. melanino-genicus* is part of the normal human oral flora and is involved in dental, oral, head, neck, and lower respiratory tract infections. *B. fragilis* group can be distinguished from other *Bacteroides* species by its growth in bile. *F. nucleatum* can be identified by its typical microscopic shape, and it is indole positive. In addition to biochemical characteristics, the speciation of anaerobes often requires metabolic end-product analysis by gas-liquid chromatography (GLC).

SPIROCHETES

Two spirochetes of clinical significance are *Treponema* species and *Borrelia burgdorferi*. Of the treponemal diseases, **syphilis** caused by *Treponema pallidum* is the most dreaded because of the devasting sequelae that could be encountered. Other treponems are *Treponema pertenue*, the etiologic agent of yaws, and *Treponema carateum*, the agent of pinta.

The course of **syphilis** begins with a 2- to 10-week incubation period. At the third to fourth week, primary syphilis is marked by the appearance of a painless chancre at the site of inoculation. By the sixth week to sixth month, the chancre is healed and the secondary stage is characterized by generalized skin and mucous membrane lesions. This is followed by a period of latency, which may last for years. In a third of these patients, late syphilis develops if left untreated, with destructive lesions in the CNS and cardiovascular systems and gummatous lesions of skin, bone, and viscera.

Diagnosis of syphilis is based on a history of exposure to individuals with syphilitic lesions, dark-field examination of all genital ulcerative lesions, and serology. Serological tests for syphilis are classified as nontreponemal and treponemal. The nontreponemal tests are based on the detection of antibodies to cardiolipin. Cardiolipin is not present on *T. pallidum*; it is the result of tissue invasion by the organism. The IgG and IgM antibodies detected by the nontreponemal assays are known as reagins. Nontreponemal assays most often used are the Venereal Disease Research Laboratory (VDRL) and rapid plasma reagin (RPR) tests. The treponemal assays include the fluorescent treponemal antibody-absorption (FTA-ABS) and microhemagglutination (MHA) tests. The sensitivity of these assays depends on the stage of the syphilitic disease (Table 4-5). The most sensitive assay in primary syphilis is the FTA-ABS. Though FTA-ABS is a highly sensitive and specific test, a patient with a positive FTA-ABS result remains FTA-ABS positive for life. On the other hand, VDRL may convert from a positive to negative result with early penicillin therapy. Thus VDRL titers may be used to monitor effective treatment. The nontreponemal assay is used in screening, and the FTA-ABS is a confirmatory test.

Laboratory diagnosis of neurosyphilis is based on pleocytosis

Table 4-5. Sensitivity of Nontreponemal (VDRL) and Treponemal (FTA-ABS) Tests Depending on the Stage of Syphilis

Stage of Syphilis	% Reactive	
	VDRL	FTA-ABS
Primary	78	85
Secondary	97	99
Latent	74	95
Late	77	95

In the FTA-ABS test, the patient serum is first absorbed with a nonvirulent strain of *T. pallidum* known as Reiter strain. This sorbent removes nonspecific interfering material.

(>4 lymphocytes/ml), elevated protein, and a reactive VDRL of the CSF. Thirty percent of patients with neurosyphilis will have a nonreactive CSF VDRL.

Early congenital syphilis corresponds to secondary syphilis; there is no incubation or primary stage. Diagnosis of congenital syphilis is difficult. The FTA-ABS test in this case is fraught with many false-positive and false-negative results. Treatment of a pregnant mother with syphilis also treats the fetus. In nontreated cases, the baby should be treated and follow-up sera should be examined by VDRL for 6 months. A decrease in VDRL titers indicates a nonsyphilitic baby, and increase in titers suggests congenital syphilis.

A single dose of 2.4 million units of penicillin G can assure effective therapy for early (primary, secondary, and latent) syphilis.

Lyme disease is a tick-borne spirochetal zoonotic disease. The tick is *Ixodes dammini* (the same tick involved in babesiosis) and other Ixodides ticks. Deer and wild rodents maintain the cycle. The spirochete is *B. burgdorferi*. Lyme disease is characterized by a skin lesion (erythema chronicum migrans [ECM]) at the site of the tick bite. As the red macule enlarges, malaise, fatigue, chills, headache, and arthralgia may accompany or precede the skin lesions. Weeks to months after the onset of ECM, neurological abnormalities (aseptic meningitis, sensory and motor abnormalities), cardiac abnormalities (atrioventricular block), and oligoarticular arthritis (especially the knee) can develop. Cases occur primarily during the summer months. Though Lyme disease has been reported throughout the country, most cases are observed in the eastern and midwestern parts of the United States. Laboratory diagnosis is serological, using ELISA or indirect immunofluorescence assay. Treatment with tetracycline, penicillin, or erythromycin early in Lyme disease often leads to rapid resolution of symptoms and prevents any sequelae.

MYCOPLASMA

Mycoplasmas do not have a cell wall. They are therefore resistant to antimicrobial agents such as penicillin whose site of action is the cell wall. Morphologically, mycoplasmas are pleomorphic in shape. Mycoplasmas of clinical significance include *Mycoplasma pneumoniae*, *Mycoplasma hominis*, and *Ureaplasma urealyticum*. *M. pneumoniae* is one of the major causes of respiratory disease (10 to 20% of total pneumonia cases), particularly among adolescents and young adults. The atypical pneumonia of *Mycoplasma* is encountered year-round. *M. hominis* and *U. urealyticum* are found in the genital tract of both asymptomatic males and females. *M. hominis* appears to be involved in pelvic inflammatory disease. *Ureaplasma* may have a role in infertility, nonspecific urethritis, and prostatitis.

Respiratory specimens submitted for *M. pneumoniae* are cultured in medium containing horse serum, yeast extract, and glucose with phenol red. The fermentation of glucose by *M. pneumoniae* will result in a color change from pink to yellow. The detection of *Ureaplasma* growth is also indicated by a change in pH; urea is hydrolyzed, resulting in an alkaline pH. Unlike the other two species, in which growth in fluid media results in no visible turbidity, *M. hominis* will show a faint haze in broth culture. *M. hominis* also produces larger colonies than *Ureaplasma*. *M. pneumoniae* resembles fried-egg colonies after 1 to 3 weeks of growth, and these may be confused with pseudocolonies formed by precipitated crystalline materials on the agar surface. Identification of *M. pneumoniae* includes the hemolysis test, which consists of overlaying agar plates containing *Mycoplasma* with a thin layer of guinea pig RBCs. After overnight incubation, a zone of hemolysis will be observed surrounding colonies of *M. pneumoniae*. Identification can also be carried out by inhibition of colonial growth with specific antiserum.

M. pneumoniae infections are diagnosed more often serologically than by culture, since growth is slow. The detection of cold agglutinins (antibodies that agglutinate human RBCs in the cold but not at 37°C) is useful in providing a tentative diagnosis of mycoplasma pneumonia. The disadvantage of this hemagglutinin test is that only half the patients with *M. pneumoniae* infections have a positive test. In addition, cold agglutinins can be detected in other diseases. Other serodiagnostic tests include the more sensitive and specific complement fixation, immunofluorescence, and ELISA tests. Treatment of *M. pneumoniae* infections is with erythromycin, and of genital mycoplasmas with a tetracycline. Tetracycline-resistant strains of *Ureaplasma* have been reported.

CHLAMYDIA

The two species of *Chlamydia* are *Chlamydia psittaci* and *Chlamydia trachomatis*. DNA homology studies show that the two species contain very little homology (10%), well below the 20% cutoff point suggested for members of the same genus. *C. psittaci* is an avian and mammalian pathogen. Psittacosis in humans almost always results from exposure to infected birds (parakeets, parrots, pigeons, turkeys, and ducks). Psittacosis presents as a respiratory infection that is usually mild or moderate. However, in untreated older individuals, the infection may be severe with a high fatality rate. Laboratory diagnosis of psittacosis is often based on serological testing.

C. trachomatis is the main cause of sexually transmitted diseases that frequently lead to serious complications. There are 15 immunotypes, which are associated with specific chlamydial disease. Immunotypes A, B, Ba, and C are usually isolated from ocular trachoma, the most common preventable form of blindness. Immunotypes L1, L2, and L3 are called the lymphogranuloma vernereum (LGV) strains of *C. trachomatis*. The LGV strains are more invasive in the human host. In tissue culture, LGV strains can also more readily infect tissue culture cells.

Infection with LGV generally begins with a small genital ulcer and development of subsequent inguinal buboes. Chronic LGV infections may lead to the complications of urethral and rectal stricture and fistulas. In the United States, LGV principally afflicts male homosexuals. Diagnosis can be made by demonstration of inclusion bodies or culture from bubo aspirate.

Immunotypes D–K have usually been associated with sexually transmitted infections and sporadic cases of conjunctivitis. *C. trachomatis* causes about half of the nongonococcal urethritis in the United States. It is the cause of 60 to 80% of postgonococcal urethritis. This is because penicillin used for the treatment of gonococcal urethritis does not kill *Chlamydia*. *Chlamydia* lacks a peptidoglycan and is thus resistant to cell wall active antibiotics. Tetracycline is used to eradicate chlamydial infection. Coinfection of gonococci and *Chlamydia* is high. Other infections associated with *C. trachomatis* are urethritis,

cervicitis, epididymitis, and salpinytitis (PID). Asymptomatic infection with *C. trachomatis* is high (20%) among women compared with men (5%). In the neonate, acquisition of *Chlamydia* via passage through an infected birth canal can lead to conjunctivitis or pneumonia in 20 to 40% of cases. *Chlamydia* is not affected by silver nitrate prophylaxis for gonococcus in newborns. Pneumonia occurs between 1 and 3 months of age. Erythromycin is the drug of choice for the treatment of neonatal chlamydial disease.

Chlamydia has an interesting life cycle. Understanding of this life cycle is vital in laboratory diagnosis of *C. trachomatis* disease. The organism is a parasite of eukaryotic cells. It cannot produce its own ATP. The cycle begins with the infectious form of the organism, the elementary body, adhering to the cell surface. It becomes ingested by phagocytosis. Within inclusion bodies of the cell, the elementary body reorganizes into a reticulate particle (also known as an initial body). The reticulate bodies divide by binary fission over the next 24 hours. The cycle is completed when reticulate bodies mature into new elementary bodies, which are released to infect new cells. The complete cycle is 48 to 72 hours.

Laboratory diagnosis of *C. trachomatis* infection includes culture of the organism in tissue culture cells (often McCoy cells), direct examination by immunofluorescence antibodies or by the less sensitive iodine stain for inclusion bodies, and ELISA for chlamydial antigens. Tissue culture cells have to be treated with diethylaminoethyl or cycloheximide, and adherence of the organism to cells requires centrifugation of the infected tissue culture cell. After 48 to 72 hours, iodine, immunofluorescence, or Giemsa stains can be used for the examination of inclusion bodies.

RICKETTSIA

Rickettsiae are bacteria, and most are obligate intracellular parasites that inhabit the alimentary canal of certain insects (lice and fleas) or arachnids (ticks and mites). Humans are an accidental host through exposure to an infected anthropod, except in the case of Q fever, which is transmitted by inhalation of dried, infected material. Five rickettsial diseases encountered in the United States are Rocky Mountain spotted fever (RMSF), Q fever, rickettsial pox, murine typhus, and epidemic typhus. RMSF is the most important of these diseases; it accounts for more than 90% of rickettsial diseases and can be the most virulent (mortality can be as high as 40% of untreated cases). The incidence of RMSF is highest in the South Atlantic states, 90% occurs between April and September, and most cases occur among children between 3 and 15 years of age. Clinical manifestations of RMSF include fever, rash, edema, headache, and thrombocytopenia. A history of tick exposure is useful. In general, laboratory diagnosis is serological demonstration of specific antibodies. These serodiagnostic assays include the Weil-Felix test and other less routinely available but more sensitive assays such as indirect hemagglutination, indirect fluorescent antibody, and latex agglutination tests. The Weil-Felix test is based on the fact that antibodies to the etiologic agent of RMSF, *Rickettsia rickettsii*, will agglutinate *P. vulgaris* strains OX19 and OX2. Weil-Felix agglutinins may be present in other rickettsial diseases (not in rickettsial pox and Q fever), as well as in patients with *Proteus* causing urinary infections, or in those with hepatic and biliary tract infections. Demonstration of rickettsial antigens in skin biopsy by immunofluorescence may be helpful in early diagnosis of the disease.

Q fever is caused by inhalation of *Coxiella burnetii*. Q fever differs from other rickettsioses clinically and resembles a typical pneumonia or influenza. Chronic infection can lead to hepatic involvement and/or endocarditis. Treatment of rickettsial infection is supportive and with tetracyclines. Q fever endocarditis may require prolonged therapy and even valve replacement.

ANTIBACTERIAL AGENTS

Antibacterial agents may inhibit bacterial growth reversibly (bacterostatic) or irreversibly (bactericidal). A given antibiotic may inhibit several reactions, with the reactions being inhibited dependent on the concentration of the antibiotic in the test medium. Most antimicrobial agents have one of the four modes of action against bacteria: They either (1) inhibit cell wall synthesis, (2) alter cell membrane permeability, (3) inhibit protein synthesis, or (4) inhibit nucleic acid synthesis.

Drugs of clinical importance that inhibit cell wall synthesis include the **penicillins, cephalosporins,** and **vancomycin.** As detailed earlier, penicillins and cephalosporins interfere with the biosynthesis of the peptidoglycan at the stage of cross-linkage between peptide chains. This results in a weakened cell wall and cell lysis.

At low concentrations of these drugs (subinhibitory or sub-MIC levels), cross-septum formation may be impaired, leading to elongated bacilli and other bizzare shapes. Different beta-lactams bind to different PBPs, which are involved in specific reactions. Thus their interference may specifically lead to filamentation (e.g., penicillin binding to PBP3) or rounded forms (e.g., mecillinam binding to PBP2).

Penicillins and cephalosporins are similar structurally (Fig. 4-16). The beta-lactam ring is crucial for antibacterial activity. Cephalosporins contain a six-membered dihydrothiazine ring, and penicillins a five-membered thiazolidine ring.

Changes in the R side chain at the six position of the penicillin nucleus and of the R_1 and R_2 side chains of

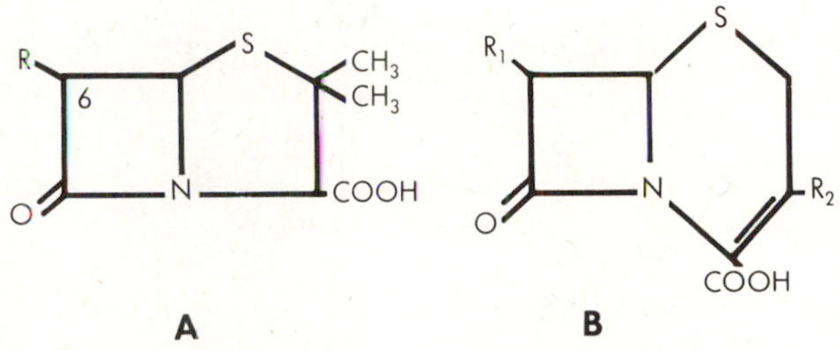

cephalosporins affect their antibacterial spectrum and pharmocologic properties. All are semisynthetic derivatives of the penicillin and cephalosporin produced by the fungi *Penicillium* and *Cephalosporium*, respectively.

Penicillin G (parenteral) and penicillin V (oral) are the most often used naturally containing penicillins. Penicillin is active against streptococci, nonpenicillinase-producing staphylococci, *T. pallidum, Neisseria*, and most anaerobic bacteria with the exception of *B. fragilis*. Broad-spectrum penicillins include ampicillin, carbenicillin, ticarcillin, and piperacillin. Ampicillin (oral or parenteral) is active against *H. influenzae* and many species of *Enterobacteriaceae*. Enterococci are also susceptible to ampicillin, but it is usually administered with an aminoglycoside for enhanced killing. Ticarcillin and carbenicillin are active against *P. aeruginosa*, indole-positive *Proteus*, and *Enterobacter* species. None of the broad-spectrum penicillins are active against *Klebsiella* and many *Serratia* strains. The new penicillin, piperacillin, has broad antibacterial activity including activity against *Klebsiella* and *P. aeruginosa*.

The semisynthetic (penicillinase-resistant) penicillins include methicillin, oxacillin, and nafcillin. Methicillin is available for parenteral use, and the latter two compounds are supplied in both parenteral and oral preparations. Their resistance to beta-lactamases is due to steric hindrance of hydrolysis of the beta-lactam bond by the acyl side chain. Methicillin is not totally refractory to beta-lactamase hydrolysis; in fact, it is hydrolyzed but at a very slow rate (0.01% of penicillin G).

Increased beta-lactamase stability is usually accompanied by a narrower spectrum of activity. The side chains may interfere with their transport across the outer membrane of gram-negative bacteria. Beta-lactam antibiotics are transported across the outer membrane or gram-negative bacteria through aqueous pores formed by specific proteins known as porins. The porins of *E. coli* are normally OmpF and OmpC. It appears that beta-lactams with increased hydrophobicity have decreased rates of diffusion through these porins.

Beta-lactamases are produced by bacteria. They hydrolyze the amide bond in the beta-lactam ring of a penicillin or cephalosporin. The beta-lactamases of staphylococci are predominantly secreted extracellularly and are inducible. The beta-lactamases of *Enterobacteriaceae* are diverse, consisting of eight major groups. Beta-lactamases of gram-negative bacteria are intracellular (located in the periplasmic space) and may or may not be inducible. Beta-lactamases have been classified by Richmond and Sykes into four main classes depending on their substrate profiles. For example, the class I beta-lactamases are predominantly active against cephalosporins, class II against penicillins. Beta-lactamases can be highly species specific (e.g., the type Id beta-lactamase of *P. aeruginosa*) or they can be found in several different bacterial species, (e.g., the R_{TEM} plasmid-mediated beta-lactamases).

Recently, beta-lactamase inhibitors (clavulinic acid and sulbactam) have been used in combination with susceptible beta-lactam antibiotics against some beta-lactamase-producing strains. These combinations extend the spectrum of susceptible beta-lactams. The structure of these inhibitors resembles that of a penicillin (Fig. 4-17).

The chief side effect of penicillins is allergic reaction. Among antimicrobial agents, the penicillins are the leading

Figure 4-16. Chemical structure of (*A*) penicillin and (*B*) cephalosporin.

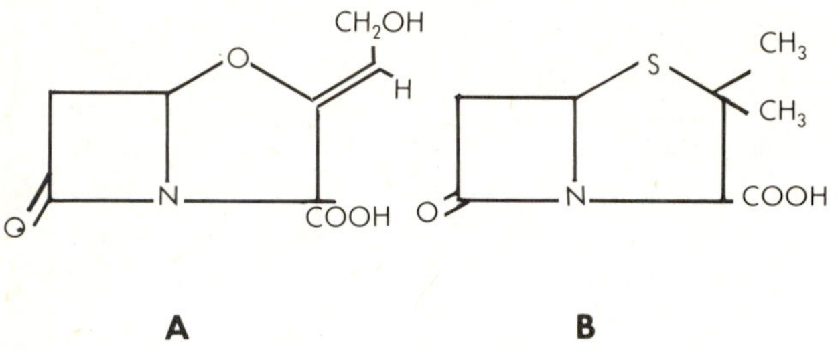

Figure 4-17. Chemical structure of (A) clauvulanic acid and (B) sulbactam.

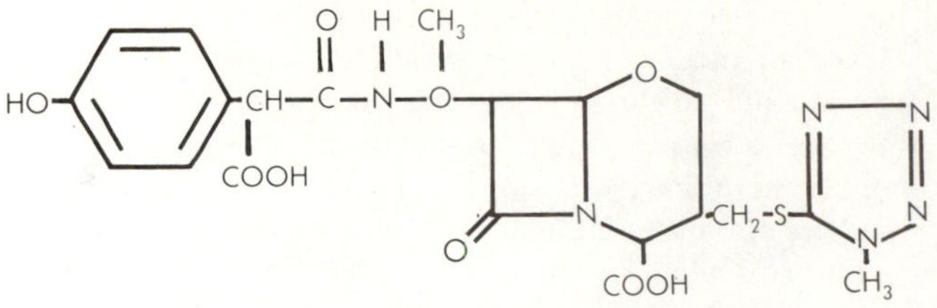

Figure 4-18. Chemical structure of moxalactam.

cause of allergy. Cross-allergic effects between penicillins and cephalosporins are observed. Cephalosporins have modes of action similar to those of penicillins; they inhibit cross-linkage of the polypeptide subunit. Both are bactericidal. The cephalosporins have often been classified by "generations" depending on their introduction and spectrum of activity. The older first-generation cephalosporins include cephalothin, cephaloridine, cefazolin, cephalexin, and cefadroxil. The later two compounds are orally administered. They are not stable to beta-lactamases and display good activity against gram-positive bacteria (except enterococci and methicillin-resistant *S. aureus*). Their activity against *Enterobacteriaceae* is variable, with no anti-*Pseudomonas* activity. The **second-generation cephalosporins** include cefamandole, cefuroxime, and cefaclor (oral). They are stable to beta-lactamases and have a broader spectrum of activity against gram-negative bacilli. Sometimes grouped as a second-generation cephalosporin is cefoxitin. Cefoxitin is not a true cephalosporin; it is a cephamycin produced by *Streptomyces lactamdurans*. It is stable to beta-lactamases and is active against most *B. fragilis* isolates.

The **third-generation cephalosporins** include ceftazidime, cefotaxime, and cefoperazone. They are stable to beta-lactamases but have poor activity against staphylococci and streptococci. They have activity against *P. aeruginosa*. It was recently observed that certain gram-negative bacilli such as *Enterobacter, Serratia*, and *Pseudomonas* containing inducible, chromosomally mediated beta-lactamases can develop resistance to broad-spectrum cephalosporins. Though these beta-lactams are supposedly resistant to beta-lactamases, the derepression of beta-lactamases in these organisms results in their resistance to beta-lactams. This resistance appears to be the result of large quantities of beta-lactamases that can bind with high affinity to many of the newer cephalosporins. This traps the cephalosporins in an enzyme-drug complex within the periplasmic space. Resistance also occurs by hydrolysis of the cephalosporin by beta-lactamases. It is observed that these newer cephalosporins are hydrolyzed by beta-lactamases at very low rates. Thus the beta-lactamase can hydrolyze or bind the beta-lactam drug, and if this inactivation exceeds the rate of drug penetration from the outside, the organism will be able to resist the drug.

Moxalactam is a semisynthetic oxacephem (Fig. 4-18). It has moderate anti-*P. aeruginosa* activity; it is not bactericidal against sensitive pseudomonads.

An added side effect of new cephalosporins possessing an *N*-methylthiotetrazole (NMTT) group at the three position of the dihydrothiazine ring (e.g., cefamandole, moxalactam, and cefoperazone) is coagulopathy. This coagulopathy is associated with prolonged prothrombin time and is reversible with vitamin K. Moxalactam, in addition, exhibits a second coagulopathy not reversible with vitamin K; this is associated with prolonged bleeding time and impairment of platelet aggregation. NMTT side chain-containing cephalosporins can also lead to a disulfiram-like reaction in individuals consuming alcohol.

Some of the most recently introduced beta-lactams are imipenem (a carbapenem) and aztreonam (a monobactam). **Imipenem** (Fig. 4-19) is stable to beta-lactamases and is active against gram-positive bacteria (except MSRA and enterococci), *Enterobacteriacae, P. aeruginosa*, and most anaerobic bacteria. Imipenem can be metabolized by renal dipeptidase. However, coadministration of a dihydropeptidase inhibitor, cilastatin, prolongs the half-life of imipenem, increases urinary recovery of imipenem, and decreases nephrotoxicity. **Aztreonam** (Fig. 4-20) lacks the bicyclic nucleus of beta-lactam antibiotics. Its activity is limited to gram-negative bacteria. It has no activity against gram-positive bacteria or against anaerobes.

Vancomycin is a glycopeptide antibiotic produced by *Streptomyces orientalis*. Its mode of action is at the cell wall (peptidoglycan biosynthesis) and at the plasma membrane. It is active against gram-positive bacteria. With the exception of *S. bovis* and enterococci, vancomycin is bactericidal. It is indicated for treatment of pseudomembranous colitis and infections with MRSA.

The **aminoglycosides** are a diverse class of antibiotics isolated from *Streptomyces* (streptomycin, tobramycin, kanamycin) or *Micromonospora* (gentamicin) or semisynthetically derived from these compounds (amikacin, a derivative of kanamycin A). They are amino sugars in glycosidic linkage.

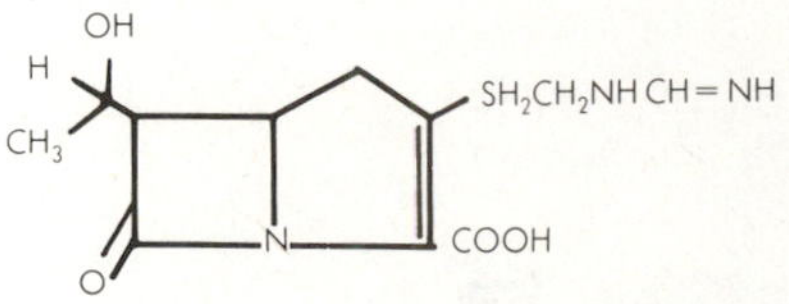

Figure 4-19. Chemical structure of imipenem.

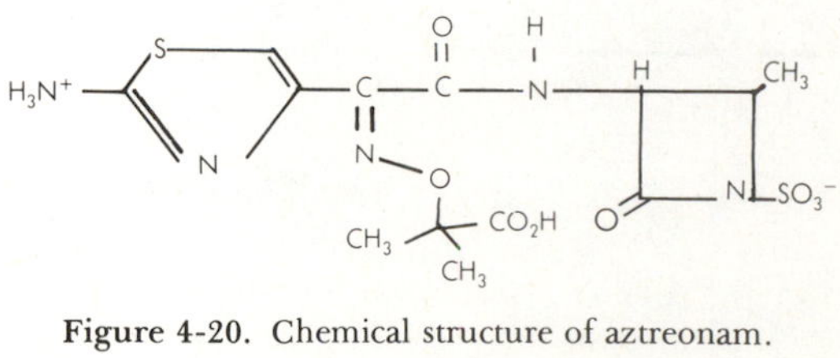

Figure 4-20. Chemical structure of aztreonam.

Their mode of action involves binding to ribosomes (rRNA) and causing misreading of mRNA to produce "nonsense proteins." They also disturb membrane function (leakiness of cell membrane and interference with the electron transport system). Modification of rRNA (e.g., single-base modification or changes in rRNA sequence) can lead to high-level resistance against specific aminoglycoside.

Aminoglycoside resistance can also be the result of a modification in the energy-dependent aminoglycoside transport system. This has been observed with *P. aeruginosa*, *E. faecalis*, and *Serratia* species. Anaerobes are resistant to aminoglycosides; they lack the oxygen-dependent transport system for aminoglycosides.

Most clinical pathogens can become resistant to aminoglycosides by obtaining plasmids that encode aminoglycoside-modifying enzymes. These enzymes include acetyltransferases (acetylation at an amino group), phosphotransferases (phosphorylation at a hydroxyl group), and adenyltransferases (adenylation at a hydroxyl group). In gram-negative bacteria, these enzymes reside in the periplasmic space. The different aminoglycosides have different susceptibility to these enzymes. Amikacin is the most resistant to enzyme in activation. Thus cross-resistance to aminoglycosides is not a rule. Aminoglycoside use in hospitals can lead to development of nosocomial strains with resistance to the aminoglycosides being used, but this does not occur with amikacin use.

The aminoglycosides are bactericidal. They have a broad spectrum of activity, including antimycobacterial activity. Not all are active against *P. aeruginosa*. Anaerobes are not susceptible to aminoglycosides. Aminoglycosides are commonly used in combination with a beta-lactam in infections in neutropenic or immunodeficient patients, in infective endocarditis, and in systemic infections with *P. aeruginosa* and resistant strains of *Klebsiella*, *Enterobacter*, and *Serratia*.

Adverse reactions to aminoglycosides include auditory and vestibular toxicity to the eighth nerve and, most important, nephrotoxicity. Aminoglycoside serum (peak and tough) levels should be monitored. Unlike with the beta-lactams, the margin between toxic and therapeutic doses is narrow for aminoglycosides.

Tetracycline, erythromycin, clindamycin, and chloramphenicol inhibit protein synthesis. The first three inhibit by binding to the 30S ribosomal subunit. This blocks aminoacyl-tRNA access to the mRNA-ribosome complex and prevents the addition of new amino acids to the growing peptide chain. Chloramphenicol competes with mRNA for ribosomal binding. These agents generally are considered bacteriostatic. All four may be orally absorbed or administered parenterally. Oral absorption of tetracycline may be impaired by dairy products. All penetrate well into body tissues. Chloramphenicol penetrates well into the CSF. Some indications for their use are (1) tetracycline in genital infections caused by mycoplasmas and chlamydia, (2) erythromycin in legionellosis and mycoplasmal infections, (3) chloramphenicol in typhoid fever, and (4) chloramphenicol or clindamycin for *B. fragilis* infections. Some adverse effects of these drugs are brown discoloration of teeth and retardation of bone growth in children with tetracycline, bone marrow suppression and "gray baby" syndrome with high doses of chloramphenicol, irreversible nondose-related aplastic anemia with chloramphenicol, GI irritation with

erythromycin, and pseudomenbranous colitis with clindamycin. Resistance to clindamycin and erythromycin can be attributed to modification of the target site (methylation of the ribosome, causing less binding of the antibiotic). Tetracycline resistance is primarily plasmid mediated and is inducible. Bacteria exposed to tetracycline may develop resistance by reducing uptake of tetracycline. Chloramphenicol acetyltransferases are the principal means of chloramphenicol resistance.

Rifamycins are isolated from *Streptomyces mediterranei*. Rifampin is a semisynthetic derivative of rifamycin B. It is bactericidal. Rifampin binds to the beta subunit of DNA-dependent RNA polymerase, to block initiation of new RNA synthesis. It has a broad spectrum of activity. Unfortunately, rifampin resistance develops quickly. This resistance may be due to single amino acid changes in the RNA polymerase, resulting in decreased binding by rifampin. Thus rifampin is rarely used alone. It is used in eradication of *N. meningitidis* carrier state and in combination with other drugs in treatment of TB.

Quinolones are bactericidal compounds that inhibit DNA gyrases, which are enzymes that control the spatial structure of DNA in vivo. The bacterial DNA gyrases are topoisomerase I and II. Topoisomerase II inserts negative supercoil into DNA without requiring ATP. This relaxes the DNA for transcription (mRNA production). Thus inhibition of DNA gyrase results in multiple effects from deregulation of gene expression and disruption of DNA supercoiling. Quinolone-resistant mutants are therefore uncommon. DNA gyrase has two subunits, A and B. Subunit A is the target of quinolones. Subunit B is the target of coumermycin and novobiocin. Resistance to DNA gyrase inhibitors is low. Resistance genes are chromosomally mediated. There is incomplete cross-resistance between nalidixic acid and the new quinolones.

Nalidixic acid is a quinolone. It is active against aerobic gram-negative bacteria. It is limited clinically to the treatment of urinary tract infections since it is poorly absorbed and has poor tissue penetration. The newer fluoroquinolones (ciprofloxacin, norfloxacin, etc.) have broader spectrum of activity including anti-*P. aeruginosa* activity, are more readily absorbed, and have good tissue and body fluid penetration. Data on the adverse effects of quinolones are still being accumulated. Possible effects may include CNS toxicity, mutagenicity, and large joint destruction. Quinolones accumulate in growing cartilage of experimental animals. At this point, quinolones should not be administered to children. Nalidixic acid has been used for years, and reports of these effects have been minimal.

ANTIBACTERIAL SUSCEPTIBILITY TESTING

Antibacterial susceptibility testing methods include the disk diffusion, agar dilution, and broth dilution tests. Several variables must be standardized in all these assays, including the test medium, the inoculum size, and the incubation period and temperature. In the disk diffusion method, a standardized inoculum (equivalent to a 0.5 McFarland standard or 10^8 cfu/ml) of the organism is plated onto the surface of an agar plate (containing Mueller-Hinton medium). Disks containing a set quantity of the antibiotic are placed on the agar and incubated overnight at 35°C. After 18 to 24 hours, a zone of (with an indefinite in vitro life span). Viruses have also been cultivated in embryonated chicken eggs (e.g., influenza virus) or in animals (e.g., arboviruses). Detection and recognition of viral infection in tissue culture can be demonstrated as cytopathic effect (CPE), in which infected cells in the monolayer are destroyed and there is inclusion body formation, hemagglutination (viral hemagglutinins on the surface of infected cells can attach to RBCs), or viral interference (interference of a cytopathic virus by a noncytopathic virus). Specimens for viral isolation yield better results if obtained within the early stage (first 3 days) of illness. The third approach is demonstration of a serological response to viral infection. In most instances, a rise in titer between acute (within 5 to 10 days of illness) and convalescent specimens (about 2 weeks subsequent to obtaining the acute specimen) is required.

DNA VIRUSES

Adenoviruses

There are 31 serotypes of **adenoviruses**. They share a group-specific complement-fixing antigen, thus allowing the detection of antibodies to this antigen and a useful means of detecting infections with these viruses. Adenoviruses are generally associated with mild upper respiratory tract illness. Acute respiratory disease (ARD) caused by adenoviruses is encountered in military recruits. Conjunctivitis with or without pharyngitis can also be caused by adenoviruses.

Herpesviruses

The herpesviruses include cytomegalovirus (CMV), herpes simplex virus (HSV), varicella-zoster virus (VZV), and Epstein-Barr virus (EBV). CMV is involved in a wide range of infections. Congenital infection with CMV (congenital cytomegalic inclusion disease [CID]) occurs from a primary or reactivation of latent CMV infection in the mother. CID may present in infants as low birth weight, microcephaly, chorioretinitis, and mental retardation or as hepatosplenomegaly with jaundice and hemolytic anemia. In adults, CMV may be acquired through blood transfusion or by saliva. The disease resembles **infectious mononucleosis** (IM) with no pharyngitis and cervical lymphadenopathy, as with the EBV infection in IM. An interstial pneumonia may occur in compromised individuals infected with CMV. CMV infection is best diagnosed by culture from urine sediments, respiratory secretion, and autopsy or biopsy tissues. Serodiagnosis includes determining rise in titer to specific anti-CMV antibodies or, in congenital infections, specific anti-CMV IgM class antibodies. Specimens for CMV culture should be kept at 4°C since freezing and thawing result in loss of CMV viability. These specimens should be cultured within 48 hours or frozen in an equal volume of 0.4-M sucrose phosphate. CMV grows best on human fibroblast cells. The CPE of CMV may not be apparent until 4 weeks of incubation. Histopathology of CMV-infected cells shows characteristic large cells with intranuclear inclusion.

There are two serotypes of HSV: HSV-1 and HSV-2. Though HSV-1 is most often associated with infections above the waist and HSV-2 with infections below the waist, this is not a strict demarcation. HSV infections of the lips (herpes labialis, or cold sores) and mouth are the most common manifestation of HSV-1. HSV-2 GU tract infections are a sexually transmitted disease. HSV-2 has been associated with cervical carcinoma. A complication of genital herpes is transmission of the virus to the fetus during passage through the birth canal. Unlike HSV infections in general, neonatal HSV infections are rarely subclinical. More than 95% of newborns infected with HSV exhibit symptoms within 1 month of birth. The disease may be disseminated, with visceral organ involvement and a high fatality rate or localized involvement of the CNS, eyes, skin, and/or oral cavity. Other HSV infections are gingivostomatis, keratoconjunctivitis, or eczema herpeticum. CNS infections include encephalitis associated with HSV-1 and meningitis with HSV-2. The laboratory diagnosis of HSV infection includes culture from skin lesions, vesicular fluid, eye specimens, and genital specimens. The virus is rarely isolated from CSF in cases of encephalitis. Cytology of these lesions shows large cells with intranuclear inclusions. CPE may be evident within 48 hours of incubation. Direct immunofluorescent antibody test on lesions may give a rapid diagnosis of HSV infection. Serology is rarely useful, though specific anti-HSV IgM detection is useful in diagnosis of congenital HSV infection. Antibodies to HSV-2 may be detected in 40 to 70% of individuals by 20 to 30 years of age.

EBV is the etiologic agent of Burkitt's lymphoma (a tumor occurring mainly in the jaws of African children), nasopharyngeal carcinoma (especially in Chinese descendants), and IM. IM is an acute viral infection usually characterized by fever, sore throat, enlarged lymph nodes, enlarged spleen, and abnormal lymphocytes in the peripheral blood. IM occurs in adolescents or young adults, although in developing countries, it occurs in young children. Virus exposure is dependent on socioeconomic status, with higher and earlier frequency of exposure in the lower socioeconomic group. As with many other viruses causing childhood infections (e.g., measles and chickenpox), the clinical manifestations are more severe among adults than children. The laboratory diagnosis of IM includes hematologic, biochemical, and serological data. The peripheral blood smear from IM patients shows an absolute increase in the number of peripheral mononuclear cells to at least 4,500/m^3 and 10% or greater atypical lymphocytes. These atypical lymphocytes are T cells cytotoxic for EBV-infected B cells. Atypical lymphocytes may be seen in other viral diseases, such as rubella, measles, mumps, adenovirus, and hepatitis, but they usually constitute less than 10% of the peripheral lymphocytes. In CMV and toxoplasmosis, atypical lymphocytes may also be increased. The chemistry of patients with IM shows liver function abnormalities, with elevated transaminase levels.

Serological diagnosis of IM includes heterophil antibodies and anti-EBV antibodies. Heterophil antibodies are found in patients with IM, serum sickness, and in some normal individuals (also known as Forssmann antibodies in normal sera). Heterophil antibodies agglutinate sheep or horse RBCs. The assay (Paul-Bunnell test) can be made more specific for IM (Davidsohn's absorption test) by differential absorption with guinea pig kidney cells or beef RBCs (Table 4-6). In most instances, a heterophil-positive IM need not be further tested for EBV serology. Rare incidences may include individuals suspected with prolonged detection of the antibody. (Heterophil antibodies are usually present for the first 3 months of illness.) EBV serology is especially useful in serodiagnosis of EBV infection in children, who often have heterophil-negative serology. Antibodies to three major EBV antigens are measured:

Table 4-6. Differentiation of Heterophil Antibodies

	Agglutination to sheep or horse RBC		
	No absorption	Absorption of serum with guinea pig kidney	Beef RBC
Normal serum (Forssmann)	+	−	+
Infectious mononucleosis	++	+	−
Serum sickness	++	−	−

1. EBV-VCA (viral capsid antigen) antibodies include IgG and IgM classes. The detection of the IgM antibodies to EBV-VCA establishes an acute EBV infection. Its profile of detection parallels that of heterophil antibodies. The IgG antibodies to EBV-VCA are present in all patients with EBV infections. Its absence rules out a diagnosis of EBV infection.
2. EBV-EA (early antigen) antibodies correlate with acute illness. High anti-EBV-EA results are also found in patients with Burkitt's lymphoma and nasopharyngeal carcinoma. There are two EA components, EA-D (diffuse) and EA-R (restricted), which describes their staining pattern in EBV-infected cells.
3. EBNA (nuclear antigen) antibody can distinguish a recent or past infection. Its absence in the presence of anti-VCA IgG indicates an acute disease process.

Varicella (chickenpox) and zoster (shingles) are two distinct syndromes of VZV. Like all herpesviruses, VZV can be reactivated, though it does so less often than HSV. Reactivation of VZV results in zoster. Primary infection with VZV results in chickenpox. The rash of varicella is characterized by a rapid progression from macule to papule to vesicle to scabs, with these various stages occurring at the same anatomic site. The lesions usually appear on the trunk. Fever accompanies the rash. Varicella in adults is often more severe, with higher fever and more profuse rashes, and it may lead to varicella pneumonia and hepatitis. Unusual types of varicella include congenital and neonatal varicella. If VZV infection occurs during the first trimester of pregnancy, congenital varicella with malformed organs may result. Neonatal varicella results if VZV infections occur within 4 days of delivery. It is characterized by hemorrhagic-like lesions, with 30% fatality rate. Hemorrhagic, progressive, disseminated varicella is observed in immuno-compromised hosts (e.g., children who have cancer and are receiving corticosteroids or chemotherapy). Disseminated VZV can result in varicella pneumonia, encephalitis, and death.

Zoster is mainly a disease of adults, afflicting immuno-suppressed patients. Chickenpox is a generalized disease. Zoster is a localized disease, with crops of lesions restricted to along the affected nerve (more than 50% involve the thoracic nerve). Recurrent zoster is not uncommon, especially among the elderly. More complications are observed with zoster than with varicella. Disseminated zoster occurs predominantly among immunosuppressed patients.

Laboratory diagnosis of VZV is by culture on human fibroblast cell line or by serology. Histologically, vesicular scrapings exhibit the same multinucleated giant cells with intranuclear inclusions seen in HSV lesions. A chickenpox vaccine is currently available for immunization of susceptible immunocompromised patients.

Poxviruses

Smallpox virus (variola) causes a highly contagious disease that has essentially been eradicated by mass immunization and intensive surveillance programs set by the World Health Organization. **Vaccinia** is a strain of cowpox. (Cowpox is believed to be a variant of the smallpox virus that has been passed through cattle). Complications of vaccinia may include encephalitis, eczema vaccinatum, and progressive vaccinia. Like smallpox, vaccinia is a disease of the past. Smallpox vaccination has been discontinued in the United States because of the elimination of smallpox; routine vaccination will give rise to more complications than the unlikely number of smallpox cases that may arise from importation. Vaccinia is one of the largest human viruses. This has made it useful as a vector in cloning large fragments of DNA or cDNA for vaccine development against a number of agents, including HIV.

Hepatitis B virus

Hepatitis B virus (HBV) belongs to the class of Hepadna viruses. It exists as a 42-nm intact virus (Dane particle) or as 20-nm spherical or tubular forms containing only hepatitis B surface antigen (HBsAg). Hepadna viruses contain a unique circular dsDNA molecule. One DNA strand has a gap missing 10 to 50% of the genome with DNA polymerase filling the gap, and the second strand is a complete strand with a nick (Fig. 4-22). The circular nature of HBV genome may facilitate its integration into host genome. HBV has the propensity to lead to chronic infection; in 10% of afflicted individuals, HBV DNA has been detected incorporated into liver cell DNA.

Hepatitis B (serum hepatitis) is transmitted via infected blood (blood transfusion, needle sticks, and wounds) and blood products, via saliva, via semen and vaginal fluids (sexual exposure), and vertically from an infected mother to infant. Individuals at risk of HBV infections include IV drug abusers, hemophiliacs, homosexual males, those receiving chronic dialysis, and multiply transfused patients. Hepatitis B may range from a mild (50% of cases) to fulminating fatal cases (1% of all cases). The incubation period of HBV is approximately 3 months. Chronic HBV antigenemia develops in 5 to 10% of cases; these individuals are HBV carriers. HBV is the cause of growth inhibition around the disk will appear for susceptible organisms. The zone diameter is measured.

Agar dilution consists of serial twofold dilutions of the antibiotic incorporated into agar plates. A bacterial inoculum of 10^4 cfu per spot is applied onto the surface of the agar. After incubation of the plates, the minimum inhibitory concentration (MIC) is determined. The MIC is the lowest dilution of the compound that inhibits visible bacterial growth. Broth dilution can be performed in microtiter trays (microdilution) or in test tubes (macrodilution). It is similar to agar dilution except that the antibiotic is diluted in broth.

To determine whether the antibiotic is bactericidal or bacteriostatic against an organism, the minimal bactericidal concentration (MBC) can be determined. After MIC determination in broth dilution, a given quantity of each tube or well with no visible growth is subcultured onto antibiotic-free agar plates. These plates are incubated and the colony counts determined. The MBC is defined as the lowest dilution of an antimicrobic that kills 99.9% of the initial inoculum. The cidal or static nature of a compound can also be determined by time-kill analysis. Time-kill curves examine the rate of killing by a given concentration of an antibiotic against a bacterial strain. Viability counts are determined versus the time of exposure to the antimicrobic. In most instances, the MBC is close to the MIC for bactericidal agents. However, when they are not (MBC/MIC ratio ≥ 32), this phenomenon is called **tolerance**. Tolerance has been observed mainly among gram-positive bacteria. Its clinical significance is uncertain; the usual practice is to treat serious infections with bactericidal agents.

Serum levels of antibiotics may be similarly analyzed by the determination of serum inhibitory concentration and serum bactericidal concentration of the antibiotic. The antibiotic-containing serum is serially diluted in broth and tested against the pathogenic bacterial strain previously isolated from the patient. Serum bactericidal titers of 1:8 and higher are desirable.

CLINICAL VIROLOGY

VIRUSES

Viruses are the smallest (20 to 300 nm) microbes infecting humans. They lack many of the enzymes required for their replication and thus depend on host enzymes for their propagation. They differ from other microorganisms in that they contain only one type of nucleic acid: either DNA or RNA. Except for Parvoviridae, which contains single-stranded DNA (ssDNA), all other DNA-containing viruses have dsDNA. The nucleic acid of RNA viruses may be either single-stranded (ssRNA) or double-stranded (dsRNA), a single molecule or segmented, and linear or circular. The nucleic acid is enclosed in a protein coat or capsid made up of subunits (capsomeres). The capsid protects the nucleic acid from nucleases. Together the capsid and nucleic acid are referred to as the nucleocapsid. The capsid symmetry may be helical (coiled), icosahedral (cubic), or complex. Figure 4-21 illustrates an enveloped virus. Envelope-containing viruses (except poxviruses) are sensitive to lipid solvents or detergents. The envelope of some viruses contains surface spikes or glycoproteins. Examples of this are the hemagglutinin and neuraminidase of influenza virus. The complete infective particle is the virion. Together, the nucleic

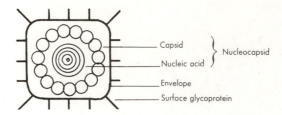

Figure 4-21. An enveloped virus.

acid, the capsid symmetry, and the presence or absence of an envelope (naked nucleocapsid) have been used in viral classification (Table 4-7).

The growth cycle of a virus starts with viral attachment to host cells. This may involve specific receptors on host cell surfaces that bind the virus. Penetration of the virion into the cell cytoplasm may occur through membrane fusion as with enveloped viruses or via endocytosis. Membrane fusion also allows virus infection of neighboring cells without the releasing of virus extracellularly. This occurs in herpesviruses, when giant syncytials are formed. Next, the viral protein coat is removed (uncoating). An eclipse follows uncoating, when infectious virus is not detectable. Synthesis of viral mRNA, viral proteins, and replication of viral genome occurs. Viral maturation occurs when all the viral components assemble. Finally the virons are released either by budding through the plasma membrane or by lysis of the infected cell.

Transcription and genomic replication vary with different viruses. In ssRNA viruses, the RNA may be positive stranded (i.e., the same sequence as viral mRNA, also known as plus stranded) or negative stranded (i.e., complementary sequence to viral mRNA). These RNA viruses encode and sometimes package a RNA-dependent RNA polymerase. Positive-stranded RNA can function as mRNA. Its replication involves the synthesis of negative-stranded RNA templates, which can be used in the synthesis of viral progeny genome or viral mRNAs. In some cases, the mRNA is translated into a single large polypeptide that is proteolytically processed into several proteins. Negative-stranded RNA must carry a virion-associated RNA polymerase that synthesizes viral mRNA at the onset of infection. Subgenomic mRNAs smaller than the genomic RNA and the full-length positive-stranded RNA are synthesized from the negative-stranded genome. The subgenomic mRNAs encode viral proteins, and the full-length positive-stranded RNA serves as a template for the synthesis of progeny viral genomes.

Retroviruses, which contain the human immunodeficiency virus (HIV), have positive-stranded RNA. They differ from other ssRNA viruses in that their nucleic acid replication involves a dsDNA intermediate. The synthesis of this DNA intermediate from RNA is carried out by a virus-coded RNA-dependent DNA polymerase, or reverse transcriptase, which is virion associated. As with the nucleic acids of dsDNA viruses, this DNA intermediate can become integrated into the host cell genome. The integrated DNA is called **provirus**. The state is known as **latency**. Under specific conditions, reactivation of the virus can occur. The only dsRNA virus of clinical significance belongs to the *Reoviridae* group. These dsRNAs are segmented. The positive-stranded RNA is synthesized from

Table 4-7. Classification of Human Viruses

Nucleic acid	Capsid symmetry	Naked or enveloped	Virus group	
DNA	Cubic	Naked	Papovavirus	Human papilloma (wart)
				JC
				BK
		Enveloped	Adenovirus	Adenovirus
			Herpesviridae	Herpes simplex virus
				Cytomegalovirus
				Varicella-zoster virus
				Epstein-Barr virus
			Hepadnaviridae	Hepatitis B virus
	Complex	Complex	Poxvirus	Variola
				Vaccinia
RNA	Cubic	Naked	Picornaviridae	Enterovirus
				Rhinovirus
			Reoviridae	Rotavirus
				Reovirus
		Enveloped	Togaviridae	Arboviruses
				Rubella
	Helical	Enveloped	Orthomyxoviridae	Influenza viruses
			Paramyxoviridae	Parainfluenza
				Measles
				Mumps
				Respiratory syncytial virus
			Rhabdoviridae	Rabies virus
			Coronaviridae	Coronavirus
	Unknown	Enveloped	Retrovirus	HIV

the genome by virion-associated RNA polymerase. This plus strand serves as mRNA and as a template for the dsRNA formation. The site of RNA virus replication is mainly in the cytoplasm, whereas for most DNA viruses (except poxviruses) this occurs in the nucleus and is dependent on host nuclear enzymes.

Host immune response to viral infection may be humoral or cellular. The type of humoral response is dependent on whether there was prior exposure to the same virus. The antibodies produced by the host to a new antigen are specific IgM, which is then switched to antibodies of the IgG class. This is known as the primary response. Subsequent exposure of the host to the same antigen results in a secondary response with more rapid and intense production of specific IgG. Specific secretory IgA is produced to virus invasion at mucosal surfaces. Antibody attachment to the virus may halt virus spread by neutralization. This attachment of antiviral antibody to viruses does not cause neutralization of all viruses. With some enveloped viruses, antibodies and complement can lead to lysis of the virus. Antibodies are an important defense against viral spread by the extracellular route. Virus spread intracellularly by cell fusion often induces viral antigens on the cell surface of infected cells. Infected cells may bind specific antibodies and complement, resulting in their lysis. Alternatively, lymphocytes sensitized to specific viral antigens will recognize viral antigens of infected cells, resulting in their destruction. T-lymophycyte recognition of virus-infected cells involves dual recognition of viral antigens and major histocompatibility antigens on the cell surface. Cytotoxicity of virus-infected cells may also involve macrophages and natural killer (NK) cells. In addition to destroying infected cells, lymphocytes release mediators. One such mediator is **interferon.**

Interferons are proteins produced by a virus-infected cell and excreted extracellularly. Other stimuli as dsRNA or polynucleotides can also induce interferon production. Interferon protects uninfected cells of the same species from viral infection. Interferon itself is not an antiviral agent. It induces mRNA synthesis and translation of an antiviral protein, which protects the cell. There are three major types of interferon: alpha, beta, and gamma, produced by leukocytes, fibroblasts, and lymphocytes, respectively. Interferons are species specific. They are not virus specific and protect cells from many viruses.

There are three approaches to laboratory diagnosis of viral infections. First, viruses can be detected directly in clinical specimens. This provides rapid diagnosis and in some cases is the only means of detecting noncultivatable viruses. Direct detection of viral antigens is often performed by ELISA and direct immunofluorescence assays. Direct detection of viral nucleic acids recently has been accomplished with DNA probes. Viruses in clinical specimens can also be detected by electron microscopy or immunoelectron microscopy. Viruses can be cultivated in living cells. Cell lines can be a primary culture (first passage of the cells in vitro), a diploid cell line (with a finite number of passages in vitro), or an established cell line

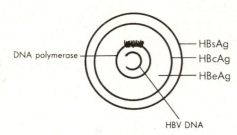

Figure 4-22. Hepatitis B virion.

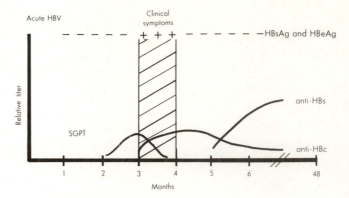

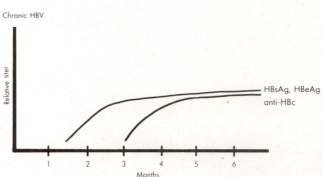

Figure 4-23. Serological profile of hepatitis B viral infection.

up to 80% of all cases of hepatocellular carcinoma. Perinatal HBV infections are likely to result in chronic HBV antigenemia.

There are several serological markers of HBV (Fig. 4-23). The HBV virus is composed of a nucleocapsid core (HBcAg) surrounded by an outer lipoprotein coat containing HBsAg (Australian or Au antigen). HBsAg has three group determinants: *a, d* or *y*, and *w* or *y*. Of the four possible combinants, serotype *adw* is the most common in the United States. The HBeAg is associated with the core.

HBsAg is produced in excess and is found in blood. It is the first serological marker of HBV infection. It peaks and falls with the aminotransferases. HBsAg detectable past 6 months of infection is diagnostic of chronic HBV infection. The disappearance of HBsAg by 3 to 4 months is followed by the appearance of anti-HBs at 4 to 5 months. Anti-HBs is protective. During the period between HBsAg disappearance and anti-HBs appearance, there is a window period when HBV infection can be diagnosed only by the detection of anti-HBc (or anti-HBe). Initially IgM anti-HBc is produced, followed by IgG anti-HBc. High IgM anti-HBc titers are indicative of a recent or ongoing HBV infection. HBeAg is almost always present only in HBsAg-containing specimens. It usually appears after HBsAg and disappears before HBsAg. Its presence indicates infectivity. Though the appearance of anti-HBe suggests less infectivity, this is not absolute.

Immunoprophylaxis of HBV infection may be passive or active. Hepatitis B immunoglobulin (HBIG) and Ig are given to newborns (at 24 hours, 3 months, and 6 months of age) born to HBeAg-positive mothers and following blood or secretion exposure to hepatitis (at 24 months and 1 month postexposure). Inactivated and cloned HBV vaccines are available and recommended to high-risk groups.

RNA VIRUSES

Hepatitis

In patients with acute or chronic HBV infections, coinfection with **delta agent** may occur. This agent is a RNA virus with antigen core encapsulated by HBsAg. It is a defective particle that replicates only in the presence of HBV. Thus the combinations of infections possible are (1) acute delta and acute HBV, (2) chronic delta and chronic HBV, and (3) acute delta and chronic HBV. The most serious of these is acute delta and chronic HBV infection, with symptoms identical to acute fulminating HBV. Patients at risk of delta infection are similar to those at risk for HBV. The serological markers of delta infections are antidelta and IgM antidelta.

Hepatitis A virus (HAV, also known as infectious hepatitis) is a picornavirus. Like all picornaviruses, it is nonenveloped, with a ssRNA containing a poly (A) tail at its 3′ end and VPg (viral protein, genome) at its 5′ end. The HAV virion is composed of four viral proteins (VP1-VP4). HAV is transmitted via the fecal-oral route, via fecal contamination (as sexual contact, especially with homosexuals, or in foodborne outbreaks involving raw oysters or food handlers). Outbreaks of HAV are common in day-care centers. Onset is usually abrupt, with fever, malaise, nausea, and abdominal discomfort. This is followed by jaundice, which resolves within 2 weeks. The disease may be more fulminant in the elderly. Serological markers of HAV include anti-HAV and IgM anti-HAV, the later being an indication of recent exposure. Passive immunization with Ig is given within 2 weeks of exposure to close contacts (family, nursery, sexual; foodborne outbreaks) of an individual with HAV.

There are two possible viral candidates categorized as non-A/non-B (NANB) hepatitis virus. It is presently responsible for 90% of posttransfusion hepatitis since no antigenic marker is available for its screening in blood. (The routine testing for HBsAg in blood has reduced its incidence of posttransfusion HBV infections.) NANB hepatitis has an intermediate incubation period between HAV and HBV. It is associated with a high rate of chronic hepatitis. At this time, diagnosis of NANB hepatitis is based on ruling out serological markers for HAV and HBV.

Influenza

Unlike other febrile respiratory illnesses, influenza occurs in widespread periodic outbreaks. The highest attack rate of influenza virus is among young children, though mortality occurs among the elderly. There are three serotypes of influenza. Influenza A consists of several subtypes determined by the two antigens present on spikes of the influenza envelope: hemagglutinin and neuraminidase. Antibodies to neuraminidase and especially to hemagglutinin antigen are protective. Antigenic drifts account for the periodic epidemics of influenza

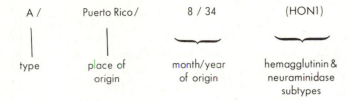

A /	Puerto Rico /	8 / 34	(HON1)
type	place of origin	month/year of origin	hemagglutinin & neuraminidase subtypes

Figure 4-24. The World Health Organization nomenclature for influenza A.

A. The World Health Organization nomenclature for influenza A is illustrated in Figure 4-24.

Influenza B is more antigenically stable, and thus outbreaks of this virus in the United States occur less frequently. Influenza C is responsible for milder and sporadic cases of influenza. Influenza C is not frequently isolated since its isolation requires embryonated hen's egg. Influenza A and B are myxoviruses. They contain eight segments of ssRNA.

A rare complication of influenza B in children (especially 5 to 16 years old) is Reye's syndrome, with CNS and liver involvement. It is characterized by vomiting and lethargy, which may progress to delirium and coma. In rare instances, there may be death and brain damage. Reye's syndrome peaks about 1 week after influenza peaks. It has been associated with salicylate use during flu and chickenpox. Thus salicylates should not be administered to children during these diseases. The laboratory diagnosis of Reye's syndrome includes liver biopsy or autopsy with microvesicular fatty metamorphosis of the liver. Liver enzymes and serum ammonia are elevated.

In temperate areas, influenza occurs during winter months. The diagnosis includes culture of throat and nasal specimens. Primary monkey kidney cells are often used, especially for isolation of influenza A. Inoculation of the amniotic and allantoic cavities of embryonated chicken eggs is not only required for influenza C isolation but may decrease the time to diagnosis of influenza A and B (2 to 3 days versus 7 to 14 days). Fluid collection from these cavities after 2 to 3 days of incubation can be examined for hemadsorption properties. (Influenza viruses are the only human viral pathogens that commonly produce hemagglutinating activity in eggs.) Serodiagnosis of influenza infections includes the hemagglutination inhibition (HI) test. Serum used for strain-specific HI testing must be pretreated to remove inhibitors or agglutinins.

Paramyxoviruses

The paramyxoviruses include parainfluenza virus, respiratory syncytial virus (RSV), measles virus, and mump virus. **Parainfluenza** viruses consist of five serotypes (1, 2, 3, 4a, 4b). They are involved in upper respiratory tract infections, bronchitis and bronchopneumonia, and croup. Parainfluenza infections are more severe in infants than in adults. Parainfluenza viruses also have hemagglutinin and neuraminidase on their envelope. Parainfluenza in tissue culture is detected by CPE and hemadsorption. Serodiagnosis is accomplished by demonstrating a fourfold rise in antibody titer to parainfluenza.

RSV is an important agent of respiratory infection (bronchiolitis and pneumonia) in infants during their first 4 to 6 months of life. The disease usually resolves within 10 days but may be fatal in infants. Primary infections and reinfections in older children and adults are mild. RSV lacks hemagglutinin and neuraminidase on its lipid envelope. RSV infections can be diagnosed by direct viral antigen detection (ELISA or immunofluorescence assay) and by culture (Hep2 or HeLa cells). Respiratory secretion specimens may be obtained by nasal wash, catheter respiration, or swab. The virus is labile and can be stored at 4°C for 48 hours prior to tissue culture cultivation. (Prolonged storage should be at −70°C.) RSV isolation may take 2 weeks before CPE (synctia) formation. Severe RSV infections in infants should receive supportive respiratory and fluid management as well as aerosol ribavirin administration.

Measles (rubeola) is a highly contagious disease. The virus enters via the respiratory tract. After a 10-day incubation period, a prodromal period (3 to 4 days) follows, with fever, coryza, conjunctivitis, and cough. Pinpoint white elevations in the buccal mocosa (Koplik's spots) are diagnostic for measles. A 5-day rash period follows, starting at the neck and progressing to the trunk and then to the feet. The maculopapular rash turns brownish, and desquamation may be noted in areas of extensive involvement. The prognosis of measles is good, though complications (otitis media and pneumonia) can occur. Subacute sclerosing panencephalitis can develop very rarely as a late sequela of measles. Measles vaccination is recommended at 15 months of age. The vaccine is an attenuated strain. An early measles vaccine contained killed measles virus; this vaccine is not protective against wild-type measles, and vaccinees may present with even more severe symptoms during measles infection. Though measles can be diagnosed clinically, laboratory diagnosis includes culture and serology. Measles virus-infected cell lines can be identified by syncytial CPE formation and their agglutination of monkey red cells. A fourfold rise in hemagglutination inhibition (HI) titer is indicative of a recent measles infection.

Mumps is an acute infection characterized by fever and swelling of the parotid glands. Complications include aseptic meningitis (10%). Severe orchitis rarely results in sterility but may decrease sperm count. Live attenuated vaccine is available to prevent mumps virus. Mump virus may be cultured. Serological tests are of value. The virus contains two distinct antigens: the V (viral) antigen associated with the hemagglutinin, which gives rise to protective antibodies, and the S (soluble) antigen, which is associated with the nucleocapsid. A patient with mumps will often have antibodies to the S antigen in an acute-phase serum. Antibodies to the V antigen appear later during convalescence. Past mumps infection is diagnosed by the detection of antibodies to the V but not S antigen.

Rubella virus

Rubella virus causes the childhood disease German measles. It is classified as a Togavirus. It is morphologically similar to group A arboviruses, which too are Togaviruses (Toga = envelope). Rubella is spread via the respiratory tract. There is a 17-day incubation period. The prodromal period is absent in children, but in adults, this 1- to 4-day period is characterized by swollen lymph nodes, malaise, and possibly low-grade fever. Postnatally acquired rubella is a very benign infection in children, with rash lasting 1 to 5 days and spreading from head to arms and trunk to extremities (25% of infected children have no rash). However, rubella is the main TORCH agent with teratogenic properties (20% of pregnant females infected with rubella during the first trimester will give birth to an infant with congenital rubella). That is, it induces failure of organ development. Intrauterine rubella infection may result in spontaneous abortion, stillbirth, live birth with single or multiple organ defects, or a normal infant. Congenital rubella results from maternal rubella viremia with subsequent placental infection and fetal viremia. Timing plays a crucial role in the pathogenesis of congenital rubella, the first trimester being the most crucial. Congenital rubella can be diagnosed by a history of possible exposure to rubella during the first trimester, presence of one or more clinical manifestations (heart defect, hearing defect, eye defect, cerebral defect, hepatitis, etc.) of congenital rubella, and viral isolation and/or serology. Specimens for culture in congenital rubella include urine, CSF, pharyngeal secretions, and tissues that may be infected. The recovery of the virus from these specimens is inversely proportional to the age of the infant. Pharyngeal secretion is the best specimen to obtain in postnatally acquired rubella. Rubella can infect a large number of cell lines, often with no CPE. The presence of rubella virus is demonstrated by the interference test (i.e., preventing CPE formation by a challenge inoculum of enterovirus).

Rubella antibodies can be demonstrated by the HI test using chick or trypsinized human O cells, passive hemagglutination test, and indirect immunofluorescence test. Serological demonstration of a fourfold rise in rubella antibodies is diagnostic of a recent infection. Congenital rubella is indicated by demonstrating the presence of rubella IgM antibodies or the presence of rubella antibodies equal to or greater than the maternal titer past 6 months of age (since maternally transferred IgG normally disappears within 6 months of birth). The prenatal screening of rubella immune status can assure immune protection to rubella. Rubella vaccination is with a live attenuated rubella virus strain.

Viral CNS diseases

Viral diseases of the CNS are categorized as either meningitis or encephalitis. Though all neurotropic viruses (except rabies) can cause both syndromes, they are more frequently associated with one syndrome or the other. For example, enterovirus and mumps cause mainly aseptic meningitis, whereas arbovirus and HSV cause mainly encephalitis. There are prognostic differences, with poorer prognosis in encephalitis. There are seasonal differences in viral meningitis; infections with enterovirus occur primarily during late summer to early fall; and mumps occurs year-round. Viral meningitis most commonly occurs in children and young adults.

Enteroviruses

Besides HAV, enteroviruses consist of coxsackie A and B viruses, echoviruses, and polioviruses. **Coxsackie A viruses** are associated with herpangina (an ulcerative pharyngitis and tonsillitis most often afflicting young children) and aseptic meningitis. **Coxsackie B viruses** have also been implicated in aseptic meningitis, neonatal myocarditis, and outbreaks of pericarditis in children and adults.

Echoviruses, especially type nine, cause aseptic meningitis. These enteroviral meningitides are often accompanied by a rubella-like rash (especially in children less than 3 years of age) and occur during the summer months. Children probably obtain the virus via ingesting feces-contaminated objects.

Poliovirus infections are often mild, with low-grade fever, headache, nausea, sore throat or constipation, and limited to 2 to 5 days. In rare instances (1% of cases), bulbar and spinal involvement occur with destruction of motor neurons, leading to flaccid paralysis.

Specimens for culture of enterovirus include throat swabs, feces, and CSF. Since these viruses are excreted in the GI tract several weeks following illness, the demonstration of the virus from feces alone does not confirm enteroviral infection. Typical enteroviral CPE consists of cell rounding and shrinking with nuclear pyknosis. Enteroviral serology is limited since there are more than 63 serotypes. There is no group antigen, so serological testing usually involves each single type.

Prevention of enteroviral infections includes good hygiene. The trivalent oral polio vaccine is recommended, with two to three doses during infancy followed by at least one booster by 5 to 6 years of age.

Arboviruses

Arboviruses (Togaviruses) can cause CNS disease and are transmitted by bites inflicted by arthropods (mosquitos or ticks). Arboviruses of importance in the United States include eastern equine encephalitis (EEE), western equine encephalitis (WEE), St. Louis encephalitis (SLE), and California encephalitis (CE). WEE and EEE can cause permanent brain damage in infants and children. The arboviruses differ in the age-group they infect, with most infected individuals in the extremities of life. In morbidity and mortality, EEE has the highest rates in geographic distribution:

Arbovirus	Geographic Distribution
WEE	Western two-thirds USA
EEE	Atlantic and Gulf coasts
SLE	Most widespread
CE	Midwest

They are similar in their arthropod transmission to humans, their occurrence predominantly in the summer to early fall months, and their ecological cycle (except CE) involving birds and small mammals. Prevention of arbovirus infection requires mosquito control. The laboratory diagnosis is rarely made by culture but is often based on serological demonstration in acute and convalescent sera.

Rabies virus

Rabies occurs after the virus enters the peripheral nerves (via rabid animal bite) or from the olfactory organs (via aerosol exposure). It is transmitted to the CNS (brain and spinal cord) and sometimes to the peripheral nerves. The incubation period is 1 to 3 months, depending on the bite site and age of the infected individual (shorter incubation period in children). Clinically, the patient presents with excitement, agitation, and ascending paralysis. Classic symptoms of rabies include hydrophobia, difficulty in swallowing, and hypersalivation. The animals most often associated with rabies include carnivorous wild animals (skunk, raccoon, fox, coyote, bobcat) and, depending on the geographic area (Mexico-Texas border and South Carolina), the domestic dog and cat. Rodents have not been implicated. Rabies has also been transmitted via corneal transplants. Airborne transmission in caves and lab accidents with rabid specimens can occur. Patients involved in an unprovoked attack (bitten or scratched) from the animal species listed above should receive prophylaxis for rabies. This includes thorough cleaning of the wound, one dose of human rabies immune globulin (RIG), and five IM doses of human diploid cell rabies vaccine (HDCV). The domestic animal involved should be confined for 10 days for observation. The head of the implicated wild animal should be decapitated, carefully refrigerated, and submitted to the State Health Department. The head is dissected, and the hippocampus, cerebral cortex, basal ganglia, and cerebellum removed for mouse inoculation and for examination for Negri bodies. Negri bodies are cytoplasmic inclusions in infected nerve cells that contain rabies antigen. Detection of rabies antigen in a corneal impression by a fluorescent antibody test may be helpful.

Retroviruses

AIDS is caused by HIV, also known as HTLV-III, human T-lymphotrophic virus, lymphadenopathy-associated virus (LAV), or AIDS-associated retrovirus (ARV). The clinical presentation of HIV infections ranges from an asymptomatic infection to persistent generalized lymphadenopathy to AIDS (characterized by lymphadenopathy, anorexia, chronic diarrhea, weight loss, fatigue, Kaposi's sarcoma, and opportunistic diseases). Opportunistic infections include diseases due to *Candida, Cryptococcus, Toxoplasma, Pneumocystis, Cryptosporidium, Stronglyloides,* CMV, HSV, and atypical mycobacteria. At present the fatality rate among patients diagnosed with AIDS is 40 to 50%. High-risk groups in the United States are homosexuals and bisexuals (70%), drug abusers (17%), Haitian immigrants (4%), and hemophiliacs (1%). The virus is transmitted via sexual contact, needles, blood transfusions, or blood products. The incubation period is thought to range from 6 months to 5 years.

HIV, like all retroviruses, is characterized by the presence of reverse transcriptase and ssRNA as its genetic material (Fig. 4-25). The genome of retroviruses contains three regions (Fig. 4-26): (1) the *gag* region coding viral internal core proteins, (2) the *pol* region coding reverse transcriptase, and (3) the *env* region coding envelope glycoproteins. It is flanked by long-terminal repeat (LTR) sequences, which allow integration of viral genome into host genome. The *gag* and *env* genes code for several proteins and glycoproteins.

1. The translational product of the *gag* gene is a p55 protein, which subsequently is processed into viral core proteins p18, p24, and p13. The p24 and p18 core proteins are moderately immunogenic, and antibodies to these proteins are observed from AIDS patients by Western blot analysis.
2. The translational produce of the *env* gene is a glycoprotein, gp150, which is processed into viral envelope glycoproteins gp41 and gp120. Both glycoproteins are immunogens and stimulate antibody production in infected hosts.

The HIV virus also possesses four genes (*tat, trs, sor,* and *3' orf*), which are involved in controlling expression of viral genes.

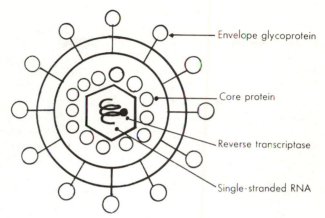

Figure 4-25. Structure of a retrovirus.

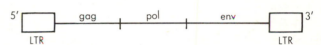

Figure 4-26. The genome of retroviruses.

At the 3' end of the genome there is more variability. This high variability explains the genetic polymorphism in HIV strains.

Human retroviruses are T-cell tropic. The receptor on host cells is T4. The T4 molecule is present on T4 helper lymphocytes. Macrophages and monocytes may also be infected by HIV, but they are seldom killed, probably because of low levels of T4 on their cell surface. HIV has been detected in the brain and spinal cord tissue of AIDS patients with dementia and neuropathy. It is hypothesized that infected macrophages transport the virus from the blood to the brain. HIV-infected brains show decreases in white matter.

HIV has affinity for T4 cells. Unlike HTLV-I and II, HIV-infected T cells are killed. Noninfected T4 cells adjacent to HIV-infected cells may participate in CPE (syncytial) formation. Subsequently, T4 lymphocyte depletion is a hallmark of HIV infection. T_H cells are characterized by surface antigens OKT4 and Leu3, and T_s cells by OKT8 and Leu2. In normal individuals, the T_H:T_s ratio is 2:3 (range 0.9 to 3.5). In AIDS patients, this ratio is less than 0:9. Other immunologic defects in AIDS are impaired delayed hypersensitivity response (i.e., anergy), low total lymphocyte count, and increased IgG and IgA levels (polyclonal stimulation, though there may be depression in some B-cell responsiveness).

The laboratory diagnosis of HIV infections is serological detection of antibodies in patient sera to HIV antigens and, recently, detection of HIV antigens themselves. The ELISA test is used in the screening of blood specimens for HIV antibodies. Presently a positive ELISA is repeated and a confirmatory test done. The confirmatory test has been either Western blot, immunofluorescence assay, or radioimmunoprecipitation assay. The serological reagents are available because of the ability of cultivating HIV in T-cell lines with added interleukin 2 (IL-2), also known as T-cell growth gactor. An immortal leukemic T4 cell line, H9, was developed to allow HIV growth without killing of the cell line. Western blot is performed by electrophorescing HIV lysate on a sodium dodecyl sulfate polyacrylamide gel. The proteins separated on the gel are then electrophoretically transferred (transblot) onto a nitrocellulose paper. Strips (lanes) of the paper are cut and soaked in the patient test serum. Antibodies specific to HIV are bound onto proteins on the paper and detected by subsequent incubation with ^{125}I or enzyme-labeled antihuman immunoglobulin.

Prevention of HIV infections includes the use of condoms, screening of blood, education about the risks of multiple sexual partners, and avoiding sharing of drug paraphernalia. Vaccines using cloned *env* genes are presently in clinical trials.

Other human retroviruses include HTLV-I (also known as adult T-cell leukemia virus [ATLV]) and HTLV-IV (also possibly related strains simian T-lymphotropic [STLV-III] virus or LAV type II). HTLV-I has been associated with adult T-cell leukemia and lymphoma. Antibodies to HTLV-IV and associated strains have been found in African patients with AIDS and among groups of Africans. The role of HTLV-II is not clear.

ANTIVIRAL AGENTS

Only a few antiviral agents are available for routine clinical use. Amantadine hydrochloride is active only against influenza A virus. Its mode of action is unclear, though it appears to be early after viral entry into host cells. It has been used both in the prophylaxis and treatment of influenza A infections. It is only 60% efficacious in its prophylactic properties, and it must be administered throughout the influenza outbreak. Amantadine can reduce the severity and duration of illness, but it must be administered early in the infection to be effective. Amantadine-resistant influenza A viruses have been isolated. Rimantadine, an amantadine analogue, is also effective, and it may have fewer CNS side effects (anxiety, insomnia, and lack of concentration) than amantadine.

Adenosine arabinoside (ara-A), also known vidarabine, is a purine nucleoside analogue with antiviral activity against the herpesviruses. In host cells, ara-A is phosphorylated by cellular kinases to a triphosphate form that inhibits DNA polymerase. It is relatively insoluble and when administered IV is given with a large fluid load, which can pose problems in patients with herpes encephalitis and cerebral edema. Recent trials have shown that acyclovir may be more effective than ara-A in the treatment of HSV encephalitis and VZV infections in severely immunosuppressed patients. Side effects of ara-A include GI (nausea, vomiting and diarrhea) and CNS (tremor, hallucination, ataxia, and dizziness) disturbances. An ophthalmic ointment of ara-A is available for herpetic keratitis. Another ophthalmic preparation available for herpetic keratitis is idoxuridine.

Acyclovir (a 2'-deoxyguanosine derivative) is the drug of choice for HSV and VZV infections. Acyclovir is activated to its monophosphate form by thymidine kinase (TK). It is then converted to the triphosphate, which is both an inhibitor and a substrate of viral DNA polymerase. HSV is the most susceptible to acyclovir; VZV is also affected but is not as susceptible. Acyclovir has little or no effect on CMV and EBV. (Some of the new acyclovir derivatives being synthesized show higher activity against CMV). This difference in acyclovir activity against herpesviruses could possibly be due to the induction of thymidine kinase levels in HSV and VZV infected cells and the lack of induction by CMV and EBV. CSF levels of acyclovir are 50% of plasma concentrations. Acyclovir resistance is primarily the result of TK-deficient strains. Side effects of acyclovir are minimal, with phlebitis noted during IV administration.

Ribavirin is a nucleoside (guanosine) analogue. It is virastatic and is incorporated into viral mRNA, leading to restricted viral protein synthesis. It is presently being used in the treatment of RSV infections in hospitalized infants and young children. The drug is given by aerosol administration. It may be effective in the prophylaxis and treatment of influenza A and B viral infection. No side effect is noted with aerosol administration.

Azidothymidine (AZT) is presently being tested and used in the treatment of HIV infections. AZT becomes phosphorylated. The triphosphate form is incorporated into DNA. However, since AZT lacks the 3'-hydroxyl group, the DNA chain is terminated. A side effect of AZT administration is bone marrow suppression.

CLINICAL MYCOLOGY

Fungi are eukaryotes. They may grow as single cells (yeasts) or multinuclear filaments (molds). Certain fungi, including many involved in systemic mycoses, exhibit dimorphism—that is, they can exist in nature as molds but in humans as yeasts. The tubular structures (or hyphae) of a mold form an intertwining filamentous mass known as a mycelium. Those hyphae that grow on or into the growth medium and absorb nutrients are the vegetative mycelium. Those hyphae that project above the medium and bear spores are the aerial mycelium. Hyphae may be septate or nonseptate. In nonseptate hyphae, there are many nuclei enclosed in the cytoplasm of a single cell wall (i.e., coenocytic). The cytoplasm of septate hyphae is also in continuous flow throughout the hyphae since their septa have fine pores.

On growth media, yeast colonies are creamy or pasty and molds are woolly or powdery. Molds reproduce by spores; yeasts reproduce by budding. The asexual spores (or conidia) aid in the identification of some fungi. Spores can exist as small single-cell microconidia or as large, single or multicellular macroconidia. Double-walled resting spores are chlamydospores. Blastoconidia arise from the budding of another cell. Arthroconidia are produced by septation of sporogenous hyphae.

A number of characteristics distinguish fungi from bacteria, including their cell wall composition. The polysaccharides of fungal cell walls are unique, such as chitin, beta-glucans, and mannan. The cytoplasmic membranes of fungi contain sterols (Table 4-8).

Fungi are identified on the basis of their growth characteristics (growth media, duration and temperature of growth), colonial morphology (color and texture, yeast versus mold), microscopic examination (conidia and hyphae), and biochemical characteristics (fermentation and assimilation). Direct microscopic examination of clinical specimens can identify fungal elements (Fig. 4-27). Some commonly used stains for detection of fungi include methenamine silver stain and periodic acid-Schiff stain. India ink has been used for the detection of *Cryptococcus neoformans* in CSF. Potassium hydroxide

Table 4-8. Characteristic Differentiation Between Fungi and Bacteria

	Fungi	Bacteria
Cell diameter (μm)	5 to 20	1 to 2
Nuclear membrane	Yes	No
Cytoplasmic membrane	Contains sterol	Lack sterol
Cell wall composition	Glucans, mannans, chitin	Muramic acid, teichoic acid

has been used for clearing specimens such as hair, skin scrapings, etc., leaving fungal elements more clearly visible.

YEASTS

Most fungi of medical importance belong to the class Deuteromycetes (Fungi Imperfecti). The sexual stages of these fungi are unknown and thus cannot be used for their classification.

Yeasts are the most common fungi infecting humans. Of these, *Candida albicans* is by far the most frequent pathogen. This yeast is part of the indigenous flora of the mucous membranes in the respiratory, GI, and female genital tracts. The most common form of candidiasis involves the mucous

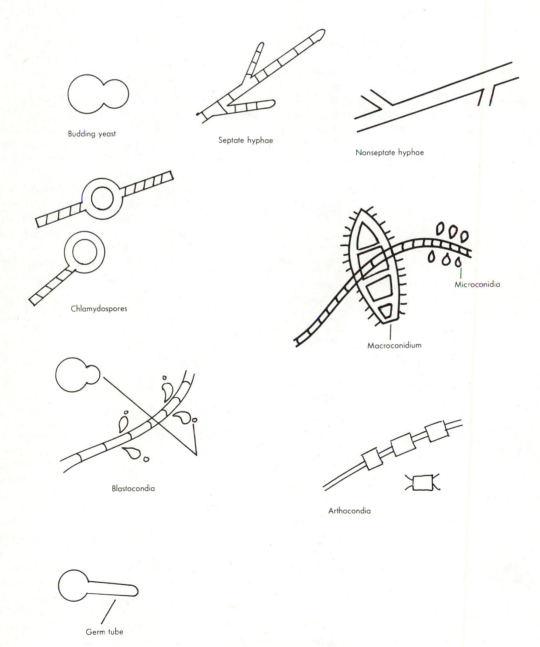

Figure 4-27. Microscopic features of fungi.

membranes, such as oral thrush and vaginitis. Patients who are on broad-spectrum antimicrobial therapy or are immunosuppressed (leukemia, lymphoma, or on immunosuppressive drugs) are predisposed to candidal colonization and invasion. Disseminated candidiasis often involves the kidneys and can also involve the lungs and other organs. Candidal invasion of the bloodstream can result from contaminated IV catheters, use of nonsterile needles or syringes (e.g., in drug addicts), and contamination during therapy. The difficulty at times in distinguishing *Candida* colonization versus invasive disease has led to the introduction of several immunodiagnostic assays involving the detection of mannan or cytoplasmic constituents in patient serum. Thus far these assays lack both sensitivity and specificity.

C. albicans exhibits dimorphism. It can exist as budding yeast cells and as hyphae. A valuable test for identifying *C. albicans* is its ability to form germ tubes in serum. Many other *Candida* species can cause disease, such as *Candida tropicalis* and *Candida krusei*.

C. neoformans (sexual stage: *Filobasidiella neoformans*) is thought to infect humans through inhalation. It is the predominant fungus found in pigeon feces. In the lungs, it causes subclinical pulmonary disease, which in the immunodeficient individual can lead to dissemination. The most common extrapulmonary cryptococcosis involves the CNS, where the disease resembles a brain tumor, brain abscess, chronic meningitis, or degenerative CNS disease. Rapid diagnosis of cryptococcal meningitis can be made by looking for encapsulated yeasts in the CSF by an India ink preparation or by an even more sensitive assay, the detection of cryptococcal antigen in CSF.

DERMATOPHYTES

Dermatophytes are filamentous fungi that invade keratin. The natural habitat of these fungi is soil (geophlilic), animals (zoophilic), and humans (anthrophilic). In general, the severity of human tinea (ringworm) is greater when caused by zoophilic and geophilic species.

Dermatophytes belong to one of three genera: *Epidermophyton, Microsporum*, and *Trichophyton*. *Trichophyton tonsurans* is responsible for greater than 90% of all tinea capitis, a scalp infection. *Trichophyton rubrum* is the primary causative agent of tinea cruris (jock itch), tinea unguium (nail plate), tinea pedis (athlete's foot), and tinea corporis (glabrous skin). *T. mentagrophytes, Microsporum gypseum, Microsporum canis*, and *Epidermophyton floccosum* are also involved in all of the dermatomycoses in North America. *E. floccosum* is not a causative agent of tinea corporis.

SYSTEMIC MYCOSES

Fungi involved in systemic mycoses include *Candida, Cryptococcus, Coccidioides immitis, Histoplasma capsulatum, Blastomyces dermatitidis*, and *Paracoccidioides brasilensis*. The latter four fungi exist as molds in soil and at 30°C but are yeasts in tissues and at 37°C. (The tissue form of *C. immitis* is spherules—spherical, thick-walled structures with numerous small endospores.) Figure 4-28 illustrates various forms of dimorphic fungi.

C. immitis is endemic in southwestern United States. Infection occurs by inhalation of its spores in dust, leading to asymptomatic pulmonary infection. In less than 1% of cases, it will disseminate with granulomatous lesions in skin, bones, and meninges. Individuals infected with or previously exposed to *C. immitis* will have a positive skin test to coccidioidin antigen. The skin test is negative in disseminated cases and is a poor prognostic sign. Serodiagnostic assays (complement fixation) can be helpful in determining the diagnosis and prognosis of coccidioidomycosis.

H. capsulatum is found in the soil in central United States in the Mississippi, Missouri, and Ohio River valleys. It is prevalent in soil fertilized with bird droppings and bat guano. Exposure to chicken houses and caves has led to *H. capsulatum* infections. Infection is via inhalation, leading to a mild respiratory tract infection. In a small number of cases the infection may disseminate, resulting in lesions in practically all tissues. Chronic pulmonary histoplasmosis resembles TB. The immunodiffusion and CIE assays may be useful in differentiating between active and inactive histoplasmosis. Two bands, h and m, may be observed. The h band is indicative of active disease. The m band is found in 70% of the sera from individuals exposed to *H. capsulatum*.

B. dermatitidis is found in Canada and the northern Mississippi and Ohio River valleys. Infection begins in the lungs and spreads to form lesions in the skin, bones, and prostate. Pulmonary blastomycosis can increase in severity over weeks to months to eventually resemble TB or carcinoma. Serodiagnosis (complement fixation test) is positive in less than 50% of patients with proven blastomycosis.

P. brasiliensis is found in South America, Central America, and Mexico. The diagnosis of systemic mycosis is made by culture and/or tissue examination. Culture identification involves the conversion of the mold to the yeast phase (in the case of *C. immitis*, the conversion to spherules may be accomplished in animals), microscopic morphology, and the exoantigen test.

Another dimorphic fungus is *Sporothrix schenckii*. Human infection results from subcutaneous inoculation via thorns and splinters. The most common form of sporotrichosis is a cutaneous lesion at the site of inoculation. This may lead, in 1 to 2 weeks, to a characteristic chain of lesions along the draining lymphatic vessel.

OPPORTUNISTIC MYCOSES

Opportunistic mycoses are fungal diseases that are not normally encountered in a healthy host but are found in persons with altered host defenses. *Candida* and *Cryptococcus* are considered opportunistic pathogens. Also, *Aspergillus, Zygomycetes* (which includes *Mucor, Rhizopus*, and *Absidia*), and other fungi cause disease in immunocompromised individuals.

Aspergillus is ubiquitous. The presence of its spores in the environment can cause contamination of clinical specimens. Thus the casual isolation of saprophytic fungi in patient specimens must be interpreted with care. The most common *Aspergillus* species isolated include *Aspergillus fumigatus, Aspergillus flavus, Aspergillus niger*, and *Aspergillus terreus*, with *A. fumigatus* accounting for over 90% of all infections. Aspergillosis can present as an allergic response (hypersensitivity) to *Aspergillus* spores, or in patients with underlying cavitary pulmonary disease (e.g., TB) the fungus can grow in these cavities into

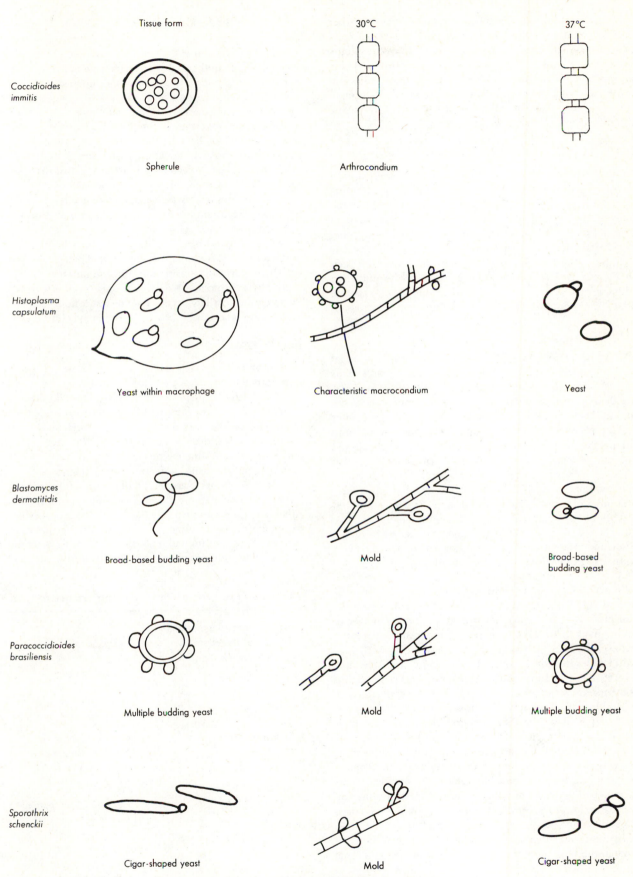

Figure 4-28. Microscopic identification of dimorphic fungi.

macroscopic fungus balls. Rarely, it can disseminate to other organs, frequently resulting in death.

Zygomycetes infection is associated with immunologic deficiency and most notably with diabetes mellitus. These fungi can directly invade blood vessels. The most common zygomycosis is the rhinocerebral form, frequently resulting in death. Diagnosis can be made by culture and by tissue examination for nonseptating, broad hyphae.

MYCETOMA

Mycetomas are chronic infections, usually of the extremities, which produce markedly deforming swelling with draining pus containing granules that are microcolonies of the invading organism. The route of infection is through the injured skin via thorns, splinters, and bites. Mycetoma may be actinomycotic, bacterial, or eumycotic. The most common cause of eumycotic mycetoma in the United States is *Pseudallescheria boydii* (previously *Allescheria*). The granules of *P. boydii* are white and when examined microscopically are seen to be interwoven, septate hyphae. These granules should be cultured.

ANTIFUNGAL AGENTS

Presently, amphotericin B (AMB) is the only antifungal agent used in the treatment of systemic fungal diseases. This polyene antibiotic is limited by its low solubility, poor stability, and high toxicity (nephrotoxic and hepatoxic). Another polyene, nystatin, is used topically for *Candida* infections. Polyenes alter fungal membranes by binding to ergosterol, the most common sterol in fungal membranes. The binding leads to altered membrane permeability. Polyenes are fungicidal. AMB-resistant fungi have decreased amounts of ergosterol.

The synthetic drug 5-fluorocytosine (5-FC) has limited use in treatment of deep-seated fungal disease. It is administered with AMB in the treatment of *C. neoformans* infections. Unlike AMB, it penetrates well into the CSF. 5-FC is taken up by fungal but not mammalian cells. Thus, it has low toxicity. 5-FC is deaminated intracellularly by fungal cells to 5-fluorouracil (5-FU). 5-FU is incorporated into RNA and thus interferes with protein synthesis. Primary resistance to 5-FC by *C. albicans* is high, and thus 5-FC cannot be used in treatment of candidosis. The primary 5-FC resistance rate to 5-FC has been reported to be as high as 42%. This high rate is the result of natural heterozygosity of 5-FC resistance in *C. albicans*.

Imidazoles include miconazole (parenteral) and ketoconazole (oral). They act by inhibiting ergosterol synthesis and thus alter membrane structure and permeability. Presently, miconazole is seldom used because of its toxicity (phlebitis, pruritus, rash, fever, nausea, diarrhea, hyperlipidemia, hematologic and hepatic toxicity). Ketoconazole is a useful alternative to amphotericin B for the treatment of infections by dimorphic fungi; it is efficacious in the treatment of chronic mucocutaneous candidosis. Ketoconazole toxicity is manifested by nausea, hepatotoxicity, and interference with testosterone and adrenocorticotropic hormone synthesis. It should not be used in CNS infections. Recently, triazoles (e.g., fluconazole) have been introduced. Fluconazole has good CSF penetration. Its efficacy in the treatment of various mycoses awaits additional data.

Griseofluvin is used in the treatment of dermatophytoses.

CLINICAL PARASITOLOGY

The Greek origin of the word *parasite* means "one who eats at the table of another." That is, a parasite is an organism that depends on another organism (the **host**) for nutritional support. A definitive host harbors the adult or sexually mature phase of the parasite. An **intermediate host** harbors the larval or developmental stages of the parasite. Some parasites have one intermediate host in their life cycle, others have two intermediate hosts. The animal that serves as a potential reservoir source of infection to humans is called the **reservoir host**. Disease in the animal itself is zoonosis.

Disease does not always accompany infection. An infected host may be asymptomatic or have a limited infection. A diseased host shows symptoms.

An understanding of the life cycle of parasites is important in the diagnosis, treatment, and control of parasitic infections.

The majority of parasites infecting humans belong to one of three phyla: Protozoa, Nemathelminthes (roundworms), and Platyhelminthes (flatworms). The classes Cestodes (tapeworm) and Trematoda (flukes) belong to the Platyhelminthes.

PROTOZOA

Protozoa are single-cell animals. Those of particular importance to humans are listed in Table 4-9.

The Mastigophora protozoa possess a whip-like filamentous structure (flagellum) for propelling the organism. Amoebas move via foot-like extensions, or pseudopodia. Sporozoa have a complex cycle with an asexual reproductive phase (schizogeny) and a sexual reproductive phase (sporogeny).

Intestinal parasitic infections are diagnosed by fecal examination. Gross examination of the stool for consistency is important. Loose stools should be examined within 1 hour of collection for motile trophozoites (i.e., amoebas), since the trophozoites may autolyse or become distorted with prolonged storage. Direct examination of the stool using a temporary stain such as iodine can yield a rapid diagnosis. Alternatively,

Table 4-9. Protozoa of Particular Importance to Humans

Mastigophora (flagellate)	
Intestinal flagellate	*Giardi lamblia*
Genital flagellate	*Trichomonas vaginalis*
Hemoflagellates	*Trypansoma gambiense*
	Trypanosoma rhodesiense
	Trypanosoma cruzi
	Leishmania donovani
Sarcondina (amebae)	*Entamoeba histolytica*
	Naelgeria fowleri
	Acanthamoeba species
Sporozoa	*Plasmodium vivax*
	Plasmodium falciparum
	Plasmodium malariae
	Plasmodium ovale
	Toxoplasma gondii
	Pneumocystis carinii
	Cryptosporidium species

trophozoites may be preserved with polyvinyl alcohol (PVA) and permanent trichrome-stained smears made. Protozoa in formed stools are more likely to be in the cyst stage. Stool preservatives for cysts include formalin-saline and Merthiolate-iodine-formalin (MIF). The formalin-saline and MIF-treated specimens cannot be used to make permanent slides. MIF-treated stools are not effective for detecting nematode ova. Thus the best stool preservatives to use are PVA and formalin-saline.

Since the passage of the organism in stools may be intermittent, at least three stool specimens at weekly intervals should be obtained. It is important that the stool be free of urine, since it could lyse trophozoites. An estimate of the number of ova present can indicate how many worms the patient harbors. It is important that stools be concentrated either by sedimentation or by flotation to detect those specimens that have low numbers of parasites or ova. In flotation, the parasite form is suspended in zinc sulfate. This causes the parasites to become buoyant and float to the surface of the fluid, where they are collected for examination.

Entamoeba

E. histolytica infection occurs in 1 to 5% of the U.S. population. It is especially common in institutions, where its transmission is aided by poor hygiene and crowding, and among sexually active male homosexuals. Epidemics of *E. histolytica* infection have been traced to cyst-contaminated water and raw vegetables.

There are two types of *E. histolytica* infections: intestinal amebiasis and extraintestinal amebiasis. Intestinal amebiasis may be asymptomatic ("carrier" state) or invasive (amebic dysentery). In some cases, the organism may invade the bowel wall, leading to its dissemination to other sites. Extraintestinal infections usually involve the liver, but abscesses may also occur in the lungs, brain, and skin. Amebic liver abscess is usually encountered in the right lobe. Pulmonary amebiasis results in 80% of cases from direct extension of liver abscess and thus afflicts the right lower lobe of the lung.

Diagnosis of intestinal amebiasis is by stool examination for trophozoites and/or cysts (Fig. 4-29). The size and the

microscopic features are important in their identification. The indirect hemagglutination test is useful in the diagnosis of extraintestinal amebiasis or invasive intestinal infections. Treatment of amebiasis is metronidazole and diiodohydroxyquin.

Giardia

G. lamblia transmission is much like that of *E. histolytica*, and infection is prevalent in institutional settings, day-care centers, and male homosexuals. It is the most prevalent intestinal parasite in the United States (1 to 16%). Outbreaks are traced to contaminated water or raw vegetables and fruits. Beavers have been implicated in waterborne outbreaks. It is also a recognized agent in traveler's diarrhea, as observed in tourists returning from Leningrad, Russia.

Most individuals infected with *Giardia* are asymptomatic cyst carriers. In others, following a 1- to 3-week incubation period, explosive, watery, foul-smelling diarrhea is accompanied by increased foul flatulence and abdominal bloating. The stool is loose and steatorrheic, with no blood or pus. Malabsorption may occur, leading to interference with fat absorption. The excessive amount of fat in the stool causes the stool to float on top of toilet paper.

Laboratory diagnosis of giardiasis is stool examination for *G. lamblia* trophozoite or cysts (Fig. 4-30). Alternatives for examination of trophozoites in duodenal fluids include duo-

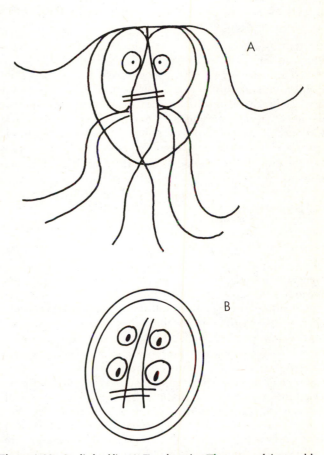

Figure 4-30. *Gardia lamblia.* (*A*) Trophozoite. The two nuclei resemble eyes. There are four sets of flagella and a sucking disk on the ventral surface. (*B*) Cyst. The oval shape contains four nuclei.

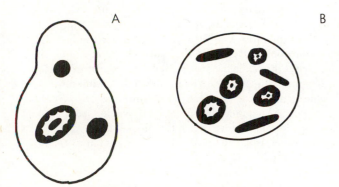

Figure 4-29. *Entamoeba histolytica.* (*A*) Trophozoite. Note the one nucleus with evenly distributed chromatin and a central karysome. The cytoplasm may contain ingested RBCs. Progressive pseudopia are seen. (*B*) Cyst. Cysts are 10 to 20 μm round. They contain 1 to 4 nuclei, like those of the trophozoite. The cytoplasm contains chromatoid bodies with rounded ends.

denal intubation or obtaining a duodenal fluid. Duodenal intubation (Enterotest) involves swallowing a gelatin capsule on a string. The string is affixed to the patient's mouth. When the gelatin dissolves, the string is released into the duodenum or jejunum. After several hours, the string is retrieved and its adherent fluid examined for trophozoites.

Treatment of giardiasis is with quinacrine, metronidazole, or furazolidone.

Crytosporidium

Cryptosporidium is a coccidial parasite that is encountered in immunosuppressed patients, homosexuals, and recently in immunocompetent individuals such as day-care attendees. In immunosuppressed patients, diarrhea may last for weeks to years. It is acquired via the fecal-oral route.

Like the malaria parasite, *Cryptosporidium* has a sexual (sporogonic) and asexual (schizontic) phase. However, unlike *Plasmodium*, *Cryptosporidium* life cycle involves only one host. The different species of *Cryptosporidium* are specific for either humans or other animals. The various developmental stages of the parasite occur on the membrane or just underneath the membrane of the small intestinal epithelial cells of the brush border.

Laboratory diagnosis of cryptospordiosis includes detecting the oocyst in stool. The acid-fast stain and auramine O stains used in mycobacteria staining are especially useful in detecting *Cryptosporidium* oocyst. There currently is no therapy for cryptosporidia infection.

Plasmodium

Approximately 638 million people live in malaria-endemic regions, and more than a million people die each year of malaria. Malaria in the United States is generally encountered in individuals who have traveled to an endemic area. Malaria was once an American disease, since the mosquito vector of malaria is abundant in this country.

The four *Plasmodium* species and their incidence affecting humans are as follows:

P. vivax	51%
P. falciparum	29%
P. ovale	3%
P. malariae	8%

Generally malaria is transmitted by the bite of a female *Anopheles* mosquito. Malaria can be transmitted by syringes shared by drug addicts, by blood transfusion, and rarely vertically (congenital malaria). In each of these cases, there is no exoerythrocytic stage so that this form need not be treated.

There are two phases in the *Plasmodium* life cycle: (1) asexual (schizogony), which occurs in humans, and (2) sexual (sporogony), which occurs in mosquitoes. When the sporozoite from the mosquito is introduced into the bloodstream of humans, the parasite undergoes schizogeny. Schizogeny has two phases: (1) exoerythrocytic, which occurs in the liver, and (2) erythrocytic. The sporozoites invade the hepatocytes, where they multiply into merozoites. When the hepatocytes rupture, the merozoites are released. In *P. vivax, P. ovale*, and *P. malariae*, the merozoites can infect other hepatocytes or RBCs, whereas in *P. falciparum* all merozoites invade only RBCs. This difference is important to remember for the following reasons:

1. Reinfection of hepatocytes may cause relapses of *P. vivax*, *P. malariae*, and *P. ovale* infections. Malaria relapses do not occur after *P. falciparum* infection.
2. *P. falciparum* illness is usually of less than 1 year duration.
3. Treatment for *P. falciparum* malaria does not require eradication of the exoerythrocytic form of the parasite, whereas with *P. vivax* and *P. ovale*, a drug has to be given for clinical cure against the circulating blood form and a second drug must be given for radical cure in eradicating the infection itself to prevent relapses.

Another difference between *P. falciparum* and the other *Plasmodium* species is the age of the RBCs they attack. *P. malariae* attacks old RBCs, *P. vivax* and *P. ovale* attack immature RBCs, while *P. falciparum* attacks all RBCs. This may explain the high density of parasitemia that occurs only in *P. falciparum* malaria and not in others.

Another difference between *P. falciparum* malaria and other malaria infections is the knob-like structures seen on the surface of the RBC infected with *P. falciparum*. This makes the RBCs sticky, resulting in their sticking to capillary endothelium. This also explains why parasitic stages are not observed beyond the early trophozoite (ring forms) in blood smears of *P. falciparum* malaria. The RBCs stick to visceral capillaries, and the parasites mature there. However, when the various stages of *P. falciparum* are observed in blood smears, the patient is generally deathly ill. This stickiness of RBCs also accounts for a fatal complication of *P. faciparum* malaria—cerebral malaria. Microscopically, the capillaries are obstructed with parasitized RBCs.

Inside the RBC, the trophozoite ingests some of the hemoglobin, resulting in a large vacuole in the parasite's cytoplasm. The resulting appearance is ring forms (nucleus stains red, cytoplasm stains blue) in Giemsa stain. The trophozoite matures into a schizont, which contains merozoites. When the schizont ruptures, the merozoites invade other RBCs and develop into the sexual forms: microgametocytes (male) and macrogametocytes (female). The release of merozoites is accompanied by high fever, chills, and sweats—all hallmarks of malaria. The parasites show synchronous growth, thus malaria shows cyclic recurrent attacks.

When the mosquito bites and feeds on human blood, the only form of the parasite that survives in the mosquito's stomach is the sexual form. The male gametocyte exflagellates by forming whip-like forms on its surface and swims toward the female gametocyte. The fertilized gamete is known as the ookinete. The ookinete penetrates the mosquito's stomach and develops into an oocyst. When the oocyst bursts, sporozoites within are released and invade the mosquito's salivary gland to complete the life cycle.

Certain population groups have some resistance to malaria:

1. Individuals with RBCs lacking the Duffy blood group. The Duffy marker is a receptor for *P. vivax*.
2. Individuals with sickle cell disease, thalassemia, and glucose-6-phosphate dehydrogenase deficiency. They are more resistant to *P. falciparum* infections, since

parasite-infected RBCs in these individuals cause potassium loss in RBCs, thereby resulting in actual physical disruption of the parasite.

Interestingly, these abnormalities are more common among African populations.

The diagnosis of malaria is primarily with peripheral blood smears. In *P. falciparum* infections, the smear usually shows ring form as the only stage. In *P. vivax* infections, the smears show *P. vivax*-infected RBCs to be slightly enlarged and with Schüffner's dots and ameboid trophozoites.

The chemoprophylaxis of individuals traveling to endemic area is chloroquine with or without primaquine. Primaquine is used for prophylaxis against the liver stages of *P. vivax* and *P. ovale*. Primaquine can cause severe hemolysis if given to individuals with glucose-6-phosphate dehydrogenase deficiencies or with Mediterranean or Oriental origins and thus is contraindicated in this group. In chloroquine-resistant malarial areas (East Africa, South America, and Southeast Asia), pyrimethamine-sulfadoxine (Fansidar) is used along with chloroquine prophylaxis. Fansidar is active only against *P. falciparum*. It is contraindicated in pregnant females and in children younger than 2 years.

Treatment of malaria includes chloroquine, chloroquine plus primaquine (*P. ovale* and *P. vivax*), or quinine plus tetracycline (for chloroquine-resistant *P. falciparum*). Vaccines containing the merozoite or sporozoite surface antigens are currently being developed.

Babesia

Babesia microti infection presents clinically like malaria. Its life cycle differs from *Plasmodium* in that the insect vector is a tick (*Ixodes dammini*) and there is no gametocyte (i.e., no sexual cycle). In the United States, babesiasis is seen in the Long Island and Martha's Vineyard regions, where deer are its natural reservoir. Infection occurs most frequently in late summer and early fall. Most *Babesia* infections are asymptomatic, but splenomegaly is a risk factor for more severe infection.

Laboratory diagnosis of babesiosis is primarily made by blood smears. It differs from *Plasmodium* in that there is no gametocyte or schizont. There is no pigment in infected RBCs. There may be many ring forms per RBC (*Babesia* 1 to 12, versus malaria 1 to 3) and three chromatin dots per parasite (*Babesia* 1 to 3, versus malaria 1 to 2). Treatment of babesiosis has been with blood transfusion. It was recently suggested that a combined therapy with clindamycin and quinine might be effective.

Toxoplasma

T. gondii is a coccidian with worldwide distribution. It can infect many mammals, but the oocyst stage occurs only in cats. Humans become infected by ingestion of cyst-containing meats that have not been properly cooked or by ingestion of or contact with oocyst-contaminated soil or cat feces.

Toxoplasma infection is generally subclinical in immunocompetent individuals. It is a major concern in neonates (congenital infection) and in immunocompromised patients. The highest rate of acquiring toxoplasmosis is during the childbearing years. Approximately one-third of females between 20 and 30 years of age have antibodies to *Toxoplasma*. *Toxoplasma* infection occurring in a seronegative pregnant female can lead to severe congenital disease, with chorioretinitis, hydrocephaly, and intracranial calcification. In the immunocompromised host (including AIDS patients), more than 50% of cases of fatal toxoplasmosis involve the CNS.

Diagnosis is mainly based on serology. The detection of IgM-specific anti-*Toxoplasma* antibodies has been useful in diagnosing congenital infection and in distinguishing between recent versus past infections in adults. Therapy of toxoplasmosis is with sulfadiazine-pyrimethamine or spiramycin.

Pneumocystis

P. carinii infection in the immunocompetent host is subclinical. By the age of 4, most children have antibodies to *P. carinii*. In immunosuppressed patients (leukemia, lymphoma, AIDS), an interstitial pneumonia results. In patients undergoing immunosuppressive therapy, the pneumonia most frequently occurs when the dose of corticosteroids is tapered. *Pneumocystis* pneumonias are also encountered in neonates and malnourished children.

Pneumocystis exists in the trophozoite cyst (contains eight sporozoites) forms. Laboratory diagnosis is primarily examination of open-lung biopsy, needle biopsy, suptum, or other respiratory specimens for sporozoite-containing cysts. Stains most often used include Gomori's silver methenamine stain and the toluidine blue O stain. Treatment of *Pneumocystis* is with trimethoprim-sulfamethoxazole or pentamidine.

Nonentamoebic amoebas

N. fowleri and *Acanthameoba* are free-living soil ameobas. Humans usually acquire *Naegleria* from swimming or other activities that may force contaminated water into the nose. After invading the nasal epithelium, the parasites migrate along the olfactory nerve and pierce the cribriform plate to the brain. *Acanthamoeba* meningoencephalitis is less common and is encountered in patients with lowered resistance.

Naegleria and *Acanthamoeba* exist in the infective trophozoite form and in the cyst form. In addition, *Naegleria* can exist also as a flagellate. Laboratory diagnosis is based on examination of CSF for motile amoebas. Both can be cultured in vitro in agar seeded with killed *E. coli*. There is no known effective treatment of amoebic meningoencephalitis.

Trichomonas

T. vaginalis is a flagellate. It is found in the vagina of 25% of all females. In about 10% of infected cases, the parasite produces vaginitis and urethritis in females and prostatitis and urethritis in males. The vaginal discharge in females with trichomoniasis is a yellowish, foul-smelling frothy discharge accompanied by itching, dysuria, and a burning sensation of the vulva and vagina. The symptoms are more severe during pregnancy and the latter part of the menstrual period. The diagnosis is made by examining a wet mount of the vaginal exudate for motile trichomonads (Fig. 4-31). Treatment of trichomoniasis is with metronidazole.

Hemoflagellates

The hemoflagellates include *Leishmania* and *Trypanosoma*. The organisms bear a free flagellum at some stage of their life cycle and are transmitted by an arthropod vector. There are four stages in their developmental cycle (Fig. 4-32).

L. donovani causes viceral leishmaniasis (also known as kala-azar) when macrophages of the deep viscera are parasitized. The disease is found in India, China, the Middle East, Africa, and South America. Visceral leishmaniasis is characterized by a grossly enlarged spleen and liver in untreated individuals. Treatment is with sodium stibogluconate.

T. gambiense and *T. rhodesiense* are the causative agents of African trypanosomiasis (also known as sleeping sickness). *T. gambiense* is present in western and central Africa and *T. rhodesiense* in eastern and central Africa. Humans are the only known natural hosts of *T. gambiense*, and the wild antelope is the reservoir host of *T. rhodesiense*. Untreated persons with *T.*

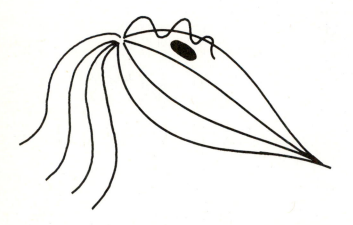

Figure 4-31. *Trichomonas vaginalis.* Note the four anterior flagella, the short undulating membrane at the anterior half of the body, the axostyle down the length of the body, the slit-like mouth, and the prominent oral nucleus.

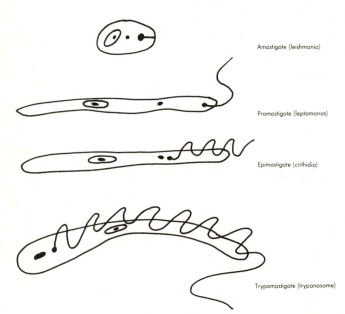

Amastigote (leishmania)

Promastigote (leptomonas)

Epimastigote (crithidia)

Trypomastigote (trypanosome)

Figure 4-32. The four stages in the developmental cycle of hemo-flagellates.

gambiense infections die a slow death involving the CNS. Untreated *T. rhodesiense* trypanosomiasis patients die more rapidly, with fulminating parasitemia and CNS involvement.

T. cruzi is the causative agent of American trypanosomiasis (also known as Chagas' disease). It is endemic in South and Central America, where the reduviid bugs inhabit the mud huts of the poor. Infection with *T. cruzi* results in enlargement of the lymphatic glands, liver, and spleen and most notably heart damage. The amastigotes invade heart muscle cells, which may eventually lead to heart failure. Diagnosis of hemoflagellate infection is made by looking for the parasitic stage in host tissue sections or body fluids.

HELMINTHS

The helminths ("worms") are divided into two phyla: (1) Nemathelminthes, containing the class Nematoda (round-worms), and (2) Platyhelminthes, containing the class Trematoda (flukes) and Cestoda (tapeworm). Some of the distinguishing characteristics of helminths are listed in Table 4-10.

Some of the differences between protozoan and helminthic diseases are as follows:

1. Eosinophilia. This does not occur in protozoan infection but may occur in helminthic infection.
2. Their multiplication. Protozoans multiply within the host. The adult helminths do not, and they have a limited life span.
3. Their elimination from the host. Treatment of protozoan disease usually requires their complete elimination from the host. This is usually not necessary or possible with helminthic infections. The amount of tissue damage and severity of symptoms in helminthic infections are usually proportional to parasite burden.

Nematodes are the only helminths containing a body cavity. Of the nematodes, only the filarial nematodes require an intermediate host. They are transmitted by (1) ingestion or inhalation of the egg stage (or in the case of *Trichnella spiralis*, ingestion of larvae in an intermediate host), (2) skin penetration of filariform larvae, and (3) the insect bite of filarial larvae.

The intestinal nematodes include *Ascaris lumbricoides*, the hookworms (*Necator americanus, Ancylostoma duodenale*), *Trichuris trichiura* (whipworm), *Strongyloides stercoralis*, and *Enterobius vermicularis* (pinworm). After being transmitted to humans, the nematodes develop into larvae that may pass through a tissue phase. The larvae then develop into adult worms in the intestine (Table 4-11).

The three most prevalent heminthic infection in the world are *A. lumbricoides*, followed by *T. trichiura*, followed by the hookworms. These are observed in tropical regions and are rarely fatal.

Ingested *A. lumbricoides* eggs hatch in the gut to release the larvae. The larvae migrate through the body (liver to heart to lung to intestine) before developing into adult worms. Clinical symptoms of ascariasis may result in heavy infections. Pulmonary symptoms resembling pneumonia can occur when large numbers of larvae migrate through the venules and capillaries of the lung. Their large size results in rupturing of small blood vessels, with resulting hemorrhage that can flood into air sacs. In some cases, hypersensitivity to larval antigens

Table 4-10. Distinguishing Characteristics of Helminths

Characteristic	Nematodes	Trematodes	Cestodes
Shape	Cylindrical, unsegmented	Leaf-like, unsegmented	Tape-like, segmented
Suckers	No	Yes	Yes
Hooklet	No	No	Usually, yes
Sexes	Separate	Not separate (except *Schistosma*)	Not separate

Table 4-11. Distinguishing Differences of Nematodes

Intestinal nematodes	Mode of transmission	Tissue phase
Ascaris	Ingestion of eggs	Gut and other tissues (liver, lung, heart)
Hookworms *Strongyloides*	Skin penetration of filariform larvae	Gut and tissues (skin, lung)
Pinworm Whipworm	Ingestion (also inhalation for pinworm)	Gut only

leads to an allergic phenomenon with eosinophilia. In children with a large worm burden, the nutrients taken by the worm from an already substandard diet can lead to malnutrition. The migratory capability of the adult worm can lead to mechanical blockage in the appendix, liver, intestine, bile ducts, and pancreatic ducts.

Diagnosis of ascariasis is made by stool examination for the unfertilized eggs and the more distinguishable fertilized eggs (Fig. 4-33*A*, *B*). Eosinophilia is present during larva migration to the lungs. Treatment of ascariasis is with pyrantel or mebendazole.

T. trichiura looks like a whip. After ingestion of the egg, the larva is released and migrates to the colon, where it matures to an adult. Most infections are asymptomatic. Heavy worm burden, especially in children, results in chronic bloody diarrhea, rectal prolapse, and anemia. Diagnosis of trichuriasis is made by stool examination for the characteristic barrel-shaped eggs with mucoid plugs at each end. Treatment is with mebendazole.

Hookworm infections are a problem in southern United States. After skin penetration due to walking barefoot, the filariform larvae make the same journey (heart to lung to intestine) as *A. lumbricoides*. The eggs released from the adult worm are unembryonated. Under favorable conditions in the soil, the larvae develop in the egg via the rhabditiform stage to the infective filariform stage.

Clinical symptoms of hookworm disease are similar to those of ascariasis, with pneumonitis when the larvae reach the lungs. In heavy worm burdens, the adult worm, which attaches to the intestine via teeth, can ingest sufficient blood to cause anemia. "Ground itch" occurs at the larval penetration site of the skin. Diagnosis of both *A. duodenale* and *N. americanus* is made by stool examination for thin-shelled ovoid eggs (Fig. 4-33*D*). These have to be distinguished from decorticated (i.e., loss of the albumin-like coat) fertilized eggs of *A. lumbricoides*. *A. lumbricoides* eggs pick up iodine, but hookworm eggs do not. If stools containing hookworm eggs are not examined and are left at room temperature, rhabditiform larvae may hatch and be confused with *Strongyloides* larvae (Fig. 4-34). Treatment of hookworm infection is the same as for ascariasis, using pyrantel or mebendazole.

S. stercoralis is unique from other nematodes in several respects:

1. It has two adult forms: one within the host and one in soil.
2. It is the only nematode whose adult can increase in number within the host.
3. It has three possible life cycles (Fig. 4-35).
   a. A cycle similar to that of the hookworm (direct or asexual cycle).
   b. A cycle involving adult worms in the soil (indirect or sexual cycle).
   c. A complete cycle within the host (autoinfection).
4. It is the only nematode that is diagnosed by the presence of larvae in the stool.

Strongyloidiasis can be asymptomatic or can present with intestinal symptoms (steatorrheic, foul-smelling stool due to the inability to absorb fat), rash (allergy to the larvae), and

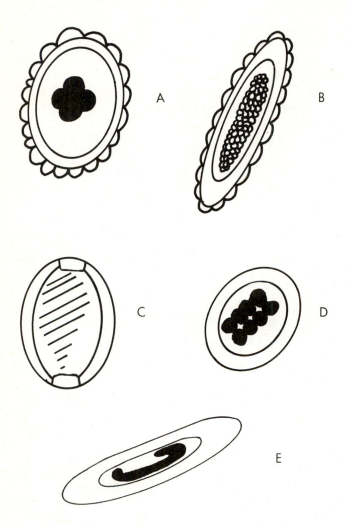

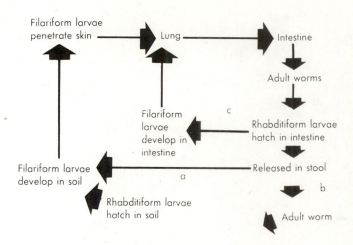

Figure 4-35. The three possible life cycles of *S. stercoralis*.

Figure 4-33. Intestinal nematodes. (*A*) Fertilized egg of *Ascaris lumbricoides,* which has a round to ovoid shape and an albuminous coat. (*B*) Unfertilized egg of *A. lumbricoides,* which is longer and narrower and has unorganized egg contents. (*C*) *Trichuris trichiura* egg, which is barrel shaped and has bipolar plugs. (*D*) Hookworm egg, which has an ovoid, thin, transparent shell. (*E*) *Enterobius vermicularis,* which has a transparent shell. One side of the egg is flat. It usually contains larvae.

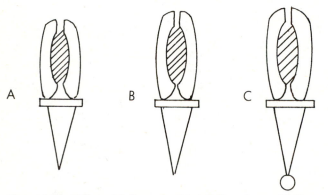

Figure 4-34. Differential diagnosis of rhabditiform larvae. (*A*) *Strongyloides stercoralis:* short buccal capsule, pointed tail. (*B*) Hookworm: long buccal capsule, pointed tail. (*C*) *Trichostrongylus:* long buccal capsule, bead-tipped tail.

pulmonary symptoms resembling pneumonia (due to migration of larvae through the lung during autoinfection). Symptoms are more severe in immunocompromised hosts. Diagnosis of *S. stercoralis* is made by examination of the stool for larvae. Treatment of strongyloidiasis is with thiabendazole.

E. vermicularis is acquired by inhalation or ingestion of parasitic eggs. Infections with this parasite often occur in institutions, in schools, or among family members. Humans are the definitive hosts. The egg hatches in the duodenum, and the larvae mature in the small intestine. Adult worms migrate to the large intestine, where they mate. The female worm lays her eggs at the perianal region, causing anal itch. Retroinfection can occur if eggs on the fingers and fingernails are transferred to the mouth. Diagnosis of enterobiasis is made by examining specimens taken from the anal area for eggs. Such specimens can be obtained by the cellophane tape test. Treatment is with pyrantel and mebendazole.

Nematode infections diagnosed by tissue examination include *Toxocara canis, Toxocara cati*, and *T. spiralis*. *T. canis* and *T. cati* are causative agents of visceral larva migrans transmitted to humans from dogs or cats, respectively. Embryonated eggs are ingested. The larvae hatch and migrate to the lungs and other tissues (such as liver, CNS, spleen, and eye). Clinically, visceral larva migrans presents with allergic pulmonary symptoms, hepatosplenomegaly, and eosinophilia. Diagnosis of larva migrans includes serology and increased eosinophilia.

T. spiralis is one of the few helminths that does not have an external host. Infection occurs by eating raw or undercooked meat containing the encysted larvae. Infected meats may include those from pigs, bears, seals, and walruses. Pigs become infected by feeding on raw garbage. In many cases, humans become infected by ingesting pork-containing "pure beef" hamburgers. In the intestine, the larva is released, molts several times, and matures to an adult. After copulation, the female bears larvae, which enter the bloodstream, travel to the heart and lungs, and are filtered out in the skeletal muscles. Here the larvae become encysted. The severity of trichinosis depends on the larvae load. In heavy infections, trichinosis is typified by myalgia, palpebral edema, and eosinophilia. Diagnosis of trichinosis is made by finding the larvae in muscle tissue biopsy or on serology (bentonite flocculation test). Treatment of trichinosis is with thiabendazole. Contaminated meat frozen for 20 days is not infective for trichinosis.

The filarial nematodes include *Loa loa, Wuchereria bancrofti, Brugia malayi,* and *Onchocera volvulus*. They are transmitted by insect vectors and are found in tropical regions. *B. malayi* is confined to southern and Southeast Asia, and *L. loa* to western and central Africa. Their life cycle is characterized by microfilarial periodicity and is of diagnostic importance for timing of blood samples taken. For example, the peak density of *W. bancrofti* in the peripheral circulation occurs between 10 P.M. and 2 A.M. and for *L. loa* during the daytime.

The microfilariae are transmitted to the arthropod during a bite and develop after several stages to the filariform stage. This is reintroduced into humans at further blood meals. Most infections are asymptomatic. However, in some cases *W. bancrofti* and *B. malayi* infections are characterized by subcutaneous swelling (including the eye) due to the parasite's migration. Eosinophilia is noted in loiasis. In each of these instances, diagnosis is made by examination of blood for microfilariae. On the other hand, *O. volvulus* infection (river blindness) is diagnosed by examining a skin snip for microfilariae. Treatment of filariasis is with diethylcarbamazine (and in *O. volvulus* also with suramin).

Trematodes include *Schistosoma mansoni, Schistosoma japonicum, Schistosoma haematobium, Clonorchis sinensis, Paragonimus westermani,* and *Fasciolopsis buski*. Except for *S. haematobium*, which is diagnosed by urine examination, the rest are diagnosed by detecting eggs in feces. The eggs of all trematodes (except *Schistosoma*) are operculated (Fig. 4-36).

The life cycle of trematodes requires the snail as an intermediate host. Except for *Schistosoma*, which can then directly infect humans, all other trematodes have a second intermediate host (fish, crab, crayfish). The miracidium larvae infect snails, and the cercariae infect the second intermediate host. In the definitive host, they inhabit specific organs (Table 4-12). Treatment of trematode infection is with praziquantel.

Schistosomiasis is the most prevalent trematode infection. It is characterized by fibrosis of the tissue, which may become obstructive. In *S. japonicum* infections, this means urinary impedence and backflow to the kidneys. In intestinal schistosomiasis, liver and intestinal fibrosis lead to impaired functions of these organs. Diagnosis of schistosomiasis is made by detecting eggs in stool; in *S. japonicum* infections, in urine.

C. sinensis (also known as the Chinese liver fluke) has fish as its second intermediate host. Humans become infected by eating raw or pickled fish. Infection is often asymptomatic, but when severe, the bile duct becomes obstructed and the liver enlarges. Diagnosis is based on the detection of eggs in a concentrated stool specimen.

F. buski cercariae do not have a second intermediate host. They encyst on aquatic vegetation. Infection in humans occurs when this vegetation is ingested. Infections are usually asymptomatic but may be severe, with diarrhea and abdominal pains. Diagnosis is based on demonstrating the presence of eggs in feces.

P. westermani is known as the lung fluke. Its second intermediate host is the crab, and humans become infected when they eat raw crabs. The metacercariae hatch in the small intestine and penetrate the intestinal wall to and through the

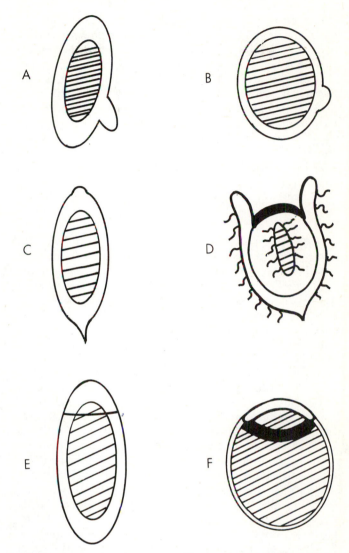

Figure 4-36. Trematode eggs. (*A*) *Schistosoma mansoni* (lateral spin). (*B*) *S. japonicum* (oval; small, lateral spine). (*C*) *S. haematobium* (terminal spine). (*D*) *Clonorchis sinensis* (operated with shoulder; terminal spine). (*E*) *Fasciolopsis buski* (operculum). (*F*) *Paragonium westermani* (flattened operculum).

**Table 4-12.
Trematodes: Their Endemic Areas
and the Organs They Afflict**

Trematodes	Organ involved	Endemic area
P. westermani	Lung, brain	Asia
C. sinensis	Liver, bile duct	Asia
F. buski	Intestinal tract	Asia
S. mansoni	Large intestine	So. America, Africa
S. japonicum	Small intestine	Asia
S. haematobium	Bladder	Africa

diaphragm to the pleural cavity. In the lungs, lesions caused by the migrating worm result in an inflammatory reaction, giving rise to TB-like symptoms. Diagnosis is based on finding eggs in stool, notably in sputum.

Cestodes are helminths that are segmented. Cestodes require at least one intermediate host. *Hymenolepis nana*, however, completes its life cycle within the same host. Cestodes include *Taenia saginata, Taenia solium, Hymenolepis* infections, and *Diphyllobothrium latum*. Infections are diagnosed by fecal examination. *T. solium* cysticercosis and *Echinococcus granulosus* infections are diagnosed by tissue examination.

T. saginata and *T. solium* usually exist as a single adult worm in humans, who are the only definitive hosts. Cattle and camels are the intermediate hosts of *T. saginata*, and pigs and humans for *T. saginata* and *T. solium*. Infection results from ingestion of undercooked or raw meat. Meats frozen at -10° C for 5 days can also prevent taeniasis. The life cycle begins with ingestion of parasitic eggs by the intermediate host. The eggs hatch in the small intestine to release the oncosphere (embryo) containing hooklets. The oncosphere circulates to the heart, diaphragm, and tongue muscles and develops into a cysticercus. Undercooked cysticercus-infected meats cause infections in humans. Once the parasite is ingested, the scolex hooks onto the small intestine and proglottids develop. Terminal proglottids containing eggs are released in fecal material, and the cycle is completed. Clinical taeniasis is mainly asymptomatic but can cause abdominal discomfort. Diagnosis is based mainly on looking for proglottids in feces (Fig. 4-37). Treatment of taeniasis is with niclosamide.

In addition to causing taeniasis, *T. solium* can cause a more severe disease known as cysticercosis. Unlike taeniasis, in which infection occurs from ingesting cysticerci, cysticerosis develops after ingesting *T. solium* eggs. Thus cysticercosis occurs from ingesting egg-containing contaminated foods or via autoinfection from poor sanitary habits. In cysticercosis, the life cycle, which was previously observed in the intermediate host, occurs in humans, resulting in the cysticercus stage in tissues (brain, eye, muscle, heart, liver, and lungs). Clinical symptoms reflect the organs affected, with brain infections being the most severe. Symptoms occur as the result of the immune response mounted from dead cysticerci. Diagnosis is based on identifying cysticerci from tissue biopsy and by serology. Treatment of cysticercosis involves either surgery or praziquantel.

Unlike *Taenia* worms, which can be 10 feet or longer, *Hymenolepis* worms are smaller. *H. nana* (dwarf tapeworm) is the smallest tapeworm (0.1 to 1 inch long). *H. diminuta* is 4 inches to 2 feet long. *H. nana* has a single host. It is transmitted from person to person, with an especially higher infection rate in children. Infection is usually asymptomatic, but in heavy infection, diarrhea is observed. Diagnosis is based on detecting parasitic eggs in stools. Treatment of *Hymenolepis* infections is with praziquantel or niclosamide. *H. diminuta* (rat tapeworm) is similar to *H. nana*, but it usually infects rodents.

D. latum (fish tapeworm) can be up to 45 feet in length. It has two intermediate hosts (a crustacean and a freshwater fish). Infections occur by ingesting raw fish (as in Japan or when Jewish housewives taste-test preparations of gefilte fish). Eggs of *D. latum* embryonate, and then the ciliated embryo (coracidium) is released and swims to a crustacean copepod ("water

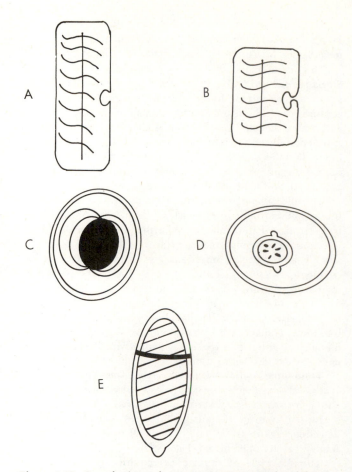

Figure 4-37. Cestodes in stools. (*A*) *Taenia saginata* proglottid (longer and narrower). (*B*) *Taenia solium* proglottid (shorter and wider). (*C*) *Hymenolepsis nana* egg (usually oval; bipolar filament; six-hooked embryo). (*D*) *Hymenolepis diminuta* (usually round; no bipolar filament; six-hooked embryo). (*E*) *Diphyllobothrium latum* (operculated; small terminal knob).

flea"), where it transforms into a procercoid. The infected copepod is ingested by a fish. The procercoid leaves the fish intestine and moves into the fish muscle (plerocercoid or sparganum stage). The infected fish (pickled or raw) is ingested by humans, and the plerocercoid develops a scolex and produces segments. The most serious consequence of *D. latum* infection is pernicious anemia. Diagnosis is based on finding the parasite's egg in stools. This is the only cestode with an operculated egg.

E. granulosus is a tapeworm of dogs. Dogs and other canines are the definitive hosts. It is found in herding communities. Eggs passed by dogs are ingested by herbivores (e.g., sheep). Here the eggs hatch, and the embryo migrates to the lungs, liver, and other organs, where it grows into a hydatid cyst. In the hydatid cyst, many daughter cysts exist.

Humans become infected by ingesting the parasite's eggs. In humans, the hydatid cyst is formed and can grow to large size in the lungs, liver, and other organs to impair vital organ functions. Diagnosis is made by examining the cyst fluid obtained by surgery and by serology. Treatment involves the surgical removal of the cyst without rupturing it.

BIBLIOGRAPHY

Campbell MC, Stewart JL: The Medical Mycology Handbook. John Wiley & Sons, New York, 1980.

Darnell J, Lodish H, Baltimore D: Molecular Cell Biology. Scientific American Books, New York, 1986.

Davis BD, Dulbecco R, Eisen HN, et al: Microbiology, 3rd ed. Harper & Row, New York, 1980.

Hoeprich PD (ed): Infectious Diseases, 2nd ed. Harper & Row, New York, 1977.

Lehninger AL (ed): Biochemistry, 2nd ed. Worth Publishers, New York, 1975.

Lennette EH, Balows A, Hausler WJ, et al (eds): Manual of Clinical Microbiology, 4th ed. American Society for Microbiology, Washington, DC, 1985.

Lorian V (ed): Antibiotics in Laboratory Medicine, 2nd ed. Williams & Wilkins, Baltimore, 1986.

Peterson PK, Verhoef J: The Antimicrobial Agents Annual. Elsevier, New York.

Rose NR, Friedman H, Fahey JL (eds): Manual of Clinical Laboratory Immunology, 3rd ed. American Society for Microbiology, Washington, DC, 1986.

Sun T (ed): Pathology and Clinical Features of Parasitic Diseases. Masson Publishing, New York, 1982.

SAMPLE QUESTIONS

DIRECTIONS: Choose the **one best** response to each question.

1. All of the following are part of the gram-negative bacterial envelope EXCEPT

   A. teichoic acid
   B. periplasmic space
   C. lipopolysaccharide
   D. lipoprotein
   E. protein

2. All of the following are true about T cells EXCEPT that they

   A. constitute 20% of peripheral lymphocytes
   B. depend on the thymus for their maturation
   C. do not have immunoglobulins on their cell surface
   D. are antigen specific
   E. produce lymphokines

3. Which of the following statements about immunoglobulin M is FALSE?

   A. Of the immunoglobulin classes, they have the longest half-life in serum
   B. They are pentamers
   C. They can fix complement
   D. They make effective agglutinating antibodies
   E. They are not transferred vertically from mother to fetus

4. All of the following are true about *Staphylococcus aureus* EXCEPT that it is

   A. coagulase positive
   B. catalase positive
   C. always sensitive to penicillin
   D. the agent of toxic shock syndrome
   E. spread by nasal and skin carriers of the organism

5. All of the following are true of methicillin-resistant *S. aureus* EXCEPT that it

   A. is a noscomial pathogen
   B. is often heterogeneously resistant
   C. is treatable with third-generation cephalosporins
   D. has an additional penicillin binding protein, PBP2a
   E. does not always produce a penicillinase

6. Detection of methicillin resistance in *S. aureus* should be done using any one of the following EXCEPT

   A. sheep blood in the test medium
   B. 24-hour incubation at 35°C
   C. 24-hour incubation at 30°C
   D. increased sodium chloride in the test medium
   E. increased inocula

7. All of the following are true of *Staphylococcus epidermidis* EXCEPT that it

   A. is often a cause of CSF shunt infections
   B. is novobiocin resistant
   C. is part of the normal flora of human skin
   D. may be methicillin resistant
   E. is coagulase negative

8. Which *Streptococcus pyogenes* cell wall component is responsible for its antiphagocytic property?

   A. Group A carbohydrate
   B. M protein
   C. T protein
   D. R protein
   E. Peptidoglycan

9. All of the following are true about *Streptococcus pneumoniae* EXCEPT that

   A. microscopically, it is a lancet-shaped diplococcus
   B. its presence in sputum cultures is always significant
   C. it contains autolysins
   D. infections may be diagnosed rapidly by the detection of their capsular polysaccharides in patient specimens
   E. it is optochin susceptible

10. Penicillin-binding proteins with decreased affinity for penicillin account for decreased sensitivity of all of the following organisms EXCEPT

A. South African *S. pneumoniae* strains
B. chromosomally mediated penicillin-resistant strains of *Neisseria gonorrhoeae*
C. intrinsically resistant *S. aureus*
D. plasmid-mediated ampicillin-resistant *Haemophilus influenzae*
E. ampicillin-resistant, nonbeta-lactamase-producing *H. influenzae*

11. Which is the most common cause of infective endocarditis?

A. Viridans streptococci
B. Enterococci
C. *Streptococcus pyogenes*
D. *Streptococcus agalactiae*
E. *Staphylococcus aureus*

12. All of the following about *N. gonorrhoeae* are true EXCEPT that it

A. requires CO_2 for growth
B. is cold sensitive
C. is a kidney-shaped, gram-negative diplococcus
D. can be grown on blood agar plates
E. may be penicillin-resistant and yet not produce penicillinase

13. Disseminated gonococcal infections are encountered most often in

A. menstruating and pregnant females
B. homosexuals
C. children
D. individuals infected with the PPNG strains of *N. gonorrhoeae*
E. infected newborns

14. All of the following about *Corynebacterium diphtheriae* are true EXCEPT that

A. all strains can cause diphtheria
B. diphtheria should be treated with antitoxin
C. laboratory diagnosis of diphtheria includes throat and nasopharyneal cultures
D. the diphtheria toxin interferes with peptide chain elongation
E. it is cultured on cysteine-tellurite agar

15. Outbreaks of *Listeria monocytogenes* infections have been associated with

A. infected food handlers
B. improperly cooked or stored meat
C. milk or milk products
D. rice
E. eggs

DIRECTIONS: The groups of questions below consist of lettered choices followed by several numbered items. For each numbered item, select the one lettered choice with which it is most closely associated. Each lettered choice may be used once, more than once, or not at all.

Questions 16–20. For each of the descriptions below, choose the immunoglobulin described.

A. IgA
B. IgD
C. IgE
D. IgG
E. IgM

16. Mainly found at mucosal surfaces

17. Mainly found early in primary immune response

18. Can pass through the placenta

19. Involved in immediate hypersensitivity reactions

20. Useful in the diagnosis of congenital infections

Questions 21–25. For each condition listed below, choose the pathogen that is most likely to be associated.

A. *Campylobacter pylori*
B. *Pasteurella multocida*
C. *Vibrio vulnificus*
D. *Salmonella* species
E. *Pseudomonas aeruginosa*

21. Dog bite

22. Peptic ulcer

23. Osteomyelitis in patient with sickle cell anemia

24. Cystic fibrosis

25. Wound infection from wading in seawater

ANSWERS

1. A	10. D	19. C
2. A	11. A	20. E
3. A	12. D	21. B
4. C	13. A	22. A
5. C	14. A	23. D
6. A	15. C	24. E
7. B	16. A	25. C
8. B	17. E	
9. B	18. D	

5

PATHOLOGY

David E. Smith

INTRODUCTION

This chapter presents an overview of the topics of pathology. It cannot be considered to be a text nor to be suitable for primary study without prior instruction in the subject. Nevertheless, it represents an attempt to include the basic concepts and information that underlie cognitive competence examinations. Within the confines of available space, it has been impossible to deal adequately with many topics that are rapidly evolving in biomedical science as they might prove relevant to the understanding of disease. An examinee should recognize that all examinations are predominantly composed of basic, well-accepted principles and related information. The ability to deal with such will be the fundamental measure of an individual's performance on the examination. Information regarding the latest topics is only cautiously and slightly included because it is evolving and subject to change within the time that the examination may be used.

As a medium for review in preparation for examinations that increasingly are designed to be multidisciplinary and problem solving, the material is mostly presented in relation to diseases organized by the systems in which their effects are greatest and by repeating categories such as congenital, inflammatory, "degenerative," neoplastic, etc. The presentations attempt to emphasize the basic concepts, paradigms, and most fundamental facts relative to each topic. As pathology pervades all of medicine and surgery, it cannot be considered that the subject ends with the coverage given here. The reader should be alert for the important presentations of pathology in the topics of other chapters that cover clinical sciences as well as for the implications regarding alterations of the normal processes discussed in the chapters on other basic sciences. The section or component relative to pathology in most examinations will certainly encompass relatively large amounts of information that the examinee is likely to have learned from such sources and may not identify as arising from his or her study of pathology itself.

One of the most common failings among medical students is that of using terms, particularly those relative to basic concepts, without a sufficiently precise awareness of their definition. This imprecision can be particularly treacherous when dealing with the analysis of problems in modern comprehensive medical examinations that are designed to project the examinee into test situations as nearly like those of clinical practice as possible. The following definitions of basic terms are presented with the purpose of encouraging readers to return to their dictionaries on frequent occasions to sharpen their acquaintance with the use of specific words.

Pus and purulent inflammation. Yellowish white, opaque fluid consisting of exudate and dead, disintegrating tissue infiltrated with numerous leukocytes or their remains.

Abscess. A localized, liquified focus of purulent inflammation surrounded by a wall of reactive and reparative tissue similar to granulation tissue.

Cellulitis. Inflammation, not necessarily purulent, of the loose subcutaneous tissue.

Phlegmon. Pyogenic inflammation that spreads through tissues along fascial planes or other natural barriers.

Caseation. A particular form of necrosis characteristic of tuberculosis that results in a stiff, plastic, white coagulum. The term is often applied to the microscopic appearance of avascular necrosis in tubercules.

Exudate. An inflammatory extravascular fluid having a high specific gravity (> 1.020) and often containing 2 to 4 g/100 ml of protein, as well as white cells that have emigrated.

Transudate. An extravascular fluid of low protein content and specific gravity less than 1.012 that is formed chiefly as a result of increased intravascular hydrostatic pressure.

Granuloma. Originally a term related to the granule-sized gross lesions of inflammations such as tuberculosis; now on a microscopic basis an aggregation of histiocytes (macrophages) that have been transformed into epitheloid cells and are surrounded by a collar of mononuclear leukocytes, principally lymphocytes and occasionally plasma cells.

Miliary. Originally a term indicating the gross size of granulomas of tuberculosis and other infections (the size of millet seed) but now implying the hematogenous spread of such infections with subsequent development of individual granulomas.

Mycotic. Usually implies a fungus as the etiologic agent, but when applied to a form of aneurysm it means less specifically any sort of microbial etiology.

Granulation tissue. Reactive inflammatory tissue that has reached the predominate stage of healing. The term is derived from the gross red granules of capillary loops visible on healing denuded surfaces but is now applied to the microscopic appearance of proliferating endothelial cells and fibroblasts with formation of new vessels and collagenous fibers.

Infarction. The localized death of tissue due to interruption of the blood supply.

Thrombus. A structured (not organized) coagulum of elements from the blood formed in association with a flowing stream of blood.

Clot. A mass formed from the elements of the blood via the coagulation mechanism; often the plasma and the cellular elements are separated by the effect of gravity before solidification of the liquid.

Embolus. Any mass, usually a thrombus but possibly fat droplets, bubbles of gas, or other substances, transported within the bloodstream from one site to another.

Tumor. Any localized swelling of tissue, although it is often used as though synonymous with neoplasm.

Neoplasia. A new growth of tissue without the normal constraints that organize tissues and organs.

Carcinoma. A neoplasm of epithelial origin capable of such unrestrained growth as to invade or spread (metastasize) to other tissues.

Sarcoma. A malignant neoplasm derived from connective tissue elements, with a growth potential similar to that of a carcinoma.

Cancer. A vernacular generic term for all malignant neoplasms, including carcinomas, sarcomas, leukemias, and gliomas.

Atypia. A term used in the description of cells that implies morphological features suggestive but not diagnostic of neoplastic transformation.

Dysplasia, carcinoma in situ, microinvasive. Terms used to indicate a conclusion regarding the degree to which a stimulated epithelium has progressed toward malignant transformation. In this use, dysplasia is considered a reversible change whereas the others are truly carcinoma. **Dysplasia** is also the name of disorderly malformation of the tissues of an organ such as the kidney.

Metastasis. The transfer of disease from one organ or part to another not directly connected with it. The term is most commonly applied to the spread of malignant neoplasms of which the ability to metastasize is a primary characteristic, but it is properly used in infectious diseases.

Hetertopia. A mass of tissue of recognizable organization displaced to other than its usual site.

Hamartoma. A benign tumor composed of an overgrowth of mature cells and tissues that normally occur in the affected part, but often with one element predominating. It may enlarge at rates and under controls similar to those of normal tissue.

Choristoma. A benign tumor composed of a mass of abnormally organized tissue histologically normal for an organ or part other than the site at which it is located.

Allergy. Originally any altered reaction of tissue due to prior exposure to a particular substance; now applied particularly to hypersensitive states such as atopic reactions.

Hypersensitivity. A state in which there are destructive effects from any immune reaction.

Sepsis. The bodily condition associated with the presence in the blood or other tissues of pathogenic microorganisms or their toxins.

Septicemia. Systemic disease associated with the presence and persistence of pathogenic microorganisms or their toxins in the blood.

Bacteremia. The presence of bacteria in the bloodstream. The term does not necessarily imply the presence of a reaction or systemic disease.

Mole. That amount of a chemical compound whose mass in grams is equal to its molecular weight or formula mass. **Mole** is also the name of pigmented skin lesions and of chorionic tumors of the uterus.

Equivalent. That weight in grams of a substance that will produce or react with 1 mole of hydrogen ion or 1 mole of electrons; the molecular weight divided by the valence.

Mean. The arithmetic average of a population of numbers; the sum of all observations divided by the number of observations.

Median. A value in an ordered set of values below and above which there is an equal number of values, or which is the mean of the two middle values if there is no one middle number.

Mode. The most frequent value of a set of data.

PRINCIPLES OF CLINICAL PATHOLOGY

Pathology is the science of the study of disease. When it was first given the status of an academic discipline, the principal available method of investigation was gross dissection, followed soon by microscopic examination. So many fundamental observations have been made with these methods that it is popular to assume that pathologists must be limited by definition to their use. In truth, such is a very narrow concept, for any investigative method derived from chemistry, biology, physics, mathematics, or any other science can be a tool for the investigation of disease and therefore a method of pathology. As knowledge was gained about the concepts of diseases, it became obvious that the methods used in their investigation might be applied to understanding the status of an individual patient. That is the essence of clinical pathology.

As scientific investigative methods developed in pathology, they seemed to take different pathways. Microbiology, for instance, became a free-standing scientific discipline but has, for the most part, left behind diagnostic bacteriology, virology, and immunology to be parts of the practice of clinical pathology. Radiology, on the other hand, arrived after the manifestations of many diseases were fairly well established, and it became a separate clinical discipline little used in clinical pathology until the arrival of radioisotopes and their participation in chemical analyses applicable to the clinical laboratory.

In this chapter and in the teaching of pathology, the various chemical, biologic, physical, and other concepts and tests used in understanding a specific disease are considered a part of the pathology of that disease and are discussed with the disease. There are, however, certain principles of laboratory medicine that are general and have less to do with the nature of diseases than with the practice of clinical pathology.

STANDARDS

The term **standards** in itself is an example of a pervasive problem for the student of clinical pathology, namely the definition and use of terms that may have a common meaning, a general meaning in science, and one or more very specific meanings relative to particular methods or problems. In analytic chemistry, a standard is a substance of known purity or concentration that can be analyzed to determine that one's method and instruments yield a result that corresponds to reality. Today, with the refined sources of supply available to all laboratories, chemical standards rarely represent a problem. However, in histology (including histochemistry), immunohistology, microbiology, and other disciplines in the laboratory in which interpretation by an operator is an important step in the process, the application of standards is less precise. For that reason, there are national programs such as the Check Sample Program of the American Society of Clinical Pathologists and the laboratory surveys of the College of American Pathologists that work actively with most laboratories to standardize analytic results. A more important meaning for clinical pathology, however, concerns the meaning or significance of a result in relation to the diagnosis of disease. **Standardization** in the clinical laboratory is a constant process of evaluation of the precision and accuracy of a method and the meaning of a positive or negative result.

Laboratory tests are performed to (1) confirm a diagnosis, (2) rule out a differential diagnosis, (3) follow the effects of therapy, (4) prognosticate, and (5) search for undetected disease. The significance of test results varies because of inherent variation in (1) the analytic method, (2) preparation of the patient and collection of the specimen, (3) the limits between which the patient experiences a state of physiological balance, and (4) the mean values obtained from different patients and groups of patients.

REFERENCE VALUES

To establish the significance of the results of a test, laboratories determine standards that are called **reference values** (note that *normal* is to be avoided because it cannot be guaranteed that the reference population does not contain some abnormal values and because it has a much more specific and valuable usage in statistics). To derive reference values there must be control of (1) the selection of the population of subjects, (2) conditions under which specimens are collected, (3) collection technique, preservation, and storage of specimens (4) the analytic method used, and (5) the collection, analysis, and presentation of the resulting data.

Reference values are usually derived by performing a test on a population of subjects judged free of relevant disease, with as much control of the other four factors as is generally exercised in the practice of the laboratory. The results will present a **normal distribution** and can be graphed as a bell curve. From them a **mean value** may be calculated and the **standard deviation** derived by summing the squares of the differences of each result and the mean, dividing the sum by the total number of results, and then taking the square root of the quotient.

$$\text{Standard deviation} = \sqrt{\frac{\Sigma\,(\text{each result} - \text{mean value})^2}{\text{number of results}}}$$

With a reasonable number of samples (usually about 30) that do not exhibit too large a standard deviation, not more than 3 to 6% of the mean, the resulting normal distribution may be represented by a bell curve that has about 95% of its area (i.e., 95% of all results of such tests) between the value that is two standard deviations below and the value that is two deviations above the mean. These two values are usually accepted as the lower and upper reference values for the test in judging its significance as a positive or negative result.

To recognize an analytic procedure capable of giving reliably reproducible and significant results, the **coefficient of variation** is calculated by expressing the standard deviation of the reference population as a percentage of the mean:

$$\text{Coefficient of variation} = \frac{\text{Standard deviation}}{\text{Mean of test results}} \times 100$$

This coefficient for the majority of laboratory tests is of the order of 5%. In the National Cholesterol Education Program, it is recommended that the goal for the coefficients of variation for cholesterol determinations in a given laboratory be 3% and for pooled results from two or more laboratories not be more than 6%. It is also suggested that reports reflect the **highest acceptable value** rather than the upper and lower limits of reference values.

It should be recognized that the coefficient of variation is a description of the application of a measurement to a population most members of which are not considered abnormal. The more critical statistic of the effectiveness of the analytic procedure itself is the **standard error of the mean**, which is calculated by dividing the standard deviation of all measurements by the square root of one less than the total number of measurements.

$$\text{Standard error of the mean} = \frac{\text{standard deviation}}{\sqrt{\text{number of measurements} - 1}}$$

SIGNIFICANCE

Even with the best possible control of every factor, the test results from a population of subjects will include some instances of positive tests from individuals who do not have the condition for which the test is being administered (**false-positives**), negative results with individuals who do have the condition (**false-negatives**), as well as the instances in which the test recognizes the condition (**true-positives**) and instances in which the test is negative and the individual is free of the condition (**true-negatives**). These events can be named and characterized mathematically as follows:

Prevalence = percentage of diseased in total population

$$= \frac{\text{true-positives} + \text{false-negatives}}{\text{total population}} \times 100$$

(In public health practice, **prevalence** is expressed as the number of diseased persons per 100,000 population. **Incidence** is the number of new cases per year per 100,000 population.)

Sensitivity = percentage of positivity in disease

$$= \frac{\text{true-positives}}{\text{true-positives + false-negatives}} \times 100$$

Specificity = percentage of negativity in health

$$= \frac{\text{true-negatives}}{\text{true-negatives + false-positives}} \times 100$$

Predictive value of a positive test = probability that a positive test is a true-positive

$$= \frac{\text{true-positives}}{\text{true-positives + false-positives}} \times 100$$

The last term, **predictive value of a positive test**, is the expression of an equation from the statistics of probability that is known as **Bayes' theorem**. Although there are difficulties in determining the actual values for true- and false-positives and negatives in addition to the difficulties in control of test administration, the calculation of the predictive value of tests is illuminating and of great value in building computerized models that approach artificial intelligence and are finding increasing application to clinical practice. An example of a startling application was supplied when it was legislated that all newborn infants should be tested for phenylketonuria. The test is remarkably specific and yields only 1 false result in 10,000, but the prevalance is only 5 to 10 in 100,000 so the predictive value is of the order of 50% and half the patients with positive tests do not have the disease.

QUALITY CONTROL

The effectiveness of the practice of clinical pathology depends on the constant reexamination of its procedures to be certain that reference, predictive, and other values do not vary or that variations are recognized and understood. This is **quality control**, and the laboratory often presents its most active and advanced practice in hospitals. However, with the advent of computers of huge capacity, **hospital information systems** are acquiring the ability to assemble, correlate, and compare information about patients and practices that make possible the easier, if not automatic, survey of the results of medical practice. Integration of laboratory results into such systems is important and facilitated by their usually quantitative expression. **Medical informatics** is the discipline that integrates such huge amounts of information and enables conclusions or judgments to be made from them. It is most interestingly applied in prospect in establishing diagnosis and determining the most efficient management of a patient's illness, as well as encompassing quality control in retrospect.

Quality control also involves techniques of personnel management and job training. Specimen collection and the reporting of results are two factors that may cancel the best of other efforts and the most sophisticated design and standardization. Inadequate sterilization of the skin is probably the most common cause of failure in blood cultures, improper specimen collection the most damaging step in urine cultures, and the lost or misdirected report destroys all other efforts at the optimal practice of clinical pathology.

UNITS OF MEASUREMENT

Quantitative biology has evolved from many sources. As a consequence, units of measurement often have been derived from the current technology of the original description of the method. As methods have become more precise and inclusive, impatience has arisen with the diverse catalogs of units of measurement and a **Système International (SI units)** is gaining wide acceptance among editors of medical publications. In due time it is to be expected that clinical practitioners will become comfortable with its nomenclature and it will replace the current diverse use of various units of volume, equivalents versus moles, grams, milligrams, kilos, etc.

The seven basic SI units are as follows:

1. Amount of substance: mole
2. Mass: kilogram
3. Length: meter
4. Time: second
5. Thermodynamic temperature: kelvin
6. Electric current: ampere
7. Luminous intensity: candela

Other units are derived from these seven. The unit of volume, for instance, is the liter. Expression of measurements in SI units often results in considerable use of exponential expressions (e.g., WBCs $72.0 \times 10^9/L$ versus $72,000/\mu L$). Tables for conversion of older conventional units into SI units are readily available.

CARDIOVASCULAR SYSTEM

BLOOD VESSELS

Because the products they deliver to and remove from other tissues are essential for cellular survival, the blood vessels are ubiquitous and participate in some way or another in all pathological processes. Their responses to injury facilitate or limit the responses of host tissues, and most of the gross features of pathological lesions are reflections of the balance of blood supply, coloration of the blood, or destruction from interruption of the integrity of the blood vessels as they affect or modify the appearance of the host tissue and its pathological response.

Congenital anomalies

Anomalies and duplications of various arteries and veins are quite common and usually do not impair the ultimate circulation in the organs served. Most—such as a **persistent left superior vena cava, a right aortic arch**, or the **esophageal arterial ring** due to absorption of the right fourth branchial arch instead of the distal right dorsal aorta with consequent origin of the right subclavian artery distal to the left—are readily understood by comparison with the normal patterns of embryologic development. Occasionally, a **duplicated renal artery** will partially obstruct the ureter or abnormalities of the circle of Willis will result in an unexpected picture in a stroke.

The most important anomalies are those that occur in vessels near the heart, and they are usually classified with congenital heart disease. Persistently **patent ductus arteriosus** is second only to ventricular septal defect among those cases and was the first to yield to surgical correction. It is life threatening because it transmits systemic pressure to the pulmonary circulation with consequent damage to pulmonary vessels, hypertension, and cor pulmonale, and it may be part of more complex anomalies of the heart itself. Hypoplasia or atresia of the pulmonary arteries and hypoplasia of the ascending arch of the aorta are respectively central to the **tetralogy of Fallot** and **hypoplastic left heart syndrome**. **Coarctation of the aorta** is a congenital defect of the media on the convex side of the descending arch with a shelf-like ridge that creates stenosis. It is usually near the insertion of the ductus, and neonatal survival depends on that relation: Significant stenosis proximal to the ductus gives no stimulation for the development of collaterals prior to birth, so severe consequences ensue when the ductus closes.

Another class of anomalies consists of hamartomatous tangles of vessels that are called **hemangiomas** or **arteriovenous malformations**. They are particularly prominent in the skin as the basis of birthmarks, and in the CNS they occur singly or as part of the **Sturge-Weber** and **von Hippel-Lindau syndromes**. Some in the skin regress spontaneously. Those in the brain tend to enlarge by opening new channels. Small lesions are frequent in viscera such as the liver and on rare occasions are large enough to result in significant hemorrhage following trauma. The occurrence of most of these lesions is random, but **Osler's hemorrhagic telangiectatic syndrome** with myriad small clusters of abnormally dilated vessels in the mucous membranes, skin, and liver is an autosomal dominant hereditary disease.

Marfan's syndrome is another disease transmitted in an autosomal dominant pattern, although with considerable variation in penetrance and expression. Although it is a generalized disease based apparently on defective collagen and elastin and possibly a metabolic defect related to the failure of crosslinkages in collagen and elastin such as occurs on exposure to beta-aminoproprionitrile in **lathyrism** and characterized by arachnodactyly, subluxation of the ocular lens, floppy mitral valves, and a variety of other malformations, a most dramatic and usually fatal feature is a **dissecting aneurysm**. These lesions are not true aneurysms in the sense of a sac formed by dilatation of the wall of the aorta but are the result of hemorrhages into the wall with tearing of its structure. The lesion might better be called **dissecting hematoma** than aneurysm. The hemorrhages are associated with a preceding degeneration of elastic lamina and the interstitial accumulation of a mucoid substance that is called **cystic medial necrosis**. In 90% of cases they are related to a transverse tear in the intima at the proximal extent of the hemorrhage and sometimes at the distal end, although in 10% there is no tear. When there are proximal and distant tears, a tract is developed in the wall of the aorta between the inner two-thirds and the outer third of the media. Being open at both ends, this tract results in a **double-barreled aorta** that is compatible with survival, but far more usually the hemorrhage ruptures through the adventitia into the mediastinum, pleura, or pericardium with fatal consequences. Sometimes the hemorrhage dissects proximally to surround and occlude a coronary artery and cause acute myocardial infarction. Others may dissect distally to sever the renal arteries or to extend into the carotid or the iliac arteries. The hemorrhages begin in the arch of the aorta (type A) in four-fifths or more of cases and, particularly when they dissect proximally, are of most severe prognosis, while those that begin beyond the ligamentum arteriosum (type B) can be treated surgically with more success. Only a minority of patients with dissecting aneurysms can be recognized to have Marfan's syndrome, but nearly all are hypertensive. The principal symptoms are sudden severe pain, often starting in the precordium and shifting to the back and even to the legs.

Inflammation

Inflammation is one of the fundamental processes of pathology. Robbins defines it as "the reaction of vascularized living tissue to local injury," and the implication is that the trigger is cell death. Cellular and serum factors play essential roles, but the principal reaction is in the blood vessels. Since Roman times, four cardinal signs have been recognized: **color** (redness), **calor** (warmness), **tumor** (swelling), and **dolor** (pain). The first three are directly the result of the changes in the blood vessels. A fifth cardinal sign added after classical times is **loss of function**.

The inflammatory process involves neutralization of injuring agents, clearing of destroyed elements, and repair of involved tissue, and these elements proceed simultaneously but with variable intensities and rates: In the earliest stages, neutralization by action of wandering cells and serum antibodies or other factors predominates, whereas the final reorganization of a scar continues long after the other factors have subsided. Four essential events are (1) **vasodilation**, opening of channels between and through endothelial cells, particularly of postcapillary venules, and passage of plasma into the injured area, (2) **attraction and migration of leukocytes**, first usually neutrophilic granulocytes and later monocytes but sometimes other cells such as eosinophils if the injurious substance is of the nature of some allergens, (3) **phagocytosis** of bacteria and other agents and cellular debris with destruction or containment of the inciting agents, and (4) **repair** by regeneration of parenchymal cells or replacement by proliferated capillaries, fibroblasts, and collagenous or other connective tissue, sometimes including heterotopic bone.

The various events are mediated by a variety of factors: **histamine** for vascular permeability; **kinins**, which stimulate vasodilatation and permeability as well as cause pain; the **complement system**, which in its various components contributes to the vascular reaction, phagocytosis, release of histamine, chemotaxis, etc.; and the **blood coagulation system**, which contributes Hageman factor, plasmin, and activators of other mediators and also plugs ruptured capillaries and facilitates the growth of endothelial buds and fibroblasts into tissue defects. **Lymphokines, prostaglandins, immunoglob-**

ulins, chalones, growth factors, the peroxide-halide-myelo-peroxidase enzymatic system, and numerous other factors play roles.

The balance of activity of the fundamental processes at any stage determines the pathological lesions themselves. With marked leukocytic migration and proteolytic activity, abscesses are formed. With pronounced stimulation of participation of macrophages, particularly under the effect of substances such as the phosphatide of the tubercle bacillus, conglomerates of such cells are large enough to be grossly visible and were called granulomas because they looked like little granules on the background of tissue such as that of the liver. The mononuclear cells crowd together into epitheloid cell patterns and may fuse to form giant cells such as the Langhan's cell of tubercles. In the late stages, the reparative growth of capillary loops, especially on exposed inflamed surfaces, give an appearance of small red granules and the name of granulation tissue to the vessels, fibroblasts, and other elements that are replacing destroyed tissue. The original applications of the terms granuloma and granulation tissue on the basis of their gross appearances have been much modified conceptually and translated into their microscopic characters of mononuclear aggregation and microvascular proliferation to such a degree as to be a constant source of sophomoric confusion. The nature of the injury, the continued action of the injurious agent, factors such as new physical distortions or other injuries, and the particular tissue involved combine to affect the rate with which inflammation proceeds to repair and in doing so will result in the accentuation of the elements of one fundamental event or another: Acute inflammation is overwhelmingly vasodilation and exudation; chronic inflammation shows prominent reparative activity and may take on elements such as mononuclear prominence and be described as granulomatous.

Although inflammation is the reaction to injury and the pathway to repair, it may itself cause or modify injury. The release of lysosomal proteases from leukocytes is destructive of tissue; immune complexes can activate complement and induce injury, a mechanism of poststreptococcal glomerulonephritis; and the inflammatory process itself seems responsible for the lesions of diseases such as rheumatic fever, rheumatoid arthritis, and the autoimmune diseases.

Vasculitis syndromes consist of a large group of illnesses with the common property of some sort of noninfectious inflammation of blood vessels. Their symptoms and clinical pictures are widely variable but characterized by systemic distribution. Arteries, veins, arterioles, venules, and even capillaries may be the principal sites of involvement or may be involved in almost any combination. The confusing classifications are probably better made on a clinical basis than pathological anatomy. Four major groups may be recognized: (1) systemic necrotizing vasculitides such as polyarteritis nodosa, with its distinctive lesions of small arteries and subsequent involvement of the kidneys, hypertension, and many other organs; (2) hypersensitivity vasculitis of the venules, usually involving predominately the skin with purpura and usually mediated by immune complex (type III) hypersensitivity reaction and including Henoch-Schölein purpura; (3) giant cell arteritides that include temporal arteritis with its headaches and systemic flu-like symptoms and Takayasu's

pulseless disease with occlusive involvement of the branches of the aortic arch; and (4) and specific disorders such as systemic lupus erythematosus, Buerger's thromboangiitis obliterans, and rheumatoid arthritis.

Infections

The vascular system is the conduit for the etiologic agent and participates in the reactions of many infectious diseases but is also the primary site of several. Small vessels, particularly capillaries, are damaged by the endothelial parasitism of rickettsia in typhus, Rocky Mountain spotted fever, and similar infections. Several viruses, particularly those of encephalitis including equine, St. Louis, and Japanese B, also target injury of small vessels. In the brain, especially the damage results in microscopic aggregates of monocytes and endothelial cells that are called glial, or typhus nodules. The human immunodeficiency virus (HIV) in acquired immunodeficiency syndrome (AIDS) causes a similar but much less prominent involvement of small cerebral vessels. *Pseudomonas aeruginosa* is notorious for infecting the walls of veins and arteries and growing there profusely, with consequent thrombosis and subsequent infarction of involved tissues. Other gram-negative bacteria occasionally behave similarly, and several fungi typically do so: *Mucor* sp and other members of the order Mucorales especially involve the brain, and the same organisms and *Aspergillus* are found in necrotizing lesions of the pulmonary vessels and lungs. Recently a spirochete, *Borrelia burgdorferi*, that has the tick *Ixodes dammini* as a host, has been identified in Lyme disease, a centrifugally spreading rash of the trunk that is followed by systemic symptoms and finally by a significant arthritis. Not much has been published regarding its microscopic lesions, but both the skin and joint manifestations strongly suggest small vascular involvement.

Syphilis is the prototypical and classic example of an infectious vasculitis. In the primary chancre, there is an intense stimulation of capillary growth; in the secondaries, the small vessels of the skin and other tissues are parasitized by *Treponema pallidum;* and in the tertiary stage, one of the most dramatic manifestations is syphilitic aortitis and its resulting aortic aneurysms. This is essentially a vasculitis of the vaso vasorum of the thoracic aorta, especially of the ascending arch. The vessels of the aortic adventitia are cuffed with lymphocytes and plasma cells and embedded in reactive fibrosis, whereas those of the aortic media have similar cellular cuffs and lie in zones in which the elastic lamina have been focally destroyed. It is destruction of this latter tissue that leads to weakening of the wall of the aorta and its saccular dilatation to form an aneurysm. Syphilitic aneurysms are strictly of the thoracic aorta, half in the ascending arch, a third in the transverse arch, and the remainder in the descending. Despite the decrease in tertiary syphilis, it can still be said that nearly all thoracic aneurysms are syphilitic rather than arteriosclerotic, which are the aneurysms of the abdominal aorta. Thoracic aneurysms may attain a remarkable size and are much more prone to produce symptoms than the abdominal variety. Pressure on surrounding structures, erosion of vertebrae or ribs, and laryngeal paralysis due to pressure on the recurrent nerve are some of the manifestations. Fatal termination is usually by rupture into the pleural space, the pericardium, and even externally through eroded ribs.

Syphilitic aortitis tends to be especially intense in the ascending aorta and overlaid by fibrosis with calcification that is similar (or maybe the same process) to arteriosclerosis. It leads to dilatation of the ascending arch, and that with laminar calcification is almost pathognomonic on radiographs. The aortitis extends into the ring of the aortic valve and involves the leaflets, with binding to the aortic wall at the commissures and consequent widening of the space between leaflets and insufficiency of the valve. This is the lesion of **syphilitic heart disease**: it is really of the aorta and aortic valve and not of the heart, except for the consequent work hypertrophy and finally failure subsequent to the aortic valvular insufficiency. Only quite rarely were cases of syphilis actively involving the coronary arteries or the myocardium reported when the tertiary disease was much more common than it is today.

Another form of inflammatory aneurysm is the so-called **mycotic aneurysm** that is due to the metastasis of an infectious, usually purulent, particle to the wall of a vessel and subsequent destruction of the wall and rupture. These are often of small vessels such as those of the brain and are false aneurysms in that the wall is not dilated but is broken and hemorrhage infiltrates the surrounding tissue until it can rupture into a zone of less resistance, with consequent dire effect. The word "mycotic" in this use is from an old meaning that included all forms of microbes, not just fungi, and these aneurysms are much more frequently due to bacteria than to fungi themselves.

Arteriosclerotic aneurysms are most important in the abdominal aorta below the renal arteries and with extension to the iliac arteries. They are lesions of the elderly and are symptomatic principally by their obliteration of branches of the aorta. **Traumatic aneurysms** that resulted from blows or knife wounds to the wall of the vessel were once an important lesion that demanded the attention of surgeons, but they are now rare.

Arteriosclerosis

Atherosclerosis is the major component of sclerotic arterial disease, and the name is often used synonymously with arteriosclerosis. Its effects, particularly ischemic heart disease, are the most important cause of mortality in the developed Western countries. Probably two-fifths of all deaths in the United States are related to this disease, almost twice as many as cancer, the second most important cause. In remarkable contrast, the rate in the Orient may be only a tenth that of the most affected countries in the West, and in South America and Africa the rates are distinctly less than in the United States, where the death rate has increased to three or four times that of 50 years ago. Major **risk factors** that have been identified are (1) **hypercholesterolemia**, (2) **hypertension**, (3) **heavy cigarette smoking**, and (4) **diabetes mellitus**, but other factors such as **obesity, age,** and **heredity** operate.

Lipid metabolism and nutrition are considered major pathogenic factors, and many present efforts to influence the incidence of the disease deal with diet. The **lipoproteins** and **lipids** involved are recognized to occur in five patterns, of which the second and fourth are most clearly related to the incidence of atherosclerosis. **Type I hyperlipoproteinemia**

consists of increased chylomicrons, markedly elevated triglycerides, and normal serum cholesterol. **Type II** involves increased low-density lipoproteins (hypercholesterolemia) and may involve normal or moderately elevated triglycerides, the former in familial cases with severe atherosclerosis and the latter presumably on a dietary basis. **Type III** consists of an increase in lipoprotein intermediates, markedly elevated cholesterol, and moderate triglycerides. **Type IV** is the most common and is marked by elevation of very low-density lipoproteins, severe hypertriglyceridemia, and normal serum cholesterol. It is considered to be importantly related to diet, obesity, and alcoholism. **Type V** shows elevated very low-density lipoproteins and chylomicrons, is familial and rare, and has uncertain relation to atherosclerosis. Despite the clear association in some groups and the theoretically attractive pathogenic relations, not all persons with atherosclerosis have hyperlipoproteinemia; less than half those undergoing surgical intervention for coronary disease are said to have abnormal lipid patterns.

The lesions of atherosclerosis involve the intima and media of elastic arteries and large and medium-sized muscular arteries. The central lesion is the **intimal plaque** that is a gray, circumscribed thickening composed of intracellular and extracellular lipids, cholesterol, fibroblasts, and smooth muscle cells. The lipids are the same as those in the serum; the smooth muscle cells, interestingly, are monoclonal. There is more or less ulceration and evidence of fibrin and cellular debris. Lesions may vary in size between a few millimeters to complete circumferential involvement of the abdominal aorta. Older lesions show calcification and more ulceration and adherent thrombus that may be the source of emboli to more distant vessels. Narrowing of the arterial lumen to the point of obliteration is the mechanism of the effect of the disease on important viscera, with subsequent parenchymous atrophy, infarction, or limitation of function as occurs in the muscles of the legs on exercise after severe narrowing of the femoral or more proximal arteries (**intermittent claudication** or **Leriche's syndrome**). Intensive extension of the process with destruction of the media of the aorta leads to **aneurysms**. Thrombosis over plaques is a most important mechanism for complete occlusion, but sometimes hemorrhages develop within the plaque from the capillaries that grow into the new tissue, and the extravasated blood causes occlusion.

Theories of **pathogenesis** emphasize (1) **disruption of the intima** with adherence of platelets and fibrinogenesis to initiate deposits, (2) **suffusion of serum components**, particularly lipids, into the site, and (3) **smooth muscle proliferation** on the basis of a monoclonal mutation as the initial event leading to abnormal attraction of lipids and platelet components. The details of these and other theories as well as the observations quoted in their support are too extensive to be reviewed here. The simplest lesion of all, the **fatty streak**, is an uncomplicated intimal accumulation of fatty macrophages with few other components of the true plaque. It is the most easily induced with experimental diets, and its incidence has the clearest correlation with caloric intake or inversely with starvation. It may be seen in the aortas of persons of all ages, but workers in the field consider that there is no conclusive evidence that it is a stage of the process of true atherosclerosis.

Mönckeberg's sclerosis consists of multiple focal calcifications in the media of medium-sized muscular arteries of older persons. It is often recognized in the radial artery and has no significance as it does not narrow the lumen or disrupt the intima. **Fibromuscular dysplasia** is a rare cause of renal ischemia and consequent correctable hypertension. It consists of hypertrophy of the muscularis with fibrosis that may give the outline of the lumen a beaded appearance of alternating stenosis and dilatation.

Other occlusive vascular diseases

Thrombosis and **embolism** are the most important manifestations of pathological vascular occlusive processes. Thrombosis is intravascular coagulation in the presence of blood flow. Virchow enunciated three fundamental conditions under which it occurs: (1) **alteration of the walls** of the vessels, (2) **stasis**, (3) and **alteration of the composition of the blood**. In all three, the initiating event must be some injury of the intima sufficient under the basic circumstance that platelets adhere and break down or tissue thromboplastin is released, and the coagulation cascade, either intrinsic or extrinsic or both, is activated. The details of the physiological processes of coagulation and its 13 or more factors should be reviewed by the student. From the point of initiation, alternating layers of platelets, fibrin, and leukocytes are built and are grossly apparent as **lines of Zahn**, which, with the adhesion to the wall, are the hallmarks of **true thrombosis** in contradistinction to **clotting**. After the mass occludes the vessel and the stream of blood flow is stopped, a "red tail" will propagate in the proximal column of static blood. Another gross characteristic of true thrombi seen at autopsy consists of their distension of the involved blood vessel because they have formed while blood pressure held the vessel open, in contrast to the collapsed vessels in which postmortem clots form.

Thrombosis of the deep veins of the legs is clinically most important, as such thrombi break away to become **emboli to the pulmonary arteries**. They are principally a result of stasis, although some inflammation of the venous wall may be apparent. Debate as to whether the inflammation came first or followed the thrombosis has led to persistence of the terms **thrombophlebitis** and **phlebothrombosis**. Although inflammation of vessels passing near sites such as a pulmonary abscess will undoubtedly lead to thrombosis, that sort of process probably plays little part in the syndrome of calf pain on stretching, chest pain, and hemoptysis that traces a venous embolus and may lead even to such dire consequences as sudden death from occlusion of the major pulmonary arteries. Thrombi in arteries are most often associated with ulcerated atherosclerotic plaques, and **mural thrombi** form over areas of infarction in the heart.

Thrombi may be **organized** by inward growth of capillaries, fibroblasts, and smooth muscle cells from the wall of the vessel with the development of **recanalization**, or they may be partially or completely **dissolved** by fibrinolysins and proteolytic enzymes from leukocytes.

The outcome of vascular thrombosis depends on the condition of the field of tissue supplied or drained by the occluded vessel. If an artery that is the sole source of oxygenation for a zone of tissue is involved, the tissue of the zone will become necrotic. The resulting process is **infarction**, which is the localized death of tissue due to interruption of the blood supply. The central region of such usually wedge-shaped lesions undergoes coagulative necrosis, is pale because of the laking and loss of erythrocytes, and swells by osmotic imbibition as the cells and their components break down. The margins are grossly red, at first because they contain damaged small vessels that are fed by surrounding collaterals and then because the surrounding tissue assumes the microscopic character of granulation tissue, sprouts of capillary loops and fibroblasts, while wandering cells infiltrate to accomplish the process of resolution of the necrotic tissue and repair. This process is clearly illustrated in infarcts of the heart and kidney, but in the liver and lung the result is modified because of their double circulation. True infarcts are rare in the liver, and they occur in the lung principally if the tissue has already been damaged by congestion from cardiac failure or inflammation. When they do occur, they are hemorrhagic rather than having ischemic centers. Venous occlusions rarely cause infarcts, but they may cause zonal congestion and make such tissues as the colonic mucosa increasingly susceptible to injury, erosion, and infection.

Cardiac failure and congestion

Heart failure develops if there is **damage to the heart** itself, or with **changes in the metabolic requirements** of the body, or with **alterations in the volume or composition of the blood**. In the first category are afflictions such as **constrictive pericarditis**, diseases of the myocardium such as **amyloid infiltration, cardiomyopathy**, or **diffuse scarring due to coronary artery insufficiency** that cause poor ventricular contraction and diastolic filling. The myocardium itself may be weakened by deficient nutrition as a result of **obstructive coronary disease, severe anemia, thyrotoxicosis**, or **deficiencies such as beriberi**. In **arrhythmias**, particularly tachycardia, there may be inadequate diastolic filling. Most frequently the problem arises because of the overwork of hypertension, under which the heart must pump against increased peripheral resistance, but overwork is also the result of decreased resistance and demand for large volume in cases of **arteriovenous fistulas** or **patent ductus arteriosus**. **Valvular insufficiency** or **stenosis** greatly increases work load.

Early inadequacy of the pump under any of the above conditions results in disproportionate reduction of renal blood flow, marked reduction in glomerular filtration rate, and retention of sodium, water, and urea. This compounds the weakness of the pump, postcapillary venous pressure increases, and **edema** fluid collects interstitially, at first in the dependent parts but then in serosal cavities and finally in the lungs. The situation is rather dynamic: During the night, when the lungs are not in the upright position, edema accumulates with consequent **orthopnea** and **paroxysmal nocturnal dyspnea**. Blood accumulates in venous beds. The veins and venules become distended so the organ enlarges, assumes a redder than normal color, is swollen, and has a moist cut surface at autopsy. Parenchymal cells between congested sinusoids or venules become atrophic and show evidence of metabolic damage, such as fatty metamorphosis, related to the sluggish circulation and hypoxia. As cardiac output falls, the arteriovenous oxygen difference rises because of increased oxygen extraction in the tissues. Severe pulmonary hypertension develops, and right ventricular hypertrophy and failure develop in addition to that of the left. Respiratory alkalosis often ensues because of the hyperventilation stimulated by the pulmonary edema.

Hypertrophy is the response of the myocardium to increased work, as it is for other muscles. Increase in protein synthesis and mass will begin very promptly—within little more than 24 hours—after the imposition of an experimental load, but the overload and the hypertrophy begin more gradually in most human disease. The mass of the myocardium is related to that of the body, and the usual normal maxima are 350 g for men and 300 g for women. The thickness of the left ventricular wall may increase from 11 mm to 15, but sometimes the thickness is not as greatly increased as the mass because dilatation is the stimulus for and precedent to hypertrophy. Both ventricles are involved, particularly in late failure, but the left will be so to a greater extent when the heart works against systemic hypertension or obstructive lesions of the systemic circulation. When the strain is primarily and principally on the right ventricle, as in fibrosing pulmonary disease or repeated pulmonary emboli, right ventricular dilatation and hypertrophy are marked (**cor pulmonale**) and congestive changes in the abdominal viscera are often extreme. Acute left ventricular failure may complicate myocardial infarcts with **cardiogenic shock**, in which there is rapid development of severe pulmonary edema and hemoconcentration.

At autopsy, **chronic congestive changes** in the liver are manifest by swelling and accentuation of the lobular markings by widened central zones. When combined with fatty metamorphosis, this gives the **nutmeg liver** that is such a diagnostic favorite of students. The spleen enlarges modestly to about 300 g and is dark red and firm. **Hypersplenism** may develop. The lungs are distended, the cut surfaces and bronchi ooze frothy fluid, and with long-standing congestion, capillaries will have leaked erythrocytes that have broken down into hemosiderin deposits to give the lung a distinctly rusty appearance. A serious and often fatal complication of failure is ischemia of enteric mucosa with subsequent devitalization and hemorrhage—**hemorrhagic, low-flow enteropathy**.

Hypertensive cardiovascular disease

Hypertension is the sustained elevation of the systolic blood pressure above 140 mm Hg and the diastolic above 90. It is a most significant risk factor in the prognosis of vascular disease and has an incidence of 25% in individuals over 50 years of age in the United States. In 90%, a specific pathogenesis cannot be recognized—**primary**, or **essential, hypertension**. The search for causes is important, however, for in several types of **secondary hypertension** due to **pheochromocytoma, coarctation, renal artery obstruction**, etc., dramatic cures may be accomplished by surgery. **Malignant hypertension** is named for its rapid progression to renal failure, often with severe neurological complications. The rest of cases are hardly benign, for half die prematurely of myocardial infarcts and others suffer heart failure, cerebral infarcts, or hemorrhage.

Hypertension can result from either **increased resistance** or **increased sodium and water retention**. The latter results first in increased cardiac output, but autoregulation of the system then increases peripheral resistance and returns cardiac output to normal at the expense of increased pressure. **Arterial** baroreceptors, **catecholamines, regulators of body fluid volume, prostaglandins, aldosterone** and **cortisol,** and the **renin-angiotensin system** are involved in the pathogenesis of hypertension. The latter system is particularly important in the hypertension of **coarctation** and **renal arterial constriction** and probably contributes to **malignant hypertension**.

The primary lesion of hypertension is **arteriolosclerosis**, a thickening of the walls of arterioles by a homogeneous, eosinophilic hyalin that results from the incorporation of plasma proteins as well as thickening of the basement membrane. The changes are prominent in the **arterioles and glomeruli of the kidneys**. In small arteries there is a proliferation of layers of smooth muscle cells to give an onionskin appearance. Fibrin, fibrinoid necrosis, and thrombosis occur as renal damage progresses into failure. The vessels of the **retina** are distinctly involved and are readily available for clinical inspection. In the benign disease there are narrowed arterioles that nick the veins where they cross. In malignant hypertension, papilledema, exudates, and linear hemorrhages are changes that are diagnostic of the condition. In the kidneys, arteriolosclerosis results in scarring of glomeruli and atrophy of nephrons. Nephrons that are not so severely affected hypertrophy, and the alternation of atrophic and hypertrophic nephrons gives the capsular surface of the organ a granular configuration. Such kidneys are diagnosed as **arteriolar nephrosclerosis** and contract by continued scarring to the point of renal failure. **Malignant hypertension**, particularly when uremia develops, is associated with striking concentric proliferation of the walls of interlobular arteries and fibrinoid necrosis of arterioles. Infarction of glomeruli and hemorrhage into tubules occurs.

Neoplasia

Blood and lymph vessels are hardly a significant source of tumors. Most that are called **angiomas** of one sort or another seem biologically to be more like malformations or hamartomas. They include **telangiectasias, capillary and cavernous hemangiomas**, and **arteriovenous malformations** that are tangled masses of vessels of various sizes, types, and degrees of mature structure. They are most obvious in the skin but most important when they occur in the CNS, although even there the majority remain symptomless or uncomplicated throughout life. **Granuloma pyogenicum** (small polypoid tumors of skin and oral mucosa) and **glomus tumors** (usually on the fingers or toes and mimicking the structure of neuromyoarterial receptor organs) are a little more like true benign neoplasms.

Hemangioendotheliomas are tumors of the skin and occasionally the liver and spleen. They are composed of vascular channels and masses of spindle-shaped endothelial cells. They are of low malignancy but are important to distinguish from the malignant **hemangiosarcoma** that is composed of more anaplastic cells, fewer and more bizarre vascular spaces, and giant cells. The latter are particularly interesting for, although rare, the tumors that occur in the liver have been clearly associated with chemical carcinogens: **Thorotrast, arsenic**, and **polyvinylchloride**. **Hemangiopericytoma** is a soft-tissue tumor of characteristic histological structure that occurs mostly in the lower extremities and retroperitoneum. Ultrastructural evidence seems to demonstrate the origin of the cells from vascular pericytes. They are of quite variable malignant potential. **Kaposi's sarcoma** has gained much attention because of its association with AIDS. It occurs as multiple blue-red nodules in the skin that increase in number and may eventually spread widely to the viscera. Histologically, the tumor is composed of spindle cells and resembles angiosarcomas. There is often an inflammatory component, and its epidemiology strongly suggests that it may be associated with a virus.

HEART

Congenital heart disease

The complex embryology of the heart offers many opportunities for missteps, and the catalog of **congenital heart disease** seems to include a syndrome for every such opportunity. Only the most common and important can be reviewed here. It should be remembered that some aortic malformations are commonly included with those of the heart and often occur in combination.

Seven of 100 live births are affected. The course and outcome are very much determined by the effect the malformation might have on the **pulmonary circulation**. If there is obstruction to pulmonary flow and **shunting from the right side to the left**, arterial blood is inadequately oxygenated and cyanosis, polycythemia, and growth retardation occur. If the **shunt is left to right**, pulmonary hypertension will become severe and obstructive, eventually to the point of reversal of the shunt with its attendant complications. **Cardiac failure**, either left or right depending on the shunted pathways, and **pulmonary infections** and **bacterial endocarditis** are the usual terminal complications. **Strokes** and **brain abscesses** occur with right-to-left shunts.

Atrial septal defects vary from persistent **probe patent foramen ovale** that is of no functional consequence and so common as to hardly be considered a malformation to less common persistent patencies of the **septum secundum** or **septum primum**, the latter usually being part of an **endocardial cushion defect**. Increased pulmonary flow and finally pulmonary hypertension are the results. **Ventricular septal defects** are the most common significant malformations. They are usually of the membranous septum just under the aortic valve. Some may close spontaneously and others may be asymptomatic throughout a normal life, but the pathological consequences are those of a left-to-right shunt. **Endocardial cushion defect** is a failure of the development of the center of the heart involving the top of the interventricular septum and the bottom of the interatrial septum resulting in a single, more or less continuous, atrioventricular valve with multiple irregular cusps. It occurs nearly always with **Down's syndrome**, which is of interesting genetic implication. **Tetralogy of Fallot** was the first malformation for which effective surgery was developed. It consists of pulmonary arterial or valvular stenosis, high interventricular septal defect, displacement of the aorta toward the deformed pulmonary valve so that the aorta overrides the septal defect, and hypertrophy of the right ventricle.

Two malformations remain most difficult to deal with. One is the **hypoplastic left heart syndrome**, in which there is **atresia of the aortic and/or the mitral valve** without a septal defect. As a consequence, blood does not flow in the left ventricle, which remains embryonic in size. The ascending aorta also fails to develop normally and is merely a common root for the coronary arteries that are fed retrograde from the arch of the aorta. Neonatal closure of the ductus is fatal. The other malformations are the **transpositions of the great vessels** that present in several varieties. In brief, the aorta and pulmonary arteries are connected to the wrong ventricles so that after closure of the foramen ovale and ductus the systemic and pulmonary circulations are completely separated. The configuration of the ventricles may also be abnormal, and there is a "**corrected**" **form** in which the arrangement is as though the right atrium were attached to the left ventricle that had migrated to the right and the ventricle led into the pulmonary artery and a similar reversal had taken place with the right ventricle. Accompanying valvular abnormalities and apparent incapacity of the structural right ventricle to maintain systemic blood pressure and flow limit the prognosis for these individuals despite the apparent correct arrangement of the circulations.

Inflammation

Significant cardiac disease results from several different kinds of inflammation: bacterial, viral, and spirochetal infections and processes that are undoubtedly of an autoimmune nature. Although their incidence in the United States has been greatly reduced by the prompt and effective treatment of streptococcal disease, **rheumatic fever** and **rheumatic heart disease** are of classic importance.

Acute rheumatic fever follows infections, usually a pharyngitis, with group A beta-hemolytic streptococci. The exact mechanism has not been completely elucidated, but there is cross-reaction between streptococcal components and myocardial fibers, and the presence of antibodies such as antistreptolysin O and others is almost constant among patients with active disease. Fever, polyarthritis, skin rashes, subcutaneous nodules, and involuntary choretic movements are features of the acute disease but are transient, whereas carditis is present in all cases and is the lesion that persists. The edges of the valves are the site of small, red nodules along the lines of closure that are called **verrucous endocarditis**. The mitral valve is most often involved (50% of cases), followed by the aortic valve, usually in combination, and a minor (10%) number involve the tricuspid or pulmonary valves. This lesion progresses to fibrosis, adhesions at the commissures, stenosis or insufficiency, and great fibrous thickening of leaflets sometimes with calcification and spread from the mitral valve to the chordae tendineae. Microscopically, the acute vegetations are composed of swollen, degenerated connective tissue covered by fibrin and platelets and overgrown by endothelial cells. These lesions in themselves are not potential sources of emboli. In the myocardium, the characteristic lesion is the **Aschoff's nodule** that lies interstitially about blood vessels. It is a focus of fibrinoid necrosis and reaction by polymorphonuclear leukocytes and plasma cells to some degree but most prominently of mononuclear cells with long, sparsely chromatic nuclei with cylindrical nucleoli called **Anitschkov's myocytes**. They are not specific for rheumatic fever, and it is debated as to whether they are reactive fibroblasts or derivatives of injured myocardial fibers. The specific components of these pathognomic nodules are the larger cells with thick cytoplasm and similar nuclei that are named **Aschoff's cells**.

Active rheumatic myocarditis is the most serious of the acute lesions, and death at that stage is usually from congestive cardiac failure. An acute **pericarditis** with deposition of fibrin on the surfaces and cellular infiltrates and even Aschoff's nodules in the interstitium occurs in early acute disease but usually resolves without sequelae. The chronic complications are those of failure arising from the overwork imposed by the stenotic and incompetent valves. The disease probably smolders, with progressive damage to the heart long after other symptoms have subsided. Certainly, Aschoff's nodules can be found in auricular appendages at the time of correction of old mitral stenosis, and the susceptibility of rheumatic valves to bacterial infection might be, at least in part, because a verrucous vegetation provides a nidus on which bacteria might lodge.

Infective endocarditis occurs when bacteria lodge and grow on the surface of the endocardium, almost always at the line of closure of the valves and in the systemic circulation. Essentially the same disease may occur in arteries at irregular sites such as the edge of a **patent ductus**. Something more than the presence of bacteria in the bloodstream is apparently necessary to initiate the disease, for it is far less frequent than bacteremia. The verrucae of rheumatic valvulitis could be such a nidus, but perhaps more commonly it might be the **thrombotic nonbacterial (marantic) endocarditis** vegetations, which are masses of fibrin, platelets, and swollen collagen similar to but usually larger and less numerous than rheumatic vegetations. The pathogenesis of this condition is not clear, its occurrence is almost occasional, but it seems related to disturbance in the coagulative mechanisms of the blood.

Many different organisms have been involved in infective endocarditis, including fungi, but the most important are *Streptococcus viridans, Staphylococcus aureus,* **enterococci** and **other staphylococci, pneumococci,** and **gram-negative rods**, with the first two formerly accounting for two-thirds of cases and the latter of growing importance among patients with immunosuppression, especially following transplants. The nature of the lesions and course of the disease depend on the balance between the virulence of the organism and the effectiveness of the healing process. Formerly, the disease was uniformly fatal and cases with organisms of low virulence, such as *S. viridans,* progressed through 6 weeks or more with fibrosis developing in the valve and over the base of the vegetation and death coming from the chronic septicemia, emboli from the vegetation, or heart failure due to the strain of additional distortion of already deformed valves that were usually the site of such **subacute bacterial endocarditis**. More virulent organisms outstripped the fibrosing process and would perforate the valves, with a higher component of acute cardiac failure. With antibiotics, the progress of the acute disease is commonly slowed, if not cured, so nearly all lesions at autopsy now have the appearance of those of the subacute disease.

The distribution of the valvular involvement is much the same as that of rheumatic valvulitis, which was the classic precedent of subacute bacterial endocarditis. A modern exception occurs in **IV drug abusers**, in whom involvement of the tricuspid valve may occur and the organisms are often common skin contaminants. Changes in the rest of the body are those of septicemia and embolization with lymphoid hyperplasia, splenomegaly, and infarcts in spleen, liver, and brain as well as the eventual cardiac failure.

Syphilitic heart disease is really the result of extension of syphilitic aortitis to the leaflets of the aortic valve. The valve is incompetent because the leaflets at the cusps adhere to the wall of the sinuses of Valsalva rather than to one another as occurs in the stenosis of rheumatic valvulitis. Marked dilatation and hypertrophy occur, and boot-shaped hearts were some of the largest seen when tertiary syphilis was more common.

Myocarditis, in addition to that of rheumatic fever, is usually acute and of viral etiology. **Coxsackievirus A and B, poliomyelitis, influenza, adenovirus, echovirus,** and **rubeola** and **rubella** viruses have been the best documented. An **idiopathic or isolated variety called Fiedler's** is also recognized. The edema and interstitial infiltrates in the myocardium in the fatal cases are rarely extensive, and most cases experience transient ECG changes and recover. More severe compromise may occur in the **toxic myocarditis of diphtheria**, and in such cases, as well as occasional cases of viral myocarditis, patients may die in acute cardiac failure. In Central and South America there is a **chronic myocarditis due to** *Trypanosoma cruzi* **(Chagas' disease)**. *Toxoplasma gondii* is a cause of acute myocarditis in the newborn and in immunosuppressed adults or in those undergoing treatment with corticosteroids.

Pericarditis may be of **viral origin**, especially with the myocarditis of coxsackievirus B and echoviruses. Other causes are **myocardial infarcts, uremia,** and **bacterial infections** such as tuberculosis when an involved tracheobronchial lymph node ruptures into the pericardium. Most acute cases due to virus heal without sequelae, except perhaps for focal fibrous thickening of the epicardium, but purulent and tuberculous pericarditis will progress to fibrous constriction and cardiac failure. The lesions vary with the etiologies, from the presence of clear fluid in the pericardial sac, to fibrinous exudates on the surface, to pus or caseous material. The combination of fluid and blood is often due to metastatic tumor growing into the pericardium.

Degenerative valvular disease

The three degenerative valvular diseases are of unknown etiology but of sufficient incidence and significance to be mentioned. The first is **mitral valve prolapse**, also known as floppy mitral valve, parachute valve, and midsystolic click syndrome, from its cardinal physical sign. It consists of a softening and interstitial mucoid alteration in the stroma of one or both leaflets, with consequent redundancy and sometimes lengthening of chordae tendineae that allows portions of the leaflet to balloon upward into the atrium under ventricular pressure. It is a common condition that is reported in 5 to 7% of the population, especially in young women. A high incidence accompanies Marfan's syndrome and, because of the similarity of the microscopic changes to some of those other tissues in Marfan's, it has been suggested without confirmation that the condition may be a forme fruste of that hereditary disease.

Isolated calcific aortic stenosis resembles the lesion of chronic rheumatic disease of that valve, but there is no other evidence that it belongs to that disorder. The valve often is bicuspid, which is considered a congenital malformation. Stenosis and enlargement of the heart are progressive to failure and begin with the appearance of a systolic ejection murmur. As in other forms of aortic stenosis, **sudden death** may occur, possibly because of interference with the bundle of His that lies in the margin of the membranous interventricular septum just beneath the involved aortic valve. It is a disease of aging, most cases appearing in the sixth or seventh decade of life, and without surgical replacement of the valve the prognosis is guarded and is for little more than 2 years of life.

Calcification of the mitral annulus consists of beaded, 5- to 8-mm masses of calcified tissue in the ring of the valve. It occurs in older people, is discovered incidentally in radiographs or at autopsy, and rarely has any significance, although individual cases of symptomatic enroachment on the valvular lumen, cardiac arrhythmia, or endocarditis have been recognized.

Ischemic heart disease

Ischemic heart disease is the most common and important of cardiac diseases. It is principally a manifestation of coronary arteriosclerosis, although sometimes the myocardium is injured by hypotension or shock, showers of emboli, or narrowing of the arteries by disorders at their ostia. It is responsible for most of the dire consequences of arteriosclerosis, is more common in men than in women, and is responsible for more deaths in the United States than cancer and infectious disease combined. Encouragingly, the rate per 100,000 men has fallen steadily from 300 in 1968 to about 250 recently. A major manifestation, **myocardial infarction**, carries a mortality of 40%, with nearly half of the deaths occurring within the first 2 hours, an observation that has motivated the development of emergency medical services throughout the country in the past decade.

Much of our knowledge and concepts of the pathology of this disease are based on clinical observations and measurements that have yielded a mass of information far too large to be adequately reviewed here. Four **clinical patterns** are most important: (1) **myocardial infarction,** (2) **angina pectoris,** (3) **chronic ischemic heart disease**, and (4) **sudden cardiac death**. Infarcts are due to severe, sudden interruption of an area of coronary blood flow and are of two kinds: (1) **transmural infarcts**, in which there is almost complete death of tissue in the distribution of the involved artery, with central yellow necrosis and surrounding red margins after 3 to 4 days, and (2) **subendocardial infarcts**, in which there are multifocal areas of ischemic necrosis limited to the inner third or half of the wall of the left ventricle, a zone of most active muscular work and farthest from the arteries in the epicardium. **Angina pectoris** consists of paroxysmal chest pain due to decreased coronary flow that is not intensive enough to cause necrosis of myocardium, although at autopsy such patients nearly always show at least microscopic evidence of **chronic ischemic heart disease** in which there are multiple, usually widely distributed small scars. Chronic ischemic heart disease leads to slowly progressive decrease of cardiac reserve and persistent failure, although the course is often interrupted by development of an infarct or arrhythmia. **Sudden cardiac death** in ischemic heart disease accounts for half its mortality and is due to arrhythmia, usually ventricular fibrillation, that appears to arise from sudden imbalance between the needs of the myocardial fiber and its available supply of oxygen. Arteriosclerosis of the coronary arteries is always present, but there is rarely anatomic evidence of a sudden change in the status of the vessels.

It has long been taught that most of significant coronary arteriosclerosis consists of lesions that narrow the first 2 cm of the major arteries, but experience with coronary angiography in connection with bypass operations has demonstrated that important narrowing or occlusion will occur in more distant sites. The significant degree of stenosis is taken to be 75% of the cross-sectional area of the vessel. Severe narrowing usually occurs in all three major trunks. The lesions are usually complicated plaques that are ulcerated, may be overlaid with thrombi, or contain hemorrhage, but in a majority of fatalities acute changes such as an occluding thrombus cannot be found and the mechanism of insufficiency seems to include a decrease in flow past a preexisting stenosis, a condition that emphasizes the importance of episodic changes in blood pressure in the pathogenesis of this disease.

Intercoronary anastomoses develop extensively with coronary arterosclerosis and may prevent infarction even when a major artery is completely occluded. They are undoubtedly responsible for the slow evolution of chronic ischemic disease. With **transmural infarcts**, patterns of distribution are associated with stenotic or occluding lesions of particular major arteries: 40 to 50% of cases involve the **left anterior descending artery** and the anterior wall of the left ventricle and anterior two-thirds of the septum; 30 to 40% involve the **right coronary** and the posterior wall of the ventricle and posterior third of the septum; and 15 to 20% involve the **left circumflex** and lateral wall of the left ventricle. The localization in the last two categories is particularly influenced by the distribution, or balance, of the left circumflex and right arteries, one of which may be disproportionately **dominant** in a particular individual, and prior collaterals are also responsible for atypical localization of infarcts in relation to the most severe lesions of the arteries.

During the first week of a transmural infarct, the softened necrotic tissue may **rupture**, with hemorrhage into the pericardium and **cardiac tamponade** or with **tearing of a papillary muscle** and sudden incompetence of the mitral valve. On healing of an extensive infarct, the scar in an inactive zone of the myocardium may be displaced during systole to give **paradoxical motion** of the outline of the heart and outward bulging to form a so-called **aneurysm**.

Cardiomyopathies

Cardiomyopathies are a category of obscure diseases characterized by gross enlargement of the heart, little in the way of microscopic changes, and progressive cardiac failure. They have been well summarized by Golden: "The cardiomyopathies are a group of disorders of the myocardium that are not relatable to coronary artery disease, hypertension, or valvular disease. Some are primary, i.e., of unknown etiology, while others are secondary to disease elsewhere in the body. All are associated with cardiac hypertrophy and slowly progressive congestive heart failure that is relatively unresponsive to therapy."

Cardiomyopathies are also categorized on the basis of their hemodynamic consequences as **restrictive, congestive**, or **obstructive**. Restrictive lesions are those that stiffen the myocardium and interfere with diastolic filling. The hemodynamic effect is comparable to that in constrictive pericarditis, and the end result is low-output failure. Congestive cardiomyopathy is the most common and is characterized by a flabby, dilated myocardium, weak pumping action, and biventricular failure. Obstructive cardiomyopathy is rare, the best-known example being **idiopathic hypertrophic subaortic stenosis**.

Examples of cardiomyopathies include (1) idiopathic congestive cardiomyopathy, (2) idiopathic hypertrophic subaortic stenosis, (3) toxic cardiomyopathy that particularly follows treatment of neoplastic disease with drugs that interfere with DNA metabolism, (4) alcoholic cardiomyopathy, (5) cardiac amyloidosis, (6) endomyocardial fibroelastosis, and (7) metabolic cardiomyopathy such as occurs in beriberi.

Neoplasia

By far the most frequent and important involvement of the heart in neoplasia is by **metastatic tumors, bronchogenic carcinoma** being the most frequent and **melanoma** interesting because a higher percentage of such tumors reach the myocardium than almost any other. Lymphomas, mesotheliomas, angiosarcomas, and other rare tumors may reach the heart by their natural extension if not by arising in the pericardium or the heart itself. **Serosanguineous pericardial effusion** should always be considered a result of neoplasia unless another cause can be proved, such as is encountered very occasionally in myocardial infarction, especially with incipient rupture.

The most frequent primary tumor is the rare, benign **myxoma**. These are masses, usually pedunculated, of soft, translucent, almost gelatinous tissue that on microscopic section are composed of stellate or globular myxoma cells, endothelial cells, macrophages, mature or immature smooth muscle cells, and other forms in a matrix of mucopolysaccharide ground substance. They occur most often in the left atrium and at any age, including infancy. It has been suggested they are organized thrombi, but most observers consider them benign tumors. Their principal effect is that of an obstructing mass, but many are apparently silent for long periods as they may be discovered only at autopsy. Far less common are **rhabdomyomas** of similar configuration and composition except for a predominance of large, often binucleate, cells with cytoplasmic glycogen vacuoles and some degree of muscle cross-striations in some cells. These occur mostly in infants and children and in association with **tuberous sclerosis**.

BLOOD, BONE MARROW, AND LYMPHORETICULAR TISSUES

NORMAL ANATOMY

The ready accessibility of the cells of the blood, bone marrow, and lymphoreticular tissues has made easy their study by more elegant staining and analysis than is usually applied to the cells of most other tissues. The application of the methods of modern cellular biology to their study has produced such large amounts of information that hematology and related oncology have become almost independent sciences, so much so that in one of the major reference texts of pathology there is hardly mention of diseases of erythrocytes in its index. As a consequence, this review cannot do justice to the large number of separate diseases and syndromes now well delimited. It will concentrate on the features, principally of pathological anatomy, common to the major classes rather than the fine differentials of the various disorders.

The student should review the concepts of **cellular development and differentiation** of the various cells of this system as well as their cytological features. The rapid turnover of these cells and the several levels of differentiation at which proliferation normally or potentially may occur present opportunities for injury and distortion that are much better recognized and understood for these tissues than for many others. The often lesser abnormalities in other members of the system in the presence of disease expressed principally in one cell line are examples of the close interrelations: the hypersegmentation of granular leukocytes in pernicious anemia, for example.

It should be kept in mind that the **bone marrow** is an organ of equal or slightly larger size than the liver. It can respond with rapid hyperplasia that easily doubles its size in adults, in whom half the marrow space is normally fatty. It is susceptible to just as rapid suppression or destruction. Also, the various techniques for ready measurement of cells add a quantitative dimension to study of these diseases that is not easily obtained with other systems. Several derived measurements are especially helpful:

Mean corpuscular volume (MCV) = hematocrit/erythrocyte count

Mean corpuscular hemoglobin (MCH) = hemoglobin/erythrocyte count

Mean corpuscular hemoglobin concentration (MCHC) = hemoglobin/hematocrit

(N.B.: Special attention is demanded for the decimal places that are not indicated here!)

ERYTHROCYTES

Congenital and hereditary diseases

The hereditary diseases of red cells are based, for the most part, on rather straightforward defects in synthesis of a particular protein. **Erythroblastosis fetalis** is an example of a congenital but not strictly hereditary disease, although the genetic status of parents regarding their blood group alleles is a hereditary prerequisite. These conditions account for the largest part of the **hemolytic anemias** that share the qualities of (1) shortened life span of erythrocytes, (2) hyperplasia of the erythoid elements of the bone marrow, and (3) accumulation of the products of erythrocytic destruction, particularly the accumulation of hemosiderin in reticuloendothelial tissues that may give organs such as the liver and kidneys a distinct, grossly apparent brown hue. Splenomegaly is often a feature, although **sickle cell disease** presents an exception with the spleen being destroyed by another feature of the disease, namely thrombosis and obliteration of blood vessels.

Hereditary spherocytosis is an autosomal dominant disease in which erythrocytes are spheroidal and inelastic and consequently subject to increased destruction. It occurs most often in persons of northern European origin and is apparently related to the metabolism of the structural protein spectrin in the cell membrane. **Sickle cell disease** is recessive and clinically important in homozygotes, the heterozygous condition apparently actually being of some survival benefit against endemic malaria in African blacks. It is due to the substitution of valine for glutamine at the sixth position of the beta chain of hemoglobin. The essential morphological defect is in the distortion of the erythrocytes induced by hypoxia. Thrombosis occurs and results in crises of abdominal pain, cutaneous ulcers (particularly on the legs), and autosplenectomy. **Thalassemia** is a heterogenous group of diseases due to deficient or absent synthesis of elements of the beta or alpha chains of hemoglobin. The homozygous condition for abnormal beta chains, called **thalassemia major**, is a very severe condition that appears early in life and is fatal without vigorous support by transfusions, which unfortunately lead to hemosiderosis and **exogenous hemochromatosis**. Inherent lesions include heterotopic bone marrow in various sites such as the spleen and retroperitoneal tissues as well as marked hyperplasia of bone marrow that may stimulate bone growth, especially in the skull, where radial spicules have a "hair-on-end" appearance on radiographs. The heterozygous condition, **thalassemia minor**, results in a mild anemia that may not require therapy but must not be confused with microcytic iron deficiency anemia, for iron therapy complicates the already increased iron stores of thalassemia. These syndromes have been called **Mediterranean anemia**, which indicates the population groups most apt to harbor the responsible genes. The **alpha-thalassemias** present a more complicated pathogenesis as there are four gene loci involved and the excess gamma-globin chains and aggregated beta chains give rise to **Bart's hemoglobin** and **hemoglobin H tetramers**, respectively. The clinical manifestations and anatomic changes are generally less marked than those of thalassemia major but in the fetus can give rise to **hydrops fetalis**, a fatal intrauterine condition expressed by severe edema, ascites, hydrothorax, and massive hepatosplenomegaly due to tissue oxygen deprivation.

Hydrops fetalis also occurs in **erythroblastosis fetalis**, in which the damage is done to the fetus by transplacental maternal antibodies against blood group factors in the fetus that are inherited from the father and not present in the mother. The major cause has been the D antigen of the Rh group, but success in preventing Rh sensitivity in Rh-negative mothers by the administration of anti-D immunoglobulin within 72 hours of delivery has not only prevented the development of erythroblastosis in the next pregnancy but has also made ABO incompatibility the more common cause. The damage to the fetus varies from the severe **hydrops** through **icterus gravis**, in which there is severe hemolysis, jaundice, and hypoxic injury to the heart and liver, to the milder **congenital anemia of the newborn**, which may be little more severe than the jaundice that accompanies the normal destruction of excess erythrocytes in the latter part of the first week of postnatal life, **icterus neonatorum**.

Infections and anemia

Many systemic infectious processes, particularly when chronic, are accompanied by an anemia that is usually mild. Some infections result in hemolysis, but the more general effect appears to be one of suppression of normal hemoglobin metabolism and erythrocyte generation, including decreased formation of erythropoietin. The increased activity of the stimulated mononuclear phagocyte system may play a part. Gross and microscopic changes related directly to the anemia are insignificant. **Malaria** is the principal example of a directly destructive infection of the red cells. Splenomegaly, visible

parasitism in the erythrocytes (the sporozoites in hepatic cells of the extraerythrocytic early asexual phase are very difficult to demonstrate with ordinary microscopy), hyperplasia of Kupffer's cells and other cells of the reticuloendothelial system and their distension with **malarial pigment** (closely similar to **hematin**), and erythrocytic debris are the principal lesions. The capillaries of the brain are particularly involved with pigment and small thrombi in the cerebral manifestation of **malignant falciparum malaria**, and the kidneys develop the lesions of acute tubular necrosis with particularly prominent hemoglobin casts in **blackfever** of infection with the same *Plasmodium falciparum*. Other protozoal infections such as **trypanosomiasis** and **leishmaniasis** also involve the erythrocytes and cause an anemia.

Acquired anemias

The outstanding acquired anemias are the **autoimmune hemolytic anemias**. Most are relatively mild, and the pathological anatomy is characterized by splenomegaly. The spleen in most is hyperactive in removing damaged or coated erythrocytes, and the **Coombs' antiglobulin test** is a principal diagnostic tool in both its direct form (animal antiglobulin, usually anti-IgG or anti-C3, reacting with globulin on the erythrocyte surface) and indirect (patient's serum utilized to coat compatible erythrocytes, which are then tested with the animal antiglobulin serums). Some of the pathological antibodies react best in **cold** and others in **warm** environments. The warm arise in response to drugs (e.g., methyldopa and penicillin) or during the course of lymphomas or collagen vascular diseases (lupus erythematosus), and the cold more commonly in response to infections (e.g., mycoplasmas, infectious mononucleosis), but a substantial number are idiopathic. The cold agglutinin group is caused by IgM antibodies, in contrast to the others. A cold hemolysin of anti-IgG is activated by the lytic C5-9 complex when the patient is exposed to cold, and massive hemolysis may occur in the disease **paroxysmal cold hemoglobinuria**.

A more direct immunologic class of hemolytic anemias are those due to isohemagglutinins that arise in response to exposure to **incompatible blood**. Acute renal tubular necrosis with prominent hemoglobin casts is prominent in severe **transfusion reactions**, and **erythroblastosis** is also an example of this group. Another type of hemolytic anemia arises in response to **trauma** to the erythrocyte. Some of these are due to the action of artificial heart valves, and others are associated with microvascular disease such as **disseminated intravascular coagulation, malignant hypertension, thrombotic thrombocytopenic purpura**, etc.

Aplastic anemia is the result of suppression of all cell lines in the bone marrow. It is most often due to exposure to chemical toxins but may follow infections, may be due to radiation, or may be idiopathic. The principal change is loss of cells in the bone marrow, even with atrophy of the fat cells, and slight reactive fibrosis and infiltration with plasma cells and lymphocytes. This should be distinguished from the fibrotic stage that develops in some myeloproliferative diseases.

Nutritional anemias

Nutritional anemias are deficiency diseases. **Iron deficiency anemia** usually arises because of unreplaced blood loss rather than a deficiency of intake or defect of absorption. The erythrocytes are small and of decreased hemoglobin content and concentration. The bone marrow presents normoblastic hyperplasia, and there is a loss of the usual stainable iron in the reticuloendothelial cells. Atrophic glossitis and atrophic gastritis develop and become symptomatic.

The **macrocytic anemias** are due to deficiencies that distort the synthesis of DNA. The paradigm is **pernicious anemia**, in which the absorption of dietary **cyanocobalamin** (vitamin B_{12}) is blocked because of the failure of gastric parietal cells to elaborate the **intrinsic factor** necessary to combine with the vitamin and promote its absorption. This is presently thought to be on the basis of an autoimmune injury to the gastric mucosa, which exhibits a typical atrophic gastritis and tendency to develop carcinoma. The bone marrow is hyperplastic, with prominent nests of distorted, enlarged erythrocyte precursors called megaloblasts. In the atrophic gastritis, the parietal cells are virtually absent. The heart and liver show fatty change, and the slightly enlarged liver and spleen are the seat of hemosiderosis. Because of its place high in the chain of metabolism from homocysteine through folate derivatives to DNA synthesis, cobalamin is also essential for the maintenance of myelin in the posterior and lateral funiculi of the spinal cord, and its deficiency results in **combined system disease** in which there is a loss of proprioceptive sensation and impairment of motor function due to demyelination in the posterior columns and the lateral corticospinal tracts of the spinal cord. Although the hematologic abnormality may be completely reversed by administration of the vitamin, the neurological damage is irreversible. The megaloblastic anemia of **folic acid deficiency** is essentially identical to pernicious anemia except for the changes in the CNS. Some other megaloblastic anemias can arise from malabsorption states associated with intestinal disease, blind loops, pregnancy, and parasitic disease (fish tapeworm) and are due to vitamin B_{12} deficiency, whereas others are folate deficiencies. An important point in therapy is to recognize that folic acid may correct the anemia, but if the deficiency is of vitamin B_{12} the neurological disease may appear and progress.

Erythrocytic proliferative disorders

The proliferative conditions of erythrocytes are less numerous and less frequent that the anemias: (1) secondary polycythemia, or **erythrocytosis**, (2) polycythemia vera, or **erythemia**, and (3) **erythroleukemia**. Hematocrit values of 50 to 55% are suggestive of polycythemia and above 60% are almost conclusive, but there must also be an increase in blood volume. Erythrocyte counts exceed 6 million and may reach almost to the "standing room only" figure of 11.5 million if there is some degree of microcytosis. Iron deficiency may result in lesser values of hemoglobin and hemoglobin concentration than would parallel the counts. **Secondary polycythemia** is a response to increased levels of erythropoietin that in turn arise from low oxygen tensions of high altitudes, respiratory and cardiac disease, some abnormal hemoglobins (e.g., methemoglobin), and some tumors, particularly renal cell carcinomas. The pathological changes are visceral congestion and the presence of thrombi due to the increased viscosity of the blood, but in general they are less advanced than in **polycythemia vera**, in

which hepatomegaly and splenomegaly with extramedullary erythropoiesis accompany the gross erythroid **hyperplasia** of the bone marrow. The latter condition is of unknown etiology, but from its cellular proliferative nature and the fact that 10 to 15% of patients develop myeloid leukemia, the accompanying stimulation of granular leukocytes, and other evidence from cell biology, it is classified with the **myeloproliferative diseases.** **Erythroluekemia** is a rare from of acute leukemia, closely related in most of its clinical and morphological features to acute myeloid leukemia. The abnormal cells in the blood and tissue infiltrates are predominately early erythroid forms.

PLATELET AND COAGULATION DISORDERS

Diseases of platelets and coagulation factors result in pathological bleeding. The final lesions are simple and similar for all: petechiae, purpura, hematomas, and bleeding, with residual lesions of scarring, hemosiderosis, and sometimes reactive hyperplasia as occurs in synovium of joints from which hemorrhage is inadequately resolved. The pathogenesis, however, involves all stages of coagulation about which tremendously detailed biochemical information is now available and should be reviewed as normal physiology and cell biology. **Platelets** can be decreased in number as a result of decreased production or increased destruction, the former occurring in diseases of the bone marrow such as leukemia and aplasia and folate deficiency and in the course of infections and by the action of cytotoxic drugs. The prototype of destructive disease is **idiopathic thrombocytopenic purpura**, in which there are autoantibodies against platelets and the organs show compensatory hyperplasias: splenomegaly and increased numbers of immature-appearing megakaryocytes in most cases. Other etiologic factors of this group are drugs, infections, mechanical injury as by prosthetic heart valves, and syndromes such as uremic hemolysis, as well as consumption in DIC and sequestration that occurs with many types of splenomegaly. Cerebral hemorrhage is a particularly dangerous outcome of this disease. Platelet function may be decreased to the point of purpura by the action of **aspirin** that suppresses prostaglandins that play a part in platelet aggregation, and a similar condition occurs in **uremia.** For all the platelet deficiency diseases, increased bleeding time is characteristic because of the failure of plug formation in the early contracted phase of injured small vessels.

Congenital deficiency underlies a complete spectrum of rare coagulation disorders that have been recognized for each of the coagulation factors. They are usually transmitted as autosomal recessive traits, but **von Willebrand's disease** (prolonged bleeding, low Factor VIII, particularly the component VIII:R that promotes platelet aggregation, and autosomal dominance) and the sex-linked **hemophilias A** (Factor VIII:C, the component that is a coagulation factor) **and B** (Factor IX, or Christmas disease) are less rare. The hemophilias are especially noted for the severity of deep hemorrhages and hemarthrosis following slight or unrecognized trauma.

Disseminated intravascular coagulation is a condition involving widespread endothelial injury that leads to coagulation within the microcirculation to such an extent that platelets and various coagulation factors, particularly fibrinogen, are consumed and the blood becomes uncoagulable. It is an important complication of shock and bacterial sepsis, particularly that due to gram-negative organisms. Petechiae and oozing hemorrhage from serious and mucous membranes are the principal anatomic features. Small thrombi of platelets and fibrin may be found in such sites as the glomerular capillaries of the kidney, but in most cases they are so small they are rapidly removed by normal fibrinolytic mechanisms. **Thrombotic thrombocytopenic purpura** and, in at least some cases, **traumatic fat embolism** are related disorders.

LEUKOCYTES

Congenital disorders

Several genetic disorders of leukocytes contribute to the spectrum of defective leukocytic function that results in increased susceptibility to infections. One example is the **Chédiak-Higashi** syndrome, an autosomal recessive disorder in which granular leukocytes have large lysosome-like granules and impaired chemotactic response, and another is chronic granulomatous disease of childhood, an X-linked enzymatic failure of the **hydrogen peroxidase-myeloperoxidase-halide** system by which phagocytized microorganisms are killed within the cell.

Infections

Leukocytes of all types are principal participants in the inflammatory process and consequently in the reaction to infections. They or their products contribute to the generation of **fever**, and their response of increased numbers in the bloodstream is the characteristic **leukocytosis** of such diseases, whereas their infiltration of infected tissues contributes to the swelling, pain, and heat of **inflammation**. In some instances, such as tuberculosis and leprosy, the infectious agent assumes an almost **symbiotic intracellular existence** in macrophages that form the characteristic granulomas of such diseases. On the other hand, it is only recently that **infections that are primarily of leukocytes** have been recognized. The **Epstein-Barr virus** is an infection of B-lymphocytes in its several manifestations of **infectious mononucleosis** and **Burkitt's tumor**, although the "atypical lymphocytes" in the blood of patients with the former condition are T-lymphocytes activated to combat the infected B cells. The RNA retroviruses known as **human T-lymphotropic viruses** (HTLV) have a recognized relation to certain leukemias but became particularly notorious when HTLV-III was discovered to be the etiologic agent of **AIDS** and was then renamed **human immunodeficiency virus (HIV)**. This virus is directed against the T-4 receptor and results in loss of the T-lymphocyte helper cells. It is of importance that the T-4 receptor is also known to occur in monocytes, macrophages, and colorectal cells.

Neoplasia

Leukemia. Leukemias are neoplastic monoclonal proliferations of stem cells of the bone marrow. They differ from other tumors in that their spread is systemic from the beginning because of the circulatory nature of the involved cells and because several etiologic factors have been well recognized in various types of the disease: ionizing radiation, chemicals such as benzene and cytotoxic drugs used in the treatment of other tumors, HTLV, and chromosomal abnormalities first recognized in Down's syndrome and the Philadelphia chromosome (translocation of the long arm of chromosome 22 to the long arm of 9 or sometimes another) of chronic myelogenous leukemia. The chromosomal factor has been particularly explored in these neoplasms, with clear demonstration of the effects of translocations of segments that include oncogenes.

Classifications have been based on recognition of the specific type of cell involved and on the malignant growth potential—that is, **acute or chronic chronology** that is a reflection of the level of differentiation of the stem cells most involved, the more acute being the less mature. It is now accepted for **acute leukemias** in the French-American-British (FAB) classification that there are essentially only **two races**, the **lymphocytic** with three subvarieties and **myelocytic** with six, including what were formerly classified separately as **myelo-monocytic, monocytic,** and **erythroleukemia**. Recognition of the various types is based on morphology and the use of certain special stains for granules and other cellular components. **Chronic leukemias** have always been easily classified as either lymphocytic or myelocytic except for the complications of terminal blastic crises, in which the cellular morphology reverts to that of the acute leukemias.

Biologically, the **acute leukemias** seem to involve defective maturation of stem cells at a level where ordinarily one of the progeny is committed to becoming the next more differentiated cell type, whereas **chronic leukemias** seem to have escaped normal mechanisms of growth regulation such as the colony-stimulating factor. In both, but particularly in the chronic form, there is less evidence of increased rates of cellular division than there is of decreased cellular maturation and destruction. With the effect of modern aggressive therapy, the completely developed morphological picture of chronic leukemia is rarely seen, but it was characterized by an **indolent course**, especially for chronic lymphocytic leukemia, **marked leukocytosis** to the level of several hundred thousand cells, and **infiltration and enlargement of organs** such as the liver, spleen, and lymph nodes. Patients with **myelocytic** disease generally had larger spleens with greater tendency to infarction, whereas the lymph nodes were prominently enlarged in the lymphocytic variety. These infiltrative phenomena tend to be suppressed nowadays, and the final lapse into a blastic crisis is a common termination. The **acute syndrome**, including the blastic crisis, is characterized by **fever, weakness, bleeding of the gums, widespread petechiae, overt hemorrhages, local pain from the bleeding and infiltrations, stroke from involvement of the brain by hemorrhages that are triggered by areas of infiltration of the leukemic cells, and finally infections by various bacteria and fungi characteristic of collapse of immunity.**

Some details of special importance include the following: (1) Acute lymphocytic leukemias rarely show B- or T-cell markers but do exhibit terminal deoxynucleotidyl transferase that is considered a marker of primitive lymphoid cells. (2) Chronic lymphocytic leukemia is mostly of B cells. (3) Myelocytic leukemic cells lose the characteristic content of alkaline phosphatase in granules. (4) The Philadelphia chromosome is present in 95% of chronic myelocytic leukemia in all bone marrow elements, as well as in the granulocytic leukemic cells.

A few special types are worth attention: (1) **Hairy cell leukemia** is a variety of B-cell lymphoid leukemia with a particular morphology of the leukemic cells, marked infiltrative splenomegaly, tartrate-resistant acid phosphatase in the cells, and a relentless chronic course in older men. (2) **Adult T-cell leukemia-lymphoma** is a T-cell neoplasm associated with human T-cell lymphotropic virus, with involvement of the T-4 marker also present in the T-cell cutaneous lymphomas. (3) The **myeloproliferative syndrome** includes chronic myelocytic leukemia, polycythemia vera, idiopathic thrombocytopenic purpura, and **agnogenic myeloid metaplasia**, in which there is fibrosis of the bone marrow with loss of myeloid cells at their normal site and prominent myeloid metaplasia in the spleen, lymph nodes, and other tissues. All cases of this syndrome tend to convert into myelocytic leukemia and undergo terminal blastic crisis.

Non-Hodgkin's lymphoma. Neoplasia of lymphocytes is called **malignant lymphoma**, the more conventional term for malignancy, **lymphosarcoma**, having been largely abandoned. For all practical purposes, there is **no benign member** of this group, but a few skin diseases are sometimes considered such. There is a growing conviction that the tumor cells are rarely derived from histiocytes or other forms of reticular cells, but categories with such names persist even if they are filled with particular forms of altered lymphocytes. With the advent of refined methods for distinguishing the races of lymphocytes, many classification schemes have been presented with the goal of distinguishing categories of therapeutic and prognostic importance, but complete success may be frustrated in that the very process of neoplasia erases differentiated characteristics that are the markers for cellular recognition and classification. To the present, all practical classifications are essentially morphological, even that of **Lukes and Collins**, which is based on functional concepts. The details by which cell forms are thus classified are beyond the responsibility of the general student or physician, but there should be an understanding of the clinical implications that can be derived from the classifications.

These tumors occur principally in patients in the sixth to eighth decade of life, with a smaller significant incidence about the second decade. **Painless lymphadenopathy**, particularly in the cervical chains, is frequently the beginning, with spread to other nodes and then to the spleen, liver, and other organs. Less commonly, the **original site may be in other tissues**, particularly those with lymphoid components such as the pharynx. **Fever, weight loss,** and **hemolytic anemia** signal systemic progression of the disease, and the GI and GU tracts may become involved, with frequent abdominal pain. The spinal nerve roots and even the cord and brain may be infiltrated. The infiltrated tissues are replaced by a homogenous, gray, usually soft tissue, but sometimes there is incited a fibrosis that results in firmness and a yellowish tint. The nodes themselves may reach 5 or 6 cm in diameter and may be matted by growth of the tumor through their capsules, but they often remain rather distinct. Infiltrates into solid organs may be prominent microscopically although difficult to discern grossly, but sometimes there are gross nodules of tumor in the spleen or liver.

Rappaport's classification has been important for recognition of the prognostic importance of two growth patterns: a **nodular form** reminiscent of lymphoid follicles that is more benign, and a **diffuse and more aggressive form**. The other element of this classification is based on cell type, with use of terms such as well or poorly differentiated, mixed, and histiocytic. The **Lukes and Collins classification** emphasizes the characteristics of individual cells, particularly the B cells that go through stages of "cleaved" nuclei and the development of "plasmacytoid" characteristics as RNA accumulates in the cytoplasm of better-differentiated cells that are producing globulins. This classification accommodates the important diffuse and nodular patterns by recognition that each has predominant cell types. What Rappaport labels **poorly differentiated lymphocytic lymphoma** is the largest group of cases, approximately 30%. His **well-differentiated lymphocytic lymphoma** includes as many as 40% of cases in which the tumor cells spill into the blood to produce a leukemia and in which there is a legitimate debate as to whether an individual case is a leukemia with prominent infiltrates or a tumor with bloodstream involvement. The same phenomenon is seen in other lymphomas to a lesser degree. **Histocytic lymphoma** as classified by Rappaport is interesting in that it includes many cases apparently of extranodal origin. The cases associated with human T-cell lymphoproliferative virus as well as a clinical group occurring especially in boys with mediastinal tumors and bone marrow and bloodstream involvement occur in Rappaport's class called lymphoblastic lymphoma. These examples are cited as reminders of rather specific syndromes that occur within the overall group and are significant in planning therapy or predicting outcome, which has very encouragingly improved in recent years. In planning chemotherapy, surgery, and radiation therapy, a clinical staging of the disease is used. The schema is essentially that employed in Hodgkin's disease as described below.

Hodgkin's disease. Hodgkin's disease accounts for about two-fifths of lymphomas. It is a neoplasm of a particular cell, probably the interdigitating reticulum cell of the framework of lymphoid tissue, a variety of histiocyte, that is manifest in a special form, the Reed-Sternberg cell, but the histological reaction includes variable mixtures of lymphocytes, eosinophilic granulocytes, plasma cells, and fibroblasts. The Reed-Sternberg cell is essential for the histological diagnosis but not absolutely specific in itself. It is a large cell, 15 to 45 μm in diameter, with often more than one bilobed or multilobed nucleus, each with a heavy nuclear membrane, translucent nucleoplasm, and prominent nucleoli that are rich in RNA and are eosinophilic or at least amphophilic.

The disease occurs principally in the third to fifth decades of life and is slightly more frequent in men. It is typically recognized to have begun in a particular group of lymph nodes, often the cervical, and there have been cases of cures by excision of localized disease. **Early symptoms** may include **fever, night sweats, weakness, weight loss, anemia, pruritus,** and **infections suggestive of altered immune status** such as herpes zoster and some fungal and less common bacterial infections. The enlarged nodes are usually painless and resemble those of other lymphomas except that they more often present a variegated appearance on cut section due to yellowish foci of necrosis or dense gray of fibrosis. Progression is typically from one group of lymph nodes to another, with eventual involvement of the mediastinal nodes in most cases. Splenic involvement is important and may grossly present a "sago" appearance in which small gray granules of tumor tissue seem to float in the soft red pulp. Large nodules of tumor in viscera are rare, but the liver and bone marrow are importantly involved in later stages.

There is fortunate agreement on the classification of Hodgkin's disease by two elements: stage and histology. The **stages** are (1) **a single group** of nodes, (2) **two or more contiguous groups** of nodes on one side of the diaphragm, (3) **nodes on both sides of the diaphragm and spleen**, and (4) additional involvement of **liver, bone marrow, or multiple extranodal tissues**. Each stage is further designated **A** (few or no systemic symptoms) or **B** (weight loss, fever, etc.). The histological **types** are (1) **lymphocyte predominant**, (2) **nodular sclerosis**, (3) **mixed cellularity**, and (4) **lymphocyte depleted**, with the first two having a very favorable prognosis and the fourth the most guarded. Using modern combined radiotherapy and chemotherapeutic programs, a 5-year survival of over 80% is achieved, with almost total success in stage 1A of lymphocyte predominant and the least success in 4B of lymphocyte depleted, symptoms in general indicating a poorer prognosis.

Plasma cell dyscrasias.   Plasma cell dyscrasias are uncontrolled proliferations of plasma cells that can result in death. In **myeloma**, tumorous masses are developed, yet they are in some ways more like hyperplasias with malignant hyperfunction than true neoplasms. A primary characteristic is abnormally high levels in the blood or urine of a **monoclonal homogeneous immunoglobulin** or one of its **constituent polypeptide chains**. The most frequent member of the group is **multiple myeloma**, in which plasma cells fill the bone marrow and create tumors that erode bone and sometimes infiltrate other organs and tissues. The abnormal globulin produced is of the IgG class in 60% of cases, of IgA in 15%, and rarely of IgM, IgD, or IgE. Very rarely have there been cases in which the abnormal, or "M," globulin has had specific antibody characteristics. In many cases in combination with the M globulin, and in about 15 to 20% of cases without the complete M globulin, free L chains are formed and freely excreted into the urine as Bence Jones protein. In addition to the destructive bone lesions, the protein precipitates in the kidney to cause tubular obstruction (**myeloma kidney**) or **immunocyte-associated amyloidosis** may develop with involvement particularly of blood vessels and destructive effects on the kidney and heart. Sometimes the lesions are solitary tumors, usually in soft tissues, that may not but usually do progress to disseminated disease.

Waldenström's macroglobulinemia is characterized by IgM and diffuse infiltrate of the bone marrow and lymphoid tissues but not tumors. It is a disease of elderly patients, and its features are dominated by the macroglobulinemia and resulting hyperviscosity of the blood. In **heavy-chain disease**, the diffuse infiltrates of plasma cells in bone marrow and other tissues synthesize only heavy chains.

Amyloidosis

This condition consists of infiltrates of a homogenous, eosinophilic, extracellular, proteinaceous substance that leads to atrophy of adjacent parenchymal cells. It is mentioned here because of the direct **association of one type with the plasma cell dyscrasias and the clear evidence in others of some degree of abnormal function of plasma cells**. The **amyloid substance** is composed of fine, 7.5- to 10-nm fibers that are aggregated into "cross-beta pleated sheets" demonstrable on x-ray crystallography. The fibers themselves are composed in one class predominately of **immunoglobulin light chains** and in the other principal class of a **unique nonimmunoglobulin** protein. The first class is associated with plasma cell dyscrasias and infiltrates in the heart, GI tract, tongue, muscles, nerves, and skin with consequent symptoms of enlargement and stiffening of the organ and malfunction such as cardiac failure, diarrhea or constipation, or peripheral neuritis. This clinical and anatomic pattern was once called **primary amyloidosis** before recognition of its relation to the function of plasma cells. The other pattern involves principally the kidneys, especially the glomeruli, the liver, and the spleen. Despite the fact that the amyloid is not from immunoglobulin, this type of **secondary amyloidosis** has long been recognized as a complication of chronic inflammatory diseases such as **tuberculosis, osteomyelitis, leprosy, rheumatoid arthritis**, and a variety of other collagen-vascular diseases. Amyloid appears in the CNS associated with degeneration of individual neurons with aging and especially in **Alzheimer's disease** and some other chronic degenerations. In older patients, amyloid infiltration of the **islets of Langerhans** is common but is not associated with any loss of function. In all types of amyloidosis, fine vessels, particularly arterioles, are infiltrated and probably are the fundamental basis of its pathogenic effects.

RESPIRATORY SYSTEM

NASAL PASSAGES, PHARYNX, AND LARYNX

The reader should consult the section on the ear, nose, and throat regarding the upper portion of the respiratory passages, including the larynx.

TRACHEA AND BRONCHI

There are hardly any diseases of the trachea that are independent of conditions in the larynx or lung, and the bronchi are so intimately a part of the lungs that they are rarely considered separately. The trachea is, of course, involved in **congenital tracheoesophageal fistulas** as discussed under the GI tract, and there are rare examples of **congenital hypoplasia**, usually associated with similar malformation of the larynx or lungs. **Congenital chondromalacia** is a condition in which the cartilaginous rings of the trachea and bronchi are poorly formed and soft so that they collapse under the effort of respiration. **Acute tracheitis** is usually an extension of acute laryngitis or a precursor of bronchitis and pneumonia but may be particularly prominent in infections with *Hemophilius influenzae* or *Bordetella pertussis*. In the former the mucosa may be inflamed to a fiery redness, and in the latter the bacilli may be so numerous as to entangle the cilia. One form of **amyloidosis** consists of submucosal plaques that may so distort the trachea and bronchi as to result in partial obstruction. Tumors of the trachea include **chondromas** that may be multiple to the extent the condition is called **chondromatosis, papillomas** similar to and often an extension from those of the larynx, tumors similar to the **pleomorphic adenomas** of salivary glands, **carcinoids**, and rarely an outright **carcinoma** that is usually squamous.

LUNGS

Congenital anomalies

Variation from the normal pattern of **segmentation** of the lungs is the most common anomaly. It is not often of clinical significance and is especially associated with cardiovascular anomalies. The lungs may be **hypoplastic**, usually in association with congenital **diaphragmatic hernias** or **osteochondrodysplastic syndromes** such as Jeune's thoracic dystrophy, and **agenesis** of one or both occurs with the unilateral condition being compatible with survival. **Bronchopulmonary sequestration** consists of a segment of lung with a separate bronchial supply and blood supply from branches of the aorta. It is important in that it leads to chronic infection. **Bronchogenic cysts** are malformations that may reach sufficient size as to interfere with respiration, as also occurs in **lobar or segmental overinflation**, which results from some form of partially obstructing lesion of a bronchus. The lesion in the bronchus may be congenital, but the overblown segment of lung is acquired and the condition may develop in adults with lately acquired lesions of the bronchi. Congenital **adenomatoid malformation** and congenital **pulmonary lymphangiectasias** are others among the total variety of congenital diseases.

Acute pulmonary injuries

A number of lung diseases of diverse and not always well-understood pathogenesis and characterized principally by their acute courses are grouped in this heading. The earliest in age of incidence is **neonatal respiratory distress syndrome** or **pulmonary hyaline membrane disease**. This is a disease of immaturity of the lung, more particularly of the ability of type II pneumocytes to produce surfactant, without which the higher-than-normal surface tension of the fluid lining of the alveoli causes collapse during respiratory efforts. Other factors such as intrapartum aspiration of amniotic fluid may also play a part, but it occurs principally in premature infants and under some conditions such as maternal diabetes. Rapidly progressive respiratory difficulty and cyanosis begin shortly after birth and may be fatal within a day or so. The lungs are poorly expanded, congested, and carnified. In the alveoli there is proteinaceous fluid; a few cells that are lymphocytes, macrophages, or pneumocytes; and the prominent and most characteristic hyaline membranes that line the walls of the alveolar ducts and alveoli. These structures are 2 to 5 μm thick, eosinophilic, and composed of fibrin, precipitated protein, and cellular debris. They are the hallmark of diffuse alveolar injury in this disease, as well as in adults when similar injury occurs. Oxygen therapy relieves the respiratory insufficiency, but often the condition becomes refractory and death occurs early. Victims may survive for days or weeks with further alveolar damage from the oxygen itself and the development of organized fibrous masses in the bronchioles with squamous metaplasia and respiratory failure, misnamed **bronchopulmonary dysplasia**.

The **sudden infant death syndrome** can be mentioned here because it is an unexpected and unexplained respiratory failure, but there are not consistent pathological changes in the lungs or in any other organs other than those such as serosal petechiae of hypoxia. It occurs in children of less than 1 year of age and most frequently in the third to fifth months of life. The incidence is said to be as high as 27 per 1,000 in premature live births, 10 times that of the remainder of the population. Of the many theories that have been and continue to be investigated is the suggestion that there is a failure of central respiratory control, possibly on a neuroanatomic basis, that results in episodic hypoventilation.

Acute interstitial pneumonia, or **diffuse alveolar damage**, was recognized in its clinicopathophysiological features, now called **adult respiratory distress syndrome**, and its pathological anatomy, which is similar to that of neonatal hyaline membrane disease. Its more prevalent and important occurrence as a complication of surgical shock, oxygen therapy, and other injuries such as aspirated substances, drugs, narcotics, and some infections, particularly viral, was not appreciated until the past decade or so. The action of oxygen-derived free radicals seems to be a common factor in many of the injuries, and the concentration of leukocytes in pulmonary capillaries with complement activation appears to play an important part. The gross lesions in the lungs may be as intense as those in the neonatal disease but are often less uniform and in later stages include bronchopneumonia of more ordinary type. The pulmonary reactions in disseminated intravascular coagulation and "traumatic" fat necrosis are related. The latter has long been explained as simply the physical embolism of fat from broken adipose cells, but closer study reveals distortions of the factors that maintain suspension of serum fat and related factors in the complement and coagulation balances.

Atelectasis is a zone of collapsed alveoli devoid of gas. It is of two principal types: (1) **compression**, which results from an impinging mass or displacement of the lung and (2) **obstructive**, which follows occlusion of an airway and absorption of the air in the alveoli. The latter process is slow if the subject is breathing room air, as the nitrogen must be removed by dissolving in the plasma, but it is more rapid with high oxygen concentrations when the hemoglobin speeds the absorption of more of the alveolar gas. Compression atelectasis is often facilitated when surfactant is decreased, and regions of the lung will collapse from pressure of the diaphragm or distension of adjacent lung. Such a mechanism is prominent in the **secondary atelectasis** of newborns. The never expanded lungs of the fetus are sometimes referred to as **primarily atelectatic**. **Pneumothorax** causes atelectasis by the increase of pressure within the pleural space. It usually arises from some fracture of the pulmonary and bronchial tissues and the creation of a flap that acts as a ball valve that allows air to be pumped into the pleural space during inspiration but does not allow its escape during expiration. The **rupture of bullae** underlies the spontaneous pneumothorax that often occurs in otherwise healthy young people. Excessive **positive pressure in artificial respiration** may force air from the terminal bronchi into the interstitium of the lung and along the bronchial trunks to a point of rupture through the pleura into the pleural space, and **needle punctures** from efforts to tap the subclavian vein or the pleura are also important causes of pneumothorax.

Edema of the lungs is of two principal types: (1) **hemodynamic** and (2) **irritative**. The first involves principles of intravascular and interstitial pressure, osmotic pressures, etc., that govern the movement of fluid between the blood vessels and the interstitial spaces. The endothelium of the alveolar capillaries has intercellular junctions like those of relatively impermeable vascular beds but are less tight than those of the alveolar epithelium. Fluid from the capillaries therefore passes in the interstitial space of the alveolar walls to lymphatics that accompany the bronchioles. This pathway will accommodate as much as a 10-fold increase in flow before the junctions of the epithelium are overcome and fluid begins to accumulate in the alveoli. As these events are within a continuous hydraulic system, this type of pulmonary edema tends to occur simultaneously throughout the lung, although its intensity may be varied by factors such as gravitational dependency and processes that alter the interstitium of the alveoli and truncal tissues. This type is predominately the result of **left-sided heart failure.** The lungs are increased to several times normal weight and are dark reddish, and their cut surfaces ooze a thin, clear fluid. When prolonged, the condition leads to small hemorrhages in the alveoli that are transformed into hemosiderin deposits, hyperplasia of type II pneumocytes that line the alveolar walls in an epithelial manner, and thickening of the interstitium. The organs are grossly firm, dark rusty colored, and less moist than in the acute condition. This is called **brown induration,** or **chronic passive congestion of the lungs. High-altitude pulmonary edema** and the edema that may develop rapidly after **head injury** are additional types of diffuse, largely hemodynamic edema, but they have additional elements of diffuse injury to the alveolar walls, probably through the mediation of released vasoconstrictor substances. **Irritative edema** arises principally from destructive influences on the alveolar walls, both epithelium and endothelium. The prototype is that of infection and the early stages of bacterial pneumonia. The involvement tends to be focal, involving lobules and zones unequally, but if the injurious agent operates sufficiently diffusely, the damage may be confluent. **Acute interstitial pneumonia** of the adult respiratory distress syndrome is an example of the latter. Both grossly and microscopically, the involved areas of lung tend to show evidence of components in addition to fluid, particularly fibrin.

Thrombotic emboli to the pulmonary arteries and pulmonary **infarcts** remain almost as frequent and as important a factor in the death of hospitalized patients as when Virchow, almost a century and a half ago, conclusively demonstrated that thrombi in the pulmonary arteries were almost always embolic from the deep veins of the legs. The incidence of significant pulmonary emboli in hospital autopsies, then and now, was 10 to 15%, and refined modern techniques have demonstrated evidence of emboli in 65% of autopsies. Important facts to be remembered are as follows: (1) Over 90% of emboli come from thrombi in the deep veins of the thighs and legs that are themselves the result of inactivity and stasis. (2) Massive thrombi that occlude the common or main pulmonary arteries are among the few causes of almost instantaneous death, but they are not common. (3) The presence of the bronchial circulation preserves the lung from necrosis and true infarction in all but 10 or 15% of pulmonary emboli, but hemorrhage, pleurisy over a peripheral lesion, and the elaboration of peptides and depressed production of surfactant result in local edema and recognizable but reversible lesions. (4) Symptoms of pain occur from irritation of the pleura, and dyspnea is related to ventilation of unperfused lung and bronchial and vasoconstriction mediated by released humoral factors and reflexes. (5) Emboli may lyse and resolve within a few days or may organize and contribute to pulmonary arteriosclerosis and hypertension. (6) Infarcts are more apt to result if there is preexisting circulatory impairment in the lung. (7) If emboli are infected, pulmonary abscesses may result. (8) Infarcts involve necrosis of pulmonary tissue and result in scars that are often almost imperceptible after all the hemorrhage is broken down and resolved. Infarcts are wedges of firm, red, swollen tissue with their apices toward the hilum and bases on the pleura that is often covered with fibrin. About three-fourths occur in the lower lobes.

Fibrosing interstitial lung disease does not fit comfortably into this topic of acute pulmonary injury, but the clinical onset of severe respiratory decompensation may be sudden and the deterioration rapid enough to justify the description as acute, which is the adjective Hamman and Rich used in the title of their article that was one of the first to call attention to what is quite apparently a group of diseases, some of recognized etiology and others idiopathic. They are characterized by markedly reduced lung volumes, decreased compliance, and ventilation-perfusion inequality but no obstruction to airflow. The lungs are heavier than normal although smaller in volume and have a stiffened consistency. The involvement is often variable in different lobes and segments, ranging from distinct scars to collections of dilated, cystic air spaces with thick and fibrous walls (honeycomb lung.) Microscopically, the alterations vary sufficiently, even in the idiopathic diseases, to be the basis of classification. A common feature is some degree of organized fibrous masses within alveoli. In the **pneumoconioses,** the irritating agent is recognizable either visually or by chemical analysis (silica, beryllium, asbestos), but the effects of **cytotoxic drugs, ionizing radiation,** and **noxious gases** are recognized by history as well as subtle histological distinctions. An important group are based on **immunologic injury** (farmer's lung due to sensitivity to fungal spores, pigeon breeder's lung due to feathers and proteins.) Systemic autoimmune disease such as lupus, rheumatoid arthritis, Wegener's granulomatosis, and Goodpasture's syndrome may be expressed in the lungs in this manner. No etiology can be proved in almost half the clinical cases, and these **idiopathic interstitial pneumonias,** or **diffuse pulmonary interstitial fibrosis,** have been subclassified in various ways such as "desquamative" and "usual" in some attempt to recognize potentials for different response to therapy such as with corticosteroids.

Primary pulmonary diseases

Asthma is a disease of small airways that are paroxysmally narrowed to cause wheezing, marked expiratory respiratory difficulty, reduced arterial oxygen due to ventilation-perfusion inequalities, and usually normal arterial carbon dioxide because of the induced reactive hyperventilation. Especially in children and young adults, a specific allergen may be identified as the precipitating cause, and the patient has elevated serum IgE. In contrast to such **atopic (allergic or extrinsic)** asthma, in older patients there is often no recognizable cause (**extrinsic or**

nonreaginic asthma), although there may be a preceding or concurrent viral infection in some cases. Still other cases arise in response to specific substances such as fungal spores, occupational dusts, or aspirin, the later apparently acting through its inhibition of the synthesis of prostaglandins. As much as 4% of the population of the United States is affected, but it is in only a very rare case that the acute attack does not subside or respond to therapy and the patient dies in status asthmaticus. The pathological alterations are in the small bronchi, which may be filled with mucus during an acute attack and show (1) increased and enlarged mucous glands, (2) hypertrophy of mural muscular fibers, (3) thickening of the epithelial basement membranes, and (4) infiltration of eosinophils. There are no intrinsic changes in the pulmonary parenchyma except that with death in status asthmaticus the mucus plugging is so extreme the lungs are hyperinflated.

The pathogenesis of chronic bronchitis is multifactorial, but the overwhelmingly recognizable cause is cigarette smoking. The pathological criteria are so nonspecific that the disease is defined functionally as the continuous presence of a productive cough for at least 3 months in each of two successive years. The symptoms in addition to cough may include dyspnea and wheezing similar to those of asthma. Morphologically, the bronchi are thickened and show evidence of hyperplasia of mucous glands, submucosal fibrosis, and often thickening of the epithelial basement membranes and variable infiltrations of granulocytes, lymphocytes, and plasma cells. The degree of mucous gland hyperplasia as a criterion has been studied by application of the Reid index, which is the ratio of the thickness in sections of the mucous glands to that of the submucosa from the cartilage to the epithelium, but it is increasingly apparent that the most significant involvement occurs when the bronchioles are involved by what seems almost to be an independent process. This bronchiolitis, or small-airway disease, shows goblet cell metaplasia of the mucosa of the bronchioles where there are normally no mucous cells, along with other evidences of mucus accumulation and other evidences of inflammation. This may progress to fibrous organization (obliterative bronchiolitis).

Both chronic bronchitis and bronchiolitis are very significantly associated with the development of chronic airflow limitation (chronic obstructive pulmonary disease [COPD]), but it is increasingly clear that the involvement of the smaller passages is pathogenically the most important. The other members of the complex included in COPD are bronchiectasis, emphysema, and asthma. All are importantly related in their etiologies to atmospheric pollution and are characterized by measurable obstruction to airflow, ventilation-perfusion abnormality, and hypoxic respiratory failure.

Emphysema of the lungs is a destructive disease of the walls of the terminal air spaces. It occurs in almost half of adults and, although usually unaccompanied by lessened pulmonary function, when severe and accompanying chronic bronchitis it is the principal cause of the ventilation-perfusion abnormality of COPD and of chronic respiratory failure. The diagnostic criteria are anatomic, and there are two major types (centrilobular and panacinar), two lesser types (distal acinar or paraseptal and irregular or paracicatricial), and some minor varieties. Centrilobular is characteristic of the damage associated with cigarette smoking. The distorted airspaces are in the center of the lobules and result from involvement of the respiratory bronchioles and their mural alveoli. Panacinar emphysema involves the entire acinus from the respiratory bronchiole to the terminal alveoli and is the form associated with alpha$_1$-antitrypsin deficiency in some, especially younger, patients. Research with patients homozygous for the Z allele at the proteinase inhibitor locus (PiZZ) who have severe enzyme deficiency has led to a general proteinase theory of the pathogenesis of emphysema: The excessive or unopposed action of proteinases is the proximate cause of the destruction of alveolar walls. The damage arising from deficiency of alpha$_1$-antitrypsin is compounded by smoking, but even persons with the more normal genotype PiMM, who tend to develop centrilobular emphysema, have increased release of elastase from pulmonary macrophages under the influence of smoking. Distal acinar emphysema exhibits blebs under the pleura and along septa, particularly adjacent to scars. Its etiology is not understood, but it occurs in young as well as older persons. Occasionally the blebs develop into cysts larger than 1 cm in diameter, referred to as bullae, which may significantly displace the adjacent lung. Rupture of blebs of distal acinar emphysema is responsible for spontaneous pneumothorax in otherwise healthy young people as well as older persons with more overt pulmonary disease. Paracicatricial emphysema is incidental to the disease that causes the scar about which it occurs.

Bronchiectasis is an abnormal, irreversible dilatation and mural distortion of bronchi accompanied by chronic, purulent inflammation and atelectasis of adjacent pulmonary parenchyma that contribute to its pathogenesis. It may develop distal to an aspirated foreign body, especially an irritative one such as an oily peanut, but many cases begin in childhood and seem to be related only to an otherwise ordinary preceding infection. Pertussis, measles, and scarlet fever were common antecedents, but with their decline adenovirus attracts more attention. Subsequent to focal bronchial obstruction, the lesion will develop wherever the obstructing body is lodged, but the more idiopathic instances are strikingly localized in the left lower lobe, particularly the basal segments. The bronchi are converted into thick-walled tubes lined with granulation tissue and pus, dilated to a centimeter or larger and extending peripherally to subpleural locations. Organized pneumonia and fibrosis develop in the atelectatic surrounding lung. A particularly vicious and widespread variety develops in patients who have cystic fibrosis of the pancreas and who survive infancy. It is almost inevitably responsible for their fatal termination.

Infections and inflammations

Pneumonia is the proper and long-established name for inflammation accompanied by some degree of consolidation of the lungs, although the term pneumonitis seems to have caught the fancy of modern students, especially when speaking of the more diffuse inflammations with less dense exudates such as the reaction to inhaled chemicals. The paradigm is that caused by types 1, 2, or 3 pneumococci. A plug of mucus containing the bacteria from an upper respiratory tract infection is aspirated into a focus in the lung, most often a lower lobe. Local injury of alveolar walls ensues, with exudation of fluid in which the organism grows rapidly. The periphery of the lesion advances into adjacent airspaces, and the earlier zones become the site of leukocytic infiltration and fibrin precipitation. Leukocytes at first are ineffective in phagocytosis of the organism, but they release endogenous pyrogens that cause the patient's typical high fever. The process proceeds rapidly until it reaches a natural barrier such as a septum or the pleura, in which it may induce edema and fibrinous exudate without penetration by the bacteria themselves. By that time, the normal host, particularly if aided by judicious administration of antibiotics, will begin to develop antibodies and the pneumonia is halted, the fever comes down by "crisis," and the exudate in the alveoli is resolved by fibrinolysis, phagocytosis, and expectoration. The usual duration is about 2 weeks. In the early stages, a blood-tinged, or rusty sputum is produced and the bloodstream is commonly invaded to produce a bacteremia. Complications include spread of the organism to the pleura to cause an **empyema, metastatic infection** to the heart valves or other sites, and failure to resolve the exudate, which progresses to **fibrous organization** or an **abscess**. At the height of the process, the involved lobe or lobes are almost uniformly involved, heavy, firm, a pinkish gray on cut section because of the high fibrin content in the alveoli, and covered by a fibrinous exudate on the pleura. Typically, the larger bronchi in the involved lobe show little sign of inflammation. This is the picture of **lobar pneumonia**. It may occasionally be caused by some other organisms such as *Klebsiella pneumoniae*, but **pneumococcal, fibrinous**, and **lobar** are practically synonymous adjectives in this application.

Bronchopneumonia is more common than lobar because it is the reaction to organisms of lower virulence, including some of the higher types of *Streptococcus pneumoniae*, and it often occurs in a patient weakened by the progress of another primary disease. The gross morphology consists of irregular foci of infiltrate, or consolidation, usually in the lower lobes or the posterior portions of the lungs, which are usually redder and more obviously congested that the uniform change of established lobar pneumonia. Microscopically, the involved lung goes through the same sequence as described above except that it does not spread as extensively. The bronchi are typically inflamed to a greater degree than in lobar pneumonia.

Some special pneumonias of current interest are those due to **gram-negative** bacteria, which account for half or more of nosocomial pulmonary infections; *Legionella pneumophila*, which causes morphological changes much like those formerly called atypical pneumonia that are often of **viral** etiology; and *Pneumocystis* pneumonia, which causes disease in immunosuppressed individuals and debilitated infants. The later causes widespread, rather light and irregular dusky gray consolidation in which there are alveolar exudates of frothy precipitate, few cells, and occasional collections of thin, disk- or cup-shaped organisms that do not stain in the usual preparations but may be demonstrated by silver impregnation.

The pathology of pulmonary **tuberculosis** is the classic and probably best-studied example of granulomatous inflammation. It has two basic forms, that which occurs in previously unsensitized individuals and that which develops in the presence of established cellular immunity. In **primary pulmonary tuberculosis**, the organism is inhaled and usually lodges in a subpleural focus in a lower lobe, conditions dictated by the

mechanics of airflow in respiration. There develops a nodule of reaction with granular leukocytes that are rapidly replaced by monocytes that lie in **epitheloid** masses and develop into **Langhan's giant cells**, surrounding fibrosis and lymphocytic infiltration, and then central **caseous necrosis**. The organisms meanwhile spread in the interstitial lymphatics to an adjacent bronchopulmonary or tracheobronchial lymph node and set up a similar tubercle. Apparently at about that time, after approximately 10 days, cellular resistance appears and the ability of organisms to spread in lymphatics is markedly inhibited and most persons heal their primary infection. These paired lesions are called **Ghon's complexes** and persist as calcified nodules. During the active phase, a few organisms escape into the bloodstream, and a few 1- or 2-mm calcified nodules in the spleen or liver are quite common in persons with calcified Ghon's complexes. In a few unfortunate individuals, the invasion of the bloodstream is massive and fatal disease develops, with many small **miliary** tubercles in many organs. A tubercle in the brain or choroid plexus may rupture into the subarachnoidal space to initiate **tuberculous meningitis**, with its thick, gelatinous exudate typically about the base of the brain and formerly of universally fatal outcome.

After primary tuberculosis is healed, the cellular immunity persists and the pattern of reactivated **secondary** disease is quite different. The hypersensitivity leads to more tissue destruction while limiting its extent to local and essentially contiguous spread. The lesions are usually in the apices of the lungs, are characterized by microscopic tubercles embedded in gross fibrosis, and become cavitary. It was formerly thought they arose from exposure to a new infectious source, but it presently appears that most may be reactivation of infection persistent from the primary episode, an explanation that would fit nicely with the characteristic prolonged positivity of tuberculin reactions. These cavities result in infectious sputum that not only is the source of contagion but may also be aspirated to set up secondary bronchogenic granulomas in the lungs or tuberculous ulcers, especially in the terminal ileum. Blood vessels traversing the foci of cavitation may be ruptured, and death from pulmonary hemorrhage is classic. Many other phenomena involving **hypersensitivity reactions** in the skin, eyes, and elsewhere, as well as granulomatous disease in other organs, are parts of tuberculous disease. Primary **GI tuberculosis** has largely disappeared with improvement of the milk supply, but it had a similar primary stage with an ulcer in the pharynx or ileum and lesions in the draining lymph nodes of the neck or the mesentery, as well as the potential of miliary spread.

Infection with **atypical tubercule bacteria** has become increasingly important. There are several important strains, but *Mycobacterium avium-intracelluare* has become quite frequent in immunodeficient patients, in whom it can cause a bacteremia, or a pulmonary picture rather like bronchopneumonia, or a more slowly progressive disease more like ordinary pulmonary tuberculosis. Other strains are associated with abscesses, ulcerative skin disease, and lymphadenitis. **Fungi**, particularly *Histoplasma* sp and *Coccidioides* sp mimic tuberculosis very closely. Particularly in the mid and lower Mississippi Valley, histoplasmosis is now probably the most common cause of Ghon's complexes.

Sarcoidosis is an idiopathic systemic granulomatous disease.

The microscopic lesions are "soft tubercles" that closely resemble those of tuberculosis but do not undergo necrosis. There is suggestive evidence that decreased T-cell function and abnormal B-cell function may be implicated. Many organs may be involved, but the worst effects can be extensive fibrosis of the lungs and hypoxic respiratory failure. Hypercalciuria, hypercalcemia, hypergammaglobulinemia, and a positive Kveim-Siltzbach skin test are features. Blacks are affected 10 times more frequently than whites.

Neoplasia

Carcinoma of the lung is clearly the greatest cancer problem in the Western world. It is the most frequent cause of death from cancer (28% of all cases) in men and women in the United States, having recently surpassed carcinoma of the breast in women. In men, the death rate increased 15-fold between 1930 and 1984. The incidence of new cases is second only to the far less malignant epithelial cancers of the skin for all persons and only behind that of breast and colorectum in women. A number of environmental factors have been clearly demonstrated as etiologic, such as asbestos, radiation, nickel, chromates, etc., but the overwhelming association is with cigarette smoking. Almost the only missing link in the chain of experimental evidence of the etiologic role of tobacco smoke is the failure to find an animal that will smoke and develop lung tumors of the type that plague human beings.

Most carcinomas of the lung arise in the epithelium of the bronchi or their glands. The principal types are (1) **squamous** (35 to 60% in surgical series), (2) **adenocarcinoma** (20 to 30%), (3) **large cell undifferentiated** (7 to 15%), (4) **adenosquamous** (1 to 3%), and (5) **small cell** (20 to 25%). It is characteristic of carcinoma of the lung that microscopic sections contain areas suggestive of different histological patterns, and the category of large cell undifferentiated varies among pathologists depending on their willingness to include or exclude lesser examples of atypical cells. The most malignant (mean survival untreated of only 4 months and 5-year survival of 1% compared with 20 to 35% 5-year survival for treated squamous carcinoma) is the **small cell carcinoma**, with the exception of the rare **giant cell variety of large cell undifferentiated**. The incidence among men is twice that of women except for the adenocarcinoma, which has no gender predilection. **Adenocarcinomas** are also the more common among nonsmokers, although most victims are smokers, and typically are tumors of the periphery of the lung and more apt to be associated with a previous scar. **Bronchioloalveolar carcinoma** is considered by some authors as a variety of adenocarcinoma that consists of mucous cells that grow along alveolar walls. The growth pattern sometimes resembles that of pneumonia more closely than a tumor, and interest has been stimulated by its occasional multicentricity and resemblence to a viral disease of sheep, **jaagsiekte**. Almost all types have been associated with **paraneoplastic endocrine syndromes**: small cell tumors with antidiuretic and adrenocorticotropic hormones, squamous with hypercalcemia, carcinoid syndrome, etc. Metastases from lung cancer are notorious for causing presenting symptoms, especially in the brain and bones, but the most frequent sites are, of course, the bronchopulmonary and mediastinal lymph nodes. Involvement of the apex of the lung and low cervical lymph nodes may spread to adjacent nerves and produce Horner's syndrome,

with ulnar nerve pain that has been called **Pancoast's tumor**. Other obscure associations are with myopathy, neuropathy, dermatologic conditions such as acanthosis nigricans, leukemoid reactions, and hypertrophic pulmonary osteoarthropathy (clubbed fingers).

Bronchial adenomas are misnamed in that they are truly low-grade malignancies. Most are of a **carcinoid** appearance and neuroepithelial derivation, with occasional associated clinical manifestations such as the carcinoid syndrome and the light and electron microscopic characteristics of GI carcinoids. Only 40% or less have metastasized to lymph nodes by the time of discovery, usually as a result of symptomatic hemoptysis or bronchial obstruction. Ten percent of "adenomas" have the appearance and characteristics of the various types of **tumors of the salivary glands**. The **chondromatous hamartoma**, composed of lobulated masses of mature cartilage rarely over 4 cm in total diameter, is a benign lesion that is discovered as a coin lesion in the lung field on radiography.

PLEURA

The pleural cavities and their linings may be involved in circulatory, inflammatory, and neoplastic processes in addition to mechanical situations due to the introduction of foreign substances, such as the **pneumothoraces** previously mentioned in connection with ruptured bullae and traumatic perforation. Circulatory disorders result in the accumulation of fluid (**hydrothorax**), blood (**hemothorax**), or lymph (**chylothorax**). The first is a **transudate** (specific gravity 1.012 or less and insignificant numbers of cells) due to circulatory failure, the second is due to rupture of a blood vessel such as the aorta due to trauma or bleeding (usually mixed with serous exudate) from metastatic tumors of the pleura, and the third (a milky fluid with significant content of fat) due to blockage or rupture of the thoracic duct or other mediastinal lymphatics by the growth of tumors, especially lymphomas. Inflammatory conditions result in a **pleurisy** with the accumulation of exudates (leukocytes, specific gravity 1.020 or higher, fibrin strands) and usually an appreciable layer of fibrin on the serous surfaces themselves. Tuberculosis, pneumonia, infarcts, abscesses, uremia, lupus, and rheumatoid arthritis are causes. If the exudate itself becomes infected, the process is converted into **empyema**, with the serous surfaces becoming a pyogenic membrane like the wall of an abscess.

Secondary or **metastatic tumors** of the pleura are by far more frequent than primary. The lung and breast are the more notorious sources. The primary tumor is the **mesothelioma**, which has attracted a great deal of attention because of its association with **asbestos** exposure. Otherwise, it is a very rare tumor that encases the lungs with thick layers of solid tumor tissue and is usually fatal in 1 to 2 years at the most. Microscopically, there is a pattern that resembles fibrosarcoma and another that has a papillary epithelial appearance, and mixtures occur. Metastatic carcinomas, particularly adenocarcinomas, may mimic the gross appearance of these malignant mesotheliomas. A **solitary, benign, or localized mesothelioma** (also called pleural fibroma) is not recognized as related to asbestos. Large fibrous pleural plaques, especially on the pleural surface of the diaphragm, result from healed postpneumonic pleurisy but when found on the parietal pleura seem to occur in patients with at least a vague history of asbestos exposure.

MEDIASTINUM

Developmental anomalies of the mediastinum consist principally of cysts (bronchial, enteric, and pericardial) hygromas and meningomyeloceles. The bronchial cyst occurs in the middle mediastinum behind the heart and the others principally in the posterior mediastinum. Inflammatory processes arise from perforation of the esophagus or trachea or from inflammation, usually granulomatous, in lymph nodes. There is a sclerosing mediastinitis sometimes associated with granulomatous foci but often idiopathic and possibly related to a similar diffuse fibrosis of the retroperitoneum or Riedel's struma of the thyroid. Tumors of the anterior mediastinum include lymphomas, teratomas, or germ cell tumors and tumors of the thyroid and parathyroids. In the middle mediastinum, tumors are usually lymphomas, and in the posterior mediastinum, neurogenic tumors predominate (schwannomas, neuroblastomas, paragangliomas).

GASTROINTESTINAL TRACT

ORAL CAVITY AND PHARYNX

Although dental disease is one of the most important causes of morbidity and the oral mucosa often reflects systemic disease such as erythema multiforme, pemphigus, measles with its Koplik's spots and Warthin-Finkeldey giant cells, and the pigmentation of Peutz-Jeghers syndrome of intestinal polyposis, the principal lesions of the oral cavity and pharynx discussed in general pathology are tumors. Leukoplakia is commonly associated with tumors of the mucous membrane. It is not necessarily precancerous, as the gross lesions may be only hyperkeratosis or acanthosis on microscopic examination, but other examples are dyskeratosis or even carcinoma in situ. Chronic irritation by chewing tobacco or ill-fitting dentures may be antecedents of this condition as well as of squamous carcinoma. Carcinomas of the lip usually occur on the lower lip and are well differentiated, but within the mouth squamous carcinomas are only moderately well differentiated and those of the base of the tongue and nasopharynx are often very poorly differentiated. These tumors spread by way of lymphatics, and definite patterns of metastasis to the triangles of the neck or the retropharyngeal space result from lesions of particular sites. Verrucous carcinoma is a special variety almost always associated with leukoplakia and tobacco chewing that invades local tissues perniciously but rarely metastasizes. Primary lymphosarcomas occur principally in the tonsil and Waldeyer's pharyngeal lymphoid ring.

Tumors of the salivary glands are a special group. The most frequent is the pleomorphic adenoma (formerly called mixed tumor) that arises in the parotid gland a dozen times more frequently than in other glands and comprises three-quarters of all salivary gland tumors. The patients are typically in their third or fourth decade of life. The histological elements are irregular epithelial and myoepithelial cells, often of rather stellate configuration, and mesenchymal elements with chondroid and myxoid characteristics. These tumors are benign but often break their capsules, and their proximity to the facial nerve complicates their complete removal so that 10% or so recur. The second most common tumor is the adenolymphoma, or Warthin's tumor, which is a benign epithelial growth with an intense lymphoid infiltrate that is not neoplastic. Less than 10% of salivary gland tumors are malignant. They are relatively more frequent among glands other than the parotid. The most important is the mucoepidermoid tumor, which varies greatly in its potential for malignancy, three-quarters being of low aggressiveness. It too presents a conglomerate histological picture, this time of a mixture of squamous, mucus-secreting, and intermediate cells. Inflammations and stones in salivary glands are the result of obstruction and infections, both viral and bacterial. Involvement particularly of the parotid is a typical component of one of the syndromes of sarcoidosis. The histopathology of these lesions is that of their expressions in other organs and tissues.

ESOPHAGUS

Congenital anomalies

Atresia is the most important congenital anomaly of the esophagus. This consists of interruption of the continuity of the esophageal tube by a fibrous strand. The distal segment of the esophagus usually communicates with the trachea near its bifurcation, but there may be no fistula or the fistula may be from the proximal segment, or the defect may be a side-by-side configuration with incomplete atresia of the esophagus itself. The condition is discovered as soon as an infant tries to swallow, and the dangerous complication is aspiration pneumonia. Diverticula are usually acquired and occur in the midportion, where they are thought to be of traction origin by fixation to a scarred tracheal lymph node, or between gaps in the pharyngeal muscles superiorly or in the muscular coat of the esophagus itself inferiorly at the diaphragm. These are considered to be pulsion diverticula due to the effect of intraesophageal pressure, particularly in cases of obstruction or achalasia. Achalasia is the result of a disturbance of the motor function. It results in a thickened and dilated organ and is an important cause of dysphagia. The cause is not understood, but there is ineffectual peristalsis in the lower segments, and the passage of food into the stomach is impeded. Hiatus hernia arises from dilation of the diaphragmatic passage for the esophagus with subsequent upward displacement of the stomach when it is distended by food or when the patient assumes certain positions. Reflux of gastric fluid occurs, and erosion of the esophageal mucosa follows, with discomforting "heartburn." It is principally a geriatric condition. In some cases, the eroded lower esophageal mucosa undergoes metaplasia to a columnar form (Barrett's esophagus).

Infection and inflammation

Esophagitis may be of many causes, including chemical (peptic reflux), viral (herpes), or bacterial of different types, but the most frequent cause, at least at autopsy, is *Candida* sp. This occurs in persons weakened by other conditions such as chemotherapy, sepsis, steroid administration, etc. Other important lesions are varices at the site of splanchnic-somatic venous collaterals in the lower esophagus, the rupture of which can be a fatal complication of the portal hypertension in cirrhotics, and the linear lacerations at the diaphragmatic level that occur with severe vomiting and can rupture, with the escape of the esophageal contents into the pleural cavity (**Mallory-Weiss syndrome**).

Neoplasia

Carcinomas of the esophagus are mostly squamous except for rather rare adenocarcinomas of the lower third. These in some instances are gastric in origin and in others may arise from a Barrett's metaplasia. Half of the squamous tumors occur in the middle third of the esophagus. Although many appear to be rather slow growing and fairly well differentiated, prognosis is grim as they seem to become symptomatic late and to invade the mediastinal lymphatics early, perhaps aided by the lack of a serosa. The epidemiology of this tumor is interesting and important, as it is much more common in some countries such as northern China and in association with various particular dietary habits, but this hint of an effect of environmental factors has not led to recognition of specific causes. Dysphagia, weight loss, hiccups, hoarseness (involvement of the recurrent laryngeal nerve), and tracheoesophageal fistula are clinical features of late cases.

STOMACH

Congeintal anomalies

Congenital anomalies are insignificant causes of disease of the stomach. The only important defect is **hypertrophic pyloric stenosis**, in which hypertrophy and hyperplasia of the circular muscle of the pylorus result in functional stenosis and obstruction of the outflow of the stomach. The condition is familial, much more common in boys than in girls, and usually becomes manifest in the second or third week of life. The exact mode of inheritance is not clear. A muscle-splitting operation is very effective in correcting the condition and preventing the otherwise relentless course of gastric obstruction, which formerly led fatally to alkalosis and aspiration pneumonia.

Infection and inflammation

The stomach is rarely the seat of bacterial or parasitic infection, and **acute gastritis** is usually related to an exogenous or an endogenous chemical influence such as alcohol and aspirin abuse, heavy smoking, uremia, drugs, and shock. The mucosa is thickened, contracted, and thrown into folds with petechiae and small erosions. The lesion is completely reversible. A rare bacterial infection and inflammation of the entire thickness of the stomach wall called **phlegmonous gastritis** is usually due to *Streptococcus* sp in patients with such infections elsewhere in the body. **Chronic gastritis** exhibits thinning of the mucosa, lymphocytic and plasma cell infiltration, and atrophic changes in the epithelium, often with a loss of parietal calls that correlates with achlorhydria. This is the gastric lesion of pernicious anemia and also of other conditions such as autoimmune thyroiditis and diabetes. A significant number of patients with long-standing chronic gastritis, perhaps 10%, develop gastric carcinoma. Hypertrophic gastritis is the name applied to the thickened, folded mucosa seen in several conditions of hyperfunction, such as results from the constant stimulation by gastrin in **Zollinger-Ellison syndrome** of

multiple endocrine tumors, or the thick submucosa infiltrated with lymphocytes that exudes serum proteins sufficiently to cause hypoalbuminemia and edema.

Peptic ulcer disease

Peptic ulcer disease requires the presence of acid pepsin in its pathogenesis but otherwise presents a confusing array of well-established but almost random features and some near contradictions. **Duodenal ulcers** accompany excess acid secretion, whereas **gastric ulcers** occur in patients with often diminished, but never absent, acid pepsin secretion—observations that lead to the thought that the predominant event in duodenal ulcers is excess action of gastric juice whereas in gastric ulcers it may be impairment of the mechanisms for maintaining mucosal integrity. The incidence of the disease has been declining for unknown reasons, and the proportion of lesions in the duodenum to those in the stomach has fallen from almost 10:1 to about 4:1. Men are affected with the duodenal lesion four times more frequently than women, but only twice so for the gastric disease. The overall incidence is now about half of the 6% observed a couple of decades ago. The peak age is about 50, and there is a distinct familial clustering of the duodenal cases but not a clear genetic pattern. Blood group O increases the risk of duodenal ulcer, group A of gastric ulcers, and HLA-B5 haplotype increases the risk for either. All of these observations lead to a strong suspicion that peptic ulcer disease is of multiple, or at least multifactorial, etiology.

The lesions are round ulcers that range from a few millimeters to 15 cm or more in diameter. The edges are rolled and contracted, with distortion of the surrounding mucosal folds into radiating ridges. The bases are denuded and covered with **fibrinoid necrosis**—in this case the morphological appearance of partially digested protein—with an underlying layer of fibrosis that increases and thickens with the chronicity of the ulcer. The ulcers may erode into surrounding structures, particularly the pancreas, or **perforate** into the peritoneal cavity with consequent disastrous release of gastric juice and stomach contents into the peritoneum. The fibrosis precedes the ulceration in its course through the wall of the stomach or duodenum and will bind arteries and veins so that when the acute digestive necrosis reaches them they are opened and bleed with sufficient vigor as to lead to exsanguination. The third important complication of peptic ulcers is gastric or duodenal **obstruction** due to the rigidity of the scar in or about the wall of the tract. Most gastric ulcers are in the antrum, with a propensity for the lesser curvature, whereas duodenal ulcers are usually within the first few centimeters beyond the pyloric ring. Rarely, peptic ulcers occur on the lip of a gastroenterostomy, in the lower esophagus with gastric reflux, in the lower duodenum or jejunum in Zollinger-Ellison syndrome, or at the mouth of a Meckel's diverticulum that contains gastric mucosa. Duodenal ulcers have no relation to carcinoma. The relation for gastric ulcers is probably coincidental but remains a topic of debate.

Neoplasia

Neoplasia of the stomach is principally **adenocarcinoma**. The incidence of this disease has fallen by a factor of 5 in the past 50 years: from 38/100,000 for U.S. men to 7 or 8 and 28/100,000 to 4 or 5 women. The reason is unknown. It remains a dismal disease with an overall 5-year survival of only 16%. The tumors tend to occur in the distal third of the stomach, often along the greater curvature. There may be polypoid, ulcerative, or superficial spreading, and there is a rather uncommon variety of diffuse infiltration of the entire wall of the stomach called linitis plastica. Histologically the patterns vary from well-differentiated glands to strands of individual cells that often contain a droplet of mucus. The latter is seen particularly in linitis plastica and in the ovaries in the metastatic tumor known as a **Krukenberg's tumor**. The spread of metastases is to the gastric, pancreatic, and hepatic lymph nodes and then to the liver, lungs, and distantly. The other principal malignant tumors of the stomach are **lymphosarcomas** and **leiomyosarcoma**. The former may give diffuse infiltration of the mucosa that can be confused grossly with hyperplastic gastritis. The latter may be difficult to diagnose, because benign leiomyomas can reach considerable size and contain large and irregular nuclei. There are also benign **adenomatous polyps** of the stomach that are even less common than significant smooth muscle tumors, although small (1 or 2 mm), smooth lentiform nodules in the submucosa and muscularis are rather frequent and may be either **leiomyomas** or **neurofibromas**.

SMALL INTESTINE

Congenital anomalies

Meckel's diverticulum is the premier congenital lesion of the small intestine. It is a remnant of the omphalomesenteric duct and is important only when it becomes obstructed and inflamed, contains functional gastric mucosa that causes peptic ulceration of the adjacent intestine (a rare circumstance), or sets up adhesions that might cause strangulation of a loop of bowel (an "internal hermia"). A sophomoric alliteration is that the diverticula are 2 inches long, occur in 2% of people, and are 2 feet from the ileocecal valve—three figures that are not strictly accurate but are close enough to keep the student reminded of the essential facts. Congenital **atresia** of any segment of the small bowel may occur, usually in company with other serious anomalies, and the small bowel participates in the relatively innocuous anomaly of malrotation of the bowel. Also, islands of pancreatic tissue in the submucosa of the upper small bowel, especially the first part of the duodenum, may form protruding masses a few millimeters to a centimeter or so in diameter. **Diverticula** of the small intestine may occur at any level and consist of herniations of mucosa and muscularis mucosae along enlarged pathways through the musuclar coats by which the blood vessels penetrate. The sac of the diverticulum consequently protrudes into the mesentery rather than into the peritoneal cavity.

Infections

The principal **bacterial infections** of the small bowel are with salmonellae, including *Salmonella typhi, Campylobacter jejuni, Vibrio cholerae*, the enterotoxic strains of *Escherichia coli, Yersinia enterocolitica,* and *Mycobacterium tuberculosis*. For most, the chief symptom is diarrhea that progresses to **dysentery** (cramps, tenesmus) and debilitating loss of fluid. The mucosa will be congested and may have an overlying light layer of fibrin and necrotic debris along with some petechiae. This part of the picture is completely reversible and is similar to that due to the acute toxic reactions of food poisoning by organisms that do not infect the intestine but exert their effect by their toxins, as well as by some chemical agents. More specific changes occur in several infections such as those of **typhoid fever** with the lymphoid hyperplasia of the Peyer's patches and subsequent longitudinal ulceration of the lower ileum, or the granulomatous transverse ulcers in the same region of **tuberculosis**. The chronology and anatomic features of both these diseases have been worked out in great detail by earlier generations of pathologists. Other infections such as with shigellae and *Clostridium difficile* exert their principal effects more on the colon.

Malabsorption

Malabsorption is an important pathological condition of the function of the small intestine. It is of varied causes that range from loss of certain enzymes necessary for the digestion of specific food substances, such as bile salts for fat absorption, through specific inborn deficiencies (e.g., **lactase deficiency**), to microbiological infection wuch as that involved in **Whipple's disease** and probably underlying **tropical sprue**. In the United States, the most common causes are **chronic pancreatitis, fibrocystic disease of the pancreas, Crohn's disease, celiac disease (gluten enteropathy or nontropical sprue)** with Whipple's disease, **small intestinal diverticulosis, disaccharidase deficiency, tropical sprue**, and **iatrogenic conditions** such as **gastrectomy** and **ileal bypass** being more rarely responsible. Only a few of these conditions have characteristic pathoanatomic changes. In **celiac disease**, the mucosa becomes atrophic and the villi and microvilli of the jejunal mucosa are blunted while the lamina propria is infiltrated by lymphocytes. These changes can be rapidly reversed on removal of exposure to wheat products, which are the major source of dietary gluten, although some patients may experience symptomatic relief without reversal of anatomic changes and are at risk for development of lymphoma or even carcinoma of the small intestine. In **Whipple's disease**, the mucosal villi are distended by macrophages that contain many bacilli that have been observed by both light and electron microscopy but have not been cultured. As in **tropical sprue**, the disease yields to broad-spectrum antibiotics even though the organisms are not characterized.

The other principal cause of malabsorption that has a specific pathological anatomy is **Crohn's disease (regional enteritis)**, which is a granulomatous disease of the intestinal wall that is of unknown etiology. Involvement is typically of the lower ileum and tends to be in one or more segments of several centimeters length with intervening skipped areas. The mucosa is ulcerated, sometimes circumferentially, and the submucosa and muscularis are thickened by fibrosis and cellular infiltrates of lymphocytes and monocytes. The latter are often concentrated into noncaseating granulomas. Involvement of the serosa leads to peritoneal adhesions, and the inflammatory process causes the formation of fistulas and abscesses. The number and length of involved segments tend to be progressive, even if attempts are made to resect all recognized lesions. In about a third of cases, the colon is also involved, and 10 to 15% of cases are limited to the colon. For the latter, the important distinction to be made is from **ulcerative colitis**. Absence or late appearance of lesions in the rectum, thickening of the wall, fistulas, and the histological granulomatous inflammation are differential features characteristic of Crohn's disease. **Perianal lesions** including fistulas and abscesses occur, especially when the colon is involved.

Ischemic lesions

Vascular disease may be the cause of destructive lesions of the small intestine particularly, although the colon may be also or exclusively involved. Occlusive arteriosclerosis of the mesenteric arteries usually underlies the condition, but the event is precipitated by an episode of splanchnic hypotension or some other catastrophe such as an embolism. Other factors such as arteritis might be involved, and some cases are triggered by venous thrombosis, particularly after abdominal surgical operations. The bowel, often over a considerable segment, is **infarcted** with necrosis and hemorrhage through the entire wall, the hemorrhage appearing, of course, because of the rich anastomoses through the arcades of mesenteric vessels that connect beyond the primary field of the occlusion or predominant insufficiency. This is a surgical emergency, for without resection the infarcted bowel not only causes intestinal obstruction but will perforate and result in peritonitis. A similar process of lesser degree and probably of greater chronicity, **acute hemorrhagic enteropathy**, results in damage only to the mucosa, with hemorrhagic necrosis and ulceration. The patient experiences acute abdominal pain, cramps, and bloody diarrhea. Complete recovery is possible, but because the underlying cause is chronic vascular insufficiency, episodes will recur with any episode of hypotension, cardiac arrhythmia, or just cardiac failure. Such cases may end in segmental scarring and chronic partial obstruction similar to Crohn's disease.

Neoplasia

Tumors of the small intestine are rare. The most common is the **carcinoid**, which, although most frequent in the appendix, where it is usually an incidental lesion of benign prognosis, has a greater potential for progressive growth and spread when it arises in the ileum. Particularly after metastasis, especially to the liver but also to the lung, a **carcinoid syndrome** may develop because of the elaboration by the tumor of 5-hydroxytryptamine and sometimes bradykinin or histamine. The syndrome consists of vasomotor disturbance (flushing), intestinal hypermotility (diarrhea, cramps, vomiting), bronchial constriction (cough, wheezing), and cardiac valvular thickening (usually in the right ventricle) that may lead to failure. Similar tumors and related phenomena occur in other organs and are part of the APUD (amine precursor uptake and decarboxylation) group of tumors.

Adenocarcinomas occur and are usually encircling lesions that are slow to cause symptoms of obstruction because of the fluid nature of the chyme. They consequently carry a poor prognosis. An exception is carcinoma of the middle third of the duodenum in the region of the ampulla; these are more properly considered tumors of the bile duct or pancreas. Benign and malignant **tumors of smooth muscle, lipomas,** and **lymphomas** also are encountered rarely, and the small intestine can be involved by **metastatic tumors** that characteristically present as raised, button-like masses in the submucosa with central ulceration of the overlying mucosa.

Hernias

The most common causes of intestinal obstruction are **hernias**. Abdominal contents, usually small bowel, protrude through a defect in the abdominal wall, usually at the inguinal or femoral canals, the umbilicus, the site of surgical incisions, or under fibrous peritoneal adhesions. **Intussusception**, the collapse of one segment into the lumen of the more distal bowel, especially at the ileocecal valve in infants and children, and **volvulus**, the twisting of a loop of bowel about its mesentery, are less common causes. In each, the peristalsis forces material into the involved loop of intestine. The loop increases in size and cannot retract, thereby becoming **incarcerated**. The flow of chyme is obstructed. Pressure at the neck of the loop obstructs veins, with consequent edema and further swelling of the loop, and eventually the arterial blood supply is occluded and the loop becomes infarcted, or **strangulated**, and peritonitis follows.

APPENDIX

The appendix is the seat of one of the most common and important GI diseases, **acute appendicitis**. The risk in this formerly important cause of death of young adults and children has been reduced from a mortality of over 35% at the beginning of the century to practically zero by improvement of diagnosis and surgical care. The exact pathogenesis of the lesion, nevertheless, is still imperfectly understood and perhaps assumes several patterns. Obstruction by a fecolith, a carcinoid tumor, or possibly lymphoid hyperplasia or *Enterobius vermicularis* seems to play a part in the initiation of the ulceration of the mucosa and development of purulent inflammation involving both submucosa and muscularis, which are histological criteria. The bacteria involved are usually those commonly present in the cecum—*E. coli* and enterococci. Complications are (1) peritonitis, at first localized but later generalized, (2) perforation, (3) abscess formation, (4) infected thrombosis of the portal vein (pylephlebitis), (5) hepatic abscess, and (6) septicemia.

A **mucocele** can develop in a chronically obstructed appendix by the metaplasia of the mucosal epithelium and accumulation of mucus. Rupture may lead to a walled-off retrocecal mass or localized chronic peritonitis. Very rarely there develops a diffuse involvement of the peritoneal surfaces with mucus-secreting epithelium, **pseudomyxoma peritonei**, similar to that which may arise from a pseudomucinous cystadenocarcinoma of the ovary. It is uncertain and debated as to whether this is due to malignant transformation in a mucocele or is the result of the appendix developing an analogue of the ovarian carcinoma.

COLON AND RECTUM

Congenital anomalies

The three principal congenital malformations of the colon and rectum are (1) **malrotation** of the colon, (2) **atresia of the anus**, and (3) **aganglionic megacolon**. **Malrotation** is a failure of the cecum to reach the right lower quadrant and persistence of the right mesocolon. It may be part of several sequences of congenital anomalies but in itself seems to be of little importance except that it has been blamed for atypical presentation of the symptoms of acute appendicitis. **Atresia** of the anus is due to failure of the proctodeum to invaginate or of the anal plate to be absorbed. In some instances it is part of a more severe maldevelopment of the cloacal septum and is associated with fistulas to the genital or urinary tracts. It is a prominent component of the **VATERS association** that is a nonrandom association of **Vertebral defects, A**nal atresia, **T**racheoesophageal fistula, **E**sophageal atresia, **R**adial and **R**enal dysplasia, and **S**ingle umbilical artery. Although the coincidence of these anomalies is definitely significant, their causation appears to be by other than a genetic mechanism. **Congenital, or aganglionic, megacolon (Hirschsprung's disease)** is due to a failure of the autonomic neurons that form the submucosal (Meissner's) and myenteric (Auerbach's) plexuses to complete their caudal migration in the embryonic hindgut. A low segment of the rectum and possibly the sigmoid colon is devoid of ganglion cells, although biopsy will often reveal prominent nerve fibers in the region. The motility of the gut is interrupted with a resultant functional obstruction and dilatation of the proximal colon. The condition becomes manifest soon after birth and can be corrected by resection of the aganglionic, undilated segment.

There is also an **acquired form of megacolon** that apparently arises on a functional basis with chronic constipation and no abnormality of the enteric nerve network. The dilatation of the colon never reaches the dimensions seen in the congenital examples. Another acquired malformation is **diverticular disease**. This occurs in older persons and is a disease of Western civilization. As many as 50% of Americans over the age of 60 may have the lesions, which consist of herniations of the mucosa and muscularis mucosae through a widened space between the fibers of the muscularis at the base of an appendix epiploicae, most commonly in the sigmoid colon. The lesions may be associated with lower abdominal pain, especially when the contents become inspissated and inflammation develops in the wall of the diverticulum. Rupture may occur, with peritonitis or pericolonic abscess, and surrounding fibrosis may cause significant intestinal obstruction. **Hemorrhoids** are the cause of much discomfort and even disability. They consist of varicosities of the superior and middle hemorrhoidal veins ("internal" hemorrhoids, which are covered with rectal mucosa) or of the inferior plexus ("external" hemorrhoids, covered by anal mucosa). They arise in conditions of increased venous pressure such as pregnancy, portal hypertension of cirrhosis, and perhaps from straining associated with chronic constipation as well as from senile weakening of the wall of the veins. They are a common cause of rectal bleeding. Much of the associated pain and itching are due to inflammation of superficial **fissures** in the perianal skin as well as over the hemorrhoids, and such fissures may be present and symptomatic without there being significant hemorrhoids.

Infections

Colitis assumes many forms. Some bacillary diseases, such as that caused by *Shigella* sp, are localized particularly in the colon. In **bacillary dysentery**, the mucosa of the colon becomes edematous, petechiae appear, a suppurative pseudo-

membrane develops over the involved mucosa, and ulceration may occur. In **cholera**, due to *Vibrio cholerae,* there is a tremendous outpouring of isotonic fluid due to activation of adenylate cyclase of the plasma membranes of the crypt epithelium of the small bowel, and the resorptive powers of the colon are overwhelmed without development of anatomic lesions. **Pseudomembranous colitis** consists of a layer of fibrin, necrotic epithelial cells and leukocytes, and fecal debris over a hyperemic mucosa with very shallow ulcers. It apparently is the result of the action of a toxin elaborated by *C. difficile*, a normal commensal, in patients who have been given broad-spectrum antibiotics, particularly clindamycin and lincomycin, and in conditions in which there seems to have been some interruption in the normal motility of the intestine, such as a postoperative ileus or in chronic debilitating diseases. In some cases, the lesion is associated with ischemic injury or infection with staphylococci or *Candida* sp.

Parasitic disease, particularly **enterobiasis** and **trichuriasis**, often involves the colon, but the most important although not the most common in the United States is **amoebic dysentery**. *Entamoeba histolytica* sets up residence in the cecum, invades the crypts of the colonic glands, and burrows through the lamina propria. There is a light leukocytic reaction, but the active lesions are characterized by liquefactive necrosis. The ulcers are flask shaped and become confluent in the submucosa, with bridges of overlying mucosa remaining. The gross and microscopic pictures can be very much like those of idiopathic ulcerative colitis. Spread occurs to other sites in the colon, including the sigmoid and rectum, and the organisms may invade venules and reach the liver to form abscesses there. They eventually may spread further to the pleura, pericardium, lung, and even to the brain by way of the bloodstream.

Inflammation

Ulcerative colitis is a chronic disease of unknown cause and significant incidence and is manifested by bloody diarrhea and variable degrees of abdominal pain, fever, and weight loss. The annual incidence in the United States is about 10 per 100,000, and it is agreed that it occurs more commonly in whites, especially Jews, and in urban populations. It occasionally is familial. The peak ages of incidence are the third and fourth decades of life, and it is slightly more prevalent in women. Extensive investigations of genetic, immunologic, infectious, and metabolic factors have yielded suggestive but never conclusive evidence of each as the etiology. It is a disease of the mucosa of the colon that begins in the rectum and may extend throughout the organ. The earliest lesions are edema and hyperemia of the mucosa and the outpouring of granular leukocytes into the mucosal crypts ("crypt abscesses"). Progression leads to ulceration of the mucosa and eventually isolation of islands of persistent mucosa that may become hyperplastic ("pseudopolyps"). The bowel becomes shortened and thickened, with loss of haustra (garden hose silhouette on barium enema).

For patients whose disease begins with a severe attack, the prognosis is of a 5-year mortality of 5 to 15%. The risk of the development of carcinoma of the colon is 10% overall and as much as four times that rate in patients whose disease begins in childhood. In general, the pathological process does not involve the deeper layers of the bowel, and perforation and peritonitis are not threats except for the catastrophic and unpredictable occurrence of toxic megacolon during an acute exacerbation. In this condition, there is a cessation of bowel motility, dilatation of the transverse colon, and septic shock. Perforation and peritonitis may occur, and the condition is an emergency that demands immediate colectomy. It may rarely occur in other ulcerative diseases of the colon such as amoebic colitis or Crohn's disease. Although the fundamental pathological process of ulcerative disease seems distinctly different from that of Crohn's disease, fibrosis and chronic changes in the bowel may make the distinction uncertain in 10 to 20% of cases when the disease is confined to the colon. Cirrhosis, biliary tract disease, arthritis, spondylitis, erythema nodosum, and pyoderma gangrenosum are systemic complications.

Ischemic colitis can have many clinical features similar to those of Crohn's disease and even ulcerative colitis. It occurs in the elderly, usually in persons who have evidence of insufficiency in other arterial beds, and predominately consists of single episodes, although a quarter may progress to scarring and stricture. The lesions are essentially submucosal hemorrhages that may resorb rapidly after some rupture with resultant colonic bleeding, whereas others ulcerate, become inflamed, and heal more slowly or rarely become gangrenous and perforate.

Irritable bowel syndrome is probably the most common GI disease in clinical practice. Despite the discomfort of the pain, watery diarrhea, and constipation and the fear that more serious disease may develop, there are no anatomic lesions or evidence of malevolent prognosis.

Neoplasia

Significant neoplasia of the colon is confined to adenocarcinoma and polyps, although carcinoids occur occasionally. There are rare examples of a variety of mesenchymal tumors. **Polyps** are localized hyperplasias of colonic epithelium that exhibit various degrees of metaplasia and argued amounts of dysplasia and anaplasia. They are distributed throughout the colon, with preponderance distally if all the smallest lesions of no clinical significance are included. They vary from 1 mm or less of flat thickening of the epithelium to berry-like masses on a drawn-out stalk of mucosa and submucosa to cauliflower-like masses intimately attached to the wall of the colon or rectum. Histologically, their epithelium is arranged in glands or gland-like structures but varies from slightly enlarged columnar cells of normal appearance to large, irregular, and hyperchromatic cells. Exactly how much of this spectrum of metaplasia is a progression toward or into neoplasia remains unsettled. The larger polyps, particularly those of villous pattern, are undoubtedly associated with the development of outright cancer, but patients have been subjected to extensive operative procedures out of unjustified fear of microscopic atypia in a polyp. Few outright carcinomas of the colon show any suggestion of origin in a polyp, yet the larger the polyp, particularly above a diameter of 2 cm, the higher the association with evidence of metastasis or the later development of carcinoma. Robbins states, "prevailing opinion now holds that most carcinomas of the colon arise in preexisting polyps." A conventional descriptive classification is (1) **hyperplastic polyps**, which are the most

frequent, small, sessile and composed of almost normal epithelium, (2a) **tubular**, usually with a distinct stalk and fair metaplasia, (2b) **tubulovillous**, larger with greater atypia, and (2c) **villous**. The latter are almost a separate entity. They are usually sessile, up to 10 cm in diameter, occur especially in the rectum, are undoubtedly precancerous if not carcinomatous, and can be associated with the secretion of copious potassium and protein-rich fluid sufficient to produce diarrhea, hypoalbuminemia, and hypokalemia. **Familial polyposis** results in transformation of almost the entire colonic mucosa into tubular or tubulovillous adenomatous polyps at an early age and practically certain development of carcinoma.

Juvenile, or retention, polyps are lesions that develop in the rectum and sigmoid of children. They may prolapse or cause rectal bleeding but are quite benign. Familial occurrence is known, but it is uncertain whether the mass of cystic and hyperplastic glands in an inflamed stroma are hamartomas or the result of inflammation.

Carcinoma of the colon and rectum is the second most frequent cancer in the United States and most Western countries. The incidence of new cases in the past few years has approached 145,000 in the United States alone. It is much less common in Africa, India, and Japan. The incidence has remained fairly steady for decades. There has been much search without totally conclusive results of possibly etiologic factors such as lack of fiber and bulk in the Western diet, bacterial toxins or their transformation of bile acids or fats into carcinogens, high meat and animal fat consumption, and the dietary level of cholesterol. **Gardner's syndrome** (familial polyposis, osteomas, fibromas, sebaceous cysts, etc.), **familial multiple polyposis, villous adenoma,** and **ulcerative colitis** are recognizably precancerous for the colon. The gross lesions are raised, ulcerated infiltrations that may project into the lumen or thicken the wall of the colon. Half or more occur in the rectum and sigmoid colon, where they are within reach of the examining finger or the sigmoidoscope. In the left colon, they tend to infiltrate and spread around the bowel so that they cause obstruction in addition to the cardinal sign of blood in the stool. In the right colon, which is of larger diameter, the lesions are more apt to be a fungating mass and may be manifest only by the anemia caused by chronic loss of blood.

The depth of penetration of the wall of the bowel is one of the most important prognostic features. In the **Dukes' classification**, originally based on a series of patients with rectal carcinoma, type A was confined to the wall of the rectum and was associated with a 98% 5-year survival, type B showed direct extension to extrarectal tissues but no lymphatic metastases and 78% survival, and type C had lymphatic or other metastases and a 32% 5-year survival. A modification of Dukes' schema to include experience with colon carcinomas defines type A as limited to the mucosa (100% survival), type B1 as limited to muscularis (67%), type B2 with penetration of the wall but no lymphatic involvement (54%), type C1 as limited to the wall and lymph nodes (43%), and type C2 as penetration of the wall with metastases (22%). Other more detailed systems have been proposed, including one based on the TNM approach (tumor, nodes, metastases). Factors such as size and location of the primary, vein or nerve sheath invasion, presence of an inflammatory reaction, and histological grade all have a bearing on prognosis to some extent or another. In general, the tumors are discovered late but are relatively slow growing. The pattern of metastasis is to local and mesenteric lymph nodes, to the liver, then to the lungs, and rarely distally to the brain and other sites. Nearly all are adenocarcinomas, and most are fairly well differentiated and contain some degree of mucus production. Adenoacanthomas occur.

Carcinoembryonic antigen (CEA) is a glycoprotein of the cell surfaces of the embryonic colon. It reappears in the serum of persons with carcinoma of the colon and sometimes of the lung, pancreas, and other sites, as well as in patients with ulcerative colitis and cirrhosis. It is of clinical value as a marker for the presence of colonic carcinoma, although its specificity and sensitivity are less than desired.

Carcinomas of the anus are largely squamous carcinomas, although a baseloid tumor and very rarely other histological patterns are encountered. Because of their location, they may metastasize to either the perirectal lymphatics or the inguinal lymph nodes. Their clinical presentation can be confusingly similar to or complicated by chronic infectious processes such as lymphogranuloma venereum and granuloma inguinale (*Calymmatobacterium granulomatis*).

LIVER

The liver, being central to so many body processes, is affected by or involved in a host of diseases. The success of the applications of cell biology and biochemistry to the study of diseases has resulted in a tremendous and varied amount of information about the pathology of the liver, yet the clinical manifestations are relatively simple because there is a tremendous physiological reserve (as much as 90% of the liver can be surgically removed with survival of the person or animal and regeneration of the liver) and the body is so dependent on hepatic function that significant failure cannot be tolerated. The syndrome of hepatic failure and jaundice, therefore, is a common clinical ground for the end stages of nearly all hepatic disease and should be reviewed as presented in clinical literature. Hepatic pathology has become a subspeciality. Probably the best summary of reasonable length is that of Edmondson and Peters in Kissane's *Anderson's Pathology*, but even it occupies 116 quarto pages and supplies almost a thousand references.

Congenital anomalies

Congenital anomalies of the liver are not numerous, probably because the organ is essential for survival and no significant malformation can be tolerated. It is sometimes distorted by inequality of lobes or even supernumerary lobes, but the mass is fairly constant in relation to the mass of the body. In the presence of a **congenital (Bochdalek's) hernia**, particularly the less frequent right-sided variety, the displaced liver may be grooved and misshapen. Other grooves and lobulations found in adults are not congenital but occur particularly when the diaphragm is displaced as a result of chronic obstructive pulmonary disease. On the other hand, there are several genetic disorders of relatively minor metabolic importance. **Gilbert's syndrome** of constitutional hyperbilirubinemia (unconjugated), **Dubin-Johnson** and **Rotor's syndromes** of conjugated hyperbilirubinemia, and the less severe

form of **Crigler-Najjar syndrome** of deficient glucuronide transferase and consequent failure of conjugation of bilirubin are examples. In each there is no structural alteration of the liver except of excess of brown pigment in hepatic cells in the Dubin-Johnson disease. In the severe form of Crigler-Najjar syndrome, the defect is so severe that the unconjugated bilirubin injures the CNS (**kernicterus**) and may be fatal. Kernicterus also occurs in conditions such as erythroblastosis fetalis when the immature enzymatic system of the liver does not efficiently conjugate bilirubin and there is also damage to the blood-brain barrier by anoxia or some other injury that allows the unconjugated bilirubin to reach and damage neurons.

The most important congenital disease of the liver is **biliary atresia**. The condition is rare and must arise late in embryogenesis after the liver is well formed. Survival is possible while the placenta clears the fetal blood and postnatally to the extent that the kidneys, lungs, and GI tract can compensate by diffusion for the lack of excretion by way of the biliary tree. The atresia may be of just a segment of the common or hepatic duct, in which case surgical anastomosis of the right or left hepatic ducts to the intestine will correct the problem, or more extensively of the intrahepatic ducts, even to the smallest tributaries in the portal spaces. Hepatic transplants have been effective in such cases.

Inflammation and infection

Inflammatory disease of the liver includes **abscesses** and **parasitic diseases**, but the most important are the varieties of viral, or presumably viral, **hepatitis**. Of these there are two distinct **hepatitis viruses, A and B**, and a third group of cases designated **non-A/non-B hepatitis** in which the etiology is not yet specifically identified and may well include two or more agents. In addition, other viruses, including **herpes simplex, cytomegalovirus, the Epstein-Barr virus**, and several other rare varieties can cause hepatic inflammation and dysfunction but are of lesser importance.

The **pathological changes in hepatitis** are similar regardless of the specific virus but vary in intensity with different agents and from case to case. Grossly, the liver may be swollen and the capsule tense with only slight congestion and no appearance of fatty change or frank necrosis. Histologically, the essential changes are (1) irregular necrosis of individual or small groups of hepatic cells, (2) swollen, "ballooned" hepatic cells, (3) ground-glass appearance of hepatic cell cytoplasm, especially in hepatitis B, (4) shrunken, eosinophilic, anuclear cells, and (5) inflammatory cellular infiltrate composed of macrophages, lymphocytes, and occasional polymorphonuclears and eosinophils, accompanied by enlargement of Kupffer's cells, that involves principally the portal triads and only occasionally appears as minute foci among the hepatic plates. In rare fatal cases, particularly due to hepatitis B, the process of cellular necrosis is overwhelming and **massive hepatic necrosis** (formerly called acute yellow atrophy) occurs, the liver being reduced to a shrunken, soft bag of its connective tissue framework. In nearly all cases of hepatitis A, the reaction resolves completely, but a minority of cases, again especially with hepatitis B but also with non-A/non-B, show continued evidence of inflammatory infiltrate (**chronic persistent hepati-**

tis) in the portal triads with minimal fibrosis that eventually subsides in several months. More extensive portal inflammation with plasma cells as well as lymphocytes and continuing piecemeal necrosis of cells in the limiting plate of hepatic cells next to the portal triads is called **chronic active hepatitis**. The later is capable of progressing into macronodular cirrhosis, but it is not clear that all cases of that irreversible damage proceed from such a process. An **autoimmune chronic active hepatitis** is not related to viral infection. It is of similar pathology, occurs principally in women, and is associated with elevated serum immunoglobulins, altered T-cell function, and other immunologic phenomena including LE cells, because of which it was formerly called **lupoid hepatitis**.

Hepatitis A is an RNA virus transmitted principally by the oral-fecal route. After an incubation period of 15 to 45 days, the virus is present in the stool, and shortly thereafter there is the onset of jaundice. IgM antihepatitis A antibody then rises for 1 to 2 months and begins to fall with the beginning of recovery. IgG antihepatitis A antibody follows the rise of the IgM by a short interval and persists as a marker of previous infection. Infectivity disappears with the rise of the IgM antibody, and the disease very rarely causes fatality and does not cause chronic hepatitis or a carrier state. **Hepatitis B** is a DNA virus transmitted mostly by blood or serum. Late in an incubation period of 1 to 6 months or longer, it appears in the bloodstream as Dane particles, which are accompanied by an e antigen (HBeAg) and the surface antigen (HBsAg, also called Australia antigen as it was first demonstrated in the blood of an Australian aborigine). The HBeAg is related in some way to the core antigen (HBcAg), an antigen that begins to rise with the onset of symptoms and is the marker of active infection. Anti-e (HBeAb) appears and rises during the recovery phase and with the HBcAb reaches its highest point when the infection is overcome and thereafter falls. Anti-surface (HbsAb) appears and rises late in recovery and persists to be the marker of prior infection.

Alcohol is a direct toxin for hepatic cells, although great variability in the intensity and duration of exposure that is injurious is observed and undoubtedly indicates the importance of other nutritional factors. The damaged hepatocytes accumulate massive droplets of fat in their cytoplasms, giant mitochondria, and tangled masses of submicroscopic filaments called **alcoholic hyalin** or Mallory bodies. Serum transaminases are elevated, and in a rare case lytic necrosis of hepatocytes occurs and the patient falls into hepatic coma and may die. In other cases, a sclerotic fibrotic process begins around the central veins and portal triads and the damage eventuates in cirrhosis of the micronodular type. Various **drugs** may also injure the liver: testosterone for instance can cause cholestasis with bile thrombi in canaliculi, erythromycin and chlorpromazine are associated with both cholestasis and hepatic cell necrosis, and methotrexate and other agents can produce more severe changes like those of viral hepatitis.

Cirrhosis is an end stage of prolonged destructive liver disease. There are several minor types, some quite specific in their pathogenesis and morphology: **Obstructive biliary cirrhosis** and **primary biliary cirrhosis** have many features similar to those of autoimmune chronic progressive hepatitis. Cirrhotic patterns occur in **hemochromatosis**, with its prominent deposition of hemosiderin in biliary and hepatic cells, in **Wilson's disease** associated with the inborn error in copper metabolism, and in **alpha₁-antitrypsin deficiency**, which is responsible for a significant proportion of childhood cirrhosis as well as severe forms of emphysema.

Efforts to develop differential diagnostic criteria for the major group of cases of cirrhosis have been frustrated by the fact that by the time clinical symptoms and hepatic failure have developed the fires of pathogenesis have reduced the organ to largely uninterpretable ashes. The two principal patterns are micronodular and macronodular. In **micronodular cirrhosis**, the injury seems to be sufficiently diffuse to involve all lobules simultaneously and to convert each into a mass of irregular regenerated plates that replace the collapsed normal lobular architecture. The central veins have been pushed into and incorporated in the enlarged and fibrotic portal spaces that reach toward and unite with their neighbors. This displacement of veins is associated with the rise in portal venous resistance, and the regenerated hepatic plates show their origin from the cord-like strands of smaller cells referred to as cholangioles. This is the prototypical pattern of alcoholic cirrhosis, and the hepatic cells usually show evidence of the preceding **fatty metamorphosis** and disruptions that create fatty cysts in the scars. **Macronodular cirrhosis** is a pattern of much larger and more irregular scars that engulf the portal spaces and surround islands of hepatic parenchymatous tissue that are 1 cm or more in diameter. The islands sometimes are composed of groups of fairly well-preserved lobules, as though the surrounding scars had resulted from destruction of large areas of the liver without parallel destruction in adjacent areas. Such might be expected in injury due to viral infections, in which case the hepatic cells would not show residue of prior fatty change. On the other hand, careful observation of the deterioration of some patients leaves little doubt that some pass from alcoholism to fatty livers to micronodular cirrhosis, to end as macronodular cirrhosis. They do not have well-preserved lobules in the totally regenerated nodules.

Neoplasia

Focal hyperplasias of the liver are not uncommon and occur as spherical masses of hepatic cells without a lobular architecture and ranging from a few millimeters to centimeters in diameter. They can be confusing in small biopsies for they resemble regenerative nodules of cirrhosis. They are sometimes called **adenomas**, but that term is better reserved for progressive lesions that reach several centimeters in diameter, are associated with the use of oral contraceptives, and have been the source of rupture and intraperitoneal bleeding in rare cases. There is also an **adenoma of bile ducts**. The most common benign tumors in the liver are **cavernous hemangiomas**.

Carcinoma of the liver is much more prevalent in parts of the world with a high incidence of chronic hepatitis B than in the United States. It usually arises in a cirrhotic liver, only one-seventh appearing in an otherwise normal liver. The incidence in patients with micronodular cirrhosis is about 5% and in macronodular cirrhosis may be as high as a fifth of cases. Eighty percent are carcinomas of hepatic cells and should be called **hepatocellular carcinoma**, although the unfortunate term "hepatoma" continues to be applied. The remaining primary carcinomas are of bile duct origin and are named **peripheral cholangiocarcinomas**. The typical gross appearance in late stages is of a large, roughly spherical mass of tumor (the "mother nodule") and multiple satellite smaller nodules. Invasion of veins is often apparent grossly as well as microscopically. The tumor may grow into the inferior vena cava, and the first site of metastasis is often the lung. Microscopically, hepatocellular tumors may look much like normal hepatocytes without a lobular arrangement, or they may be quite pleomorphic and undifferentiated. Many contain some amount of cholangiole-like strands, which is the predominant pattern in cholangiocarcinomas. Seventy percent of hepatocellular carcinomas secrete alpha-fetoprotein (AFP).

Angiosarcoma of the liver is a rare malignant tumor that forms large hemorrhagic masses that may bleed into the peritoneal cavity. Its occurrence has been associated with Thorotrast or arsenic and more recently with vinyl chloride. There are reports of successful resection of these tumors as well as very rare cases of early primary carcinoma confined to the mother nodule.

BILE DUCTS AND GALLBLADDER

Congenital anomalies

Diseases of the biliary system, other than malformation, are very predominately diseases of women. **Congenital conditions**, in addition to **atresia** mentioned above as it affects the liver, consist of **absence, duplication, or malposition of the gallbladder** that are of more importance to the surgeon than to the patient.

Cholelithiasis

Cholelithiasis is present in many as a fifth of adults and is closely associated with metabolic imbalances in the composition of the bile and with inflammation of the gallbladder. Metabolic stones are purely cholesterol or pigment and are little associated with inflammation. Mixed stones contain cholesterol, calcium bilirubinate, and calcium carbonate and are multiple, faceted, and usually accompanied by chronic cholecytitis. Major complications are passage of the stone with biliary colic, acute inflammation, or obstruction. Rarely a stone may erode through the gallbladder into other structures bound by fibrous adhesions.

Infection and inflammation

Acute cholecystitis is initiated by impaction of a stone in 9 of 10 cases. The primary injury seems due to the effect of the chemicals of the bile on the mucosa, but if bacterial infection is added, the wall may become **gangrenous** from the intense inflammation, and sometimes the obstructed gallbladder is converted into a bag of pus (empyema). Perforation and peritonitis are complications.

Neoplasia

Carcinoma of the gallbladder is usually an adenocarcinoma of insiduous onset. It nearly always occurs in an organ scarred by chronic inflammation and in the presence of stones. The incidence is low, only 1 to 3% of cancers, and is four times more common in women than in men. **Carcinomas of the external bile ducts** may give earlier symptoms of obstruction but are nevertheless of poor prognosis. The **carcinoma of the ampulla of Vater** is a variety. Because carcinoma is not as regularly associated with chronic cholecystitis and consequent inelastic fibrosis of the gallbladder, that organ may be distended in obstruction due to cancer in contrast to that due to stones, but this **law (Courvoisier's)**, like a 55-mile-per-hour speed limit, is more often violated than complied with.

EXOCRINE PANCREAS

Congenital anomalies

The most common **congenital abnormalities** of the pancreas are (1) **heterotopias** that are small, benign, usually insignificant aberrant masses that lie under the mucosa of the stomach, duodenum, or other parts of the GI tract and (2) various **anomalies of the ducts** that have been accused of importance in the pathogenesis of pancreatitis. The most important anomaly, however, arises from failure of the two parts of the embryonic pancreas to fuse properly. In some cases, the head of the pancreas then surrounds the duodenum (**annular pancreas**) and can cause obstruction.

Cystic fibrosis

Cystic fibrosis has outgrown its original designation as a disease of just the pancreas as appreciation has developed of its genetic nature and widespread effects on the lung, skin, and other organs. It is the most common lethal genetic disease of white people, the gene being present in 5% of the population and the homozygous clinically expressed condition appearing about once in 1600 live births. There are abnormalities of mucus secretion in many organs with consequent obstructive phenomena in ducts. Ciliary action is disturbed in the bronchi. High concentrations of sodium, potassium, and chloride are excreted in the sweat glands and salivary glands. The autonomic nervous system displays increased responses to alpha-adrenergic and cholinergic and decreased response to beta-adrenergic stimuli. In the fetus, meconium is thick and sufficiently plastic to cause **meconium ileus** and even perforation, with subsequent **meconium peritonitis**. The pancreas is atrophic, fibrotic, or destroyed in association with dilated, microcystic ducts filled with inspissated secretions. Loss of exocrine pancreatic function is very serious in infancy, but islets survive and diabetes mellitus is a late complication. Most serious are the effects on the lungs, where a very severe chronic purulent bronchitis and bronchiectasis develop and are the usual cause of death, which can now be postponed until about the third decade of life. Involvement of the biliary tree may lead to cirrhosis. The nature of the fundamental metabolic defect or defects is still unknown.

Infection and inflammation

Pancreatitis is of varied character and mostly disputed pathogenesis. There is clearly an acute form associated with viral infections (e.g., mumps) that seems usually to be transient but may have an unappreciated role in chronic progressive disease. The principal **acute pancreatitis** causes pain, nausea, vomiting, and abdominal tenderness of acute onset and is due to activation by some mechanism or another of the pancreatic proteases with consequent necrosis, erosion of blood vessels, thrombosis, and hemorrhage. Lipases are activated, split triglycerides in surrounding adipose tissue and cause the precipitation of white chalky calcium soaps (**fat necrosis**). Amylase is also released into the bloodstream and peritoneal fluid and with the lipase is an important clinical marker of recent necrosis in the pancreas. The process can be catastrophic, with the induction of shock, dehydration, hypocalcemia, and death, or it can result in walled-off masses of hemorrhage and necrotic tissue (**pseudocysts**), or it can subside only to recur and become **chronic pancreatitis** with eventual scarring and destruction of the gland and the formation of stones in the dilated and obstructed ducts. The latter results in malabsorption, steatorrhea, and eventually diabetes, although the islets resist the destructive process far longer than the acini. Alcoholism and biliary tract disease, particularly cholelithiasis, are definitely associated with the genesis of pancreatitis, as are other conditions such as the hypercalcemia of hyperparathyroidism and the metabolic disturbances of Cushing's syndrome and some forms of hyperlipidemia.

Neoplasia

Carcinomas of the pancreas constitute about 3% of cancers in both men and women. They are nearly all adenocarcinomas of different degrees of anaplasia and usually of distinct scirrhous tendency. Many seem to be rather slow growing, but by their situation, especially in the body and tail, they are clinically silent until they reach a considerable size. Even in the head, where obstruction of the bile duct tends to be the first symptom, the retroperitoneal and acapsular configuration of the pancreas apparently allows early spread to retroperitoneal lymphatics and disposes toward a dismal prognosis. It is rare before the age of 40, and etiologic associations are similar to those of carcinoma of the biliary tract, plus a recent accusation against coffee that seems to be of questionable statistical design.

ENDOCRINE GLANDS

The most important diseases of the endocrine glands are conditions that alter their normal physiological functions—for example, increases or decreases in normal control and feedback mechanisms, destructive processes involving the glands, benign or malignant neoplasia, and alterations in the response of target tissues as occurs in **testicular feminization** and **obesity-related maturity-onset diabetes**. The underlying pathological processes, in addition to neoplasia, may be infectious, autoimmune, genetic, nutritional, or rarely traumatic as in **postthyroidectomy hypoparathyroidism**.

In general, the lesions of the endocrine glands are far less complicated than their functional effects. The physiology of the endocrine system and the clinical manifestations of its diseases should be reviewed in conjunction with the following paragraphs.

HYPOTHALAMUS

The endocrine effects of the hypothalamus are manifested in conjunction with or through action of the pituitary gland. It secretes peptide hormones that reach the adenohypophysis through a portal system of small veins along the pituitary stalk or the neurophyophysis by way of neurons. The hormones of the first type are secreted by nuclei in the medial basal hypothalamus, are regulated by neurotransmitters and feedback from target organs, are trophic hormones for various functions of the adenohypophysis, and comprise the **tuberohypophyseal group**. The **neurohypophyseal group** are vasopressin (antidiuretic hormone [ADH]) and oxytocin, which are elaborated in the supraoptic and paraventricular nuclei and stored in the posterior pituitary.

Pathological conditions of the neurohypophyseal endocrines arise from (1) neoplastic or inflammatory involvement of the axis by pituitary tumors, metastatic tumors, and localized inflammation such as abscesses or meningitis, (2) surgical or radiation injury, or (3) trauma. The manifestations are those of **diabetes insipidus** due to deficiency of ADH and are characterized by polyuria and polydipsia with subsequent elevation of serum sodium and osmolarity. The syndrome of **inappropriate ADH secretion** is just the reverse, with expansion of extracellular fluid volume and dilutional hyponatremia. It occurs more often as a result of inappropriate ADH secretion by tumors such as oat cell carcinoma of the lung and in some nonmalignant pulmonary disease than from direct involvement of the neurohypophyseal system, although it may appear in CNS disorders such as encephalitis, hemorrhage, meningitis, and trauma and can also be a side effect of drugs. No distinct syndrome has been recognized to be derived from the action of oxytocin.

The syndromes associated with the tuberohypophyseal group intimately involve the pituitary itself and are usually associated with hyperplasias, atrophy, or neoplasia of the adenohypophysis.

The principal **neoplasm** directly associated with the hypothalamus, or more precisely with the infundibulum, is the **craniopharyngioma**. It is a vestige of Rathke's pouch and may be found within the sella but is usually suprasellar and may sometimes invaginate into the third ventricle. It is most common in children and young adults but sometimes is first manifested in older persons. Craniopharyngiomas are encapsulated and usually cystic or multiloculated but occasionally solid and partially calcified. The tissue resembles that of primitive oropharynx or tooth buds with a background of loose stellate cells around islands and cysts of epithelial cells. The lesions are biologically benign and produce symptoms by obstruction of the ventricular system or by pressure on surrounding nervous tissue. Other neoplasms or hamartomas associated with Rathke's pouch result in glandular remnants along the pituitary stalk or pharyngeal pituitary tissue and are rarely functional or large enough to be symptomatic. **Gliomas, germ cell tumors, epidermoid inclusion cysts**, and **lipomas** also occur and may give rise to a hypothalamic syndrome.

PITUITARY GLAND

Diseases of the pituitary, like those of other endocrine glands, are usually discussed in functional terms: **hypopituitarism** or **hyperpituitarism**. The causes of the former are destructive lesions, except for the rare instances of failure of hypothalamic secretion of trophic releasing factors. Hyperpituitarism, on the other hand, is usually associated with overgrowths of one or more types of cells of the anterior hypophysis, referred to as **adenomas**. With the use of sensitive analyses for hormones in blood and immunocytochemistry, the importance of small (less than 10 mm) **microadenomas** has been emphasized. These may as well be thought of as **focal hyperplasias**, for they are recognized by their functional effects rather than characteristics of a true tumor. Invasion of surrounding structures is a late effect, and rapid growth and potential for metastasis characteristic of true **carcinomas** is very rare.

Adenomas of the pituitary have conventionally been classified as acidophilic, basophilic, or chromophobic on the basis of the reaction of their cells to conventional stains. However, ultra-microscopy and more critical methods of examination have enabled tumors, as well as the normal cells of the gland, to be more specifically classified in terms of the hormones with which they are associated. Many tumors previously classified as chromophobic have been demonstrated to belong to specific types, although the cells do not reveal sufficient specific granules to be recognized by regular stains. Chromophobic adenoma, composed of true null cells, occurs much less frequently than seemed to be indicated by collected statistics of a few years ago, and puzzling cases of clinical syndromes of clearly specific hyperfunction with tumors so classified are now understood.

Pituitary tumors have accounted for about 10% of intracranial tumors in neurosurgical experience, but recent emphasis on microadenomas, particularly very small foci, has resulted in reports of adenomas in as many as 25% of pituitaries at routine autopsies. Perhaps two-thirds of the tumors secrete prolactin (PRL), growth (somatropic) hormone (GH), or both, with the lactotropes being the most common cell recognized today in pituitary tumors. The remainder of adenomas are about equally distributed between the basophilic group that secrete follicle-stimulating hormone (FSH), luteinizing hormone (LH), thyrotropin (thyroid-stimulating hormone [TSH]), adrenocorticotropic hormone (ACTH), and melanocyte-stimulating hormone (MSH) and the chromophobic adenomas, composed of inactive null cells.

The symptoms of adenomas of significant size are those of increased intracranial pressure and local compression of the optic tracts; third, fourth, and sixth cranial nerves; and of the hypothalamus. The endocrine syndromes of functional adenomas are **acromegaly** or **gigantism** with GH, **amenorrhea-galactorrhea** with PRL, **hyperthyroidism** with TSH, and **Cushing's syndrome** (adrenocortical hyperfunction) and **Nelson's syndrome** (basophilic adenoma and hyperpigmentation after resection of hyperplastic adrenal cortex) associated with ACTH and MSH.

THYROID GLAND

Congenital disorders of the thyroid include **thyroglossal duct cysts** due to persistence of some part of that embryonic structure, abnormal configuration such as the otherwise insignificant midline **pyramidal lobe** and **heterotopias** of thyroid tissue, and **cretinism**. The latter is of two principal types: a hypoplasia due to prenatal iodine deficiency, called endemic cretinism, and sporadic cretinism due to agenesis or dysplasia of the thyroid or genetic defects in thyroid hormone synthesis.

Inflammation of the thyroid may rarely be due to bacterial infection. More importantly, **granulomatous** or **subacute**

thyroiditis is thought to be due to viral infection, causing disruption of follicles with reactive infiltrations of lymphocytes, neutrophils, and giant cells. **Autoimmune (Hashimoto's) thyroiditis** is characterized by infiltrations of plasma cells and lymphocytes, the latter forming distinct follicles. **Riedel's fibrous thyroiditis** is probably a manifestation of idiopathic fibrosclerosis, as it exhibits a fibrosis that not only destroys the thyroid tissue but infiltrates surrounding muscle, but the diagnosis has sometimes been used for the end stages of other thyroid inflammations. In general, thyroiditis causes mild hyperthyroidism, local tenderness, and fever in acute stages and may cause hypothyroidism in chronic or late stages.

Hyperplasia of the thyroid is a reaction to stimulatory influences that may be of several types. The action of TSH during metabolic cycles, because of deficient iodine intake or in response to goitrogens (drugs as well as foods), causes thickening of the follicular epithelium, accumulation of colloid, and increased mass of the gland. As the stimulus may not be constant and different areas of the gland may vary in their response, focal areas of overgrowth or nodules may develop over time. These **goiters**, which may be either **diffuse** or **nodular**, are **nontoxic**. Another form of stimulation is by abnormal immunoglobulins that combine with TSH receptors to cause both hyperplasia and hyperfunction of the thyroid epithelium. This results in **Grave's disease** (diffuse toxic goiter), which also includes an exophthalmos-producing factor among its abnormalities. The symptoms are those of marked hyperthyroidism, and the enlarged gland is composed of thick, folded epithelium and little stored colloid.

Adenomas are benign tumors that are usually well circumscribed, encapsulated, solitary lesions in which the follicular architecture is preserved although it may be distorted, and a variety of histological patterns are described. Distinction from nodules of hyperplasia may be difficult. The epithelium may take up radioactive iodine, but hyperthyroidism is not a feature. Carcinomas are of three main types: (1) **papillary**, which is the most frequent, remains under hormone control, occurs in young persons, and is rarely fatal, (2) **follicular**, with a greater potential for distant metastasis, especially to lung and bone, and a 5-year survival of 65%, and (3) **undifferentiated**, which is highly malignant and tends to occur in older persons. The rare **medullary carcinoma** is of interstitial C cells that are of neurocrest origin, secretes calcitonin, and exhibits amyloid in its stroma but produces no endocrine syndrome.

PARATHYROID GLANDS

A very rare but most interesting congenital anomaly of the parathyroid glands is their **agenesis associated with absence of the thymus**. Afflicted infants have severe hypoparathyroidism as well as absence of cellular immunity. Recognition of the combination and the common embryologic origin of the glands from the third and fourth branchial pouches enabled **Di George** to clarify the role of the mammalian thymus in immunity.

The glands are most important because of the roles they play in the metabolism of calcium and phosphorus and in renal disease and metabolic bone disease. The changes in the glands themselves are **hyperplasia, adenomas,** and **destruction,** the latter mostly iatrogenic as a result of thyroidectomy. **Hyperplasia** is usually the result of renal failure to excrete phosphorus with consequent stimulation of calcium metabolism, but it can occur in vitamin D deficiency, in intestinal malabsorption, and in end-organ failure of response to parathyroid hormone (**pseudohypoparathyroidism**). All glands are affected, and the overgrowth of cells crowds out the fat cells that are dispersed throughout normal parathyroid tissue. There is also a **primary hyperplasia** that accounts for about 15% of cases of primary hyperparathyroidism. The remainder of such cases are due mostly to adenomas. Histological distinction between adenomas and hyperplasia is often difficult. Adenomas are almost always single, may compress and cause atrophy of a surrounding zone of parathyroid tissue, and are usually without effect on the other glands. **Carcinomas** are rare and very difficult to distinguish from thyroid carcinoma unless there is accompanying hyperparathyroidism.

Secondary results of **hyperparathyroidism** are most important in the diseases of these glands. They consist of **osteitis fibrosa, nephrocalcinosis, renal calculi,** and **metastatic calcification** in many tissues, particularly sites of acid excretion such as pulmonary alveolar walls, gastric mucosa, and the kidneys. In primary hyperparathyroidism, the osteoclastic fibrosing lesions particularly can become large enough to result in deformities and fractures.

ADRENAL GLANDS

The functional aspects, or pathophysiology, of disease of the adrenal glands are considerably more complicated than the pathological anatomy. The normal and clinical physiology of **adrenal cortical insufficiency, Cushing's syndrome, hyperaldosteronism,** and **pheochromocytomas** should be reviewed.

Congenital disorders include **ectopic distribution** of adrenal tissue, principally cortex but sometimes medulla, in many different retroperitoneal sites, including the capsule of the kidneys. They can rarely assume importance when an attempt is made to completely eradicate cortical steroid secretion in the control of cancer. There is also **congenital hypoplasia,** one type of which occurs in anencephalic fetuses, a demonstration of the intimate association between the hypothalamic-pituitary axis and the adrenals.

The **adrenogenital syndrome** is due to an inborn enzymatic (autosomal recessive) deficiency, most often of 11-hydroxylase, that blocks formation of cortisol and results in feedback diversion of steroid synthesis to pathways that result in increased amounts of gonadal-type hormones. The results are virilization or feminization, and the former can be particularly prominent in infants with associated distortions of the external genitalia and **pseudohermaphroditism.** In slightly older children, early muscle development results in the "**infant Hercules.**" The adrenals themselves have diffuse cortical hyperplasia or may appear normal.

Inflammations result in destruction of the gland and **hypoadrenocorticism** (Addison's disease) when bilateral. **Tuberculosis** was formerly the principal etiologic condition and remains important but shares responsibility with other granulomatous processes such as **histoplasmosis** and especially with an apparently **autoimmune adrenalitis,** formerly called primary adrenal cortical atrophy, which is the cause of most modern cases. Hyponatremia, hyperkalemia, and hypoglycemia are cardinal manifestations, and weakness, anorexia,

weight loss, and darkening of the skin and mucous membranes are prominent symptoms.

The adrenals are sometimes the **site of acute hemorrhagic destruction in cases of disseminated intravascular coagulation** arising in acute pyogenic septicemia due to meningococci, or less commonly *S. pneumoniae, Staphylococcus* sp, and *H. influenzae.* The syndrome is named **Waterhouse-Friderichsen's,** and the loss of cortical function may add to the drastic effects of the infection and the DIC, but the syndrome certainly cannot be induced directly by surgical adrenalectomy and is hardly worthy of the name of acute adrenocortical insufficiency.

Diffuse and nodular hyperplasia and **adenomas** of the adrenal cortex constitute a confusing anatomic classification of cases of **hyperadrenocorticism.** The cells of the three zones of the cortex are associated with secretion of different steroids: hydrocortisone (cortisol) from the predominate zona fasciculata, aldosterone from the zona glomerulosa, and androgens and estrogens principally from the zona reticularis. Histological identification of the specific cell type is difficult, if not impossible, so the hyperplasias or "adenomas" associated with the various hyperfunctions look very much alike. **Diffuse hyperplasia** is more common in **Cushing's syndrome** because most cases are the result of hyperfunction of the pituitary, whereas **adenomas** are recognized in 90% of cases of **aldosteronism.** When the lesion is solitary and large it is easy to accept as a benign neoplasm or adenoma, but more commonly at autopsy there are multiple, small foci that have incomplete or no encapsulation and that are better considered nodular hyperplasias. Rarely a true **adrenocortical carcinoma** occurs and is the cause of hyperfunction. These lesions tend to be expressed especially with feminization or virilization.

The only important lesions of the adrenal medulla are the **pheochromocytoma,** which occurs in adults, produces catecholamines, and is associated with episodic or sustained hypertension, and the **neuroblastoma,** which occurs in infants and is an important example of a malignant tumor that may undergo spontaneous or induced maturation.

AMINO PRECURSOR UPTAKE AND DECARBOXYLATION (APUD) TUMORS AND SYNDROMES

A family of tumors derived from endocrine tissues has been recognized because of the proclivity of the tumors to occur in multiple organs and to secrete low-molecular-weight peptide hormones. Various combinations have been given eponyms such as **Wermer's syndrome** for adenomas of the pituitary, islets, and parathyroid and **Zollinger-Ellison syndrome** for multiple gastrin-secreting islet adenomas. **Carcinoids** occur throughout the GI tract and in the bronchi and excrete serotonin, resulting in vasomotor and smooth muscle-related symptoms. **Pheochromocytomas** are also APUD tumors, and the embryonic origin of the cells of many members is from the neuroectoderm, but some arise from the entoderm, such as the **enterochromaffin cells.** The tumors in the various syndromes are sometimes carcinomas.

ENDOCRINE PANCREAS

Perhaps because of the early isolation and clinical application of insulin and the triumphs of biochemistry in understanding carbohydrate metabolism, there seems to be more specific information regarding the **islets of Langerhans** than any other gland, including the pituitary. Four cell types have been identified with four active hormones: A with glucagon, B with insulin, D with somatostatin, G with gastrin, and another, F, with an identified pancreatic polypeptide of yet unknown function. Additional hormones have been identified without having yet been associated with a specific cell, including serotonin and vasoactive intestinal polypeptide. The principal disease associated with this intricate situation is, of course, **diabetes mellitus**, which is well understood to be far from a simple hormone deficiency. Lesions of the islets, such as **amyloid infiltration, congenital hyperplasia**, and **lymphocytic** and **eosinophilic infiltration**, are considerably although not exclusively associated with diabetes. The latter, observed in early juvenile diabetes, is interesting because of the parallel of a virus-induced lesion in animals. **Adenomas** and **rare carcinomas** of islet cells are recognized by their specific endocrine hyperfunctions.

Diabetes mellitus could be classified as a genetic disease because of the strong association of the juvenile form with HLA haplotypes B8, B15, Dw3, and Dw4, as well as strong familial incidence in all types and almost 100% concordance of the maturity type in identical twins. The two types, **juvenile** and **maturity**, differ in that the first is associated with a loss of B cells and responds to insulin replacement in doses similar to those necessary after pancreatectomy while the maturity type has many features of a target tissue, or insulin receptor, disease. In the latter, for instance, there are often increased stores of insulin in the islets, effective therapeutic doses of insulin may have to be many times the size of those in juvenile diabetes, and antibodies to insulin receptor sites and to insulin itself complicate the picture. Obesity is particularly important in decreasing the receptor sites on the cell membrane. It should be noted that the terminology of juvenile and maturity onset does not signify absolute chronologic criteria, for each type occurs within the age period of the other although in decreased incidence.

The pathology of diabetes mellitus is essentially that of its effects on other organs than the pancreas. The demonstration of **absence of granules in the B cells** of the islets is the only diagnostic lesion that can be recognized. The fundamental generalized lesion is a **microangiopathy** that results in thickening and hyalinization of the basement membranes of capillaries, venules, and arterioles. The process proceeds to typical **"intercapillary" sclerosis** in the renal glomeruli, a quite specifically diagnostic appearance first described by Kimmelstiel, and **microaneurysms** in the retina that accompany sclerotic vessels, and exudates that produce a typical appearance recognized as **diabetic retinopathy** through the ophthalmoscope. **Atherosclerosis** is accelerated and intensified in diabetics. It involves large and small arteries and leads to gangrene of extremities and myocardial infarcts. Arterioles become sclerotic and, particularly as the kidneys become involved, **hypertension** and **cerebral hemorrhage** result. **Cataracts** are another complication in the eyes. **Peripheral neuritis** develops in association with sclerosis of vasa nervorum and may be markedly debilitating. All these changes exhibit a wide range of incidence and intensity in various patients. In general, arteriosclerotic changes are more prominent in maturity diabetes, renal in juvenile, and

eye changes in all cases. None shows an absolute correlation with duration of the diabetes itself.

GONADS

Various lesions, particularly tumors, of the ovary are associated with abnormal secretion of androgens or estrogens or both. The **polycystic ovary (Stein-Leventhal) syndrome** involves hirsutism, infertility, amenorrhea, and obesity but not actual masculinization. The ovaries are enlarged and have thick capsules under which there are multiple small follicular cysts. There are elevated androgen levels and low levels of testosterone-binding protein, facilitating increased effect of the hormone. Another lesion and syndrome are **hyperthecosis** and **stromal hyperplasia**, and the enlarged ovaries with increased and luteinized stroma may cause actual masculinization with clitoral hypertrophy, frontal balding, deepening of the voice, etc. Among the ovarian tumors, the **granulosa-theca cell tumors** produce estrogen with clinical effect, **Sertoli-Leydig cell tumors** produce androgens to various degrees, and in children the Sertoli type is associated with estrogenic phenomena. **Gynandroblastoma** sometimes produces significant androgen. The germ cell tumors, particularly **choriocarcinoma**, produce gonadotropin in sufficient amount to serve as a marker for the persistence of the tumor. The remainder, including the important malignant carcinomas, do not have endocrine activity.

Atrophy or dysgenesis of the testis with subsequent eunuchoid status is the more prominent clinical endocrinopathy of the testis. This occurs in genetic disorders such as **Klinefelter's syndrome** and rarely after bilateral **orchitis**. **Gynecomastia** develops in 2 to 10% of cases of testicular tumors, but it is often difficult to ascertain the presence or nature of abnormal levels of hormone. The germ cell tumors, particularly **choriocarcinoma**, secrete gonadotropin. **Sertoli and Leydig cell tumors** cause estrogenic or androgenic effects, respectively, especially in children, in whom the Leydig cell tumor, although essentially benign, results in macrogenitosomia and premature closure of epiphyses.

GENITOURINARY TRACT AND BREASTS

KIDNEYS

Congenital anomalies

The kidneys arise embryologically by the upward migration of ureteral buds to meet the nephroblastoma. Failure of this union results in **agenesis of the kidney**, which may be either unilateral or bilateral. When bilateral, it is accompanied by the facial deformities of wide-set eyes, parrot-beak nose, receding chin, and low-set ears that is called Potter's syndrome. Unilateral agenesis, although twice as common as bilateral, is compatible with normal development and life. These and other abnormalities of position and configuration such as **bifid ureters** or **pelves** and **horseshoe kidneys** are not genetic, in contrast to several varieties of polycystic kidneys. **Adult polycystic disease** is autosomal dominant and consists of cysts that result from blocks of some of the collecting tubules. The cysts gradually enlarge and by the fourth or fifth decade have compressed surrounding nephrons sufficiently to cause renal failure. The kidneys meanwhile have grown as large as a football, and cysts develop in other organs, particularly the liver, pancreas, and spleen. The disease is inevitably bilateral, but it may progress more rapidly in one kidney than the other. There is an **infantile form** that seems to be similar except that more collecting tubules are involved and the uninvolved nephrons are compromised more rapidly. This occurs as a result of a homozygous phenotype of an autosomal recessive gene. **Dysplastic kidneys** are not the result of genetic mechanisms. They are small, do not show normal papillae and cortex, and microscopically contain incompletely formed tubules and glomeruli and hamartomatous tissue. They may be unilateral or partial, especially in patients with bifid or duplicated ureters. Other congenital diseases include **medullary sponge kidney, medullary cystic disease**, and **hereditary nephropathy**.

Simple cysts of the kidneys are single or few. They may represent a mechanism similar to that in adult polycystic disease but are not hereditary and often occur in kidneys afflicted by other scarring diseases such as pyelonephritis or arteriolar nephrosclerosis. The cysts may attain considerable size and can deform the pelvis, with resulting obstructive phenomena. Patients who have end-stage renal disease and whose life is prolonged by renal dialysis often develop multiple moderate-sized cysts throughout their kidneys. The cysts in this **acquired (dialysis-associated) cystic disease** often contain oxalate crystals or small, nodular epithelial hyperplasias.

Primary renal disease

The application of modern research methods of electron microscopy, immunohistology, cellular physiology, and genetics has made our knowledge of renal diseases so precise that their classification has outgrown the boundaries of any licensing examination. Two reference texts of pathology each list 60 diseases of the kidneys with at least a 12% lack of concordance. In glomerular disease, particularly, the nomenclature is a complicated mixture of terms based on etiology, morphology, and eponyms. A quick review is best approached with emphasis on renal pathophysiology, for most of the inflammatory or degenerative diseases share many clinical features that are essentially those of renal failure.

The physiological reserve of renal function is very large. Loss of half of the normal renal mass is barely perceptible by carefully performed tests of function, of which creatinine clearance is one of the most sensitive. Nephrons have considerable capacity to hypertrophy in compensation for loss of other nephrons. The unit hypertrophy or loss is of entire nephrons so that preservation or decrease of glomerular and tubular functions are balanced. As a consequence, progressive renal disease—which is ultimately a matter of losing nephrons—may be masked or undetected until as many as 90% of nephrons are rendered nonfunctional. Under such circumstances, the course of renal failure may appear to present with sudden onset and rapid progression, and the clinical features from case to case have much in common regardless of the underlying pathogenesis. The kidneys themselves are scarred and shrunken to such a degree that originally specific morphological changes are obliterated. For this condition, **end-stage renal disease** is a commonly applied descriptor.

Several syndromes constitute a foundation for understanding the pathophysiological features of the course and final outcome of various renal diseases: the **uremic syndrome**, the **nephrotic syndrome**, and the **nephritic syndrome**. To review these entities, the reader should first review the normal physiology of the nephron, for in their early stages the functional changes can be closely correlated with the presence of lesions of particular parts of the nephron. **Uremia** consists of azotemia (elevation of blood urea concentration), the retention of other substances normally excreted by the kidneys, and distortion of metabolic and endocrine functions subserved by normal renal function. Hypertension and anemia develop early. There are many and various symptoms: weakness, weight loss, poor appetite, headache, lethargy, and occasionally convulsions. Water intoxication, sodium depletion, petechiae in skin and GI mucosa, fibrinous pericarditis, and a respiratory distress syndrome (uremic pneumonia) are other features. The **nephrotic syndrome** consists of proteinuria (over 3 g/24 hours), hypoproteinemia, edema, lipiduria, and hypercholesterolemia. Hypertension and azotemia are not features. It occurs in various types of glomerular disease, particularly **lipoid nephrosis**, and in other conditions such as **amyloidosis, renal vein thrombosis**, and **diabetic glomerulosclerosis**. Especially in children there is susceptibility to infection by organisms such as *S. pneumoniae* and *Staphylococcus* sp. Depending on the nature of the underlying renal disease, the syndrome may subside or may evolve into progressive and chronic renal failure. The **nephritic syndrome** is characterized by hematuria, red cell casts, proteinuria (usually less than 2 g/24 hours), hypertension, oliguria, and azotemia. It is symptomatic of primary glomerular injury, and acute **poststreptococcal glomerulonephritis** is prototypical. Depending again on the nature of the primary renal disease, recovery is often complete, but congestive cardiac failure or uremia may supervene.

Glomerulonephritis

The essential lesion of glomerulonephritis is acute injury of the glomerulus and subsequent reaction of its components. The mechanism of injury is usually by deposition of immune complexes that may involve IgA, IgM, IgG, C3, and C4. In one variety, **rapidly progressive glomerulonephritis**, the injury is done by antiglomerular basement antibodies and there is also injury to pulmonary alveolar basement membranes with hemorrhages (**Goodpasture's syndrome**). Other important types are **acute postreptococcal glomerulonephritis, membranoproliferative glomerulonephritis, lipoid nephrosis, focal segmental sclerosis, membranous glomerulonephritis**, and **Berger's disease (IgA nephropathy). Chronic glomerulonephritis** may be the result of progression of several of the acute syndromes but most often has no recognizable predecessor. It is a progressive, extreme destruction of glomeruli and tubules that is likely the result of exposure to small doses of antigen over a prolonged period.

The renal diseases of **systemic lupus erythematosus** (SLE) and of chronic bacteremia (**focal embolic glomerulonephritis**) are also forms of glomerulonephritis with immune complex injury. **Disseminated intravascular coagulation, thrombotic purpura**, and **eclampsia** exhibit glomeruli injured by fibrin deposits and thrombi. **Diabetic glomerulosclerosis** is a diffuse and nodular increase of basement membrane substance that is part of the general microangiopathy and often results in a nephrotic syndrome. **Amyloidosis** also affects glomeruli by heavy deposits of amyloid fibrils along the capillaries.

Infections

Pyelonephritis is the principal infectious disease of the kidney. It is classified as a **tubulointerstitial** disease by the authors of a major textbook to emphasize the destructive involvement of both epithelial and interstitial structures as well as other features common to the infectious disease and to others of toxic or immunologic origin such as **analgesic nephritis**, **urate nephropathy** of gout, **radiation nephritis**, **transplant rejection**, and **myeloma kidney**. Unfortunately, the term seems to have been applied by others rather specifically to **acute tubular necrosis**, discussed in a following paragraph.

For **pyelonephritis**, the principal bacteriologic cause is *E. coli*, but *Aerobacter aerogenes*, *P. aeruginosa*, *Proteus* organisms, or *Streptococcus faecalis* may be the agent. The other essential pathogenic factor is obstruction in the urinary tract. Prostatic disease, pregnancy, and probably vesicoureteral incompetence are important, and the latter may be the rather common condition of young girls that is associated with bacteriuria.

Acute pyelonephritis usually (but not always) is accompanied by fever, leukocytosis, flank pain, dysuria, leukocyte casts, and proteinuria. In the **chronic** form, the symptoms are more apt to be those of insidious renal failure and anemia. The acute lesions begin in the interstitium and rapidly involve groups of nephrons, filling the tubules with pus. Whether the organisms arrive by retrograde extension along lymphatics or interstitial spaces communicating with the pelvic calyces or by way of the bloodstream has been hotly debated. Different cases may well represent involvement by either or both pathways. The chronic form may evolve from the acute but in many cases seems to arise de novo. The inflammation tends to be focal and to result finally in depressed, flat-based scars, but it may be total or diffuse, particularly in the end-stage chronic form. Bacteria may persist within the kidney, but it is also likely that they stimulate antibodies that evoke a tissue-destructive autoimmune process. Generalized sclerotic vascular changes and hypertension are features of chronic pyelonephritis, as is ultimate uremia.

Abscesses, or **carbuncles**, arise from bacteremia of *Staphylococcus* sp and other organisms and do not progress into the more general disease of pyelonephritis, nor is the peripelvic tissue necessarily involved. The other diseases mentioned above as tubulointerstitial share many of the features of chronic pyelonephritis such as the interstitial infiltrates of lymphocytes and plasma cells and the atrophic tubules filled with dense protein casts as well as the scarring. They may have specific features such as extruded casts of Bence Jones and Tamm-Horsfall protein in **multiple myeloma**, acute vasculitis in **transplant rejection**, urate crystals in **gout**, etc.

Acute tubular necrosis

States of shock or exposure to nephrotoxins result in selective necrosis of renal tubular epithelium and are the underlying cause of most cases of acute renal failure. The shock may result from traumatic injury, bacteremia, burns, transfusion reactions, and many other causes. It appears to operate through local ischemia of the renal tubule with consequent focal necrosis of epithelium and disruption of the basement membrane (**tubulorrhexis**). The nephrotoxins, of which **mercuric chloride** is the classic and **sulfonamides, glycols,** and **aminoglycoside antibiotics** are examples, result in more diffuse necrosis of epithelium, particularly of the proximal tubule. The lesions of tubulorrhexis are difficult to recognize in ordinary sections and were first conclusively demonstrated by microdissections of entire nephrons. In addition to the epithelial changes, there are interstitial edema, dilation of tubules, protein casts that may contain hemoglobin, and leukostasis in thin-walled interstitial veins.

The disruption of tubular epithelium destroys the function of the nephron, and the glomerular filtrate is almost reabsorbed, resulting in an initial oliguria followed by signs of fluid overload and uremia. Potassium retention is characteristic and life threatening. If the patient is maintained by dialysis and other means, diuresis begins in a few days to several weeks when the tubular epithelium regenerates, but it is much longer before normal renal function returns, with the gradual reacquisition of normal differentiated functions of the tubular cells.

Arteriolar nephrosclerosis

Associated with **benign**, or **essential, hypertension** the kidneys develop a diffuse atrophy of nephrons and scarring of glomeruli and the interstitium—termed **arteriolar nephrosclerosis** because of the prominent thickening and hyalinization of intrarenal arterioles. Some nephrons become atrophied and shrunken while others dilate and hypertrophy. This is the basis for the granular gross configuration of the cortical surface, while the total process results in the loss of sufficient substance so that the final appearance is that of the contracted end-stage kidney. The interlobular and arcuate arteries undergo fibroelastic hyperplasia and fibrosis. Although some cases of early hypertension are not accompanied by morphological changes in the kidneys, late cases inevitably develop nephrosclerosis. If renal vascular changes are not the basis of all hypertension, they at least contribute to its irreversibility and must in some instances be primarily causative, especially when the principal lesion is **constriction of major renal arteries** by **fibromuscular hyperplasia** or fortuitous localization of atherosclerotic plaques.

Malignant hypertension may develop in a patient with the more benign form or may develop rapidly in a previously normotensive individual. The kidneys contain **fibrinoid necrosis** of arterioles, particularly the afferent glomerular arterioles, and a **hyperplastic arteriolitis** of interlobular arterioles. The latter are probably the result of a thrombotic process and have an onionskin appearance in sections. The glomeruli show thrombosed capillaries and necrotizing inflammation. The amount of scarring and contraction depends on the extent of prior disease in cases developing from benign, or essential, hypertension. Uremia may be fulminant, papilledema and retinal hemorrhages develop, and cerebral symptoms of headache, vomiting, and convulsions indicate the widespread effects of the disorder.

Urolithiasis

Calculi, or **stones**, may form in any part of the urinary tract, particularly at sites of stasis and infection, but most originate in the calyces of the renal pelves. They are composed of a matrix of mucoprotein in which there are embedded crystals of calcium oxalate, calcium phosphate, magnesium ammonium phosphate, urate, cystine, or other substances rarely. The calcium-containing compounds in various combinations account for three-quarters or more of all stones. The underlying causes may be conditions such as hyperparathyroidism that result in increased urinary concentration of the minerals that form the stones. Colicky pain in the flank and hematuria are classic symptoms.

Neoplasia

The most common tumors of the kidneys are **cortical adenomas**. They occur especially in previously scarred kidneys. Their histological appearance is remarkably similar to that of some renal cell carcinomas, and it may be impossible to be certain a moderate-sized lesion is not cancerous, but the vast majority of those less than an inch in diameter have no evidence of potential for metastasis. They are spherical, yellow or gray, discrete nodules in the cortex that may appear to be papillae filling a cyst. Some authors have termed them **nodular hyperplasias of tubules**.

Another common benign tumor at autopsy is the medullary **hamartoma** that is a mass of fibrous and muscular tissue 1 to 2 mm in diameter and appears as a small pale sphere in a medullary papilla.

The important malignant tumors of the kidney are (1) **renal cell carcinoma** of adults (2) **Wilms' tumor (nephroblastoma)** of children, and (3) **carcinoma of the renal pelvis**. The latter is usually of transitional epithelium and identical with the more common tumors of the bladder. Like them, they may be multicentric. A true **squamous carcinoma** occurs rarely.

Wilms' tumor is a tumor that usually occurs in children 1 to 4 years of age. From the organoid appearance of its histological elements and a number of coincident phenomena such as aniridia, urogenital anomalies, hemihypertrophy, and chromosomal abnormalities such as deletion in the short arms of of chromosome 11, it is considered a tumor of embryonic origin and derived from the mesonephric mesoderm. Sections may contain muscle, bone, and cartilage as well dark, small epithelial cells that form poorly developed tubules and aborted glomeruli. Modern chemotherapy, radiotherapy, and surgery have raised the survival rate to 90% from its previous mortality of 60 to 90% with surgery alone.

Renal cell carcinoma is the most frequent malignant tumor of the kidney in adults but accounts for only 2 or 3% of all cancer other than that of skin. It is predominant in men. Most tumors are of considerable size when discovered, and the progress of metastatic disease is usually slow. Successful resection of solitary metastases in lung or brain has occurred. The tumors are usually spherical masses in the cortex of a pole of the kidney. Frequently there are areas of necrosis and hemorrhage, but hematuria is often a late symptom because the tumor does not involve the pelvis. Invasion of veins, sometimes with extension of the tumor into the vena cava and even into the right atrium of the heart, is characteristic and an indication of metastatic potential. Fever, perhaps from the tumor necrosis, hypertension from renin production, and polycythemia due to erythropoietin production have been observed in various cases.

URINARY BLADDER

Congenital anomalies

The urinary bladder is derived from the embryonic urogenital sinus that in turn is the anterior portion of the cloaca attached to the allantois and thus to the yolk sac. It is lined by a particular epithelium adapted to great distension, **transitional squamous epithelium** or **urothelium**. A relatively minor anomaly is persistence of a lumen in the derivative of the allantois, the **urachus**, that extends into the umbilicus and gives rise to a **fistula**, a **cyst**, or a draining **sinus**. More extensive malformation results in an opening of the anterior wall with **exstrophy** of the mucosa and failure of the pubic symphysis. The mucosa is then the seat of infection, undergoes metaplasia, and may give rise to a rare **adenocarcinoma**, which may also arise from an urachal remnant in the apex of an intact bladder. As there is formation of urine during fetal development, an infant with an obstructive anomaly of the urethra may be born with **hypertrophy of the bladder**, which is actually a work hypertrophy just as develops in adult males from urethral obstruction due to prostatic disease. Diverticula are usually acquired and result from such obstruction, but they can be congenital. Complete agenesis of the bladder is very rare, and the bladder usually does not participate in the posterior cloacal malformation of **imperforate anus**.

Infections

Cystitis is one of the most common diseases of humanity, especially of women. Antecedent conditions are obstruction, urinary stasis, or trauma. Instrumentation almost inevitably leads to infection. The most common agents are the intestinal bacteria, especially *E. coli*. Prolonged inflammation leads to local thickening and metaplasia of the epithelium that may become cystic and lined with columnar epithelium (**cystitis cystica** or **cystitis glandularis**). A rare and peculiar form of metaplasia that must be distinguished from carcinoma is **malacoplakia**, in which plaques and polyps contain structures named **Michaelis-Gutmann** bodies. The bladder is almost inevitably involved in cases of renal **tuberculosis** and can be infected by fungi, especially *Candida* sp and *Actinomyces* sp. Parasites such as *Echinococcus* and *Stronglyoides stercoralis* may infect the bladder, but the most notorious of this group is *Schistosoma haematobium*, which is a widespread cause of disease in northern Africa and the Middle East. It is associated with extensive metaplasia of the bladder and carcinoma.

Calculi form in bladders with urinary stasis and infection. They usually are of calcium oxalate, perhaps mixed with calcium phosphate, and sometimes of ammonium magnesium phosphate (struvite) when associated with urea-splitting bacteria.

Neoplasia

Carcinoma of the bladder is an important cause of death of men over age 75. Painless hematuria is the classic symptom. Nearly all tumors of the bladder are of its transitional epithelium and should be considered as a single class. Intractable recurrence after operative removal is frequent, and the most important application of pathological principles in this disease is the careful grading and staging of the lesions, which vary from quite benign to highly malignant, especially in the less common squamous carcinomas. The elaborate systems of evaluating these tumors incorporate assessment of a number of factors. One of the more popular is the **TNM** classification (**tumor, nodes, metastases**).

Surface antigens of normal bladder cells cross-react to blood group isoantigens. This reactivity is preserved in the better-differentiated tumors and lost in the more malignant. Although there are many polypoid lesions of the bladder in both neoplastic and inflammatory diseases, truly benign epithelial polyps are very rare. These cancers were one of the first to be recognized as related to exposure to carcinogens, especially aniline dyes, and also to cigarette smoking and abused analgesic drugs, but not to saccharin in human beings.

URETERS

Everything said about obstructive, infective, and neoplastic diseases of the bladder can also be applied to the ureters and renal pelves. The phenomenon of recurrent separate neoplasms in the bladder or the ureters or pelves is a basis for considering the lower urinary tract as a unique unit and the designation of the epithelium as **urothelium** by some writers. Bifid or duplicated ureters are relatively common anomalies of little significance and few complications, but anomalous relations to blood vessels can be important in initiating obstruction and infection.

The ureter is protected from back-flow of urine during micturition by the valve-like action of its angulated course through the muscular wall of the bladder. If the angle is not sufficiently acute or there are other causes of patency of the ureterovesical junction, urine will be forced back up the ureter and into the renal pelves (**vesicoureteral reflux**), carrying with it such bacteria as may be present in the urine. From the pelves there are entry points around the calyces into the lymphatics and interstitium of the renal papillae. This pathway is considered important in the development of pyelonephritis and has been particularly studied in the frequent, although mostly benign, bacilluria of young girls.

PROSTATE

Congenital anomalies

The most important anomalies of the prostate are more properly considered anomalies of the prostatic urethra in which folds and redundancies cause partial or complete obstruction that leads to urinary retention and infection.

Infections

Acute and chronic prostatitis are predominantly bacterial diseases due to the same organisms that infect the bladder. An element of trauma quite often precedes acute prostatitis, but the chronic disease is more insidious, and there is evidence that agents such as *Chlamydia trachomatis* might be involved. Leukocytes are quite commonly present in the acini of the prostate and must be accompanied by infiltrations of the surrounding stroma if the histological diagnosis is to be made. Abscesses may develop. The prostatic urethra is involved in gonorrhea, and the inflammation will spread into the adjacent ducts, but the formation of chronic fistulas occurs in the penile urethra. Granulomatous prostatitis is a common part of renal and disseminated tuberculosis and rarely of systemic fungal disease, but there is also a form of disease with discrete microscopic granulomas that contain no bacteria and that are apparently reactions to prostatic secretions extruded from inflamed and broken acini.

Neoplasia

The prostate ranks right behind the lung, colon and rectum, and breast in the list of sites of significant **cancers** (other than skin). It is a disease of men over 50 years of age and practically never occurs before the latter fourth decade. It has been stated that 50% of men over 70 years old harbor the lesion, but that figure includes a very low-grade **latent cancer** about which there remains some uncertainty as to its true malignant potential. It originates in the posterior lobe of the gland, rapidly penetrates the capsule, and reaches the walls of the seminal vesicles, at which point it is surgically unresectable without intolerable sacrifice of vesical and sexual function. The more malignant grades metastasize to regional lymph nodes, the lungs, and particularly to bone (especially sacrum and vertebrae), where the reactions are usually osteoblastic. Significant involvement of the bladder is late and rather unusual. Like the normal epithelium, the cancerous cells produce **acid phosphatase**. When the cancerous cells break out of the prostate, the enzyme levels are elevated in the serum of at least 60% of patients and can serve as a sensitive marker for the progress of the disease. Histologically, the tumors are nearly all adenocarcinomas, but they vary from small, well-differentiated acini to diffuse infiltrations of single cells. There are several systems to express the grade and stage of the tumor, and their careful application gives very significant insight into prognosis. Epithelium of a carcinoma, like that of the prostate itself, requires androgen for maintenance, and orchiectomy and the administration of estrogens will retard the progress of metastatic disease.

Nodular hyperplasia (**benign hypertrophy**) is likewise a disease of older men and is rarely encountered in persons younger than 40. It is also endocrine related in that it does not occur in eunuchs. The lesions arise in the periurethral portion of the gland and involve the median and then the lateral lobes. They consist of spherical proliferation of groups of acini and accompanying stroma, with markedly heightened epithelium that folds into papillary structures. Urinary obstruction is related to distortion of the internal vesicle sphincter by the encroaching glands. As the incidence is much the same as that of carcinoma, there is considerable overlap in the occurrence of the two diseases, but there is little convincing evidence of any significant causal relation.

TESTES

Congenital anomalies

Anorchidism and **monorchidism** (undoubtedly fetal resorption of testis rather than truly an absence) are rare anomalies. More important is **cryptorchidism**, which may be unilateral or bilateral and results in malmaturity of the involved organ at puberty and an increased incidence of testicular tumors in the undescended testis. Also, anomalies of the gubernaculum, mesorchium, or tunica probably underlie **torsion of the testis**, which develops suddenly in young men and is marked by rapid obstruction of the twisted veins, engorgement, and then infarction. The condition often follows straining or violent exercise and is always unilateral.

Several genetic syndromes result in failure of complete development of gonads. The most conspicious of these in men is **Klinefelter's syndrome**, which is XXY intersexuality. The testicular tubules are sclerotic and hyalinized and show very little or no spermatogenesis, but the interstitial cells are prominent and apparently increased. The patients are eunuchoid and often mentally retarded.

Infectious disease

Bacterial veneral disease may involve the epididymis in acute inflammation but rarely spreads to the testes. Granulomatous disease such as **tuberculosis** can involve testes as well as the epididymis, while **tertiary syphilis** results in interstitial inflammation and fibrosis. A fifth of cases of **mumps** in adults result in an **interstitial orchiditis** that may be severe enough to lead to testicular atrophy that is usually unilateral.

Neoplasia

Nearly all tumors of the testes are derived from germinal epithelium. They are of five main types: (1) **seminoma**, (2) **yolk sac tumors**, (3) **teratoma**, (4) **embryonal carcinoma**, and (5) **choriocarcinoma**, in ascending order of malignancy. The **seminoma** is the most common of these tumors (40%), is radiosensitive, and is curable in 90% of cases without visceral metastases. The **yolk sac tumor** is a disease of infants, and survival is 80%. Its cells contain large amount of alpha-fetoprotein, which is a sensitive marker in serum for the presence or persistence of the tumor or related cells, as there are sometimes detectable levels in cases of other tumors of the testis. **Teratomas** are of variable degrees of differentiation, but most of the tissue usually appears quite mature. **Embryonal carcinoma** has undergone a marked change in prognosis with modern chemotherapy, and survival has risen from almost zero to over half of cases in which the tumor is confined to the testis by pathological examination. Pure **choriocarcinoma**, which is fortunately rare, remains the most malignant and intractable of the tumors. Unlike the similar tumor of the placenta, it is not sensitive to methotrexate. It is composed of both cytotrophoblasts and syncytiotrophoblasts, and the latter secrete **human chorionic gonadotropin**, which is the other sensitive marker in testicular tumors. Two-thirds of testicular tumors have some mixture of types, and the presence of one of the markers in tumors of other than those of its primary cell is probably indicative of syncytiotrophoblasts or yolk sac cells that are not necessarily malignant. The staging of these tumors deals principally with search for involvement of the tissues of the spermatic cord, retroperitioneal lymph nodes, and distant viscera. With modern therapy, the stage of the disease is as important as the histological typing, with the possible exception of seminomas.

VULVA AND VAGINA

Inflammations due to various organisms but particularly to fungi (*Candida albicans*) and *Trichomonas* in the vagina are common. These are particularly troublesome in diabetics and the aged, when they may be preceded by **atrophic vaginitis**.

The important **neoplasms** are **squamous carcinoma** of the vulva, again predominately a disease of the elderly, a rare similar carcinoma in the vagina, and **adenosis** and **clear cell carcinoma** of the vagina. Adenosis is the occurrence of glands and columnar epithelium in sites normally of squamous epithelium in the vagina. It has occurred in increased incidence in women whose mothers received **diethylstilbestrol** (DES) during their pregnancy with the patient. The lesion is common (perhaps as high as 90%) in such patients and may be a precursor of the quite malignant clear cell carcinoma, but the latter seems to have arisen in less than a fifth of 1% of cases. These diseases have become apparent in the second and third decades among exposed patients. As DES therapy of pregnant women has been discontinued for 15 or more years, the development of these lesions in their offspring is becoming rare.

Embryonal rhabdomyosarcoma (sarcoma botryoides) is a rare, highly malignant tumor, usually of infants. Microscopically it has a stroma of stellate cells and a hypercellular cambium zone of spindle cells beneath a normal epithelium. It may occur in older women, but it is then important to distinguish it from the **benign stromal polyp** that has a more mixoid stroma and no cambium.

UTERUS

Congenital anomalies

Various partial and even complete duplications of the uterus are the principal uterine malformations, whereas vestiges derived from the mesonephric ducts and heterotopias of müllerian epithelium are histological anomalies. The uterus remains infantile in Turner's syndrome (45 XO).

Infections

Acute cervicitis is caused by pyogenic bacteria, *Neisseria gonorrhoeae*, as a venereal infection, or by staphylococci or streptococci in postpartum women. **Chronic cervicitis** is of less specific and mixed etiologies. It may result in enlargement of the cervix, distortion, erosions, and blocked glands that become **Nabothain cysts**. Other agents such as herpesvirus type 2 (HSV-2) and *C. trachomatis* may be involved in the chronic process, and the possible relation of the prolonged inflammation, infection, and metaplasia of repair to the genesis of carcinoma is being considered. Because of the inherent high resistance of the endometrium, a membrane that is renewed every month, **acute endometritis** exists almost exclusively in postpartum uteri, where it is the central lesion of classic **puerperal** or **childbed fever**, the entity whose solution by Ignaz Semmelweis in Vienna in 1849 opened the modern era of asepsis. The predominant causative organism has been *Streptococcus pyogenes*, but gram-negative bacteria and *Bacteriodes* sp have been involved, and there have been cases of postpartum tetanus due to *Clostridium tetani*, particularly in postabortive cases. Contamination and the retention of gestational fragments are principal pathogenic elements. **Chronic endometritis** is a less well-defined entity based principally on symptoms of menorrhalgia and menorrhagia and the finding of plasma cells in the endometrial stroma. The etiologic agent is often not apparent, but there have been associations with intrauterine contraceptive devices. There are also cases of tuberculosis of the endometrium and some other such specific infections. The fallopian tubes, on the other hand, are very susceptible to acute and chronic infection by gonococci (60% of cases), streptococci, staphylococci, and coliform organisms. **Acute salpingitis**, a purulent inflammation of the lining and muscular wall of the tube, spreads to the adjacent peritoneum and has a very painful and devastating clinical effect. The tube often becomes obstructed, and the inflammation sequestrates about the tube and ovary to form **tubo-ovarian abscesses**. Fever, bacteremia, intestinal obstruction from adhesions, dysmenorrhea, and infertility result. The inflammation may subside to leave the dilated tube filled with sterile fluid (**hydrosalpinx**) or the old abscess presenting as a mass that can suggest an ovarian tumor.

Endometriosis

The pathogenesis of endometriosis is obscure. The condition consists of the development of endometrial tissue, including both the epithelial and glandular elements and the stroma, at sites on the pelvic peritoneum. The tissue, like true endometrium, is responsive to the menstrual cycle, and the implants enlarge and bleed, with resultant pain and subsequent fibrosis and adhesions that result in much discomfort. A similar condition, **adenomyosis**, consists of the presence of endometrial glands and stroma between the muscle bundles of the myometrium deep to the basal zone of the normal endometrium. The uterus is enlarged and is the source of pain, but in many cases the aberrant tissue does not undergo cyclic changes and hemorrhage.

Neoplasia

Carcinoma of the uterus has decreased in 40 years from first rank to sixth as the cause of cancer deaths in American women. Of its two components, **carcinoma of the endometrium** has remained almost constant, but **cervical carcinoma** has declined dramatically. This has been coincident with the development of the diagnostic technique of **exfoliative cytology**, which has also contributed greatly to the understanding of the genesis of these cancers, even if its effective application in the recognition and cure of early cases might not be the entire explanation for the changes in incidence of the disease. Several epidemiologic observations regarding carcinoma of the cervix have been well established: greater incidence in women with earlier and more active sexual practices, in those with more children, in prostitutes, in those infected with herpes simplex virus type 2, and in those of lower economic status. The tumors are of squamous type and begin at the columnar-squamous junction in the lower endocervix. There is a well-recognized sequence of increasing numbers and extent of cells with malignant appearance: **dysplasia, carcinoma in situ, microinvasive carcinoma,** and **invasive carcinoma**. From that point, staging based on the extent and spread of the tumor is most important in evaluating its prognosis. Histological grading is not of much value. Not all cases with dysplasia progress, but most patients with carcinoma in situ develop invasive disease, although it appears that most take certainly more than 2 years and perhaps as long as 10 to do so. Early symptoms are subtle and consist mostly of slight hemorrhage. Late complications consist of tumor infiltration of pelvic tissues more than a prominence of distant metastases. In times past, most patients died of either infection from the ulcerated tumor mass in the vagina or from renal failure following obstruction of the ureters. With modern therapy, cure rates are expected to be 100% for cases of in situ disease, 85% for stage I cases, but only 15% for stage IV.

Carcinoma of the endometrium is an adenocarcinoma predominantly of postmenopausal women, although other risk factors include (1) obesity, (2) hypertension, (3) diabetes mellitus, and (4) prolonged exposure to excessive estrogens. Fat tissue is the site at which androstenedione, which continues to be secreted by the adrenal and ovarian stroma after the menopausal ovary ceases to produce estradiol, is converted to estrogens, and this may be the link between these risk factors. Postmenopausal bleeding is the primary symptom. Most cases are recognized while still confined to the corpus of the uterus (stage I) and have a prognosis of 90% 5-year survival. **Adenomatous hyperplasia** of the endometrium also is associated with abnormalities of estrogen secretion, and from 3 to 25% of patients are said to progress to endometrial carcinoma if not treated. In this lesion, which occurs in premenopausal or early menopausal women, there is proliferation of glandular epithelium with atypia and without increased stroma. **Cystic hyperplasia** occurs in the same age-group but consists of equal or greater proliferation of stroma and less atypia of epithelium and is not thought to be of malignant potential. In both cases, the primary symptoms are menorrhagia and menometrorrhagia. Most **endometrial polyps** are essentially focal hyperplasias but may occur without more diffuse involvement of the surrounding endometrium.

Leiomyomas are the most common tumors of the uterus, developing in a fourth of women during their reproductive years. They may enlarge rapidly during pregnancy and regress after menopause. The tumors arise within the myometrium of the corpous of the uterus but may be displaced toward the cavity, where they cause bleeding; into the cervix, where they may cause obstruction that may be particularly difficult during delivery; or toward the serosa, where they may become attached to the omentum and a piece of intestine and eventually obtain a new blood supply from the implanted area and sever their attachment to the uterus (**migratory fibroid**). They are composed entirely of whorls of muscle and fibrous tissue and may contain dramatic areas of necrosis, fibrosis, calcification, and some atypia of muscle cells, but they are probably not the source of malignant tumors. **Sarcomas** of various types, including the **malignant mixed müllerian tumor** that is exclusively of this site, are quite rare.

OVARIES

Congenital anomalies

The "streak ovaries" of Turner's syndrome (45, XO chromosomal abnormality), the dysplasias of hermaphroditism, and developmental heterotopias or hamartomas are almost the only congenital ovarian lesions.

Neoplasia

Almost all the important pathological conditions of the ovary are in this category. Exceptions might be made for conditions such as **polycystic ovarian syndrome (Stein-Leventhal)**, but even in that condition the organ is enlarged, thickened, and cystic. Although the incidence of new cases of ovarian cancer is only two-fifths that of uterine cancer, the low overall survival rate of 37% places the number of fatalities about equal to that of pancreatic carcinoma and is exceeded only by fatalities due to lung, breast, and colon carcinoma. The tumors, particularly the epithelial carcinomas, are clinically silent in their early development, and their exposure to the peritoneum results in a very high percentage not being diagnosed until after they have spread beyond the ovary. The same relation of the surface of the ovary to the peritoneum may also contribute to the high incidence of bilateral occurrence of ovarian tumors, particularly of the malignant serous variety, which reaches two-thirds or more. The spread of ovarian carcinomas is predominantly to the peritoneal surfaces, with complications of adhesions and intestinal obstruction. Visceral and bony metastases are late and usually not very prominent.

The ovaries have potential for a large variety of tumors. The accepted classification scheme divides the 40 or so types into four classes: (1) **epithelial**, (2) **germ cell**, (3) **stromal**, and (4) **metastatic**. The **epithelial** account for two-thirds of the total, the **germ cell** tumors a fifth, and the **stromal** an eighth. Nearly all the malignant tumors (95%) are of the epithelial variety, with the **serous cystadenocarcinoma**, the **mucinous cystoadeno-carcinoma**, and the **endometroid carcinoma** being the principal types. Each of these tumors has a form of "borderline" malignancy, with a prognosis that is very difficult to predict from histological examination, as well as a benign and a clearly malignant form. The germ cell tumors are most prominently represented by the **teratomas** that are tumors of girls and young women and mostly benign. Like the epithelial tumors, they are often cystic. Rarer members of this group are analogues of the testicular germ cell tumors. The stromal tumors include the **granulosa-theca cell** group, which may cause hyperestrogenism, and the **Sertoli-Leydig cell tumors** (**arrhenoblastoma**, etc.), which may masculinize the patient. **Fibromas** are sometimes associated with mysterious hydro-thorax that clears after removal of the ovarian tumor. Of the **metastatic tumors**, those from the breast are most common, and a variety composed of dispersed, mucin-containing, signet ring cells that usually arise from the stomach and bear the eponym **Krukenberg's tumors** are the most infamous.

PLACENTA

Ten to 15% of pregnancies end in **spontaneous abortion** during the first trimester. It is thought that abnormalities of the fetus or placenta (**"blighted ovum"**) underlie these events, but demonstration of such lesions in the gestational debris is rarely successful.

Neonatal death is often associated with various disorders of the placenta: (1) infarcts, scarring, and hypoplasia in the **pla-cental insufficiency syndrome**, (2) inflammation along with **amnionits** and pneumonia in the fetus from infections, and (3) **hematomas and tears** of the placenta in premature separation.

Toxemia of pregnancy is dependent on the presence of the placenta, although the details of pathogenesis are far from completely understood. **Preeclampsia** consists of hypertension, proteinuria, and edema and develops in the third trimester in 5 or 6% of pregnancies. **Eclampsia** consists of the additional features of coma and convulsions. The pathological lesions of the full syndrome include those of disseminated intravascular coagulation with fibrin thrombi in renal glomeruli and other small vessels, particularly at the periphery of the hepatic lobules, where focal necrosis will develop, and petechiae in the brain and many other organs.

Neoplasia

For unknown reasons, tumors from the placenta occur in widely varying incidence in various parts of the world. In the United States, **hydatidiform mole** complicates 1 in about 2,000 pregnancies, but in India it is 10 times more common. **Choriocarcinoma** is rare (10 to 20 times less common than mole) in this country. The **mole** consists of proliferating, malformed, cystic, avascular, and edematous villous structures that invade the myometrium. A fifth invade so deeply (**invasive mole** or **chorioadenoma destruens**) that hysterectomy is necessary for their removal. Not more than 2 or 3% harbor or progress to choriocarcinoma. For moles, invasive moles, and choriocarcinoma, elevated serum **human chorionic gonado-tropin (HCG)** level is a sensitive marker of persistence of the tumorous syncytiotrophoblasts. Hemorrhage and rupture of the uterus are complications of invasive mole. **Choriocarci-noma** is the malignant tumor of placental elements, both cytotrophoblasts and syncytiotrophoblasts. The tumor does not form villi, and both cellular elements metastasize widely to other viscera. Formerly the disease was uniformly fatal, but the results of chemotherapy with methotrexate and actinomycin of these gestational (in contradistinction to gonodal) tumors have been spectacular, with cure rates as high as 100%.

BREASTS

Congenital anomalies

The principal malformations of the breast consist of exten-sion of glandular tissue into the anterior anxillary fold or the presence of **supernumerary nipples** or **small breasts** along the embryonic ventral, or mammary, ridge. These lesions may be the seat of tumors or cystic changes. Enlargement of the breasts, either bilateral or unilateral, will result from hyper-estrogenism in either women or men. The unilateral lesions are thought to be due to abnormal sensitivity of the local tissue. In **gynecomastia** of boys or men, the excess tissue is largely periductal fibrous tissue with hyperplasia of the ductal epithe-lium but without any lobular development. The tissue in **virginal hypertrophy** of young women is excessive but histo-logically normal.

Inflammatory disease

Infections in the breast occur principally in the lactating breast, usually in the first few weeks of nursing, when *Staphylococcus* sp and less commonly *Streptococcus* sp gain access through cracks and fissures in the nipple to cause **lactational mastitis**, which is a purulent inflammation in the ducts or the lobules and sometimes interstitially, especially with strepto-cocci. The involvement is segmental, may progress to the formation of an **abscess**, and only occasionally results in a contracted scar on healing. **Fat necrosis** is often called "traumatic" but, like some other forms of panniculitis, may not be preceded by an injury. The lesions are firm and fibrous and contain lipid-filled macrophages, foreign body giant cells, and sometimes focal calcification. They are of importance not just because they may be painful but because they may be confused with carcinoma.

Fibrocystic disease

This degenerative lesion in the breasts of women of reproductive age is usually bilateral and causes nodularity or lumpiness of the breasts that is often painful or tender, especially in the premenstrual period. The principal pathological change consists of irregular dilatation or cyst formation in the ducts, presumably due to some sort of focal obstruction, with surrounding fibrosis that is often accompanied by foci of benign overgrowth of lobular epithelium, myoepithelium, and stromal connective tissue of the lobule (**sclerosing adenosis**). There may be foci of calcification that can be identified on mammography and must be biopsied to rule out carcinoma. Fibrocystic disease of this **nonproliferative type** is not associated with any increased risk of cancer, but other cases contain hyperplasia, atypia, and dysplasia of the epithelium of the ducts and lobules. This type, called **proliferative fibrocystic disease**, is less common and is apparently associated with a severalfold increased risk of cancer.

Neoplasia

There are several benign neoplasms of the breast, of which two are most important. The **fibroadenoma** is a solitary, discrete, firm nodule that is the most common tumor of women in their third decade of life. Histologically, they are composed of great proliferations of loose periductal-type fibrous tissue with entrapped, enlarged, and compressed ducts. A variety known as **cystosarcoma phyllodes** reaches great size and appears to have a very active stroma but despite its name is nearly always benign. The other significant benign lesion is **intraducatal papilloma**, which is also most common in women in their third and fourth decades. It consists of an epithelial polyp with a fine fibrous stroma that arises from the wall of a duct, projects into and may occlude the lumen, and is responsible for painless bleeding and discharge from the nipple.

Many valiant efforts have been made to interpret changes within the epithelium of the breast that might be precancerous. At present, **atypical proliferative changes, carcinoma in situ,** and **intraductal carcinoma** are generally recognized and considered stages that develop into **ductal carcinoma**, although most cases present as completely developed **infiltrating ductal adenocarcinoma. Lobular carcinoma** is a less frequent variety, and **in situ lobular carcinoma** is a particularly interesting lesion that is being recognized by x-ray mammography followed by biopsy as it does not cause a palpable or grossly visible lesion. Patients are apparently cured by biopsy in a third of cases, but it is reported that a fifth will eventually develop more manifest disease, often in the other breast. Such behavior emphasizes the complexity of factors involved in neoplasia in this endocrine-sensitive tissue.

Breast cancer is the most common cancer of the women in the United States. The risk of a woman's developing the disease during her fifth or sixth decade is about 1 in 30. Although it is commonly asserted that the total risk is 1 in 11, that figure assumes constancy of present age-specific incidence rates for an entire lifetime of 85 years. Unlike a number of other cancers, the incidence and mortality have remained almost unchanged during the past five decades or longer. The 5-year survival rates have improved slightly, from 63 to 75% for white women and 46 to 62% for black in the past 25 years. Familial, geographic, nutritional, and endocrine (prolonged exposure to estrogenic stimuli by early menarche, late menopause, etc.) are suggestive factors that have been intensively studied.

Histological types are of some relevance in prognosis, **scirrhous** and **lobular** being less favorable in the long run than **medullary, colloid,** and **papillary.** Most important for the individual is the status of the axillary lymph nodes: Patients with no nodal involvement have had 65% 20-year survival, whereas those with level III, or high axillary, involvement have experienced only 12%. **Axillary lymph node status, tumor size,** and **histological types** are of decreasing order of influence on estimated prognosis. The detection of **estrogen receptor protein** in tumor cells has been useful in predicting endocrine sensitivity of the tumor, especially in the treatment of metastases, and shows some suggestion of value in prognosis, with the positive tumors being more favorable. The regional lymph nodes, lungs, and bone are common sites for **metastases,** some of which may be as late as 20 years in appearing. Local extension into the lymphatics of the overlying skin gives **inflammatory carcinoma** that is of very poor prognosis, while extension into the epidermis of the nipple results in an eczematoid lesion (**Paget's disease**) that does not affect prognosis unfavorably. Bilateral occurrence varies with the type of cancer, being about a quarter in lobular and comedo cancer, about 5% in low-grade ductal carcinoma, and as high as 15% for all types combined.

CENTRAL AND PERIPHERAL NERVOUS SYSTEMS, MUSCLES, AND ORGANS OF SPECIAL SENSE

NERVOUS SYSTEM

Unique features of the normal gross anatomy of the nervous system consist of (1) the internal functional organization that results in local lesions in the brain and spinal cord manifesting themselves in disturbed functions in other parts of the body to which the involved neurons project and (2) the physical effects of the encasement within the rigid skull and vertebral column. The projected localized dysfunctions may be the result of loss of function or of hyperactivity. In the first case, paralysis such as the hemiplegia following an infarct of the internal capsule is prototypical. In the second, jacksonian epilepsy with its progressively spreading clonic movements beginning in one group of muscles and spreading to others innervated by motor cortex adjacent to the primary irritative focus is illustrative. The pathological nature of the causative lesions is not generally indicated by such localized projections and may be neoplastic, infectious, metabolic, ischemic, toxic, metabolic, or of any other origin capable of destroying or irritating neurons.

Confinement within unyielding bony cases gives the brain and spinal cord limited abilities to accommodate (1) the swelling of inflammation and vasodilatation, as may occur with the hypercapnia of acute respiratory failure, or (2) the displacement of surrounding structures by mass lesions such as tumors or abscesses. For the spinal cord, the result is usually a rapidly progressive paralysis bilaterally involving those structures innervated from the segments of the cord caudal to the compressing lesion. In the brain, the principal effects, besides those that may arise from the specific location of the causative lesion, are the result of **increased intracranial pressure**. Headache, recurrent vomiting, papilledema, confusion, dementia of varying degree, and eventually coma are major symptoms.

A particularly devastating consequence of the bony excasement is **herniation**, which may occur between its compartments when the contents of one swells. The structures that pass through the incisura of the tentorium and the foramen magnum are most likely to be involved, and the former are much more important than the latter. In the midbrain, the pressure of displaced parts interferes with the blood supply of the tectum of the pons, leading to destructive **hemorrhages (Duret's lesions)**, compression and insufficiency of the posterior cerebral artery with infarction of the medial portions of the occipital lobes, and disruption of function of the abducens nerve or tracts in the cerebral peduncle opposite to the enlarging lesion. At the foramen magnum, where disproportionate pressures may arise because of masses in the cerebellum or in more superior parts of the brain or because of decreased pressure in the spinal canal subsequent to the removal of spinal fluid, the cerebellar tonsils surround and compress the medulla. This is sometimes accepted as a mechanism for central cardiorespiratory failure, but more often the true explanation will be associated with other changes in the status of the patient. A third herniation is that of the cingulate gyrus beneath the free edge of the falx, but it rarely causes significant effect by compression of the supracallosal portion of the anterior cerebral artery. Other important herniations with circulatory impairment of involved tissue may occur at openings through the skull, particularly traumatic or even surgical defects.

For the peripheral nervous system, symptoms are directly related to the function and distribution of the nerves that are involved. In many instances such as the **peripheral neuritis** of diabetes mellitus, the picture depends on some factor common to several nerves, such as the vulnerability of longer nerves to degenerations in their periphery in contrast to the preservation of function in more proximal segments and in shorter nerves. The functional disturbance and the consequent symptoms may be either sensory or motor and manifested by increased or distorted activity such as paresthesias or loss of function. Localized lesions such as tumors may be remarkably silent as far as clinically detectable effect on the involved nerve might be concerned.

The reader should refer to other sections of this book that deal with neuroanatomy, neurophysiology, and clinical neurology and neurosurgery for details in addition to this brief reference to the general symptomatology of lesions of the CNS and their causes. This will be particularly important in the review of specific diseases for which the pathological lesions are discussed.

The histological components of the nervous system are of three important categories: (1) the neurons, (2) the glia, and (3) supportive tissues such as blood vessels, connective tissue, and histiocytes. Remarkable properties of the neurons relative to

their participation in pathological processes are (1) the lack of growth or regenerative capacity of any significant degree, (2) reactivity of either hyperactivity or loss of function depending on the nature of the pathological process and manifest variability in symptoms because the normal function of particular groups of neurons may be either stimulatory or inhibitory, and (3) susceptibility or vulnerability to ischemia, atrophy, the distorted storage of metabolic products, and degeneration of intracellular components such as neurofilaments resulting in fibrillary tangles or inclusions of various types, among other things.

The principal true glial cells are **astrocytes** and **olgiodendroglia**. **Microglia** are resident representatives of the mononuclear phagocyte system, and **ependymal cells** are differentiated remnants of the original neural tubular cells whose residual function is the lining of the ventricular system. These cells, to greater or lesser degrees, have the capacity for multiplication and are the source of tumors as well as reaction to injury. The astrocytes will hypertrophy in reaction to injuries such as infarction or chronic infection. The reaction is slow and not easily evident histologically for 4 to 6 weeks. They form the equivalent of scars for the CNS. They are the source of the majority of primary tumors (60 to 70% of gliomas). Oligodendroglia are important in the formation and maintanance of myelin. As such they participate in the various conditions in which myelin is damaged by metabolic, toxic, or infectious actions, but they are otherwise not prominent in many other pathological processes and are the source of only a minority (about 3%) of glial tumors. Ependymal cells participate in few reactions but form tumors a little more frequently (approximately 5% of gliomas).

Microglia are the equivalent of histiocytes rather than being actual glia, despite their name. Augmented by bloodborne macrophages, they are the principal scavenger cells that respond to destructive lesions and are rare sources of tumors. The scanty fibroblastic reactions that may occur in wounds, abscesses, and a few other lesions are derived from the coats of blood vessels. More specific cells in the meninges that are derived, like glia and neurons, from the embryonic neuroepithelium may increase in size and number, especially with age, but are pathologically important principally for the tumors with which they are related: meningiomas and nevi or the very rare melanoma.

Congenital anomalies

The most important and frequent anomalies of the nervous system are those that derive from failure of normal closure and development of the embryonic neural tube. These range from **lumbosacral meningomyeloceles** to **anencephaly** to **craniorachischisis**. The gross lesion consists of substitution of a thin vascular membrane for the missing segment of the cord or brain. Histologically, the tissue is a mixture of connective tissue, blood vessels, glial tissue, and occasionally distorted neurons. Functional defects and symptoms depend on the segment involved and range from a motor defect of the lower extremities and pelvic musculature that can be tolerated with lumbosacral meningoceles to fatal deficiency incompatible with postnatal survival in the cases of more cranially situated major malformations. **Encephaloceles** and **nasal gliomas** (which are more choristomas than neoplasms) are examples of less severe lesions of this category.

Other malformations involve segments in which closure of the neural tube seems to have occurred but later development is faulty. A large variety of specific names are applied to these lesions depending on their location and character. **Porencephaly** is cavitation of the cerebral hemispheres with communication between the subarachnoidal space and the ventricles; **arrhinencephaly** is failure of development of the primitive olfactory portions of the brain. In **hydranencephaly**, the centrum semiovale is missing and the overlying cortex deficient. **Agyria, lissencephaly, micropolygyria, agenesis of the corpus callosum**, and a number of other conditions are of this same category. In the cerebellum, the **Arnold-Chiari malformation** is a deformity of the brain stem that accompanies spinal myeloceles and leads to ventricular obstruction and hydrocephalus, whereas the **Dandy-Walker syndrome** is a failure of development of the vermis of the cerebellum. In the spinal cord, **syringomyelia** is the presence of longitudinal cavities that may be congenital or secondary to tumors or other conditions. The lesions create a disassociated loss of pain and temperature while touch is preserved because of the neuroanatomy of the decussation of the spinothalamic tracts within the cord.

Hydrocephalus is the dilatation of a portion of the ventricular system. It often involves obstruction at a narrow segment such as the aqueduct, which may be congenitally narrowed and branched or forked. In many other instances, it is acquired and secondary to deformity of the canal by tumors or interference with the absorption of CSF due to changes in the subarachnoidal space or villi such as might follow meningitis. The CSF pressure is usually increased, but there is a syndrome of **normal-pressure hydrocephalus** associated with reversible mental disturbances that apparently is the result of a slowly progressive process that can be relieved by a ventricular shunt. **Atrophy** of the brain results in increased intracranial space that will be filled with CSF. If the deformity results principally in enlargement of the ventricles, it is called **hydrocephalus ex vacuo**. If atrophy of the cortex is more prominent, the term **external hydrocephalus** is sometimes applied. **Hydromyelia**, the corresponding process in the spinal cord, is uncommon and rarely significant.

Numerous diseases of the CNS are of a genetic nature and in that sense congenital. Most involve degeneration of neurons over a period of time, such as the loss of cells in the basal ganglia, especially the caudate nucleus, and the frontal cortex in **Huntington's chorea**, which exhibits autosomal dominant inheritance and a delayed onset of chorea and dementia in the third to fifth decades of the patient's life. Several conditions incorporate the inherited proclivity to develop benign or even malignant tumors that may involve several types of tissue as well as multiple sites. These are called **phacomatoses** and include **neurofibromatosis**, in which there are multiple tumors of Schwann's cells, increased activity of melanoblasts giving pigmented lesions of the skin (café au lait spots), and sometimes tumors of the meninges. **Von Hippel-Lindau disease** includes a special sort of tumor of blood vessels called a **hemangioblastoma**, which occurs in the cerebellum or other sites in the brain stem and spinal cord and in the retina along with a vari-

able incidence of tumors in other organs such as angioma of the liver, pheochromocytoma of the adrenal, and carcinoma of the kidney. **Tuberous sclerosis** is characterized by astrocytic tumors or malformations that incorporate malformed neurons in the cortex, astrocytic glial masses beneath the ventricular ependyma, adenoma sebaceum of the facial skin, and sometimes rhabdomyoma of the heart, angiomyolipoma of the kidney, or pancreatic cysts. Symptoms of phacomatoses are related to the localization and nature of their tumors and will involve dementia, motor deficiencies, or seizure disorders if there are abnormalities of the neurons.

Several disorders of blood vessels of the nervous system are essentially malformations. These are discussed in the paragraphs on vascular diseases.

Infections

The pathways of access for infections of the CNS are limited by the encasement of the brain and spinal cord. The principal portal is through the bloodstream, but it may be by way of involvement of adjacent structures such as the ethmoid sinuses, the mastoid cells, or destructive lesions of the skull that are usually the result of trauma. In rare instances such as rabies, the infectious agent may spread to the brain by way of the axons of peripheral nerves themselves. Within the brain and spinal cord, the involvement may spread freely within the fluid-filled pia-arachnoid and ventricles (meningitis) or may be localized within the nervous substance in the form of abscesses, granulomas, or cysts. Finally, there may be diffuse inflammation of the brain substance (encephalitis), which is often associated with primary involvement of small blood vessels and particular effect on neurons, either diffusely or with accentuation of damage to particular nuclei or structures.

Meningitis, or more properly **leptomeningitis**, is manifested by the exudation of inflammatory cells into the pia-arachoidal space. It is characteristically due to bacterial infection, and the cells are first polymorphonuclear leukocytes but will later include many mononuclear macrophages. There are, of course, exceptions. For example, *Listeria monocytogenes* and some viruses, such as that of **lymphocytic choriomeningitis**, incite principally a mononuclear reaction. Other agents such as spirochetes, fungi, and parasites can invoke a chronic meningitis and are also not likely to cause the exudation of granulocytes. Acute meningitis causes sensitivity of the nerves along blood vessels in the meninges, especially the dura, and will result in pain or reflex reaction when the meninges are stretched as by flexing the head or raising the legs. There are systemic signs of infection such as fever and tachycardia, and depression of mental function will result in the development of coma.

Various clinical features are characteristic of specific bacteria. For example, neonates fall victim to *E. coli*; infants and young children are especially susceptible to *H. influenzae,* and young adults (especially in crowded conditions that promote epidemics) to *Neisseria meningitidis*; pneumococcus may appear in either the very young or the aged and is especially apt to complicate spread as a result of sinusitis or trauma; and other forms of stretptococci spread from middle ear and mastoid infection.

Increased pressure, increased protein, decreased sugar, and pleocytosis are characteristic of the CSF in meningitis. Grossly, the brain and spinal cord are swollen, the gyri flattened, and there is congestion of the fine meningeal blood vessels and recognizably purulent exudate that collects particularly in the basal cisterns and along the larger blood vessels. Microscopically the pia-arachnoid is filled with leukocytes, typically intact and fragmented granulocytes, fibrin, and protein-rich fluid. Complete recovery may be obtained with effective antibiotics, but the more natural course is to a fatal termination or fibrous scarring in the fluid pathways and blood vessels of the pia-arachnoid, with subsequent complications of hydrocephalus and ischemic damage to the parenchyma of the brain.

Localized infections of the brain generally partake of the gross and histological character of abscesses, granulomas, or cysts in other organs, caused by the etiologic agent involved. The fibroblastic reaction with deposition of collagen in an abscess wall or about a granuloma in the brain is distinctly less than that which occurs in other tissues but is nevertheless distinct and greater than for almost any other lesion in the CNS. Symptoms tend to be those of a space-occupying lesion with local defects of function and secondary pressure effects. Fever may not be prominent, but a fatal terminal development may be the rupture of the lesion into the subarachnoidal space or a ventricle with a subsequent acute meningoventriculitis.

The bacterial etiology of abscesses depends on that of the mastoiditis, wound infection, or other lesion from which it arises, with the significant addition of organisms, including anaerobic bacteria, typical of pulmonary infections. Tubercle bacilli are the most significant cause of granulomas and the source of tuberculous meningitis by their typical rupture. Helminthic diseases such as echinococcosis and cysticercosis cause space-occupying cysts in the brain.

Fungal diseases tend to be expressed principally as a meningitis, although they probably begin as localized lesions. Of these, cryptococcosis is most important and is characterized by a dissolution of small areas of brain substance with hardly any reaction (the organism was once called *Torula histolytica*), although the most extensive part of the reaction is a chronic meningitis. In this condition, the original infection is probably in the lung and may be silent, but for other fungi such as *Histoplasma, Coccidioides, Candida, Phycomycetes,* etc. involvement of the nervous system occurs principally as part of disseminated disease.

Encephalitis, or encephalomyelitis, is usually of viral etiology. The arboviruses include agents with predominant or exclusive effects in the CNS, such as equine, St. Louis, Japanese B, and others, whereas herpes and related cytomegalic inclusion viruses are also important, the latter especially as a complication in AIDS. Rabies, poliomyelitis, and measles round out the list of most frequent and important viral encephalitides. The clinical picture is usually that of a devastating destruction of neurological function accompanied by systemic signs such as fever and sometimes by localizing symptoms that are the result of the proclivity of some viruses for specific localities in the nervous system (e.g., poliomyelitis for motor cells in the spinal cord and cortex, herpes for the temporal lobes). Grossly, the brain is swollen but may show few other indications of destruction, although the temporal necrosis in herpes simplex and the ependymitis of neonatal cytomegalic inclusion disease are examples of grossly apparent lesions.

Microscopically, the lesions are more impressive. Again, they vary with the etiologic agent to some specific extent. The cytoplasmic inclusions or Negri bodies of rabies, the type A inclusions of the herpesviruses, and the glial nodules of St. Louis and equine encephalitis are examples. Glial nodules are small collections of microglia and other mononuclear cells apparently about local areas of capillaries. They are prominent in the encephalitis of rickettsial disease such as typhus and Rocky Mountain spotted fever. The nodules are prominent features, along with giant cells probably of macrophage origin, in the encephalitis that is being increasingly recognized in fatal cases of AIDS. Some protozoal diseases, such as malaria, trypanosomiasis, and toxoplasmosis cause an encephalitis, and the latter is also increasingly recognized in association with AIDS.

Creutzfeldt-Jakob disease is a rapidly progressive dementia with spongiform degeneration of the cortex and basal ganglia. Its natural mode of transmission is essentially unknown, although cases have developed from inoculation through corneal transplantations or into primates. It and some related diseases such as kuru of the Fore tribe of New Guinea and scrapie of sheep are of great interest because their etiologic agents are apparently small proteins rather than viruses with nucleic acids. They are called prions and are resistant to most of the usual disinfective agents such as formalin but are destroyed by autoclaving, hypochlorite, and other agents that denature proteins.

There are several inflammations of the nervous system that follow other infectious diseases but are not due to the direct action of the infectious agent. The mechanism of the damage, which is usually a process destructive of myelin, is generally not understood, although some seem to involve the development of autoimmune antibodies. Landry-Guillain-Barré syndrome is predominantly a rapidly progressive motor paralysis due to axonal and myelin damage in peripheral nerves. It attained particular notoriety because of its appearance in association with a national campaign for vaccination against swine influenza. Acute disseminated encephalomyelitis is a rare sequela to measles, mumps, or chicken pox and has followed vaccination against these diseases, smallpox, rabies, and even typhoid.

Vascular disease

Brain damage from vascular disease is nearly always part of systemic conditions, of which arteriosclerosis and hypertension are the most important. It occurs as a result of rupture or occlusion of a vessel. The hemorrhages that occur in hypertensives are usually massive infusions of blood into the substance of a cerebral hemisphere, nearly always in the region of the lentiform nucleus but elsewhere in a hemisphere or into the cerebellum or pons in 10 to 20% of cases. Progression to death is usually a matter of hours or a day or so. Pathological examination is rarely successful in demonstrating involvement of a particular artery. The hemorrhage may rupture into the ventricle but rarely through the cortex. Few more than 10% of patients survive. Another group of massive hemorrhages arise from rupture of a small arteriovenous malformation that may be demonstrable clinically by arteriography and by careful dissection in fatal cases. These patients are not as apt to be hypertensive, and the location of the lesion is more frequently in sites other than the basal ganglia, with a greater tendency to rupture into the subarachnoidal space to some degree. Of the other vascular malformations, **cavernous angiomas** rarely bleed and **capillary hemangiomas** are never the source of significant hemorrhage.

Saccular aneurysms occur on the larger arteries in the subarachnoidal space and are the cause of almost all massive subarachnoidal hemorrhages. Ninety percent arise at branches of vessels derived from the internal carotid artery and rarely more than 2 or 3 cm from the circle of Willis. The etiology of these aneurysms is uncertain, although they develop at sites of congenital malformation of the arterial wall and are associated to some degree with hypertension. The bleeding is usually a massive effusion into the subarachnoidal space but can dissect into the cerebral substance.

In conditions associated with bacteremia and embolization, such as infectious endocarditis, local infection of an arterial wall may occur with the development of a "mycotic" aneurysm and rupture. These lesions are distributed more widely than the typical locations of either saccular aneurysms or hypertensive cerebral hemorrhages.

Ischemic lesions are associated with the narrowing of arteries by arteriosclerosis and the formation of thrombi. Temporary decrease in flow as may occur during a hypotensive episode is often a precipitating cause of damage in a vascular field served by a narrowed but otherwise patent vessel. Cerebral vascular spasm can be demonstrated by arteriography and may play a part in decreasing local blood flow below a critical level. The principal vascular lesion may be in the carotid artery in the neck rather than intracranial. Emboli from the heart or from ulcerated plaques in the aorta or carotid artery may occur. Whatever the mechanism of decreased or interrupted blood flow, the effect is that of ischemia with destruction of neurons, especially in the field served by the vessel. In cases of the involvement of very small vessels, the damaged area may be simply one of loss of neurons and focal hypertrophy of astrocytes, forming a small solid scar interrupting the microscopic architecture of the cortex or a nucleus. Such are the lesions of **"little strokes"** (transient ischemic attacks [TIAs]) that cause usually transient confusion and a minor loss of functions, usually in elderly patients. Larger lesions result in greater defects, which may be more clearly demonstrated by neurological examination and from which recovery, although usually to some degree, may not be complete. Edema without neuronal death in peripheral portions of the focus of ischemia is responsible for the extent of initial symptoms from which recovery may occur. These infarcts resolve over a period of months by liquefactive necrosis into cystic areas of gliosis in the white matter and collapse of cortex, from which the neurons are completely lost. If the initial lesion is large enough, there may be a fatal outcome, and a large area of the brain, such as that served by the middle cerebral artery, may be softened and almost fluid, a condition called **encephalomalacia**.

Vascular disease of the spinal cord is not common. Vascular malformations bleed, and occlusion of a major spinal artery is apt to result in destruction of a segment of the cord with consequent loss of function in all the involved tracts. This is called **transverse myelitis** despite its not being an inflammation at all. In peripheral nerves, diffuse disease of small vessels, such

as occurs in diabetes mellitus, results in segmental demyelination and distorted function, especially sensory. Again, this is termed "peripheral neuritis" without being an inflammation, but modern practice favors **peripheral neuropathy**.

Demyelinating disease

Demyelinating diseases are assigned to this category because their most prominent feature is loss or poor development of myelin. Their pathogenesis is poorly understood, and etiologies are unknown or uncertain. Some may be toxic, as **central pontine myelinolysis** was originally considered to be of alcoholic etiology. Others such as the **leukodystrophies** have been demonstrated to be associated with an inborn error of metabolism, and the **disseminated perivascular encephalitides** show much evidence of autoimmune reaction. The study of most of these uncommon diseases is so specialized that they are not generally considered appropriate subjects for general licensing examinations. For that reason, only the most frequent and important of these diseases is mentioned here.

Multiple sclerosis (disseminated sclerosis) is characteristically a disease of young adults. It is a little more frequent in women and distinctly more frequent in northern climates than in southern. The clinical course consists of the repeated onset of neurological deficits of many types, indicating that the characteristic lesions have developed in unpredictable sequence in widely dispersed regions of the CNS. The optic tracts, cerebellum, and spinal cord are sites where involvement is often appreciated, but the periventricular white matter is almost constantly involved on postmortem examination. Scotomata, diplopia, paresthesias, tremors, speech difficulty, and many other disabilities may initiate relapses. The course is characteristically one of an attack followed by reacquisition of most lost function and then another attack with more loss of function, with a gradual progression in the amount of permanent disability. It may be prolonged over 20 years with long periods of inactivity, but about 10% of cases are continuously progressive, and some may be fulminant. The lesions consist of pinkish blot-like foci in the white matter that on microscopic examination show active or old destruction of myelin sheaths. Axons are first preserved, but they are gradually lost, and an astrocytic gliosis slowly permeates the area of destruction. Multiplicity and variety of site and size are pathognomic, but symmetry can sometimes be distinct. Paralysis and urinary tract infection are usual late complications. The etiology remains unknown, although there are repeated observations of direct or indirect association with infections or infectious agents.

Degenerative diseases

This category is again a collection of relatively rare diseases that have been the subject of very specialized study and are hardly appropriate for this book or for general licensing examinations. Many of its members have a strong hereditary, or at least familial, character. Quite a few have been recognized to be associated with inborn errors of metabolism and with disease in other organs. **Wilson's disease** involves abnormal accumulation of copper, usually associated with decreased ceruloplasmin and cirrhosis. **Amaurotic familial idiocy** (Tay-Sachs disease) is due to a deficiency of hexosaminidase A with accumulation of ganglioside in neurons. **Gaucher's disease** shows accumulation of its characteristic cerebroside in neurons as well as in the systemic reticuloendothelial system. Three diseases of this category are of significant incidence: Alzheimer's disease, parkinsonism, and amyotrophic lateral sclerosis.

Alzheimer's disease is a gradual and generalized deterioration of cerebral neurons. It was originally described as a dementia beginning in or prior to the sixth decade of life, but it is now recognized as indistinguishable from similar disease of later onset, although the cases in older patients are sometimes designated as senile dementia, Alzheimer type. The clinical progression is gradual, beginning with loss of recent memory and progressing to deterioration of all mentation and loss of motor coordination and function. It may run a course of 2 to 10 years. The brain is diffusely atrophic, with hydrocephalus ex vacuo. Microscopically, the lesions are an accumulation of irregular tangled masses of neurofibrils in neurons of the cortex, plaques of amyloid fibrils and argyrophilic masses in the neurophil, intraneuronal bodies called granulovacuolar bodies, and Hirano bodies in the dendrites. The hippocampus is a site of particular involvement, and recent studies emphasize the early involvement of the nucleus basalis of Meynert. None of these changes is specific or pathognomic. The differences between the lesions of Alzheimer's disease and changes in the brains of other aged and senile patients is largely a matter of degree and localization of the most intense damage. In some cases, there is a familial occurrence, and a genetic defect has been located on chromosome 21.

Parkinsonism is a syndrome rather than a specific disease, as it occurs in several conditions that have in common destruction in the dopaminergic neurons of the corpus striatum and globus pallidus. The functional deficiencies are pill-rolling tremor, akinesia, cogwheel rigidity, and related motor disorders of coordination. Grossly, no lesions may be apparent, or there may be small old infarcts if the syndrome is related to that etiology. Sometimes depigmentation of the substantia nigra can be appreciated. Microscopic changes may involve disruption of the pigmented cells of the substantia nigra, the presence of cytoplasmic inclusions (Lewy bodies) in remaining cells of the substantia nigra, or changes that are essentially those of depopulation of neurons in the other sites of principal involvement mentioned above. Neurofibrillary tangles similar to those in Alzheimer's disease may be found. Of particular interest has been the development of the syndrome in some individuals who engaged in the recreational use of "tailored drugs," resulting in permanent damage to the dopaminergic neurons of the basal ganglia. In many cases of the naturally occurring syndrome, considerable clinical improvement follows the administration of levodopa, a precursor of dopamine.

Amyotrophic lateral sclerosis (Lou Gehrig's disease) is a progressive degeneration and loss of central motor neurons of unknown etiology. Some atypical cases among natives of Guam appear to be infectious. It is better called **motor neuron disease**, for there is a constellation of variants that involve spinal anterior horn cells at different times of life, motor cortex neurons, motor neurons of the brain stem, and the lateral corticospinal tracts. The gross changes in the CNS are rarely striking, but there may be appreciable shrinkage of the anterior gray horns of the spinal cord, thinning of the cerebral motor cortex, and sometimes a chalky whiteness of the lateral funiculus of the spinal cord. The latter is due to demyelinization and gliosis of the corticospinal tracts and justifies the name "lateral sclerosis." Microscopically, the neurons are lost without reaction except for some degree of astrocytic gliosis. Clinically and anatomically, the degree and sites of greatest involvement are variable. The classic symptoms are those of gradual and progressive denervation of skeletal muscle with the development of fasciculations, tremors, weakness, and finally paralysis. The disease became infamous when the baseball great Lou Gehrig fell victim.

Nutritional, metabolic, and genetic disorders

As was noted above, there are many hereditary diseases of the nervous system that involve recognized inborn errors of metabolism. These include **lipid storage diseases; mucopolysaccharidoses; amino acid disturbances**, of which **phenylketonuria** may be the most widely recognized; **glycogen storage diseases**; and **mineral storage diseases** such as Wilson's. In most of these, the gross pathological changes are subtle, inconstant, or nonexistent. Microscopically, accumulations of abnormal metabolites, particularly in neurons, are the hallmarks. These can be identified with greater or less success by the use of histochemical methods, but chemical analysis is the definitive determination.

Deficiencies of several vitamins have direct or indirect effects on the nervous system. **Thiamine deficiency**, particularly as it occurs in chronic alcoholics, results in **Wernicke's polioencephalitis** that is associated with **Korsakoff's psychosis**. The lesion is seen as an erythema and interstitial hemorrhages in the region of the hypothalamus, the mamillary bodies, and about the aqueduct. Microscopically, the most prominent change is the thickening and endothelial hyperplasia in small blood vessels along with the interstitial hemorrhage that results in hemosiderosis. The disorder can be so acute that the dementia and ocular paralysis progress to coma and death. A less severe manifestation of thiamine deficiency in alcoholics is a **peripheral neuropathy**.

Deficiency of cobalamin, or vitamin B_{12}, will lead to **combined system disease** that is so called because it is a demyelination of the posterior and lateral funiculi of the spinal cord. The symptoms are those of proprioceptive deficiency and paralysis. The progress of the loss can be arrested by correcting the vitamin deficiency, but repair of the lesions does not occur. The changes are a destruction and loss of myelin and axons in the involved tracts. A spongy appearance develops in the demyelinated areas, but there is little cellular reaction.

The changes in other metabolic disorders with serious effects on the CNS are often nonspecific or inapparent. **Niacin and riboflavin deficiencies** cause demyelination, particularly in peripheral nerves. The unconjugated bilirubin of **erythroblastosis** causes neuronal necrosis, particularly in the basal ganglia and cerebellum. **Lead poisoning** causes edema of the brain, and intranuclear inclusions may be found in neurons as they are in hepatic cells. **Hypertensive encephalopathy** is more a physiological reaction than metabolic and is principally diffuse edema that may be accompanied by small hemorrhages and ischemic foci.

Some genetic diseases, especially **Down's syndrome**, cannot be recognized as having an anatomic change that is in any way indicative of the neurophysiological deficiency, although various subtle and inconstant alterations have been reported in several series of cases.

Neoplasia

Primary tumors of the CNS comprise slightly less than 10% of all tumors, whereas the experience with metastatic tumors seems to vary widely but is probably at least half as frequent as primary tumors as a cause of clinical disease. **Metastastic tumors** increase in incidence the longer the clinical course of a primary carcinoma, and the nervous system involvement in such cases tends to be eclipsed by the other features of the case. Carcinoma of the lung is the most common primary source of metastatic carcinoma of the brain, and the breast is second. Almost any other type of malignancy can also be the primary source, but renal cell carcinoma, melanoma, and carcinomas of the GI tract are most notorious. Metastatic tumors are more common in adults, and the sites are dependent on the size and vascularity of the target areas of the nervous system. The cerebellum is consequently involved in 10 to 15% of cases, quite in contradistinction to the absence of gliomas of that organ in adults. In children, **retinoblastoma, neuroblastoma,** and leukemia are principal causes of metastatic involvement.

Lymphomas occur as both metastases and primary tumors. The former are often predominantly in the dura or leptomeninges and have probably spread from adjacent disease in the vertebrae or skull and are part of generalized systemic disease of the various types of this tumor. Primary lymphomas are also typed according to the classification used for tumors elsewhere in the body. Most of the tumors that can be typed by the use of immunologic cell surface markers are of B cells, but half or so cannot be successfully classified by such techniques. Primary lymphomas occur as tumors principally in the cerebral hemispheres of adults, but it is of particular interest that increased numbers have recently been recognized in patients of altered immunologic status such as those with renal transplants or AIDS.

Tumors that arise from cells unique to the nervous system constitute a special category in the study of cancer. They are malignant in their growth and effect on the patient but do not metastasize outside the nervous system. Their symptoms share the phenomena of space-occupying lesions and increased intracranial pressure, but their sites of origin and age incidence are characteristically associated with their cell types.

Grossly, the tumors may be soft or firm, gray or pink masses that may be uniform or may contain foci of hemorrhage and necrosis. The latter are signs of more rapid growth that outstrips the blood supply and are therefore indications of higher malignancy. The borders may appear to be diffuse and indefinite or sometimes sharp and clear. The latter may occur in the more malignant tumors because the speed of growth compresses surrounding brain, but there is never a true plane of cleavage and operative experience proves that gliomas cannot, for all practical purposes, be completely excised. Microscopically, the tumors are classified by the types of cells that can be recognized. The degree of malignancy in some types is judged by the amount of anaplasia, the evidence of necrosis, the stimulation of blood vessels to endothelial proliferation, and evidence of mitotic activity. Between tumor types, however, the application of such criteria of malignancy is not always comparable: Medulloblastomas, for instance, are quite malignant in their behavior but show few of the criteria of malignant growth characteristic of glioblastomas.

The **glioblastoma** is a highly malignant tumor of astrocytes. On a scale of I to IV, they are III and IV. The constitute about half of all gliomas and are characteristically tumors of the cerebral hemispheres in adults. The less malignant **astrocytomas** are only half as frequent but have about the same incidences. A special case is a slow-growing, relatively benign astrocytoma of the cerebellum in children that is often associated with the formation of cysts. It is so distinct in its biologic and histological characteristics as to justify separate classification. Sometimes called **pilocytic juvenile astrocytoma,** this lesion may have a long course and can apparently be cured by excision in a few instances. The more common astrocytoma of adults has a mean prognosis of 2 to 6 years, whereas the malignant glioblastomas lead to death in 6 months to a year, with little response to even the most vigorous therapy.

Oligodendrogliomas are rather rare tumors, predominantly of the cerebral hemispheres of adults. They account for about 3% of gliomas and are of intermediate malignant prognosis. **Ependymomas** are a little more frequent and variable in both their sites of occurrence and malignancy. In children, they occur as one of the three cerebellar tumors, along with astrocytomas and medulloblastomas. In adults, they are hemispheric tumors. Their grade varies from relatively benign to quite malignant.

Medulloblastomas are tumors of primitive cells that are now considered to present potential for differentiation into either neuronal elements or glia, although most tumors are composed so completely of small, dark, round cells that recognition of these potentials can only be made by special and intensive study. They account for about 3% of intracranial tumors and are now included in a class of **primitive neuroectodermal tumors** that includes differently differentiated tumors that have formerly been referred to by other names suggestive of a primitive embryologic origin. The less typical tumors may occur in sites other than the cerebellum and in patients other than children. Growth of the tumor is usually rapid, but intensive therapy, particularly with irradiation, will give encouraging results.

Tumors of Schwann's cells occur on peripheral nerves and on those portions of spinal or cranial nerves with peripheral-type myelination within the skull or vertebral canal. Their cells contain the S-100 protein that is specific for an origin from neuroepithelium. The most important sites are the eighth (auditory) nerve and the long roots of the spinal nerves. They are classified as **schwannomas,** or **neurilemomas,** when they have characteristic histological structures called Antoni A and B substance and Verocay bodies. They are encapsulated benign tumors that grow on the side of nerves. On the eighth nerve, they and meningomas are the principal posterior fossa tumors of adults and cause tinnitus followed by signs of vestibular disturbance and deafness and then increased intracranial pressure. They tend to occur singly but may occur in the phakomatosis of **von Recklinghausen's disease.** The more typical tumor of that disorder is the **neurofibroma** that is also derived from Schwann's cells but infiltrates the nerve diffusely, does not have the characteristic histological structures of the schwannoma, and is associated with the occurrence of sarcomas of similar origin.

Meningiomas are the third most frequent primary intracranial tumors. Although tumors of cells of various types such as lymphocytes, osteoblasts, etc. very rarely occur in the meninges and are included in the general classification as meningioma, the characteristic tumor owes its essential properties to its derivation from the arachnoidal cap cell, which is of neural crest origin. Histologically, four patterns are recognized: meningothelial, fibroblastic, transitional, and angioblastic. Grossly, the tumors tend to occur where there are normal arachnoidal villi (i.e., along the sagittal sinus, on the falx cerebri, along the sphenoid ridge, in the olfactory groove, and in the cerebellopontile angle), with a fair number lying laterally over the cerebral hemispheres at some distance from the sagittal sinus itself. The location is one of the most important factors that influence the course of this essentially benign tumor. About 10% have some cellular irregularity and even mitotic figures, which forecast a greater tendency for recurrence after surgical removal. In all, about 15% recur because of the impossibility of adequate removal or heightened growth potential. In the histological patterns, the angioblastic is more often indicative of a poor prognosis. The whorled arrangement of cells is a highly characteristic histological feature, and small, spherical, laminated calcified bodies called psammomas occur in many tumors. A very interesting feature of meningiomas is that 90% are reported to have an abnormality involving chromosome number 22. True sarcomas do occur but are very rare.

MUSCLES

The histology and physiology of muscle are topics that are of very specialized importance for relatively few diseases. Skeletal muscle has two types of fibers: (1) the slow, red fibers that have predominantly oxidative metabolism and are rich in mitochondria and myoglobin and poor in phosphorylase and adenosine triphosphatase (ATPase) and (2) the fast, white fibers with glycolytic metabolism, fewer mitochondria, less myoglobin, and rich phosphorylase and ATPase. Special histochemical techniques that demonstrate phosphorylase under different conditions of pH are useful in studying the distribution and changes in proportion of these fibers for the diagnosis of several degenerative disorders: **polymyositis** is characterized early by perifascicular atrophy of both types of fibers, **myotonic dystrophy** and the **myopathy of rheumatoid arthritis** by involvement principally of slow (type I) fibers. The small, angulated fibers in groups (fasicular atrophy) of **motor neuron disease** and the subsequent reinnervation with groups of fibers of the same type are well demonstrated by these methods.

Congenital diseases of muscles are insignificant and consist mostly of the failure of development of a muscle or group of muscles. Hereditary disease, on the other hand, is most important and manifested in the **muscular dystrophies** and **congenital myopathies**. The former are classified by their typical distribution of the principally involved muscles (e.g., lower limb girdle in **Duchenne's type**) as well as the modes of inheritance—sex-linked or autosomal dominant or recessive. The histology of the dystrophies generally is not specific for the various types. However, the congenital myopathies have a variety of relatively specific histological changes (e.g., rod bodies, abnormal mitochondria, glycogen storage), although their dysfunctions are all quite similar and are principally a generalized hypotonia that results in the **floppy infant syndrome**.

Inflammatory muscular disease is of two types: (1) that due to specific bacterial, viral, or parasitic etiologies (e.g., **abscesses, Coxsackie A and B, trichinosis**) and (2) idiopathic or possibly autoimmune. In the latter, **polymyositis** is most important. It has a wide age distribution, may be associated with skin manifestations (when it is known as **dermatomyositis**), and has an interesting association with coincident visceral carcinomas, especially in patients in their 60s or older. **Myositis ossificans** is a peculiar degeneration of muscle with the focal replacement by fibrous tissue that undergoes ossification. It occurs in two forms: (1) a progressive, probably hereditary disease of children and (2) posttraumatic, particularly following hemorrhage into muscle.

The specific malignant tumors of striated muscle are **rhabdomyosarcomas**. They are one of the most common soft-tissue tumors of children, presenting as embryonal and alveolar types. The pleomorphic type with typical giant cells is a tumor of adults, whereas the botryoid is a rhabdomyosarcoma, usually of embryonal type, that protrudes into a cavity such as that of the uterus or the nasal passages. These are highly malignant tumors, but improved radiotherapy and chemotherapy as well as surgery have raised prognosis to the level of 85% survival. Other soft-tissue tumors such as **liposarcomas** and **osteosarcomas** occur in muscle. **Desmoid tumors, nodular fasciitis,** and **palmar fibromatosis** occur in muscles but are composed of essentially benign fibroblasts, although their growth can be aggressive and persistent.

EYES

Ophthalmologic pathology, like ophthalmology itself, is a highly specialized science, and only a few of its aspects can be mentioned for examination review. The eye has its share of congenital malformations and hereditary diseases. It is involved in syndromes that involve other organs, such as the vascular malformations of **Sturge-Weber syndrome** and glial hamartomas on the retina in **tuberous sclerosis. Retrolental fibroplasia** is a condition that develops in premature neonates, not because of heredity but because of the susceptibility of the vessels of the premature retina to high levels of oxygen that might be administered because of the respiratory insufficiency. Vascularization of the retina is first inhibited, and then there is pathological neovascularization and organization in the retina and finally retinal detachment.

Various infectious diseases may afflict the eyes. **Toxoplasmosis** and **cytomegalic inclusion virus disease** have recently received much attention in association with AIDS. In medical history, **sympathetic ophthalmia** is of great importance as it was one of the very first recognized examples of autoimmunity. When the natural isolation of the uveal tract is broken by trauma and inflammation, antibodies develop that then create destrictuve inflammation in the other eye, often with resultant blindness.

The eye is importantly involved secondarily to systemic disease. Retinal changes in **diabetes** are the major causes of blindness in the middle decades. They consist of capillary microangiopathy similar to that in the kidneys and elsewhere, saccular microaneurysms, and hemorrhages and exudates in the retina. In **hypertension**, retinal changes seen through the ophthalmoscope are basic to recognition of the malignant phase of the disease. They consist of attenuated retinal arterioles, focal retinal ischemia, flame-shaped hemorrhages, and cotton-wool spots that occur in the ganglion and nerve fiber layer. The latter are actually focal ischemic necrosis with a characteristic debris called cytoid bodies.

The principal tumors of the eye are the **melanoma** that occurs especially in white adults and the **retinoblastoma** that is a disease of children. The melanoma grows relatively slowly and metastasizes late. When it occurs in the iris, it is especially curable, perhaps because it is recognized early. There are histological patterns of spindle and epithelioid cells, and predominance of the former is associated with a more favorable prognosis than the latter. Retinoblastoma is a tumor with many similarities to neuroblastoma. It occurs in very young children and is thought by some to be congenital. Some have been shown to secrete catecholamines, qualifying them as **APUD cells**. The majority of cases are sporadic but seem to represent a mutation, as the condition may be passed genetically. In the familial cases, 90% are bilateral, 50% of offspring will develop the tumors, and there is often a deletion on the long arm of chromosome 13. The tumors are well differentiated and histologically are characterized by regular, small cells that are frequently arranged in well-differentiated rosettes. With modern therapy, cure rates of 90% can be achieved, but survivors bear the burden of their heredity, even if the patient's tumor was spontaneous, and an increased incidence of later osteosarcoma.

EAR, NOSE, AND THROAT

The midline of the face and the nose is the seat of a number of congenital malformations related to the embryonic fissures of that region. The ear may also be deformed, especially in several syndromes associated with chromosomal abnormalities. **Thyroglossal cysts** and **branchial cleft cysts** are thought to originate in embryonic malformations, although they often do not become manifest until the second or third decade of life. Each has a characteristic histological structure.

The common **carcinomas** of this region are squamous and especially in the larynx are associated with chronic irritation such as that due to excessive smoking. The latter show chronic **keratosis** and **carcinoma in situ** that apparently precede the invasive malignancy. Another special tumor of note is the **verrucous carcinoma**, which is nonmetastasizing despite its proliferative redundancy and local invasiveness. The nose is afflicted with a unique tumor, the **olfactory neuroblastoma**, derived from the reserve cells of the olfactory epithelium and much like other neuroblastomas except for a less malignant growth potential. The nasopharynx is the seat of **malignant lymphomas** as well as poorly differentiated squamous tumors mixed with lymphocytes formerly called **lymphoepitheliomas** and characteristically quite malignant. A particularly unusual tumor is the **midline malignant reticulosis**, which often is a challenging histological diagnosis because it is overlaid by inflammation and granulation tissue.

Another malignant midline condition of this region is **Wegener's granulomatosis**, a condition apparently of auto-immune etiology and malignant course. It is essentially a vasculitis that may or may not be accompanied by a granulomatous reaction. It may also affect the lungs, kidneys, and other viscera.

Tumor-like conditions are **juvenile laryngeal papillomatosis**, which is an epithelial overgrowth due to a virus of the papova group and capable of being so extensive as to cause respiratory obstruction in the larynx; the **vocal nodule**, which is a localized, degenerative proliferation of submucosal connective tissue of the vocal cords ("singer's node"); and **nasal polyps**, which are edmatous enlargements of submucosal tissue with eosinophilic infiltrations and overlying epithelial hyperplasia that are the result of chronic allergic rhinitis.

Pathology of the inner ear is most often concerned with infection. **Otitis media** is a purulent inflammation due to pneumococcus, *H. influenzae*, or beta-hemolytic streptococci in most instances. It may lead to **osteomyelitis** of the mastoid cells, infected thrombosis or emboli of the emissary veins, and **brain abscess. Serous otitis media** is a sterile, hydropic inflammation that follows infection or an allergic response. **Keratomas** (sometimes called **cholesteatomas**) are keratotic accumulations due to epithelial stimulation by inflammation and sequestration. Of the degenerative diseases of the ear, **otosclerosis** is of interest because of its hereditary nature, its early onset in the third decade, and its importance as the cause of deafness in early adulthood. The pathological process is one of fibrous adhesion of the foot plate of the stapes to the oval window followed by osteosclerosis of the surrounding temporal bone and the foot plate, but not the other parts of the stapes.

SKIN, MUSCLE, JOINTS, AND BONE

SKIN

Dermatopathology, like dermatology itself, is a science of precise classification and Latin nomenclature. The specialized classifications are beyond the purpose of this presentation, but there are a number of conditions of frequent incidence and considerable general clinical importance.

Congenital and hereditary diseases

Several diseases of the skin are hereditary, and some are so dominant as to develop soon after birth although not truly congenital. The various forms of **ichthyosis** are characterized by hyperkeratosis and fissuring of the epidermis and microscopically by hyperkeratosis of the superficial layer and various changes in the deeper layers, including loss of the granular layer in **dominant ichthyosis vulgaris**, with rapid keratinization and intracellular edema and ballooning of squamous cells in **dominant ichthyosis congenita**. A hyperplasia of elastic fibers in the dermis characterizes **cutis hyperelastica (Ehlers-Danlos syndrome)**, the "rubber man" disease. The underlying defect seems to be in any of a number of biochemical processes involved in the formation of elastin and collagen and even platelets. Abnormalities of other structures such as the joints, sclerae, trachea, and arteries sometimes accompany the skin disease. **Pseudoxanthoma elasticum** is another hereditary disorder of elastic tissue. In this the abnormal tissue appears as plaques on the neck and areas of skin folds such as the axilla. The elastic fibers in these lesions undergo calcification and occasionally incite the development of granulomas. Abnormalities of pigmentation include the **Peutz-Jeghers syndrome**, in which melanotic spots are present on the lips, oral mucosa, and digits in association with polyps of the small intestine. The **vitiliginous loss of pigment** may sometimes be segmental and follow the distribution of a nerve.

Infections

The catalog of infectious diseases that involve the skin is too exhaustive to be repeated here. Bacteria, viruses, spirochetes, fungi, and protozoa are etiologic agents. The skin manifestations may be the most prominent and characteristic features of systemic infection, as in measles, or may be almost the only lesions, as in most infections with herpes simplex. The dermatologic lesion may be considerably modified by immune phenomena of the primary disease, as is recognizable in the manifold dermal lesions of tuberculosis. In many other conditions, such as that of **common acne**, the bacterial involvement may be a purely secondary complication or may play a part in development of more advanced lesions after a fundamental alteration has occurred, illustrated in the example of acne by the growth of lipolytic *Propionibacterium acnes* in the sebaceous glands prepared by the special physiology of adolescence.

Autoimmune and hypersensitivity diseases

The skin participates prominently in many types of allergic and immune phenomena. Conditions considered autoimmune include **systemic lupus erythematosus**, in which a rash develops on the face (butterfly distribution) and chest, with edema of the dermis and liquefactive degeneration in the basal cell layer of the epidermis. The skin in **progressive systemic sclerosis (scleroderma)** exhibits atrophy of the epidermis and its appendages and a thickening of the collagen of the dermis, although neither chemical analysis nor a search for antibodies in the skin elucidates the mechanism by which that organ participates in the systemic disease.

Pemphigus is a primary skin disease with several types in which there is the development of widespread bullae of the skin and mucous membranes. These bullae are fluid-filled spaces that split the epidermis just above the basal layer by dissolution of squamous cells (acantholysis). Antibodies adherent to the intercellular bridges can be demonstrated by IgG immunofluorescence. Treatment by immunosuppression has reversed the former almost total mortality in this condition.

Erythema multiforme is a manifestation of hypersensitivity to various foreign materials including drugs and fungi. The histology is as variable as the clinical aspects and includes various cellular infiltrates in the subepidermis. **Erythema nodosum** occurs in patients with tuberculosis and Crohn's disease, as well as in response to drugs including sulfonamides and penicillin. The lesions are predominantly on the anterior aspects of the legs and are necrotizing vasculitis surrounded by granulomatous reaction in the panniculus or subdermis. **Urticaria** is a focal, intense edema in the dermis accompanied by itching. It is a direct response to histamine, and through the release of that substance locally or even distantly the lesions develop in response to drugs, allergenic foods, infections, ultraviolet light, or emotional disturbance.

Neoplasia

Malignant tumors of the skin are the most common of all cancers. Each year enough skin cancers develop in the United States so that one person in five would be affected if the distribution were uniform for all ages and population groups. Probably half the population will eventually develop one or more skin cancers. About a third are **squamous carcinomas**, a bit more than half are **basal cell carcinomas**, only a fiftieth (2%) are **malignant melanomas**, and the remainder are of a wide variety, including **lymphomas** and recently the notorious **Kaposi's sarcoma** that has complicated about a fifth of cases of AIDS. Fortunately, more than 90% of the squamous and basal cell carcinomas are curable by local excision and even the melanomas are cured in 100% of the less advanced cases and almost half the cases with tumors of the highest stages.

Of the three principal types of tumors, there are benign and malignant varieties that seem to cause confusion on both clinical and histological bases. These are (1) basaloid cell tumors that have benign forms called **seborrheic keratosis** or **verruca senilis** and a malignant form called **basal cell carcinoma** that has invasive capabilities despite its inability, for all practical purposes, to metastasize, (2) squamous cell tumors of which the benign, although premalignant, form is the **senile** or **solar keratosis**, and (3) pigment cell tumors that include the **benign nevi** and the **malignant melanomas** as well as some intermediate, premalignant types such as the **lentigo maligna**.

Seborrheic keratosis occurs principally on the forehead and trunk of older patients. It is a raised plaque, often pigmented rather darkly, that has a greasy texture. It consists of elevated, broad areas of acanthosis with the cells predominately small, dark, irregularly pigmented, and lacking the clear intercellular bridges of pure squamous cells. The papillomatous masses surround islands or "pearls" of retained keratin. The basement membranes are smooth and intact. The **basal cell carcinoma** occurs mostly on the upper face, including the upper lip, of middle-aged or older patients, especially blonds and persons exposed to much sunlight. The proliferating basaloid cells undermine the epidermis at the edges of the lesion, and there is a tendency for central ulceration that is the basis for the name "**rodent ulcer**." Left unattended, the lesion will erode deeply into cartilage and bone, causing disfiguring destruction. Very rare examples of distant metastases have been reported, but the early lesions especially are readily eradicated by excision or irradiation. Some tumors contain foci of squamous cells and are labeled **basosquamous** or **transitional**, with an implication of increased aggressiveness, but the evidence for greater malignancy is equivocal. Basal cell carcinomas are the most common of all malignant tumors of the skin.

The **solar** or **senile keratosis** is a plaque that occurs on skin exposed excessively to sunlight, including the hands as well as the face, neck, and especially the lower lip. It is characterized by dyskeratosis as well as acanthosis, and the lower margins in histological sections are frayed and resemble invasion into the underlying dermis that is usually infiltrated by some amount of lymphocytes and monocytes. Certainly, squamous carcinomas occur in the same patients and at the same locations, and it is generally considered that the keratosis is premalignant, although the associated squamous carcinomas rarely metastasize. These lesions also occur in response to exposure to x-radiation and chemicals such as arsenicals. **Squamous** or **epidermoid carcinomas** occur in the same types of patients. Their growth is more aggressive, ulceration is common, and metastasis occurs, although not frequently (2% of cases), as long as the lesion arises from the skin proper. With involvement of the mucous membranes, including the vermillion border of the lower lip, or in the scars of old burns or on the genitalia, the prognosis is less favorable and more aggressive therapy is required.

Nevus is a generic term for stable, nonneoplastic, presumably congenital lesions of the skin, but it is most commonly applied to tumors that are local masses of melanotic cells. These lesions may occur at any site and have a variety of appearances to which specific names are applied. The essential feature is the presence of melanocytes, or nevus cells, in the subepidermal connective tissue or the lower layers of the epidermis. When the cells are exclusively in subepidermal nests, the lesions are benign. Involvement of the basal layer of the epidermis is called **junctional change** and is associated with a low incidence of malignant transformation. The **compound nevus** has both conjunctional change and underlying nests of nevus cells, and it is in the recognition of atypia and invasiveness of the cells of these nests or pegs that a diagnosis of malignant melanoma is made. **Malignant melanomas** occur in several growth patterns or types: (1) nodular, (2) superficial spreading, (3) lentigo maligna, and (4) acral-lentiginous, each with characteristic prognostic implications. The most important criterion of prognosis is the depth of invasion, which is reported as being at one of five levels that vary from confinement of the melanoma cells to the epidermis to invasion of subcutaneous fat but is more meaningful when measured in millimeters below the stratum granulosum. The more superficial tumors are easily cured by excision, but the deeper lesions carry a mortality of 50% or more despite the most aggressive surgical and other therapies.

JOINTS

There are a number of conditions that can be considered congenital deformities or diseases of joints, such as the various forms of **talipes**, the complex deformities of **arthrogryposis multiplex**, and the abnormal mobility of **cutis hyperelastica (Ehlers-Danlos syndrome)**. As many as 6% of newborns exhibit some degree of abnormalities of joints, but most are corrected by normal growth. The most important diseases of joints are the inflammations.

Arthritis

The major forms of arthritis are (1) **degenerative**—osteoarthritis, posttraumatic, neuropathic; (2) **infectious**—pyogenic, tuberculous; (3) **idiopathic**, possibly immunologic—rheumatoid, rheumatic fever; and (4) **metabolic**—gout.

Degenerative arthritis is essentially a wear-and-tear phenomenon, although from case to case there are signs of the interplay of inflammatory, metabolic, or other factors. **Osteo-**

arthritis is characteristically a disease of older persons that involves the larger, weight-bearing joints. The early lesion is a fraying and splitting of epiphyseal cartilage followed by erosion and then a reaction of overgrowth (eburnation) of the underlying bone. The latter reaction may extend laterally to form spurs or lips at the edge of the joint surfaces. Those that form on the distal interphalangeal joints are called **Heberden's nodes**, and involvement of these small joints has a hereditary characteristic. The joints are painful and motion becomes limited, but fusion does not occur. Trauma that disrupts the normal surfaces of a joint will initiate the process in younger patients and in joints less commonly involved in the naturally occurring disease. The loss of proprioception in degenerative disease of nerves such as **tabes dorsalis** and some cases of **peripheral neuritis** is thought to lead to repeated small traumas from which reflexes to pain and other sensation protect normal joints and the joint erodes and degenerates. **Charcot's joint**, which is usually an involvement of one knee but can occur in other sites, is the paradigm.

Infectious arthritis results from many different etiologic agents, including bacteria, viruses, and fungi. The agent may be introduced into the joint by open trauma or by way of the bloodstream. Factors that determine the occurrence of arthritis in the course of various diseases or the sometimes characteristic involvement of a particular joint are unknown (e.g., the occurrence of purulent involvement of the sternoclavicular joint in some cases of **gonorrheal urethritis**). **Viruses**, especially those of the common exanthems, cause an acute arthritis that heals completely. The same can be seen in **Reiter's syndrome**, which is thought to be due to infection by *Chlamydia* sp accompanying urethritis, although there is also a high association with HLA-B27. The **purulent arthritides** exhibit histological reactions typical of infection in other tissues and can lead to permanent impairment of the joint depending on the amount of destruction of cartilage that occurs. The opposing, eroded surfaces may fuse by bony ankylosis. Involvement is usually of only one joint, and the larger ones are most frequently involved. **Tuberculous arthritis** has much the same pathogenesis. It is typically in the hip or knee and tends to be latent and slowly progressive.

The arthritis of **rheumatic fever** is acute and tends to involve a succession of different joints. The reaction is nonspecific and does not cause destruction of tissue, so there is no residual on subsidence. **Rheumatoid arthritis** is a polyarticular disease that is usually symmetrical, particularly involves the wrists and proximal interphalangeal joints, and is three times more frequent in young women than men. The etiology is highly associated with the HLA-Dw4 or HLA-DRw4 antigen and is characterized by the development of rheumatoid factor that is IgM, and sometimes IgG and IgA, antibodies to the Fc fragment of IgG heavy chains. Infections, especially viral, may play an initiating role. The essential lesion is a heavy inflammatory infiltrate of the synovium by lymphocytes and plasma cells accompanied by a vasculitis and less regularly by granulomas. The same vasculitis and granulomas occur in the subcutaneous tissue, especially over pressure points, in a fifth of patients and are called **rheumatoid nodules**. They may occur in other viscera. In the joints, the synovial inflammation leads to proliferation and the growth of a **pannus** that covers the articular cartilage, which then undergoes dissolution. The underlying bone thins, the joint cavity is obliterated, and in the most advanced lesions bone invades the pannus and the joint undergoes bony ankylosis and obliteration. Among several related diseases is **ankylosing spondylitis**, which fuses the vertebral and sacroiliac joints of young men, 95% of whom have an HLA-B27 haplotype. Involvement of the root of the aorta with development of aortic insufficiency is part of this disease. Another is **juvenile rheumatoid arthritis**, in which the joint involvement is similar to rheumatoid arthritis itself but the patients are younger and do not exhibit the serological phenomena.

Gout is a hereditary disease, principally of men, that involves the deposition of crystals of monosodium urate in the synovial tissues and fluid and focally in other tissues, especially subcutaneously and in the kidney. The crystals invoke a foreign body reaction, which together with the sheaves of needle-like crystals forms the **gouty tophus**. The first metatarsophalangeal joint is notoriously the site of early involvement, and the episodes are acute and very painful. Tophi often develop on the helix of the ear and in the kidney, where, along with the effect of stones of urate precipitated from the urine, they predispose to destructive pyelonephritis. Episodes are recurrent and involve increasing numbers of joints, with destructive changes similar to those of osteoarthritis. Hyperuricemia (above 7 mg/100 ml, the saturation point of plasma at 37°C) is an essential part of the disease but is not primarily causative as it occurs 50 to 100 times more frequently than gout itself. **Primary gout** is associated with diabetes mellitus, atherosclerosis, hypertriglyceridemia, and hypertension. **Secondary gout** is a part of other syndromes of abnormal metabolism of nucleic acids. The mode of inheritance is apparently multifactorial.

Neoplasia

Many tumors that involve the joints are primary in adjacent bone. Benign tumorous diseases include **xanthofibroma** (also called **villonodular synovitis, giant cell tumor of tendon sheath**, and **benign synovioma**), in which slowly growing nodules of spindle cells, macrophages, and giant cells develop, and **osteochondromatosis**, in which multiple nodules of cartilage fill the joint cavity. **Synovioma**, or **synovial sarcoma**, is a malignant tumor, more often of periarticular tissue than of the synovium itself, that most commonly arises in the knee of young men. Microscopically, this is one of the few malignant tumors with a characteristically biphasic cell pattern: spindle cells and synovioblastic cells that resemble epithelium.

BONE

Hereditary and congenital diseases of bone and the skeleton are too numerous and varied to be cataloged for review in preparation for general examinations. Smith and Jones, a popular reference on human malformations, list 18 syndromes under **facial-limb defects**, 29 under **osteochondrodysplasias**, and an additional 4 under **osteochrondodysplasia with osteosclerosis**.

Infections

Involvement of bone is not a prominent feature of most infectious diseases. Bacterial infection can be introduced by direct inoculation in compound fractures, but the two most important pathways are by way of the bloodstream to the marrow cavity and by spread from an abscess or granuloma of adjacent soft tissue.

Osteomyelitis, although a generic term for infections in bone, is classically a bloodborne infection, usually by staphylococci but more recently by gram-negative bacteria in an increased number of cases. The organisms lodge in the marrow of the metaphysis and set up purulent inflammation that spreads into the haversian and Volkmann's canals, leading to necrosis of segments of bone called **sequestra**. The periosteum is stimulated by the inflammation and rapidly forms a surrounding layer of new bone called the **involucrum**. This physical arrangement of encapsulated necrotic bone is responsible for the chronicity typical of the condition. Modern antibiotics have greatly modified the incidence and progression of this disease, although at the same time greater variety is recognized among the bacterial causes: significant numbers of group B streptococci in children and *Salmonella* sp, especially in persons with sickle cell disease. A **Brodie's abscess** is a form of localized, self-contained but persistent osteomyelitis, usually with very little formation of pus. The long-standing draining sinuses that develop in chronic active osteomyelitis are associated with a significant incidence of particularly malignant squamous carcinoma of the surrounding skin. Hematologists quite commonly observe small foci of acute infection or granulomas in biopsies of bone marrow of patients with various conditions, but such patients rarely develop osteomyelitis or other progressive infection of bone.

Tuberculosis of bone is also due to hematogenous spread of the bacilli to the marrow during the course of infection elsewhere, although in old series half the cases presented no other evidence of active infection by the time the bone disease became manifest. The long bones and spine are most frequent sites. The general incidence is now greatly reduced, and the disease occurs principally in cases of chronic progressive pulmonary tuberculosis. The lesions are chronic and destructive without the productive proliferative bone reaction of pyogenic osteomyelitis. Lesions may spread into adjacent soft tissue to form "cold" abscesses, the paradigm of which occurs in **Pott's disease** when the tuberculosis destroys vertebral bodies to cause kyphosis and extends into the psoas muscle, where it may dissect along the sheath to present in the inguinal region.

Metabolic bone disease

Because the skeleton is a great reservoir of minerals that is constantly undergoing revision in response to metabolic needs, physical stresses, and alterations in the physiological internal environment, it becomes involved in a great many metabolic diseases, often with quite characteristic lesions but other times with changes that are more clearly manifested in the chemical constituents of the blood and body fluids. Knowledge of the normal processes and histology of bone formation and growth are essential to understanding bone lesions. This topic is of such large dimension that it can be little more than outlined here.

Hormones.   The activity of **parathyroid hormone** is fundamental in normal calcium metabolism. When levels of the hormone are abnormally increased either because of the secondary effects of renal disease operating through distortions of the balance of phosphorus and calcium or because of the primary hypersecretion by tumors of the parathyroid, osteoclastic activity is stimulated, calcium is removed from matrix, osteoid is poorly calcified, and fibroblastic proliferation occurs in the marrow space. These changes are called **osteitis fibrosa**, and in advanced cases of primary hyperthyroidism they may result in sufficient resorption of foci of bone as to create demineralized and fibrotic foci termed **osteitis fibrosa cystica** that can be confused with giant cell tumors. **Von Recklinghausen's disease of bone** is the name given to these extreme examples of the effects of hyperparathyroidism. The effects of the hormone on bone are intertwined with those of vitamin D because both substances are essential components of calcium metabolism. **Calcitonin** is the hormone of the parafollicular cells of the thyroid. Although it has inhibitory effects on osteoclasts and levels are increased in patients with medullary carcinoma of the thyroid, there are no recognizable lesions in bone. **Pituitary growth hormone** stimulates bone growth to **gigantism** or **acromegaly** in a histologically nonspecific manner; **thyroid hormone** stimulates bone remodeling and in excess can result in negative calcium balance and osteoporosis. Diabetics develop diminished bone mass because of a physiological effect of **insulin** on bone collagen synthesis and mucopolysaccharide production. **Adrenal corticosteroids** in excess cause demineralization of bone, a feature of **Cushing's disease**, but the more important hormone related to clinical **senile osteoporosis** is estrogen. This disorder, most importantly manifest in postmenopausal women although it occurs to a lesser extent in aged men, has little characteristic histological change other than a decrease in the amount of bone. The decline with age in the amount of stress stimulus of exercise is another important factor in this disease, and there are undoubtedly others, although a deficiency of calcium correctable by increased intake is not one of them.

Vitamins. **Vitamin D**, of all the vitamins, is most importantly involved in normal metabolism and disease of bone. A great deal of its effect is in conjunction with that of parathyroid hormone. In excess, which occurs mostly with excessive intake by faddists although lesser amounts may be excessive for infants, it causes demineralization of bone, hypercalcemia, hypercalciuria, and metastatic calcification of soft tissues. In deficiency it causes **rickets** before the epiphyses are closed and is associated with **osteomalacia** in adults. In the former there is failure of calcification of the epiphyseal cartilage and osteoid with weakening of the bone structure and displacement. The weight-bearing bones become bowed, and sites of frequent motion such as the costochondral junctions become enlarged (**rachitic rosary**). In osteomalacia there is failure of calcification of the osteoid of normal bone turnover and the changes of hyperparathyroidism that arise because of the decreased calcium absorption from the GI tract. **Vitamin C deficiency** (**scurvy**) is also manifest in the epiphyses of infants. The defect there is a failure of proper formation of osteoid, not of calcification, and a fragility of capillaries. The epiphyses become disorganized, bony trabeculae are poorly formed and broken, and there is interstitial hemorrhage. **Vitamin A** in experimental deficiency results in inhibition of enchondral bone growth but probably does not contribute to human bone disease.

Renal osteodystrophy results from chronic renal failure and uremia. It is of increasing frequency because of the maintenance of patients on dialysis. The common denominator of the lesions is osteitis fibrosa of hyperparathyroidism, but many other features of vitamin D deficiency and disturbed calcium and phosphorus balance appear. High levels of aluminum accumulate in the bones of dialyzed patients and influence the development of osteomalacia.

Osteitis deformans (**Paget's disease**) is probably not properly considered a metabolic bone disease although it is a disorder of distorted remodeling of bone. Respiratory syncytial virus is speculated to be an important etiologic factor. It is a disease of later life, resulting first in hyperactivity of the resorptive phase of bone remodeling with hyperfusion. The bone becomes deformed, bowed, and thickened. The pattern then passes into one of accelerated bone formation and sclerosis. A **mosaic pattern** of partially reorganized haversian systems overlaid by others is characteristic of the sclerotic phase. Such complications as deafness may arise from involvement of the temporal bone. The most conspicious changes are enlargement and thickening of the skull (an increase in hat size) and bowing of the legs, with decrease of stature. The disease is the most frequent antecedent of osteosarcoma in adults.

Neoplasia

The pathology of tumors of bone is a subspecialty unto itself. Rosai has compiled a very informative table of facts of site, incidence, and prognosis that lists 25 varieties, whereas the International Histological Classification provides for 38 classes. Principal divisions are tumors of (1) **bone**, (2) **cartilage**, and (3) elements of the **marrow** other than hematopoietic tissue. Most bone tumors have quite characteristic sites and ages of occurrence, which, with the structure of the tumor as revealed by radiographs, are often as helpful as histological examination in identification and statement of prognosis.

The eight varieties of malignant tumor are (1) **osteosarcoma**, principally of the long bones of youths, with less than 50% 5-year survival, (2) **juxtacortical osteosarcoma**, a subvariety of middle-aged persons and of 80% survival, (3) **chondrosarcoma**, which occurs in middle age in the axial skeleton as well as the femur and humerus and has malignancies of four-fifths, half, or one-fifth that are predictable from the histological grading of the tumor, (4) **mesenchymal chondrosarcoma**, a uniformly more malignant variety of slightly younger people, (5) **Ewing's sarcoma** of the long bones and pelvis of children and of only a quarter survival even with the best modern therapy (there is a suggestion this tumor be classified with the primitive neuroectodermal tumors), (6) **malignant lymphoma**, (7) **plasma cell myeloma**, which is of either a diffuse type that is uniformly fatal and a focal type that can be eradicated by radiotherapy, and (8) **fibrosarcoma**, a tumor of the long bones and jaws occurring in youth to middle age. Osteosarcoma, chondrosarcoma, and myeloma are more common in males, and the others are of approximately equal distribution. Two tumors, the **giant cell tumor**, a tumor of the ends of the femur, tibia, and radius of young adults, and **chordoma** are of lesser malignant prognosis although the latter is characterized more by the chronicity of its course than by any potential for cure. The benign lesions include **osteomas, osteoblastomas, chondroblastomas, chondromas, fibromas, fibrous dysplasia, bone cysts, eosinophilic granulomas**, and other tumors of rare incidence.

BIBLIOGRAPHY

Braunwald E, Isselbacher KJ, Petersdorf RG, et al: Harrison's Principles of Internal Medicine, 11th ed. McGraw-Hill, New York, 1987.

Galen RS, Gambino SR: Beyond Normality: The Predictive Value and Efficiency of Medical Diagnoses. John Wiley & Sons, New York, 1975.

Golden A: Pathology: Understanding Human Disease. Williams & Wilkins, Baltimore, 1982. A general and sufficient beginning textbook that, with its selective presentations, readability, brevity (480 pages), and good illustrations is an adequate general review of pathology that can be accomplished in a continuous reading.

Henry JB: Clinical Diagnosis and Management by Laboratory Methods, 17th ed. WB Saunders, Philadelphia, 1984.

Kissane JM: Anderson's Pathology, 8th ed. CV Mosby, St. Louis, 1985. The nearest thing to a handbook of the subject readily available in the United States.

Love RR: The risk of breast cancer in American women. JAMA 257:1470, 1987.

Ravel R: Clinical Laboratory Medicine; Clinical Application of Laboratory Data. Year Book Medical Publishers, Chicago, 1984.

Robbins SL, Kumar Y: Basic Pathology, 4th ed. WB Saunders, 1987.

Robbins SL, Cotran RS, Kumar V: Pathologic Basis of Disease, 3rd ed. WB Saunders, Philadelphia, 1984. The most popular textbook in most medical schools.

Rosai J: Ackerman's Surgical Pathology, 6th ed. CV Mosby, St. Louis, 1981.

Smith DW, Jones KL: Recognizable Patterns of Human Malformation, 3rd ed. WB Saunders, Philadelphia, 1982.

Speicher CE, Smith JW Jr: Choosing Effective Laboratory Tests. WB Saunders, Philadelphia, 1983.

SAMPLE QUESTIONS

DIRECTIONS: Each question below contains five suggested answers. For **each** of the five alternatives of **each** item, you are to respond either YES (Y) or NO (N). In a given item, all, some, or none of the alternatives may be correct.

1. Celulitis is correctly described as

   A. pyogenic inflammation that spreads through tissues along natural barriers
   B. surrounded by a wall of reaction and reparative granulation tissue
   C. inflammation of the loose subcutaneous tissue
   D. sometimes of viral etiology, although usually due to hemolytic streptococci
   E. not necessarily purulent

2. Granulation tissue is correctly described as

   A. a healing stage of inflammation
   B. containing proliferating endothelial cells and fibroblasts
   C. presenting granules of loops of new vessels and connective tissue on a denuded surface
   D. an aggregation of histiocytes that transform into epitheloid cells
   E. a stiff, plastic mass of necrotic coagulum

3. Progressive pulmonary hypertension is responsible for the fatal outcome of

   A. patent ductus arteriosus
   B. interventricular septal defect
   C. tetralogy of Fallot
   D. hypoplastic left heart syndrome
   E. postductal coarctation of the aorta

4. At autopsy of an adult who died relatively suddenly, the aorta has a three-cornered tear in the intima 5 cm above the aortic valve and hemorrhage within its wall extending from the tear down to compress the right coronary artery at its origin.

   A. The etiology of the lesion is syphilitic
   B. The cause of death is cardiac arrhythmia secondary to coronary insufficiency
   C. Long, thin hands and feet and redundant leaflets of the mitral valve, if present, are significantly related to the aortic lesion
   D. A similar aortic lesion develops in rats fed sweat pea meal that contains a chemical that blocks cross-linkage in collagen and elastin
   E. Prothrombin and partial thromboplastin times were probably prolonged before the onset of the aortic lesion

5. A young person dies after a couple of weeks of fever, progressive loss of cerebral faculties, and finally coma. At autopsy the brain is swollen, with flattened gyri and bilateral uncinate grooves. In microscopic sections, there are small collections of a dozen or so histiocytes about venules with thickened endothelium scattered throughout, but predominately in gray matter. These findings are compatible with

   A. Rocky Mountain spotted fever
   B. infection with human immunodeficiency virus
   C. St. Louis encephalitis
   D. tuberculosis
   E. infection with *Hemophilus influenzae*

6. Major risk factors for the development of atherosclerosis include

    A. a high-fat diet and serum cholesterol greater than 260 mg/100 ml of serum

    B. consumption of more than a six-pack (72 ounces) of beer or 5 jiggers (½ pint) of whisky per day

    C. blood pressure higher than 130/95 mm Hg

    D. smoking more than 30 cigarettes a day

    E. signs and symptoms of osmotic diuresis and fasting plasma glucose greater than 140 mg/100 ml

7. A 55-year-old man undergoes gastric resection for carcinoma. On the second postoperative day, he has sharp right-sided thoracic pain and slight hemoptysis. His left calf is 38 cm in circumference and the right 36 cm. On the fourth day, he collapses while walking and dies within a few minutes. Expected findings at autopsy based on these data include

    A. a gray firm area about a cavity 1 cm in diameter in the apex of the right lung

    B. a cerebral hemorrhage 5 cm in diameter in the left external capsule

    C. left ventricular hypertrophy and a heart weight of greater than 450 g

    D. swollen kidneys with thickened pale cortices in which there are scattered red foci 1 mm or less in diameter

    E. dark red, uniform, soft coagula of blood lying loosely in both pulmonary arteries

8. A man is found dead in January, huddled beneath newspapers over a heating vent in the sidewalk. Postmortem examination by the medical examiner reveals on the leaflets of the tricuspid valve a couple of masses 5 and 10 mm in diameter of fibrin, platelets, and swollen collagen. In the lungs there are birefringent 1- to 3-μm crystals in the alveolar and peribronchiolar tissues and eosinophilic precipitate, polymorphonuclear leukocytes, and fibrin in the alveoli. The sections of the liver have a nutmeg appearance. These findings support diagnoses of

    A. rheumatic cardiac disease

    B. infection, most likely by gram-positive cocci

    C. asbestosis

    D. chronic alcoholism

    E. intravenous drug abuse

9. Stages of acute inflammation include

    A. transient arteriolar vasoconstriction

    B. vasodilatation of arterioles, opening of capillaries, dilatation of venules

    C. increased permeability of microvasculature

    D. microvascular thrombosis

    E. leukocytic emigration

10. A patient dies after a long course of congestive cardiac failure. At autopsy the heart is dilated and enlarged to 600 g, the myocardium is flabby, and a uniform red-brown (normal) color throughout. All coronary arteries contain raised yellow plaques that cover 15% of the intimal surface and occlude 25% of the cross-sectional areas at the scattered sites of maximal involvement. The clinical history is most likely to include

    A. episodes of chest pain radiating to the left arm

    B. syphilis

    C. alcoholism

    D. repeated streptococcal pharyngitis in childhood

    E. blood pressure above 130/95 mm Hg

11. Which of the following are correctly paired statements of relations among the anemias?

    A. Malaria: hematin-like pigment in cerebral capillaries

    B. Erythroblastosis fetalis: incompatibility of parental ABO antigens

    C. Hypochromic microcytic anemia: folic acid deficiency

    D. Thalassemia minor: valine substituted for glutamine at the sixth position of the beta chain of hemoglobin

    E. Autoimmune hemolytic anemia: positive Coombs' antiglobulin test

12. In patients with which of the following diseases is demonstration of a cell-destructive antibody pathognomonic?

    A. Paroxysmal cold hemoglobinuria

    B. Sickle cell anemia

    C. Thrombotic thrombocytopenic purpura

    D. Hereditary spherocytosis

    E. Transfusion reactions

13. A 45-year-old patient had a leukocyte count of 200,000/mm^3, predominately segmented or band neutrophils that did not stain for alkaline phosphatase, a palpably enlarged spleen and liver, and solidly hyperplastic iliac bone marrow. Response to therapy was excellent for 3 years, but then over a period of 4 months, he developed fever, weakness, bleeding of the gums, and widespread petechiae that progressed until a fatal cerebral hemorrhage occurred. During those last months, many large, agranular mononuclear cells appeared in the blood.

    A. During the original episode and before therapy the Philadelphia (Ph$_1$) chromosome was probably demonstrable in monocytes

    B. The final months represent transformation to acute lymphocytic leukemia

    C. Platelets were probably increased at the beginning, normal during remission, and decreased terminally

    D. The liver at death was likely of near normal size or slightly enlarged and devoid of cellular infiltrates

    E. The terminal cerebral hemorrhage was probably related to the development of hypertension

14. A patient 30 years old has fever, night sweats, weight loss, and enlargement of the left cervical lymph nodes. On biopsy, the architecture of the nodes is obliterated by lymphocytic infiltrates and fibrosis. A characteristic giant cell establishes the diagnosis. You would expect it to be described as having

A. uniform eosinophilic cytoplasm and multiple, regular, small nuclei that have delicate chromatin and are distributed along the periphery of the cell
B. scanty clear cytoplasm, more than one bilobed or multilobed nuclei with heavy nuclear membranes, translucent nucleoplasm, and prominent amphophilic nucleoli
C. uniform eosinophilic cytoplasm of irregular outline containing a few needle-shaped refractile inclusions, together with multiple small regular nuclei with delicate chromatin that are scattered throughout the cell
D. dark, epithelial appearing cytoplasm with basophilic, granular inclusion masses and a huge single nucleus with all chromatin condensed along the nuclear membrane, clear nucleoplasm, and a single large spheroid eosinophilic body
E. scanty irregular cytoplasm and several large and irregular nuclei with dark and clumped chromatin and several nucleoli

15. A microscopic section of lung from the autopsy of an adult who died with acute respiratory failure shows plugging of small bronchi with mucus, hyperinflation of alveoli, increase and enlargement of bronchial mucous glands, hypertrophy of bronchial muscle, thickened bronchial epithelial basement membranes, and infiltrates of eosinophils. It may be concluded from these observations that

A. the patient had emphysema
B. serum IgE was probably abnormal
C. the diagnosis is bronchopneumonia
D. serum IgG was probably elevated because of this disease
E. death was probably due to pulmonary emboli rather than the described changes

16. Which of the following statements regarding the pathogenesis of pneumococcal lobar pneumonia are true?

A. The "crisis" occurs when opsonins appear
B. The first event is aspiration of a bacteria-laden mucous plug into a terminal bronchiole
C. Fibrin in the alveolar exudate usually provides a framework for the ingrowth of fibroblasts
D. The alveoli around the site of bacterial inoculation are first filled with a cell-poor fluid exudate
E. Bacteria spread from alveolus to alveolus by growing in fluid that passes through the pores of Kohn

17. A 39-year-old man develops hemoptysis and on radiographic examination has an irregular density at the apex of the right lung. Biopsy of an enlarged firm right subclavicular lymph node demonstrates a squamous carcinoma.

A. Five-year survival with modern therapy is expected to be 60%
B. A history of heavy cigarette smoking is very likely
C. This is the tumor type most commonly associated with symptoms and signs of hyperparathyroidism
D. Ptosis, pupillary constriction, anhidrosis, and pain in the distribution of the ulnar nerve, if present, all could be explained by the tumor in this case
E. Microscopic sections of the tumor in the lung would be expected to show mucus-filled alveoli lined by tumor cells that have undergone globlet cell metaplasia

18. A 32-year-old man develops a nodule in his right parotid gland that slowly enlarges over 2 years. Surgical pathological examination after resection showed it to be composed of irregular epithelial and myoepithelial cells, often of stellate configuration, buried in mesenchymal elements with chrondroid and myxoid characteristics.

A. This tumor may cause drooping of the right side of the face and inability to close the right eye
B. Wide excision must be performed to prevent metastases
C. Capsular penetration accounts for a 10% recurrence rate and nerve involvement
D. A history of chewing tobacco is to be expected
E. Similar tumors occur in the trachea and other salivary glands

19. A colectomy for chronic ulcerative disease yields a specimen that has longitudinal mucosal ulcers along the taenia throughout, with extension into the rectum. Within the ulcers are protruding masses of mucosa. The wall is dilated but not much thickened. The accompanying 10 cm of distal ileum is normal. Microscopically, the ulcers undermine adjacent mucosa, but the inflammation, both acute and chronic, is largely confined to the crypts of the glands and the interstitium of the upper submucosa. Findings that mitigate against a diagnosis of Crohn's disease are

A. involvement of the entire colon
B. involvement of the rectum
C. lack of involvement of the ileum
D. thinness of the colonic wall
E. lack of microscopic granulomas

20. In some states, it has been legislated that all newborn infants be tested for phenylketonuria. The sensitivity and specificity of the test are each of the order of 99.99. The prevalence of the disease is about 0.01, or 10/100,000 population. The predictive value of a positive test is of the order of

A. 99%
B. 95%
C. 50%
D. 5%
E. 1%

21. An 18-year-old patient with chronic renal failure has depressed serum calcium and elevated serum inorganic phosphorus. He develops a swelling of the femur just above the knee and on radiological examination there is a round, sharply bounded area of radiolucency. On biopsy the lesion contains fibroblasts and tumor giant cells that replace the normal marrow and erode the surrounding bone. From these data, which of the following statements are probably true?

    A. The most likely diagnosis is giant cell tumor of bone
    B. The thyroid gland will be enlarged
    C. The serum creatinine will be elevated
    D. One parathyroid will be enlarged and hyperplastic and the others atrophic
    E. The patient will develop a flapping tremor on holding his arms extended forward while his eyes are closed

22. A 48-year-old woman with no complaints has a 1-cm focus of sparse granular calcification in each breast on mammography performed as a routine on a physical checkup.

    A. Both lesions should be considered carcinoma until diagnosed by biospy
    B. There is a fair possibility that the lesions are fibro-adenomas
    C. Fat necrosis can account for the findings
    D. The story is typical for intraductal papillomas
    E. Bilaterality strongly suggests a benign process

23. Which of the following statements regarding nodular hyperplasia of the prostate are true?

    A. It occurs in patients in the fifth decade and older
    B. It can be prevented by early orchiectomy
    C. The ureterovesical valve prevents hydronephrosis and pylonephritis from being complications
    D. It is a precancerous condition
    E. It is readily diagnosed by digital rectal examination because it principally involves the posterior lobe

24. A 45-year-old woman has a long history of poor and irregular diet accompanying considerable alcohol abuse. She gradually develops fatigability, anorexia, increased abdominal girth, ankle edema, and a slight yellow tint of her sclerae.

    A. The increased waistline is a result of obstruction of hepatic venules
    B. She is at risk for peptic ulcer, esophageal bleeding, and fatal coma
    C. Needle biopsy of the liver will show hepatic cells filled with large droplets of neutral fat and arranged in lobules of single-cell-thick plates about central venules
    D. Impairment of hepatic protein metabolism contributes to the ankle edema
    E. She probably also has pulmonary emphysema due to an enzyme deficiency that is also responsible for the hepatic damage

25. The prognosis for children of parents, each of whom are heterozygous for cystic fibrosis, has many dismal features.

    A. Two-thirds of the children of these parents will have the clinical disease
    B. A pregnancy may result in a child born with intestinal obstruction
    C. Pancreatic insufficiency, unless corrected by therapy, is life threatening in the first decade
    D. Diabetic coma is a common complication
    E. Cirrhosis is the principal cause of a fatal outcome in patients who survive to the late second or third decades.

ANSWERS

1. A-N, B-N, C-Y, D-N, E-Y
2. A-Y, B-Y, C-Y, D-N, E-N
3. A-Y, B-Y, C-N, D-N, E-N
4. A-N, B-Y, C-Y, D-Y, E-N
5. A-Y, B-Y, C-Y, D-N, E-N
6. A-Y, B-N, C-Y, D-Y, E-Y
7. A-N, B-N, C-N, D-N, E-N
8. A-N, B-Y, C-N, D-N, E-Y
9. A-Y, B-Y, C-Y, D-N, E-Y
10. A-N, B-N, C-Y, D-N, E-N
11. A-Y, B-Y, C-N, D-N, E-Y
12. A-Y, B-N, C-N, D-N, E-N
13. A-Y, B-N, C-Y, D-Y, E-N
14. A-N, B-Y, C-N, D-N, E-N
15. A-N, B-Y, C-N, D-N, E-N
16. A-Y, B-Y, C-N, D-Y, E-Y
17. A-N, B-Y, C-N, D-Y, E-N
18. A-Y, B-N, C-Y, D-N, E-Y
19. A-N, B-Y, C-Y, D-Y, E-Y
20. A-N, B-N, C-Y, D-N, E-N
21. A-N, B-N, C-Y, D-N, E-N
22. A-Y, B-N, C-Y, D-N, E-N
23. A-Y, B-Y, C-N, D-N, E-N
24. A-Y, B-Y, C-N, D-Y, E-N
25. A-N, B-Y, C-Y, D-N, E-N

6

PHARMACOLOGY

Margaret A. Reilly

The objective of this chapter is to review the major principles of pharmacology and the major information regarding most drugs commonly in use today in the United States. This is not an exhaustive compendium of drug knowledge, nor is it meant as a textbook for first-time learners. These two types of publications are in ample supply. Of necessity, long lists of adverse effects and drug interactions have not been included. The author has attempted to focus on possible serious adverse effects and on frequently observed adverse effects. Great effort has been made to be both precise and concise. The reader is cautioned that more extensive knowledge of a drug's actions and effects, its precautions and contraindications, must be obtained before any drug is prescribed for or administered to any person. *Unless otherwise noted, drug doses in this chapter represent the range of recommended oral adult doses over 24 hours.* All drugs are potentially toxic. They must be used carefully and skillfully to enable patients to derive the greatest benefit with the least amount of harm.

DRUG EFFECTS

Drugs are chemical substances that can modify the physiological activity of living cells. All drugs produce many effects, some that are beneficial and others that are harmful. The beneficial or therapeutic effects are those desired actions for which the drug is administered. Other undesired effects are **adverse drug reactions**, the most common of which is the **side effect**. These are expected effects that occur at normal therapeutic doses of the drug, such as constipation when opiate (narcotic) analgesics are administered. If the drug dose is reduced, side effects can be alleviated but therapeutic effects also may disappear.

It should be pointed out that side effects can be relative. They can become the therapeutic effect in some clinical situations. For example, the constipating effect of the opiates becomes the desired effect when these agents are used as antidiarrheal drugs. Patients should be alerted to side effects, especially those that warn of impending drug toxicity, such as anorexia and nausea in persons receiving a digitalis glycoside. Particular attention must also be paid to side effects that can endanger the patient's well-being. Sedation makes driving a car hazardous; orthostatic hypotension can cause severe falls, especially in the elderly. If side effects become too severe or troublesome, drug administration may have to be terminated.

A type of adverse effect that is referred to as **primary toxicity** occurs when the administered dose of drug is too large. (The actual dose given may be "normal," but the patient's response can be excessive.) Primary toxicity is a continuation or exaggeration of the therapeutic effect, such as spontaneous hemorrhage in persons receiving anticoagulant medication. This type of toxicity is alleviated by discontinuation or reduction of drug dosage, and it can often be avoided by initiating therapy with low doses that are gradually increased until the desired effects are obtained (**titrating** the dose to the patient's response). Persons with decreased hepatic and/or renal function (e.g., the elderly) are especially susceptible to primary toxicity from drugs that are hepatically or renally inactivated. Other preexisting pathology can alter responsiveness to drugs—for example, hyperthyroidism sensitizes myocardial cells to the stimulant effect of catecholamines.

Tolerance is an adverse reaction that causes some drugs to lose their therapeutic effectiveness when they are used for a period of time. (However, tolerance to side effects may occur while the beneficial effects persist.) As tolerance develops, ever increasing doses of drug are required to achieve the original desired effects. Some drugs induce the activity of enzymes that inactivate them; thus, tolerance occurs because the drug is more rapidly degraded. This is **pharmacokinetic tolerance**. Other drugs seem to promote adaptive changes in cells that result in **pharmacodynamic tolerance**. Cross-tolerance among drugs can occur. Persons who consume large amounts of alcohol frequently require greater than normal doses of barbiturates or general anesthetics.

Drug dependence or **addiction** is an adverse effect that is sometimes related to tolerance. Some drugs, taken over a period of time, lead to a person's inability to control his or her use of the drug. When dependence is physical or physiological, the continuous presence of the drug has induced functional changes that render some cells incapable of "normal" activity when the drug is absent. Withholding drug administration will produce a withdrawal or abstinence syndrome, which consists of well-defined physiological signs and symptoms. Psychological dependence refers to an intense craving for and habitual use of a drug for some pleasurable or mood-altering effect. In this type of dependence, withholding the drug does not result in a well-defined abstinence syndrome, although persons often report subjective feelings such as headache, anxiety, or irritability.

Another adverse effect of some drugs is **organ toxicity**. This can be a direct interaction of the drug with cells, or it may occur as the result of *allergic* (hypersensitivity) or *idiosyncratic* reactions. Many drugs (e.g., several of the antibiotics) induce renal damage as they are excreted. Hepatic injury can occur as the liver attempts to detoxify or inactivate some drugs. Depression of bone marrow activity or destruction of cells in the blood can lead to serious blood dyscrasias such as leukopenia, thrombocytopenia, or anemia. Destruction of the auditory nerve by the aminoglycoside antibiotics causes deafness and vestibular dysfunction. The occurrence of organ toxicity can be reduced by determining organ activity before drug therapy is initiated. Decreased function of an organ usually suggests that drugs toxic to that organ be withheld. Organ function tests should be continued throughout drug administration to detect early indications of tissue damage.

Teratogenicity is damage to fetal tissues. Most drugs have some degree of lipid solubility, thus cross the placenta and enter fetal tissues. *Teratogenesis occurs especially during the first trimester of pregnancy*, when the greatest differentiation of organ systems takes place. Retardation of growth and development can be the result of drugs taken later in pregnancy. Most drugs, including alcohol, nicotine, and over-the-counter preparations, are contraindicated during pregnancy unless they are essential to maintain the health of the mother and the fetus. All drugs discussed in this chapter should be considered hazardous in pregnancy. This topic is discussed further in a later section.

Drug allergy is an adverse reaction due to individual persons' immune responses to drugs. Drugs, which are usually small molecules, complex with larger protein molecules in the circulatory system to form haptens, which then provoke the formation of antibodies. When the drug is given again, even in minute amounts, an allergic response that can be very severe will result. Persons who have other allergies are especially prone to develop drug allergies and are usually quite sensitive to histamine, thus to drugs that release this endogenous amine from mast cells and basophils. Allergy to inert components of drug formulations can occur. Tartrazine, a yellow dye, is included in many medications; persons allergic to aspirin are especially prone to hypersensitivity reactions to this chemical. Some tartrazine-containing preparations do not show the characteristic yellow coloring.

Allergic responses can take several different forms. Immediate reactions that occur within minutes of exposure to a drug include life-threatening asthma (difficulty in breathing as histamine constricts bronchioles and causes them to swell with edema) and anaphylactic shock (histamine-induced vasodilation leading to circulatory collapse). Dermatologic reactions such as itching and urticaria are milder forms of immediate reactions; some dermatologic responses develop gradually over several hours. A more slowly developing type of allergic reaction is *serum sickness*. The appearance of lymph node enlargement, pain in the joints, and fever or rash 1 to 2 weeks after exposure to a drug are among the manifestations of this delayed reaction. Persons who have shown allergic symptoms after drug administration should usually not be given that drug again and should carry some medical identification that warns of their allergy. There are however some occasions when drugs (e.g., penicillin) are required by persons who are allergic to them. Such administration demands great caution. Mechanical means for resuscitation must be available, as well as IV forms of epinephrine and corticosteroids to counteract asthma and anaphylaxis should they occur.

Drug idiosyncrasy refers to certain unusual and abnormal reactions to normal doses of drugs that appear to be caused by individual physiological characteristics rather than by the pharmacology of the drug. Some idiosyncratic reactions occur because of genetic variations in enzymes that metabolize drugs. A deficiency of glucose 6-phosphate dehydrogenase (G6PD) in erythrocytes predisposes persons to hemolytic anemia when certain drugs (e.g., antimalarials) are administered. Persons with abnormally low plasma levels of pseudocholinesterase are at risk of prolonged respiratory depression from succinylcholine. In some persons, barbiturates induce abnormal increases in hepatic synthesis of porphyrin. Malignant hyperthermia provoked by general anesthetics such as halothane appears to be a genetically determined drug idiosyncrasy.

RECEPTORS

Many drugs appear to exert their effects by selectively interacting with structures called receptors, which are located on cell membranes or on organelles within cells. **Agonists** are drugs (and endogenous substances) that bind to receptors and thus cause some alteration in the physiological activity of cells. Agonists have both affinity (ability to bind to receptors) and intrinsic activity (ability to directly cause some effect to occur). **Antagonists** have affinity only. They bind to receptors but have no direct effects of their own. Their usefulness as drugs is based on their ability to prevent agonists from binding to the receptors. Agonist-receptor interactions initiate cellular activity such as activation of enzymes and formation of second messengers like cyclic adenosine monophosphate (cAMP). Agonists exhibit marked stereoselectivity for receptors, suggesting that these sites of action are structural components of cells. The blocking activity of many antagonists can be overcome by increasing the concentration of agonist at the receptors. In this competitive type of inhibition, dose-response curves are shifted to the right but the maximum effect is not suppressed. In noncompetitive antagonism, the antagonist binds irreversibly to the receptor. The maximal effect of the agonist is reduced irrespective of the concentration of agonist at the receptor sites. It has been suggested that agonists stimulate receptors only at the initial interaction (**rate theory** of drug action) and must continuously rebind to receptors to sustain drug effects. In contrast, the **occupancy theory** of drug action postulates that drug effects depend on the number of receptors that combine with the agonist.

Intrinsic activity, or **efficacy**, refers to the maximum effect produced by a drug. For example, the loop diuretics such as furosemide have greater efficacy than the potassium-sparing diuretics. Furosemide causes much more intense diuresis. **Potency** refers to the activity per unit weight of a drug. Those agents that are therapeutically effective in small doses are said to be more potent.

In addition to interaction with receptors, drug mechanisms of action include inhibition of enzymes and alterations in cellular membrane permeability.

STRUCTURE-ACTIVITY RELATIONSHIPS

The relationship of the structure of many drugs to their pharmacologic actions suggests that the configuration of receptors confers considerable selectivity on drugs. Slight alterations in the structure of a drug molecule can significantly affect its potency and even convert it from an agonist to an antagonist. These observations have prompted development of numerous new drugs and classes of drugs, such as the histamine H_2 receptor antagonists. In many instances, the congeners or analogues possess important advantages over the original or prototype drugs. For example, the beta-adrenergic antagonists metoprolol and atenolol have greater selectivity for $beta_1$ receptors in the heart thus are somewhat safer for use in persons susceptible to asthma. Similarly, atenolol and nadolol, which are renally excreted as unchanged drug, are safer in the presence of liver dysfunction than are the hepatically inactivated propranolol and metoprolol.

PHARMACOKINETICS

Pharmacokinetics describe the fate of a drug once it has been administered. It is the interaction of the drug with the physiology of the patient. The onset, intensity, and duration of action of drugs are modified by the physiological and pathological status of each individual.

All apsects of pharmacokinetics are influenced by the ability of drug molecules to cross biologic membranes. Passive movement across membranes is achieved most easily by lipid-soluble molecules. Solutions of drugs consist of both nonionized (lipid-soluble) and ionized (water-soluble) molecules. The drug's **pKa** is that pH at which one-half of the molecules in solution are in each state. Variations in the pH of solutions will change the ratio of nonionized to ionized molecules and thus will affect the passage of drugs across membranes. Drugs that are weak acids become less ionized at acid pH; those that are weak bases are less ionized at alkaline pH.

Small water-soluble molecules appear to diffuse passively through pores in cell membranes. Active systems that transport naturally occurring substances such as glucose and amino acids can facilitate the passage of similarly structured drugs.

Drugs that are systemically administered (i.e., that must be transported from the site of administration to the site of action) must gain access to the circulatory system. This process is **absorption**. Drugs administered PO must be dissolved in the GI tract. Here absorption generally occurs by passive diffusion of nonionized molecules along a concentration gradient. The acidic pH of the stomach reduces the ionization of weak acids such as salicylates and promotes their passage across the gastric mucosa. As intestinal contents become increasingly alkaline, weakly basic drugs become nonionized and are absorbed. Drug molecules are rapidly transported away by the flow of blood, thus maintaining the gradient of higher drug concentrations in the GI lumen. Absorption after parenteral administration (IM, SC) is affected by the solubility of the drug and by perfusion at the site of administration. Muscle, which is highly vascular, provides for rapid absorption of most drugs. There is less blood flow through subcutaneous tissue; thus, drugs administered by this route will be more gradually absorbed and will usually have a longer onset and duration of action.

Absorbed drug is then transported throughout the body by the circulatory system, with molecules leaving the vasculature and entering various tissues including those where the site of action is found. This phase of pharmacokinetics is **distribution**. Lipid-soluble molecules are most rapidly distributed as they encounter little resistance to passage across biologic membranes. The **volume of distribution** (V_d) is the ratio of the total amount of drug in the body to that remaining in the circulatory system. Highly lipid-soluble drugs that distribute quite evenly throughout the body and drugs that are sequestered in various tissues will have a relatively large apparent volume of distribution. Other drugs (e.g., large, highly water-soluble molecules) remain concentrated in the plasma. Drugs that bind extensively to plasma proteins such as albumin will concentrate temporarily in the vascular compartment, since only the unbound molecules can be distributed to body tissues. As drug leaves the circulatory system, bound molecules move off the protein binding sites and become free. Protein binding of molecules reduces their access to sites of action but also slows their inactivation by the liver or kidneys.

Distribution of drugs is also affected by the permeability of capillary walls in various tissues. The tight junctions of cells in the small vessels of the CNS (the blood-brain barrier) impede the entry of lipid-insoluble substances into the brain and spinal column.

Dependent on absorption and distribution is the concept of **bioavailability**, or the relative amount of an administered drug dose that is able to reach sites of action. This is usually estimated in terms of the concentration of drug reaching the circulatory system within a predetermined time interval after administration. **Bioequivalence** compares the bioavailability of similar drug formulations. Differences in bioavailability can result in serious fluctuations in serum concentrations of drug when preparations from various sources are substituted in a patient who has been stabilized on one product. Some generic forms of drug appear to lack bioequivalence with trade-name formulations. The bioavailability of some agents administered PO is greatly reduced by first-pass hepatic extraction of drug. The portal circulation carries much of the blood from the GI tract directly to the liver, where drugs such as propranolol and lidocaine are rapidly removed and inactivated so that a significant portion of the dose never reaches the general circulation.

All drugs are eventually eliminated from the body. Some are renally excreted as unchanged drug, and others are hepatically biotransformed into inactive water-soluble molecules. **Biotransformation** is especially important for the elimination of agents that are nonionized at normal urinary pH. Several types of enzymatic reactions contribute to the hepatic inactivation of drugs. The microsomal or mixed-function oxidase enzymes catalyze deamination, N-oxidation, N- and O-dealkylation, and aromatic and aliphatic hydroxylation of a large number of drugs. The nicotinamide adenine dinucleotide phosphate (NADPH)-dependent cytochrome P450 is part of this system. The activity of the microsomal drug-metabolizing enzymes can be enhanced or induced by many drugs, most notably the sedative-hypnotics. Enzyme activity may be reduced in infants, the elderly, and persons with liver dysfunction, thus caution is required when hepatically inactivated drugs must be administered. Lower than normal drug doses are usually effective.

Other hepatic enzymes confer increased water solubility by conjugation of drug molecules to form glucuronides and sulfate and glycine conjugates. Acetylation, important to the inactivation of drugs such as isoniazid, is genetically deficient in some persons ("slow acetylators"), who are thus at greater risk of drug toxicity. *S*-adenosylmethionine is the methyl donor for the *N*- and *O*-methylation of substances such as nicotinic acid.

Hepatic biotransformation usually destroys the pharmacologic activity of drugs but can yield metabolites that are nevertheless toxic. The renal route is important for the excretion of these substances, as well as for those drugs that are ionized and thus water soluble at urinary pH. Less than optimal renal function, again not uncommon in infants, older adults, and persons with renal disease, increases the risk of adverse reactions to such drugs. Most substances are filtered into the nephron at the glomerulus, although some drugs are actively secreted by the tubule into the forming urine. Manipulation of urinary pH can alter the degree of ionization and thus the excretion of many substances. Treatment of overdose of alkaline drugs such as the amphetamines can include administration of a urinary acidifier such as ammonium chloride to enhance ionization and excretion of drug. Raising urinary pH with sodium bicarbonate will promote removal of drugs that are acids.

A minor pathway for drug excretion is by way of the bile and the feces. However, as these agents pass through the intestine they are often reabsorbed into the circulatory system. This enterohepatic circulation can prolong the action of drugs.

The elimination of drugs from the body usually follows first-order kinetics. The biologic half-life is that time interval required for one-half of the drug present at time zero to be removed. Drugs with short biologic half-lives must be administered more frequently than those with a longer half-life. A time span somewhat longer than four half-lives is needed for the plasma level of drug to reach its steady state or for drug to be entirely eliminated from the body once administration has ceased. However, if absorption or elimination is altered—for example, by delayed gastric emptying, hepatic enzyme induction, or hepatic or renal dysfunction — then the characteristic drug half-life may be shortened or prolonged.

DRUG INTERACTIONS

Effects of drugs can be modified by the simultaneous or recent previous administration of other drugs or ingestion of foods. Therapeutic effects can be enhanced, and some clinical conditions (e.g., hypertension and cancer) are treated with drug combinations that permit administration of doses lower than would be effective if just one agent were given. This can reduce the incidence and severity of side effects. Drug combinations are also used to counteract adverse reactions, as in the administration of antiemetics concurrently with antineoplastic agents to reduce the severe nausea and vomiting characteristic of chemotherapy.

Drug interactions can also occur inadvertently. Although many are mild and of little clinical consequence, some drug interactions can be severe enough to be fatal. Examples of the latter are the severe respiratory depression that can be induced by two CNS depressants given simultaneously and the tyramine or "cheese" reaction that produces hypertensive crisis in persons taking monoamine oxidase (MAO) inhibitors.

All persons who take drugs are at risk of drug interactions. Hospitalized patients are given large numbers of drugs; many persons experience adverse interactions that prolong their hospitalization. Persons at home also use many drugs, both prescription and over-the-counter preparations, and are often not aware that drugs can interact adversely or that certain foods or alcohol should be avoided.

There are many mechanisms by which drug interactions develop. Some occur even before drugs are administered. In vitro incompatibilities are chemical or physical interactions between drugs combined in solution. Diazepam will not mix with IV fluids or solutions of other drugs. Because of its alkaline pH, sodium bicarbonate inactivates or precipitates a large number of drugs in solution. The compatibility of drugs to be mixed in solution must always be considered.

Similar incompatibilities can occur when drugs are taken PO. Chemical complexation of tetracyclines with calcium from dairy products prevents absorption of the antibiotics from the GI tract. Mineral oil will reduce absorption of fat-soluble vitamins and drugs. Changes in gastric pH, induced by antacids or by drugs such as cimetidine (Tagamet) or the anticholinergics, which reduce acid secretion, will alter the degree of ionization of some drugs.

Changes in urinary pH also will affect the ionization and tubular reabsorption of drugs. Urinary pH is normally acid, thus acidic drugs are nonionized and reabsorbed whereas basic drugs are in their water-soluble ionized form. Drugs and dietary constituents such as fruit juices and proteins can modify pH and drug reabsorption in the nephrons. Renal drug interactions occur also by way of competition for active tubular secretion. Salicylates, probenecid, penicillins, methotrexate, and the oral hypoglycemics are some of the drugs that are inactivated at least partly by renal secretion.

Competition for hepatic drug-metabolizing enzymes may result in slower inactivation of some drugs. MAO inhibitors enhance the effects of many drugs including the barbiturates and opiates. The reduced clearance of drugs such as diazepam, propranolol, and oral anticoagulants given concurrently with cimetidine is thought to involve reduced enzyme activity.

Drug interactions occur when there is increased activity (induction) of the hepatic enzymes. The barbiturates and sedative-hypnotics are among the drugs that induce enzyme activity resulting in more rapid biotransformation of drugs such as lidocaine, oral anticoagulants, and other lipid-soluble agents. Close observation of patients is required when the inducing drug is terminated, since doses of other drugs may have to be decreased as enzyme activity returns to normal levels. The hepatic enzymes are also induced in persons who smoke or who consume significant amounts of alcohol.

Competition among drugs for plasma protein binding sites can result in enhancement of drug effects. Among the agents that bind extensively to these sites are digitoxin, nonsteroidal anti-inflammatory drugs including the salicylates, oral anticoagulants and hypoglycemics, and some antineoplastics.

Some drug interactions occur at the level of receptors. Simultaneous administration of two drugs with anticholinergic activity, as either the intended therapeutic effect or a side effect, can produce additive suppression of the cholinergic nervous system. Receptor antagonists will reduce the effectiveness of agonists. The presence of propranolol or other beta-blockers can interfere with the ability of epinephrine to stimulate cardiac activity. This competitive receptor blockade can be overcome by increasing doses of the agonist.

There are additional mechanisms of drug interactions, some of which are included in later sections of this chapter under discussions of individual drugs. The possibility of interactions should always be considered whenever drugs are administered. A change in the clinical status of patients who are receiving drugs may be an interaction. This should be investigated before additional drugs are prescribed. To reduce the risk of drug interactions, only those drugs that are absolutely necessary should be prescribed. A thorough medical and drug history should be obtained before drug therapy is initiated. The physician should be familiar with sites and mechanisms of drug actions and interactions. Patients should be made aware of the possibility of drug interactions and that over-the-counter preparations, certain foods, and alcohol must at times be avoided.

GUIDELINES FOR DRUG ADMINISTRATION

Before administration of any drugs, a thorough medical history should be obtained from the patient. Individual characteristics such as allergies, current or previous diseases, family history of disease, use of alcohol or tobacco, diet, and capacity for self-care can all significantly influence the consequences of drug administration.

The potential for interindividual as well as intraindividual variations in persons' responses to drugs must always be considered. Elderly persons and infants, especially premature neonates, have greater than normal responsiveness to many drugs. Women have a greater sensitivity than men to many drugs since their higher ratio of adipose to muscle tissue favors sequestration and longer plasma half-life of lipid-soluble agents. In men, exposure to endogenous testosterone promotes a higher level of activity of the hepatic drug-metabolizing enzymes. Body size also influences individual responsiveness. Prescribing drugs based on body weight (e.g., mg/kg) helps to reduce the risks of overdose in small persons and insufficient dose in large persons. The clinical status of a patient affects his or her response to drugs. Hepatic or renal disease can interfere with drug inactivation; cardiovascular disorders alter patterns of blood flow and affect distribution of drugs to sites of action or inactivation. Circadian variations in the effects of some drugs (e.g., general anesthetics, corticosteroids) as well as in the course of some pathological conditions have been reported.

To ensure safe and effective administration of drugs, consideration of all the factors that contribute to patients' responsiveness must guide drug dosage selection. Drug orders must be written legibly and must provide complete instructions for administration. The vast number of similar drug names (e.g., metoprolol and metaproterenol) foster confusion and inadvertent administration of incorrect drugs. Units and amounts of drugs must be clearly specified.

ROUTES OF ADMINISTRATION

Drugs are administered locally (topically), with intended effects in one area of the body, or systemically for widespread effects or for transport to a site of action inaccessible to local application. Application to the skin or into the eye or ear and injection into a confined area are types of local administration. Systemic administration may be enteral, with absorption from the GI tract, or parenteral, which bypasses GI absorption.

The PO route is most frequently used for systemic effects. Dry drug formulations (capsules and tablets) and liquid forms (syrups, elixirs, etc.) can be given by this route. Drugs must become dissolved in the stomach in order to be absorbed—thus the importance of advising patients to take sufficient amounts of water (or other liquid if compatible) with dry oral drug forms. Absorption from the PO route is influenced by many factors, including presence of food in the GI tract and motility of the tract (which can be altered by drugs such as opiates, anticholinergics, and laxatives). Onset of action is slow, and duration of action is prolonged as drug is absorbed gradually over a period of time. Oral medications may cause GI upset with vomiting and diarrhea, and they present the risk of aspiration. The PO route is not used in unconscious or uncooperative patients.

The sublingual route of administration differs from the PO in that the drug is not swallowed but rather is placed under the tongue so that absorption occurs across the sublingual capillary membranes. The patient must understand that the drug is not to be swallowed and that eating, drinking, and smoking should be avoided until the drug has been completely absorbed.

Inhalation of drugs can be used for both local and systemic administration. Bronchodilators delivered from a nebulizer or other pressure device act locally on the bronchioles, whereas anesthetics such as halothane must be absorbed across pulmonary surfaces and transported to their CNS site of action. In medical emergencies such as myocardial infarction and cardiac arrest, some systemic drugs (epinephrine, atropine) can be instilled into the lungs via endotracheal tube.

Injection of drugs is most commonly into muscle (IM), subcutaneous tissue (SC), or directly into the venous circulation (IV). Intrathecal (into the spinal column) and intra-arterial administration are occasionally used. Absorption from muscle is rapid for most drugs, since this tissue is highly vascular. Drugs in oily suspensions (emulsions) can be given IM for gradual absorption and a prolonged duration of action. SC absorption is slower, and some drugs produce severe tissue damage when given by this route. IV administration provides for the most rapid and complete drug action but is a more hazardous route. Only those drug solutions that are labeled for IV administration should be given by this route. All injections must use sterile drug preparations and equipment to reduce the risk of infection.

The transdermal route allows systemic administration of drug through the skin. Nitroglycerin, which is ineffective orally, is available in several transdermal dosages. Disks of the anticholinergic scopolamine, which prevents motion sickness, provide a prolonged duration of action and reduced intensity of side effects. Also available in transdermal form are estrogen and clonidine.

GERIATRIC PHARMACOLOGY

Elderly persons (age 65 and older) consume a large number of drugs, both prescription and over-the-counter preparations. Elderly persons also experience a large proportion of adverse drug reactions and interactions. As the size of the elderly population increases, it becomes ever more apparent that drug effects often are altered in this age-group and that physicians must consider these changes when treating and prescribing drugs for the elderly. Unfortunately, research in this area has been sparse and the exact mechanisms of altered drug responsiveness in the elderly are not completely understood.

There are many physiological changes that take place with advancing age. Because these changes are quite prevalent, they are usually considered to be part of the normal physiology of aging. However, some authorities propose that they are pathological alterations resulting from less than prudent lifestyles or less than adequate health care in younger years. The reasons for such changes are inconsequential for those elderly persons in whom the changes have already occurred (although knowledge of the mechanisms of these changes could be of much benefit to younger persons). It must be recognized that changes that modify drug actions in the elderly do occur.

In elderly persons, the pharmacokinetics of some drugs may be altered. There are several changes in the GI tract that could influence absorption of drugs administered PO. Motility along the GI tract and blood flow in the mesenteric vessels decrease. Reduction in gastric acid secretion can influence the degree of ionization of drug molecules. Most studies, however, have found little evidence for changes in GI absorption of drugs, although that of vitamins and nutrients may be decreased.

Changes in body composition alter the volume of distribution for drugs. There is a reduction in lean body mass and concomitant increase in adipose tissue in the elderly. Lipid-soluble drugs will be sequestered and have prolonged plasma half-lives, whereas water-soluble agents may initially be present in higher amounts in the plasma but can be more rapidly excreted by the kidneys. Dehydration occurs frequently in elderly persons as the kidneys become less able to conserve water. This further reduction in total body water will influence the plasma concentrations of drugs.

Changes in hepatic function occur with advancing age. Synthesis of some plasma proteins (e.g., albumin) decreases, reducing the available number of binding sites for drugs such as warfarin (Coumadin) and phenytoin (Dilantin). As plasma free-drug concentrations increase, there is more rapid delivery of drug to sites of action as well as to sites of inactivation such as the liver and kidneys. Activity of the hepatic enzymes that biotransform drugs may be altered, resulting in a slower rate of drug metabolism.

Reduced cardiac output and alterations in blood flow can hinder transport of drugs. Reduced hepatic blood flow decreases the efficiency of hepatic biotransformation, and reduced renal perfusion interferes with renal clearance of drugs. Glomerular filtration declines significantly, but this is not indicated by serum creatinine levels because muscle mass is also reduced. Decreased filtration results in higher plasma

levels of such drugs as digoxin and many of the antibiotics, which are excreted as unchanged drug. Secretion and reabsorption by the nephrons are also reduced. These changes in renal function influence not only the clearance of drugs but also the maintenance of electrolyte balance in the elderly. Decreased reabsorption of potassium and magnesium can enhance digitalis toxicity and antagonize the effectiveness of antiarrhythmics.

Altered responsiveness to drugs in the elderly may also be pharmacodynamic. There is some evidence that beta-adrenergic receptors become less sensitive and that benzodiazepine receptors (i.e., those for diazepam [Valium]) are increasingly responsive with advancing age.

In addition to age-related physiological changes, many other factors contribute to geriatric responses to drugs. Older persons have a greater incidence of disease, both acute and chronic. Pathological consequences of congestive heart failure and hepatic and renal disease can alter the disposition of drugs. Concomitant with an increased incidence of disease is an increase in the number of drugs used, enhancing the risk of drug interactions. Malnutrition reduces hepatic synthesis of plasma proteins and influences drug-metabolizing enzyme activity.

There is much interindividual variation in drug responsiveness among the elderly. Physiological changes of aging occur at varied rates, and superimposed pathological factors differ among individuals. Thus "proper" drug doses are hard to define for this population, and it is recommended that drug administration in the elderly be initiated at lower (by one-third to one-half) than the usual amounts. After adequate intervals of time for drug effects to appear, increments can be made cautiously. Only those drugs that are absolutely necessary should be given; drug regimens should be periodically reviewed and those agents no longer required should be terminated. Special consideration must be given to the possibility of drug interactions. Patterns of alcohol consumption should be determined. Elderly persons appear to metabolize ethanol quite slowly, enhancing the risk of severe CNS depression when other psychopharmacologic agents (heavily prescribed for the elderly) are given. All drugs should be considered hazardous for use in geriatric patients; some of those that are especially deleterious are indicated in subsequent sections of this chapter. Elderly patients, like all patients, must be given adequate information to enable them to use drugs safely and effectively. Special assistance may have to be given to those who have hearing, sight, or memory deficits or who are easily confused.

DRUGS AND PREGNANCY

Most drugs cross the placenta (those most lipid-soluble will cross most easily) and are carried by the umbilical vein directly into the fetal circulation. Drugs readily enter all fetal tissues including the brain. The fetus has no capacity to inactivate drugs. The hepatic drug-metabolizing enzymes are not completely developed until after birth. Drugs excreted into the amniotic fluid can be swallowed and reabsorbed into the fetal circulation. Plasma protein levels are low, thus drugs are not held in the circulatory system by protein binding.

Many drugs are known or suspected teratogens. When administered to a woman during the first trimester of pregnancy, they can cause fetal damage or death. The severely cytotoxic antineoplastic drugs are teratogenic, as are many hormones administered exogenously. Fetal alcohol syndrome, the result of maternal alcohol consumption, consists of developmental abnormalities ranging from minor structural characteristics of the facial bones to severe CNS aberrations and mental retardation.

In later pregnancy, drugs have a broad spectrum of adverse pharmacologic and developmental effects on the fetus and neonate. Oral hypoglycemics can cause suppression of blood glucose levels that persists after the birth of the infant. Iodides induce neonatal hypothyroidism. Maternal smoking of cigarettes retards fetal development, increasing the risk of spontaneous abortion,, stillbirth, and infants of smaller than average birth weight. The vasoconstrictive action of nicotine is believed to reduce blood flow to the placenta. Placental abnormalities occur more frequently in women who smoke. In addition, blood levels of carbon monoxide are elevated in smokers and can interfere with the transport of oxygen.

Although drugs in general are contraindicated during pregnancy, it is at times necessary to administer drugs to a pregnant woman. Disorders such as diabetes mellitus, epilepsy, and hypertension must be carefully controlled to protect the health of both the mother and the fetus. When drugs are required, the woman should be under close medical supervision throughout her pregnancy. Drug doses should be as low as possible—just sufficient to maintain control of the disorder. The woman should be informed of the potential adverse effects, both of her medical condition and of the drug she is receiving, on her infant. At the time of birth, the physician should be aware of the medical condition and of the drugs that were administered during pregnancy and should have available means to manage possible adverse consequences.

Women who have regularly used physiologically addictive drugs during their pregnancy will often give birth to an infant who is drug dependent and who may undergo withdrawal after birth. In this context, it must be remembered that methadone maintenance is an opiate dependency. Barbiturates, opiates, and other CNS depressants taken by the mother just previous to labor and delivery can cause marked respiratory and cardiovascular depression in the neonate.

Many of the drugs administered during labor and delivery are CNS depressants. Opiate analgesics, phenothiazines, the antihistamine hydroxyzine, and general anesthetics are used to reduce pain and anxiety. These should be used in doses just sufficient to be effective. Epidural anesthesia (usually with lidocaine or procaine) may not cause neonatal depression but can produce severe hypotension in the mother, leading to fetal oxygen deprivation and bradycardia. Epidural anesthesia also reduces the mother's ability to assist in delivery by "pushing" the fetus through the birth canal. If the drug is administered before fetal descent has occurred, a cesarean delivery may become necessary.

Some drugs are given to affect labor, either to inhibit (tocolytic agents) or to enhance (oxytocic agents) its progress. The most frequently used tocolytic is ritodrine (Yutopar), a beta-adrenergic agonist that relaxes uterine smooth muscle. Ritodrine is given IV to suppress uterine contractions, then PO therapy is substituted to prevent the recurrence of contractions. Threatened preterm birth may be delayed briefly by ritodrine

to permit administration of corticosteroids to hasten fetal lung maturation. However, this drug combination can cause maternal pulmonary edema. Ritodrine is contraindicated in hyperthyroidism, eclampsia, uncontrolled diabetes mellitus, hypertension, and other cardiovascular disorders. Adverse effects in both the mother and the fetus/neonate include tachycardia, changes in blood pressure, and fluctuations in blood glucose and potassium levels.

The use of oxytocics is discussed under "Endocrine Pharmacology." More routinely they are used to control postpartum uterine hemorrhage and occasionally to induce abortion.

PEDIATRIC PHARMACOLOGY

Administration of drugs to infants and children requires great caution. Immaturity of the kidneys and of the hepatic drug-metabolizing enzymes results in delayed inactivation of drugs. In the infant, low levels of plasma proteins reduce the available sites for drugs that bind to these molecules. Hemoglobin degradation products can cause hyperbilirubinemia or neonatal jaundice; drugs compete with bilirubin for plasma protein binding sites. Young children generally are more responsive to drugs than are teenagers and adults. The safety and efficacy of most drugs have not been determined in children, thus doses must be carefully selected and patients closely observed for drug effects.

Unintentional administration of drugs to infants can occur when nursing mothers receive medications that are excreted in breast milk. Research has not yet adequately identified those maternal drugs that are hazardous to the nursing infant. Evidence suggests that anticoagulants can cause prolonged clotting time in the infant, and antithyroid drugs will suppress release of the hormones vital to early growth and development. Antineoplastics and radioactive isotopes are too severely cytotoxic to risk injury to the infant. CNS depressants cause excessive sedation and interfere with feeding. Diuretics can cause dehydration in the infant and can reduce maternal secretion of milk. Nursing mothers should be encouraged to avoid all medications, especially during the first few weeks after birth. When drugs are required and the mother continues to nurse, the infant must be closely observed for drug effects.

DRUG TESTING AND LEGISLATION

Drugs arise from various sources. Substances developed from studies of structure-activity relationships, those few of the thousands of natural and synthetic compounds screened for therapeutic effectiveness, and those whose action is serendipitously discovered all may become useful drugs or may be discarded in the process of testing and evaluation.

Drugs are tested initially for therapeutic potential in animal models of various diseases or in in vitro systems such as receptor binding assays. Acute and chronic toxicity are determined in several species of animals. Those agents that appear to have some therapeutic action and a relative degree of safety may be presented to the Food and Drug Administration (FDA) for Investigational New Drug (IND) status. This permits clinical testing to begin in humans, under closely controlled conditions. Phase I, often conducted in young healthy volunteers, attempts to delineate a safe dose range for humans. Phase II involves testing for drug efficacy in carefully selected and closely observed patients. In Phase III, the drug being evaluated is administered to a larger and usually more diverse patient population than that involved in Phase II. Careful observation for both therapeutic response and adverse reactions continues to be important. Drug effects are compared with those produced by placebo, often in the same patient who is alternately given both "drug" forms. Testing can be done in a double-blind manner that reduces the possibility of unconscious bias regarding the drug's effects. New drugs are also compared with standard drugs to determine whether they have greater efficacy or lower toxicity.

When clinical studies are completed, drugs that appear to be safe and effective for humans are presented again by the manufacturer to the FDA in a New Drug Application (NDA). After review of the clinical data included in the NDA, the FDA may release the drug for general marketing. Often it is in this phase that many adverse drug effects become apparent. Physicians must be observant for such responses and must report them to the drug's manufacturer. If evidence of significant toxicity accumulates, the FDA may withdraw the drug from the market or may recommend its use only in certain persons (e.g., those that are refractory to all other forms of therapy).

Federal legislation provides for regulation of the manufacture and sale of drugs in the United States. The Pure Food and Drug Act of 1906 established the FDA to enforce laws designed to protect consumers from ineffective or dangerous drugs. The FDA has the power to approve or deny administration of drugs to humans. Some drugs can be dispensed only with a physician's prescription, whereas others are available without prescription (over-the-counter drugs). Manufacturers cannot make false or misleading claims about their products and must provide adequate instructions for the safe and effective use of all drugs.

In reaction to the alarming increase in drug abuse and addiction that occurred in the 1950s and 1960s, the federal government passed the Comprehensive Drug Abuse Prevention and Control Act of 1970. Also referred to as the Controlled Substances Act, this law classified many drugs into schedules according to their addiction liability and established guidelines regarding the possession, availability, and use of these substances.

The Orphan Drug Act of 1983 has established principles and incentives for the development and marketing of drugs that promise no financial return to the manufacturer. Included are substances that are not subject to patent laws and those that will alleviate rare disorders and thus have a limited market.

The Drug Price Competition and Patent Term Restoration Act of 1984 has reduced the requirements for approval to market generic forms of drugs. A single-dose bioequivalency test in a small number of healthy volunteers can be sufficient, although the FDA can demand more extensive studies. The bioequivalency of the generic form must be between 80 and 120% of the standard drug.

DRUG CLASSIFICATIONS AND GROUPS

CENTRAL NERVOUS SYSTEM DRUGS

Antidepressants

Major psychiatric depressions are categorized into bipolar and unipolar affective disorders. In bipolar disorders, periods of depression alternate with periods of mania and with periods of relatively normal mood. In unipolar disorders, depression and normal mood alternate. Depressive disorders are often seasonal or cyclical, with spontaneous remissions. The etiology of major affective disorders is not fully understood. Environment, heredity, and CNS biochemistry all appear to be factors. Some depressions are triggered by major life events, although most reactive depressions remit over time and should not be treated with drugs unless they are persistent and incapacitating. Many major depressions seem to arise from within. There is no apparent external reason for the sadness and hopelessness felt by the patient. The fact that the drugs useful in treating depression are agents that alter CNS neurotransmitter systems supports the hypothesis that brain chemistry is involved.

The antidepressant drugs (Table 6-1) are grouped into three categories: the tricyclics and the MAO inhibitors, which have been used for many years, and several second-generation drugs, which bear some similarities to the tricyclics. Early theories on the mechanism of action of antidepressants were

Table 6-1. Antidepressant Drugs

Generic name	Trade name	Recommended adult doses (mg PO/day)
Tricyclic drugs		
Amitriptyline	Elavil	75–150
Desipramine	Norpramin Pertofrane	75–200
Doxepin	Adapin Sinequan	75–150
Imipramine	Tofranil	75–200
Nortriptyline	Aventyl Pamelor	75–100
Protriptyline	Vivactyl	15–40
Trimipramine	Surmontil	75–200
MAO inhibitors		
Isocarboxazid	Marplan	30
Phenylzine	Nardil	30–60
Tranylcypromine	Parnate	10–20
Second-generation drugs		
Amoxapine	Asendin	200–300
Maprotiline	Ludiomil	75–150
Trazodone	Desyrel	150–400
Benzodiazepines		
Alprazolam	Xanax	0.75–4

based on their ability to inhibit synaptic inactivation of the neurotransmitters norepinephrine and serotonin. However, the immediate effect on neurotransmitters was difficult to reconcile with the delayed onset (2 to 3 weeks) of clinical antidepressant effects. Current theories stress the ability of these drugs to alter CNS receptors, in particular to reduce the sensitivity of (to "down regulate") beta-adrenergic receptors.

The **tricyclic antidepressants**, so called because of their three-ring molecular nucleus, are the most commonly used antidepressants. Because of their considerable lipid solubility, these drugs are generally biotransformed in the liver and thus must be administered cautiously in the presence of hepatic dysfunction. Most tricyclics cause some degree of sedation and anticholinergic effects such as dry mouth, constipation, and urinary retention, which can be especially troublesome in the elderly. Great caution must be used if tricyclics are administered to persons with glaucoma or prostate enlargement. Cardiovascular side effects occur, most notably orthostatic hypotension and tachycardia. Overdose of a tricyclic can be fatal; ventricular fibrillation and atrioventricular block can occur. These drugs have been used as agents for committing suicide, and children who accidentally injest a few tablets are in great danger of dying. The cholinomimetic physostigimine has been used to reverse many of the effects of tricyclic toxicity.

Because of the potential for additive effects, anticholinergic drugs and CNS depressants should be administered cautiously to persons receiving a tricyclic antidepressant. The tricyclics inhibit the presynaptic amine pump, which recaptures norepinephrine into adrenergic nerve terminals, thus the action of sympathomimetic drugs will be enhanced. However, drugs such as guanethidine, which require the amine pump for transport to their site of action, will be less effective. The H_2-receptor antihistamine cimetidine can enhance the effects of the tricyclics. The combination of a tricyclic and a MAO inhibitor, long considered absolutely contraindicated, has recently been found to be effective in many refractory cases of depression. Extreme caution and careful adjustment of doses by a physician experienced in the use of antidepressants are necessary.

The **MAO inhibitors** fell into disrepute when their ability to induce hypertensive crisis after ingestion of tyramine became apparent. However, these drugs are often of great benefit to persons who do not respond to the other antidepressants.

The MAO inhibitors reduce the enzymatic degradation of catecholamines and other monoamines. The major toxicity of these drugs occurs because of the inhibition of intestinal and hepatic MAO, which normally metabolizes monoamines (e.g., tyramine) from dietary sources. These amines, which are potent vasopressors, are able to reach postsynaptic alpha receptors and cause potentially fatal hypertension. For this reason, persons taking MAO inhibitors must avoid certain foods (Table 6-2). Persons who will not adhere to dietary restrictions should not be given MAO inhibitors. The concurrent ingestion of most other drugs, both prescription and over-the-counter agents, also is contraindicated. Because they have a long duration of action, 7 to 14 days must elapse between drug termination and relaxation of restrictions.

Additional adverse effects of MAO inhibitors are cardiac arrhythmias and orthostatic hypotension. Both the tricyclics

Table 6-2. Dietary Restrictions With MAO Inhibitor Therapy

Cheeses except for cream and cottage

Red wines and beer

Yogurt

Brewer's yeast

Fava and broad beans

Bananas

Liver

Pickled and smoked fish

Fermented foods

Excessive amounts of caffeine

Chocolate

and the MAO inhibitors can lower the seizure threshold and can induce hypomanic episodes.

Lithium is currently the only drug widely used for the control of mania in bioplar depression. Its safety margin is narrow, and patients must be closely monitored for signs of drug toxicity. Serum levels of lithium should be maintained between 0.6 and 1.4 mEq/L, although some patients, especially the elderly, will have adverse effects at lower levels. Doses administered to gain control during manic episodes can be reduced for maintenance therapy. Early symptoms of toxicity include GI disturbance, ataxia, thirst, polyuria, confusion, and drowsiness. Severe effects include convulsions, coma, fatal cardiac arrhythmias, and circulatory collapse.

Lithium is inactivated totally by renal excretion, thus must be administered very cautiously in persons with renal dysfunction. Lithium is excreted or reabsorbed by the renal tubules in parallel with sodium, so adequate intake of salt and fluids should be maintained. Lithium itself can induce sodium depletion. Diuretic therapy causes salt and water depletion, resulting in enhanced lithium retention and increased risk of toxicity. This drug combination should therefore be avoided. Lithium is contraindicated during pregnancy, since cardiovascular toxicity and suppression of thyroid function in the fetus and neonate can occur.

Although the **second-generation antidepressants** have many similarities to the tricyclics, they also possess characteristics that set them apart. Trazodone appears to work through serotonergic activity. It is both an agonist and an antagonist, and it inhibits synaptic uptake. Trazodone causes less cardiotoxicity and cholinergic suppression than the tricyclics. Its therapeutic and sedative effects are marked in some patients and absent in others. Priapism and increased sexual drive have been reported. Maprotiline resembles desipramine in structure and activity. The incidence of seizures and dermatologic reactions appears to be more frequent than with other tricyclics. Nomifensine inhibits synaptic uptake of dopamine and norepinephrine. It has little effect on the cardiovascular system, thus it is considered safer than the tricyclics in persons with cardiovascular disorders. Anticholinergic and sedative effects also appear to be fewer than for other antidepressants. Amoxapine blocks dopamine receptors and thus has antipsychotic efficacy as well as the potential to induce extrapyramidal movement disorders. Severe seizures have occurred in persons receiving amoxapine. Sedative and anticholinergic activity are frequent. Alprazolam is a benzodiazepine with antianxiety and antidepressant efficacy. Sedation is the most common adverse effect.

Antipsychotic drugs

Used in the management of schizophrenia, agitation, and other behavioral and personality disorders, antipsychotic drugs (Table 6-3) are also called **neuroleptics** or **major tranquilizers**. Although these agents do not cure psychotic illness, they can control many of the symptoms and enable patients to lead relatively normal lives.

The **phenothiazines**, of which chlorpromazine is the prototype and is the agent against which the potency of other antipsychotics is measured, are the most widely used. Other

Table 6-3. Antipsychotic Drugs

Generic name	Trade name	Recommended adult doses (mg PO/day)
Phenothiazines		
Chlorpromazine	Thorazine	30–200 (25 mg IM)
Fluphenazine	Prolixin	0.5–10
Mesoridazine	Serentil	100–400
Perphenazine	Trilafon	12–24 (5–10 mg IM)
Prochlorperazine	Compazine	15–50 (5–10 mg IM)
Promazine	Sparine	60–800 (50–150 IM)
Thioridazine	Mellaril	150–800
Trifluoperazine	Stelazine	2–40
Thioxanthines		
Chlorprothixene	Taractan	75–600
Thiothixene	Navane	6–60
Butyrophenones		
Haloperidol	Haldol	1–10 (2–5 mg IM)
Additional drugs		
Molindone	Moban	15–225
Loxapine	Loxitane	20–100

drugs effective in alleviating psychotic illness (listed in Table 6-3) all produce similar therapeutic and adverse effects. Patients refractory to one antipsychotic drug may respond to an alternate agent. Blockade of CNS dopamine receptors appears to be the mechanism of action for these drugs. This observation has given rise to a dopaminergic hypothesis for the etiology of schizophrenia. Additional support for this hypothesis is that dopamine agonists such as the amphetamines can induce a syndrome very similar to schizophrenia.

The antipsychotic drugs alleviate all of the symptoms of psychotic disturbance. Some are used to manage hyperactivity and aggression in children (e.g., chlorpromazine) or to reduce emotional symptoms such as fear and depression in the elderly (e.g., thioridazine) and to achieve rapid control in psychiatric emergencies. Haloperidol is effective in Tourette's syndrome. Some of the phenothiazines are used as antiemetics, and some will control refractory hiccups.

In general, the antipsychotics have antihistaminic, anticholinergic, and antiadrenergic activity. Drowsiness is a common side effect of many, although tolerance may develop. Blockade of alpha-adrenergic receptors causes hypotension, especially orthostatic, which can be severe. Hypertension also occurs as well as changes in heart rate. Sudden death apparently due to cardiac arrest has been reported. Caution is required in patients with cardiovascular disorders. Agranulocytosis and other changes in blood constituents develop. Preexisting blood dyscrasias are contraindications to the antipsychotic drugs. Photosensitivity is common. Anticholinergic exacerbation of glaucoma and urinary retention make these drugs hazardous in some persons. Altered control of body temperature, possibly through inhibition of sweating, presents the risk of fatal hyperthermia in warm environments. The elderly seem especially sensitive to this effect. A neuroleptic malignant syndrome includes fever, altered levels of consciousness, and muscle rigidity. Depression of the cough reflex predisposes to the danger of choking on foods.

A major adverse effect of the antipsychotic agents is **tardive dyskinesia**. Characterized by abnormal involuntary movements of the facial muscles in particular, this disorder develops slowly during chronic drug administration and is usually irreversible. Abrupt termination of drug may precipitate or worsen tardive dyskinesia. Patients should be closely observed for appearance of subtle indications of this adverse effect, and drug treatment should be stopped by gradual reduction of doses if it develops. Tardive and other dyskinesias (parkinsonism, akathisia, and dystonias) that occur with antipsychotic medications appear to be the result of blockade and subsequent hypersensitivity of dopamine receptors in the extrapyramidal region of the brain. Some acute reactions can be eased with anticholinergic agents; however, tardive dyskinesia may be exacerbated. Anticholinergic drugs should not be given concurrently with antipsychotics. They do not prevent dyskinesia but can suppress early warning symptoms that drug administration should cease.

Several preexisting clinical conditions necessitate cautious use of the antipsychotics. A lowering of seizure threshold provokes convulsions, especially in persons with seizure disorders. In the elderly and in persons with pulmonary disease, severe and even fatal pneumonia can develop. Gastric ulcer and cardiovascular diseases may be aggravated. Changes in renal function or blood components suggest that drug be gradually terminated. The antiemetic effect can hide drug toxicity and other disturbances such as intestinal obstruction and increased intracranial pressure, which usually produce vomiting. Antipsychotic drugs are contraindicated in Parkinson's disease, in which the deficits in dopaminergic transmission are worsened by dopamine receptor blockade. Preexisting CNS depression can be deepened.

The antipsychotic drugs are hepatically metabolized and can induce a hepatitis-like syndrome. Caution is required in the presence of liver disease. The plasma half-life of these agents is long (up to 20 hours). They are sequestered in many tissues, are highly protein bound, and are enterohepatically circulated. The onset of antipsychotic effect is prolonged; 3 to 6 weeks of continued administration may be required before a good therapeutic response is obtained. In contrast, sedation occurs much more rapidly, within hours or even minutes depending on route of administration (which can be IV, IM, or PO). Drug doses should be increased only very gradually. Chronic doses, which may be continued for many years, should be reduced to levels that just maintain control of symptoms. Although the antipsychotics all produce similar effects, there are some differences in degree of sedative, extrapyramidal, and anticholinergic action.

Numerous other adverse responses have been attributed to the antipsychotics. Endocrine changes, allergic reactions, bronchospasm, increase in appetite, decrease in thirst, vision disturbances, constipation due to reduction in GI motility, confusion, depression, and worsening of psychosis are a few of the effects that must be continually observed for in persons taking these drugs.

Many drug interactions can occur. Anticholinergic drugs add to the suppression of cholinergic activity. Alpha-adrenergic blockade by the antipsychotics prevents a pressor response to epinephrine. MAO inhibitors reduce the inactivation of these drugs, whereas hepatic enzyme inducers increase the rate of biotransformation. Antipsychotic agents interfere with presynaptic uptake of guanethidine and amphetamines and reduce the efficacy of levodopa and other dopamine agonists. Effects of CNS depressants can be potentiated. There have been some reports of increased haloperidol toxicity when lithium is given concurrently. The phenothiazines can elevate plasma levels of beta-blockers such as propranolol and metoprolol.

Sedative-hypnotics

Sedatives produce a relaxed, calm state of mind. Hypnotics induce sleep. The sedative-hypnotic drugs are sedative at low doses and hypnotic at higher doses. Used in particular to relieve insomnia, this category of drugs includes benzodiazepines, barbiturates, and several miscellaneous agents. Insomnia can be transient or chronic and can markedly affect general health and well-being. Sedative-hypnotics provide short-term alleviation, as tolerance to their effects develops rapidly. The causes of each incidence of insomnia should be investigated, and nonpharmacologic therapy should be considered. Sleep disturbance can be a symptom of an underlying disorder like depression. Sleep patterns change with advancing age. Drugs such as caffeine, alcohol, nicotine, alpha-adrenergic antagonists (e.g., over-the-counter decongestants) and some of the antidepressants can interfere with sleep. It is ironic that sedative-hypnotics, by altering patterns of rapid-eye-movement (REM) sleep, also can cause sleep disturbances.

Barbiturates. The barbiturates (Table 6-4) are a large group of drugs having several therapeutic applications. An important difference among them, related to their degree of ionization and lipid solubility at physiological pH, is their onset of action. The ultrashort-acting barbiturates (e.g., thiopental) are used for induction and supplementation of general anesthesia. Intermediate-acting agents, (e.g., pentobarbital) are used in particular as sleeping aids and for preanesthetic sedation. Long-acting barbiturates (e.g., phenobarbital) are anticonvulsants effective in the control of acute and chronic seizure disorders.

The barbiturates are well-absorbed after parenteral or PO administration. Those that are most lipid soluble are most rapidly and widely distributed to all parts of the body including the CNS. As acids thus largely nonionized at normal urinary pH, the barbiturates readily diffuse out of the renal tubules and back into the circulatory system. The barbiturates are metabolized in the liver by the microsomal oxidizing-enzyme system and have the ability to induce the activity of these enzymes. Some barbiturates can also be excreted unchanged in the urine.

The barbiturates are general CNS depressants. Overdose will produce coma and fatal respiratory failure. They appear to work by stabilizing nerve cell membranes, thus making neurons less responsive to stimuli. Their sedative and hypnotic effects seem mediated by depression of the reticular activating system in the brain stem. Recent evidence suggests that the inhibitory CNS neurotransmitter gamma-aminobutyric acid (GABA) may be involved in the mechanism of action of the barbiturates.

Because they are CNS depressants, the barbiturates can cause drowsiness, fatigue, dizziness, and, in increasing doses, respiratory depression. They can also produce paradoxical CNS stimulation with restlessness and excitement, especially in elderly persons. (Barbiturates are best not used at all in the elderly, since they can also produce severe CNS depression.)

The barbiturates are highly addictive drugs, and all are controlled substances. Tolerance to their effects develops rapidly, thus inducing patients to use larger and larger doses. Psychological dependence occurs first, and continued use rapidly produces physiological dependence. Abrupt termina-

Table 6-4. Barbiturate Sedative-Hypnotics

Generic name	Trade name	Recommended adult doses (mg PO/day)
Amobarbital	Amytal	45–100
Butabarbital	Butisol	45–100
Hexobarbital	Sombulex	30–200
Pentobarbital	Nembutal	90–120 (150–200 mg IM)
Secobarbital	Seconal	30–200

tion of drug administration results in an abstinence syndrome that can include restlessness, anxiety, tremors, and convulsions, which can be severe.

Withdrawal from barbiturate dependence is most safely accomplished under hospitalization, using gradually reduced doses of a long-acting agent (e.g., phenobarbital). Close observation of the patient is necessary as doses are carefully adjusted to amounts just sufficient to prevent the development of withdrawal symptoms.

Because the barbiturates are often used as agents of suicide, they should be dispensed with great caution if at all to persons suffering mental depression. (Benzodiazepine hypnotics are somewhat safer in this respect.) Emergency treatment of barbiturate overdose consists most especially of supporting respiration and blood pressure until the drug effects disappear. Alkalinization of the urine (e.g., with sodium bicarbonate) can alter the degree of drug ionization and thus enhance the excretion, especially of the longer-acting barbiturates. Long-term care of persons who have deliberately taken barbiturate (or any other) overdoses should include assistance in identifying and alleviating the causes of such actions.

The barbiturates are involved in two major groups of drug interactions. The first is with any drug that has CNS depressant activity. Significant enhancement of CNS depression can occur, rapidly leading to respiratory depression and failure. The second group of interactions involves drugs that are hepatically metabolized. The barbiturates induce the acitvity of the microsomal enzyme-oxidizing system, thus many drugs are inactivated more rapidly and must be given in larger doses to be effective. When barbiturate administration is terminated, the enzyme activity will return to normal levels and the dose of the continued drug will probably have to be reduced. Close observation of the patient is necessary at such times. Barbiturates also induce the hepatic synthesis of porphyrins, which precludes their use in persons susceptible to porphyria.

Barbiturates in small doses are sometimes administered together with (nonnarcotic) analgesics. Their sedative effect may decrease the emotional response to pain and may also help to induce rest. Barbiturates themselves are not analgesic and in fact can be hyperalgesic.

Benzodiazepines.   The use of barbiturates as sedative-hypnotics has largely been replaced by the **benzodiazepines**. Three are used as hypnotics: flurazepam (Dalmane, 15 to 30 mg), which has a long plasma half-life and duration of action; triazolam (Halcion, 0.125 to 0.5 mg), with a short half-life; and temazepam (Restoril, 15 to 30 mg), with an intermediate half-life. The longer duration of flurazepam is due in part to the formation of pharmacologically active metabolites. Daytime sedation is a hazardous side effect. Persons must be warned to use caution when driving or operating other machinery.

The benzodiazepines interact with highly specific receptors that are most abundant in the limbic system and the cerebral cortex. The inhibitory effects of the neurotransmitter GABA are enhanced by the benzodiazepines, which produce more selective and less marked CNS depression than the barbiturates and thus have a wider safety margin when administered alone. Concurrent administration with other CNS depressants (e.g., alcohol) can cause extreme enhancement of respiratory depression, which can be fatal.

The hepatic microsomal enzymes inactivate the benzodi-azepines, thus the elderly and persons with decreased liver function may rapidly develop excessive sedation when normal drug doses are administered. The H_2-receptor antihistamine cimetidine decreases the biotransformation of diazepam and may have the same effect on all benzodiazepines.

Psychological and physiological drug dependence develops with continued use of the benzodiazepines, which are controlled substances (Schedule IV). Abrupt termination of administration, especially of those agents having a short plasma half-life, results in rebound insomnia and anxiety. (The pharmacology of the benzodiazepines is discussed further under "Antianxiety drugs.")

Additional sedative-hypnotics.   **Chloral hydrate** (0.5 to 2 g) and **triclofos** (1.5 g) are metabolized to trichloroethanol, which has hypnotic activity. The final inactive metabolite, trichloro-acetic acid, binds strongly to plasma proteins and thus can potentiate the effects of other drugs that are protein bound. Both hepatic and renal function are important for elimination of chloral hydrate and triclofos. Tolerance, as well as psychological and physiological dependence, may occur and withdrawal can be severe. Chronic high doses cause renal damage. These drugs must be administered cautiously to persons with cardiac disease.

Ethchlorvynol (Placidyl, 0.5 to 1 g) and **glutethimide** (Doriden, 250 to 500 mg) should be used only for therapy lasting less than 1 week. Hepatic enzymes extensively metabolize these drugs. Glutethimide induces the hepatic microsomal enzymes and has signficant anticholinergic activity. Both drugs produce psychological and physiological dependence and in overdose can cause respiratory failure.

Paraldehyde (4 to 8 ml) is usually administered PO despite its objectionable odor and taste. IM injection sites must be chosen carefully, as paraldehyde can damage nerve fibers. Hepatic enzymes are important for drug inactivation, although 20 to 30% of a dose can be excreted unchanged by the lungs. Overdose can result in prolonged coma. Like all sedative-hypnotics, paraldehyde is a controlled substance.

Antianxiety drugs

The **benzodiazepines** (Table 6-5) are currently the most widely used antianxiety agents. Additional uses for benzodiazepines include diazepam in the management of seizures, alcohol withdrawal, muscle spasm, and presurgical anxiety; chlordiazepoxide in alcohol withdrawal and presurgically; chlorazepate in alcohol withdrawal and seizure disorders; lorazepam presurgically and for insomnia; and oxazepam in alcohol withdrawal and for anxiety and tension in the elderly. Alprazolam appears to be especially effective in alleviating anxiety accompanying depression. (Benzodiazepines are also discussed under "Sedative-hypnotics" and "Anticonvulsants.")

The mechanism of action of the benzodiazepines appears to involve interaction with the CNS inhibitory neurotransmitter GABA. In contrast to the barbiturates, which were previously used to alleviate anxiety disorders, the benzodiazepines produce less widespread CNS depression. Their action is relatively specific for the limbic and reticular activating systems.

The benzodiazepines are hepatically metabolized, some (e.g., diazepam and chlordiazepoxide) to active metabolites, which extends their duration of action. Lorazepam and oxazepam yield inactive metabolites and are safer for use in the elderly and in persons with hepatic dysfunction. Benzodiaze-

Table 6-5. Benzodiazepine Antianxiety Drugs

Generic name	Trade name	Recommended adult doses (mg PO/day)
Alprazolam	Xanax	0.75–4
Chlordiazepoxide	Librium	15–100 (50–100 mg IM)
Chlorazepate	Tranxene	30–60
Diazepam	Valium	4–40 (2–20 mg IM, IV)
Halazepam	Paxipam	20–160
Lorazepam	Ativan	2–6 (0.05 mg/kg IM)
Oxazepam	Serax	30–120

pines are most commonly given PO. IV administration of diazepam, chlordiazepoxide, or lorazepam is used when an immediate onset is needed or the PO route is not suitable. However, this route can cause respiratory and cardiac arrest, especially in the elderly and in seriously ill patients. IM administration of these drugs is painful, and absorption is poor. The benzodiazepines bind extensively to plasma proteins. Because of their lipid solubility, they readily cross biologic membranes and are sequestered in adipose tissue.

The benzodiazepines have a notably wide margin of safety when they are used in recommended doses for brief periods of time and when other CNS drugs are avoided. The most common adverse effect is sedation, to which tolerance frequently develops within a few days. Other reported CNS effects include headache, confusion, ataxia, sleep disturbances, fatigue, dizziness, syncope, depression, and occasional extrapyramidal motor dysfunction. Blood dyscrasias and hepatic dysfunction can develop with long-term administration. Fever, rash, and vision disturbances may occur. Paradoxical CNS stimulation has been reported, especially in psychiatric patients. This reaction requires termination of drug administration. The possibility of respiratory depression and changes in cardiovascular function necessitates cautious administration in persons with pulmonary or cardiovascular disorders, especially when a parenteral route is used. Means for resuscitation must be available before IV or IM administration is begun. Additional adverse effects that can occur with the parenteral route are cough, laryngospasm, hyperventilation, and chest pain during peroral endoscopy. Local anesthetics can reduce this last effect. Tonic status epilepticus has occurred after IV administration of diazepam in persons with petit mal. Severe hypotension may occur, especially if barbiturates, opiates, or alcohol is taken simultaneously. Thrombophlebitis or lactic acidosis can develop following IV administration. The benzodiazepines are contraindicated in coma or shock.

The benzodiazepines do produce psychological and physiological drug dependence and must be given cautiously if at all to persons with history of drug abuse (with the exception of short-term management of alcohol withdrawal). To terminate long-term administration, drug doses should be reduced gradually. Abrupt cessation of drug can induce a withdrawal syndrome similar to that in alcohol and barbiturate dependence. Anxiety, insomnia, tremor, cramps, vomiting, diarrhea, and convulsions can occur. In the treatment of anxiety, benzodiazepines should be administered only for short periods of time. Nondrug means for alleviating or coping with anxiety and stress should be encouraged.

Benzodiazepines may be teratogenic. Habitual use throughout pregnancy can result in muscle flaccidity and physiological drug dependence, with subsequent withdrawal in the neonate. Accumulation of drug in breast milk may induce sedation and weight loss in the nursing infant. Children and the elderly are particularly sensitive to the CNS depression produced by benzodiazepines. Therapy should be instituted with low drug doses that can be gradually increased as necessary. Patients should be observed for cumulative effects arising from the long plasma half-lives of many benzodiazepines. The presence of hepatic or renal dysfunction requires cautious administration.

Under usual circumstances, the benzodiazepines are most dangerous when they are administered simultaneously with other CNS depressants, including alcohol. Patients must be instructed to avoid such drugs. Marked depression of the CNS can develop, resulting in extreme lethargy, respiratory failure, brain damage, and death. Benzodiazepines should not be given to persons acutely intoxicated with alcohol. Opiates given concurrently should be at reduced dosage. The benzodiazepines are somewhat anticholinergic and can add to that action of other drugs. Cimetidine prolongs the plasma half-life of diazepam and possibly of other benzodiazepines; isoniazid and disulfiram (Antabuse) also have been reported to reduce the clearance of these drugs. Rifampin and smoking of cigarettes induce hepatic biotransformation of the benzodiazepines. Both increased and decreased effectiveness of benzodiazepines in women taking oral contraceptives have been noted. Administration of PO doses with food will decrease both GI disturbances and drug absorption. Antacids also reduce oral drug absorption. IV benzodiazepine solutions are incompatible with many fluids and drugs.

Several additional agents are available for use in the management of anxiety. **Meprobamate** (Equanil, Miltown, 0.75 to 1.6 g), which was the first of this type of drug to be used extensively, did not produce the same degree of CNS depression as the barbiturates. Similarly to the benzodiazepines, meprobamate induces drug dependence and is a Schedule IV controlled substance. Drug administration should be gradually tapered, especially after long-term use. Meprobamate appears to selectively depress activity in the thalamus and limbic system. It is hepatically inactivated. Teratogenicity and neonatal drug dependence may occur if meprobamate is used during pregnancy. Administration to persons with seizure disorders can precipitate convulsions, which can also occur during drug withdrawal. Meprobamate can induce all the symptoms of CNS depression (sedation, ataxia, dizziness, weakness, confusion) but can also cause paradoxical stimulation (panic reactions, insomnia). Hypersensitivity responses include rash, fever, blood dyscrasias, hyperpyrexia, bronchospasm, renal failure, anaphylaxis, and severe dermatologic reactions.

There is usually cross-sensitivity among meprobamate and

the skeletal muscle relaxants carbromal and carisoprodol. GI disturbances and cardiovascular effects such as arrhythmias and severe hypotension have occurred. Meprobamate is contraindicated in porphyria, which can be exacerbated. Overdose can cause fatal cardiovascular and respiratory collapse. Combination with other CNS depressants results in intensification of effects.

Hydroxyzine (Atarax, Vistaril, 50 to 100 mg, 25 to 100 mg IM) has antihistaminic, anticholinergic, antiemetic, muscle relaxant, and local anesthetic activity. It is used in the management of anxiety concomitant with many disorders. Used both pre- and postsurgically, it reduces anxiety and emesis and will potentiate analgesic activity, allowing reduction in drug dosage. Hydroxyzine alleviates the severe itching of allergic and other dermatologic reactions. It is administered only by the PO and IM routes, the latter into a large muscle mass. The drug can induce severe nerve and subcutaneous tissue damage, and injection sites should be alternated. The most common adverse effects are sedation and dry mouth. Patients must be observed for changes in the oral mucosal lining. Tremor and seizures will occur at high dosages. Hydroxyzine may be teratogenic. Other CNS depressants should be avoided, as their effects can be potentiated.

Buspirone (Buspar) represents a new, nonsedating type of antianxiety agent.

Antiparkinson drugs

Parkinsonism is the result of defective dopaminergic transmission in the nigrostriatal pathway that terminates in the basal ganglia of the extrapyramidal system. Idiopathic Parkinson's disease develops in a small percentage of the population, usually with onset after the age of 50 years. Parkinsonism can also occur after manganese and carbon monoxide poisoning or viral encephalitis and can be induced by drugs like reserpine, which depletes neuronal dopamine content, by neuroleptics, which are dopamine receptor antagonists, and by methylphenyltetrahydropyridine (MPTP), a contaminant found occasionally in synthetic "street" opiates. The progression of the syndrome is usually slow, with gradual appearance of resting tremor, muscle stiffness, and akinesia (difficulty in initiating voluntary movement).

The decrease in dopaminergic activity is accompanied by an increase in cholinergic influence. (Evidence suggests that other neurotransmitter systems, e.g., noradrenergic, serotonergic, and opioid, are also affected). The drugs used to treat parkinsonism interact with these CNS neurotransmitters to alleviate the symptoms of the disease. The progression of the syndrome is not affected. One of the major disadvantages of the currently available antiparkinson drugs is the gradual loss of their efficacy.

Levodopa (Larodopa, Dopar, 0.5 to 8 g), the precursor of dopamine, is most frequently employed in the treatment of parkinsonism. Dopamine itself is not useful because it does not cross the blood-brain barrier. Levodopa enters the CNS and is taken up by dopaminergic neurons and converted by dopa decarboxylase to dopamine. Levodopa is also peripherally transformed into dopamine, necessitating either administration of large doses or coadministration of a dopa decarboxylase inhibitor that does not cross the blood-brain barrier. In current practice, carbidopa is usually given with levodopa. Sinemet is a commercial preparation that combines both drugs in one dosage unit.

Nausea and vomiting are frequent adverse effects of levodopa that can be ameliorated by reducing doses and by administering the drug immediately after meals. The latter measure, however, can reduce the amount of levodopa that reaches the CNS. Protein ingestion should be limited, as dietary amino acids seem to compete with levodopa for passage across the blood-brain barrier. Levodopa can also cause hypotension and hypertension, cardiac arrhythmias, involuntary movement of skeletal muscles (dyskinesias), hallucinations, and euphoria.

The optimal onset of levodopa therapy (i.e., early or late in the course of the disease) is controversial. Once levodopa has lost its effectiveness, the other currently available drugs are also ineffective. Loss of levodopa activity is characterized by the "on-off" effect: rapid alternation between control and exacerbation of symptoms. This may be partly related to fluctuations in the amounts of drug entering the brain. Measures such as IV administration or giving the drug shortly before meals will occasionally ameliorate the loss of response.

Bromocriptine (Parlodel, 2.5 to 15 mg) is a dopamine receptor agonist used in the treatment of parkinsonism. Like endogenously formed dopamine, it directly stimulates dopamine receptors, thus reducing the deficit that causes parkinson symptoms. However, it is not effective in all patients. Because of its similar mechanism of action, its adverse effects resemble those of levodopa. Concomitant administration of a dopa decarboxylase inhibitor is not required, however.

Amantidine (Symmetrel, 100 to 200 mg), developed as a virucidal agent, appears to stimulate release or to reduce reuptake of neuronal dopamine. In parkinsonism, its efficacy is low and tends to diminish further after a few months of treatment. Its adverse effects are similar to those of levodopa, with the addition of livedo reticularis (a black and blue mottling of the skin on the legs).

Anticholinergic drugs, including some that are also antihistaminic (Table 6-6), have a different antiparkinson action from the drugs just described. Anticholinergics reduce the cholinergic hyperactivity that is presumed to occur as inhibitory

Table 6-6. Antiparkinson Anticholinergic Drugs

Generic name	Trade name	Recommended adult doses (mg PO/day)
Benztropine	Cogentin	0.5–6
Biperiden	Akineton	4–8
Diphenhydramine	Benadryl	75–200 (10–100 mg IM, IV)
Ethopropazine	Parsidol	50–600
Orphenadrine	Disipal	150–250
Procyclidine	Kemadrin	7.5–15
Trihexyphenidyl	Artane	1–10

dopamine influence decreases. (The pharmacology of these drugs is described under "Autonomic Nervous System Pharmacology.")

Combinations of these drugs can be used in the management of parkinsonism. However, additional levodopa should not be administered to persons taking a dopa/carbidopa combination, and caution must be used when transferring patients from levodopa alone to levodopa plus a decarboxylase inhibitor. Side effects of the antiparkinson agents are occasionally alleviated with other drugs—for example, the reduction of postural hypotension by methylphenidate (Ritalin). Vitamin B_6 (pyridoxine) is a dopa decarboxylase cofactor that can increase the rate of inactivation of levodopa. Administration of antipsychotic drugs such as the phenothiazines and haloperidol should be avoided in parkinsonism since their dopamine blocking properties will reverse the efficacy of antiparkinson agents. Levodopa is contraindicated in persons taking MAO inhibitors, as hypertensive crisis can occur.

General anesthetics

General anesthetics include IV drugs as well as gases and volatile liquids administered by inhalation. Anesthesia is achieved in distinct steps ("stages" and "planes") that are similar for all agents. During recovery from anesthesia, these steps occur in reverse order. **The first stage** is induction, lasting from onset of drug administration to loss of consciousness. IV barbiturates produce an extremely brief induction and are often used to carry the patient rapidly through this stage and the second to the surgical stage, which is then maintained with inhalation anesthetics. The latter drugs produce a more gradual induction in which the patient is somewhat aware of changes in mentation. Some surgery can be performed in this stage, although in such instances deeper anesthesia is usually induced and then lightened. Even though pain and other sensations are suppressed, the patient's sense of hearing is often quite acute at this level of consciousness.

The second stage of anesthesia is delirium, characterized by loss of voluntary control. Depression of higher cerebral centers seems to disinhibit subcortical regions. This is a dangerous stage, for the patient may struggle violently or vomit. On recovery, patients will not remember their actions or the events that occurred during this time.

The third stage, that of surgical anesthesia, is divided into four planes of gradually deepening loss of involuntary activity. Ocular and respiratory signs delineate these planes. The patient's pupils, widely dilated in the delirium stage, return to normal. The eyes wander in plane 1 but become fixed in plane 2 as the pupils constrict. In plane 3, pupillary dilation begins as CNS hypoxia develops; the pupils become nonreactive to light, and the blinking reflex is lost.

Respiration also changes during the deepening planes of stage III. Usually relatively normal in planes 1 and 2, breathing grows shallow as the intercostal muscles are paralyzed by the spinal depression that occurs in plane 3. Respiration becomes abdominal as the diaphragm assumes a greater role in breathing. When this diaphragmatic breathing lessens and becomes irregular, then plane 4 has been reached. This plane is dangerously close to stage IV, characterized by respiratory failure and death unless anesthesia is terminated and supportive measures are begun immediately. Stage IV and plane 4 of stage III can be avoided by careful administration of anesthesia and by close observation of the patient. Most surgical procedures can be performed at plane 3. Spinal depression produces virtually complete relaxation of all skeletal muscles. If further paralysis of muscle is required, neuromuscular blocking drugs can be administered while the patient's respiration is mechanically assisted.

On completion of the surgical procedure, anesthesia administration is terminated and the patient gradually recovers consciousness as the drug is eliminated from the body. One of the greatest dangers during recovery is vomiting and aspiration; patients should not be left unattended until full return of consciousness. Some anesthetic agents are sequestered in adipose tissue and prolong recovery as they are slowly released back into the circulation.

Anesthetic agents are usually combined with each other and with other drugs to minimize dangerous adverse reactions. This is called **mixed** or **balanced anesthesia**. The stages and planes of anesthesia become less distinct when multiple agents are used. For example, preanesthetic opiates and anticholinergics can obscure some of the characteristic ocular changes.

Inhalation anesthetics. Volatile liquid anesthetics include the **fluorinated agents** halothane (Fluothane), methoxyflurane (Penthrane), isoflurane (Forane), and enflurane (Ethrane). All are nonflammable and nonexplosive. The fluorinated anesthetics cause varying degrees of myocardial depression and hypotension.

Halothane produces rapid induction that can quickly progress to a dangerously deep level of anesthesia. Administration of this agent requires caution and skill. Halothane dilates bronchioles and does not stimulate respiratory secretions. Neuromuscular blocking agents usually must be given to achieve adequate relaxation. Halothane produces extreme uterine atonia that can be refractory to oxytocic agents. Hypotension and cardiac arrhythmias can occur; the latter can be reduced by avoiding both hypoxia and concurrent administration of catecholamines. Potentially fatal hepatotoxicity is a characteristic adverse effect of halothane. Patients should be observed for jaundice, leukocytosis, and fever. Repeated administration of this agent should be avoided or spaced at prolonged intervals. Recovery from halothane is relatively free from nausea and vomiting.

Methoxyflurane produces slow induction and recovery. Other agents can be used for more rapid induction to stage III anesthesia; skeletal muscle relaxants frequently are required. Opiates are contraindicated when this agent is used, since respiratory failure can occur. Methoxyflurane may cause hepatotoxicity, although renal toxicity is more frequent. Administration of large or prolonged doses of this drug should be avoided, and patients must be observed for changes in renal function.

Isoflurane achieves greater skeletal muscle relaxation and less myocardial sensitization to catecholamines than other fluorinated agents. **Enflurane** is less likely to cause liver and kidney damage. Induction and recovery are rapid. Depression of respiration can be significant. A relatively good degree of muscle relaxation can be achieved with enflurane, although large doses can stimulate the CNS, causing muscle twitching similar to seizure activity.

The fluorinated agents, like most inhalation anesthetics, can produce **malignant hyperthermia** in patients with genetic predisposition to this potentially fatal reaction. Muscle biopsy can predict susceptibility, and dantrolene (see "Skeletal muscle relaxants") can be given to reduce elevated body temperature or prophylactically before surgery. Increases in heart and respiratory rate are additional symptoms of this syndrome.

Gas anesthetics include cyclopropane, nitrous oxide, and ether. **Cyclopropane** produces good anesthesia with rapid induction and skeletal muscle relaxation. Oxygen must be administered concurrently, making a combination of gases that is highly explosive. Cardiac arrhythmias, postsurgical hypotension, laryngospasm, and vomiting during recovery can occur. Concurrent administration of anticholinergics or catecholamines increases the risk of arrhythmia. This anesthetic is frequently used in high-risk patients, since it does not markedly affect blood pressure.

Nitrous oxide produces no skeletal muscle relaxation and relatively light anesthesia (plane I of stage III is the deepest attainable). Induction and recovery are rapid. It is frequently used as a component of balanced anesthesia, enhancing the efficacy of other gas anesthetics such as halothane. Nitrous oxide is analgesic and can be used alone for brief surgery (1 to 2 minutes) and for dental and obstetric procedures that do not require deep loss of consciousness. Adequate oxygen must be given with nitrous oxide to avoid serious hypoxia. Brief procedures can be performed under 70 to 80% nitrous oxide. With administration for more than a few minutes, lower concentrations of anesthetic must be used. After prolonged nitrous oxide administration, patients should breathe 100% oxygen for 5 to 10 minutes. Caution must be used in the presence of disorders adversely affected by hypoxia and by administration of high levels of oxygen. In general, nitrous oxide is quite safe in moderate concentrations. It does not produce nausea or organ toxicity. Alone it is nonflammable, but it will support combustion, as will the high concentrations of oxygen used simultaneously.

Ether induces good anesthesia and muscle relaxation for most surgical procedures, including those of long duration. It also produces analgesia and can be used with no supplementary drugs. The classic stages and planes of anesthesia are most distinct with ether. Induction is slow (10 to 20 minutes). Administration of drug can be decreased once surgical anesthesia is attained. Recovery is prolonged, and vomiting frequently occurs. Ether induces little change in cardiovascular activity, and the risk of catecholamine-induced arrhythmias is low. Reflex respiratory stimulation helps to maintain normal spontaneous breathing. Irritation of the respiratory tract produces a significant increase in secretions that can be reduced by anticholinergic premedication. Postsurgical atony of the GI and urinary tracts can be alleviated with cholinomimetics. Drugs with neuromuscular blocking effects, including several antibiotics, can add to the skeletal muscle relaxation of ether. Ether is both explosive and flammable. Vinyl ether (Vinethene) is similar to ether but produces rapid induction and recovery and is used only for surgical procedures that are of short duration. Skeletal muscle relaxation is not as good as that produced by ether, and the potential for organ toxicity is greater.

Systems for administration of inhalation anesthetics can be open, semiclosed, or closed. In open systems, vapors from the anesthetic mix with ambient air, and additional oxygen and respiratory support are not necessary as long as spontaneous breathing occurs. In a semiclosed system, vapors mixed with oxygen are administered by face mask and expired gases are removed from the system. Expired gases are not vented from a closed system. Carbon dioxide is removed and oxygen is added to the anesthetic vapors, which the patient rebreathes. A closed system reduces both the danger of fire and the exposure of medical personnel to the anesthetic.

Inhalation anesthetics in general are not biotransformed. They are eliminated as they were absorbed—that is, across the alveolar surfaces.

Intravenous anesthetics. The ultrashort-acting barbiturates **thiopental** and **methohexital** are frequently used for induction of anesthesia, which is then maintained with inhalation agents. Barbiturates do not produce analgesia or muscle relaxation. The use of adjunctive drugs can make barbiturate anesthesia suitable for some procedures that are of short duration. Recovery from barbiturates is usually rapid and free of nausea and vomiting. However, the marked lipid solubility of these drugs promotes sequestration in adipose tissue, and the subsequent slow release after termination of anesthesia can cause prolonged sedation. Since respiratory depression or arrest can occur, means for support of respiratory and cardiovascular function must be available. Because laryngospasm and bronchospasm can develop, the barbiturates are given cautiously if at all to asthmatic patients. Barbiturates potentiate the effects of other CNS depressants.

Ketamine is an IV agent that produces analgesia and a "dissociative" state in which the patient is awake but lacks awareness. It is used for brief surgical or painful procedures. It does not produce skeletal muscle relaxation. Cardiovascular and respiratory activity usually increase (severe hypertension and stroke are contraindications to the use of ketamine), although hypotension, bradycardia, and apnea also occur, the latter especially after rapid administration. Recovery from ketamine anesthesia is characterized by delirium and hallucinations that may persist for several hours. These symptoms can be reduced by placing the patient in an environment free of sensory stimuli or by administering diazepam or a barbiturate. Premedication with an opiate also decreases the risk of such unpleasant experiences. Ambulatory patients must remain under observation until recovery from ketamine is complete. The street drug phencyclidine (PCP) is related to ketamine.

A combination (called **Innovar**) of the opiate fentanyl and the neuroleptic droperidol is administered IV to produce a state known as neuroleptanalgesia. Pain sensation is markedly depressed, and the patient is sedated but conscious. Innovar is used for induction and as an adjunct to maintain anesthesia. It can be used alone for some surgical and diagnostic procedures that are facilitated by the patient's ability to respond. Innovar can produce adverse effects of both fentanyl and droperidol. Respiratory depression or failure can occur and can be alleviated by a narcotic antagonist. Patients should be closely observed for 24 hours after drug administration. Marked muscle rigidity, restlessness, changes in blood pressure and heart rate, laryngospasm, bronchospasm, delirium, and hallucinations can occur.

Although the IV agents are more easily administered than the inhalation anesthetics, they are not as readily excreted. In general they must be hepatically inactivated, and severe adverse reactions may require support of vital functions until the drug is metabolized.

Adjunctive drugs. Many drugs are used in conjunction with general anesthetics. Preanesthetic medications to reduce anxiety and facilitate achievement of surgical anesthesia include the benzodiazepines (e.g., diazepam; midazolam [Versed]), the barbiturate sedative-hypnotics, and the antianxiety antihistamine hydroxyzine. Opiates may be given presurgically if needed for supplemental anesthesia. However, they can increase nausea and vomiting during recovery. Opiates are used briefly after surgery to alleviate severe pain. Phenothiazines produce sedation and can suppress vomiting caused by general anesthetics. They also potentiate hypotension during surgery, thus are more safely administered only during recovery, when the occurrence of vomiting is most frequent.

Skeletal muscle relaxants are frequently employed during surgery. **Succinylcholine** provides brief paralysis for intubation. **Tubocurarine** has a longer duration of action and will prevent reflex muscle response to painful stimuli. The effects of the nondepolarizing neuromuscular blockers can be reversed by cholinesterase inhibitors such as neostigmine. Anticholinergic drugs can be given presurgically when the use of anesthetics that cause laryngospasm, bronchospasm, bradycardia, or respiratory secretion is planned. Cholinomimetics are used postsurgically to stimulate the urinary and GI tracts. Antiarrhythmic drugs should be readily available when agents such as cyclopropane and halothane, which promote catecholamine-induced rhythm disturbances, are used.

Anticonvulsants

Seizures can arise from a number of causes that provoke abnormal firing of cells in the CNS. Hypoglycemia, head injury, tumors, cerebral anoxia or edema, drug ingestion or withdrawal, and high fever especially in children are among the disorders that may generate convulsions. Epilepsy is a common neurological disturbance of which the major symptom is convulsions. Seizures are classified into several types. **Partial seizures** begin in one body area and may remain localized or become generalized. Included are **jacksonian** and **psychomotor seizures**. **Generalized seizures** are bilateral throughout and may be **tonic-clonic** (grand mal), **myoclonic** (involving certain muscle groups), or brief alterations in consciousness called **absence seizures** or **petit mal**. **Status epilepticus** is a rapid series of grand mal seizures.

There are several groups of anticonvulsant drugs, each being effective against certain types of seizures. The decision to initiate a course of drug therapy after a first seizure should be based on thorough examination to rule out secondary causes that can be treated and to assess the risk of further seizures against the potential adverse effects of the anticonvulsant drugs. If drug therapy is begun, doses should be increased gradually until seizure control or adverse reactions appear. If one drug fails, another appropriate drug should be gradually substituted. A large percentage of patients can attain seizure control with a single drug. Combinations of drugs should be used only if no single agent is effective. Some patients will be refractory to all drug treatment. Administration of anticonvulsants should never be terminated abruptly, since exacerbation of seizures, including status epilepticus, may occur. Patients must be made aware of this and should carry medical identification outlining their drug regimen. Although drugs do not cure epilepsy, some patients do not require lifelong therapy. After several years of complete seizure control, drugs may be gradually withdrawn to determine if seizures will recur.

Although the anticonvulsants represent several pharmacologic groups, they share some common characteristics. All cause CNS depression, resulting in drowsiness, slowed reflexes, ataxia, and other symptoms. Alcohol should be avoided by persons with seizure disorders since it may potentiate drug-induced CNS depression, can interact with the biotransformation of many anticonvulsants, and also increases the risk of seizure activity (i.e., it lowers the seizure threshold). Many anticonvulsants are folate antagonists and can induce megaloblastic anemia. Several anticonvulsants have been linked with birth defects and neonatal hemorrhage. However, convulsions can cause temporary fetal anoxia, and women with seizure disorders who are or want to become pregnant require special care.

Barbiturates are among the earliest drugs recognized to have anticonvulsant action. The long-acting **phenobarbital** (100 to 300 mg, 200 to 300 mg IM, IV) is widely used in the management of tonic-clonic and partial seizures. It is effective in status epilepticus and in convulsions secondary to disorders such as tetanus, eclampsia, and drug toxicity. **Mephobarbital** (Mebaral, 400 to 600 mg) and **metharbital** (Gemonil, 100 to 600 mg) control both grand and petit mal. **Amobarbital** (Amytal, 60 to 150 mg) and **secobarbital** (Seconal 100 to 300 mg) may be used in acute convulsive episodes. The barbiturates produce CNS depression by stabilizing neuronal cell membranes, in particular in the reticular activating system. Administered PO, IM (deep to prevent tissue damage, although blood vessels and major nerves must be avoided), or IV (avoid extravasation), the barbiturates are inactivated by and also strongly induce the hepatic microsomal enzymes. Some barbiturates bind to plasma proteins.

The most common adverse effect of barbiturates is drowsiness; other symptoms of CNS depression may also appear. Respiratory depression occurs, especially at higher doses, and coma and death may follow. The barbiturates have been used as agents of suicide. Support of vital functions is usually the most effective treatment of overdose. GI upset, cardiovascular depression, and allergic reactions may occur. Barbiturates are contraindicated in porphyria and respiratory depression. Caution is required in the presence of hepatic or renal dysfunction (e.g., in the elderly), pain (barbiturates can be hyperalgesic), severe anemia, diabetes mellitus, asthma, and cardiovascular disease. Administration during pregnancy can result in fetal malformation, decreased levels of vitamin K-dependent clotting factors, and neonatal drug dependency and withdrawal. The barbiturates produce psychological and physiological addiction and should not be given to persons with history of drug abuse. Abrupt discontinuance may precipitate withdrawal symptoms (possibly severe) and sleep disturbances, as well as exacerbation of seizures. Barbiturates may provoke "paradoxical" excitement in children and in the elderly. Drug interactions are numerous. Potentiation of other CNS depressants including alcohol can be lethal. The hepatic inactivation of many drugs (e.g., theophylline, oral anticoagulants, corticosteroids, estrogens) is increased, necessitating larger doses. When barbiturate administration is terminated, patients must be observed for development of drug toxicity, and doses may have to be reduced as enzyme activity returns to normal. MAO inhibitors, valproic acid, and disulfiram reduce the inactivation of barbiturates. Foods or drugs containing calcium interfere with the GL absorption of barbiturates.

The **hydantoins** are a second group of drugs that have long been used as anticonvulsants. **Phenytoin** (Dilantin, 300 to 400 mg), **mephenytoin** (Mesantoin, 50 to 600 mg), and **ethotoin** (Peganone, 1 to 3 g) are most effective in generalized grand mal and in partial seizures. They reduce cellular excitability by stabilizing cell membranes, in particular in the motor cortex and brain stem. Phenytoin is also used as an antiarrhythmic. Because of the cardiodepressant activity of the hydantoins, IV administration is contraindicated by such cardiovascular disorders as sinus bradycardia and heart block. The usual route of administration for the hydantoins is PO. Phenytoin may be given IV in emergencies (e.g., status epilepticus and neurosurgical seizures), although hypotension, arrhythmias, and respiratory arrest can occur. Administration should not exceed 50 mg/minute. The IV line should be flushed with saline after phenytoin, which is alkaline and thus incompatible with other drugs in solution. Because of tissue irritation and erratic absorption, the IM route should be used only if an IV line cannot be established. The hydantoins are hepatically metabolized and renally excreted. Caution is required during administration to the elderly or to persons with decreased liver or kidney function. Adverse effects are numerous. Blood dyscrasias occur in particular with mephenytoin, which also causes more CNS adverse effects such as sedation and is usually used only for patients who have not responded to other drugs. Porphyria is a relative contraindication. Megaloblastic anemia may develop. Lymph node hyperplasia, usually reversible but occasionally progressing to malignancy, has been reported. Rashes of several types, including potentially fatal dermatologic manifestations, may occur. Hyperglycemia, hepatitis, GI disturbances, and gingival overgrowth are but a few of the many adverse effects that can be expected.

Drug interactions also are numerous. Many drugs (e.g., cimetidine, disulfiram, dicumarol, isoniazid, and several antibiotics) interfere with inactivation of phenytoin. Salicylates in high doses can displace hydantoins from plasma protein binding sites. Antacids, foods or drugs containing calcium, and some chemotherapeutic agents interfere with oral absorption. Hepatic enzyme inducers decrease hydantoin effectiveness. Phenytoin itself is an enzyme inducer, thus can decrease the effects of other hepatically metabolized drugs. Phenytoin may displace oral anticoagulants such as warfarin from protein binding sites and can add to the effects of other cardiac depressants. Phenytoin depletes folic acid, yet administration of this vitamin can enhance phenytoin metabolism.

Two groups of drugs, the **succinimides** and the **oxazolidinediones**, are especially useful in reducing the incidence of absence seizures. The succinimides are **ethosuximide** (Zaron-

tin, 500 mg), methsuximide (Celontin, 0.3 to 1.2 g) and phensuximide (Milontin, 1 to 3 g). Ethosuximide is considered by many to be the drug of choice for petit mal, whereas methsuximide is generally reserved for patients refractory to other drugs. The succinimides depress the motor cortex activity that is characteristic of petit mal. Inactivation of these agents appears to be both by hepatic biotransformation and by renal excretion of unchanged drug, thus caution is necessary in persons with hepatic or renal dysfunction. Patients who experience other types of seizures in addition to petit mal will require additional drug therapy. The succinimides can provoke grand mal seizures. There are many adverse effects. Blood dyscrasias that can be fatal, personality changes such as depression and aggression, dermatologic disorders, renal damage, GI upset, CNS symptoms such as drowsiness, and alterations in mental activity are just a few. The succinimides may enhance the effects of other anticonvulsants such as valproic acid, phenytoin, and primidone. As with all anticonvulsants, abrupt termination of drug may increase seizure occurrence.

The oxazolindinediones **paramethadione** (Paradione, 0.9 to 2.4 g) and **trimethadione** (Tridione, 0.9 to 2.4 g) have greater toxicity than the succinimides, thus are reserved for refractory patients. Among their serious adverse effects are potentially fatal renal damage (kidney function should be monitored, changes usually require drug termination), dermatologic disturbances that can become life-threatening (appearance of any rash requires cessation of therapy), blood dyscrasias (observe for signs of anemia or abnormal bleeding), GI and CNS symptoms, syndromes similar to lupus erythematosus and to myasthenia gravis, fatigue or drowsiness, and vision changes (hemeralopia). The oxazolidinediones are teratogenic, thus contraindicated in pregnancy. Other contraindications include preexisting hematologic disorders, hepatic or renal dysfunction, and ophthalmic conditions that might be exacerbated by spontaneous bleeding. All patients must be closely observed for appearance of adverse effects. Administration of the oxazolidinediones can provoke grand mal seizures; abrupt withdrawal of drug can provoke petit mal. Although few specific drug interactions have been reported, the concurrent administration of any drug having similar adverse effects could result in additional toxicity.

Some of the **benzodiazepines** are effective anticonvulsant agents. **Clonazepam** (formerly Clonopin, the trade name has been changed to Klonopin to reduce confusion with similar drug names) is useful in some types of petit mal and partial seizures and can be effective in persons refractory to succinimides. **Clorazepate** (Tranxene) is occasionally combined with other drugs to control partial seizures. Oral **diazepam** (Valium, 2 to 40 mg) may be used as an adjunct in seizure disorders; given by slow IV bolus (5 to 10 mg), this benzodiazepine will terminate status epilepticus. The benzodiazepines can provoke grand mal seizures; clonazepam combined with valproic acid may increase the occurrence of petit mal. Diazepam should not be administered to persons who have recently ingested alcohol, because severe CNS depression can occur. Phlebitis and thrombosis may develop with IV administration; extravasation should be avoided. Diazepam should not be combined with other drugs in IV solutions. Benzodiazepines are addictive, thus are contraindicated in persons with history of drug abuse.

(The many additional adverse effects and precautions of these drugs are discussed under "Antianxiety drugs.")

Paraldehyde (Paral) also will terminate status epliepticus and may be used to control seizures secondary to eclampsia, tetanus, and drug ingestion. It can be given rectally or by IV bolus or infusion. Paraldehyde is hepatically inactivated, thus is administered cautiously if at all in persons with liver dysfunction. The drug is also excreted partly through the lungs and is contraindicated in respiratory disorders. Paraldehyde can produce physiological dependence. IV administration may provoke pulmonary hemorrhage or edema, cardiovascular failure, coughing, and tissue damage at the injection site. Given rectally, paraldehyde can damage the mucosal lining of the bowel. Metabolic acidosis may occur. Cardiovascular and respiratory depression caused by overdose can be fatal. The effect of other CNS depressants can be enhanced. Disulfiram given within the previous 10 to 14 days contraindicates paraldehyde administration, since inactivation of the latter drug will be reduced. [Paraldehyde is discussed further under "Sedative-hypnotics.")

Valproic acid (Depakene, 15 to 60 mg/kg) is used alone or in combination with other drugs in the treatment of petit mal, and it may also be effective in other types of seizures including grand mal. Its mechanism of action may involve elevation of the amounts of the inhibitory neurotransmitter GABA in the CNS. Valproic acid is metabolized in the liver and has been reported to cause hepatic damage that can be fatal. Liver function should be determined before drug is begun and should be monitored frequently, especially during the first 6 months when risk of hepatotoxicity is greatest. Patients, especially those having preexisting liver disease, should be closely observed for any signs of deteriorating hepatic function. Valproic acid, like most anticonvulsants, may be teratogenic. Other adverse effects include GI disturbances, impaired blood coagulation, mental changes, sedation, and pancreatitis. Valproic acid is often used in combination with other anticonvulsants, although adverse interactions have been reported. Valproic acid with clonazepam can control petit mal but may also exacerbate it. Valproic acid can decrease or elevate plasma levels of phenobarbital and can potentiate the effects of all CNS-depressant drugs. The effect of valproic acid on platelet function can add to the action of anticoagulant drugs. Salicylates may displace valproic acid from plasma protein binding sites.

Carbamazepine (Tegretol, 0.4 to 1.2 g) has potentially serious side effects, and its use as an anticonvulsant is frequently reserved for those patients with generalized tonic-clonic or partial seizures refractory to other drugs. Carbamazepine is also used to relieve glossopharyngeal and trigeminal neuralgia and certain other types of pain (it is not a general analgesic, however) and it has investigational use in the treatment of psychiatric disorders. The mechanism of action of carbamazepine is not known. The drug is hepatically biotransformed, and one metabolite is pharmacologically active. both the parent drug and metabolites bind to plasma proteins. Plasma levels of drug should be monitored to decrease the risk of toxic effects: 5 to 12 mcg/ml is the recommended range.

Carbamazepine can cause potentially lethal bone marrow depression. Complete baseline blood counts should be obtained before therapy is begun and repeated weekly for 3 months, then monthly. Patients must be observed for any evidence of anemia, infection, or bleeding. Any sign of blood dyscrasia requires that drug administration be terminated (with the precaution that abrupt cessation of anticonvulsant medication may precipitate seizures). Persons with previous history of blood dyscrasias should not be given carbamazepine. This drug may impair hepatic and renal activity. Tests to determine function of these organs should precede therapy, and drug administration in persons with decreased function requires caution. Jaundice or proteinuria may develop. Structurally related to the tricyclic antidepressants, carbamazepine has similar anticholinergic and sedative properties and can provoke confusion or psychotic symptoms, especially in the elderly. Other CNS side effects include dizziness, loss of coordination, vision disturbances including lens opacity, tinnitus, and hallucinations. Nausea and vomiting are common but can be reduced by initiating therapy with low doses. Cardiovascular effects such as changes in blood pressure, thrombophlebitis, aggravation of cardiac failure, or vascular insufficiency can be severe. Administration to persons with cardiovascular disorders requires caution. Dermatologic reactions can be serious. Carbamazepine stimulates secretion of antidiuretic hormone, making it useful in the treatment of diabetes insipidus but giving it the potential to cause water intoxication. The hepatic inactivation of many drugs such as the oral contraceptives and anticoagulants, theophylline, and possibly other anticonvulsants is enhanced by carbamazepine. Conversely, anticonvulsants such as phenytoin and phenobarbital may increase carbamazepine metabolism. Cimetidine and propoxyphene (Darvon) may reduce the inactivation of carbamazepine. Because of its tricyclic nature, this drug should not be given concurrently with MAO inhibitors. CNS depression may be potentiated by other depressant drugs. Concomitant administration of drugs that suppress bone marrow activity should be avoided.

Primidone (Mysoline, 0.75 to 2 g), used in the treatment of partial and generalized tonic-clonic seizures, is hepatically metabolized partly to phenobarbital. A second metabolite, phenylethylmalonamide, has anticonvulsant activity. Both metabolites have a long plasma half-life. Primidone can be effective against seizures refractory to other drugs including barbiturates. Primidone can cause dizziness, ataxia, emotional changes, and marked sedation; tolerance may develop to these effects. Other adverse responses include dermatologic reactions, nausea, vision disturbances, and occasionally megaloblastic anemia that can be reversed by folic acid administration.

Phenacemide (Phenurone, 1.5 to 3 g) is reserved for patients who are refractory to other drugs; it is especially effective in controlling psychomotor seizures. Phenacemide is hepatically inactivated and must be given cautiously to persons with decreased liver function. Severe mental changes may require termination of drug. Other adverse reactions include GI upset, sedation, hematologic disorders (blood counts should be determined frequently), hepatic and renal damage, and allergy. Phenacemide is considered to be one of the more toxic anticonvulsants, and patients should be closely observed for appearance of adverse effects. Drugs with similar adverse effects should not be concurrently administered.

The carbonic anhydrase inhibitor **acetazolamide** (Diamox, 0.35 to 1 g) can be combined with other anticonvulsants to aid in the control of grand mal, petit mal, and partial seizures. The exact mechanism by which this drug reduces abnormal CNS activity is not known. The rapid development of tolerance to the efficacy of acetazolamide can be reduced by intermittent drug administration. (The pharmacology of acetazolamide is discussed under "Diuretics.")

Magnesium sulfate can be used as an anticonvulsant and is discussed under "Electrolytes and Trace Elements."

Central nervous system stimulants

The CNS stimulants have very limited clinical application, although some like the amphetamines are widely misused and abused. Caffeine and the analeptics doxapram and nikethamide are discussed under "Respiratory stimulants."

The **amphetamines** (Table 6-7) are sympathomimetic amines that have greater effect in the CNS than in the periphery. Their legitimate consumption has declined significantly in recent years. The anorectic action of amphetamines makes them useful for initiating weight-reduction programs. Tolerance rapidly develops to this effect, and administration of drug should not be continued beyond 2 to 3 weeks. Amphetamines, in particular **dextroamphetamine**, are indicated in the management of narcolepsy. In this disorder, tolerance does not develop to the beneficial effects of these drugs. Amphetamines also have sustained activity in the treatment of juvenile behavioral abnormalities characterized by hyperactivity and short attention span. The exact mechanism by which amphetamines exert their therapeutic effects is not known. They appear to release norepinephrine from sympathetic neurons and also to directly stimulate adrenergic receptors. Although they are generally considered cerebral stimulants, their anorectic effect is probably exerted in the hypothalamus and their counteraction of narcolepsy in the reticular system. Several theories have been proposed for the alleviation of behavioral disorders. Amphetamines are hepatically inactivated.

Amphetamines have significant potential for abuse and are Schedule II controlled substances. Feelings of euphoria and great energy and alertness are contributing factors in their misuse. Larger and larger doses are consumed as tolerance develops to these effects. Amphetamines should not be administered to persons with history of drug misuse. Signs of abuse are hyperactivity, irritability, confusion, hallucinations, insomnia, and psychosis resembling schizophrenia. Termination of drug use provokes depression and fatigue ("crashing"). Amphetamine administration should never be continued unless the patient is clearly obtaining therapeutic benefit from the drug and shows no indication of misuse. For weight reduction, other methods should be tried first and amphetamines used only briefly and as a final resort. Reduction in caloric intake and modification of eating habits must be included in the patient's regimen.

In the treatment of hyperkinesis, drugs should not be administered to children merely for the benefit of parents or teachers. In children, amphetamines can suppress food intake sufficiently to interfere with growth and if taken late in the day can interfere with proper rest. In some children, amphetamines exacerbate the symptoms of hyperkinesis. These children may respond to the antihistamines hydroxyzine or diphenhydramine or to the tricyclic antidepressant imipramine. Periodically, drug administration should be reduced or stopped to determine whether the child has yet outgrown his or her disability.

Because they are sympathomimetic, amphetamines have a marked stimulatory effect on the cardiovascular system. Dextroamphetamine appears to have weaker cardiovascular action than other amphetamines. Vasoconstriction results in elevated blood pressure; heart rate may be increased or reflexly slowed. Amphetamines are contraindicated in hypertension, in arteriosclerosis and other cardiovascular disorders, and in hyperthyroidism, which sensitizes the myocardium to sympathomimetic influence. Overstimulation of the CNS can occur; at high doses convulsions may be followed by coma and death. GI effects include vomiting, diarrhea, constipation, and dry mouth. Amphetamines cause pupillary dilation, thus are hazardous in persons with glaucoma. Patients should be cautious in such activities as driving, since amphetamines can obscure extreme fatigue. Doses should be given at times that will not interfere with patients' normal sleep patterns. To discontinue long-term administration, drug dosages should be gradually reduced.

Amphetamines should not be administered concurrently with MAO inhibitors, since the hypertensive action of the latter can be potentiated. Drugs that alkalinize the urine will promote amphetamine reabsorption; those that acidify urine (e.g., ammonium chloride) favor its excretion and have been used to treat drug overdose. Since amphetamines can elevate blood glucose levels, caution is required when these drugs are administered to diabetics. Hypoglycemic drug doses may have to be increased. However, amphetamine-induced reduction in food intake will decrease the antidiabetic drug requirements. Antihypertensive drugs also may be less effective when amphetamines are administered simultaneously.

The slight elevation of mood and energy obtained with low doses of amphetamines is occasionally considered beneficial in persons suffering mild or reactive depression that produces apathy and fatigue. Amphetamines may potentiate opiate analgesia and can modify persons' responses to chronic painful disorders.

The **anorexiants** phenmetrazine (Preludin, 50 to 75 mg), mazindol (Mazanor, 1 to 3 mg), diethylproprion (Tenuate, 75 mg), phendimetrazine (70 to 105 mg), and phentermine (15 to 37.5 mg) have actions quite similar to the amphetamines. They are effective only for a brief period of time (up to 12 weeks) and have sympathomimetic cardiovascular effects. They are subject to abuse. Phenylpropanolamine (PPA) is a similar drug available in over-the-counter appetite suppressants. Its efficacy is ques-

Table 6-7. Amphetamines

Generic name	Trade name	Recommended adult doses (mg PO/day)
Amphetamine		5–30
Benzphetamine	Didrex	25–150
Dextroamphetamine	Dexedrine	5–30
Methamphetamine	Desoxyn	10–15

tioned, and it has been reported to cause psychotic symptoms and marked cardiovascular stimulation. Persons taking MAO inhibitors must be warned against this type of medication. Fenfluramine (Pondamin, 60 to 120 mg) is an anorexiant that depresses the CNS, thus causing sedation.

Pemoline (Cylert) is a CNS stimulant used in the management of hyperkinesis. It has minimal cardiovascular effects. Pemoline appears to work by way of stimulation of central dopaminergic pathways. It is both hepatically metabolized and renally excreted as unchanged drug. The presence of hepatic or renal dysfunction requires cautious drug administration. Drug-induced alterations in hepatic function, sometimes developing gradually, have been reported. Liver function should be monitored. Anorexia and insomnia, usually transient, are frequent adverse effects. Once-a-day dosing early in the morning can reduce interference with sleep. Paradoxical drowsiness, dyskinesia, seizures, and other CNS symptoms may occur. The onset of action is long; alleviation of hyperactivity often develops gradually over 3 to 4 weeks.

Methylphenidate (Ritalin) is used mainly in the management of hyperkinesis or attention deficit disorders in children, and its mood-altering action may be of benefit in some instances of mild depression. The drug is hepatically inactivated. Its actions are similar to those of the amphetamines. Changes in heart rate and blood pressure can occur, thus caution is required in persons with hypertension and other cardiovascular disorders. Abdominal pain and suppression of growth can be especially troublesome side effects in children. Methylphenidate lowers seizure threshold and should be discontinued if convulsions occur. Anxiety, agitation, and psychotic behavior may be exacerbated and require that the drug be discontinued. Dermatologic disorders, indicative of hypersensitivity, have occurred, as have alterations in blood constituents. Blood counts should be monitored. The most frequent adverse effects are nervousness and insomnia. In overdosage, hyperpyrexia and other symptoms of severe CNS and cardiovascular stimulation can develop. Severe hypertension may result if methylphenidate is combined with MAO inhibitors or sympathomimetic agents. Methylphenidate inhibits biotransformation of antidepressants, anticonvulsants, and anticoagulants.

AUTONOMIC NERVOUS SYSTEM PHARMACOLOGY

Adrenergic agonists

Drugs that stimulate sympathetic or adrenergic activity are also called **sympathomimetics**. These drugs interact with the four types of receptors in the sympathetic nervous system: alpha$_1$ postsynaptic receptors; alpha$_2$ presynaptic receptors, which seem to inhibit further release of the adrenergic neurotransmitter norepinephrine; beta$_1$ receptors in the heart, and beta$_2$ receptors in various other tissues including bronchiolar smooth muscle.

The naturally occurring agonists, which are also catecholamines, are epinephrine, norepinephrine, and dopamine. Epinephrine activates alpha- and beta-adrenergic receptors. Norepinephrine has greater effects on alpha receptors in blood vessels, although it also strongly stimulates beta$_1$ receptors in the heart. Dopamine (the precursor of the other two catecholamines) interacts with both alpha and beta receptors, and also with receptors that are specific for dopamine itself.

Some synthetic adrenergic drugs activate both alpha and beta receptors, whereas others stimulate only one receptor type. Some agonists interact directly with the receptors (direct-acting). Others cause the release of norepinephrine and/or epinephrine, which then stimulate receptors. Such agents are called indirect-acting agonists. A few drugs appear to act both directly and indirectly.

The adrenergic drugs have many therapeutic uses, some of which are discussed more extensively in other sections of this chapter. In anaphylactic shock, **epinephrine** rapidly reverses vasodilation, stimulates cardiac activity, and dilates bronchioles. In cardiac arrest, epinephrine alone may restore heartbeat, or it can be used to enhance cardiac responsiveness to electric shock. Epinephrine must be administered parenterally. It is available in solutions of various concentrations, and great care must be taken that the correct amount (0.5 to 1 mg/5 minutes IV) is given since an overdose can be lethal. The bronchodilator action of epinephrine makes it especially useful in alleviating asthma. Epinephrine is one of the many types of drugs used to treat glaucoma. The mechanism by which it reduces intraocular pressure is not completely understood. Epinephrine is frequently combined with intraspinal and local anesthetics to induce vasoconstriction, which will slow absorption and prolong drug action. When epinephrine is administered in this manner, care must be taken not to inadvertently inject the drug into a blood vessel, and the patient must be closely observed for systemic signs of adverse reactions.

The major clinical use for **norepinephrine** (levarterenol [Levophed], 2 to 4 mcg/minute IV) is in the treatment of hypotension resulting from vasodilation. Alpha-receptor stimulation causes vasoconstriction and an increase in blood pressure. Reflex bradycardia can occur. **Dopamine** (Intropin) also is used to alleviate hypotension that occurs in myocardial infarction, congestive heart failure, and other clinical conditions. Although low doses activate dopamine receptors and cause dilation of renal and splanchnic vascular beds, high doses stimulate alpha-adrenergic receptors to produce vasoconstriction. Dopamine is most effective when administration is begun soon after the onset of shock. Any depletion of blood volume must be corrected when norepinephrine or dopamine is used. Both drugs are given by closely controlled IV infusion.

The synthetic adrenergic agonist **isoproterenol** (Isuprel, 10 to 60 mg sublingual, 0.5 to 5 mcg/minute IV) selectively activates beta receptors. It is useful in treating many cardiovascular disorders and some types of shock and in relieving bronchoconstriction. Terbutaline (Brethine, 7.5 to 15 mg) and albuterol (Proventil, Ventolin, 6 to 32 mg) are relatively selective for beta$_2$ receptors, causing relaxation of bronchioles and dilation of blood vessels. The use of ethylnorepinephrine and metaproterenol treatment of asthma is discussed under "Bronchodilators." Phenylephrine is a synthetic agonist that activates alpha receptors. The resulting increase in blood pressure can provoke a reflex bradycardia and terminate paroxysmal atrial tachycardia. Some alpha agonists (e.g., pseudoephedrine) are used as nasal decongestants. Metaraminol (Aramine, 2 to 10 mg IM, SC; 0.5 to 100 mg IV infusion) is an alpha agonist that alleviates hypotension accompanying hemorrhage, spinal anesthesia, anaphylactic reactions, and other types of shock. Ephedrine stimulates alpha and beta receptors by direct action and also by release of norepinephrine.

Its indications include hypotensive states and broncho-constriction.

Dobutamine (Dobutrex, 2.5 to 15 mcg/kg/minute IV) is similar to dopamine. It stimulates beta$_1$ receptors, thus improving cardiac function following myocardial infarction, congestive heart failure, or cardiac surgery. It is administered by IV infusion titrated to the patient's closely monitored response. Hypertropic subaortic stenosis or other obstructions to cardiac output are contraindications to dobutamine.

Many of the adverse effects of the adrenergic drugs are the result of their actions on alpha and beta receptors: arrhythmias (both increase and decrease in rate), chest pain, alterations in blood pressure, pulmonary edema, cerebral hemorrhage, restlessness, headache, anxiety. There are many drug interactions. Adrenergic antagonists will reduce the effectiveness of the agonists. The MAO inhibitors will potentiate effects, and the risk of hypertensive crisis is great. Combinations of these two types of drugs are contraindicated. Concomitant administration of digitalis, inhalation anesthetics, phenothiazines, and tricyclic antidepressants increases the risk of cardiovascular arrhythmias. Aerosol bronchodilator combinations that include corticosteroids have caused sudden death, especially in children. Oxytocics and thyroid hormones administered with sympathomimetics can provoke severe hypertension. Some drug interactions are dependent on whether the sympathomimetic drug is direct or indirect acting. For example, the tricyclic antidepressants, which inhibit presynaptic uptake of amines, will enhance those drugs that directly stimulate receptors but will reduce the effects of indirect-acting agents, which must enter the nerve terminals to release norepinephrine.

All adrenergic drugs must be administered cautiously in the presence of any cardiovascular disorder. Parenteral administration is hazardous in all persons. Close attention to drug dose and patient response is required. Infiltration of norepinephrine can cause severe vasoconstriction and tissue necrosis. The alpha antagonist phentolamine injected locally may help to reduce this damage. Blood volume depletion must always be corrected in hypotensive states before sympathomimetic therapy can be effective. Norepinephrine is contraindicated, and epinephrine and metaraminol must be used cautiously when additional vasoconstriction might further compromise tissue perfusion.

Adrenergic antagonists

The adrenergic antagonists are selective for either alpha or beta receptors. The alpha antagonists are used to manage disorders exacerbated by adrenergic vasoconstriction. Phenoxybenzamine (Dibenzyline, 20 to 80 mg) has a longer duration of action and is used longer term to manage pheochromocytoma and vasospastic disorders such as Raynaud's syndrome. Phentolamine (Regitine, 200 to 300 mg, 5 mg IM, IV) is a diagnostic agent for pheochromocytoma and helps to control its symptoms before and during surgery. Hypertensive crises resulting from MAO inhibitor interactions and rebound hypertension after withdrawal of propranolol or clonidine usually respond to phentolamine.

Phenoxybenzamine should not be administered when a fall in blood pressure could be hazardous, and it must be used with caution in the presence of coronary and cerebral arteriosclerosis and renal dysfunction. Adverse effects such as postural hypotension are the result of adrenergic blockade. Phentolamine is

contraindicated in patients with coronary insufficiency (e.g., myocardial infarction, angina pectoris) and must be administered cautiously in the presence of GI ulcer or inflammation. Epinephrine should not be given concurrently with alpha receptor antagonists, since unopposed beta effects on blood vessels can cause severe hypotension and reflex tachycardia.

The ergot alkaloids ergotamine and dihydroergotamine are alpha receptor antagonists but also have a direct vasoconstrictor effect. They are used mainly to relieve cluster and migraine headaches. The ergot alkaloids are hepatically inactivated, and a large portion of each dose is lost on the first pass through the liver. These drugs are contraindicated in hypertension, cardiovascular disease, and other disorders exacerbated by vasoconstriction that can be severe enough to cause gangrene. Other adverse effects include reflex bradycardia, chest pain, and GI disturbances. Caffeine enhances the absorption of ergotamines administered PO.

The beta-adrenergic antagonists (Table 6-8), or beta-blockers, have in recent years grown considerably both in number and in clinical uses. Angina pectoris and some cardiac arrhythmias respond to beta antagonists, which decrease myocardial contraction and the rate of depolarization of the sinoatrial node and prolong conduction through the atrioventricular node. Beta-blockers are used extensively in the treatment of hypertension and are discussed in that section of this chapter. Recent investigations indicated that administration of beta-blockers (e.g., propranolol and timolol) following myocardial infarction will reduce the risk of reinfarction and sudden death. Timolol is used topically to control glaucoma. Beta-blockers also have some efficacy in reducing the occurrence of migraine headaches and in controlling the symptoms of acute anxiety (e.g., stage fright). Propranolol can be used to control some of the symptoms of pheochromocytoma but should be given only as an adjunct to alpha-adrenergic blockade.

Some beta-blockers are highly lipid soluble, thus will cross the blood-brain barrier, and they are inactivated by the liver, which clears a large portion of each dose by the first-pass effect. Others are water soluble, thus do not enter the CNS and are renally excreted. Some like metoprolol are somewhat "cardioselective"—that is, they usually produce less stimulation of

Table 6-8. Beta-Adrenergic Antagonists

Generic name	Trade name	Recommended adult doses (mg PO/day)
Acebutolol	Sectral	200–800
Atenolol	Tenormin	50–100
Labetolol	Normodyne, Trandate	400–800
Metoprolol	Lopressor	100–450
Nadolol	Corgard	40–240
Pindolol	Visken	15–60
Propranolol	Inderal	30–320 (1–3 mg IV)
Timolol	Blocadren	20–60

beta$_2$ receptors. Some beta-blockers have local anesthetic or membrane-stabilizing action.

Beta antagonists have many adverse effects. Blockade of beta$_1$ receptors in the heart can cause severe bradycardia, heart block and heart failure, hypotension, pulmonary edema, and exercise intolerance. Blockade of beta$_2$ receptors in the lungs will result in bronchospasm. Those blockers that cross the blood-brain barrier cause severe mental depression, fatigue, sleep disturbances, and other CNS aberrations. GI disorders, bone marrow depression, and changes in blood glucose levels occur. Administration of beta-blockers should never be abruptly terminated as rebound hypertension may result.

Most beta-blockers are contraindicated in persons with asthma and similar respiratory diseases. Those that are cardio-selective may be administered cautiously, although close observation is necessary since these drugs at higher doses or in sensitive persons can cause bronchoconstriction. Administration of beta-blockers to persons with diabetes is hazardous. These drugs inhibit insulin release and mobilization of stored glucose and fatty acids and will precipitate hypoglycemia. In addition, they block the symptoms (e.g., tachycardia) of inadequate blood glucose levels. Beta-blockers were long considered to be contraindicated in congestive heart failure but are now used when there is evidence of adverse excessive adrenergic influence. These drugs must be administered cautiously in the presence of any cardiovascular disorder. Beta-blockers are contraindicated in persons taking MAO inhibitors, since unopposed alpha stimulation can result in hypertensive crisis. Beta-blockers administered concurrently with digitalis increase the risk of atrioventricular depression and heart block. Cardiac depressant drugs like antiarrhythmics can add to the depressant effects of beta-blockers, and hypotensive agents can contribute to a severe fall in blood pressure.

Cholinergic agonists

There are two types of receptors in the cholinergic nervous system: **muscarinic** in the heart, glands, and smooth muscle and **nicotinic** in the neuromuscular junction, the ganglia of both the sympathetic and parasympathetic system, and the adrenal medulla. The CNS appears to have both muscarinic and nicotinic receptors. Both types are stimulated by the cholinergic neurotransmitter acetylcholine and by some cholinergic drugs. Other drugs act more selectively on only one type of receptor. Some cholinergic agonists (cholinomimetics or parasympathomimetics) directly stimulate receptors, whereas others (the anticholinesterases) act indirectly by inhibition of neurotransmitter inactivation by the acetylcholinesterase enzyme.

One of the major uses of the direct-acting cholinomimetics such as pilocarpine and carbachol is in the management of glaucoma. These drugs cause miosis and promote drainage of fluid from the inner chamber of the eye. Bethanechol (Urecholine, 20 to 120 mg, 2.5 to 10 mg SC) directly stimulates muscarinic receptors, making it useful for alleviating postsurgical GI and urinary atony.

The cholinesterase inhibitors prolong the action of acetylcholine, thus enhance both muscarinic and nicotinic effects. Edrophonium (Tensilon, 2 to 10 mg IV) is a short-acting anticholinesterase used mainly for diagnosis of myasthenia gravis and to differentiate between cholinergic and myasthenic crises. Neostigmine (Prostigmin, 15 to 375 mg), pyridostigmine (Mestinon, 0.6 to 1.5 g), and ambenonium (Mytelase, 15 to 50 mg) are administered chronically to improve neuromuscular function in myasthenia patients and to reverse some neuromuscular blocking agents. Physostigmine (Eserine, Antilirium), which crosses the blood-brain barrier, is used to reverse the anticholinergic effects of overdose of antihistamines, benzodiazepines, psychotherapeutics, anticholinergics, and other drugs with cholinolytic activity. Some of the anticholinesterases are also used in the treatment of glaucoma.

Because they activate a system that influences many vital physiological functions, the cholinomimetic drugs have many side effects. Bradycardia, hypotension, increased secretion of saliva and gastric juices, stimulation of intestinal and urinary smooth muscle, bronchoconstriction, vision disturbances, respiratory depression, and convulsions are some of the effects that may occur. These can be reversed by atropine. In myasthenic patients, cholinergic overdose must be distinguished from possible myasthenic crisis before an anticholinergic is administered. Topical (i.e., ophthalmic) administration occasionally results in absorption of sufficient drug to produce systemic effects.

Contraindications to the cholinergic agonists include peptic ulcer, myocardial infarction, asthma or similar respiratory disorders, pregnancy, and hyperthyroidism. These drugs are administered cautiously if at all to persons with Parkinson's disease or seizure or cardiovascular disorders. Bethanechol is contraindicated when intense stimulation of the GI or urinary tract is hazardous, such as in the presence of obstruction or recent surgery in these tracts. Other cholinergic agonists require extreme caution in these situations.

Excessive cholinergic activation can be caused by exposure to toxins such as organophosphate insecticides, nerve gases, and mushrooms containing muscarine and similar substances. Symptoms of poisoning include salivation and tearing, diarrhea, vision disturbance, bradycardia, restlessness, delirium, convulsions, respiratory difficulty, and shock. Atropine, pralidoxime (Protopam), and other anticholinergic agents are used as antidotes.

Cholinergic antagonists

The anticholinergic or parasympatholytic drugs (Table 6-9) that block postganglionic cholinergic transmission have a wide range of therapeutic uses. Atropine, originally derived from the belladonna plant, is an antiparkinson agent and preanesthetic medication to reduce respiratory and salivary secretions and prevent bronchospasm and laryngospasm. It is used in the management of acute myocardial infarction and other disorders characterized by vagal bradycardia. Atropine is an antispasmodic in the GI, biliary, and urinary tract and is used topically to produce mydriasis and paralysis of accommodation for ocular examinations. Several other anticholinergics, trihexyphenidyl (Artane), orphenadrine (Disipal), ethopropazine (Parsidol), benztropine (Cogentin), and biperiden (Akineton), are used in particular to alleviate idiopathic and drug-induced Parkinson's symptoms. Like atropine, scopolamine is used as preanesthetic medication; combined with an opiate such as morphine it produces analgesia and amnesia that is called twilight sleep. Scopolamine prevents motion sickness and is available in a transdermal form (Transderm Scōp). Anticholin-

Table 6-9. Cholinergic Antagonists

Generic name	Trade name	Recommended adult doses (mg PO/day)
Atropine		0.4–0.6 (parenteral also)
Clidinium	Quarzan	10–30
Hyoscyamine	several	0.75–1.5
Methantheline	Banthine	200–400
Methscopolamine	Pamine	10–12
Propantheline	Pro-Banthine	22.5–75
Scopolamine		0.32–0.65 mg SC, IM

ergics are used frequently as GI antispasmodics and as adjuncts in peptic ulceration to reduce gastric secretion.

The anticholinergic drugs have numerous side effects including vision disturbances, dry mouth, constipation, paralytic ileus, urinary retention, thickening of bronchial secretions, and tachycardia. Following administration of ocular solutions, contact dermatitis, conjunctivitis, and localized edema may occur. Anticholinergic overdose produces a potentially fatal syndrome characterized by CNS stimulation, delirium, hypertension, hyperthermia, and respiratory depression. Contraindications to the anticholinergics include cardiovascular disease that involves or would be exacerbated by an increase in heart rate, narrow-angle glaucoma, obstruction or hypoactivity of the GI tract, severe ulcerative colitis, prostatic enlargement, and myasthenia gravis except for the reversal of cholinergic crisis. Caution is required in the presence of respiratory disorders that may be aggravated by increased viscosity of bronchial secretions. Anticholinergics interfere with temperature regulatory mechanisms, thus in hot environments, body temperature can rapidly rise to fatal levels. Anticholinergics may suppress lactation, and, as for all drugs, pregnancy should be considered a relative if not absolute contraindication. The effects of anticholinergics can be greatly exaggerated in the elderly, in whom therapy should always be instituted with low drug doses.

Anticholinergics must be administered cautiously to persons receiving any other drug with cholinolytic action. Antihistamines, benzodiazepines, tricyclic antidepressants, antipsychotics, and many other drugs given concurrently can add to the suppression of the cholinergic system. MAO inhibitors interfere with the hepatic inactivation of the anticholinergics. Corticosteroids given concurrently can provoke elevations in intraocular pressure. Anticholinergics will reduce the effectiveness of cholinomimetics. IV administration of anticholinergics during cyclopropane anesthesia can induce arrhythmias. Anticholinergics prolong gastric emptying time, thus may alter absorption of drugs administered PO. Atropine can be used to reverse bradycardia caused by beta-adrenergic blockers.

SOMATIC NERVOUS SYSTEM PHARMACOLOGY

Skeletal muscle relaxants

Skeletal muscle spasm due to increased muscle tone results from damage to nerve, muscle, or related tissue such as ligaments and is characteristic of bone fractures, spinal cord and brain injuries and tumors, strains and sprains, cerebral palsy, multiple sclerosis, and many other disorders. Administration of muscle relaxants to alleviate spasticity should yield some benefit to the patient's physical or psychological well-being. For some persons, spasticity serves to support the ability to function—for example, increased tone in weak leg muscles may assist in walking.

Several skeletal muscle relaxants decrease efferent stimulation from the CNS. **Meprobamate** (Equinil, Miltown 1.2 to 2.4 g), **carisoprodal** (Rela, Soma 1.4 g), and **diazepam** appear to suppress neuronal activity in the brain. This reduces muscle tone but also causes such adverse effects as drowsiness, ataxia, and vertigo. Drug dependence, both psychological and physiological, can occur, and a withdrawal syndrome including anxiety, tremor, hallucinations, and seizures may follow abrupt termination of drug administration. All three drugs are hepatically inactivated, and all can potentiate other CNS depressant drugs. Meprobamate and carisoprodal are contraindicated in persons with acute intermittent porphyria; all patients should be observed for allergic reactions. Overdose of meprobamate or carisoprodal can produce fatal cardiovascular and respiratory depression, and these drugs have been used as agents for suicide. In such occurrences, unabsorbed drug should always be removed from the stomach to prevent delayed overdose. (The pharmacology of diazepam is discussed under "Antianxiety drugs.")

Mephenesin (Tolserol, Tolseram) and the related drugs chlorphenesin (Maolate, 1.6 g), chlorzoxazone (Paraflex, 0.7 to 2 g), methocarbamol (Robaxin, 4 g), and metaxalone (Skelaxin, 2.4 to 3.2 g) may work in both the brain and the spinal cord. These also cause central symptoms such as drowsiness and can potentiate other CNS depressants. They do not generally induce drug dependence. Methocarbamol can be given parenterally (IM or IV); however, the drug vehicle (polyethylene glycol) precludes such administration to persons with renal dysfunction.

Baclofen (Lioresal, 15 to 80 mg), an analogue of the inhibitory neurotransmitter GABA, is an effective skeletal muscle relaxant that has been used in particular in the treatment of multiple sclerosis. In patients with convulsive disorders, baclofen can lower the seizure threshold. Drowsiness, vertigo, and muscle weakness are the most common side effects. Abrupt termination of administration can provoke hallucinations. Baclofen is renally excreted, thus administration in the presence of kidney impairment requires caution. Potentiation of CNS depressants can occur.

Cyclobenzaprine (Flexeril, 20 to 40 mg), structurally and pharmacologically related to the tricyclic antidepressants, is a centrally acting muscle relaxant generally recommended only for short-term (2 to 3 weeks) administration. (The tricyclic drugs are discussed under "Antidepressants.")

Dantrolene (Dantrium, 25 to 400 mg, 1 to 10 mg/kg IV) is a direct skeletal muscle relaxant. It interferes with calcium mobilization, thus uncouples contraction from excitation.

Dantrolene is used in the management of anesthetic- and neuroleptic-induced malignant hyperthermia. The drug appears to be hepatically inactivated and can induce fatal hepatic dysfunction. Liver function should be monitored; liver dysfunction is a contraindication to chronic administration. Dantrolene binds extensively to plasma proteins. Several days of PO dosing may be required before reduction of spasticity is noted. Administration should be stopped if therapeutic effects do not occur within 6 to 7 weeks. Side effects are numerous and include drowsiness, extreme muscle weakness at high doses, diarrhea severe enough to require cessation of therapy, changes in blood pressure, and photosensitivity. Dantrolene may be carcinogenic. Potentiation of CNS depressant drugs can occur.

Neuromuscular junction blockers

There are two types of neuromuscular junction blockers, and, although both reach the same endpoint (i.e., flaccid paralysis of skeletal muscle), there are important pharmacologic differences that must be understood to ensure safe administration. The **competitive** or **nondepolarizing blockers** bind to nicotinic receptors on the motor end plate and prevent the interaction of the neurotransmitter acetylcholine with its receptors. The effects of the competitive blockers can be overcome by increasing the amount of acetylcholine in the junction. The **noncompetitive** or **depolarizing blockers** initially depolarize the postjunctional membrane to produce muscle contraction (fasciculations) followed by paralysis. The membrane appears to repolarize but does not respond to neurotransmitter. Increased amounts of acetylcholine in the junction will not overcome noncompetitive blockade and may in fact intensify paralysis.

Gallamine (Flaxedil, 1 mg/kg IV), **pancuronium** (Pavulon, 0.04 to 0.1 mg/kg IV), atracurium (Tracrium), vecuronium (Norcuron), and the **curare derivatives** metocurine (Metubine, 0.2 to 0.4 mg/kg IV) and tubocurarine are competitive blockers; **succinylcholine** (Anectine, 0.3 to 1.1 mg/kg IV) and the seldom-used **decamethonium** (Syncurine) are depolarizing agents. Both types are used to produce muscle relaxation during surgery and antidepressant shock therapy, for endotracheal intubation, and to facilitate cooperation with mechanical respirators. The neuromuscular junction blockers are administered parenterally; all except succinylcholine are renally excreted. Both types of blockers can paralyze respiratory muscle (although most other skeletal muscles are affected earlier and at lower doses), thus should be administered only when resuscitative means including mechanical ventilation are immediately available. Prolonged respiratory failure can occur; patients should not be left unattended until they have fully recovered from drug effects. These drugs do not alter pain perception or the level of consciousness. When they are used for surgery, the physician must ensure an adequate level of anesthesia since paralyzed patients will not be able to communicate their discomfort. Although patients appear to be asleep or unconscious, their sense of hearing may be unaffected.

Neuromuscular junction blockers must be used with great caution in persons already having some degree of respiratory depression. Cardiovascular disorders also require caution, since some degree of ganglionic blockade may result (especially with curare derivatives), causing changes in blood pressure and heart rate. The curare derivatives can provoke histamine release followed by bronchoconstriction and vasodilation. Persons with a history of allergy are especially sensitive to these effects. Metocurine and gallamine are available as iodides, which are contraindicated in persons with iodide allergy. Reduction in body temperature and electrolyte and acid-base imbalances can alter patient responsiveness to the neuromuscular junction blockers. Potassium reverses the competitive agents but intensifies the paralysis of the depolarizing drugs. Magnesium itself has a neuromuscular blocking action and will enhance both types of blockers. In general, these drugs are contraindicated in myasthenia gravis, when neuromuscular transmission is already severely deficient. However, tubocurarine may be used diagnostically when cholinergic testing has been inconclusive. Neuromuscular blockade will strongly intensify myasthenic symptoms.

Drug interactions of the neuromuscular junction blockers are numerous. Inhalation anesthetics like ether and halothane intensify neuromuscular blockade, as do drugs such as the diuretic furosemide and the aminoglycosides and certain other antibiotics that have an inhibitory effect of their own on neuromuscular transmission. Diazepam, the ganglionic blocker trimethaphan, and beta-adrenergic antagonists (especially those that have a membrane-stabilizing effect) also can add to the blockade of transmission. The competitive blockers can be antagonized and the depolarizing blockers intensified by cholinergic agonists. A competitive blocker administered first will prevent the effects of a depolarizing blocker; however, administration of a competitive agent after a depolarizing one can intensify paralysis.

The administration of succinylcholine requires additional precautions. This drug is inactivated, usually quite rapidly, by a plasma cholinesterase. However, some persons genetically lack this enzyme and can experience prolonged intense paralysis with succinylcholine administration. Succinylcholine can elevate intraocular pressure, thus is contraindicated in glaucoma, open eye injuries, and usually in ocular surgery. Because succinylcholine initially produces contraction of muscles, myoglobinuria and muscle soreness can occur. When succinylcholine is used in cesarean delivery, the infant may be born with severe respiratory depression and require artificial respiration. Succinylcholine has been implicated in occurrences of malignant hyperthermia and is contraindicated in persons with a history or risk of this disorder. All patients should be closely observed for early warning signs such as jaw muscle spasm and generalized rigidity. All drug administration should be stopped immediately. IV dantrolene can help to control body temperature.

Local anesthetics

Local anesthetics reduce the permeability of neuronal membranes, interfering with ionic fluxes required for transmission of impulses. Their greatest effect is on small unmyelinated (e.g., pain) fibers. Local anesthetics are administered by several methods. Lotions, creams, and other dermatologic forms are applied to the skin. Solutions are applied to mucous membranes, such as in the mouth and respiratory and urinary tracts. Rectal suppositories and ophthalmic solutions are available. Injectable solutions are administered around peripheral nerve terminals (infiltration) or injected into the epidural or subarachnoid space of the spinal cord. Specific regions of the body can be anesthetized without altering the patient's level of consciousness.

There are numerous local anesthetics; the most frequently used include procaine (Novocaine), bupivacaine (Marcaine), lidocaine (Xylocaine, also used as an antiarrhythmic drug), dibucaine (Nupercainal), and benzocaine (used mainly in dermatologic preparations). Cocaine preparations are available for dermatologic and mucous membrane application (except in the urinary tract, from which absorption is too rapid). Local anesthetics are used topically to relieve pain, itch and irritation of skin (e.g., poison ivy, insect bites, minor burns and injuries), and mucous membrane (e.g., hemorrhoids) disorders. (Many topical preparations are available as over-the-counter drugs.) Injectable forms provide anesthesia for dental, obstetric, and surgical procedures. Some injectables contain epinephrine, which produces vasoconstriction to reduce systemic absorption and to prolong the local action of the drug. Great care must always be taken to avoid intravascular administration of local anesthetics. Even with careful administration, sufficient drug may be absorbed to cause systemic effects. This risk is increased if the skin or mucous membrane is not intact.

Adverse effects of local anesthetics include CNS stimulation and/or depression, which can progress to convulsions (controlled with diazepam or short-acting barbiturates) and respiratory arrest. Means for resuscitation must always be immediately available when local anesthetics are administered. Cardiovascular depression, changes in blood pressure, and cardiac arrest also can occur, as can fetal and neonatal bradycardia when local anesthetics are used during labor and delivery. High doses of local anesthetics can paralyze skeletal muscle. Spinal anesthesia can produce headache and backache, profound hypotension, and respiratory arrest. Potential drug interactions include enhancement of neuromuscular blockade and changes in blood pressure when preparations with epinephrine are administered to persons receiving MAO inhibitors or drugs that affect adrenergic receptors. All local anesthetics contain either an ester or an amide linkage. The esters are inactivated by a plasma esterase, the amides by the hepatic enzymes. Anesthetics injected into the spinal cord are inactivated quite slowly. Preparations containing preservative agents should not be administered by this route.

HISTAMINE AND ANTAGONISTS

Histamine is an endogenous amine that is stored in mast cells and basophils and can be synthesized by certain cells in brain and gastric mucosa. Histamine modulates gastric acid secretion and is probably a CNS neurotransmitter. It may have a physiological role in cardiovascular function. In allergic reactions, histamine (and other mediators) released from mast cells and basophils causes bronchoconstriction, vasodilation, and increased capillary permeability leading to urticaria, nasal congestion, asthma, and anaphylactic shock.

The actions of histamine are mediated by two types of histamine receptors. H_1 receptors are most involved in allergic responses, H_2 receptors mediate gastric acid secretion. Both types appear to be present in the cardiovascular system and the CNS.

Histamine is used pharmacologically as a diagnostic agent. Administered IV (0.01 to 0.05 mg), histamine stimulates the release of catecholamines from pheochromocytomas. Hista-

mine (0.05 mg SC) is also used as a secretagogue for gastric acid, to aid in the identification of pernicious anemia and gastric carcinoma. Close observation with monitoring of blood pressure and heart rate is necessary. Histamine can provoke asthma and anaphylactic shock. Persons who have allergies are especially sensitive to both exogenous and endogenous histamine. **Betazole** (Histalog, 0.5 mg/kg IM SC) is an analogue of histamine that also stimulates gastric secretion and is reported to have lower potential for adverse reactions. The life-threatening allergic manifestations of both drugs can be reversed by epinephrine.

Just as there are two types of histamine receptors, there are two groups of histamine receptor antagonists, each having distinct clinical usefulness. The H_1 receptor blockers, also called "classic" or "conventional" antihistamines (Table 6-10), have long been used for a variety of indications, and several are available without prescription. They are frequently used to alleviate milder allergic symptoms. In this context, antihistamines are of greatest benefit when taken prophylactically. They do not prevent histamine release and have little efficacy for reversing histamine actions already occurring. The life-threatening aspects of asthma and anaphylactic shock are more rapidly alleviated with adrenergic drugs and corticosteroids. Topical antihistamine preparations can cause allergic dermatitis. Most H_1 antihistamines have marked anticholinergic activity, giving them some use in the treatment of parkinsonism but also conferring on them such adverse effects as dry mouth and thickening of bronchial secretions. Antihistamines, in particular as over-the-counter preparations, are used as sleeping aids and for the prevention of motion sickness. The most prominent side effect of most H_1 antihistamines is sedation, which can be sufficiently severe to result in vehicular and industrial accidents. Other CNS depressants, including alcohol, can potentiate this

Table 6-10. Histamine H_1-Receptor Antagonists

Generic name	Trade name	Recommended adult doses (mg PO/day)
Azatadine	Optimine	2–4
Brompheniramine*	Dimetane	16–24
Chlorpheniramine*	several	12–24
Clemastine	Tavist	2.6–8
Diphenhydramine*	Benadryl, others	75–200
Phenindamine*	Nolahist	100–150
Promethazine*	Phenergan	25–50
Pyrilamine*	Albatussin, Histan, Triaminic, others	50–200
Terfenadine	Seldane	120
Tripelennamine	PBZ	75–600

*Also available in an over-the-counter form.

effect. A recently developed group of H_1 antihistamines, represented by terfenadine (Seldane) and azatadine (Optimine), do not cross the blood-brain barrier in significant amounts, thus are reported not to cause sedation. Paradoxically, large doses of antihistamines can cause CNS stimulation resembling anticholinergic toxicity. The H_1 antihistamines have a relatively rapid onset of action and are metabolized by the hepatic microsomal enzymes.

The usefulness of histamine H_2 receptor antagonists is based on their ability to suppress gastric acid secretion. **Cimetidine** (Tagamet, 0.4 to 2.4 g) provided a new approach to the prevention and treatment of duodenal and gastric ulcers, including those that are stress induced and those that occur in Zollinger-Ellison syndrome. Cimetidine is renally excreted. The blood-brain barrier is reported to be impermeable to cimetidine, yet there are some side effects (e.g., confusion and hallucinations) that appear to be centrally mediated. These are more likely to occur in the elderly and in the presence of pathology that may alter the blood-brain barrier.

An important adverse effect of cimetidine is its interaction with many drugs that are hepatically inactivated (e.g., propranolol, lidocaine, theophylline, diazepam, oral anticoagulants). Cimetidine decreases the rate of biotransformation, thus increasing the serum levels of these drugs. The exact mechanism of this effect is not known. Cimetidine may decrease hepatic perfusion or it may interact at the level of the hepatic enzymes. Cimetidine can reduce serum levels of digoxin; antacids can reduce the absorption of cimetidine.

Ranitidine (Zantac 200 to 300 mg), an H_2 antihistamine quite similar to cimetidine, may have fewer side effects and fewer drug interactions. However, the adverse effects of cimetidine became apparent only after the drug was approved for general use, and in a similar manner, reports of adverse effects of ranitidine are accumulating. Famotidine (Pepcid, 20 to 40 mg) may have a longer duration of action than the other H_2 antagonists.

RESPIRATORY TRACT PHARMACOLOGY

Bronchodilators

Narrowing of the bronchioles (bronchoconstriction) impedes the flow of air into the alveoli. Often referred to as asthma, this condition can be life threatening and must be quickly treated with drugs that open the bronchioles (bronchodilators). Changes in airway resistance also occur in other pulmonary disorders such as bronchitis and emphysema. Two types of agents, the sympathomimetics and the methylxanthines, increase the availability of cAMP in the bronchiolar smooth muscle, causing it to relax. Increased levels of cAMP may also inhibit allergic release of bronchoconstrictive mediators from mast cells.

The **sympathomimetics** stimulate beta$_2$ receptors in the lungs, activating adenyl cyclase, which converts adenosine triphosphate (ATP) to cAMP. Various sympathomimetics (discussed under "Autonomic Nervous System Drugs") can be administered PO, parenterally, or as aerosols. However, the catecholamines epinephrine, isoproterenol (Isuprel), and isoethrine (Bronkosol) generally are not orally effective. Albuterol (Proventil, 6 to 32 mg) appears to have a high degree of selectivity for beta$_2$ receptors. Isoetharine, metaproterenol

(Alupent, 60 to 80 mg), and terbutaline (Brethine, Bricanyl, 7.5 to 15 mg) are somewhat selective for beta$_2$ receptors, thus have less cardiovascular effect than isoproterenol, which activates both beta$_1$ and beta$_2$ receptors. Epinephrine and ephedrine stimulate both types of beta receptors and also alpha receptors, thus causing vasoconstriction. Bitolterol (Tornalate) is a prodrug that is converted to the beta agonist colterol; it appears to have a longer duration of action than other inhaled sympathomimetics. Isoproterenol is probably the most efficacious of the sympathomimetic bronchodilators. Tolerance can develop to the effectiveness of the aerosols; excessive use can cause bronchospasm. Sudden death due to cardiac arrest has occurred with isoproterenol. All sympathomimetics must be used with caution in the presence of cardiovascular disease and thyroid hyperactivity. Beta$_2$ stimulation results in glycogenolysis, which can be hazardous in diabetics. Patients must be carefully instructed in the use of self-administered aerosols.

The **methylxanthines** elevate cAMP levels by inhibiting its catabolism by the phosphodiesterase enzyme. Methylxanthines may also interact with adenosine receptors. Theophylline and aminophylline (theophylline ethylenediamine) are available in several forms under numerous trade names. (Caffeine also is a methylxanthine.) These drugs are administered PO (0.5 to 1 g), rectally (suppositories and retention enemas, the latter being more effective), IM (which can be painful), and IV (aminophylline, up to 0.9 mg/kg/hour). Many adverse effects occur: cardiovascular stimulation, CNS stimulation (especially in children), hypotension, diuresis, increased gastric secretion, and GI upset. The margin of safety is narrow, and life-threatening arrhythmias and seizures may develop without warning. For this reason, serum levels of drug should be monitored, and guidelines established by the FDA followed to reduce the risks inherent in methylxanthine administration. Particular caution is required in the presence of cardiovascular disease, peptic ulcer, seizure disorders, liver dysfunction (the methylxanthines are hepatically inactivated), and renal dysfunction (which can be exacerbated). Methylxanthine metabolism is reduced in infants and the elderly, by low-protein diets, and by many pathological states. Drugs such as cimetidine prolong the half-life, whereas factors (including cigarette smoking) that induce hepatic enzymes shorten the duration of action. Concurrent administration of methylxanthines and beta agonists produces a marked elevation of cAMP. Methylxanthines increase the risk of digitalis toxicity. Aminophylline in solution is incompatible with many other drugs.

Corticosteroids

Inflammation and localized edema can contribute to narrowing of the bronchioles. This effect, which occurs particularly in allergic reactions, is often alleviated with corticosteroid administration. Hydrocortisone, methylprednisolone, and prednisone are given systemically, whereas beclomethasone (Vanceril), betamethasone (Valisone), and dexamethasone (Decadron) are available in aerosols. Because of the numerous severe adverse effects of the corticosteroids (discussed under "Endocrine Pharmacology"), these drugs should be used only when bronchoconstriction is not adequately controlled with other drugs. Systemic administration can induce a degree of adrenal insufficiency that is not compensated after transfer to aerosol forms of drug and that may be fatal. Withdrawal from systemic corticosteroids must always be accomplished slowly to allow hypothalamic-pituitary-adrenal function to return to normal. Periods of stress usually require additional amounts of exogenous steroid. Adverse effects characteristic of aerosol administration are hoarseness and oral infections. Systemic absorption of aerosols can be sufficient to suppress adrenal function. Patients using inhalant beta agonists and inhalant corticosteroids should administer the bronchodilator first. This will enable the corticosteroid to penetrate deeper into the airways. However, several minutes should elapse before administration of the corticosteroid, because the hydrocarbons used as propellants may interact adversely.

Decongestants

Histamine is a potent bronchoconstrictor stored in mast cells found in lungs, skin, and other tissues and released by allergic reactions, tissue injury, and extreme cold. Histamine is also a vasodilator that increases capillary permeability and can cause nasal congestion and bronchiolar edema. These effects require the interaction of histamine with H_1 histamine receptors, thus the H_1 antihistamines are another group of drugs that affect the respiratory system. The H_1 antihistamines are used to reduce the symptoms of allergic seasonal rhinitis. They do not prevent histamine release, and they are less effective if given after symptoms have occurred—that is, after histamine has interacted with its receptors. (The pharmacology of the antihistamines is discussed under "Histamine and Antagonists.")

Alpha-adrenergic vasoconstrictors also are used as nasal decongestants and are discussed under "Autonomic Nervous System Drugs."

Cromolyn sodium

Cromolyn sodium (Intal) prevents the release of histamine and leukotrienes (slow-reacting substance of anaphylaxis) from mast cells in the lungs. Administered by inhalation (20 mg q.i.d.), it is used only prophylactically in patients at risk of severe bronchial asthma. It is of no use, and should not be administered, once an acute asthmatic reaction has begun. The adverse effects of cromolyn include bronchospasm, allergy including serum sickness and anaphylaxis, nasal irritation, and drowsiness. Some of the drug is absorbed systemically and is inactivated both renally and hepatically. Patients must be instructed in the administration of this drug.

Mucolytics

Thick mucous secretions also contribute to narrowing of the bronchioles (e.g., in cystic fibrosis) and may form dry, hard plugs in the smaller airways. Acetylcysteine (Mucomyst, 0.2 to 1.0 g q.i.d.) is nebulized into a mist that is inhaled to reduce mucus viscosity. The drug may cause bronchospasm, thus it is also available in combination with the bronchodilator isoproterenol. A large volume of watery mucus may have to be suctioned, especially if the patient cannot cough. (The use of acetylcysteine as an antidote to acetaminophen overdose is discussed under "Analgesics.")

Expectorants

Several drugs are used to promote a productive cough. Potassium iodide, terpin hydrate, and guaifenesin (glyceryl guaiacolate, 0.4 to 2.4 g) are available in many oral preparations, some without prescription. Although their efficacy is not proven, these drugs appear to stimulate respiratory secretions and reduce mucus viscosity. Potassium iodide can suppress thyroid function and is contraindicated during pregnancy (see "Thyroid Pharmacology"). Terpin hydrate is also available in combination with the opiate antitussive codeine (discussed under "Narcotic analgesics.") Inhaling vaporized distilled water helps to dislodge viscous mucus; increased intake of liquids PO may also help to reduce mucus viscosity. Drugs with anticholinergic activity (e.g., antihistamines) should be avoided, as these promote thickening of respiratory secretions.

Antitussives

Although coughing serves the physiological purpose of removing matter from the respiratory tract, it is at times desirable to suppress a cough, such as one of a dry nonproductive nature caused by irritation of the respiratory tract. Antitussives are used for this purpose. The most potent are the opiates (narcotics) such as codeine (60 to 120 mg). (The pharmacology of these drugs, which suppress the cough center in the medulla, is discussed under "Narcotic analgesics.")

Dextromethorphan (40 to 120 mg) and levopropoxyphene are related to the opiates but produce less CNS depression and appear not to be addictive. Benzonatate (Tessalon, 300 to 600 mg) depresses the responsiveness of the respiratory tract stretch receptors. Diphenhydramine (100 to 150 mg) is an antihistamine with antitussive effects; its anticholinergic action, however, can increase mucus viscosity. Noscapine is a nonnarcotic antitussive with potency similar to codeine. Most of these drugs produce drowsiness and can potentiate the effects of other CNS depressants such as alcohol. Some interact adversely with MAO inhibitors. It must be noted that chronic cough can be a symptom of serious underlying disorders.

Respiratory stimulants

The analeptics or respiratory stimulants **doxapram** (Dopram, 0.5 to 4 mg/kg IV) and **nikethamide** (Coramine, 0.5 to 2.5 g IV) are seldom used because of their potential for serious adverse effects. The best treatment for respiratory depression, including that caused by drug overdose, is mechanical support of ventilation until spontaneous breathing resumes. Doxapram may be administered IV for brief periods of time to increase the rate and depth of respiration in persons with chronic obstructive pulmonary disease and to hasten recovery from general anesthesia. Nikethamide has been used to alleviate respiratory depression in carbon monoxide poisoning, ingestion of alcohol, general anesthesia, and cardiac arrest. It can be given IV, IM, and PO. The mechanism of action of the analeptics involves stimulation of the respiratory center in the medulla and of the peripheral arterial chemoreceptors. Both drugs have a narrow safety margin. Adverse effects include CNS stimulation that produces restlessness, anxiety and convulsions, decreased cerebral blood flow, bronchospasm, and increased gastric acid secretion. Catecholamines are released, blood pressure and cardiac activity can increase, and arrhythmias may develop. The analeptics are never administered intra-arterially, since vasospasm and thrombosis can occur. Because of their potential for toxicity, these drugs are administered only to hospitalized persons under close observation.

The numerous contraindications to the administration of analeptics (doxapram in particular) include seizure disorders, certain respiratory and cardiovascular disorders, cerebrovascular accident, and head injury. Both drugs are metabolized in the liver, and MAO inhibitors will decrease the inactivation of doxapram. Concurrent administration of sympathomimetics increases the occurrence of hypertension. Administration of anesthetics that promote catecholamine-induced arrhythmias should be terminated at least 10 minutes before an analeptic is given. Diazepam or a short-acting barbiturate can be used to control analeptic-induced seizures.

The carbonic anhydrase inhibitor **acetazolamide** has investigational use in the prevention of high-altitude "mountain sickness." It induces a mild metabolic acidosis that increases the rate and depth of respiration. Acetazolamide should not be administered in the presence of electrolyte imbalances, renal dysfunction, or pulmonary disturbances that may preclude response to the drug-induced acidosis. (Acetazolamide is discussed under "Diuretics.")

Oxygen

Oxygen is essential for life, yet its administration must be carefully undertaken to avoid serious consequences. Concentrations of oxygen greater than 40% administered for several days can cause pulmonary infiltrates, interstitial pneumonitis, and atelectasis. Oxygen administration is hazardous in persons with chronic lung disease. Long-term elevations in carbon dioxide reduce the effectiveness of the hypercapnic stimulus and increase the dependency on low oxygen levels to maintain respiration. In such persons, increased levels of oxygen will suppress breathing and can lead to respiratory arrest. In premature infants, high oxygen concentrations can cause retrolental fibroplasia progressing to retinal detachment.

GASTROINTESTINAL TRACT PHARMACOLOGY

Antiulcer drugs

Several types of drugs are used in the treatment of peptic ulceration, which probably occurs as the result of the combined action of pepsin and gastric acid on the mucosal lining of the upper GI tract. Since pepsin is active only below pH 3.5 to 4.0, the administration of antacids to neutralize gastric acid will reduce the activity of this digestive enzyme. **Antacids** relieve the pain and discomfort of peptic ulcers and also promote healing. Many antacids are available without prescription and unfortunately are misused by consumers. Most antacids stay within the GI tract, although the absorption of the metal ion components can have adverse consequences. One antacid, sodium bicarbonate, is extensively absorbed and can lead to systemic alkalosis. This substance, in the form of "baking soda," is widely used by the public for self-medication. It causes a rapid and pronounced but short-lived rise in gastric pH that is often followed by rebound hypersecretion of acid. The high sodium content of this substance makes it hazardous in persons with congestive heart failure, hypertension, and other disorders exacerbated by sodium. Ingestion of significant amounts of calcium (e.g., from dietary sources or other antacids) concurrently with sodium bicarbonate can lead to milk-alkali syndrome, characterized by elevated blood levels of calcium, deposition of this ion in tissues, and development of renal stones or dysfunction.

Nonsystemic antacids contain aluminum, calcium, or magnesium salts. Some also contain sodium, although many

have been reformulated to contain less of this ion. A wide variety of antacids is available without prescription. Aluminum antacids (aluminum phosphate, carbonate, and hydroxide) have the greatest acid-neutralizing capacity and also have demulcent (soothing) activity on the GI tract. Aluminum hydroxide is also used in the management of hyperphosphatemia. Phosphate ion in the GI tract is bound into a nonabsorbable complex excreted in the feces. Adverse effects of aluminum antacids include hypophosphatemia and constipation. Calcium carbonate also causes constipation, can contribute to the development of systemic alkalosis and milk-alkali syndrome, and can cause rebound hyperacidity. Magnesium antacids (magnesium carbonate, hydroxide, oxide, and trisilicate) cause diarrhea and may be used as laxatives (e.g., magnesium hydroxide or milk of magnesia). Electrolyte and water imbalances may occur if diarrhea is severe. Systemic absorption of magnesium can result in hypermagnesemia, especially in persons with inadequate renal function. The constipating aluminum or calcium antacids are often combined or alternated with magnesium preparations to alleviate the diarrheal effect of the latter.

The most frequent adverse effects of antacids are alkalosis and other electrolyte imbalances. Drug interactions occur because changes in pH induced by the antacids can alter absorption from the GI tract (formation of insoluble complexes can also occur) and excretion in the urine. Hypermagnesemia can add to the depressant effects of the neuromuscular junction blockers. Antacids must always be administered with care in persons with renal dysfunction, cardiovascular disorders (preparations containing sodium are especially hazardous), and systemic alkalosis.

The H_2 receptor antihistamines **cimetidine** and **ranitidine** are relatively new and extremely effective therapeutic agents in the prevention and treatment of peptic ulcers. These drugs block the apparent final common pathway of gastric acid secretion, that of histamine action on H_2 receptors in the gastric mucosa, and are discussed under "Histamine and antagonists."

Anticholinergics are also used in the management of peptic ulcer. Cholinergic stimulation by way of the vagus nerve induces secretion of many digestive juices, including pepsin and gastric acid. (The pharmacology of these drugs is presented under "Cholinergic antagonists.")

A unique drug for the treatment of peptic ulcer is **sucralfate** (Carafate), which binds with protein at the ulcer site to form a protective covering. It is administered up to 8 weeks to promote healing of the ulcer. Very little of the drug is systemically absorbed. Adverse effects are minimal. Constipation, diarrhea, GI discomfort, and vertigo have been reported. One gram of drug must be given 1 hour before meals and at bedtime. Antacids interfere with its activity and should not be given within 1/2 hour before or after sucralfate administration. Sucralfate reduces the absorption of orally administered phenytoin, tetracycline antibiotics, and cimetidine.

Antidiarrheals

In addition to being an annoying inconvenience that can interfere with a person's daily activities, diarrhea if severe or chronic can cause life-threatening dehydration and electrolyte imbalances, especially in infants and in the elderly. There are a variety of causes for diarrhea, such as viral infection, drug reactions, food poisoning, anxiety, and malabsorption syndrome. Chronic diarrhea should be investigated to determine whether there is an underlying disorder that requires treatment.

The most effective antidiarrheals are the **opiates**: codeine, paregoric (2 to 4 mg), loperamide (Imodium, 4 to 16 mg), and diphenoxylate (15 to 20 mg, one of the components of Lomotil). The opiates interact directly with receptors in the GI tract to increase muscle tone in sphincters and decrease GI motility. Transit time through the bowel is prolonged, allowing better reabsorption of water and electrolytes from the feces. The opiates can produce drug dependency, thus should be used only for acute therapy. Opiates (and other antidiarrheals) should not be administered to persons with microorganism-induced diarrhea or with drug-induced pseudomembranous colitis. This would increase the penetration into or irritation of the intestinal wall by microroganisms and their toxins retained in the bowel. Like all opiates, these antidiarrheals can cause CNS depression and can potentiate other depressant drugs. Overdose or exaggerated response to an opiate can be reversed by a narcotic antagonist. (The pharmacology of the opiates is discussed under ''Narcotic analgesics.'')

Anticholinergics, because they also decrease intestinal motility, may be combined with opiates for the treatment of diarrhea. Lomotil is diphenoxylate plus atropine. Donnagel-PG (15 to 30 ml q 3 hours) contains opium, atropine, hyoscine (scopolamine), plus two locally acting agents, kaolin and pectin. (Donnagel is also available without opium). Side effects and precautions are the same as for anticholinergics in general (discussed in this chapter).

Locally acting agents are less effective as antidiarrheals. Many are available without prescription. Adsorbents (activated charcoal, attapulgite, bismuth salts, kaolin, pectin) work by binding to toxins and irritants and by soothing the GI mucosa. These agents can also adsorb and remove many nutrients, intestinal enzymes, and drugs (e.g., digoxin), and antibiotics should not be administered within 2 hours either before or after these antidiarrheals. They may cause greater fluid and electrolyte depletion than diarrhea itself, thus their use in young children should be under medical supervision. Their efficacy in alleviating diarrhea is not proven, although administration of large amounts can result in constipation.

Antibiotics can be used to treat diarrhea caused by microbial infections. It must be noted, however, that antibiotics may also eradicate normal intestinal bacteria and cause diarrhea to occur. This effect can be alleviated by administration of agents that promote recolonization of the intestine, e.g., Bacid and other acidophilus preparations which contain *Lactobacillus*. Milk, buttermilk, and yogurt also enhance the growth of this bacillus and of *Escherichia coli*.

Laxatives

Recurrent constipation can be a symptom of an underlying pathological disorder. It is a frequent complaint in the elderly and in physically inactive persons. Laxatives are also used to evacuate the bowel for surgery or diagnostic tests, to remove toxins or parasites, and to reduce painful irritation of hemorrhoids during defecation. Laxatives act locally in the bowel by several different mechanisms. Two types, **saline** and **bulk forming**, increase the bulk of the feces. Saline laxatives are nonabsorbable salts such as sodium and potassium phosphate, magnesium citrate, sulfate, and hydroxide. By osmotic pressure they draw large amounts of fluid into the intestine. Their action is rapid; bowel evacuation may begin within 1 to 2 hours. Ions from these drugs may be absorbed, accumulating to toxic levels in persons with renal dysfunction. Bulk-forming laxatives such as methylcellulose and psyllium are indigestible materials that remain in the intestinal tract to add bulk to the feces. They have a slower, more gentle action.

Several laxatives such as bisacodyl, cascara, castor oil, phenolphthalein, senna, and glycerin suppositories work by **direct stimulation** of peristalsis. In general, these require 6 to 8 hours before an effect occurs. Still other laxatives are used to soften the feces. These **emollient** or **surface-active agents**, which include docusate (dioctyl) salts and poloxamer, promote absorption of water and fats into the feces. They are used especially in postmyocardial infarction patients, in whom the elevated intrathoracic pressure (''Valsalva's maneuver'') of straining to defecate can be hazardous. Mineral oil can be used to soften and lubricate the feces.

An agent used to treat both constipation and diarrhea is **calcium polycarbophil**, which has the capacity to bind a large volume of water. It relieves constipation by retaining water and adding bulk to the feces and alleviates diarrhea by slowing the passage of water through the intestine.

The laxatives in general have a variety of adverse effects. Many preparations are available without prescription and are frequently abused by consumers who become both psychologically and physiologically dependent on them. Nausea and vomiting are not uncommon. Dehydration and electrolyte imbalance can occur, the latter by excretion of ions and by absorption of components of the drug. Preparations containing sodium are hazardous in persons with cardiovascular disease; all preparations containing absorbable ions must be used cautiously in the presence of renal dysfunction. Laxatives are contraindicated in intestinal obstruction, appendicitis, ulcerative colitis, and some other intestinal disorders. The cause of abdominal pain should always be determined before laxatives are administered. Stimulant and bulk-forming laxatives should not be given if feces are impacted. Mineral oil decreases the intestinal absorption of fat-soluble vitamins and carries the risk of aspiration pneumonia. Laxatives shorten transit time through the intestine, thus can decrease the absorption of many drugs, including digitalis. Anticholinergics, which slow intestinal transit, can promote the systemic absorption of laxatives. The docusate salts enhance absorption of mineral oil. Exercise and proper diet, including adequate consumption of fluids, can help to alleviate constipation and should be encouraged in persons who have this complaint.

Digestants

Insufficient endogenous amounts of enzymes and other substances essential for digestion of food will lead to malnutrition and can cause diarrhea due to undigested or unabsorbed foods. Digestants are used to replace gastric acid, bile salts, and pancreatic enzymes.

Gastric acid provides the proper pH for the enzyme pepsin, which digests protein. Hypochlorhydria occurs frequently in elderly persons; achlorhydria is a symptom of pernicious anemia. **Hydrochloric acid** can be administered as capsules or tablets of glutamic acid hydrochloride (325 mg before meals) or betaine hydrochloride. These must be accompanied by a large glass of water. Dilute hydrochloric acid solution is also available. It should be sipped during meals through a straw to prevent contact of acid with tooth enamel. These preparations can cause acidosis and are contraindicated in persons with acidosis or peptic ulcer.

Bile salts, which are necessary for the digestion of fats and for absorption of fat-soluble vitamins, may be deficient in patients with a variety of hepatic and biliary disorders. Bile salts in the form of ox bile extracts (150 to 600 mg) can be administered, or hydrocholeretics such as dehydrocholic (250 to 500 mg after meals) and ketocholanic acids can be used to promote the flow of low-viscosity bile. Bile salts and hydrocholeretics may be given concurrently. All of these preparations have a laxative effect and may be used for this purpose. All are contraindicated in biliary obstruction, nausea, undiagnosed abdominal pain, and certain hepatic disorders. Ox bile is contraindicated in persons allergic to beef protein.

Pancreatic enzymes digest starches (amylase), protein (trypsin), and fats (lipase). They are deficient in cystic fibrosis, pancreatitis, and after pancreatectomy. Pancrelipase (Cotazym) and pancreatin (Viokase) are derived mainly from porcine pancreas, thus are contraindicated in persons allergic to protein from this species. Some forms are enteric coated and should be swallowed whole; concurrent administration of drugs that raise gastric pH will cause early disruption of the coating, exposing some enzyme to destruction by gastric acid but also liberating enzyme high in the intestinal tract. Adverse effects, usually occurring only at high doses, include nausea and diarrhea. Patients should have a well-balanced diet, and enzyme doses should be adjusted to food intake.

Emetics

The emetics apomorphine and ipecac are used to induce vomiting to evacuate poisons from the stomach. Whenever possible, a poison control center should be consulted before these drugs are given. Emetics are contraindicated when the ingested toxin is strong acid or alkali or a petroleum product, substances that can do additional harm on a second passage through the esophagus. Ingestion of convulsants such as strychnine also precludes the use of emetics, as convulsions would greatly increase the risk of aspiration of vomitus. Emetics should never be given to a person who is not fully conscious and alert, because of the risk of aspiration. Persons who have received emetics should not be left unattended until vomiting has ceased. Ipecac induces vomiting by stimulating the medullary vomiting center and also by local irritation of the gastric mucosa. Ipecac syrup (15 to 30 ml) is administered PO with a large glass of water. (It should be noted that ipecac is also available as a highly concentrated fluidextract.) If the first dose is ineffective, a second dose may be given. If vomiting still does not occur, the ipecac should be removed from the stomach by gastric lavage or activated charcoal. Systemic absorption of ipecac can cause intestinal bleeding, arrhythmia, and convulsions. Apomorphine works centrally by stimulating the chemoreceptor trigger zone. A large glass of water should be ingested by the patient just before SC injection of 2 to 10 mg of apomorphine. Only one dose should be given; vomiting should begin within 15 minutes. Apomorphine is an opiate and will produce CNS depression, which can be reversed with the narcotic antagonist naloxone (Narcan), as can the violent persistent emesis that may occur. Apomorphine can cause hypotension and tachycardia, thus requires caution in the presence of cardiovascular disease.

Antiemetics

Antiemetics are used to relieve the physiological and psychological discomfort of nausea and vomiting and to reduce the risk of ensuing dehydration, electrolyte imbalance, and malnutrition. Vomiting is a complex response that can be caused by local irritation, drug side effects or toxicity, middle ear disturbances including motion sickness, anxiety, increased intracranial pressure, intestinal obstruction, and many other disorders. The cause for persistent vomiting must be diagnosed. In patients receiving drugs with antiemetic action (including antihistamines and neuroleptics that are used for other indications), this warning signal of potentially life-threatening disorders may be suppressed. Brief episodes of nausea are probably best not treated as they serve to remove toxic or irritating substances from the GI tract. A variety of drugs are available to help control more prolonged and severe vomiting; in general these are more effective if administered before vomiting has begun.

Antihistamines (discussed previously) are most effective in alleviating vestibular disturbances (e.g., motion sickness). Dimenhydrinate (200 to 400 mg) and meclizine (25 to 100 mg) are available without prescription. Hydroxyzine (25 to 100 mg IM) has use as a postsurgical antiemetic. The most prominent side effects are drowsiness and anticholinergic effects such as dry mouth. Controversy still surrounds the possible teratogenic action of the antihistamine doxylamine combined with vitamin B$_6$ and sold as Bendectin for the treatment of nausea in early pregnancy (morning sickness). Trimethobenzamide (Tigan) is a weak antihistaminic antiemetic that is seldom used because it is hepatotoxic. The anticholinergic **scopolamine** is also effective for motion sickness. It is available in a transdermal system (**Transderm Scōp**) with a long duration of action. The pharmacology of this drug, which should not be administered to children, is discussed under "Autonomic Nervous System Pharmacology."

Phenothiazines (used also for psychiatric disturbances and discussed under "Antipsychotic drugs") help to reduce vomiting induced by general anesthetics, antineoplastic chemotherapy, and radiation. Their marked side effects (e.g., extrapyramidal dystonia, akinesia and parkinsonism, anticholinergic effects, sedation, and hypotension) limit their usefulness to short-term administration or to nausea not controlled by other therapy. The phenothiazines and the antihistamines are CNS depressants and will potentiate this effect of other depressant drugs.

Some drugs are used in particular as antiemetics. **Diphenidol** (Vontrol, 150 to 300 mg) is effective in vestibular and more centrally caused emesis. Its side effects include disorientation and hallucinations, limiting its use to persons under close medical supervision. **Benzquinamide** (Emete-con, 50 mg IM q 3 to 4 hours) is used mainly for anesthesia-induced vomiting. It has anticholinergic action and can cause either drowsiness or CNS excitation. Because it may stimulate cardiac activity and elevate blood pressure, IV administration is contraindicated in cardiovascular disease. **Metoclopramide** (Reglan, 40 mg) is a relatively new dopamine receptor blocker (as are the phenothiazines) that appears to reduce the severe refractory vomiting that can accompany chemotherapy with such agents as cisplatin. Because it speeds GI transit time, it may also be useful in reducing gastroesophageal reflux and in facilitating GI diagnostic procedures. GI hemorrhage and obstruction are contraindications. In addition to the centrally acting antiemetics, several agents are used for their local actions on the GI tract. Many of these (e.g., antacids and phosphorated carbohydrate solution) are available without prescription.

Centrally acting antiemetics should be used very cautiously in children. These drugs may be implicated in the development of Reye's syndrome following viral illnesses such as chicken pox and influenza. The presence of liver dysfunction also dictates caution in the use of the centrally acting drugs that are hepatically inactivated.

DIURETICS

Diuretics promote renal excretion of sodium and water. They are used clinically in the management of cardiovascular disorders such as congestive heart failure and hypertension, of hepatic disorders when ascites (fluid in the peritoneal cavity) is present, and of certain renal disorders. Some diuretics also have more specialized uses, such as reduction of cerebral edema and intraocular pressure.

There are several groups of diuretics, and they share many characteristics. These will be presented first, then the individual groups will be discussed. Although diuretic efficacy does vary, all diuretics can cause dehydration and reduction in blood volume severe enough to cause thromboembolism and cardiovascular collapse. Fluid intake and output must be monitored. Peripheral (i.e., lower extremity) edema is more readily mobilized than is ascites; thus fluid loss in persons with hepatic cirrhosis must not be allowed to occur too rapidly. Because the kidneys play a major part in electrolyte excretion, all diuretics have the potential to cause electrolyte and acid-base imbalances. Diuretics work at different points along the renal tubules, thus will affect ions in various ways. All except the potassium-sparing diuretics can cause hypokalemia. This is of special concern in persons receiving digitalis, for potassium depletion enhances digitalis toxicity. (See further discussion under "Cardiotonic drugs"). Hypokalemia and alterations in blood pH can also precipitate or aggravate hepatic encephalopathy. Diuretics are usually contraindicated in the presence of electrolyte or acid-base imbalances that might be exacerbated.

Diuretic administration to persons with renal disease or dysfunction requires great caution. Some diuretics can compound kidney damage. In addition, the efficacy of all diuretics is dependent on the working capacity of the nephrons. Diuretics should be used only under medical supervision and require special caution in the elderly, who are at increased risk of electrolyte depletion and dehydration. Diuretic administration should be scheduled so that sleep is not affected. For example, those with rapid onset should be given early in the day so that diuresis is over by evening.

In addition to that with digitalis, there are several drug interactions common to many of the diuretics. Most potentiate the effects of antihypertensive agents. (Several groups, in particular the thiazides, potassium-sparing, and furosemide,

are frequently used in antihypertensive combination therapy.) The renal excretion of lithium is reduced by concurrent administration of a diuretic; this drug combination is generally contraindicated. Administration of corticosteroids or adrenocorticotropic hormone (ACTH) will increase the risk of hypokalemia. The occurrence of orthostatic hypotension is increased by the use of barbiturates, opiates, and alcohol.

Individual groups of diuretics

Carbonic anhydrase inhibitors (acetazolamide [Diamox], 0.25 to 1 g; dichlorphenamide [Daranide], 25 to 200 mg; methazolamide [Neptazane], 100 to 200 mg) block the reaction of carbon dioxide with water to form carbonic acid, which dissociates into hydrogen and bicarbonate ions. This reaction occurs in particular in the epithelial cells of the proximal portion of the nephron, where much bicarbonate is reabsorbed to maintain acid-base balance. The carbonic anhydrase inhibitors thus promote excretion of bicarbonate along with sodium and potassium; chloride is reabsorbed. Systemic hyperchloremic acidosis, which reduces the efficacy of the carbonic anhydrase inhibitors, develops. For this reason, these drugs are often given on an alternate-day schedule. The carbonic anhydrase inhibitors produce mild diuresis, thus in the treatment of edema they are used only in combination with other drugs. They are also adjuncts in the treatment of some types of epilepsy (e.g., petit mal) and some types of glaucoma. (They are contraindicated, however, in chronic closed-angle glaucoma). Acetazolamide may reduce the symptoms of mountain sickness, as respiration is stimulated by the resulting mild acidosis.

Additional adverse reactions to the carbonic anhydrase inhibitors include paresthesias, photosensitivity, bone marrow depression, and CNS effects such as dizziness, drowsiness, anxiety, and confusion. These drugs are sulfonamide derivatives and should not be given to persons who are allergic to such agents. They may be teratogenic. Drug interactions can occur as urine becomes alkaline. Basic drugs such as quinidine, amphetamines, and tricyclic antidepressants will be less ionized thus more readily reabsorbed. Acidic drugs will be excreted. Administration of sodium bicarbonate will alleviate systemic acidosis and restore efficacy to the carbonic anhydrase inhibitors. Antidiabetic medications may become less effective, since the carbonic anhydrase inhibitors can promote hyperglycemia.

Osmotic diuretics also work in the proximal portion of the nephrons. They are filtered but poorly reabsorbed, and the resulting elevation in osmotic pressure in the tubule prevents reabsorption of water. Mannitol (Osmitrol, 1.5 to 2 g/kg IV over 30 to 60 minutes) is the osmotic diuretic most frequently used for the reduction of cerebral edema, to measure glomerular filtration rate, and to prevent acute renal failure from progressing to an irreversible stage. Other osmotic agents such as urea (Ureaphil, up to 4 ml of 30% solution per minute) may be used acutely to reduce elevated intraocular pressure. Mannitol and urea are administered only IV; they are confined intravascularly and attract a large volume of water, which is carried to the kidneys. Drug administration must be terminated if diuresis fails to occur. The expanded blood volume can precipitate or aggravate congestive heart failure. A urinary catheter may be inserted to facilitate diuresis and measurement of urinary output. Inadequate renal function is a contraindication to the administration of these drugs; a test dose of drug may be given to determine renal responsiveness. Additional contraindications include severe dehydration, intracranial hemorrhage, and pulmonary edema. Osmotic diuretics can cause hypernatremia if fluid loss is excessive; other electrolyte imbalances and renal damage can develop. Mannitol solutions are available in five concentrations ranging from 5% to 25%. Concurrent blood infusions must be undertaken cautiously as agglutination can occur. Extravasation can cause tissue necrosis. If steroids are given concurrently to reduce cerebral edema, patients must be observed for hypokalemia.

The **mercurial diuretics** inhibit renal reabsorption of sodium and chloride in the loop of Henle. These drugs are seldom used today. Only mersalyl is available, in combination with theophylline (Mercutheolin, Theo-Syl-R), which potentiates diuretic action and promotes renal excretion of the nephrotoxic mercury ions. Mersalyl is most effective at acid pH; tolerance develops but can be reversed by administration of ammonium chloride. One to 2 ml/day is given parenterally, usually IM. Slow IV injection may be used in emergencies but can cause sudden death. SC injections are painful. Rapid intense diuresis occurs; as with all diuretics, dehydration and electrolyte imbalances can develop. Hypersensitivity to mercury is a contraindication and can be determined by administration of a test dose of drug. Mercury poisoning may occur, especially in persons with renal dysfunction. Dimercaprol (BAL) can be used as antidote.

The **organic acid** or **"loop" diuretics** (furosemide [Lasix], 20 to 120 mg, 20 to 40 mg IM, IV; ethacrynic acid [Edecrin], 50 to 400 mg; and bumetanide [Bumex], 0.5 to 2 mg) interfere with sodium and chloride reabsorption throughout the length of the nephron. The greatest influence occurs, however, at the loop of Henle, where decreased ion transport reduces the medullary "countercurrent mechanism," which reabsorbs water from the collecting ducts. The loop diuretics are also called "high ceiling" because of their marked diuretic efficacy, which carries the potential for severe electrolyte and water depletion. These drugs are orally and parenterally effective and are used to alleviate a variety of edematous states. Furosemide, one of the most widely prescribed drugs in the United States, is used in the management of hypertension. Additional adverse effects include ototoxicity, hyperuricemia, agranulocytosis, thrombocytopenia, orthostatic hypotension, and GI upset. Ethacrynic acid can cause severe watery diarrhea that contraindicates further administration. It may also be teratogenic. Severe dehydration and electrolyte imbalance of hepatic coma must be alleviated before a loop diuretic is administered. These drugs require special caution in elderly or debilitated persons. There are many drug interactions in addition to those listed for diuretics in general. Concurrent administration of aminoglycosides (e.g., streptomycin) increases the risk of ototoxicity. The loop diuretics bind extensively to plasma proteins and may displace drugs such as warfarin from binding sites. Salicylate excretion can be inhibited. Nonsteroidal anti-inflammatory drugs such as indomethacin reduce the antihypertensive action of furosemide.

Thiazide diuretics (there are several; hydrochlorothiazide is the most widely prescribed drug in the United States) are used to alleviate edema and hypertension, the latter with a 2- to 4-week onset of action. They also (paradoxically) relieve diabetes insipidus and interact with calcium metabolism to reduce calcium excretion and formation of renal stones. The thiazides reduce reabsorption of sodium and chloride in the distal tubule of the nephron. Many have a sufficient duration of action to be effective with once-daily administration. Thiazides produce somewhat less intense diuresis than the loop diuretics, yet they carry most of the risks of diuretics in general. Thiazides can cause hyperuricemia, hyperglycemia, photosensitivity, and bone marrow depression. They bind extensively to plasma proteins. Most of the thiazides are sulfonamide derivatives, thus are contraindicated in persons sensitive to these substances. These drugs are administered PO or IV; extravasation must be avoided. Thiazides can prolong the action of some skeletal muscle relaxants.

Potassium-sparing diuretics, as their name implies, are the only diuretics that do not induce hypokalemia. They can, however, lead to hyperkalemia. Spironolactone (Aldactone, 25 to 200 mg) is an aldosterone antagonist; amiloride (Midamor, 5 to 10 mg) and triamterine (Dyrenium, 100 to 200 mg) have a similar effect (i.e., inhibition of sodium reabsorption in exchange for potassium and hydrogen in the distal tubule) but do not interact with aldosterone. These drugs produce mild diuresis; they are usually combined with other diuretics to enhance sodium and water loss and reduce potassium excretion. They have a long onset and duration of action. Spironolactone, which may be teratogenic, is also used to diagnose and manage hyperaldosteronism. Triamterene may contribute to the formation of renal stones. The potassium-sparing diuretics are contraindicated in persons with hyperkalemia. They should not be administered concurrently with each other or with potassium supplements. The angiotensin-converting enzyme (ACE) inhibitors captopril and enalapril inhibit the synthesis of aldosterone, thus increase the risk of hyperkalemia. Hyperkalemia can be alleviated by IV administration of insulin, glucose, or bicarbonate. The potassium-sparing agents, like all diuretics, have many adverse effects and drug interactions, and their administration dictates caution and observation.

CARDIOVASCULAR PHARMACOLOGY

Familiarity with cardiovascular physiology is of utmost importance to understanding cardiovascular pharmacology. The many compensatory mechanisms that come into play in cardiovascular disease can influence and/or be influenced by the administration of drugs. Cardiovascular disease is prevalent in the United States and most other highly developed countries, thus the cardiovascular drugs are among the most widely used.

Antihypertensive drugs

Hypertension (persistent elevation of systolic and/or diastolic blood pressure) is a common disorder. Some occurrences (about 10% in the United States) are the result of other disorders such as eclampsia and renal artery disease. Treatment of such secondary hypertension is usually aimed at the underlying disease, for when this remits then blood pressure returns to normal levels. However, in most cases there is no apparent reason for the elevation in pressure, thus these cases are considered primary or essential hypertension. The cause of essential hypertension is not known, although many risk factors like heredity and smoking have been identified. The objective of drug treatment in essential hypertension is to induce changes in the cardiovascular system that will result in a fall in blood pressure. There are several types of antihypertensive agents, having diverse mechanisms of actions. Refractory hypertension often responds to combinations of antihypertensive agents. "Step therapy" refers to the stepwise addition of drug(s) to gain control of blood pressure.

Drugs do not cure essential hypertension, and they usually must be taken chronically to maintain control. It is important that measures, including drug administration if necessary, be taken to reduce high blood pressure. Hypertension can lead to myocardial infarction, blindness, stroke, and kidney and other organ damage. Essential hypertension is often asymptomatic. Thus once-yearly monitoring of blood pressure is recommended for all adults. Compliance with drug regimens is a frequent problem because of the numerous adverse effects of the antihypertensive agents. The patient often feels better when he or she is not taking medication.

Diuretics, in particular the thiazides and furosemide, are among the drugs most frequently used in the treatment of high blood pressure. Mild hypertension will often respond to a diuretic alone; moderate and severe cases are controlled with a diuretic plus one or two other antihypertensive agents. The exact mechanism by which diuretics lower blood pressure is not understood. They reduce blood volume and sodium content, although the volume frequently returns to normal with no increase in blood pressure. The decrease in sodium may lower vascular responsiveness to endogenous vasoconstrictors, or diuretics may have a direct relaxant effect on blood vessels. (The pharmacology of the diuretics is discussed under "Diuretics.")

The sympathetic nervous system probably contributes to the etiology of essential hypertension, since many of the effective drugs reduce the activity of this autonomic branch. Some drugs appear to work in the CNS, inhibiting outflow of sympathetic stimulation. **Clonidine** (Catapres, 0.2 to 2 mg) and **guanabenz** (Wytensin, 8 to 64 mg) stimulate alpha$_2$ receptors, which in turn reduce adrenergic release of norepinephrine. Drowsiness and dry mouth are frequent side effects. Retention of sodium and fluid can be offset by administration of a diuretic. Alpha-adrenergic antagonists including the tricyclic antidepressants will reduce clonidine's efficacy. Interestingly, clonidine can cause severe mental depression and is usually contraindicated in persons with a history of this disorder. These drugs can add to the bradycardic activity of other cardiovascular depressant drugs, and caution must be used when they are administered to persons with cardiovascular disorders. Clonidine and guanabenz will enhance the depressant effects of other CNS depressants. Administration of clonidine should never be abruptly terminated, as there can be a rapid recurrence of severe high blood pressure.

Methyldopa (Aldomet, 0.5 to 3 g) appears to act in the CNS after it is converted to the alpha$_2$ receptor stimulant, alpha-methylnorepinephrine. Methyldopa may also be a peripheral vasodilator. The drug has a slow onset and long duration of action. It is renally excreted. Side effects include drowsiness, vertigo, fever, and sodium and fluid retention. Hemolytic anemia and fatal hepatic failure can occur. Frequent monitoring of blood counts and liver function can reduce the incidence of these effects. Hepatic disease can be a contraindication to the administration of methyldopa. Methyldopa interacts with

many drugs, potentiating the effects of other antihypertensive agents and of CNS depressants.

Some antihypertensive drugs inhibit sympathetic activity by reducing the amount of norepinephrine stored in the peripheral nerve terminals. **Reserpine** (Serpasil), the first such drug to be used, is today generally a second-line drug because it produces severe mental depression and GI irritation. It is thus contraindicated in depression and GI ulceration. Reserpine can aggravate preexisting asthma or cardiovascular disease. Drowsiness and diarrhea are frequent side effects. Reserpine lowers the seizure threshold, thus can reduce the efficacy of anticonvulsant drugs. Tricyclic antidepressants interfere with the action of reserpine, possibly by blocking its transport into the nerve terminals. Reserpine can add to the effects of cardiac and CNS depressants. The hepatic enzymes inactivate reserpine.

Guanethidine (Ismelin, 25 to 50 mg) also depletes peripheral norepinephrine stores. It does not cross the blood-brain barrier, thus does not produce the CNS side effects observed with reserpine. It has a slow onset of antihypertensive action. Guanethidine is given only by the PO route. A large percentage of each dose is lost on the first pass through the liver. Orthostatic hypotension and sodium and fluid retention are frequent side effects; the drug is contraindicated in congestive heart failure. Many drugs like alcohol and cardiac depressants add to the hypotensive effect of guanethidine. Some drugs such as MAO inhibitors and tricyclic antidepressants reverse the effect of guanethidine. **Guanadrel** (Hylorel, 20 to 75 mg) is an analogue of guanethidine with similar pharmacology but a shorter onset and duration of action.

Another group of drugs widely used in the treatment of hypertension as well as many other disorders is the **beta-adrenergic antagonists** or **beta-blockers** (discussed under "Autonomic Nervous System Pharmacology"). The beta-blockers probably have both a central and a peripheral mechanism of antihypertensive activity. They appear to decrease sympathetic outflow from the brain, and they also block sympathetic stimulation at beta receptors in peripheral tissues. Beta-blockers decrease heart rate and conduction velocity and suppress the renin-angiotensin system. Sodium and fluid retention and exercise intolerance are common adverse effects.

Several **vasodilators** are used in the management of chronic hypertension and of hypertensive crises. Important adverse effects common to all of these are orthostatic hypotension, reflex tachycardia that can be sufficiently severe to cause angina, and retention of sodium and water. These drugs must be administered cautiously in the presence of other cardiovascular disorders. Diuretics should be given concurrently, and beta-blockers can be used to reduce reflex cardiovascular stimulation.

Prazosin (Minipress, 1 to 20 mg) is a vasodilator that appears to reverse alpha-adrenergic vasoconstriction. It causes a lower incidence of tachycardia than other vasodilators. Prazosin causes orthostatic hypotension, especially at the initiation of therapy. Given PO, a large percentage of each dose is lost on the first pass through the liver, which is the site of drug inactivation. Prazosin binds extensively to plasma proteins.

Diazoxide (Hyperstat) and **hydralazine** (Apresoline, 40 to 300 mg) cause direct vasodilation of arteries. They are given PO in chronic hypertension and IV to control hypertensive crisis. Diazoxide is a nondiuretic thiazide that suppresses insulin release and can elevate blood glucose levels. It is extensively bound to plasma proteins, thus IV administration of 1 to 3 mg/kg is by rapid bolus or "IV push." In the presence of renal failure, protein binding may be decreased and the hyperglycemic effect may be greatly intensified. Competition for protein binding can elevate free plasma levels of the oral anticoagulants. Hydralazine is rapidly lost in the first pass through the liver. It is biotransformed mainly by acetylation, thus in persons who are "fast acetylators" the inactivation of this drug is especially rapid. Hydralazine can cause drug fever, blood dyscrasias, and a lupus-like syndrome. These effects require that administration be terminated.

Minoxidil (Loniten, 5 to 100 mg) is an oral arterial vasodilator that is used only for refractory hypertension. It appears to inhibit sympathetic vasoconstriction, but it causes less orthostatic hypotension than many of the other antihypertensive agents. Among the more severe adverse effects are pulmonary hypertension and pericardial exudation. An interesting side effect is stimulation of hair growth, and topical preparations to reverse baldness are under investigation. A beta-blocker and a diuretic are usually concurrently administered to reduce the side effects and to potentiate the antihypertensive activity of minoxidil.

Nitroprusside (Nipride) is a direct vasodilator that is given only by the IV route (3 mcg/kg/minute). It is especially useful in the management of hypertensive crisis. It is very rapidly inactivated by the liver. A slow infusion continuously titrated to the patient's response will provide close control of blood pressure. Nitroprusside is also used to induce hypotension during some surgical procedures. The metabolites of this drug include cyanide, which can accumulate to toxic levels, and thiocyanate, which interferes with thyroid function by inhibiting uptake of iodine. Hypothyroidism and hepatic and renal dysfunction require cautious administration of nitroprusside.

The **vasodilators** are also used in the management of heart failure, to reduce the vascular resistance to blood flow. The combination of hydralazine and isosorbide dinitrate (Isordil, a nitrate vasodilator) has been shown to prolong survival in patients with congestive heart failure.

Captopril (Capoten, 75 to 450 mg) and **enalapril** (Vasotec) represent a new group of antihypertensive agents called converting enzyme inhibitors. They inhibit ACE, which synthesizes angiotensin II, a powerful endogenous vasoconstrictor. A diuretic is usually coadministered to potentiate antihypertensive activity. Since the ACE inhibitors can produce serious adverse effects such as agranulocytosis, renal toxicity, and exacerbation of autoimmune disease, they are used only after other drugs have proved unsuccessful. Food in the GI tract reduces the absorption of the ACE inhibitors, which are given only by the PO route and are inactivated by renal excretion. These drugs reduce renal excretion of potassium by inhibition of aldosterone secretion, thus coadministration of potassium salts or potassium-sparing diuretics can cause hyperkalemia. Captopril is also used together with diuretics and digitalis in the management of congestive heart failure.

The **calcium channel blockers** or antagonists are another relatively new group of cardiovascular drugs that may be effective antihypertensive agents. Verapamil (Isoptin, Calan, 240 to 480 mg), nifedipine (Procardia, 40 to 120 mg), and diltiazem (Cardizem, 120 to 240 mg) are in general use, and several are in various stages of clinical trial. These drugs block the slow inward flow of calcium into cells. Calcium is required for muscle contraction; lower levels of the ion produce less contraction (i.e., less vascular constriction and less forceful myocardial contraction). Renin release is dependent on intracellular flow of calcium. The calcium channel blockers also decrease conduction velocity in the heart. They have been especially effective as antiarrhythmics and antianginal drugs and are covered in those sections of this chapter.

The MAO inhibitor **pargyline** (Eutonyl) is a second-line antihypertensive drug. Its potential for toxicity, including hypertensive crisis when combined with certain foods or drugs, requires that it be administered skillfully. (The pharmacology of the MAO inhibitors is discussed under "Antidepressants.")

The alpha-adrenergic antagonist phentolamine is useful in the control of hypertensive crisis. It reduces the vasoconstriction caused by sympathomimetics and by MAO inhibitor interactions and is used in the treatment of pheochromocytoma. Its major adverse effects are tachycardia and extreme hypotension, thus its use in patients with cardiovascular disease requires caution. Epinephrine should not be administered concurrently with this or any alpha antagonist, as unopposed beta stimulation will result in severe vasodilation and fall in blood pressure. Norepinephrine, which does not have beta activity in blood vessels, can be used to counter overresponsiveness to phentolamine.

The **ganglionic blockers** have limited use in hypertension. Transmission through sympathetic and parasympathetic ganglia is impeded, thus these drugs have numerous side effects. Trimethaphan (Arfonad), which has a brief duration of action, is given IV to control hypertensive crisis and also to produce hypotension in brain and heart surgery. Trimethaphan releases histamine, making it hazardous in persons with history of allergy. Mecamylamine (Inversine) may be used PO in some instances of moderate to severe chronic hypertension. Abrupt discontinuance can result in rebound hypertension.

Cardiotonic drugs

After 200 years, the **digitalis glycosides** are still virtually synonymous with cardiotonic drugs. One drug recently approved, amrinone (Inocor), is reserved for short-term use in persons who have not responded to other therapy. Cardiotonic drugs increase the force of cardiac contraction (positive inotropy). This increases the cardiac output of the failing heart and greatly improves cardiovascular hemodynamics, resulting in renal excretion of sodium and water, decreased peripheral vascular resistance, and slower heart rate. There are several digitalis preparations (Table 6-11), all having the same steroid nucleus and pharmacologic (therapeutic and adverse) effects but differing in onset and duration of action, binding to plasma proteins, and route of inactivation.

The mechanism of action of digitalis appears to be inhibition of ATP-dependent exchange of Na^+ and K^+ across the myocardial cell membrane, causing increased intracellular levels of sodium and subsequently of calcium. Digitalis exerts several cardiac effects in addition to positive inotropy. There is a decrease in conduction velocity (an increase in conduction time) through the atrioventricular node. For this reason, digitalis is frequently used as an antiarrhythmic agent in the management of atrial tachycardias. Ventricular rate is decreased

Table 6-11. Digitalis Glycosides

Generic name	Trade name	Route	Onset of action	Recommended adult* doses
Ouabain	—	IV	3–10 min	0.25–1 mg total/24 hours
Deslanoside	Cedilanid-D	IV	10–30 min	0.8–2 mg total dose
Digitoxin†	Crystodigin, Purodigin	PO	1–4 hours	0.05–0.2 mg/24 hours maintenance
Digoxin	Lanoxin	IV	5–30 min	0.125–0.5 mg/24 hours
		PO	1–2 hours	0.125–0.5 mg/24 hours maintenance

*Drug doses must be individualized to factors including patient's age, hepatic and renal function, serum electrolytes, and previous administration of digitalis.

†Hepatically inactivated. Other glycosides are renally excreted.

because fewer impulses are conducted through the atrioventricular node. However, this effect can also cause varying degrees of heart block progressing to complete block with cardiac arrest or ventricular escape rhythm. Digitalis is administered cautiously if at all to persons with decreased atrioventricular conduction, and doses should be withheld if the pulse rate falls below 60 beats per minute.

Digitalis also increases ventricular automaticity, resulting in characteristic ECG changes and ventricular arrhythmias (tachycardia and fibrillation) that can be fatal. Digitalis has a very narrow safety margin. Patients must be observed closely for signs and symptoms (including anorexia and nausea, vision aberrations, and, in the elderly especially, depression and confusion) that can signal impending digitalis toxicity. Serum levels of digitalis must be monitored by radioimmunoassay: 15 to 25 ng/ml for digitoxin and 0.5 to 2.0 ng/ml for digoxin are considered optimal, although some persons, especially the elderly, will have toxic effects within this range. Hypokalemia must be avoided. Decreased serum potassium potentiates digitalis toxicity, as do hypomagnesemia and hypercalcemia. Serum electrolytes must be monitored. The possibility of digitalis intoxication should be considered in any clinical change in persons receiving this drug. Some of the arrhythmias provoked by digitalis are difficult to distinguish from those that are treated with digitalis.

Digitalis administration should be discontinued at the first appearance of toxicity. In the presence of hypokalemia and adequate renal function, potassium may be administered with caution. Arrhythmias can be controlled with phenytoin, lidocaine, or propranolol, but it must be remembered that beta-adrenergic blockers will add to the depression of atrioventricular conduction. Recently approved for the reversal of digitalis toxicity is the use of antigen-binding protein fragments (digoxin immune Fab [Digibind]), which bind and neutralize digoxin and digitoxin.

Because of the slow onset of action of some digitalis preparations, large initial doses may be administered to rapidly achieve therapeutic serum levels (digitalization). Lower doses are subsequently used to maintain drug effects. Digitalis must be administered with special caution to the elderly and to infants. Premature neonates are very sensitive to its effects; older infants are much less sensitive and require proportionally larger doses. Changing from one digitalis preparation to another must be done carefully because of the variations in plasma half-life.

Digitalis is involved in many drug interactions. In the treatment of congestive heart failure, diuretics that deplete serum potassium and magnesium are often administered concurrently. Corticosteroids and physiological events such as vomiting, diarrhea, and excessive perspiration can waste potassium. Patients should be encouraged to eat foods rich in potassium, and/or potassium supplements may have to be given. Intravenous calcium is contraindicated during digitalis administration. Interactions with digitoxin can occur by way of displacement of this glycoside, which binds extensively to plasma proteins, and also by induction of hepatic enzymes, which results in more rapid biotransformation. Quinidine and calcium antagonists can increase serum levels of digoxin. The absorption of digitalis administered PO is reduced by antacids, by cimetidine, and by hypolipemic resins. Sympathomimetic agents increase the risk of digitalis-induced arrhythmias.

Amrinone, representing a new type of inotropic agent ("nonglycoside noncatecholamine"), is reserved for short-term IV administration in patients with refractory congestive heart failure or for patients in whom other drugs are contraindicated. Amrinone differs from digitalis in several ways. It increases intracellular calcium content by inhibiting cAMP phosphodiesterase. Amrinone seems to enhance rather than suppress atrioventricular conduction, and it is a direct vasodilator.

Amrinone is hepatically inactivated and can also be excreted unchanged by the kidneys. The plasma half-life can be as long as 12 hours in patients with congestive heart failure. PO administration has proved unfeasible because of GI and CNS side effects. Milrinone, an analogue currently in clinical trial, appears to cause fewer adverse reactions. The effectiveness of these drugs is enhanced by concomitant administration of catecholamines such as epinephrine and is reduced by calcium channel blockers (e.g., verapamil) and by cholinomimetics.

The use of **catecholamines** (e.g., dopamine and dobutamine) in the treatment of congestive heart failure is discussed under "Autonomic Nervous System Pharmacology."

Drugs affecting blood coagulation

Anticoagulants are used in the management of clinical

situations (e.g., deep venous thrombosis, pulmonary embolism, disseminated intravascular coagulation, postsurgery) that carry the risk of intravascular formation of blood clots (thrombosis) and breaking off of particles (emboli) that can lodge in vessels of and impede blood flow to vital organs such as the heart, lungs, and brain.

Heparin (5,000 to 40,000 units IV/24 hours) is different in several ways from the oral or coumarin-type anticoagulants. Heparin is derived from animal sources, thus allergic reactions in persons sensitive to bovine or porcine proteins are not uncommon. Heparin must be administered parenterally. Since it interferes directly in clot formation by preventing conversion of precursors to thrombin and fibrin, heparin has an immediate onset of action. However, the duration of action is relatively short. Inactivation occurs by way of hepatic enzymes and also by renal excretion. The plasma half-life of heparin is prolonged in persons with renal dysfunction. Partial thromboplastin time (PTT) should be monitored to evaluate individual persons' responses to heparin. Overdosage of the drug is treated with protamine sulfate administered by slow IV infusion. (Protamine itself has anticoagulant activity.) Paradoxically, heparin can cause platelet aggregation resulting in thrombocytopenia and thromboembolism.

The **coumarin-type anticoagulants** (Table 6-12) are administered PO. They inhibit the hepatic synthesis of several clotting factors, thus their onset of action is prolonged (72 to 96 hours for full anticoagulation). The oral anticoagulants are metabolized by hepatic enzymes. Their plasma half-life is longer in the presence of liver disease and shorter when hepatic enzyme-inducing drugs are concomitantly administered. Vitamin K is an antidote to oral anticoagulant overdose. Persons depleted of vitamin K (e.g., those on antibiotics that eradicate intestinal bacteria synthesizing vitamin K) will have an exaggerated response to these anticoagulants. Additional interactions occur because the oral anticoagulants bind extensively to plasma proteins and can be displaced by other drugs. Patients' responses to the oral anticoagulants should be monitored with prothrombin time (PT) determinations.

Heparin and the oral anticoagulants share several characteristics. For both, the major adverse effect is severe hemorrhage (either spontaneous or following injury) due to excessive suppression of blood coagulation. Drug doses must be carefully adjusted to each individual, with frequent monitoring of clotting time. Drug interactions are numerous. In addition to those already mentioned, many drugs enhance the effect on

Table 6-12. Oral Anticoagulants

Generic name	Trade name	Recommended adult doses (mg PO/day)
Anisindione	Miradon	25–150
Bishydroxycoumarin	Dicumarol	25–200
Phenprocoumon	Liquamar	0.75–6
Warfarin	Coumadin, others	2–15

coagulation (e.g., salicylates and other nonsteroidal anti-inflammatory drugs) and many drugs antagonize that effect (e.g., oral contraceptives and corticosteroids). The potential for interaction must be considered whenever any drug is added to or removed from the regimen of a person receiving an anticoagulant. Anticoagulants are contraindicated when there is active bleeding or great risk of hemorrhage (e.g., gastric ulcer, severe hypertension, eye or CNS surgery) and must be administered cautiously to elderly persons, who for several reasons are especially sensitive to the anticoagulants.

Heparin and the oral anticoagulants do not disrupt clots already present. This is accomplished with thrombolytic agents such as streptokinase and urokinase, which activate plasminogen, an enzyme that dissolves fibrin. Streptokinase is derived from streptococci and can be inactivated by antistreptococcal antibodies, which are frequently present in patients' blood. A large loading dose may be given to overcome this effect. However, streptokinase itself can provoke the formation of antibodies, resulting in allergic reactions and in reduction of effectiveness. Urokinase, derived from human cells, does not have these disadvantages, but it is much more costly than streptokinase. Tissue plasminogen activator (tPA) is an endogenous antithrombotic agent.

Thrombolytic agents are used when thrombi or emboli are known or highly suspected to be present, such as in pulmonary embolism, deep venous thrombosis, and early in acute myocardial infarction. These drugs are administered IV or intra-arterially. Blood coagulation must be monitored continuously, and the patient observed for signs of hemorrhage (especially at the site of injection) during administration and for at least 24 hours thereafter. Contraindications include recent cerebrovascular accident or neurosurgery and active bleeding or significant potential for bleeding. Anticoagulants should not be given concurrently with thrombolytics but are often used subsequently to prevent further thrombosis.

Hemostatic agents are used to reduce bleeding. Those used topically to control bleeding from small vessels include thrombin and human fibrin, gelatin foam (Gelfoam), and cellulose (Oxycel). Aminocaproic acid (Amicar) is a systemic (PO or IV) hemostatic used to control excessive bleeding resulting from fibrinolysis, hemophilia, or overdose of thrombolytic agents and to prevent disruption of clots after cerebral aneurysm. Aminocaproic acid must not be administered to persons with disseminated intravascular coagulation unless heparin is also given.

Hemophilia can be treated also by the administration of missing **clotting factors**. Antihemophilic Factor VIII is available in several preparations, all of which are administered IV. Because this factor is derived from human blood, there is the risk of transmission of hepatitis and/or acquired immunodeficiency syndrome (AIDS). (The transmission of AIDS may be reduced by testing of donor blood for HTLV-III or HIV—human immunodeficiency virus—antibodies.) Administration of Factor VIII can induce production of inhibitors to its action and may cause hemolysis in patients having blood types other than O. Erythrocyte replacement may be required. Allergic reactions also have been reported. Anti-inhibitor coagulant complex (Autoplex) reduces the action of the Factor VIII inhibitor. Human-derived coagulant factor IX (Konyne) is available for the control of bleeding in Christmas disease.

Antianginal drugs

Angina pectoris is chest pain that arises in the myocardium when narrowing of the coronary arteries renders the oxygen supply to the heart inadequate. Angina is classified as stable (or "classic") and unstable. The chest pain of stable angina is induced by stress or exercise and is of short duration if the cause of increased oxygen demand is removed. Persons having unstable angina will experience unpredictable chest pain, even at rest, and are considered to be at risk of acute myocardial infarction. In Prinzmetal's angina, the cause of the diminished myocardial oxygen supply appears to be coronary artery spasm. Drugs that alleviate angina (nitrite/nitrate vasodilators, beta-adrenergic antagonists, and calcium channel blockers) either decrease myocardial oxygen demand, increase myocardial oxygen supply, or do both.

The **nitrite/nitrate vasodilators** continue to be the drugs of choice for initiating the treatment of angina. Direct relaxation of vascular smooth muscle causes both venous and arteriolar dilation. This reduces "preload" or the amount of blood returning to the heart. Arterial dilation decreases "afterload," or the resistance to blood flow. Both effects decrease myocardial oxygen demand. Nitrite/nitrate vasodilators also appear to channel increased amounts of blood to previously underperfused myocardial regions, thus improving oxygen supply. Nitrite/nitrates are rapidly inactivated, especially by the hepatic first-pass effect after oral administration. The sublingual and transdermal routes are frequently used to enhance the action of these drugs. The onset of action is rapid, and the duration (except for sustained-release forms) is usually short.

Sublingual nitroglycerin tablets can be used to prevent angina. One tablet is taken 5 to 10 minutes before any activity expected to provoke chest pain. Sublingual tablets are also taken to relieve acute attacks. The onset of action is within 2 minutes. If one tablet does not provide relief from pain, two more may be taken each at 5- to 10-minute intervals. If this fails to reduce pain, the patient should immediately contact the physician as an acute myocardial infarction may be in progress. Nitroglycerin must be protected from heat, light, and moisture, which inactivate it. Supplies should be discarded after 6 months. Tablets will cause a mild burning sensation sublingually if the drug is still active. Also used to relieve acute attacks of angina is amyl nitrite, a vapor provided in small glass ampules. It begins to act within seconds after inhalation.

IV nitroglycerin (Tridil, Nitro-Bid IV) is used in acute angina and also to reduce cardiac work load in congestive heart failure (e.g., after myocardial infarction) and occasionally to control blood pressure during surgery. Several concentrations are available. The usual dose is 5-20 or more μg/minute. Special containers and tubing must be used, since nitroglycerin adsorbs to polyvinylchloride.

Other nitrite/nitrate preparations with longer onset and duration of action are administered chronically to reduce the occurrence or severity of angina attacks. Nitroglycerin in an oral sustained-release tablet (Nitro-Bid), isosorbide dinitrate (Isordil, Sorbitrate, 20 to 120 mg) in sublingual and oral forms, and erythrityl and pentaerythritol tetranitrate (Cardilate, 30 to 90 mg, and Peritrate, 30 to 160 mg) in oral tablets are used. Transdermal nitroglycerin is prepared as an ointment (Nitro-Bid) and as transdermal patches (Nitro-Dur, Nitrodisc) containing various dosages. The effectiveness of the patches has been controversial. Also available are a sublingual aerosol spray (Nitrolingual) and a buccal tablet form (Nitrogard) of nitroglycerin. Many of these preparations are also used in the management of congestive heart failure. Combinations of nitrates plus a sedative, an antianxiety agent, or ethaverine to reduce arterial spasm are available.

Nitrite/nitrates are contraindicated in the presence of anemia and of conditions that may be aggravated by a decrease in cardiac output. Vasodilation and subsequent cerebral underperfusion can lead to increases in intracranial pressure, which can be hazardous in the presence of head injury. Increased intraocular pressure may occur. Common side effects of the nitrite/nitrates include hypotension, tachycardia (which can precipitate angina), dry mouth, vision disturbances, and headache due to cerebral vasodilation. Tolerance does develop to both therapeutic and adverse effects. Headache can be relieved with an analgesic such as aspirin if not otherwise contraindicated. Other drugs that cause vasodilation and/or decrease in blood pressure (including alcohol) will add to the hypotensive effect of the nitrite/nitrates.

Beta-adrenergic antagonists are used in the management of angina, both for their own ability to reduce myocardial oxygen demand by inhibiting sympathetic stimulation and to prevent reflex tachycardia induced by reductions in blood pressure. (The pharmacology of these drugs is discussed under "Autonomic Nervous System Pharmacology.")

The **calcium channel blockers** are a relatively new group of drugs effective in the control of both stable and unstable angina. They are frequently combined with the nitrite/nitrate vasodilators, and are also used experimentally in the treatment of uterine hyperactivity, migraine, hypertension, myocardial infarction, and many other cardiovascular disorders. As their name implies, these drugs reduce the slow inward flow of calcium into cells. This influences both myocardial and vascular smooth muscle contraction, causing vasodilation and reducing coronary artery vasospasm. (The calcium channel blockers have much less effect on skeletal muscle contraction, which uses calcium stored within the cell.) There are important pharmacologic differences among the calcium channel blockers that affect their therapeutic usefulness and their adverse effects.

Verapamil prolongs conduction and the refractory period in the atrioventricular node. It is administered IV and PO to control many supraventricular arrhythmias. In some situations it is preferred to digitalis; however, it is contraindicated in second- and third-degree heart block and also in Wolff-Parkinson-White reentrant arrhythmias. Oral verapamil is used to alleviate angina. Verapamil is rapidly metabolized in the liver; its half-life is prolonged by hepatic dysfunction and congestive heart failure. It binds extensively to plasma proteins. Verapamil can depress sinoatrial activity, thus requires caution in persons with nodal dysfunction such as sick sinus syndrome. It also has a negative inotropic effect and is contraindicated in congestive heart failure.

Verapamil frequently causes hypotension, which can be reversed with calcium or sympathomimetic amines. Preexisting severe hypotension is a contraindication, and hypotensive drugs can add to that effect of the calcium channel blockers. Some ventricular tachyarrhythmias may worsen after verapamil administration. Persons with cardiomyopathies are especially at risk of adverse reactions to verapamil. Heart block, extreme slowing of heart rate, and cardiac arrest may occur. Cardioversion and electric pacing can be used to manage these adverse effects. Beta-adrenergic blockers should not be administered IV within 2 hours of IV verapamil, as excessive myocardial depression can occur. Oral administration of these two types of drugs requires close observation for myocardial depression, especially at the atrioventricular node. Concurrent administration of verapamil and digitalis results in elevated serum levels of the latter drug and may severely depress atrioventricular conduction. The antiarrhythmic disopyramide (Norpace) should not be given within 48 hours before to 24 hours after verapamil.

Diltiazem also depresses atrioventricular conduction (it is contraindicated in second- and third-degree heart block), but its greatest effect is to reduce constriction in the coronary arteries. Caution is required in persons with sinoatrial dysfunction, as further suppression of activity may occur. Diltiazem is hepatically metabolized with extensive first-pass extraction. Adverse effects, although infrequent, can include arrhythmias, hypotension, bradycardia, edema, congestive heart failure, and headache. Bradycardia and heart block may be relieved with atropine, hypotension with sympathomimetics. Other drugs that depress atrioventricular conduction (e.g., digitalis and beta-blockers) may add to this effect of diltiazem.

Nifedipine appears to have its greatest effect on peripheral blood vessels. In addition to its use in angina, nifedipine is administered experimentally in hypertension to reduce cerebrovascular spasm and congestive heart failure. Nifedipine is hepatically metabolized, although not as rapidly as other calcium channel blockers. It is highly protein bound. Adverse effects that are frequent although usually not serious include hypotension, dizziness, headache, edema, and respiratory difficulty. Congestive heart failure, myocardial infarction, and arrhythmias that may be drug induced have been reported. Hypotensive agents such as beta-blockers can enhance the fall in blood pressure caused by nifedipine and may increase the risk of congestive heart failure.

Pharmacotherapy of acute myocardial infarction

Myocardial infarction refers to the destruction of cardiac tissue that follows interruption of coronary artery blood flow. Thrombosis, embolism, and arterial spasm are the usual causes of myocardial ischemia. Damage to the myocardium can produce arrhythmias or asystole, with inadequate cerebral perfusion resulting in brain damage. Since myocardial infarction can be rapidly fatal, emergency measures must be taken if life is to be preserved. Several types of drugs (summarized here and covered elsewhere in this chapter) are used in the management of myocardial infarction and its accompanying complications. Because an immediate effect is required, drugs are usually given IV and often by rapid bolus. Some drugs can also be given via endotracheal tube for absorption through the lungs. The patient should subsequently be hyperventilated for 30 seconds to deposit the drug well into the alveoli. IM administration is rarely used, as resulting elevations in serum creatine phosphokinase (CPK) would interfere with the measurement of this enzyme to assess the extent of myocardial damage.

Arrhythmias frequently occur in myocardial infarction. Premature ventricular contractions or ventricular tachycardias are usually treated with **lidocaine**, which reduces ventricular automaticity and irritability. Lidocaine is administered by IV bolus and/or continuous IV infusion. It is rapidly biotransformed in the liver (making it ineffective if given PO), thus requires extra caution in persons with decreased hepatic function or perfusion. Adverse effects include excessive depression of the ventricular conducting system, decreased responsiveness to defibrillation, and CNS symptoms such as headache, altered level of consciousness, dizziness, tremors, convulsions, respiratory arrest, and coma. Lidocaine is ineffective in supraventricular arrhythmias.

Procainamide (Pronestyl) can be used to control both ventricular and supraventricular tachyarrhythmias. Automaticity, irritability, and conductivity in all regions of the heart are suppressed. It is usually administered by IV bolus in emergencies and is used PO to prevent recurrence of arrhythmias. Adverse effects include severe hypotension due to the vasodilatory action of the drug (especially after IV administration), and significant depression of myocardial activity is evidenced by prolonged P-R intervals and widened QRS complexes. Hypotension can be reversed by fluid replacement and pressor amines. Chronic administration can provoke formation of antinuclear antibodies and development of a reversible lupus-like syndrome. Procainamide must be given cautiously in the presence of decreased atrioventricular conduction, including that caused by digitalis. Because it has anticholinergic activity, procainamide can cause an increase in heart rate.

Calcium channel blockers, verapamil in particular, may be administered by IV push to reduce atrial arrhythmias. The greatest effect of verapamil is to slow atrioventricular conduction velocity, thus it must be used carefully if some degree of heart block already exists. Sinus node function may also be decreased. Hypotension and bradycardia, the latter reversible by atropine, isoproterenol, or electric pacing, are notable adverse effects of verapamil. Concurrent administration of disopyramide is contraindicated.

If other drugs fail to terminate severe ventricular tachyarrhythmias, **bretylium** (Bretylol) by IV push may be successful. Additional doses can be given. Bretylium reduces the release of norepinephrine in response to sympathetic stimulation. Its onset of action can be slow. Initially there may be a burst of norepinephrine release causing vasoconstriction and an increase in heart rate. The drug has positive inotropic effects and, in contrast to lidocaine and procainamide, it increases myocardial responsiveness to defibrillation. The use of bretylium in management of acute myocardial infarction is rapidly increasing. Continuous IV infusion will reduce the risk of ventricular fibrillation. Hypotension, including orthostatic, is a significant adverse response. The initial release of norepinephrine can enhance digitalis toxicity. Nausea and vomiting occur, especially after rapid IV administration.

As a result of decreased sinus activity or reduced atrioventricular conduction, bradycardia can also occur during myocardial infarction. The safest management of bradycardia is via electrical pacemaker. However, **atropine**, which blocks parasympathetic slowing of heart rate and conduction, will often alleviate bradycardia and accompanying hypotension. The dose should be at least 0.5 mg; lower doses can enhance bradycardia. All of the adverse anticholinergic effects must be considered when atropine is used. Slow heart rate may also be reversed with the beta-adrenergic stimulant **isoproterenol**, although an increase in myocardial oxygen demand and in ventricular irritability can be hazardous in myocardial infarction. Slow IV infusion with constant monitoring of cardiac activity is required. The appearance of premature ventricular contractions requires immediate reduction in dose or termination of administration. As with all catecholamines, the effects of isoproterenol are enhanced by digitalis.

Acidosis often accompanies myocardial infarction. Circulatory failure slows the delivery of venous blood to the lungs and impedes excretion of carbon dioxide. Acidosis reduces myocardial responsiveness to defibrillation and to many drugs. **Sodium bicarbonate** is often the first drug (after oxygen) administered in circulatory failure, although its safety and efficacy have been questioned. Administration should be repeated only if determination of arterial blood gases indicates that acidosis persists. Potassium or calcium deficits should be corrected before or concurrently with bicarbonate administration. Overdose of bicarbonate produces alkalosis and sodium and fluid overload. Sodium bicarbonate must not be allowed contact with any other drugs in the IV system, or precipitation and inactivation will occur. Extravasation must be avoided, as severe tissue necrosis may develop. Sodium bicarbonate is not administered by endotracheal tube, because alveolar collapse can result.

Cardiac arrest or ventricular fibrillation that fails to circulate blood can develop as ventricular cells are damaged or destroyed. Electrical defibrillation is usually the most effective means for restoring normal heartbeat. The beta-adrenergic agonist **epinephrine** (Adrenalin, available in several concentrations) may help in controlling cardiac activity and can increase myocardial responsiveness to defibrillation. Once the heartbeat is restored, this drug will increase the rate and force of contraction. If circulation has ceased, IV administration will be ineffective since distribution to sites of action will not occur. Thus intracardiac injection may be deemed necessary despite its hazards. Catecholamines inadvertently deposited into the myocardium rather than the ventricular chambers can cause irreversible fibrillation. Isoproterenol and epinephrine given simultaneously increase the risk of arrhythmias, as does the administration of catecholamines to digitalized patients. Extravasation of epinephrine will cause tissue necrosis.

A group of drugs used almost routinely in the acute phase of myocardial infarction is the **narcotic analgesics**, morphine and meperidine (Demerol) in particular. Their purpose is to reduce pain and apprehension, both of which activate the sympathetic nervous system and increase myocardial oxygen demand. Morphine is also effective in reducing pulmonary edema that develops subsequent to left ventricular failure. Its mechanism is thought to be via vasodilation and reduction of venous return to the already overloaded cardiac chambers. Vasodilation also facilitates ventricular emptying. Narcotic analgesics, however, carry the risk of hypotension and of significant respiratory depression.

Diuretics also can be used to correct pulmonary edema. IV administration of the loop diuretics such as furosemide causes rapid diuresis and reduction of intravascular volume. Care must be taken, however, that reduction in blood pressure and volume does not adversely affect myocardial perfusion or result in hemoconcentration that will provoke thrombosis.

"Pump failure" and **cardiogenic shock** are potential complications of myocardial infarction. Ventricular wall damage reduces the strength of contraction and may lead to myocardial rupture. Pharmacotherapy of this heart failure is hazardous (and controversial) but if undertaken carefully can be lifesaving. Small IV doses of **furosemide** may sufficiently ease the work load of the heart; however, electrolyte and fluid imbalances must be avoided. Small doses of digitalis may be useful, although hypoxia sensitizes the myocardium to the arrhythmogenic effects of the cardioactive glycosides. Hypokalemia must be avoided as it will increase the risk of adverse responses. Vasodilators can reduce the resistance to cardiac outflow but can also compromise perfusion of the myocardium and may induce tachycardia and increased oxygen consumption.

Cardiogenic shock is often fatal, thus warrants aggressive treatment, usually with adrenergic agonists. The drugs of choice were previously **metaraminol** and **norepinephrine**. These increase the force of contraction of undamaged myocardial cells and also cause constriction of blood vessels. This latter action can further reduce perfusion of vital organs in patients who are already vasoconstricted. There is also the risk of catecholamine-induced arrhythmias. **Dopamine** and **dobutamine** strengthen contraction with less increase in myocardial oxygen demand. Dopamine is rapidly becoming the preferred drug for increasing blood pressure and cardiac output during acute myocardial infarction. Dopamine is always given by infusion, and its actions are dose related. Low (0.5 to 2 mcg/kg/minute) doses stimulate dopamine receptors to dilate renal and mesenteric blood vessels, improving perfusion of the kidneys. Doses of 2 to 10 mcg/kg/minute cause norepinephrine release and exhibit beta-stimulating properties. Alpha-adrenergic effects, especially vasoconstriction, appear at 10 to 20 mcg/kg/minute. Dopamine can cause an increase in heart rate and blood pressure and a reduction in myocardial oxygen supply. Extravasation will result in tissue necrosis.

In the **early stages** of acute myocardial infarction, **thrombolytic agents** such as streptokinase and tissue plasminogen activator may be useful. Calcium chloride may be administered when cardiac arrest is associated with hypocalcemia, hypokalemia, or excessive response to calcium channel blockers. The administration of anticoagulants during the recovery phase is controversial. Sedatives are used to promote rest and recovery. Administration of beta-adrenergic blockers such as propranolol and timolol begun soon after myocardial infarction has been shown in several studies to significantly reduce the occurrence of reinfarctions and sudden death.

Antiarrhythmic drugs

A variety of drugs are used in the management of cardiac arrhythmias; several attempts to classify these agents have been made. One that has been widely accepted with some modification is that of Vaughn Williams (Table 6-13).

Class I drugs, which are further divided into groups A, B, and C, have membrane-stabilizing effects. They reduce the inward sodium current, thus slowing phase O depolarization. Class II drugs are the beta-blockers, competitive antagonists of beta-adrenergic stimulation. Class III agents prolong the duration of the action potential, thus of the effective refractory period. Class IV agents are the calcium channel blockers, which interfere with calcium influx into cells. Because the antiarrhythmics work by varied mechanisms, they are each effective

Table 6-13. Antiarrhythmic Drugs

Generic name	Trade name	Recommended adult doses
Class IA		
Disopyramide	Norpace	400–800 mg PO/24 hours
Procainamide	Pronestyl, others	50 mg/kg PO/24 hours
Quinidine	Cin-Quin, others	10–20 mg/kg PO/24 hours
Class IB		
Lidocaine	Xylocaine	1–4 mg/min IV
Mexiletine	Mexitil	0.2–1 g PO/24 hours
Phenytoin	Dilantin	300–400 mg PO/24 hours
Tocainide	Tonocard	1.2–2.4 g PO/24 hours
Class IC		
Flecainide	Tambocor	100–400 mg PO/24 hours
Encainide	Enkaid	25–200 mg PO/24 hours
Class II		
Beta-adrenergic blockers (see Table 6-8)		
Class III		
Amiodarone	Cordarone	0.4–1.6 g PO/24 hours
Bretylium	Bretylol	5–10 mg/kg slow IV q 6 hours
Class IV		
Verapamil	Calan, Isoptin	240–480 mg PO/24 hours

in particular types of arrhythmias. Unfortunately, all antiarrhythmic agents are also arrhythmogenic. They may exacerbate existing rhythm disturbances or cause new ones to develop. Thus persons receiving these drugs must be closely monitored.

The **Class IA agents—quinidine, procainamide,** and **disopyramide**— prolong the P-R, QRS, and Q-T intervals by slowing both depolarization and repolarization of myocardial cells. They are effective for ventricular and supraventricular arrhythmias. All of these agents have anticholinergic activity and can cause an increase in sinoatrial activity. Quinidine and disopyramide can induce paroxysmal ventricular fibrillation or torsade de pointes; procainamide prolongs the Q-T interval to a lesser extent but may still cause such arrhythmias.

Quinidine is rarely administered IV because its marked vasodilatory effect produces severe hypotension. It may be given IM, although the usual route is PO, for the control of several types of arrhythmias. An initial test dose should be given to determine the patient's responsiveness to this drug. Quinidine is metabolized mainly in the liver, although a small amount is renally excreted unchanged. Several types of cardiac dysfunction, in particular conduction disorders, as well as renal dysfunction, are contraindications to quinidine. Its anticholinergic action makes it unsuitable for use in persons with myasthenia gravis. Adverse effects are numerous; they may occur rapidly after the first dose or appear gradually with chronic administration. Significant depression of conduction occurs, and this can progress to ventricular fibrillation manifested as "quinidine syncope," which can be fatal. All adverse effects should be reported by the patient, who may require a reduction in dosage. A characteristic adverse response is cinchonism. GI disturbances are common. Drug interactions also are numerous. Quinidine can elevate serum levels of digoxin and can enhance digitalis toxicity, although administration of quinidine in atrial flutter may be preceded by digitalis to produce a mild degree of atrioventricular depression and prevent ventricular tachycardia. Quinidine increases the effects of the oral anticoagulants and adds to the cardiodepressant activity of other antiarrhythmics. Quinidine concomitant with verapamil can produce severe hypotension in persons with hypertrophic cardiomyopathy. Hypokalemia reduces the effectiveness of quinidine (and of most Class I agents). Acid urine facilitates quinidine excretion, alkalinization promotes renal reabsorption.

Procainamide is quite similar to quinidine, although it is safer for IV administration. It is used for many of the same types of arrhythmias. It is often effective in controlling lidocaine-resistant ventricular arrhythmias (see "Pharmacotherapy of acute myocardial infarction"). A major portion of procainamide is excreted unchanged by the kidneys, with approximately 25% biotransformed by a plasma enzyme to the active N-acetyl metabolite. Some persons are genetically deficient in this enzyme. Heart or renal failure prolongs the drug's half-life. The most frequent side effect is hypotension. Increased ventricular rate or atrioventricular heart block can develop. Agranulocytosis, occasionally fatal, and thrombocytopenia have occurred. A lupus-like syndrome, reversible if drug is discontinued, may appear with chronic administration. The N-acetylprocainamide may have lower potential to cause this adverse effect; however, some persons do not respond therapeutically to the metabolite, and its electrophysiological properties are somewhat different and may include greater prolongation of the Q-T interval. Procainamide adds to the fall in blood pressure produced by other hypotensive agents and to the anticholinergic effects of other drugs that block the parasympathetic nervous system. Procainamide also enhances the skeletal muscle relaxation produced by magnesium, succinylcholine, and the aminoglycoside antibiotics. Alkalinization of the urine may reduce renal excretion.

Disopyramide is included in Class IA yet is not completely similar to quinidine and procainamide. It is especially effective against ventricular arrhythmias, including occasionally those resistant to quinidine or to lidocaine. Frequently administered PO, disopyramide is renally excreted both as unchanged drug and as metabolites. Cardiac, renal, and hepatic dysfunction can prolong its plasma half-life. It has strong anticholinergic activity and a marked negative inotropic effect, and can cause hypotension and congestive heart failure. Concomitant administration of other antiarrhythmics requires close observation to prevent severe myocardial depression. Disopyramide can be used in digitalized patients. It prolongs the Q-T interval, thus may provoke serious ventricular arrhythmias. Disopyramide has oxytocic acitivity. Drugs that induce hepatic enzymes can reduce the effectiveness of disopyramide, as can hypokalemia.

Hyperkalemia potentiates toxicity. Loading doses are contraindicated in cardiomyopathies, as circulatory collapse may result. Occasional hypoglycemia has been reported.

Class IB antiarrhythmics, of which **lidocaine** is the prototype, shorten action potential duration and effective refractoriness of Purkinje's fibers and have little effect on the contractility or the P-R, QRS, and Q-T intervals. Lidocaine (discussed under "Pharmacotherapy of acute myocardial infarction") is effective against ventricular arrhythmias, but its rapid hepatic inactivation precludes PO administration. The newer antiarrhythmics tocainide (Tonocard) and mexiletine (Mexitil) are very similar to lidocaine and are orally effective. Food in the GI tract will delay the absorption of tocainide and will also minimize adverse GI effects. Alkalinization of the urine or decreased renal and hepatic function will prolong the plasma half-life of this drug. Arrhythmias refractory to lidocaine usually do not respond to tocainide. Mexiletine is hepatically inactivated, with a prolonged plasma half-life in the presence of liver dysfunction or cardiac failure. Mexiletine also causes GI disturbances and adverse CNS effects such as dizziness, fatigue, headache, and convulsions. This drug has been combined with propranolol, quinidine, or amiodarone to enhance their effectiveness in refractory ventricular arrhythmias.

Phenytoin is a Class IB antiarrhythmic that is especially effective in reversing digitalis toxicity, and may be used also for other ventricular arrhythmias. Phenytoin is hepatically inactivated; its plasma half-life is affected by drugs that induce or inhibit the hepatic enzymes. Some patients are genetically deficient in the parahydroxylation enzyme, thus are at great risk of drug toxicity. Phenytoin itself can increase liver enzyme activity, thus decreasing the effectiveness of other drugs. It binds extensively to plasma proteins; this may be decreased in patients with renal and hepatic disease. Phenytoin can be given IV or PO. The former requires special caution, as rapid IV administration may result in marked hypotension and cardiac and CNS depression. The drug has a narrow margin of safety; serum concentrations must be monitored. (Phenytoin is further discussed under "Anticonvulsants.")

Several drugs in various stages of development have prompted the additional classification of **IC agents.** These drugs markedly depress conduction in the His-Purkinje system, with less effect on refractoriness. They prolong the P-R and QRS intervals but have less effect on the Q-T interval. **Flecainide** (Tambocor) is administered PO and is inactivated both renally and hepatically. It is arrhythmogenic, can depress sinus node activity, cause atrioventricular heart block, and precipitate congestive heart failure. Its use is recommended only for severe refractory ventricular arrhythmias.

The **Class II antiarrhythmics,** the **beta-blockers,** are used especially in arrhythmias arising from adrenergic activity. The pharmacology of these agents is discussed under "Autonomic Nervous System Pharmacology."

Class III agents, which prolong the duration of the cardiac action potential and thus of the refractory period, are often effective in controlling ventricular fibrillation. **Bretylium** is discussed under "Pharmacotherapy of acute myocardial infarction." It is used frequently in the treatment of this medical emergency.

Amiodarone is administered PO to ameliorate refractory ventricular arrhythmias. This drug has a markedly long (3 weeks to 3 months) plasma half-life and a long onset of action (up to 21 days). It is excreted in the bile. Adverse effects include pulmonary fibrosis, depression of sinus node activity, atrioventricular heart block, ataxia, tremor, corneal microdeposits, bluish-gray skin discoloration, nausea, occasionally fatal hepatitis, and changes in thyroid function due to its iodine content. Amiodarone enhances the actions of oral anticoagulants, digitalis, and the Class IA antiarrhythmics.

The **Class IV antiarrhythmics,** the calcium channel blockers, are used in the treatment of angina pectoris and are discussed under "Antianginal agents." **Verapamil,** which depresses atrioventricular conduction, has been found to be especially effective against atrial arrhythmias. Verapamil causes vasodilation and a decrease in the force of cardiac contraction. The resultant fall in blood pressure provokes reflex sympathetic stimulation that improves cardiac function. Verapamil is more effective than digitalis in slowing atrioventricular conduction under conditions of increased sympathetic activity such as exercise and stress. **Diltiazem,** which has actions similar to verapamil, may also be an effective antiarrhythmic.

The **digitalis glycosides,** used in the management of certain atrial arrhythmias, were previously discussed under "Cardiotonic drugs."

Antilipemic drugs

Antilipemic drugs lower serum levels of triglycerides and cholesterol, which circulate in transport forms called lipoproteins. Lipoproteins are classified as very low density (VLDL), low density (LDL), intermediate density (IDL), high density (HDL), and chylomicrons. VLDL, IDL, and chylomicrons are composed mainly of triglycerides, whereas LDL and HDL contain a larger proportion of cholesterol. High LDL levels correlate with a greater incidence of atherosclerosis and coronary heart disease, high HDL levels with reduced risk. Hyperlipemia may be secondary to such disorders as hypothyroidism, nephrotic syndrome, or diabetes mellitus. Alterations in diet (reduction in fat, cholesterol, and caloric intake) and a program of moderate exercise should be the initial therapy for persons with primary elevations in serum lipids. Antilipemic drugs should be reserved for those who do not respond adequately to dietary measures. Other controllable risk factors such as hypertension, obesity, and cigarette smoking should receive attention. Unfortunately, elevated blood lipid levels often go undetected until the occurrence of a severe, possibly fatal, myocardial infarction. Measurement of blood lipoproteins should be included in routine physical examinations.

Hyperlipidemia has been classified ("Fredrickson Types") according to blood lipid content. In Type I, chylomicrons are elevated; alterations in diet are the therapy for this hereditary disorder. In Type II, LDL and VLDL are increased; IDL are higher in Type III; and Types IV and V are characterized by elevations of VLDL. Several groups of antilipemic agents that work by various mechanisms are available; dietary modifications should accompany drug therapy.

The bile acid sequestrants **cholestyramine** (Questran, 4 g with each meal) and **colestipol** (Colestid, 15 to 30 g) bind bile acids and reduce their enterohepatic recirculation. This promotes conversion of cholesterol to bile acids and a reduction in serum LDL, usually within 4 weeks of daily administration. Sequestrants are especially effective in Type II hyperlipidemia.

Cholestyramine is also used to reduce blood and tissue levels of bile acids in persons with partial biliary obstruction. The sequestrants are not systemically absorbed. They are given PO before meals, always mixed with liquids or high-moisture foods. Constipation is a frequent side effect; fecal impaction may occur. Laxatives or stool softeners can be used to prevent these effects. Other GI symptoms, reduced blood coagulation due to vitamin K depletion, and bone demineralization due to vitamin D deficiency can occur. The sequestrants bind many substances, thus reducing their GI absorption. Nutrients, fat-soluble vitamins, and many drugs (e.g., digitalis, oral anticoagulants, chlorothiazide, and several antibiotics) are affected. For this reason, vitamin supplements may be required, and administration of any other drugs should be at least 1 hour before or 4 to 6 hours after a sequestrant is taken. When sequestrant administration is terminated, close observation for possible dose reduction is required, since ensuing greater absorption of drugs may result in toxicity. Because the sequestrants exchange chloride ions for bile acids, hyperchloremic acidosis may develop, especially in children.

Niacin (nicotinic acid, 1 to 2 g with each meal) reduces hepatic synthesis of VLDL and inhibits mobilization of free fatty acids from adipose tissue. It is most effective in hyperlipidemia Types III, IV, and V. A major side effect is cutaneous vasodilation with marked flushing and itching, especially of the face. Tolerance often develops to this effect. Taking the drug with meals or as a sustained-release form may also decrease its incidence and severity, as can reduction in prostaglandin synthesis by administration of aspirin. Other adverse effects include hypotension, abdominal pain, increased gastric secretion, hyperglycemia, and hyperuricemia. Caution is required if niacin is administered to persons with peptic ulcer, diabetes, or gout; doses of drugs used to control these disorders may have to be increased or niacin terminated. Hepatic dysfunction can be a contraindication, since niacin itself is hepatotoxic. Liver function should be monitored throughout therapy. Niacin may enhance the hypotensive action of drugs that induce a fall in blood pressure.

Dextrothyroxine (Choloxin, 1 to 8 mg) lowers serum lipids by enhancing the catabolism of LDL. It is most effective in Type II hyperlipidemia. Dextrothyroxine is contraindicated in persons with cardiovascular disease because it may increase the occurrence of angina and the risk of myocardial infarction. Dextrothyroxine has all the effects of thyroid hormones, and cardiac stimulation and arrhythmias may occur. Insomnia, weight loss, hyperthermia, nervousness, and GI disturbances are some of the numerous side effects that can develop. Hyperglycemia may necessitate higher doses of insulin or oral medication in diabetics. Dextrothyroxine increases the risk of digitalis- and anesthesia-induced arrhythmias. The therapeutic effect of oral anticoagulants is enhanced. Pregnancy and hepatic or renal disease are additional contraindications. In general, dextrothyroxine should be used only when response to other drugs has been inadequate.

Clofibrate (Atromid-S, 2 g) is effective in the treatment of hyperlipidemia Types III, IV, and V. It appears to decrease the synthesis and enhance the catabolism of VLDL. It can elevate levels of LDL. Adverse effects include nausea and other GI symptoms, arrhythmias, increased incidence of angina, renal and hepatic dysfunction, and muscle pain and stiffness (myosi-

tis). GI malignancy and formation of biliary stones have been reported. Clofibrate is contraindicated in pregnancy and used only with caution in the presence of renal or hepatic disease. Clofibrate binds extensively to plasma proteins, displacing oral anticoagulants (and potentially other drugs) if administered concurrently. **Gemfibrozil** (Lopid, 0.9 to 1.5 g) has pharmacologic effects quite similar to clofibrate; its action appears to be inhibition of hepatic synthesis of lipoproteins. Serum levels of HDL may increase. Gemfibrozil is contraindicated in the presence of gallbladder disease.

Probucol (Lorelco, 1 g) inhibits cholesterol synthesis and may reduce absorption of dietary cholesterol. It is used for Type II hyperlipidemia. It must be administered cautiously in the presence of cardiovascular dysfunction. The ECG should be monitored; marked changes especially in the Q-T interval indicate that drug administration should be terminated. Additional adverse effects frequently noted are GI disturbances.

Beta-sitosterol (24 to 36 g) has had limited use in the treatment of Type II hyperlipidemia. It appears to reduce absorption of dietary cholesterol. Its major adverse effects are GI disturbances.

Because antilipemic agents work by various mechanisms, combinations of drugs are often effective when a single drug has failed to lower serum lipids or has produced intolerable side effects. Drug therapy of hyperlipidemias should always be preceded by dietary attempts to lower serum lipids and should always be accompanied by continued restrictions of dietary fat intake. Antilipemics have a long onset of therapeutic effect. However, if 3 to 4 months of administration fail to significantly lower lipoproteins, drugs should be discontinued.

ANALGESICS

Pain is a symptom of an underlying disturbance. Severe and/or persistent pain must be investigated to determine whether the cause itself requires or will respond to treatment. Analgesics are used to alleviate pain. The two major categories of analgesic drugs are the narcotic (or opiate) analgesics and the nonnarcotic agents.

Narcotic analgesics

The narcotic analgesics are used to control severe pain. **Opium**, its derivatives (e.g., **morphine** and **codeine**), and numerous synthetic opiates including some with both agonist and antagonist properties are available. All are Schedule II controlled substances. **Heroin**, a Schedule I substance, is diacetylmorphine. Some opiates are also used as antitussives, antidiarrheals, general anesthetics, and preanesthetic sedatives. The opiates exert their effects by interacting with highly specific opiate receptor sites in several CNS regions and in the GI tract. The narcotic analgesics suppress transmission of pain sensation and also produce euphoria and apathy, which alter the patient's emotional response to pain. Analgesics are most effective if administered before pain becomes intense.

Although there are differences in potency and efficacy, the opiates possess several characteristics in common. They all depress respiration, even at therapeutic doses. In overdose they can cause severe depression leading to respiratory arrest. With repeated use, the opiates all produce physiological drug dependence, often preceded by psychological dependence on their euphoriant effect. Opiate abuse is not uncommon among physicians and other health-care personnel who have access to legal supplies of narcotics. Drug tolerance is a characteristic common to all opiates. Increasing doses are needed to produce analgesia or euphoria or to prevent the appearance of withdrawal symptoms. Because tolerance and dependence occur, the opiate analgesics should be used only for severe pain (mild to moderate pain is treated with nonnarcotic agents) of brief duration, such as following surgery or during myocardial infarction. The only exception is severe pain associated with terminal illness such as cancer, when the reduction of pain and suffering should take precedence over concern that drug dependence will occur. However, tolerance to analgesia also will develop, necessitating larger drug doses, which will cause greater sedation and respiratory depression. Additional adverse effects common to the opiates include hypotension (especially orthostatic), changes in heart rate, urinary retention, and biliary tract spasm. GI complaints include nausea, vomiting, and constipation. Peristalsis is suppressed. Opiates cause miosis or pupillary constriction, which can be diagnostic of narcotic use or misuse. (It must be noted, however, that as respiratory depression and cerebral anoxia develop, pupillary dilation will appear.) Some opiates, morphine in particular, provoke histamine release that can result in symptoms ranging from rash to anaphylactic shock. Persons with history of allergy are especially sensitive to the effects of histamine. Respiratory distress such as asthma or chronic lung disease can be exacerbated by the bronchoconstrictive action of histamine, as well as by the respiratory depressant effect of the opiate.

IV administration of opiates requires extreme caution, as the risk of respiratory depression and cardiovascular failure are great. A narcotic antagonist and some means for mechanical respiration should be available before an opiate is administered. Opiates are contraindicated in head injury and other disorders that predispose to elevated intracranial pressure. Respiratory depression resulting in increased blood levels of carbon dioxide will cause CNS vasodilation and an additional increase in pressure. Furthermore, the depressant effects of the opiates can conceal the symptoms of progressive brain injury. Administration of opiates during labor and delivery can result in neonatal respiratory depression. This is especially hazardous in premature infants, who are already at great risk of respiratory distress. Chronic use of opiates (e.g., heroin, methadone) by a woman during pregnancy can result in the delivery of a drug-dependent infant who will experience abstinence symptoms soon after birth. Opiates require caution in the presence of abdominal pain, as some disorders can be aggravated by the ensuing increase in smooth muscle tone. In addition, the nature and location of pain can assist in diagnosis. The opiates are hepatically inactivated, thus liver dysfunction prolongs their plasma half-life.

Probably the most common type of drug interaction involving the opiates is potentiation of other CNS depressant drugs. Concurrent administration of antihistamines, general anesthetics, antidepressants, sedative-hypnotics (e.g., barbiturates), and antianxiety agents can produce severe CNS depression, coma, and death. Meperidine has produced severe, even fatal, reactions when given simultaneously with MAO inhibitors. Exaggerated narcotic effects have occurred, as have hyperpyrexia, hypertension, and convulsions. Cimetidine can inhibit the inactivation of narcotics. Drugs that suppress respiration can add to that depression caused by the opiates. General anesthetics and other drugs or factors that reduce blood pressure will increase the risk of severe hypotension. Narcotic antagonists, including partial agonists, will provoke withdrawal in persons physiologically addicted to opiates. Narcotic analgesics are included in numerous combinations with various types of other drugs such as nonnarcotic analgesics.

In addition to their common properties, the opiates have individual characteristics and uses. **Morphine** is the most widely used parenteral (SC, IM: 5 to 20 mg q 4 hours; IV: 4 to 10 mg over 4 to 5 minutes; and rectal: 10 to 20 mg q 4 hours) analgesic for severe acute pain; it is not well absorbed after PO administration. Morphine is used in the management of acute myocardial infarction to reduce pain and apprehension and also to alleviate the pulmonary edema that frequently accompanies this medical emergency. Morphine is administered before surgery to reduce apprehension and to enhance induction of anesthesia. **Meperidine** (Demerol, 50 to 100 mg q 3 to 4 hours), which is orally effective, is used in much the same manner as morphine.

Methadone (2.5 to 10 mg q 6 hours), also orally active, has a characteristically long plasma half-life. In therapeutic doses, it produces less sedation and euphoria than other opiates. It is an effective analgesic and has special use in the treatment of opiate addiction. Detoxification can be achieved by administering gradually reduced doses of methadone over several days, or maintenance consisting of substitution of methadone for other opiates may enable persons to resume a more stable life-style. Abrupt termination of methadone produces gradually developing, more prolonged but less severe withdrawal than other opiates. Severe and persistent constipation often occurs in persons taking maintenance doses of methadone.

Codeine (15 to 60 mg q 4 to 6 hours) has lower efficacy than morphine but is widely used as an analgesic and an antitussive. It is administered PO and parenterally and is frequently combined with nonnarcotic analgesics. Large doses of codeine can cause restlessness and cough. **Fentanyl** has a rapid onset and short duration of action; it is used especially as adjunct medication for surgery (50 to 100 mcg IM). **Alphaprodine** is often used for obstetric analgesia and for brief surgical, dental (especially in children), and diagnostic procedures. **Paregoric** is an opium tincture used as an antidiarrheal. **Brompton's mixture** is an oral solution of varied composition. In addition to an opiate (usually morphine), ingredients may include sedatives, stimulants, antidepressants, nonnarcotic analgesics, and ethanol. It is administered to alleviate severe chronic pain, such as in terminal illness. Continuous infusion or intermittent bolus of opiates via indwelling IV, intrathecal, or epidural catheter has been reported to control severe acute pain while causing fewer adverse effects. **Propoxyphene** has lower analgesic efficacy than most other opiates, yet it produces similar effects including drug dependence and respiratory depression that can be reversed by narcotic antagonists.

Some narcotic agonist-antagonists (partial agonists) are effective analgesics. **Pentazocine** (Talwin, 50 to 600 mg), **butorphanol** (Stadol, 1 to 4 mg q 3 to 4 hours), **nalbuphine** (Nubain, up to 160 mg/24 hours parenterally) and **buprenorphine** (Buprenex) are used in much the same manner as morphine and meperidine and produce similar adverse effects including respiratory depression. Abuse potential may be less than that of pure narcotic agonists. The partial agonist analgesics are contraindicated in known or suspected opiate abusers, as they can precipitate a withdrawal syndrome.

Narcotic antagonists.   The narcotic antagonists reverse the effects of opiates only and not of other drugs such as alcohol and barbiturates. **Levallorphan** (Lorfan, 1 to 3 mg IV over 30 minutes) is an agonist-antagonist, whereas **naloxone** (Narcan, 0.4 to 10 mg IV) is a "pure" antagonist and the drug of choice for reversing opiate effects (e.g., in drug overdose or in postsurgical patients). (Naloxone is also used investigationally to improve circulation in some types of shock, such as after spinal cord injury.) Levallorphan and naloxone can be diagnostic in opiate overdose. However, levallorphan may deepen respiratory depression caused by opiates or by nonopiate drugs. The narcotic antagonists compete with opiates for receptor binding sites and have a rapid onset of action. However, the antagonists have a short duration of action, thus patients must be closely observed for signs of return of opiate overdose. In persons who are physiologically dependent on opiates, administration of an antagonist can rapidly provoke severe withdrawal symptoms, thus these drugs require caution when given to known or suspected addicts. Rapid reversal of narcotic effects, such as in postsurgical patients, may cause vomiting, cardiac arrhythmias, pulmonary edema, and changes in blood pressure, especially in persons with preexisting cardiovascular disorders. The narcotic antagonists can be administered IM, IV, or SC. They are hepatically inactivated.

In addition to respiratory depression, levallorphan in large doses can produce dysphoria, disorientation, hallucinations, drowsiness, and other opiate responses. Because naloxone is a pure antagonist, it is relatively free of side effects. Addition of other drugs or substances to IV solutions of naloxone may inactivate the antagonist.

Naltrexone (Trexan) is a pure narcotic antagonist with a long duration of action, which makes it well suited for the rehabilitation of addicts. It prevents opiates from binding to receptors, thus blocks opiate-induced euphoria. Since it can provoke withdrawal, naltrexone administration should begin only after the patient has been withdrawn from opiate dependence—that is, is opiate free for at least a week to 10 days. When therapy is begun, observation for signs of withdrawal is necessary.

Nonnarcotic analgesics

The oldest and most widely used nonnarcotic analgesics are the salicylates such as aspirin. Also useful in the management of mild to moderate pain are acetaminophen, the nonsteroidal anti-inflammatory drugs (NSAIDs), and several miscellaneous agents. In contrast to the opiates, many nonnarcotic analgesics also reduce fever and inflammation. Persistent fever or inflammation can be symptomatic of serious underlying disorders.

Salicylates.   In addition to their analgesic activity, salicylates are antipyretic and in higher doses are anti-inflammatory. Because of its ability to reduce platelet aggregation, aspirin is used to decrease the risk of myocardial infarction in men with unstable angina and of recurrent transient ischemic attacks in men. In men, platelets appear to be more responsive to factors that affect aggregation. The salicylates appear to exert their effects through inhibition of prostaglandin synthesis. Salicylates

are well absorbed after PO administration. They are acids and thus are nonionized at normal gastric pH. Salicylates bind extensively to plasma proteins and are hepatically biotransformed to a glycine conjugate. Alkalinization of urine promotes ionization and enhances excretion of the salicylates, whereas acidification increases their tubular reabsorption.

Although they are available without prescription, the salicylates can produce severe, even fatal, adverse effects. Aspirin overdose is lethal, especially in children, and continues to be the cause of several hundred deaths every year in the United States. Aspirin has marked effects on blood coagulation (chronic administration can induce anemia) and is irritating to the gastric mucosa. Extreme caution is required if this drug must be administered to persons with ulcers, other GI damage, or coagulation deficiencies or to those requiring surgery. Adverse effects associated with aspirin use during pregnancy include extended gestation and labor, teratogenicity, maternal and neonatal hemorrhage, and low birth weight. Although still controversial, administration of salicylates to children with chicken pox or influenza has been strongly linked to subsequent development of Reye's syndrome. Many authorities now recommend against any use of aspirin in children, preferring acetaminophen for analgesic or antipyretic action. Symptoms of Reye's syndrome include lethargy, vomiting, and personality changes. Early detection and treatment can be lifesaving. Salicylates can inhibit renal function, and large doses may induce hepatic damage and alter blood glucose levels. Allergy to aspirin, especially in asthmatic children, is not uncommon. Cross-reactivity to other NSAIDs may be present.

Symptoms of salicylate toxicity include tinnitus, tachycardia, nausea, confusion, fatigue, and dizziness progressing to hyperthermia, hemorrhage, dehydration, alterations in acid-base balance, convulsions, failure of respiration and of the renal and cardiovascular systems, coma, and death. Treatment of toxicity must include evacuation of unabsorbed drug, support of cardiovascular and respiratory function, restoration of fluid and electrolyte balance, and reduction of elevated body temperature. Convulsions are best controlled with diazepam. Alkalinization of the urine will enhance drug excretion.

Salicylates are involved in many drug interactions. The risk of GI irritation and ulceration is increased by concurrent administration of alcohol, corticosteroids, and NSAIDs. Antidiabetic agents become less effective. Aspirin should not be given simultaneously with other drugs that decrease blood coagulation. Alterations in renal excretion and competition for plasma protein binding sites can result in drug interactions. Acetazolamide induces systemic acidosis, which enhances the lipid-solubility of acid drugs. Salicylates reduce the effectiveness of uricosuric agents. (Large doses of salicylates are uricosuric; low doses inhibit uric acid excretion.) Salicylates are present in a large number of over-the-counter drug preparations.

Diflunisol (Dolobid, 1 to 1.5 g) has structural and pharmacologic similarities to salicylates. It is a prostaglandin synthetase inhibitor and is analgesic, antipyretic, anti-inflammatory, and uricosuric. GI irritation occurs, requiring caution and close observation in patients with ulcer and similar disorders. Platelet aggregation is reduced; this can enhance the effects of anticoagulants. Diflunisol has a long duration of action. It binds extensively to plasma proteins and is renally excreted; renal dysfunction prolongs plasma half-life. Fluid retention and ophthalmologic and hepatic changes may occur. Neither aspirin nor acetaminophen should be given concurrently, and pharmacokinetic interactions occur with the NSAIDs.

Acetaminophen. Acetaminophen is the only aminophenol analgesic now in use. Phenacetin was removed from the market because of its significant toxicity. Acetaminophen is equal to aspirin in analgesic and antipyretic potency and is an acceptable substitute in persons who are allergic to aspirin or who cannot tolerate aspirin because of side effects or coagulation deficiencies. Acetaminophen has no anti-inflammatory efficacy. The exact mechanism of action of this drug is not known, although it appears to work at least in part through inhibition of prostaglandin synthesis.

Acetaminophen (0.3 to 2.6 g) is hepatically inactivated. One metabolite is hepatotoxic and can produce severe, even fatal, liver damage when the drug is taken in large doses. Acetaminophen has been used as an agent of suicide. Liver dysfunction and chronic alcohol consumption significantly predispose patients to acetaminophen hepatoxocity, which develops over several days and causes death by way of gradual hepatic failure. If administered soon (possibly up to 18 hours) after drug overdose, acetylcysteine enhances inactivation of the toxic metabolite by providing sulfhydryl groups for conjugation.

In recommended doses, acetaminophen has few adverse effects. Compared with aspirin, acetaminophen causes virtually no GI irritation and very little suppression of platelet aggregation. (However, persons receiving anticoagulants should be observed for excessively impaired coagulation.) Acetaminophen can cause methemoglobinemia resulting in anemia. It is contraindicated in persons with preexisting oxygen transport deficits. Acetaminophen may also decrease platelet and leukocyte counts. CNS stimulation, sedation, allergy, and decreased blood glucose levels can occur.

Acetaminophen does not alter the action of uricosuric drugs and has no influence on the excretion of uric acid. Many drug formulations, both prescription and over-the-counter preparations, contain acetaminophen plus a variety of other agents including narcotic analgesics such as codeine. Drugs that induce hepatic enzymes can enhance the metabolism of acetaminophen.

Nonsteroidal anti-inflammatory drugs. The major indication for the NSAIDs (Table 6-14) is arthritis, which occurs in several different forms that cause inflammation and pain in the joints. (Aspirin is still the drug of choice for initial therapy of many forms of arthritis and is the preferred drug for those who respond to and can tolerate salicylates.) Aspirin and the NSAIDs relieve the symptoms but do not slow the progression of arthritic disease. Some NSAIDs are used for musculoskeletal sprains and strains, for severe menstrual discomfort, and for other types of mild to moderate pain.

The NSAIDs have many characteristics in common. They inhibit prostaglandin synthesis and have therapeutic efficacy similar to aspirin. Most NSAIDs appear to cause less GI irritation than aspirin, although **indomethacin** has been associated with a significant incidence of bleeding and ulceration. NSAID influence on platelet aggregation is less than that of aspirin yet can be hazardous in persons with coagulation deficits. Sodium and water retention can occur, thus caution is required if these drugs are administered to persons with hypertension or other cardiovascular disorders. Most NSAIDs

Table 6-14. Nonsteroidal Anti-Inflammatory Drugs

Generic name	Trade name	Recommended adult doses (PO/day)
Fenoprofen	Nalfon	0.9–3.2 g
Ibuprofen	Motrin, others	0.9–2.4 g
Indomethacin	Indocin	50–200 mg
Ketoprofen	Orudis	150–300 mg
Meclofenamate	Meclomen	200–400 mg
Naproxen	Anaprox	0.5–1.25 g
Piroxicam	Feldene	20 mg
Sulindac	Clinoril	300–400 mg
Tolmetin	Tolectin	1.2–2 g

are hepatically biotransformed to renally excreted metabolites, but a few are excreted unchanged. The elderly and persons with hepatic or renal impairment often require greatly reduced doses. NSAIDs cause alterations in hepatic function and have been associated with kidney damage, especially in patients with decreased renal function. Kidney function should be monitored and patients observed for signs of failure. Because of their interactions with prostaglandin synthesis, the NSAIDs can be hazardous during pregnancy.

NSAIDs are involved in many drug interactions. They bind extensively to plasma proteins and can displace other drugs from binding sites. Alterations in hepatic inactivation of other drugs have been reported in particular with phenylbutazone. NSAIDs reduce the effectiveness of antihypertensive agents, including beta-blockers, thiazides, and furosemide. Competition for renal tubular secretion appears to be the mechanism by which NSAIDs enhance the toxicity of the antineoplastic drug methotrexate. Concomitant administration of salicylates can reduce the effectiveness of the NSAIDs. Administration with food will slow absorption but reduce GI irritation. Indomethacin reduces lithium excretion.

NSAIDs also have individual characteristics. **Indomethacin** irritates gastric mucosa and can aggravate CNS disorders; this agent in particular depends on renal elimination. Therapy for dysmenorrhea is usually with **naproxen, mefenamic acid,** or **ibuprofen.** Ibuprofen can be obtained without a prescription. Indomethacin has been used experimentally to inhibit premature labor and to promote closure of the ductus arteriosus in neonates. **Piroxicam** has a relatively long plasma half-life and duration of action. Because of its apparently greater toxicity, **phenylbutazone** is reserved for persons who do not respond to any other therapy. **Meclofenamide** often causes GI disturbances, including severe diarrhea.

Additional antirheumatic agents. **Gold compounds** can be administered parenterally (Myochrysine, Solganal) or orally (auranofin [Ridaura]); the latter route appears to cause fewer adverse effects. These agents slow the development of joint degeneration and are of most benefit if administered early in the course of disease. Gold accumulates in many tissues, including the kidneys, liver, and bone marrow. Its apparent mechanism of action is inhibition of lysosomal enzymes. Therapeutic action and some adverse effects develop slowly. Drug elimination is slow, and injectable forms (10 to 50 mg/dose) are usually administered once each week. Gold salts bind extensively to plasma proteins. Dermatologic and mucous membrane reactions occur, and pruritus and a metallic taste can be early symptoms. Bone marrow suppression can result in severe hematologic disorders. GI, hepatic, renal, and pulmonary function may be affected. Significant toxicity such as the appearance of protein or blood in the urine requires termination of drug therapy. Corticosteroids can be used to reverse some of the adverse effects, and dimercaprol will enhance inactivation of gold compounds.

Penicillamine (Cupramine, 1 to 4 g) has anti-inflammatory action, possibly by interaction with immune responses. Onset of effect requires several weeks. This drug is also used to alleviate cystinuria and to chelate excessive amounts of copper in Wilson's disease. Adverse reactions are numerous, and some can be severe. The drug should be taken when the stomach is empty. It is renally excreted and requires caution in the presence of kidney dysfunction. Penicillamine is teratogenic. Renal, pulmonary, and hematologic toxicity, GI disturbances, skin fragility, allergic reactions, and many other adverse responses can occur. In the treatment of rheumatoid arthritis, penicillamine is used only for refractory disease.

The antimalarial drug **hydroxychloroquine** (Plaquenil) is occasionally used as an anti-inflammatory agent. Ophthalmologic damage may develop; patients should be observed for changes in vision. Hematologic and hepatic toxicity occur. Persons with deficient G6PD are at increased risk of hemolysis.

Costicosteroids are also used to reduce inflammation in arthritis. These drugs are discussed under "Adrenal pharmacology."

Additional antigout agents.   In gout, inflammation occurs as the result of elevated blood levels of uric acid. Thus, agents that reduce urate synthesis or enhance its excretion (the latter are uricosuric agents) are often used in the treatment of this painful disorder. Many of these drugs can also precipitate acute attacks of gout. Hyperuricemia can be a complication of other diseases and can be caused by administration of some drugs such as anticancer agents.

Allopurinol (Zyloprim, 200 to 600 mg) inhibits xanthine oxidase and reduces the synthesis of uric acid. It is the drug of choice in chronic gout. Maintenance of a slightly alkaline urine and increased fluid intake (unless otherwise contraindicated) reduce the risk of renal damage. Dosages should be reduced in the presence of renal impairment. Dermatologic reactions occur and may precede more serious toxicity, including exfoliative dermatitis, vasculitis, and fatal hepatotoxicity. Allopurinol enhances the effects of oral anticoagulants, theophylline, azathioprine, and mercaptopurine.

Probenecid (0.5 to 2 g) promotes urate excretion by suppressing tubular reabsorption. Increased fluid intake and an alkaline urine reduce the formation of renal stones. GI disturbances and aggravation of peptic ulcer may occur. G6PD deficiency predisposes patients to hemolysis. Probenecid binds to plasma proteins and is renally excreted. Renal dysfunction

can prolong the drug's half-life and can also interfere with its therapeutic effectiveness. Probenecid inhibits the renal excretion of many drugs including methotrexate, some NSAIDs, and several antibiotics such as the penicillins. The latter may be combined with probenecid to prolong their duration of action.

Sulfinpyrazone (Anturane, 200 to 800 mg) is a uricosuric agent often effective when gout is refractory to other treatment. GI irritation is a frequent adverse effect that can be reduced by administration with milk or food. The drug is contraindicated in the presence of gastric ulcer or GI inflammation. Because blood dyscrasias may develop, blood counts should be monitored. Salicylates can interfere with the action of uricosuric drugs. Sulfinpyrazone binds extensively to plasma proteins and may displace oral anticoagulants.

Colchicine (4 to 8 mg) alleviates inflammation in gout by inhibiting leukocyte activity. It is the drug of choice in acute attacks of gout; administration should begin at the first appearance of symptoms. The drug is severely toxic, and patients must be observed for early symptoms such as GI pain, vomiting, and diarrhea. When these effects appear, drug administration must be stopped in order to prevent progression to renal damage, bone marrow depression, muscle weakness that can lead to respiratory failure, and other serious reactions. Colchicine is given PO or IV; the IM or SC routes produce unacceptable irritation of tissues. Drug administration can be terminated once the gout attack is under control, although chronic administration of small doses will reduce the occurrence and severity of attacks. Special caution is required in the elderly and in persons with cardiovascular, renal, or hepatic disease. Colchicine can damage GI mucosa and reduce the absorption of drugs given PO. The effects of CNS depressants and of sympathomimetics can be enhanced. Acidifying agents reduce the action of colchicine; alkalinization increases it.

Additional analgesic agents. **Methotrimeprazine** (Levoprome) is a phenothiazine derivative and produces many of the same types of effects as that group of psychotherapeutic agents. The drug is given IM only, usually for periods not longer than 1 month. Because of its potential to cause severe and prolonged orthostatic hypotension, methotrimeprazine is usually given only to hospitalized or nonambulatory patients. It is useful in obstetrics when respiratory depression would be hazardous, and as pre- and postsurgical sedation and analgesia. The drug is hepatically inactivated. Elderly persons and those with cardiovascular, renal, or hepatic disorders are most sensitive to its actions. The effects of CNS depressants are enhanced. Concurrent administration of MAO inhibitors and antihypertensive agents is contraindicated. The drug can be mixed with scopolamine or atropine but is incompatible with other agents. The dose of anticholinergic should be reduced, however, as additive effects can result in tachycardia and other exaggerated parasympatholytic responses.

DRUGS USED IN TREATMENT OF MIGRAINE

Ergotamine is frequently used to alleviate migraine and other vascular headaches. Suppository, sublingual (2 to 6 mg/24 hours) and aerosol (0.36 mg up to 5 times in 24 hours) forms have a more rapid onset of action than oral tablets. Ergotamine is a vasoconstrictor and is also a serotonin and alpha-adrenergic receptor antagonist. It is contraindicated in hypertension, peripheral vascular disease, and other disorders exacerbated by vasoconstriction, and also during pregnancy because of its oxytocic action. Ergotamine is most effective if taken at the first sign of headache. The side effects of ergotamine derive in particular from its vasoconstrictive action: muscle weakness, changes in heart rate and blood pressure, numbing of fingers and toes, even development of gangrene. Vomiting may also occur, although this can be a consequence of the migraine attack, and can preclude PO administration of drugs. Ergotamine is often combined with caffeine, which increases its vasoconstrictor efficacy and may enhance its absorption. Some drug formulations also include belladonna for its antiemetic effect and a barbiturate for sedation. The ability of ergotamine to prevent the development of headaches has been questioned. Dihydroergotamine given IM is used in particular to terminate cluster headaches.

Methysergide (Sansert, 4 to 8 mg) is used prophylactically in persons who have frequent or severe headaches. It is not always effective, and administration should be terminated if there is no clear benefit. Chronic administration can provoke inflammation and fibrosis of many tissues including the heart, lungs, and structures in the peritoneal cavity. The latter can obstruct the ureters and lead to urinary retention. The drug is given in 6-month courses, with doses tapered during the last month, followed by one drug-free month. Methysergide is an antagonist of serotonin, which has been implicated in migraine, yet the exact mechanism of methysergide's effectiveness is not known. This drug can cause vasoconstriction, thus is contraindicated in pregnancy and in cardiovascular disorders exacerbated by resistance to blood flow. Drowsiness, dizziness, and vomiting can occur. Vomiting can be reduced by administering the drug with food.

Propranolol is also used in the prevention of migraine. Its efficacy may be related to inhibition of calcium flux. (The pharmacology of propranolol is discussed under "Autonomic Nervous System Pharmacology.") Calcium channel blockers are also being investigated for antimigraine efficacy.

ANTI-INFECTIVE DRUGS

Anti-infective drugs include naturally occurring and semisynthetic substances (e.g., the penicillin and aminoglycoside antibiotics) and synthetic agents (e.g., the sulfonamides). Although this is a large and diverse group of agents, there are several common characteristics that must be considered when any one is administered.

Secondary infections or superinfections are a potentially serious adverse effect of all anti-infective therapy. These occur when the normal microorganism content of the intestinal, GU, or respiratory tracts is reduced, allowing those organisms not susceptible to the drugs being administered to flourish. The resulting overgrowth produces an infection that may prove quite resistant to available agents. Prolonged administration of drugs and use of broad-spectrum agents present the greatest threat of superinfection. In patients at risk, frequent monitoring of the flora of the intestinal, GU, and respiratory tracts will detect the presence of overgrowth of microorganisms that would require changes in anti-infective therapy.

Another serious problem that has grown out of the excessive and indiscriminate use of anti-infectives is the appearance of resistant strains of microorganisms. Many bacteria have natural resistance to several of the antibiotics. Other strains of microorganisms, once susceptible to drugs, have acquired a resistance to those agents. Anti-infective drugs destroy first those cells that are least resistant to them, allowing the survival of mutants that have greater resistance. If drug therapy is terminated before all of the microorganism is eradicated, the less-susceptible cells flourish and give rise to a drug-resistant strain. Transfer of genetic material between microorganisms can also foster the emergence of resistant strains.

Allergy is frequently encountered with the use of anti-infective drugs. Immediate responses such as asthma and anaphylaxis as well as delayed hypersensitivity can occur.

Tissue toxicity, renal damage in particular, can be induced by many anti-infective agents. Renal excretion is the route of inactivation of most of these drugs. Persons with decreased kidney function, including the elderly, are at greater risk of drug toxicity. Renal function should be monitored to detect deterioration that would require termination or reduction of drug dosage. Most anti-infective agents do not readily penetrate the blood-brain barrier but do cross the placenta and enter fetal tissues.

The risk of adverse effects can be decreased by careful selection and administration of the anti-infective. These drugs should be used only when they are absolutely necessary. Diagnosis and identification of the invading microorganism will reduce the use of inappropriate drugs. Sensitivity testing of microorganisms that may have acquired drug resistance can identify the anti-infective agent that will be most effective. Material for culture must be obtained before drug administration is begun. The course of treatment must be sufficiently long to eradicate all microorganisms yet should be terminated once that has been accomplished. Complete removal of the microorganism does not coincide with the disappearance of symptoms; drug administration must continue for a longer period of time. Anti-infectives work best when the patient's immune system is active. Persons with immune responses that are suppressed by disorders such as leukemia, lymphoma, or AIDS or by drugs such as antineoplastics, corticosteroids, or immunosuppressants will be less responsive to anti-infective agents.

Concurrent administration of two anti-infective agents is appropriate in a limited number of clinical situations. Peritonitis, endocarditis, and septicemia are occasionally most responsive to carefully chosen drug combinations. Some anti-infective combinations have reduced efficacy. For example, those agents that are most effective against actively dividing bacteria will be impeded by bacteriostatic drugs that slow cellular growth.

Administration of anti-infectives to prevent infection also is appropriate in a limited number of situations—for example, the use of penicillin to prevent streptococcal endocarditis in persons who have a history of rheumatic heart disease and who undergo tooth extraction. Prophylactic use of some anti-infective agents may reduce the recurrence of infection in AIDS patients. Use of anti-infectives in persons who are not at great risk of serious infections is usually unnecessary and can be hazardous. Anti-infective agents have no use in the prevention or treatment of viral infections such as the common cold.

Antibacterial drugs

Penicillins. Penicillin was the first antibacterial discovered, but its clinical applications emerged only after the development of the early sulfonamides. Several semisynthetic forms (Table 6-15) of this drug have proved superior to the original penicillin G (benzylpenicillin). Agents resistant to destruction by gastric acid and the beta-lactamase enzyme penicillinase and drugs with a broader spectrum of antibacterial activity have been developed.

The penicillins interfere with the formation of the bacterial cell wall. Microorganisms thus affected are not able to protect themselves against the influx of fluid from their hypotonic environment. The cell wall is a structure specific to nonmammalian cells, thus the toxicity of penicillins to mammalian cells is relatively low. The action of the penicillins is bactericidal, i.e., susceptible bacteria are completely destroyed by these drugs. Microorganisms that are rapidly dividing are most easily eradicated by penicillin.

Penicillins G and V are useful against gram-positive bacteria such as streptococci, pneumococci, listeriae, clostridia, and *Corynebacterium diphtheriae.* Actinomycetes and spirochetes, including those that cause syphilis, are quite susceptible to penicillins. The broad-spectrum penicillins like **ampicillin** will attack gram-negative bacteria including shigellae, salmonellae, *E. coli,* and *Hemophilis influenzae.* Scarlet fever, endocarditis, pneumonia, and meningitis are disorders frequently treated with penicillins. Staphylococcal invasions must be tested for penicillinase activity. Many strains, especially those responsible for nosocomial infections, have acquired resistance to penicillin

Table 6-15. Penicillins

Generic name	Trade name	Recommended adult doses
Penicillin G	several	400,000–600,000 units q 4–6 hours, PO
Penicillin V	several	125–500 mg q 6 hours, PO
Amoxicillin	Amoxil	250–500 mg q 8 hours, PO
Ampicillin	Omnipen	250–500 mg q 6 hours, PO
Bacampicillin	Spectrobid	400–800 mg q 12 hours, PO
Carbenicillin	Geocillin	200–400 mg/kg/24 hours, IV
Cloxacillin	Tegopen	250–500 mg q 6 hours, PO
Methicillin	Staphcillin	1 g q 4–6 hours, IM, IV
Mezlocillin	Mezlin	200–300 mg/kg/24 hours, IM, IV
Nafcillin	Unipen	250–500 mg q 4–6 hours, IM, IV, PO
Oxacillin	Prostaphlin	0.5–1 g q 4–6 hours, PO
Piperacillin	Pipracil	6–18 g/24 hours, IV
Ticarcillin	Ticar	150–200 mg/kg/24 hours, IV

G and must be treated with a penicillinase-resistant drug such as **oxacillin.** Penicillin G is still the drug of choice for most susceptible organisms, especially when parenteral administration is indicated. For mild infections, penicillin V is preferred for the PO route because of its resistance to destruction by gastric acid.

Treatment of staphylococcal infections is often initiated with a combination of penicillin G and a penicillinase-resistant penicillin. Established staphylococcal infections are difficult to treat, and strains that do not produce penicillinase are less responsive to the semisynthetic drugs. Once the susceptibility of the invading organism has been identified, one of the forms of penicillin can be terminated if responsive staphylococci are not present.

Ampicillin is used for many pediatric infections of the meninges, GI tract, throat, and middle ear. This penicillin can be administered PO or parenterally. It is not resistant to penicillinase. **Amoxicillin** and **bacampicillin** are similar to ampicillin and may be preferred for PO administration because they are more completely absorbed from the GI tract and produce less diarrhea.

The broad-spectrum penicillins are active against *Pseudomonas aeruginosa* and several strains of *Proteus.* These drugs should be used only for infections that are not susceptible to other treatment, to decrease the risk of acquired bacterial resistance. Aminoglycoside antibiotics are frequently given concurrently with the broad-spectrum penicillins. However, the two drugs should not be mixed in solution.

The most severe adverse reaction to the penicillins is drug allergy. Up to 10% of persons treated with these antibiotics can be expected to exhibit some symptom of hypersensitivity. Those with other allergies are at greatest risk. Existing hypersensitivity can be determined by dermal and subdermal testing with a small amount of a penicillin or of benzylpenicilloyl polylysine (Pre-Pen). Hypersensitive persons afflicted with infections that are most responsive to penicillin may be carefully "desensitized" by administration of gradually increasing amounts of drug. These procedures should be undertaken only with close observation for signs of allergic reactions and only when means for controlling such reactions are readily available. Cephalosporin hypersensitivity is often observed in persons with penicillin allergy. Penicillin G procaine should not be given to persons with procaine allergy.

Blood dyscrasias that may represent bone marrow depression or hypersensitivity reactions are associated with the penicillins. Reduction in coagulation has been reported especially with nafcillin, carbenicillin, and ticarcillin. Thrombophlebitis can occur following IV administration.

Adverse GI effects include nausea, cramps, diarrhea, and superinfections manifested as colitis, stomatitis, and glossitis. The penicillins are relatively nontoxic to the kidneys, although allergic reactions can induce renal dysfunction and damage. The major route of inactivation for the penicillins is by glomerular filtration and tubular secretion, thus caution is required when these drugs are administered to infants, the elderly, and other persons with decreased renal function. Penicillins that are excreted in bile (e.g., nafcillin and cloxacillin) may be safer in these patients. Hypernatremia or hyperkalemia can occur in persons receiving high doses of sodium or potassium salts of penicillin. Persons with renal dysfunction are at greatest risk. Some penicillins (e.g., ticarcillin, carbenicillin, and piperacillin) may cause hypokalemia.

Although the blood-brain barrier is relatively impermeable to the penicillins, high serum levels or inflammation of the meninges can facilitate sufficient entry into the CNS to cause symptoms such as confusion, anxiety, hallucinations, and seizures. Damage to nerves and blood vessels can occur following inadvertent intravascular administration.

Oral penicillins are best absorbed from an empty stomach, except for those that are stable in the presence of gastric acid. Probenecid can prolong the plasma half-life of penicillins by reducing tubular secretion of the antibiotic. Some antibacterial agents work synergistically with penicillins. However, other antibiotics, such as those that are bacteriostatic, can reduce the effectiveness of the penicillins. Penicillin V and ampicillin may interfere with the GI absorption of oral contraceptives. Amoxicillin and ticarcillin are available in combination with **clavulanic acid** (Augmentin and Timentin) to provide resistance to penicillinase.

Cephalosporins.   Closely related in structure and mechanism of action to the penicillins, the cephalosporins (Table 6-16) are a rapidly growing group of antibiotics. The first generation of cephalosporins is largely susceptible to beta-lactamase destruction, whereas the second- and third-generation agents have increased effectiveness against gram-negative microorganisms. Some cephalosporins are effective against nosocomial infections unresponsive to other antibiotics. However, penicillins are usually the preferred drugs for susceptible infections. Cross-allergenicity with penicillins occurs, although for some patients cephalosporins are suitable alternatives to pencillin.

Cephalosporins are more acid stable than penicillins, and PO administration is better tolerated when these drugs are taken with milk or food. Cephalosporins usually are given parenterally, either IV (thrombophlebitis may develop) or deep IM (pain and subcutaneous necrosis can occur). Inactivation of the cephalosporins (except for cefoperazone, excreted in the bile) occurs mainly by renal excretion. These agents are nephrotoxic, so renal function should be determined before administration and monitored during therapy. Third-generation cephalosporins readily cross inflamed meninges and are especially effective in controlling gram-negative bacillary meningitis. Many types of osteomyelitis respond to cephalosporins, which penetrate bone. The first-generation drugs treat pneumococcal and staphylococcal invasions, some second- and third-generation agents control *H. influenzae* and *E. coli.* Some urinary tract infections unresponsive to penicillin and sulfonamides are alleviated by cephalosporins.

Pseudomembranous colitis, a clostridial superinfection induced during broad-spectrum antibiotic therapy, has occurred with cephalosporins. Diarrhea can be the first symptom of this potentially fatal intestinal inflammation. Cephalosporin-resistant bacterial strains have emerged. The second- and third-generation agents, **moxalactam** in particular, cause hypoprothrombinemia and hemorrhage that is responsive to vitamin K administration.

Bacteriostatic antibiotics can reduce the effectiveness of the cephalosporins. Aminoglycosides administered concurrently for some infections will increase the risk of nephrotoxicity. Probenecid interferes with the renal secretion of cephalosporins. A disulfiram-like interaction following alcohol ingestion has been reported for cefoperazone, cefamandole, and moxalactam.

Imipenem is a beta-lactam antibiotic similar to penicillins and cephalosporins. It is resistant to beta-lactamase enzymes and has a very broad spectrum of antibacterial action. Imipenem is available in combination with cilastatin (Primaxin) which inhibits the renal inactivation of the antibiotic. Renal impairment prolongs the plasma half-life of both drugs. Persons allergic to penicillin are usually also hypersensitive to imipenem.

Tetracyclines.   These broad-spectrum agents (Table 6-17) are effective against gram-positive and gram-negative bacteria as well as chlamydiae, mycoplasmae, and rickettsiae. Many

Table 6-16. Cephalosporins

Generic name	Trade name	Recommended adult doses
First-generation		
Cefadroxil	Duricef	1–2 g/24 hours
Cephalexin	Keflex	1–4 g/24 hours
Cephradine	Anspor	500 mg q 12 hours
Cephapirin	Cefadyl	0.5–1 g q 4–6 hours
Cephalothin	Keflin	0.5–1 g q 4–6 hours
Cefazolin	Ancef	0.25–1 g q 6–8 hours
Second-generation		
Cefaclor	Ceclor	250 mg q 8 hours
Cefamandole	Mandol	0.5–1 g q 4–8 hours
Cefotixin	Mefoxin	1–2 g q 6–8 hours
Cefuroxime	Zinacef	0.75–1.5 g q 8 hours
Third-generation		
Cefotaxime	Claforan	1 g q 6–8 hours
Ceftizoxime	Cefizox	1–2 g q 8–12 hours
Cefoperazone	Cefobid	1–2 g q 12 hours
Moxalactam	Moxam	2–6 g/24 hours

Table 6-17. Tetracyclines

Generic name	Trade name	Recommended adult doses (mg PO/day)
Doxycycline	Vibramycin	100
Methacycline	Rondomycin	600
Minocycline	Minocin	200
Oxytetracycline	Terramycin	1,000–2,000
Tetracycline	several	1,000–2,000

strains of microorganisms have acquired resistance to the tetracyclines. Long-term use of these antibiotics is usually not advisable. These agents interfere with bacterial synthesis of proteins and are bacteriostatic rather than bactericidal. Infections frequently treated with tetracyclines include Rocky Mountain spotted fever, trachoma, psittacosis, brucellosis, typhus, Lyme disease, and mycoplasmal pneumonia. Tetracyclines are alternatives to penicillin in the treatment of syphilis, gonorrhea, and other venereal diseases. They are occasionally used to prevent respiratory infections in persons with chronic pulmonary disease.

Tetracyclines are given enterally and parenterally. Administration with food reduces the incidence of GI disturbances; however, calcium, magnesium, and iron form insoluble complexes with the tetracyclines and prevent their absorption. (Doxycycline and minocycline can be taken with dairy products.) With the exception of doxycycline, these drugs are not metabolized but are excreted unchanged in urine and bile. Doses should be decreased in the presence of impaired renal function.

The tetracyclines are contraindicated during pregnancy and early childhood. They chelate with calcium in developing bones and teeth, interfering with skeletal growth and causing permanent discoloration of tooth enamel.

Because of their broad spectrum of activity, the tetracyclines induce superinfections. Invasions of *Candida albicans* can be treated with antifungal drugs such as nystatin. Diarrhea during tetracycline therapy can be a symptom of pseudomembranous colitis or of staphylococcal enterocolitis. Tetracyclines should be terminated and oral administration of vancomycin instituted to control these secondary infections.

Decomposed tetracyclines can cause renal dysfunction resembling Fanconi's syndrome, with glucose, protein, and amino acids appearing in the urine. These drugs must be stored away from heat and humidity. Expiration dates should be checked before use. Tetracyclines can be hepatotoxic, especially at high doses. Photosensitivity and hypersensitivity reactions occur in persons receiving these drugs. Increased intracranial pressure, vertigo, ataxia, and nausea have been reported. Vestibular disturbances are most common with minocycline, which also causes bluish-gray skin discoloration.

The tetracyclines can increase the bioavailability and thus the toxicity of digoxin. The action of the anticoagulants is enhanced by the reduction in prothrombin activity induced by the tetracyclines. The effectiveness of oral contraceptives is decreased. Drugs that induce hepatic enzymes will shorten the plasma half-life of doxycycline. The bacteriostatic action of the tetracyclines will interfere with the bactericidal action of the penicillins.

Aminoglycosides.   The aminoglycosides (Table 6-18) have a broad spectrum of activity but are used mainly for control of infections caused by gram-negative bacteria including *Serratia, Klebsiella, Enterobacter, E. coli,* and *Proteus.* Gentamicin and tobramycin are effective against *P. aeruginosa.* The aminoglycosides inhibit protein synthesis by disrupting ribosomal function. Acquired resistance appears frequently. The sensitivity of invading microorganisms to aminoglycosides should be determined before drug therapy is begun.

The aminoglycosides are used in several ways. They are poorly absorbed when administered PO. This makes them

Table 6-18. Aminoglycosides

Generic name	Trade name	Recommended adult doses (parenteral, per day)
Amikacin	Amikin	15 mg/kg
Gentamicin	Garamycin	3 mg/kg
Kanamycin	Kantrex	15 mg/kg
Neomycin	Mycifradin	15 mg/kg
Netilmicin	Netromycin	3–4 mg/kg
Streptomycin		1–2 g
Tobramycin	Nebcin	3–5 mg/kg

quite suitable for controlling bacteria in the GI tract. **Kanamycin, neomycin,** and **paromomycin** are used to prepare the intestine for surgery or to eradicate ammonia-forming bacteria that exacerbate the clinical course of hepatic coma. Intestinal amebiasis responds to paromomycin. Neomycin will alleviate *E. coli* infections of the bowel and is also used topically for skin and eye infections and to reduce the risk of bacterial invasion of the urinary bladder in catheterized patients. PO administration of the aminoglycosides usually causes few adverse effects other than nausea, vomiting and diarrhea, and malabsorption or clostridial colitis with prolonged treatment. However, if the intestinal mucosa is damaged or renal function is impaired, blood levels of the antibiotic may rise sufficiently to produce adverse effects characteristic of parenteral aminoglycosides (see below).

Parenteral administration of the aminoglycosides is used to control susceptible strains of bacteria causing septicemia, peritonitis, or meningitis or that have invaded tissues such as bone and the respiratory or urinary tract. Streptomycin is used especially in the management of tuberculosis. The aminoglycosides are inactivated by glomerular filtration. Doses should be reduced in infants, the elderly, and persons with renal impairment. These drugs are also nephrotoxic, and patients should be well hydrated to reduce the concentration of the aminoglycosides in the renal tubules. Renal function should be determined before and throughout therapy. Deterioration of function suggests dosage reduction or termination. A characteristic adverse effect of the aminoglycosides is ototoxicity or damage to the auditory (eighth cranial) nerve, leading to loss of hearing and vestibular function. Aminoglycosides should not be administered to persons with preexisting hearing deficits. Renal impairement increases the risk of irreversible deafness. Audiometric testing before and during therapy can detect early loss of function. Administration should be terminated if hearing loss appears or if dizziness or tinnitus develops. The aminoglycosides are contraindicated in pregnancy. Monitoring of blood levels of drug can reduce the risk of toxicity.

The aminoglycosides cause a wide range of additional adverse effects such as GI upset, changes in blood pressure and electrolyte elvels, allergic reactions, agranulocytosis, thrombocytopenia, pain following IM administration, and muscle weakness that can result in respiratory failure. Superinfections can occur. Although these drugs do not readily enter the CNS, they can cause symptoms such as confusion, headache, and depression. These effects occur in particular when inflammation of the meninges has increased the permeability of the blood-brain barrier. Aminoglycosides, **gentamicin** in particular, can be given by the intrathecal route to treat CNS infections.

Because of their potential for nephrotoxicity and ototoxicity, the aminoglycosides should not be administered concurrently with other drugs that have similar adverse effects. Mannitol and the loop diuretics can enhance aminoglycoside toxicity. Concomitant administration of general anesthetics, neuromuscular blockers, skeletal muscle relaxants, or other drugs that depress muscular activity will increase the risk of respiratory paralysis. (This risk is greater also in the presence of Parkinson's disease or myasthenia gravis and also with the use of neomycin and streptomycin.) In certain infections like pseudomonal septicemia, aminoglycosides and penicillins work synergistically. Aminoglycosides enhance the action of penicillins by weakening bacterial cell walls, and penicillins destroy cell walls, allowing greater entry of aminoglycosides into the cells. However, mixture of these drugs in the same injection solution will result in loss of aminoglycoside activity.

Sulfonamides. This group of anti-infective drugs consists entirely of synthetic rather than naturally occurring or semisynthetic agents. The sulfonamides have a broad spectrum of activity that includes streptococci, staphylococci, meningococci, *E. coli,* chlamydiae, hemophili, klebsiellae, plasmodia, and toxoplasmae. Because many strains have acquired resistance, sensitivity testing should be used to determine responsiveness to drug therapy. The sulfonamides interrupt bacterial uptake and utilization of para-aminobenzoic acid (PABA), thus prevent the synthesis of folic acid and subsequently of DNA. Since human cells utilize folic acid from dietary sources, their metabolism is not affected by sulfonamides. The efficacy of the sulfonamides can be reduced by the presence of large amounts of pus and tissue debris that contain PABA. Trimethoprim, which also interferes with PABA metabolism, combined with sulfamethoxazole (co-trimoxazole [Bactrim; Septra]) has enhanced efficacy and broader activity. Sulfonamides are most frequently given by the PO route. Hepatic acetylation is an important route for inactivation; genetic deficiency of this enzyme increases the risk of toxicity in slow acetylators. Metabolites are renally excreted. Some sulfonamides bind extensively to plasma proteins.

The sulfonamides have a variety of clinical uses. The short-half-life agents **sulfamethizole** (Thiosulfil, 2 to 4 g) and **sulfisoxazole** (Gastrisin, 2 to 8 g) are effective for many urinary tract infections, and their marked water solubility reduces the risk of renal damage. **Co-trimoxazole** has the same range of activity, and its longer plasma half-life reduces the required frequency of drug administration. The venereal diseases chanchroid and chlamydial lymphogranuloma are susceptible to sulfisoxazole and sulfadiazine (2 to 4 g). Several of the sulfonamides are used to alleviate *Hemophilus* infections of the middle ear (otitis media). Prophylactic administration of sulfonamides will reduce the incidence of pharyngeal streptococcal infections in persons with a history of rheumatic fever. Crohn's disease and ulcerative colitis may respond to **sulfasalazine** (Azulfidine, 3 to 4 g). A large portion of this drug remains in the GI tract and is converted in the colon to sulfapyridine and

aminosalicylic acid, the latter having anti-inflammatory action. Some meningeal infections are treated with IV sulfisoxazole or sulfadiazine. The increased permeability of the inflamed meninges allows substantial entry of drug into the CNS. Nocardiosis can be controlled with high doses of sulfonamides or co-trimoxazole. Sulfonamides are included in the therapy of some protozoal infections. Chloroquine-resistant malaria is treated with quinine and pyrimethamine plus a sulfonamide such as sulfisoxazole. Pyrimethamine combined with sulfadoxine (Fansidar) is used to prevent chloroquine-resistant malaria. Pyrimethamine combined with sulfadiazine will alleviate toxoplasmosis.

Sulfonamides are also used topically. Sulfisoxazole and sulfacetamide are available in ophthalmic ointments and solutions for the treatment of eye infections. Silver sulfadiazine (Silvadene Cream) is applied to burns to prevent infection. This preparation has largely replaced mafenide (Sulfamylon), which carried greater risk of metabolic acidosis and allergy and produced intense pain on application.

The sulfonamides can cause renal dysfunction and damage that occasionally is fatal. Crystals of drug precipitate in urine and produce mechanical injury. This occurs less frequently with the highly water-soluble sulfamethizole, sulfisoxazole, and the triple sulfa preparations that contain low doses of sulfadiazine, sulfamerizine, and sulfamethazine. Alkalinization of the urine and ingestion of sufficient fluids enhance the solubility of sulfonamides. Frequent urinalysis will indicate the presence of drug crystals or blood in the urine.

Blood dyscrasias occur in persons receiving sulfonamides. Bone marrow depression leads to anemia, agranulocytosis, and thrombocytopenia. Persons with G6PD deficiency may develop hemolytic anemia. Close observation for signs and symptoms of hematologic changes is necessary.

Disturbances of both CNS and peripheral nervous system activity including neuritis, depression, drowsiness, hearing loss, vertigo, and convulsions have been reported. GI upset, hepatitis, pancreatitis, and photosensitivity can occur. Allergic reactions can be severe, ranging from anaphylaxis to delayed dermatologic responses. Symptoms of Stevens-Johnson syndrome require that sulfonamides be terminated immediately to avoid injury to internal organs. Diuresis, goiter, or hypoglycemia may develop. The sulfonamides are structurally related to the thiazides, thyroid suppressants, and oral antidiabetic agents, thus are contraindicated in persons with allergy to any of these drug groups. Sulfasalazine is contraindicated in persons allergic to salicylates. Sulfonamides are quite hazardous during pregnancy and lactation and in infants. In susceptible persons, these drugs can provoke porphyria.

Sulfasalazine appears to be involved in several drug interactions. The effects of digoxin and of folic acid are decreased; the action of sulfasalazine may be reduced by ferrous sulfate and by some antibiotics. Local anesthetics that are PABA derivatives may reverse the effectiveness of the sulfonamides. Drugs that bind to plasma proteins can be displaced by sulfonamides. Competition with methotrexate and tolbutamide for renal tubular secretion can increase blood levels and effects of these drugs. Sulfamethizole may inhibit hepatic biotransformation of phenytoin and oral hypoglycemic agents.

Macrolides. **Erythromycin** is the most frequently used drug of this group. Troleandomycin has great potential for hepatotoxicity and is used only for streptococcal and gonococcal infections unresponsive to other agents. Erythromycin is available in several forms for PO (base, stearate, estolate, and ethylsuccinate) and IV (lactobionate and gluceptate) administration for treatment of various infections, including syphilis and gonorrhea in persons allergic to penicillin. Erythromycin is also effective against diphtheria, legionnaires' disease, and mycoplasmal pneumonia. Some upper respiratory *Hemophilus* infections are treated with erythromycin together with a sulfonamide. Erythromycin can be used to prevent bacterial endocarditis in persons who have a history of rheumatic fever and who must undergo oral surgery or dental procedures.

Erythromycin is usually administered PO in doses ranging from 1.0 to 4 g/day. The IV forms are given by slow infusion only when high serum levels of antibiotic must be attained rapidly or when PO administration is not possible. Erythromycin base is available in enteric coated forms that protect the drug from acid degradation. The conjugated forms are acid stable. Inactivation is by way of hepatic concentration into the bile, thus impaired liver function can prolong the plasma half-life of erythromycin. These drugs, especially the estolate, are hepatotoxic. Patients should be observed for signs of decreasing liver function. Jaundice may develop 2 weeks or more after treatment has begun. Renal impairment can also prolong the action of erythromycin. Loss of hearing, which is usually reversible, and GI disturbances can accompany erythromycin administration. Pseudomembranous colitis and severe allergic responses also occur. Erythromycin potentiates the effects of digoxin, theophylline, and carbamazepine.

Clindamycin and lincomycin. These antibiotics inhibit protein synthesis in many penicillin-resistant microorganisms but are usually used only in penicillin-intolerant persons or for penicillin-resistant infections. They are especially effective against *Bacteroides fragilis,* which can cause peritonitis and female pelvic infections. The sensitivity of invading microorganisms should be determined before these antibiotics are given. Superinfection with clostridia can progress to potentially fatal colitis. Diarrhea or blood or mucus in the feces requires that erythromycin be discontinued. Vancomycin and corticosteroids can help to reduce bowel infection and inflammation. Antidiarrheals that reduce peristalsis will exacerbate this type of colitis, thus are contraindicated. Clindamycin and lincomycin can increase the paralysis caused by neuromuscular blocking drugs.

Additional antibiotics. Several additional antibiotics have very limited use, usually for those strains of microorganisms that are resistant to other drugs. **Chloramphenicol** is especially effective against salmonellae, tularemia, and *B. fragilis.* Its relative ease of entry into the CNS makes it useful in meningitis. Chloramphenicol severely depresses bone marrow and can cause fatal vascular collapse in neonates (gray baby syndrome). This drug is hepatically inactivated.

Vancomycin is not absorbed PO but is administered by this route to control bowel infections such as clostridia. It can be given parenterally to combat resistant strains of microorganisms or as a substitute antibiotic in persons allergic to penicillin. IV administration can cause thrombophlebitis. Vancomycin is nephrotoxic and ototoxic. In the presence of renal dysfunction, this drug rapidly reaches toxic blood levels.

Nalidixic acid, nitrofurantoin, cinoxacin, and the **methen-**amine preparations are used mainly in the treatment of urinary tract infections. **Phenazopyridine** is often combined with sulfonamides and other drugs for its local anesthetic effect on the urinary bladder. This dye produces red urine.

The **polymixins** are effective against gram-negative bacteria. Parenterally they are used to treat pseudomonal urinary tract infections. The polymixins are nephrotoxic. Topical forms are available for ophthalmic, otic, and dermatologic infections. Bacitracin, frequently combined with polymixin B and neomycin, is used mainly for dermatologic infections.

The **sulfones** such as **dapsone** are used in the management of Hansen's disease (leprosy). Long-term drug administration is required. Hemolytic anemia may develop in persons deficient in G6PD.

Pharmacotherapy of tuberculosis

Drugs available today can cure tuberculosis, although long-term (up to 2 years) treatment is required to completely eradicate the infection. Combinations of drugs are used to decrease the development of resistant bacteria and also to allow reduction in drug dosages, thus lowering the incidence of adverse reactions. The combination of choice is **isoniazid** (INH, 5 mg/kg) and **rifampin** (Rifadin, 600 mg).

Isoniazid interferes with bacterial lipid and nucleic acid synthesis and is bactericidal. It is effective in preventing as well as in curing tuberculosis. Isoniazid is well absorbed from the GI tract. It easily enters the CNS. Inactivation is by acetylation and renal excretion. Slow acetylators will require lower doses than rapid acetylators and must be observed for signs of drug toxicity. Impaired renal function also prolongs the plasma half-life of isoniazid.

Hepatitis that can be fatal is a serious adverse effect of isoniazid. This can develop after several months and occurs most frequently in patients over the age of 40. Consumption of alcohol increases the risk of liver damage. Monthly measurement of hepatic function is required in persons receiving isoniazid. Administration must be stopped if deterioration is detected, and alternative antitubercular drugs are given. When hepatic function returns to normal, isoniazid may be reinstated cautiously and continued only if hepatic function remains normal.

Isoniazid causes a peripheral neuritis that may be subsequent to its ability to induce pyridoxine (vitamin B_6) deficiency. Routine administration of vitamin B_6 will help to prevent this effect. Persons who are malnourished or who consume large amounts of alcohol are at greatest risk of neuropathy. Hypersensitivity reactions and blood dyscrasias are also reported with isoniazid.

Isoniazid enhances the effects of carbamazepine, phenytoin, and the benzodiazepines. The MAO enzyme can be inhibited, leading to hypertensive reactions if sympathomimetics or foods containing tyramine are ingested. Diamine oxidase also is inhibited, resulting in potentiation of the action of histamine.

Rifampin, employed in antitubercular drug combinations, kills the causative bacteria by interfering with nucleic acid synthesis. It is administered PO, and food will decrease its absorption. Rifampin is hepatically inactivated. Some of the drug is excreted in bile and undergoes enterohepatic circulation. The drug binds to plasma proteins and enters the CNS. It may be teratogenic and can be hepatotoxic. Renal dysfunction and failure can occur, as well as blood dyscrasias, GI disturbances, and hypersensitivity reactions. Intermittent administration of large doses can produce a flu-like syndrome. Rifampin induces the hepatic drug-metabolizing enzymes, enhancing its own biotransformation and that of methadone, corticosteroids, oral anticoagulants, hypoglycemics, and contraceptive, and some beta-blockers. Rifampin causes body secretions such as tears and urine to be orange.

Ethambutol (Myambutol, 15 mg/kg) is often added to the antitubercular regimen. It causes bacterial cell destruction by interfering with metabolic processes. Administration with food helps to prevent GI side effects. Ethambutol is excreted in the urine and feces, largely as unmetabolized drug. Its characteristic toxicity is optic neuritis. Patients must be observed for changes in vision and the drug discontinued if deterioration occurs.

Other drugs used in the treatment of tuberculosis include ethionamide (Trecator-SC), cycloserine (Seromycin), para-aminosalicylic acid (PAS), and the antibiotic streptomycin. These agents generally are toxic to the liver and to the nervous system.

Antiviral agents

Antibacterial drugs are not virucidal. Their misuse in attempting to cure common colds and influenza has facilitated the appearance of drug-resistant strains of bacteria and the occurrence of many secondary infections or superinfections. There are very few drugs that are effective against viruses. Unlike bacteria, these microorganisms live within host cells and are thus somewhat protected from pharmacologic assault. Fortunately, many viral diseases (e.g., polio, smallpox, and yellow fever) can be prevented with the proper use of vaccines.

Amantadine (Symmetrel, 200 mg) is used both to prevent and to reduce the severity of influenza A infections. It is most often administered to persons who are at great risk of severe consequences from this viral infection, such as the elderly and persons with pulmonary diseases. Persons exposed to the influenza A virus can be given influenza vaccine plus amantadine. The drug appears to interfere with viral invasion of host cells. It is also an effective antiparkinson agent.

Amantadine has anticholinergic side effects and can add to the cholinergic suppression induced by other drugs. Depression, confusion, and psychotic symptoms can occur. The seizure threshold is lowered, particularly in persons with convulsive disorders. Hypotension (especially orthostatic), congestive heart failure, and blood dyscrasias can develop. Amantadine is inactivated mainly by renal excretion of unchanged drug, thus doses must be adjusted carefully in persons with decreased kidney function.

Some drugs that resemble pyrimidine and purine bases and appear to inhibit synthesis of viral DNA are effective against herpes simplex types 1 and 2. **Acyclovir** (Zovirax) and **vidarabine** (Vira-A) can be given systemically. Acyclovir is administered PO (600 mg/day) or IV (5 mg/kg) to reduce the severity and promote healing of initial genital herpes simplex infections. Chronic administration may decrease the frequency of recurrences, but the extent of acyclovir's long-term toxicity is not known. This drug is also used to treat mucocutaneous herpes simplex infections (cold sores) in immunosuppressed persons. Common adverse effects include vomiting, diarrhea, and

dizziness. IV administration increases the risk of nephrotoxicity from this drug. Acyclovir-resistant strains of herpes simplex have appeared.

Vidarabine administered IV (15 mg/kg) early in the course of herpes simplex encephalitis can reduce the severity of this potentially fatal infection. The drug is not well absorbed after IM or SC injection. Its poor solubility necessitates the infusion of large fluid volumes, posing the risk of overhydration. Vidarabine is hepatically metabolized and renally excreted. Dysfunction of either of these organs prolongs the drug's plasma half-life. GI symptoms such as vomiting and diarrhea can occur. Confusion, tremor, hallucinations, fatal metabolic encephalopathy, and at high doses bone marrow depression are additional adverse effects. Because of its possible carcinogenicity, vidarabine is used only when the invading microorganism is known to be herpes simplex.

Idoxuridine and **trifluridine** (Viroptic) as well as acyclovir and vidarabine are available as ophthalmic preparations for the suppression of herpes simplex keratitis. Infections resistant to one agent may be responsive to an alternate drug. Inflammation, pain, pruritus, and photophobia can accompany the application of these drugs. Genetic mutation and carcinogenesis may occur.

The rapid evolution of AIDS and the identification of the virus that causes this usually fatal illness have prompted extensive research for virucidal drugs. Zidovudine (Retrovir, previously azidothymidine [AZT]) has been approved for some patients. Suramin, alpha-interferon, phosphonoformate, and other drugs are in various stages of clinical trials.

Antiprotozoal drugs

Antimalarials. Malaria continues to be endemic in many of the underdeveloped areas of the world. The most severe occurrences are caused by *Plasmodium falciparum*. The parasite, which is spread by the *Anopheles* mosquito, thrives in human hepatocytes and erythrocytes, which are destroyed in the course of the disease. The most commonly used antimalarials are **chloroquine** (Aralen, 300 mg), **hydroxychloroquine** (Plaquenil, 310 mg), **primaquine** (15 mg), and **pyrimethamine** (Daraprim, 25 mg), the latter also in combination with sulfadoxine (Fansidar) to treat chloroquine-resistant strains. Quinine also is used to control infections unresponsive to chloroquine. Primaquine attacks those schizonts in hepatocytes (exoerythrocytic forms), whereas those in erythrocytes (erythrocytic forms) are most susceptible to chloroquine. The *P. falciparum* microorganism can be completely eradicated, although fatal hypoxia can occur during an acute attack. In contrast, *Plasmodium vivax* is not eliminated and relapses develop periodically over many years. Drugs can be used to alleviate and also to prevent acute attacks. Weekly administration of chloroquine and primaquine to travelers in Anopheles-infested areas helps to prevent malaria. Sulfadoxine is added to the prophylactic drug regimen in areas where there is chloroquine-resistant disease.

The chloroquines can be given PO or parenterally. These drugs can cause blood dyscrasias and irreversible retinal damage. In persons with G6PD deficiency, hemolytic anemia can develop. GI disturbances, hypotension, and headache occur, as can the appearance of muscle weakness that requires termination of drug. Adverse effects occur most frequently with the larger drug doses that are required to control acute attacks. Overdose can cause convulsions and cardiac arrest.

Primaquine is ineffective in acute malarial attacks. It is used to eliminate the parasite from hepatocytes and thus to prevent relapse. Blood dyscrasias, idiosyncratic reactions in persons with G6PD or methemoglobin reductase deficiencies, and GI disturbances occur with administration of this drug. Primaquine and quinacrine potentiate the toxicity of one another; therefore, administration of one drug should be terminated several days before the other is given.

Pyrimethamine is used mainly to suppress malarial attacks, and in large doses to control toxoplasmosis infections. It is a folic acid antagonist; leucovorin can be given to reverse agranulocytosis and thrombocytopenia. Patients must be monitored for signs of blood dyscrasias. G6PD deficiency predisposes to hemolytic anemia. Pyrimethamine is administered PO and causes glossitis and GI disturbances, which can be decreased by taking the drug with food. Overdose produces marked CNS stimulation, and caution is required in patients with seizure disorders.

Quinine, the first antimalarial agent, is now rarely used. It is effective against many plasmodial strains that are resistant to other drugs. Since it is a skeletal muscle relaxant, it is used occasionally in the treatment of nocturnal cramping of the legs. Because of its teratogenic and oxytocic actions, it is contraindicated in pregnancy. Quinine has cardiovascular effects similar to those of the antiarrhythmic quinidine. Hemolytic anemia occurs in the presence of G6PD deficiency. Other blood dyscrasias, vision and GI disturbances, tinnitus, confusion, syncope, restlessness, and convulsions can occur. Overdose can cause fatal depression of respiratory and cardiovascular function. The effects of neuromuscular blocking drugs, oral anticoagulants, and digitalis glycosides are potentiated by quinine. The drug binds extensively to plasma proteins and is hepatically inactivated. Urinary alkalinization will enhance the toxicity of quinine.

Other protozoal infections. Trypanosomes cause such diseases as African sleeping sickness, pneumocystic pneumonia, and Chagas' disease. A variety of drugs, including pentamidine and suramin, are used in the treatment of these potentially fatal diseases. Leishmanial infections are usually controlled with sodium stibogluconate.

Intestinal amebiasis is caused by *Entamoeba histolytica*. The liver, intestinal tract, and other internal organs can be severely damaged by this protozoal infection. **Metronidazole** (Flagyl) is especially useful in controlling amebiasis as well as trichomoniasis and serious infections caused by several susceptible strains of anaerobic bacteria. It is administered PO and IV. Impaired hepatic function can prolong the plasma half-life of this drug. Metronidazole may be carcinogenic and teratogenic. GI disturbance is the most frequent adverse effect. Vertigo, confusion, headache, convulsions, paresthesias, changes in renal function, leukopenia, hypersensitivity reactions, and overgrowth of candidae can occur. Metronidazole potentiates the action of the oral anticoagulants and produces a disulfiram-like reaction following alcohol ingestion. It is less effective when hepatic enzyme-inducing drugs are concurrently administered.

Also used in the management of amebiasis are **diloxanide**, the antibiotics tetracycline and paromomycin, and **emetine**, which has a more rapid onset of action. Emetine administration requires caution in elderly persons and should be avoided in the presence of cardiovascular and renal disease. Patients must be observed for signs of congestive heart failure. The older antiamebic drugs carbasone and diiodohydroxyquin have largely been replaced by the newer drugs, which are considered to be more effective and less toxic.

Giardiasis is a protozoal infection of the intestine that can cause severe diarrhea and malabsorption of vitamins, carbohydrates, and fats. Metronidazole, furazolidone (Furoxone) and quinacrine (Atabrine) are effective in alleviating giardiasis. MAO inhibitors and sympathomimetic amines as well as alcohol are contraindicated in persons receiving furazolidone.

Anthelmintic drugs

The anthelmintics are used in the treatment of worm infestations. Since there are several types of worms that can thrive in human intestine and other organs, there are many drugs in this category. All have significant toxicity, although agents such as hexylresorcinol and quinacrine are being replaced by apparently safer drugs including niclosamide (Niclocide) and mebendazole (Vermox). The parasite should be identified before drug therapy is initiated so that the most effective agent can be selected. Persons with worm infestations may be malnourished and anemic and may have fluid and electrolyte imbalances if diarrhea has occurred.

Niclosamide is effective against pork, beef, fish, and dwarf tapeworms that infest the intestines. It causes partial digestion of the worm and can release larvae that invade other tissues. Disintegration of the worm head (scolex) hinders identification and assurance of complete elimination of the parasite. Niclosamide (2 g) should be administered after an overnight fast. Tablets are chewed then swallowed with water. A mild laxative can be used to facilitate bowel evacuation and worm identification. Niclosamide causes few adverse effects because little is absorbed systemically. Nausea, vomiting, and other GI symptoms occur occasionally. Examination of feces must continue for 3 months to assure complete removal of worms.

Mebendazole eradicates a broad spectrum of intestinal parasites: roundworm (*Ascaris*), pinworm (*Enterobius*), hookworm, and whipworm (*Trichuris*). The drug blocks glucose uptake, causing depletion of glycogen stores and death of the worm. Very little drug is absorbed systemically, thus adverse effects are mainly GI. Mebendazole is contraindicated in pregnancy. The drug is taken twice daily for 3 days.

Piperazine (Antepar, 0.65 to 3.5 g) eradicates roundworms and pinworms by paralysis and release of the intact worm from the intestine. This drug is absorbed from the GI tract and is renally excreted. CNS symptoms such as vertigo, headache, and lowering of seizure threshold in persons with convulsive disorders have been reported. GI and vision disturbances occur. Hypersensitivity reactions may require termination of therapy, which usually lasts 2 (roundworms) to 7 (pinworms) days.

Thiabendazole (Mintezol, 25 mg/kg) has a broad spectrum of activity. Threadworm (*Strongyloides*), whipworm, pinworm, roundworm, and cutaneous larva migrans are responsive. This drug also is somewhat effective in alleviating trichinosis. It is systemically absorbed and is hepatically inactivated. GI disturbances and CNS symptoms such as drowsiness, fatigue, and headache occur. Hypersensitivity reactions require that the drug be terminated, since dermatologic reactions (erythema multiforme) can be severe and fatalities have been reported.

Pyrantel (Antiminth, up to 1 g) is used frequently to eradicate roundworms and pinworms by paralysis and release from the intestine. Some of the drug is absorbed and can provoke CNS symptoms including drowsiness and headache. GI disturbances occur more frequently. Elevations in serum glutamic-oxaloacetic transaminase (SGOT) have been reported, prompting caution when the drug is administered to persons with impaired hepatic function. Hypersensitivity, usually manifested as a skin rash, requires that the drug be discontinued.

Pyrvinium (Povan, 5 mg/kg) is especially effective against pinworms. The drug will stain bedding and clothing, and feces and vomitus will be colored bright red. Tablets should be swallowed whole to avoid staining of tooth enamel.

Diethylcarbamazine and **suramin** are used to eradicate filarial infestations of various tissues. Suramin can cause circulatory collapse and is contraindicated in renal dysfunction.

Schistosomiasis, which invades the liver and other organs, is treated with a variety of drugs. The most useful is **praziquantel** (Biltricide), which has relatively low toxicity and is effective against the four species of schistosome that infest human tissue.

Antifungal drugs

Amphotericin B (Fungizone) is administered IV (0.25 to 1 mg/kg/day) and intrathecally to control infections including histoplasmosis, coccidioidomycosis, cryptococcosis, blastomycosis, and candidiasis. The drug alters fungal cell wall permeability. It is extensively bound to plasma proteins and slowly inactivated by renal excretion, with a plasma half-life of 24 hours. Systemic administration is appropriate only for hospitalized patients who can be closely observed for serious adverse reactions. Nephrotoxicity and electrolyte imbalance frequently occur. Renal function and serum electrolytes must be monitored. Renal tubular acidosis can be alleviated with systemic alkalinizers. Blood dyscrasias and hepatic failure have been reported. Fever, headache, malaise, GI disturbances, thrombophlebitis, cardiac arrhythmias and arrest, changes in blood pressure, loss of hearing, and convulsions are some of the varied and occasionally severe adverse effects of amphotericin B. Antiemetics, aspirin, antihistamines, and maintenance of plasma sodium levels can reduce the severity of some of these responses. Amphotericin B can cause hypokalemia, which will potentiate digitalis toxicity and reduce the efficacy of antiarrhythmic agents. Concurrent administration of corticosteroids or of other nephrotoxic drugs should be avoided. Amphotericin is also available for topical administration.

Miconazole (Monistat), like amphotericin B, is usually administered by slow IV infusion (0.2 to 3.6 g/day) or intrathecally. It is effective against a broad spectrum of fungi. It can be instilled into the bladder to treat susceptible urinary infections. Miconazole is hepatically inactivated and has an elimination half-life of 20 to 24 hours. It appears not to cause serious renal or hepatic toxicity. However, the first dose (of no more than 200 mg) must be given cautiously as cardiac and respiratory arrest can occur. Frequently reported adverse effects are pruritus, phlebitis, nausea (which can be alleviated with antiemetics), fever, and hyperlipidemia, probably due to the drug vehicle. Miconazole reverses the antifungal efficacy of amphotericin B and can enhance the action of the oral anticoagulants. Miconazole is available in topical forms for treatment of athlete's foot (tinea pedis) and vaginal candidiasis. Rash, itching, and burning may occur.

Flucytosine (Ancobon, 50 to 150 mg/kg) is effective in cryptococcal and candidal infections, including some that are resistant to amphotericin B. It is administered PO and is less toxic than amphotericin. The drug is renally excreted, thus the greatest risk of adverse reactions occurs when kidney function is inadequate. Bone marrow depression occurs, requiring frequent measurement of blood components and avoidance of other drugs that induce blood dyscrasias. Additional adverse effects include vomiting, diarrhea, and alterations in liver function, which should be monitored. Development of resistant strains occurs.

Ketoconazole (Nizoral, 200 to 400 mg) is administered PO and is not useful for CNS infections. It has a broad spectrum of antifungal activity. Absorption is best accomplished from an acid environment, thus administration of drugs that alter gastric pH (e.g., cimetidine, antacids, anticholinergics) must be scheduled carefully. Ketoconazole can cause fatal hepatotoxicity. Liver function should be monitored. The most frequent adverse effects are GI disturbances. Headache, photophobia, pruritus, fever, and drowsiness also occur.

Nystatin (Mycostatin) is used topically in the treatment of candidial infections of the skin and mucous membranes. Administered PO, the drug remains within the GI tract, where it ameliorates or prevents candidial overgrowth. GI disturbances are the most frequently reported adverse effects.

Griseofulvin (0.5 to 1 g) is effective against dermatophytes that cause infections of the skin, nails, and hair. It is used only for severe infections that do not respond to topical treatment. Griseofulvin is administered PO and is incorporated into the lowest keratin layers, which are not accessible to topical preparations. Absorption varies greatly and can be enhanced by foods with high fat content. Administration for several weeks or months may be required. Hepatic, renal, and bone marrow function should be monitored. Toxicity is usually low. The most commonly reported adverse effects are GI disturbance, hypersensitivity, fatigue, and mental confusion. Blood dyscrasias and paresthesias can occur, especially with chronic administration of high doses. Griseofulvin can cause a disulfiram-type reaction after ingestion of alcohol and may decrease the efficacy of oral anticoagulants. Hepatic enzyme inducers such as the barbiturates can enhance the biotransformation of griseofulvin. Persons allergic to penicillin may also show hypersensitivity to this drug.

IMMUNOLOGIC AGENTS

Active immunity against many infectious diseases can be induced by administration of vaccines and toxoids that contain killed or attenuated microorganisms or their by-products. These agents act as antigens to stimulate the production of antibodies by the human immune system. Subsequent exposure to the microorganism provokes a rapid immune response, which prevents the development of infection. Smallpox was the first disease successfully controlled by a vaccine, and has been almost completely eradicated from the earth. Infections such as measles and poliomyelitis, not uncommon two or three decades ago, now appear only in populations that have avoided active immunization with vaccines.

In the United States, infants are routinely inoculated with DPT antigen, which contains diphtheria and tetanus (lockjaw) toxoids and pertussis (whooping cough) vaccine, and with polio vaccine. Many children receive additional vaccines against measles, rubella (German measles), and mumps. Some vaccines are reserved for use in persons at increased risk of developing infections such as rabies, influenza, and hepatitis.

Diphtheria toxoid imparts long-lasting immunity to this bacterial infection that can damage the myocardium and cause suffocating pharyngeal inflammation. Booster inoculations can be given every 5 to 10 years to persons at risk of exposure. As with most vaccines, there is danger of allergic reactions. Fever, malaise, and soreness at the injection site may develop. The Schick test uses this toxoid to determine immunity to diphtheria. A positive response indicates lack of endogenous protection against the bacteria. Nonimmune persons exposed to diphtheria can be rapidly immunized with diphtheria antitoxin, which neutralizes the damaging bacterial toxin. The diphtheria bacterium (*C. diphtheriae*) is also susceptible to penicillin.

Tetanus toxoid also provides long-lasting immunity. Booster inoculation should be given every 10 years or after tissue injury with risk of tetanus exposure. Caused by clostridial bacteria that thrive in soil, tetanus attacks the CNS. The release of the inhibitory neurotransmitter glycine is blocked, resulting in potentially fatal convulsions. Rapid immunity with a duration of several weeks can be provided by tetanus immune globulin. Administration of the toxoid may produce generalized malaise, a localized reaction at the injection site, and occasional damage to the nervous system. The toxoid should not be given when there is risk of concurrent exposure to polio.

Pertussis vaccine is not administered to persons beyond the seventh birthday, to children who have reacted adversely to previous doses of vaccine, nor to persons with disorders of the nervous system. Pertussis immune globulin is of human origin, thus carries little risk of allergic reactions.

Poliomyelitis vaccines are available for PO or parenteral administration, the latter used only for immunosuppressed persons. These vaccines are contraindicated in the presence of respiratory infections. Three doses of the oral vaccine are given to infants, and one booster dose when the child enters school. Occurrence of paralytic polio in inoculated persons and close contacts has been reported.

Rubella vaccine is usually administered at the age of 12 to 15 months, in combination with measles and mumps vaccines (MMR II). The vaccine can also be given to adults who lack rubella immunity. It is contraindicated during pregnancy, and women receiving inoculation must agree to avoid pregnancy for at least 3 months. Generalized malaise and localized soreness at the site of injection can occur. Thrombocytopenia has been reported.

Measles is a childhood disease that can lead to serious complications including fatal encephalitis. **Measles vaccine** should not be administered during pregnancy, and conception should be avoided for at least 3 months following administration.

It is also contraindicated in persons allergic to protein from poultry. Fever and convulsions in children may occur. Rare instances of encephalitis after inoculation have been reported. Measles immune globulin can be administered for rapid protection and will reduce the severity of the disease.

Administration of the **mumps vaccine** occasionally causes mild fever and inflammation of the parotid glands. Febrile seizures, encephalitis, and allergy may occur, especially in persons hypersensitive to poultry.

Hepatitis B inoculation is advised for laboratory and health-care personnel, institutionalized persons, hemodialysis and oncology patients, drug abusers, and other persons at significant risk of exposure to this virus. The incubation period for hepatitis is prolonged (up to 6 months), and exposure may occur long before the active disease becomes apparent. An immune globulin also is available.

Influenza is a viral respiratory infection that can be especially dangerous in diabetics, the elderly, and persons with chronic lung or heart disease. **Flu vaccines** must be administered each year, usually at the start of the winter flu season. Inoculation and natural immunity do not always provide protection, as the influenza virus is capable of undergoing rapid mutation. Local tenderness, fever, and allergic reactions can occur, particularly in persons with poultry hypersensitivity. Neurological disorders including encephalopathy and Guillain-Barré syndrome have appeared after administration of influenza vaccines.

Rabies is a rare but serious viral infection spread by wild animals and occasionally by domestic animals. Unless treated early in the course of disease before symptoms appear, rabies is fatal. Widespread inoculation of household animals has helped to control this disease, but recent years have seen a gradual increase in its incidence in humans. Prophylactic use of **rabies vaccine** is recommended only for persons at significant risk of exposure to the virus, such as veterinarians and laboratory personnel. Persons who have been exposed to the saliva of an animal known or suspected to be rabid should be given rabies immune globulin (antirabies serum) as soon as possible by the IM route and by local infiltration around the area of the injury. Cleaning of the bite will also aid in the removal of the virus. Rabies vaccine, derived from human cell cultures, is then administered in a series of injections over 4 weeks.

Other vaccines are available for persons traveling to areas where diseases such as **cholera** and **typhoid fever** are endemic. A tuberculin vaccine is used to test for present or past infection with tuberculosis. **BCG** (bacillus Calmette-Guérin) vaccine derived from the bovine bacteria is occasionally used to attempt to immunize persons at significant risk of exposure to tuberculosis. This vaccine is also used to stimulate the immune system in some cancer patients. Human gamma-globulin can be given to provide temporary passive immunity to persons exposed but possibly not immune to various infectious diseases. Injection of gamma-globulin can produce severe pain.

Successful active immunization with vaccines and toxoids depends on the response of the patient's own immune system. Thus these agents should not be administered to persons with disease- or drug-induced immunosuppression. The safety of these agents during pregnancy is not known. All vaccines and toxoids, except those derived from human sources, carry the risk of allergic responses to animal protein contaminants. Mild adverse effects, ranging from local reactions at the site of injection to generalized malaise, are the most common following administration of immunizing agents.

IMMUNOSUPPRESSANT AGENTS

Drugs that suppress the immune system will prevent rejection of organ transplants. Administration of these agents in diseases such as rheumatoid arthritis and lupus erythematosus, which may have an autoimmune etiology, is largely experimental. The potential for carcinogenicity and unopposed infections makes the use of immunosuppressants extremely hazardous.

Azathioprine (Imuran) is a purine analogue related to the antineoplastic 6-mercaptopurine. It is usually administered together with the corticosteroid prednisone to prevent rejection in renal transplantation. Severe refractory rheumatoid arthritis may be alleviated with azathioprine. The drug is biotransformed, partly to mercaptopurine, in the liver and in erythrocytes. Reduced renal function prolongs the plasma half-life of the drug and its metabolites, requiring reduction in dosage. Azathioprine can provoke marked bone marrow depression, resulting in thrombocytopenia, leukopenia, and anemia. Secondary infections can be severe. Nausea and vomiting, characteristic of the antineoplastic drugs, occurs with azathioprine. This drug can be hepatotoxic and may induce malignancies, including lymphomas and acute myelogenous leukemia. **Allopurinol**, which may be administered concurrently to reduce serum uric acid, inhibits the inactivation of azathioprine. Administration of the latter drug should be reduced to no greater than one-third of the usual dose.

Cyclosporine (Sandimmune) suppresses immunity by altering the activity of T-lymphocytes. It usually is not myelosuppressive, although some reductions in platelets and leukocytes have been noted. Cyclosporine is relatively water insoluble. It is prepared in olive oil and ethanol for PO administration (absorption is slow and variable) and in ethanol for IV administration. The drug, which binds extensively to plasma proteins, has a plasma half-life of almost 20 hours. It is biotransformed and excreted in the bile. Cyclosporine has been effective in suppressing rejection in renal, hepatic, and cardiac transplantation, and it reduces graft-versus-host disease following bone marrow transplantation. The most frequent adverse effect of cyclosporine is nephrotoxicity that can produce symptoms quite similar to renal transplant rejection. Secondary infections, in particular viral invasions, can occur. Additional adverse effects include allergic reactions, hepatotoxicity, fluid retention, hypertension, and the appearance of lymphomas. Corticosteroids can be administered concurrently with cyclosporine, but other immunosuppressant drugs are contraindicated.

Muromonab-CD3 (Orthoclone OKT3) is a monoclonal antibody preparation that suppresses T-lymphocyte activity in acute renal transplant rejection. Administered by IV bolus for 10 to 14 days, the drug provokes the development of antibodies that can reduce the efficacy in subsequent use and may result in allergic responses. Pulmonary edema and meningitis have occurred.

Other drugs that are used to suppress immunologic responsiveness are the antineoplastics **methotrexate** and **cyclo-phosphamide** (discussed under "Antineoplastic Drugs") and the corticosteroids (discussed under "Endocrine Pharmacology"). Antithymocyte globulin can be used as an adjunct in immunosuppressant therapy.

ANTINEOPLASTIC DRUGS

Significant advances have been made in the chemotherapy of some forms of cancer, whereas other forms have remained resistant to drug treatment. Antineoplastic drug combinations are employed against some malignancies, and drugs are used in conjunction with surgery and radiation.

Antineoplastic drugs are toxic not only to malignant cells but also to normal cells, especially those that proliferate rapidly. Thus these drugs produce many serious adverse effects. Suppression of bone marrow activity depletes all the formed elements of the blood. Leukopenia leaves the patient vulnerable to infection. Drugs should be terminated if granulocytes fall to less than $1,000/mm^2$. Severe spontaneous hemorrhage can develop as the result of thrombocytopenia. Platelet counts below $40,000/mm^2$ require that drug therapy be discontinued. When myelosuppressant drugs are combined, careful attention must be paid to their additive effects on the bone marrow.

Cells of the GI tract also are rapidly proliferating and are susceptible to damage from the antineoplastic drugs. Inflammation and ulceration of the mucosa can develop at any site along the tract, including the mouth and the esophagus.

Perhaps of less physiological significance but of great psychological importance to the patient is the hair loss (alopecia) induced by some of the antineoplastics. Cooling of the scalp or the use of a tourniquet during drug administration may reduce the amount of drug reaching the hair follicles, another area of rapid cell proliferation. Hair growth usually resumes, although the color and texture may differ from the original hair.

Embryonic and fetal cells proliferate rapidly, thus are subject to damage by the antineoplastic drugs. Fetal abnormalities have been attributed to several of these agents, although normal infants also have been born following maternal treatment for cancer. Suppression of ovarian and testicular function often occurs during antineoplastic therapy.

A severe and frequent adverse effect of the antineoplastics is nausea and vomiting. This may be due to direct GI toxicity or to toxic by-products of cellular destruction, which stimulate the chemoreceptor trigger zone. Antiemetics can be administered concurrently, although they have limited ability to suppress this effect. The phenothiazines and metoclopramide (Reglan) are occasionally effective, as are tetrahydrocannabinol (dronabinol, Marinol) and its synthetic analogue nabilone (Cesamet). Vomiting that accompanies chemotherapy can be so devastating both physically and psychologically that some patients refuse further treatment. Dehydration and electrolyte imbalances can result, necessitating fluid and ion replacement.

The destruction of cells by antineoplastic agents can lead to hyperuricemia. In patients with lymphomas and acute lymphoblastic leukemia, rapid turnover of malignant cells also liberates uric acid, producing considerable risk of renal damage from precipitated urate crystals. Persons receiving chemotherapy should be well hydrated to enhance the solubility of urates and to promote rapid elimination from the kidneys. Allopurinol (Zyloprim), which inhibits xanthine oxidase, thus reduces the formation of uric acid, and systemic alkalinizers can help to reduce plasma and urinary levels of urates.

Antineoplastic drugs work by a variety of mechanisms. Some, called cell cycle-specific agents, are especially toxic to rapidly proliferating cells, thus have their greatest effect in rapidly growing neoplasms. Cell cycle-nonspecific agents are most useful in the treatment of more slowly proliferating malignancies. Cancer cells often develop drug resistance, causing agents once effective to become useless. Combinations of drugs can reduce the recurrence of malignancy due to drug-resistant cells. *Because of their marked cytotoxicity, antineoplastic drug doses are individualized, thus are not included in this review.*

Alkylating agents

Alkylating agents interfere with DNA replication and are cell cycle nonspecific. They are toxic to both rapidly and slowly proliferating malignancies and are effective in many types of cancers including Hodgkin's disease, acute lymphocytic leukemia, ovarian and breast tumors, multiple myeloma, melanoma, and mycosis fungoides. These drugs are generally carcinogenic, mutagenic, and potentially teratogenic.

Mechlorethamine or **nitrogen mustard** (Mustargen) was the first widely used antineoplastic agent. Usually administered IV, it is also given intraperitoneally and intrapleurally to alleviate accumulation of fluid (effusion) induced by carcinomas. Mechlorethamine is a vesicant, causing blistering of the epidermis, thus like most antineoplastics must be prepared and administered with great care to avoid injury to the patient and to health-care personnel. Thrombophlebitis can occur with IV administration, and extravasation will damage subcutaneous tissue. Immediate infiltration with sodium thiosulfate will reduce this injury. Mechlorethamine is particularly toxic to bone marrow. Preexisting anemia, thrombocytopenia, and leukopenia can be exacerbated, especially in persons with chronic lymphatic leukemia. Severe hemorrhage and infections can be fatal, and concomitant use of other myelosuppressive therapy requires extreme caution. Mechlorethamine is probably teratogenic. Its use during pregnancy and lactation is contraindicated unless no alternative antineoplastic agent is suitable. Hyperuricemia, nausea and vomiting, alopecia, diarrhea, amenorrhea, impaired spermatogenesis, and hearing loss can occur in persons receiving mechlorethamine.

Cyclophosphamide (Cytoxan) is a frequently used alkylating agent, often in combinations with other antineoplastics. It is effective in a wide range of malignancies and has been used investigationally in alleviating severe rheumatoid arthritis and lupus erythematosus. It can prolong remission in children with acute lymphoblastic leukemia. Cyclophosphamide is administered PO and IV. Like most antineoplastics, it is contraindicated in mothers who are breast-feeding and relatively contraindicated in pregnancy, particularly during the first trimester. Cyclophosphamide can produce all of the characteristic adverse effects of chemotherapy: bone marrow depression with immunosuppression (anemia and thrombocytopenia are less frequent), vomiting and diarrhea, alopecia, inflammation and ulceration of the GI mucosa. The risk of potentially fatal hemorrhagic cystitis can be reduced by adequate hydration and frequent emptying of the urinary bladder. Drug adminis-

tration must be interrupted if cystitis develops. Pulmonary, ovarian, and bladder fibrosis have been reported, mainly in persons receiving large drug doses. Hepatic dysfunction and jaundice can develop. Cyclophosphamide can cause inappropriate secretion of antidiuretic hormone (ADH), leading to water intoxication. Cyclophosphamide inhibits the inactivation of succinylcholine, thus will enhance its respiratory depressant activity.

Chlorambucil (Leukeran) is orally effective in the treatment of Hodgkin's disease, chronic lymphocytic leukemia, and other lymphocytic malignancies. It is somewhat less toxic than other nitrogen mustard derivatives, although bone marrow depression can be severe and irreversible. The drug should not be administered to persons already myelosuppressed following radiation or other chemotherapy. Frequent monitoring of formed blood elements throughout therapy will indicate whether dosage reduction or termination is required. Chlorambucil may be teratogenic and mutagenic and can induce hyperuricemia. Nausea and hepatotoxicity occur with less frequency than with most other antineoplastic agents.

Melphalan (Alkeran) is used in the treatment of several cancers including multiple myeloma and ovarian tumors. It is administered PO, although absorption is quite variable and is best achieved when food is not present in the GI tract. Like chlorambucil, this drug can induce severe myelosuppression. Patients must be observed for signs of abnormal bleeding and infection, and frequent blood counts will help to indicate whether reduction or termination of drug administration is necessary. Vomiting can occur with high drug doses. Occasional pulmonary fibrosis has been reported. Melphalan can be particularly toxic in the presence of renal failure, and dosages may have to be reduced. The drug can be given intermittently or continuously and may require several months to produce therapeutic effects.

The **nitrosourea** antineoplastics are alkylating agents that are especially effective in treating CNS malignancies. These drugs produce most of the adverse effects of antineoplastic therapy. Carmustine (BiCNU) is administered IV over 1 to 2 days every 6 weeks. Myelosuppression can be gradual but severe. Bone marrow activity must recover to adequate levels before a subsequent dose is given. Vomiting occurs frequently, and hepatotoxicity and renal damage have been reported. Pulmonary infiltration or fibrosis can occur with chronic administration. Extravasation or contact with skin can cause burning and hyperpigmentation. Pain at the injection site can result from venospasm. **Lomustine** (CCNU, CeeNU) is similar to carmustine, although it is administered PO on an empty stomach.

Dacarbazine (DTIC), like the other alkylating agents, can produce fatal myelosuppression, with thrombocytopenia and leukopenia occurring more frequently than anemia. Vomiting occurs in a large percentage of patients given dacarbazine, although tolerance does develop. Anaphylactic reactions and hepatotoxicity, which can be fatal, are occasionally induced by this drug. A characteristic syndrome similar to influenza has been observed, especially after large doses of dacarbazine. Administered by IV bolus or infusion, extravasation will cause intense pain and severe tissue damage.

Busulfan (Myleran) often produces remission of chronic myelogenous leukemia in adults. It is not effective in children, who usually do not have the Philadelphia chromosome, nor is it active against acute or lymphocytic leukemia. The most severe adverse effect is extensive myelosuppression. Disease-induced hyperuricemia can be exacerbated. Bronchopulmonary dysplasia and subsequent pulmonary fibrosis occasionally develop as late as 10 years after therapy and are usually fatal. Fever, cough, and respiratory difficulty suggest termination of busulfan. Cataracts and a syndrome of adrenal suppression have occurred during chronic administration of this drug.

Streptozocin (Zanosar) is used in the treatment of pancreatic carcinoma. Renal toxicity including anuria, tubular acidosis, and glycosuria are characteristic effects of this alkylating agent. Renal function should be determined before therapy is initiated and then monitored carefully to detect early signs of potentially fatal renal damage. Severe myelosuppression, hepatotoxicity, and frequent nausea and vomiting occur with streptozocin administration. Changes in glucose metabolism have been reported.

Antimetabolites

Antimetabolites have structural similarities to vitamins and other substances required for the survival of cells. They suppress cellular growth by altering various metabolic processes. They are cell cycle specific, being most toxic to cells during the S phase of DNA synthesis and the G2 phase of RNA and protein synthesis. The antimetabolites are particularly effective against rapidly proliferating malignancies. Like all antineoplastic drugs, these agents are toxic to normal cells also.

Methotrexate (amethopterin), the first chemotherapeutic antimetabolite, is effective in suppressing choriocarcinoma and various leukemias. It is frequently used to maintain remission in childhood lymphoblastic leukemia. Methotrexate is used alone and in combined chemotherapy for mycosis fungoides, hydatidiform moles, and for other rapidly progressive tumors of the lungs, breast, and head. Although it is highly toxic, this agent is also used to alleviate symptoms of severe refractory psoriasis. Methotrexate inhibits the enzyme dihydrofolate reductase so that folic acid cannot be converted to tetrahydrofolate, which is required for protein synthesis. This action can be detrimental to normal cells also. "Leucovorin rescue" can reduce the degree of cytotoxicity. After allowing some time for a dose of methotrexate to influence the activity of rapidly dividing malignant cells, leucovorin (folinic acid) is administered to replace tetrahydrofolate and enable normal cells to resume growth before they are irreversibly damaged.

Methotrexate is given PO and parenterally, including intrathecally. The drug binds to plasma proteins. It is renally excreted, and impaired kidney function retards elimination. Methotrexate may exacerbate renal damage. It accumulates in liver cells and can cause severe hepatotoxicity, including cirrhosis and fibrosis. Hepatic function should be measured before drug administration is begun and throughout therapy. Myelosuppression, GI irritation and ulceration, alopecia, rashes, photosensitivity, vomiting, diarrhea, pneumonitis, obstructive pulmonary disease, and CNS symptoms including convulsions are among the numerous severe adverse effects of this drug. Patients receiving methotrexate must be closely observed. Toxicity may appear suddenly and be rapidly fatal. Alcohol and other hepatotoxic agents can enhance this toxicity, thus should be avoided. Salicylates, NSAIDs, and probenecid reduce the renal excretion of methotrexate. Phenylbutazibem salicylates, and sulfonamides can displace methotrexate from protein binding sites.

Mercaptopurine (6-MP, Purinethol) and thioguanine, purine analogues that disrupt nucleic acid synthesis, are used to induce and maintain remission of acute leukemias. Severe and delayed myclosuppression with depletion of all formed clements of blood occurs. Close monitoring of blood counts is necessary; with any marked decrease the drug should be terminated. Continued observation will indicate whether hematopoietic changes are drug or disease induced, and drug therapy may be resumed. Toxic drug doses may be required to induce remission. Supportive therapy such as isolation, antibiotics, and platelet transfusions will contribute to patients' survival. Hyperuricemia often accompanies the use of the purine analogues. Allopurinol can reduce the production of uric acid but also suppresses the inactivation of mercaptopurine, which must be given in greatly reduced dosage (one-fourth to one-third of normal) when these drugs are combined. The inactivation of thioguanine is much less affected. These drugs are hepatotoxic. Patients require frequent monitoring of liver function and observation for anorexia, jaundice, and abdominal pain. This effect occurs most frequently with large doses and has been reported up to 8 years after therapy. GI ulceration and nausea are occasional adverse effects. Decreased renal function prolongs the plasma half-life of mercaptopurine but does not appear to affect that of thioguanine.

Pyrimidine antimetabolites such as fluorouracil (5-FU), floxuridine (FUDR), and cytarabine (ara-C) inhibit synthesis of DNA and are effective against several types of malignancies. These agents are usually administered IV, although the intra-arterial route is used for floxuridine in the treatment of hepatic metastases. Cytarabine can be given SC and is most useful in leukemias. As with many of the antineoplastics, severe myelosuppression is a frequent adverse effect of the pyrimidine analogues. These drugs have a narrow margin of safety. Marked changes in blood counts or symptoms of GI damage require that therapy be terminated. Nausea, vomiting, diarrhea, myocardial ischemia, alopecia, GI hemorrhage, and hyperuricemia are among the many adverse reactions. Fluorouracil is available in topical preparations for treatment of solar keratoses.

Vinca alkaloids

Vincristine (Oncovin) and vinblastine (Velban) are plant derivatives that disrupt the formation of the mitotic spindle, thus are cell cycle specific. Vincristine is effective against childhood leukemia and is a component of MOPP (mechlorethamine, Oncovin, procarbazine, and prednisone) combination therapy, which is used particularly for Hodgkin's disease. The characteristic toxicity of vincristine is neurologic: paresthesias, difficulty in walking, neuritic pain, loss of deep tendon reflexes, paralytic ileus, ataxia, and convulsions occur. Vomiting and alopecia are frequent, but myelosuppression rarely develops. Constipation with fecal impaction in the upper colon requires careful diagnosis and alleviation. Occasionally, inappropriate secretion of ADH leads to hyponatremia. Vincristine is administered IV, and extravasation must be avoided as this drug is highly toxic to subcutaneous tissue. Infiltration with hyaluronidase can help to minimize damage.

Vinblastine, in contrast to vincristine, produces significant myelosuppression. It is highly effective against Hodgkin's disease and is used singly and in combination for several types of malignancies including lymphomas, Kaposi's sarcoma, and testicular cancer. Leukopenia and nausea and vomiting are frequent adverse effects. Neurotoxicity has been reported occasionally. Vinblastine is administered IV once weekly, although doses are withheld if leukocyte counts remain depressed. Extravasation can cause marked tissue damage.

Antibiotics

Bleomycin, mitomycin, plicamycin, doxorubicin, and daunorubicin are by-products of various *Streptomyces* strains and have activity against several types of cancers.

Bleomycin (Blenoxane) is used alone and in drug combinations against lymphomas and squamous cell and testicular carcinomas. It is cell cycle specific and appears to inhibit synthesis of DNA. Pulmonary toxicity is characteristic, manifested as pneumonitis and fibrosis occurring most frequently in the elderly and in persons receiving large doses of drug. Chest x-rays, monitoring of pulmonary function, and close observation for respiratory difficulty are recommended. Dermatologic disturbances, often delayed until 2 to 3 weeks into the course of therapy, and nausea and vomiting are frequent. Anaphylactoid reactions, which occur immediately or several hours after administration, are observed usually following the first or second drug dose. Occasional instances of hepatic and renal toxicity have been reported. Bleomycin is renally excreted, and its half-life is prolonged by renal impairment. Myelosuppression is infrequent.

Mitomycin (Mutamycin), which alkylates DNA and prevents its replication, is used in drug combinations for several types of carcinomas. Myelosuppression is frequent and severe. Subsequent doses must be withheld until bone marrow activity recovers. Mitomycin is administered IV, and extravasation should be avoided. Renal and pulmonary damage, GI irritation, vomiting, and alopecia are frequent adverse effects.

Plicamycin (Mithracin) is used in the treatment of testicular cancer and will alleviate refractory hypercalcemia and hypercalcuria induced by malignancies. Characteristic is a "hemorrhagic syndrome" that can begin with hematemesis or epistaxis and may progress to severe hemorrhage. Patients should be monitored for clotting abnormalities. Myelosuppression, thrombocytopenia in particular, occurs and can increase the risk of extensive blood loss. Renal and hepatic dysfunction and electrolyte imbalances have been reported. Vomiting can be severe. Administration is by the IV route; thrombophlebitis can occur, and extravasation will produce tissue damage.

Doxorubicin (Adriamycin) is effective against several types of malignancies including solid tumors, lymphomas, and leukemias. Cardiac toxicity is characteristic. Congestive heart failure detected early may respond to digitalis and diuretics. However, cardiac toxicity frequently develops rapidly and does not respond to treatment. Life-threatening arrhythmias can occur. Preexisting heart disease may predispose to this cardiotoxicity. Doxorubicin suppresses bone marrow activity, in particular the production of leukocytes. Alopecia, vomiting, and GI ulceration can be severe. The drug is administered IV at 3-week intervals; extravasation destroys subcutaneous tissue. Doxorubicin is excreted in the bile, and its half-life is prolonged by hepatic dysfunction.

Daunorubicin (Cerubidine) is effective against acute non-lymphocytic leukemia. Cardiotoxicity and myelosuppression can be severe. Vomiting and alopecia are common. Extravasation results in tissue damage.

Hormones

Estrogens such as diethylstilbestrol and ethinyl estradiol are effective in metastases of prostatic cancer and of breast cancer in postmenopausal women. Side effects are those characteristic of estrogen. Androgens are administered to premenopausal women with breast cancer. Nausea, fluid retention, and masculinization are frequent side effects. (The pharmacology of the hormones is discussed under "Endocrine Pharmacology.")

Tamoxifen (Nolvadex) is a competitive antiestrogen that suppresses growth of estrogen-dependent breast tumors. Vomiting and hot flashes are common side effects. Occasional temporary exacerbation of symptoms of bone and skin metastases seems to be an indication of the therapeutic activity of the drug. Vision disturbances have been reported, as well as occasional thrombocytopenia.

Estramustine (Emcyt) combines an estrogen with nitrogen mustard for use in estrogen-resistent prostatic metastases. Vomiting and estrogenic side effects occur frequently.

Corticosteroids are frequent adjuncts in the treatment of cancer. They are antineoplastic in some lymphatic malignancies and breast cancer. They alleviate the cerebral edema that often occurs with radiation therapy and cranial tumors. Corticosteroids also produce euphoria that relieves some of the psychological discomfort of cancer patients. Mitotane is an antiadrenal that concentrates in the adrenal cortex and destroys both normal and malignant cells. It is administered in inoperable adrenal cortical carcinoma.

Additional antineoplastic agents

Cisplatin (Platinol) used alone and in drug combinations has been effective against testicular, ovarian, bladder, and squamous cell tumors and lymphomas. It alkylates DNA and is cell cycle nonspecific. Nausea and vomiting, which occur in almost 100% of patients treated with cisplatin, may be alleviated with metoclopramide. Cisplatin is renally excreted and has a plasma half-life of up to 72 hours. Severe nephrotoxicity occurs frequently. Drug doses are withheld if renal function is impaired. Pretreatment IV infusion of fluids and slow IV administration of drug concomitant with mannitol may somewhat reduce the risk of renal damage. Hyperuricemia and ototoxicity can occur, especially in children. Symptoms of the latter include tinnitus and dizziness. Myelosuppression induces leukopenia, thrombocytopenia, and anemia. Immediate anaphylactic reactions have been reported. Aluminum needles cannot be used for administration, as this metal inactivates cisplatin. Peripheral neuropathy, hypertension, and electrolyte imbalances are additional adverse effects of cisplatin. Ototoxic antibiotics should be avoided, although furosemide, which has ototoxic activity, may be administered instead of mannitol to promote elimination of drug from the kidneys.

Procarbazine (Matulane) is particularly useful as a component of MOPP therapy. Vomiting and myelosuppression are the most frequent adverse effects. Procarbazine crosses the blood-brain barrier and induces CNS symptoms including ataxia, anxiety, depression, and hallucinations. This drug inhibits MAO, thus patients are at risk of hypertensive crisis if sympathomimetic drugs or foods containing tyramine are taken concurrently. Alcohol ingestion can provoke a disulfiram-like reaction. CNS depressants may exacerbate some of the neurological effects of procarbazine.

L-**Asparaginase** (Elspar) is an enzyme derived from *E. coli,* which inactivates asparagine that is essential for the survival of leukemic cells. Nonmalignant cells are capable of synthesizing asparagine, thus are less susceptible to the cytotoxicity of this drug. Asparaginase is cell cycle specific, exerting its effect at the G1 phase of the cycle as the cell prepares for DNA synthesis. Hypersensitivity reactions can include fatal anaphylasix; allergic patients may be carefully desensitized. Marked hyperuricemia can occur as large numbers of cells are disrupted. Hyperglycemia, hepatotoxicity, renal failure, and CNS symptoms can develop.

Interferon, synthesized by recombinant DNA technology, is effective against hairy cell leukemia in adults. Both direct antineoplastic activity and immune system modulation are believed to contribute to its efficacy. Administration is by the IM or SC route. Inactivation seems to occur in the renal tubules. A flu-like syndrome that includes fever, chills, and fatigue is the most frequently reported adverse effect. Nausea, diarrhea, hypertension, arrhythmias, myelosuppression, and CNS symptoms (dizziness, depression, vision and sleep disturbances, and decreased mental status) can occur. Administration to persons with renal or hepatic impairment or cardiovascular or CNS dysfunction requires caution.

Radioactive isotopes

Isotopes of iodine (^{131}I), phosphate (^{32}P), and gold (^{198}Au) emit beta particles that destroy both malignant and normal cells. ^{131}I localizes in the thyroid and is effective in treating tumors of that gland. ^{32}P is occasionally used in leukemias and bone metastases, and ^{198}Au for pediatric brain tumors. Patients should be isolated to protect others from irradiation; urine and bedding will be contaminated until the isotope is eliminated.

ENDOCRINE PHARMACOLOGY

Hormones are biochemicals secreted by endocrine glands into the circulatory system for transport to other tissues ("target tissues"), where they regulate physiological activity. Most hormones appear to work by way of interaction with receptors either on cell membranes or on intracellular structures. Hormones may be administered in small doses to replace those that are lacking because of disese or injury to endocrine glands (e.g., administration of insulin to diabetics). In the management of some disorders, hormones are administered in larger than physiological amounts (e.g., corticosteroids to alleviate inflammation).

Many hormones are destroyed in the GI tract or inthe first pass through the liver, thus must be administered parenterally. Most hormones are inactivated, and the metabolites are renally excreted. Alterations in hepatic or renal function can influence the plasma half-life of these substances. The secretion of many hormones is under negative feedback control. Decreased plasma levels result in increased synthesis and release; elevated plasma levels have the opposite effect. Thus, exogenously administered hormones will suppress endogenous hormone production. Endocrine systems that have been suppressed require time to resume normal physiological activity. Secretion of a few hormones is under control of plasma levels of other substances (e.g., insulin release responds to blood glucose content).

Pituitary pharmacology

The pituitary has been called the "master gland" because it secretes hormones that influence the physiological function of many other glands and tissues (Table 6-19). Both the anterior and posterior pituitary are endocrine glands, and pituitary insufficiency may be of one or several hormones. Some pituitary hormones stimulate the activity of other endocrine glands. Inadequate secretion from these glands must be diagnosed as primary or secondary failures. For example, corticosteroid insufficiency can be due to inability of the adrenal cortex to synthesize and release hormone (primary failure) or to inadequate ACTH synthesis and release from the pituitary to stimulate the activity of the adrenals (secondary failure).

Anterior pituitary.   **ACTH** is used mainly as a diagnostic agent for adrenal insufficiency (e.g., Addison's disease). The treatment of adrenal insufficiency, either primary or secondary, usually entails replacement therapy with adrenal hormones (see below). ACTH is used occasionally to alleviate the muscle weakness of myasthenia gravis. Exaggerated muscle weakness can occur early in this therapy, resulting in respiratory depression or arrest.

Growth hormone (GH, also called somatostatin) promotes release of free fatty acids and entry of amino acids and glucose into cells. It is essential for proper growth and attainment of normal height. GH has long been derived from human pituitary, but recent evidence indicating a risk of its causing

Table 6-19. Target Tissues for Pituitary Hormones

Hormone	Target tissue
Anterior pituitary	
Adrenocorticotropic hormone (ACTH)	Adrenal gland
Growth hormone (GH, somatostatin)	Various body tissues
Thyroid-stimulating hormone (TSH)	Thyroid gland
Follicle-stimulating hormone (FSH)	Ovaries, testes
Luteinizing hormone (LH)	Ovaries, testes
Posterior pituitary	
Antidiuretic hormone (ADH, vasopressin)	Kidneys
Oxytocin	Ovaries, mammary glands

Creutzfeldt-Jakob disease (a slow, fatal viral infection of the CNS) led to the removal of human GH from the market. Recombinant DNA techniques show promise of providing a new and safe source. GH must be administered parenterally (IM). Its ability to stimulate skeletal growth is lost after closure of the epiphyses of the long bones. Hypercalciuria and renal stones may develop during GH therapy. There is also the risk of hyperglycemia, especially in diabetics.

Thyroid-stimulating hormone (TSH) is used only as a diagnostic agent to determine thyroid function. Both primary and secondary hypothyroidism are treated by replacement administration of thyroid hormones (see below).

Sexual development and the ensuing synthesis of the sex hormones by the testes in males and by the ovaries in females are under the regulation of the gonadotropic hormones follicle-stimulating hormone (FSH) and luteinizing hormone (LH) or interstitial cell-stimulating hormone (ICSH), which are secreted by the anterior pituitary. FSH stimulates spermatogenesis or follicle maturation and estrogen release. LH promotes synthesis of androgens by the Leydig's cells in the testes or of estrogen and progesterone by the corpus luteum. (Small amounts of sex hormones are also released from the adrenal cortex but usually produce no observable effects except in adrenal hypersecretion, when the amounts become physiologically significant.)

These hormones or substances with similar activity have special pharmacologic applications. The urine of postmenopausal women has high levels of FSH and LH because the negative feedback influence of estrogen on the pituitary is absent. These are extracted for use as **human menopausal gonadotropins** (HMG, menotropins, Pergonal). **Human chorionic gonadotropin** (HCG) extracted from the urine of pregnant women has strong LH-like activity. HMG and HCG can be used to treat infertility in women with secondary ovarian failure—that is, when the reproductive organs are normal but do not receive appropriate stimulation from the pituitary. Several days of IM administration of HMG to stimulate follicle maturation is followed by injection of HCG if increased estrogen activity is detected. This will cause ovulation. Pregnancy occurs in approximately one-fourth of women thus treated. The possibility of multiple fetuses is significant. Hyperstimulation of the ovaries can also cause rupture of the ovarian cyst and severe hemorrhage. Abdominal pain may be a warning that this has occurred.

These hormones can also treat male infertility. If sexual development and testosterone levels are inadequate, HCG is administered to bring these to maturity. Then HCG and HMG are coadministered to promote spermatogenesis. HCG is used in cryptorchidism (undescended testicle). If this treatment fails, the presence of androgens should be tested for. If absent, the primary failure of the testes will necessitate the administration of testosterone. Administration of HCG in young boys must be undertaken carefully, as premature sexual development can occur. The appearance of penile erections indicates that drug dosage should be reduced. HCG is also used to diagnose testicular failure.

Clomiphene (Clomid, Serophene) is a synthetic oral fertility drug for women with secondary pituitary and ovarian failure. Clomiphene appears to compete for estrogen receptor binding, thus decreasing negative feedback suppression of gonadotropin release from the pituitary. The increased production of FSH and LH by the anterior pituitary brings about ovulation and pregnancy in approximately one-fourth of patients. Overstimulation of the ovaries and multiple fetuses can occur, as well as vision aberrations and vasomotor symptoms similar to those of menopause. Clomiphene is used in males to diagnose testicular function. Clomiphene and HMG are contraindicated in pregnancy and in neoplastic disease.

Danazol (Danocrine) suppress release of FSH and LH from the pituitary. It is a second-line drug in the treatment of severe fibrocystic breast disease and of endometriosis and is being tried as an oral contraceptive in males. Because it is weakly androgenic, danazol can cause increased facial hair, deepening of the voice, and other masculine effects. It is inactivated in the liver, thus must be used with caution in persons with decreased hepatic activity. Pregnancy is a contraindication.

Posterior pituitary. **Oxytocin** causes contraction of the smooth muscle of the uterus and the mammary glands. During pregnancy, the myometrium gradually changes from relative insensitivity to extreme responsiveness to this hormone. Oxytocin should not be used to induce or hasten normal labor and delivery. It is reserved for abnormal circumstances such as uterine inertia, maternal diabetes mellitus, eclampsia, completion of spontaneous abortion occurring after the fifth month of pregnancy, or when rupture of the amniotic sac is not followed by onset of labor within 12 hours. The adverse effects of oxytocin can be fatal to both mother and fetus. Maternal hypertension, water intoxication, cardiac arrhythmias, and rupture of the uterus can occur, as well as fetal arrhythmias and cerebrovascular rupture. Sustained contraction of the uterus can reduce blood flow to the placenta and interfere with fetal oxygenation.

Oxytocin is frequently used after completion of the second stage of labor—that is, after delivery of the infant. This stage is often characterized by severe uterine bleeding and marked atony of the myometrium. Administration of oxytocin or drugs with similar uterine-stimulating action (oxytocics) at this time causes strong contractions, which exert pressure on open vessels, helping to stanch the flow of blood. The **ergot alkaloids** (ergonovine and methylergonovine) are oxytocics that may be used to reduce postpartum hemorrhage. They are never administered before delivery of a live infant. The ergot alkaloids are also used in the treatment of migraine headaches, which may result from cerebral vasodilation. These drugs induce severe constriction of blood vessels that can lead to gangrene of toes and fingers.

Some of the **prostaglandins** have oxytocic activity in early as well as later pregnancy and are used to induce abortion.

ADH increases the permeability of the distal tubule and collecting duct of the nephron to water, thus allowing its reabsorption. ADH is released from the pituitary in response to decreased blood volume or increased plasma osmolarity. Also called **vasopressin**, this hormone in larger amounts is a vasoconstrictor and will stimulate contraction of the smooth muscle of the GI tract and the uterus. These effects demand caution when ADH is administered during pregnancy or to persons with cardiovascular disease. (Conversely, oxytocin in large amounts has an antidiuretic effect.)

Exogenous ADH is used for replacement therapy in the management of diabetes insipidus that is central in origin—

that is, when the endogenous hormone is absent. ADH must be administered parenterally. Forms are available for intranasal instillation. **Desmopressin** (DDAVP) and **lypressin** (Diapid) are synthetic ADH analogues that have much lower pressor and oxytocic activity and a longer duration of action. Doses must be adjusted to each individual, and fluid intake and output should be monitored. ADH and desmopressin are also used to control hemorrhage in von Willebrand's disease and some cases of hemophilia.

Thyroid pharmacology

Drugs are used in the management of overactivity (hyperthyroidism) and underactivity (hypothyroidism) of the thyroid gland. Hyperthyroidism may also be treated with surgical removal of a portion of the gland. Since the overactive thyroid is often highly vascular and presents the risk of marked hemorrhage, antithyroid drugs may be administered before surgery to reduce the activity and the size of the gland.

Methimazole (Tapazole) and **propylthiouracil** (PTU) inhibit the synthesis but not the release of triiodothyronine (T_3) and tetraiodothyronine (T_4). These drugs are always given PO and have a gradual onset of action. Several days may elapse before significant reduction in thyroid activity is noted.

Adverse effects, which occur in a small percentage of patients, include nausea, skin rash and pigmentation, headache and joint pain, and bone marrow suppression with thrombocytopenia and agranulocytosis. Patients must be observed for signs of infection and of abnormal bleeding. Blood tests may be used to monitor cell counts. Thyroid suppressant drugs can cause hypothyroidism that may require replacement therapy with thyroid hormones.

Methimazole or PTU may be administered concurrently with **iodine solutions** in the preparation of patients for surgery. Three nonisotopic preparations of iodine are available: sodium iodide, potassium iodide, and Lugol's solution. All suppress the release of thyroid hormones and are also used in the management of thyrotoxicosis, or thyroid storm. This crisis of thyroid hyperactivity is often characterized by cardiac arrhythmias, since thyroid hormones sensitize the myocardium to the beta-stimulating effects of catecholamines. For this reason, the beta-blocker propranolol is also used in the treatment of thyrotoxicosis. Adverse effects of the iodides include allergic reactions, serum sickness, hemorrhage, and laryngeal edema that can be fatal. Skin rashes, swelling of the parotid glands, and soreness of the mouth, throat, and gums occur.

Radioactive iodine (sodium iodide 131) is used in the treatment of thyroid tumors, of hyperthyroidism in the elderly, and also diagnostically to determine thyroid function and to detect malignancy. It is given PO, and it concentrates in the thyroid, where it is cytotoxic. TSH may be coadministered to enhance uptake of the isotope by the gland. A frequent consequence of this treatment is hypothyroidism. Occasionally, inflammation of the thyroid (thyroiditis) occurs a few weeks after ^{131}I administration. This also can result in destruction of the gland. Administration of ^{131}I may temporarily increase circulating levels of hormone; propranolol can be used to suppress cardiac stimulation.

All antithyroid drugs are contraindicated during pregnancy. They suppress fetal gland activity and can produce persistent underactivity in the infant. Hypothyroidism in infants and children must be diagnosed and treated without delay by replacement of physiological amounts of T_3 and T_4. These hormones are essential to proper physical and mental growth and development; their absence in children results in the irreversible retardation of cretinism. In older children and adults, hypothyroidism (myxedema) is much less devastating, but the symptoms (e.g., cold intolerance and fatigue) are easily alleviated by replacement administration of a thyroid hormone preparation.

The thyroid gland produces three hormones. Calcitonin interacts with parathyroid hormone to regulate calcium metabolism (discussed in a later section). T_4 and T_3 influence many aspects of vital physiological function (e.g., metabolism, respiration, cardiovascular activity, and temperature regulation). These two hormones are usually present in a ratio of 4 to 1. Many tissues have the ability to convert T_4 to T_3, which is the more potent of the two.

There are several natural and synthetic thyroid preparations. **Thyroid** USP, **thyroglobulin** (the storage form of these hormones, called Proloid) and liotrix (Euthyroid) contain both T_3 and T_4; **levothyroxine** (Synthyroid) is T_4; **liothyronine** (Cytomel) and **dextrothyroxine** (Choloxin) are T_3. They are all orally active and have a slow onset of effect. Levothyroxine can be given IV when a more rapid response is needed. All are highly bound to plasma proteins such as thyroxine-binding globulin (TBG) and thyronine-binding prealbumin (TBPA). The thyroid hormones are metabolized in the liver and excreted in bile, from which they are subject to enterohepatic circulation. Side effects resemble the symptoms of hyperthyroidism: weight loss, nervousness, insomnia, and increased heat production. Cardiovascular stimulation resulting in tachycardia, angina, and congestive heart failure requires extreme caution when thyroid preparations are administered to the elderly and to persons with cardiovascular disease. Drug dosage should be adjusted to each patient and decreased at the first sign of toxicity. Thyroid hormones should not be administered to euthyroid persons for the purpose of weight reduction, as exogenous administration leads to reduction in endogenous hormone production.

The administration of thyroid hormones enhances the cardiovascular effects of sympathomimetic amines and tricyclic antidepressants. Increased metabolism of clotting factors potentiates anticoagulants. Phenytoin and the salicylates compete for plasma protein binding sites, increasing the levels of free hormone. Resins such as cholestyramine (Questran) reduce the enterohepatic circulation. Effects on metabolism may necessitate increased amounts of corticosteroids and hypoglycemic agents.

Parathyroid pharmacology

Parathyroid hormone (PTH) is secreted in response to decreased blood levels of calcium. PTH promotes calcium absorption from the GI tract and calcium resorption from bone and also increases renal excretion of phosphate. The thyroid hormone calcitonin opposes PTH by reducing bone resorption. These two hormones plus vitamin D regulate calcium metabolism. Symptoms of hypocalcemia include tetany and convulsions. Long-term treatment usually consists of administration of calcium salts and vitamin D. PTH may be used acutely to alleviate hypocalcemia; it must be injected, and the appearance of antibodies reduces its efficacy.

Vitamin D, available as **calcitriol** (Rocaltrol) and **dihydrotachysterol** (Hytakerol), increases bone resorption and intestinal uptake of oral calcium. Calcium salts (carbonate, lactate, gluconate, chloride) can be administered PO or parenterally. These preparations enhance the cardiovascular effects of digitalis. Thiazide diuretics can add to the hypercalcemic effect, whereas corticosteroids reduce it.

The adverse effects of therapy intended to elevate blood levels of calcium most frequently are due to hypercalcemia. Renal stones and renal failure may occur, as can osteoporosis, muscle weakness, hyporeflexia, confusion, cardiac arrhythmias, nausea, and other GI symptoms. Treatment of hypocalcemia requires caution in persons with cardiovascular or renal dysfunction. Calcium levels can be reduced by administering phosphates, which bind serum calcium, loop diuretics, which enhance calcium excretion, or synthetic salmon calcitonin (Calcimar).

Calcitonin, a thyroid hormone, has effects opposite to those of PTH. It inhibits bone resorption and promotes renal excretion of calcium. Calcitonin is administered parenterally (SC or IM) to alleviate hypercalcemia and will reduce the rate of bone metabolism in Paget's disease. Calcitonin is contraindicated in pregnancy and lactation. Relatively abundant amounts of serum calcium are needed in these physiological states. Nausea, allergic reactions, inflammation at injection sites, and antibody formation resulting in decreased efficacy can occur.

Other drugs that are used occasionally in the treatment of calcium disorders include sodium cellulose phosphate, which binds calcium and magnesium ions in the GI tract, thus preventing their absorption (there are many contraindications to the use of this drug), and etidronate disodium, which slows bone metabolism. The latter drug is especially useful in Paget's disease. Both drugs are contraindicated in pregnancy and lactation.

Pancreatic pharmacology

The pancreas is both exocrine and endocrine. It secretes digestive enzymes, which it releases directly into the upper intestine, and it also synthesizes the hormones insulin and glucagon. Failure of the exocrine pancreas causes digestive disorders. (The pharmacotherapy of these conditions was previously discussed under "Gastrointestinal Tract Pharmacology.")

The endocrine pancreas contributes to the regulation of carbohydrate, protein, and fat metabolism. **Insulin**, synthesized in the beta cells of the islets of Langerhans, is secreted in response to blood levels of glucose, amino acids, or ketone bodies and to some GI hormones. This hormone is required for the transport of glucose into most cells (liver and brain are notable exceptions). It promotes synthesis of glycogen (the storage form of glucose) and subsequent glycogenolysis to mobilize stored glucose when it is needed by the body. Insulin inhibits conversion of proteins to carbohydrates (gluconeogenesis) and promotes storage of free fatty acids. In the absence of insulin, increased metabolism of fatty acids produces "ketone bodies," which accumulate in the circulatory system and cause ketoacidosis, which can be fatal. **Glucagon**, synthe-

sized in alpha cells, opposes many of the actions of insulin and can be administered to reverse severe insulin reactions.

Failure of the endocrine pancreas results in **diabetes mellitus.** Juvenile-onset (insulin-dependent) diabetes usually begins early in life and involves a complete lack of insulin production. Treatment requires lifelong insulin replacement. Maturity-onset diabetes (noninsulin-dependent) develops later in life. The pancreas retains its ability to synthesize insulin but appears to secrete insufficient amounts. There is also evidence that insulin receptor sensitivity is altered in maturity-onset diabetes. Treatment involves combinations of dietary restrictions, weight loss if the patient is obese, and administration of hypoglcemic agents or insulin.

There are several forms of insulin (Table 6-20). The major differences among them are in onset and duration of action. All must be administered parenterally. Regular insulin has a rapid onset of action and can be administered IV in diabetic crises. The long-acting insulins help to prevent hypoglycemia during sleep. Insulins with varied onsets and durations are usually combined in order to provide more consistent control of blood glucose levels. Dosages and administration schedules must be individualized; variations in mealtimes should be avoided. Hypoglycemia is a constant danger, as glucose deprivation can damage brain cells. Diabetics must always be alert for signs of hypoglycemia (e.g., fatigue, hunger, tremor, weakness, and tachycardia). Orange juice, sugar, or candy can be used to counteract hypoglycemia. Dextrose or glucagon administered IV is especially useful if consciousness has been lost. Much research currently focuses on the development of infusion pumps that will supply insulin in response to physiological stimuli such as increases in blood glucose levels. Disease, renal dysfunction, stress, exercise, and many drugs can alter insulin requirements. The presence of protein in insulin derived from animal sources can provoke allergic reactions, as well as the production of antibodies and resistance to insulin's actions. (All endocrine preparations obtained from animal sources carry these risks.) Recombinant DNA techniques have now

Table 6-20. Insulin Preparations

Type	Onset (hours)	Duration (hours)
Rapid-acting		
Insulin (regular)	1/2–1	6–8
Insulin zinc (prompt or semilente)	1/2–1 1/2	12–16
Intermediate-acting		
Isophane insulin (NPH)	1–1 1/2	24
Insulin zinc (lente)	1–2 1/2	24
Long-acting		
Protamine zinc insulin (PZI)	4–8	36
Insulin zinc (ultralente)	4–8	36

provided a source of insulin (Humulin) that is free of these adverse effects.

Repeated SC injections of insulin lead to hypertrophy and atropy of subcutaneous fat (lipodystrophies). Injection sites should be alternated to minimize this effect. Dosage errors due to the availability of three insulin concentrations and three syringe types have decreased with the discontinuance of the U-80 form. In addition to U-40 and U-100 (40 and 100 units/ml, respectively), a highly concentrated form (U-500) is available for persons with resistant diabetes who require large doses of insulin.

The oral hypoglycemic agents (the **sulfonylureas**, Table 6-21) stimulate functional pancreatic cells to synthesize and secrete insulin and may also have a direct influence on the uptake of glucose by various tissues. In some persons, the response to these drugs may be lost after several months. In addition, stressors such as surgery or infection may temporarily necessitate administration of insulin. Transfer from insulin to oral agents must be done carefully. These drugs generally are hepatically metabolized; many bind extensively to plasma proteins. They are contraindicated during pregnancy. (Pregnancy in diabetic women is always high risk and must be closely monitored. Insulin is used to control blood glucose levels.)

As with insulin, the most prominent adverse effect of the oral antidiabetic agents is hypoglycemia. Suppression of bone marrow function and GI upset may occur. There are many drug interactions; alterations in hepatic metabolism and competition for protein binding in plasma are two of the mechanisms involved. The sulfonylureas interfere with the degradation of alcohol, causing a disulfiram-like reaction. Drugs that alter glucose kinetics (e.g., thiazide diuretics) will affect the requirements for hypoglycemic agents.

A controversial but well-publicized study (University Group Diabetes Program, published in 1970) reported that administration of tolbutamide increased the risk of cardiovascular incidents and that diabetic control by dietary measures was as effective as that obtained with pharmacotherpy. As with all drugs, the hypoglycemic agents should be used only when nondrug measures will not control disease.

Adrenal pharmacology

The adrenal cortex produces **glucocorticoid hormones**, which affect fat, carbohydrate, and protein metabolism, and **mineralocorticoids**, which affect electrolyte and water balance. These hormones together with epinephrine and norepinephrine secreted by the adrenal medulla mediate physiological responses to stress.

Endocrine disturbances of the cortex take the form of both hypo- and hyperactivity. Glucocorticoids, secreted in a negative feedback manner in response to plasma levels of corticotropin (ACTH), modulate utilization and storage of fatty acids, glucose, and proteins and also influence cardiovascular and CNS activity. Glucocorticoids (cortisol is the principal glucocorticoid in humans) are essential to survival and must be replaced when there is adrenal insufficiency (Addison's disease). Glucocorticoids may also be administered in greater than physiological amounts in the management of clinical conditions such as inflammatory and allergic disorders. The naturally occurring glucocorticoids have some mineralocorticoid activity, which is absent in most synthetic forms.

Glucocorticoids (Table 6-22) are administered PO, parenterally (IM, IV), and topically (including inhalation and intra-articular). Doses should be the lowest possible, and termination of therapy must always be done cautiously. Exogenous glucocorticoids suppress endogenous hypothalamic-pituitary-adrenal function, which recovers gradually as hormone administration is tapered. Abrupt withdrawal results in adrenal insufficiency, which can be life threatening. Endogenous secretion of cortisol follows a distinct circadian pattern with the highest levels occurring around the time of awakening. Administration of glucocorticoids once daily at this time causes much less suppression of the adrenal axis than do equally divided doses given throughout the day.

Glucocorticoids, both endogenous and exogenous, influence many physiological functions. Thus, administration of these substances, especially in large amounts, will cause numerous side effects. Alterations in metabolism result in redistribution of stored fat, increased blood levels of triglycerides

Table 6-21. Oral Hypoglycemic Agents

Generic name	Trade name	Recommended adult doses (mg PO/day)
Acetohexamide	Dymelor	250–1,500
Chlorpropamide	Diabinese	100–250 ,
Glipizide	Glucotrol	2.5–40
Glyburide	DiaBeta, Micronase	1.25–20 ,
Tolazamide	Tolinase	100–1,000
Tolbutamide	Orinase	1,000–2,000

Table 6-22. Glucocorticoids

Generic name	Trade name	Recommended adult doses (mg PO/day)
Cortisone	Cortone	20–300 (also IM)
Hydrocortisone	Cortef	20–240
Betamethasone	Celestone	0.6–7.2
Dexamethasone	several	0.75–9
Methylprednisolone	Medrol	4–48
Prednisolone	several	5–60
Prednisone	several	5–60
Triamcinolone	Aristocort	4–60

and glucose, muscle weakness and wasting, capillary and epidermal fragility, impaired healing of wounds, osteoporosis, and in children suppression of skeletal growth. Other adverse effects include development of gastric ulcers, decreased resistance to infections, electrolyte imbalance, and aberrations in CNS function.

There are many contraindications to the administration of glucocorticoids, such as gastric ulcer, hypertension, and osteoporosis. Drug interactions are numerous. Agents that induce hepatic enzymes will enhance the inactivation of glucocorticoids. Coadministration with anticholinergics increases the risk of elevated intraocular pressure. Salicylates and other drugs that are gastric irritants increase the risk of ulcer development. Severe hypokalemia can result when diuretics add to the potassium-wasting mineralocorticoid activity. The risk of hemorrhage in persons receiving anticoagulants may be either reduced or increased. Elevation of blood glucose levels may necessitate higher doses of hypoglycemic agents.

Adrenal dysfunction will also affect endogenous levels of the mineralocorticoids. The major one of these is **aldosterone**, which acts in the distal tubule of the nephron to increase the excretion of potassium and hydrogen ions and promote reabsorption of sodium, chloride, and water. Plasma volume and levels of sodium and potassium all influence the action of the renin-angiotensin-aldosterone system. The mineralocorticoids **desoxycorticosterone** (Doca, Percorten) and **fludrocortisone** (Florinef) must be used with caution in the presence of cardiovascular disease, since excessive fluid retention and hypertension may occur. (It is not always necessary to administer mineralocorticoids in adrenal insufficiency. Ingestion of sodium chloride plus the inherent mineralocorticoid activity of many glucocorticoids often provides sufficient replacement.) The mineralocorticoids can induce hypokalemia that can increase the risk of digitalis toxicity and decrease the efficacy of some antiarrhythmic drugs.

Cushing's syndrome or excessive adrenocortical influence can result from tumors that secrete ACTH or corticosteroids or can be iatrogenic (from administration of large amounts of corticosteroids). Endogenous hypersecretion may be amenable to surgical removal of tumors or to administration of **aminoglutethamide** (Cytaden) and **trilostane** (Modrastane), which inhibit synthesis of corticoids. These drugs are contraindicated in pregnancy. Care must be taken that adrenocortical function is not overly suppressed, especially in times of stress. **Metyrapone** (Metopirone) is an inhibitor of corticosteroid production that is used diagnostically to assess function in the adrenal axis.

Reproductive pharmacology

Testosterone is the major androgen produced by the testes. Its synthesis increases sharply in the early teens (at puberty). Testosterone regulates and maintains the development of the male sex organs and secondary sex characteristics. Together with inhibin and small amounts of estrogen synthesized in the seminiferous tubules, testosterone inhibits the release of pituitary gonadotropins (discussed under "Pituitary pharmacology") in a negative feedback manner. Testosterone enters cells of target tissues and is there enzymatically converted to its active form, dihydrotestosterone, which stimulates synthesis of RNA and thus of protein. Testosterone promotes growth in

many tissues (anabolic effect), but it also causes closure of the epiphyses of the long bones. Several androgenic drugs including orally active analogues (Table 6-23) are available for replacement therapy when endogenous testosterone is insufficient and for treatment of other clinical indications. Testosterone is rapidly inactivated by the hepatic enzymes and is not orally effective.

Several esters of testosterone are prepared in oil or implantable pellets so that absorption from IM or SC sites is prolonged and the interval between drug administrations can be extended. Testosterone and methyltestosterone are available in buccal tablets; **fluoxymesterone** (Halotestin) is given PO.

Hypogonadism (failure of the testes to synthesize testosterone) may become apparent before or after sexual development. In the former instance, exogenous testosterone replacement will promote normal development; in the latter, replacement prevents loss of masculine characteristics. When administration of testosterone has been used to induce sexual development, larger maintenance doses are needed than when development has occurred during natural puberty. Testosterone is not very effective in treating male infertility or impotence. In cryptorchidism, failure to respond to pituitary hormones may require that testosterone be administered. However, care must be taken not to induce premature puberty.

Androgenic drugs, in particular those with a short duration of action, are used in the treatment of advanced breast cancer in women. The major effects of euphoria and pain reduction are often accompanied by masculinizing side effects. The occurrence of hypercalcemia requires immediate cessation of drug therapy and administration of fluids to prevent precipitation of calcium in the kidneys.

Table 6-23. Androgens

Generic name	Trade name	Recommended adult doses
Testosterone	several	10–100 mg IM 2–3 times/week
Testosterone propionate	several	200–400 mg IM every 2–4 weeks
Testosterone enanthate	several	10–100 mg IM 2–3 times/week
Danazol	Danocrine	100–800 mg PO/day
Fluoxymesterone	Halotestin	2–30 mg PO/day
Methyltestosterone	several	10–200 mg PO/day
Nandrolone	Deca-Durabolin, others	25–100 mg IM every 1–4 weeks
Oxandrolone	Anavar	2.5–20 mg PO/day
Stanozolol	Winstrol	4–6 mg PO/day
Testolactone	Teslac	1 g PO/day

Androgens are effective in treating severe anemia. They stimulate renal production of erythropoietin and may also have a direct effect on bone marrow activity. Several synthetic testosterone analogues have marked anabolic activity and reduced androgenicity. These may be administered in clinical conditions characterized by negative nitrogen balance (e.g., after surgery, debilitating illness, or extensive burns). Their efficacy is not proven, however, and patients often convalesce just as well when adequate nutrition is provided.

The androgens, including those used as anabolics, have serious adverse effects in addition to those already noted. Retention of sodium and fluid can lead to congestive heart failure and/or elevation of blood pressure. For this reason, caution is required in persons who have preexisting cardiovascular disease. Hepatitis and hepatic carcinoma may occur. Androgens are contraindicated in pregnancy (they are teratogenic) and in enlargement or cancer of the prostate gland.

Androgens increase the therapeutic effectiveness of anticoagulants and antidiabetic agents. Anabolic androgens can be used to reduce corticosteroid-induced osteoporosis, but the combination may result in severe edema. Drugs such as barbiturates, which induce the hepatic enzymes, can reverse the effects of the androgens.

Secretion of the **female hormones (estrogens** and **progestins)** begins during puberty and continues in a marked cyclical pattern (menstrual cycle) until about the age of 50, when menopause occurs. As in males, the anterior pituitary in females begins in the early teens to release large amounts of gonadotropins. FSH stimulates growth of ovarian follicles, which begin to secrete estrogens. LH is secreted in small amounts until the second week of each cycle, when a rapid increase in hormone causes ovulation or release of the ovum from the follicle. The ovum is carried to the uterus, which, under the influence of estrogens, has been prepared for embryo implantation if the ovum is fertilized. During this time, LH has converted the empty follicle into the corpus luteum, which secretes progesterone. Progesterone inhibits gonadotropin secretion in a negative feedback manner. As LH levels fall, the corpus luteum loses its capacity to function. Since the endometrium (lining of the uterus) requires progesterone to remain intact, it begins to slough off as the menstrual flow. However, if ovum fertilization and implantation into the endometrium have occurred, the cells that will become the placenta begin to secrete HCG, which enables the corpus luteum to continue secretion of progesterone so that the uterus will remain in the pregnant state. The continued presence of progesterone suppresses FSH and LH secretion from the pituitary, thus the menstrual cycle is temporarily interrupted until pregnancy has ended. The placenta also synthesizes estrogens.

In addition to causing proliferation of the uterus lining, estrogens affect many other tissues and cause the characteristic changes that occur in girls in puberty: development of the reproductive organs and breasts, calcification of bone, and closure of the epiphyses. The ovary produces estradiol-17β, estrone, and estriol; there are several synthetic forms of these hormones. Progesterone suppresses uterine contractility and prepares breast tissue for lactation.

Estrogens and **progestins** (Table 6-24) have several clinical uses. Combinations of various forms and in various doses are

Table 6-24. Estrogens and Progestins

Generic name	Trade name	Recommended adult doses (mg PO/day)
Estrogens		
Estradiol	Estrace	1–2
Estradiol valerate	several	10–20 mg IM, every 4 weeks
Conjugated estrogens	Premarin	1.25–7.5
Diethylstilbestrol		0.2–0.5
Estrone	Bestrone	0.1–0.5 mg IM, 1–3 times/week
Ethinyl estradiol	Estinyl	0.02–0.05
Chlorotrianisene	TACE	12–25
Progestins		
Progesterone		5–10 mg IM/day
Hydroxyprogesterone	Delalutin	1 g IM/week
Medroxyprogesterone	Provera	5–10 mg
Norethindrone	Norlutin	10–30 mg

used as oral contraceptives that suppress release of FSH and LH so that ovulation does not occur. The inclusion of estrogen causes uterine proliferation, and changes in the progesterone content of the tablets taken later in each cycle allow sloughing comparable to the menstrual flow. Concern over the possible carcinogenicity of long-term exposure to estrogen led to the development of oral contraceptives containing progestins only ("mini-pill"). However, these do not suppress gonadotropin secretion as completely as the combination contraceptives, and unwanted pregnancy can occur. The synthetic estrogen diethylstilbestrol is a postcoital ("morning after") contraceptive. Administration must be started within 72 hours of intercourse, and it is not recommended for frequent therapy.

Estrogens are used to reduce many of the symptoms of menopause, which are the result of decreasing levels of female hormones and unopposed secretion of pituitary gonadotropins. Progestins alleviate symptoms of endometriosis and endometrial cancers. Estrogens are somewhat effective in the treatment of prostate cancer and of breast cancer, especially after menopause has occurred.

The estrogen-progesterone oral contraceptives have been used in the treatment of painful menses (dysmenorrhea). However, the relief from a few days of discomfort each month requires chronic exposure to these drugs. Recent advances in the knowledge of female physiology have led to the use of the NSAIDs such as naproxen (Anaprox) and ibuprofen (Motrin) to reduce prostaglandin synthesis and thus alleviate many menstrual symptoms.

All dosage forms of the estrogens and progestins are relatively rapidly metabolized in the liver and are given cautiously if at all to persons with hepatic dysfunction. The naturally occurring hormones are too quickly destroyed to be active after PO administration. Estrogen is available in transdermal form (Estraderm). Because of their effect on blood coagulation, estrogens increase the risk of thromboembolism (especially in women who smoke cigarettes) and are contraindicated in persons with hypercoagulation disorders. The therapeutic efficacy of anticoagulants is reduced. Estrogens cause retention of sodium and water, which can lead to elevation in blood pressure. Estrogens and progestins are teratogenic, and their use during pregnancy is contraindicated. Thus if a woman desiring to take oral contraceptives has any possibility of being pregnant, that must be ruled out before drug administration is begun. Estrogens are carcinogenic and are contraindicated in certain forms of cancer.

Coadministration of drugs that induce hepatic enzymes can reduce the effectiveness of estrogens and progestins, leading to failure of contraception. Estrogens may increase or decrease requirements for anticonvulsant drugs, and they inhibit the hepatic inactivation of corticosteroids. Women who both smoke and use oral contraceptives often require larger than usual amounts of vitamin C. Women over the age of 35 who smoke should not use oral contraceptives.

VITAMINS

Vitamins are organic compounds required for normal physiological function. Healthy persons who consume a well-balanced diet of fresh and properly prepared foods usually do not require supplemental vitamins. However, deficiencies can cause serious illness. The **fat-soluble vitamins** (A,D, E, and K) are stored in adipose and hepatic tissue, and deficiencies appear gradually. **Water-soluble vitamins** (B complex and C) are not stored, thus lack of these substances rapidly produces characteristic symptoms. Replacement forms of most vitamins can be administered both PO and parenterally.

Vitamin A (retinol) is essential to proper growth and skeletal development, for synthesis of steroid hormones, and for night vision. It is obtained from carotenoid precursors in yellow and leafy vegetables and organ meats. To be absorbed from the GI tract, fat-soluble vitamins require the presence of bile salts. Administration of mineral oil or bile acid sequestrants such as cholestyramine can induce deficiencies of the fat-soluble vitamins. Clinical conditions such as cystic fibrosis, hepatic cirrhosis, and GI surgery can reduce the absorption and storage of vitamin A. Symptoms of deficiency include dryness of the skin and mucous membranes, night blindness, and corneal changes that can lead to loss of vision. Diarrhea and renal stones can develop as the integrity of the intestine and kidney epithelium is lost. Overdose of vitamin A ("hypervitaminosis A") can cause toxic symptoms including increased intracranial pressure, fatigue, headache, hepatic dysfunction, and premature epiphyseal closure in children.

Vitamin D (cholecalciferol), together with parathyroid hormone, regulates calcium and phosphate metabolism. It is obtained from egg yolks and animal and fish oils. Most milk sold in the United States has added vitamin D. In addition, ultraviolet irradiation (e.g., with sunlight) of the skin converts the inactive precursor 7-dehydrocholesterol to vitamin D. Symptoms of vitamin D deficiency are softening of bone (rickets in children, osteomalacia in adults) and infantile tetany.

Serum calcium and phosphate levels are reduced, and alkaline phosphatase is elevated. Impaired renal function can reduce the conversion of vitamin D to its active form. Pancreatitis or malabsorption syndrome hinders the absorption of vitamin D administered PO. This vitamin is contraindicated in hypercalcemia and hyperphosphatemia. Excessive amounts of vitamin D produce nausea, drowsiness, muscle weakness, thirst, and polyuria. Calcium is mobilized from bone and deposited in soft tissues. Irreversible renal damage can develop. Hypercalcemia can precipitate arrhythmias, especially in persons with cardiovascular disease.

Vitamin E (the tocopherols) is an antioxidant that appears to influence many physiological functions (e.g., steroid and muscle metabolism, heme and porphyrin synthesis, utilization of vitamin A, and reproduction). Dietary sources include vegetable oils, nuts, eggs, whole grains, and milk. Drugs and pathological conditions that hinder absorption of fats can contribute to vitamin E deficiency. Skeletal muscle lesions similar to muscular dystrophy and anemia due to fragility and disruption of erythrocytes occur when vitamin E is inadequate. Administration is usually PO, although in severe deficiency the parenteral route can be used. The toxicity of vitamin E is low. GI and genital tract disturbances and muscle weakness have been reported. Vitamin E may increase the effectiveness of the oral anticoagulants.

The hepatic synthesis of clotting factors is dependent on adequate amounts of **vitamin K**, which can be administered to reverse the action of the oral anticoagulants. A significant proportion of this vitamin is derived from intestinal bacteria and absorbed in the same manner as other fat-soluble vitamins. Persons receiving antibiotics that reduce the endogenous flora may begin to show signs of hypoprothrombinemia and prolonged clotting time. This vitamin can be obtained from dietary sources such as nuts, cheese, organ meats, and leafy vegetables. Phytonadione, or vitamin K_1, administered IV can provoke severe anaphylactoid reactions; the solution must be carefully diluted and administered by slow infusion. Hemolytic anemia has been reported in G6PD-deficient persons receiving menadione. For vitamin K to be effective, hepatocytes must have the capacity to synthesize clotting factors. Large doses of vitamin K can suppress hepatic function, and in infants can cause hyperbilirubinemia and fatal brain damage.

The **B vitamins** are a series or "complex" of water-soluble substances that influence several aspects of metabolism. They do not accumulate in tissues, thus must be replenished regularly. Deficiencies are usually to more than a single B vitamin.

Vitamin B_1 (thiamine) is essential for nerve conduction, carbohydrate metabolism, and energy production. Dietary sources for this vitamin include unprocessed cereal grains, meat, nuts, and yeast. B_1 deficiencies produce changes in nerve function that are manifested as beriberi, Wernicke's syndrome, and Korsakoff's psychosis. Alcoholics and persons on a limited diet frequently are deficient in thiamine. Changes in GI pH produced by antacids and gastric secretion suppressants lead to the destruction of dietary vitamin B. A diet high in carbohydrates increases the need for this vitamin. Anaphylactoid reactions have been reported following IV administration of thiamine.

Vitamin B_2 (riboflavin) is required in the function of the mitochondria. It is found in eggs, milk, yeast, leafy vegetables, liver, and meat. Symptoms of deficiency include corneal vascularization with burning and photophobia, dermatitis, and deterioration of the oral mucous membranes. IM injection sites for riboflavin should be rotated to avoid irritation.

Vitamin B₃ (niacin or nicotinic acid) is incorporated into nicotinamide adenine dinucleotide (NAD) and nicotinamide adenine dinucleotide phosphate (NADP), which are hydrogen acceptors in the oxidation-reduction reactions of energy production. This vitamin is derived from yeast, nuts, liver, and meats. Pellagra develops in niacin deficiency. This disorder is characterized by skin eruptions, red swollen tongue, and CNS disturbances ranging from confusion and depression to hallucinations and dementia. Niacin causes vasodilation and flushing, especially of the face and neck. A fall in blood pressure may occur, causing dizziness and adding to the hypotensive action of other drugs. Excessive amounts of niacin can produce vomiting, peptic ulceration, hepatic damage, and cardiac arrhythmias. Administration requires caution or may be contraindicated in persons with history of any of the latter three disorders. During therapy with this vitamin, hepatic function should be monitored and diabetics observed for blood glucose control.

Vitamin B₅ (pantothenic acid) deficiency is rare and appears only when pantothenic antagonists are administered. Symptoms include fatigue, GI disturbances, and psychosis. Pantothenic acid is a component of coenzyme A, necessary for carbohydrate and fatty acid metabolism. It is available for PO administration.

Vitamin B₆ (pyridoxine) is required for the metabolism of amino acids and carbohydrates. Deficiencies can be induced by such drugs as hydralazine, isonicotinylhydrazine (isoniazid, INH), and oral contraceptives. Lack of vitamin B₆ can produce seizures in children and neuritis, irritability, and depression in adults. Dermatologic and mucous membrane changes and anemia may occur. Dietary sources of pyridoxine include liver, whole grains, yeast, and meats. Administration of vitamin B₆ can cause flushing, paresthesias, and pain following injection. Pyridoxine is a cofactor for the dopa decarboxylase enzyme, thus can reduce the efficacy of levodopa.

Vitamin B₉ (folic acid) is required for production of the formed elements of blood. Deficiency of this vitamin results in megaloblastic anemia. Green leafy vegetables and eggs are the major source of folate, which is converted to the tetrahydrofolate active form. The action of this vitamin is blocked by methotrexate. Folic acid reduces serum levels of the anticonvulsant phenytoin, which in turn may suppress folate levels. The oral contraceptives can induce a mild folate depletion.

Vitamin B₁₂ (cyanocobalamin) is essential for hematopoiesis and myelin synthesis. It is found in egg yolk, fish, and organ meats. Deficiency results in anemia, neurological symptoms, and spinal cord degeneration. The parenteral route (IM or SC) is preferred, since it provides more complete absorption of the vitamin, especially in the presence of pernicious anemia. Administration of vitamin B₁₂ can cause thrombosis, peripheral edema, hypokalemia, congestive heart failure, and allergic responses including anaphylactic shock.

Vitamin C (ascorbic acid) is important for carbohydrate metabolism, for synthesis of collagen and healing of burns and wounds, and for the formation of folinic acid. Stressors such as infections and chronic illness increase the utilization of vitamin C. Citrus fruits, tomatoes, and green vegetables are especially rich in this water-soluble, heat-labile vitamin. Ascorbic acid deficiency produces scurvy, characterized by anemia and spontaneous bleeding of mucous membranes. Excessive amounts of this water-soluble substance are renally excreted and can cause renal stones. Urinary pH may be lowered, promoting reabsorption of acidic drugs and crystallization of the sulfonamide antibiotics. Hemolytic anemia can occur in G6PD-deficient persons. Smoking of cigarettes shortens the plasma half-life of vitamin C.

ELECTROLYTES AND TRACE ELEMENTS

The major electrolytes, required for proper physiological function, are the cations calcium, magnesium, potassium, and sodium and the bicarbonate, chloride, and phosphate anions. Body content of these ions is finely controlled in particular by the kidneys, which excrete or reabsorb electrolytes in response to many stimuli, and by the lungs, which participate in bicarbonate metabolism by excreting carbon dioxide. The possibility of electrolyte imbalance must be considered after any loss of body fluids: excessive vomiting or diarrhea, gastric suction, hemorrhage, and extensive burns. Diseases such as diabetes mellitus, renal dysfunction, and hypo- or hypersecretion of adrenocortical or parathyroid hormones will alter electrolyte levels, as will the administration of certain drugs, most notably the diuretics.

Sodium is the most abundant extracellular ion. It is replaced daily by dietary ingestion and is actively conserved by the kidneys, often at the expense of potassium and hydrogen. Intake of large amounts of fluid either by mouth or by IV infusion will dilute body sodium, resulting in hyponatremia. Sodium can be replaced by increasing dietary salt (NaCl) consumption or by IV administration of isotonic (0.9%) or hypertonic sodium chloride solution.

Calcium is important for many physiological actions like muscle contraction, blood coagulation, and CNS function. Bones and teeth are composed of calcium. (Calcium metabolism is discussed under "Parathyroid pharmacology.") Milk and other dairy products are rich sources of calcium; several calcium salts are available for PO or IV administration. Adequate calcium amounts are essential during pregnancy and lactation. Intake of calcium is often advised for postmenopausal women to counteract bone resorption and osteoporosis. Calcium salts may be used in the management of acute myocardial infarction, to increase myocardial contraction and responsiveness to defibrillation. Calcium increases both the therapeutic and toxic effects of the digitalis glycosides. In susceptible individuals, increased calcium intake can lead to renal stones.

Potassium is an intracellular ion involved in muscle contraction, nerve impulse transmission, and many other physiological processes. It must be replaced daily by dietary intake. Under aldosterone influence, potassium is excreted in exchange for reabsorbed sodium in the distal tubule of the nephron. Administration of diuretics can cause hypokalemia (low blood levels of potassium), although under most circumstances intracellular levels remain sufficient. However, persons receiving digitalis are at increased risk of drug toxicity. The potassium-sparing diuretics can cause hyperkalemia (retention of potassium). Marked increases or decreases in myocardial potassium can cause cardiac arrest. Liquid and tablet forms of potassium salts are available for PO administration; GI upset and ulceration are frequent side effects. IV solutions must be well diluted and administered slowly, preferably in a large vein. Renal dysfunction, Addisons's disease, and potassium-sparing diuretic therapy are contraindications to the administration of potassium salts, and caution is required in patients with cardiovascular disease. Hyperkalemia can be treated with sodium polystyrene sulfonate (Kayexalate), a resin that exchanges sodium for potassium in the GI tract. Since this drug adds to sodium intake, it must be used cautiously in the elderly, in congestive heart failure, hypertension, and other conditions sensitive to sodium overload or potassium depletion. Calcium and magnesium are also bound by this resin. GI symptoms, including fecal impaction in the elderly, can occur. Most ion exchange occurs in the large intestine, thus this drug may be administered rectally. The suspension should be retained in the colon for 3 to 4 hours.

Magnesium is an intracellular ion that acts as cofactor for many enzymes. Like potassium, it is protective against digitalis toxicity. Magnesium sulfate may be administered PO or IV. Magnesium depresses CNS activity and neuromuscular transmission, thus is used occasionally to control convulsions. Excessive elevation of magnesium will cause severe CNS depression (CNS depressant drugs can add to this effect), hypotension, and cardiovascular and respiratory depression. Loss of the knee-jerk reflex requires that magnesium administration be stopped. IV calcium salts may be used to reverse magnesium toxicity, but in patients receiving digitalis this combination may result in complete heart block. Magnesium is contraindicated in the presence of heart block or myocardial infarction, and extreme caution must be used in other cardiovascular disorders and in renal dysfunction. The action of neuromuscular blocking drugs (e.g., succinylcholine) may be enhanced by magnesium.

Chloride is an extracellular ion important in the regulation of acid-base balance. Chloride loss occurs together with sodium loss, thus hyponatremia is always alleviated with sodium chloride. Depletion of chloride results in retention of bicarbonate ion and metabolic alkalosis.

Bicarbonate ion depletion results in acidosis. Any factor that influences renal function, such as disease, alteration in urinary pH (which influences ionization of carbonic acid), changes in potassium excretion, and administration of diuretics (which remove chloride ions together with sodium), can alter acid-base balance. Sodium bicarbonate can be administered to correct bicarbonate deficit. IV administration during acute myocardial infarction may correct acidosis caused by respiratory depression. This salt is also used as an antacid and as a urinary alkalinizer to promote excretion of acid drugs. Self-mediation (e.g., with household baking soda) can lead to systemic alkalosis. Administration is contraindicated in congestive heart failure, edema, and other disorders aggravated by sodium excess. Extravasation during IV administration will cause severe tissue damage. Sodium lactate, occasionally used to correct metabolic acidosis, is hepatically converted to bicarbonate. **Tromethamine** (Tham) corrects acidosis by binding hydrogen ions; it is administered only by the IV route. Extravasation can cause tissue necrosis as a result of local

vasoconstriction. Phentolamine or procaine with hyaluronidase can be used to restore tissue perfusion. Renal function must be adequate before administration of any agent intended to correct electrolyte or acid-base imbalance. Blood gases and electrolytes should be measured before and throughout therapy.

Phosphate ions are involved in skeletal development, in leukocyte and platelet function, and in maintaining acid-base balance. Hypophosphatemia can be corrected by administration of potassium phosphate or sodium phosphate (PO administration can cause diarrhea). Excessive phosphate levels, which may occur in renal failure or exposure to organophosphate insecticides, can be reduced by administration of antacids containing calcium or aluminum, which bind to phosphate. Similarly, phosphate ion administered in hypercalcemia will bind calcium and promote its transport to bone. (Phosphate and calcium metabolism are discussed under "Parathyroid pharmacology.")

Several **metal ions** are needed in minute or trace amounts for various physiological actions.

Iodine is required by the thyroid gland for the synthesis of the hormones thyroxine and triiodothyronine. This element is found in many foods and is routinely added to table salt ("iodized salt"). Excessive amounts of iodine can produce hypersecretion or suppression of release of thyroid hormones. Iodine is well absorbed from the GI tract, thus increased dietary intake or PO administration of iodide salts is usually therapeutic in iodine deficiency if the thyroid gland is functional. Iodine is excreted in the urine. Allergic reactions to iodine can occur. Some radioactive and radiopaque diagnostic agents contain iodine.

Copper is cofactor for many enzymes and is essential for blood coagulation and for hemoglobin function. Copper is present in many foods and in drinking water, and deficiencies are uncommon. Copper excess reverses the utilization of zinc and iron and causes cardiovascular changes that can be fatal. Copper is stored in liver and kidney; it is excreted in bile. Wilson's disease is retention of excessive amounts of copper.

Iron is essential for hemoglobin synthesis; a deficiency will produce anemia. Large amounts of iron are required during pregnancy, otherwise iron deficiencies usually occur only when there is significant blood loss. Iron is present in many foods and is absorbed from the GI tract, especially in the less-ionized ferrous form. Vitamin C (ascorbic acid) promotes absorption of iron. Hypersensitivity to iron should be ruled out before it is administered. Several iron salts are available for PO administration but are contraindicated in peptic ulcer and require caution in the presence of other GI disorders since they cause GI irritation and bleeding. This can be reduced if the drug is taken with a small amount of food. However, food will interfere with the absorption of the iron. Antacids and tetracyclines also decrease the absorption of iron salts administered PO. Iron with dextran is available for parenteral administration when the PO route is unacceptable. Subcutaneous tissue may be stained or damaged, thus injection should be deep IM. The IV route may be used in severe deficiency but is quite hazardous. Accumulation of excessive iron, as might result from overdose of iron preparations, from frequent blood transfusions, or in thalassemia can be treated with deferoxamine (Desferal), which preferentially chelates the ferric ion. The complex is renally excreted. Kidney dysfunction is a contraindication to administration. Deferoxamine can cause red discoloration of the urine. Slow SC infusion appears to be most efficient because it provides prolonged contact with body iron stores. IM and slow IV infusion are also used. Adverse effects include pain at the injection site, allergy, cataracts, GI upset, tachycardia, and vision changes. Shock can occur with rapid IV administration. Deferoxamine may be teratogenic.

Chromium, cobalt, manganese, and zinc are additional trace elements. Chromium affects glucose metabolism by modulating the action of insulin. Cobalt is essential for vitamin B_{12} function; excessive levels cause polycythemia. Manganese is cofactor for many enzymes. Zinc is important for the activity of several enzymes required for normal growth and development. Zinc salts, including the oxide ointment that can be purchased without prescription, have been used to enhance the healing of wounds.

Excessive levels of some metal ions can be reduced by pharmacologic agents. Deferoxamine, which removes iron, has been discussed. **Calcium disodium EDTA** will combine with chromium, copper, zinc, lead, nickel, and manganese. Administration is IM or IV. The latter enhances elevated intracranial pressure if cerebral edema is present. Renal damage and bone marrow suppression can occur by either route. **Disodium EDTA** binds calcium, zinc, and magnesium and promotes potassium excretion. It is given IV and can cause thrombophlebitis, hypoglycemia, convulsions, arrhythmias, and respiratory arrest. **Dimercaprol** removes arsenic, gold, and mercury. Overdose of the latter two ions may be iatrogenic after the administration of mercurial diuretics or gold salts. Dimercaprol must be given by deep IM injection, which can be painful. Tachycardia, hypertension, and kidney damage may occur. The latter can be minimized by maintaining urine at alkaline pH. Dimercaprol may be given concurrently with calcium disodium EDTA in lead poisoning. It should not be used in cadmium, iron, or selenium toxicity. The drug is hepatically inactivated.

BIBLIOGRAPHY

Two books are excellent resources for extensive information on all drugs:

Gilman AG, Goodman LS, Rall TW, et al (eds): The Pharmacological Basis of Therapeutics, 7th ed. Macmillan, New York, 1985.

American Medical Association: AMA Drug Evaluations, 6th ed. American Medical Association, Chicago, 1986.

The Medical Letter on Drugs and Therapeutics, published biweekly by the The Medical Letter, Inc., New Rochelle, NY, contains reports of new drugs, new indications and adverse effects, and frequent reviews of pharmacologic interest.

Reviews and Reports on specific topics:

Abramowicz M (ed): Acute drug abuse reactions. Med Lett Drugs Ther 27:77, 1985.

Abramowicz M (ed): The choice of antimicrobial drugs. Med Lett Drugs Ther 28:33, 1986.

Bader A, Hunt CO, Ostheimer GW: Systemic medications during labor and delivery. Res Staff Physician 32:41, 1986.

Bruni J, Albright PS: The clinical pharmacology of antiepileptic drugs. Clin Neuropharmacol 7:1, 1984.

Bullingham RES: Optimum management of postoperative pain. Drugs 29:376, 1985.

Carter SK: Adjuvant chemotherapy of cancer: A review of its current status. Drugs 31:337, 1986.

Cohen JL: Pharmacokinetic changes in aging. Am J Med 80(Suppl 5A):31, 1986.

Ferguson RK, Vlasses PH: Hypertensive emergencies and urgencies. JAMA 255:1607, 1986.

Gerber JG, Nies AS: Beta-adrenergic blocking drugs. Annu Rev Med 36:145, 1985.

Hill RM, Tennyson LM: Drug-induced malformations in humans. In Stern L (ed): Drug Use in Pregnancy. Williams and Wilkins, Baltimore, 1984.

Lant A: Diuretics: Clinical pharmacology and therapeutic uses. Drugs 29:57 (part I), 162 (part II), 1985.

Peachy JE, Naranjo CA: The role of drugs in the treatment of alcoholism. Drugs 27:171, 1984.

Vaughn Williams, EM: Classification of antiarrhythmic drugs. In Sandoe et al (eds): Cardiac Arrhythmias. Ad Astra, Södertälje, Sweden, 1970. pp. 449–473.

SAMPLE QUESTIONS

DIRECTIONS: Each question below contains four suggested answers of which **one** or **more** is correct. Choose the answer:

A if **1, 2, and 3** are correct
B if **1 and 3** are correct
C if **2 and 4** are correct
D if **4** is correct
E if **1, 2, 3, and 4** are correct

1. Enhancement of cholinergic activity in the neuromuscular junction will reverse the effects of

1. decamethonium
2. pancuronium
3. succinylcholine
4. tubocurarine

2. Which of the following drugs can be administered by IV bolus during acute myocardial infarction?

1. Bretylium
2. Dopamine
3. Verapamil
4. Isoproterenol

3. In the treatment of Parkinson's disease, the efficacy of levodopa is reduced by

1. progression of the disease
2. vitamin B_6 administration
3. a high-protein diet
4. dopa-decarboxylase inhibitors

4. Mental depression is a frequent adverse effect of the administration of

1. propranolol
2. methylphenidate
3. cimetidine
4. lithium

5. Opiate drugs are used clinically for their

1. antiemetic effects
2. antidiarrheal effects
3. ability to relieve cerebral edema
4. antitussive effects

6. All persons living in the United States should be inoculated against

1. poliomyelitis
2. hepatitis
3. diphtheria
4. rabies

DIRECTIONS: Each group of questions below consists of lettered choices followed by several numbered items. For each numbered item select the **one** lettered choice with which it is **most** closely associated. Each lettered choice may be used once, more than once, or not at all.

Questions 7–10. For each of the drugs listed below, choose the condition for which it provides relief.

A. Grand mal seizures
B. Petit mal seizures
C. Insomnia
D. Depression
E. Parkinsonism

7. Triazolam

8. Ethosuximide

9. Maprotiline

10. Primidone

Questions 11–13. For each of the dopamine doses listed below, choose the desired effect.

A. Positive inotropy
B. Vasoconstriction
C. Increased renal blood flow
D. Decreased blood pressure
E. Decreased stroke volume

11. 0.5 to 2 mcg/kg/minute

12. 2 to 10 mcg/kg/minute

13. 10 to 20 mcg/kg/minute

Questions 14–16. For each of the drug interactions listed below, choose the pair of drugs in which the first drug would have that effect on the second.

A. Imipramine/guanethidine
B. Furosemide/lithium
C. Allopurinol/azathioprine
D. Phenobarbital/warfarin
E. Cimetidine/diazepam

14. Impedes distribution to site of action

15. Reduces renal excretion

16. Enhances biotransformation

Questions 17–19. For each of the effects on calcium metabolism listed below, choose the agent that produces that effect.

A. Parathyroid hormone
B. Sodium cellulose phosphate
C. Cyanocobalamin
D. Calcitonin
E. Calcitriol

17. Binds calcium in the GI tract

18. Increases renal excretion of phosphate

19. Reduces bone resorption

Questions 20–23. For each of the infectious diseases listed below, choose the related characteristic.

A. Prevented by oral vaccine
B. Responsive to amantadine
C. Responsive to penicillin
D. Responsive to isoniazid
E. None of the above

20. Hepatitis B

21. Poliomyelitis

22. Syphilis

23. Tuberculosis

Questions 24–26. For each of the possible causative factors of vitamin deficiency listed below, choose the vitamin most likely to become deficient.

A. Vitamin A
B. Vitamin B_1
C. Vitamin B_5
D. Vitamin B_9
E. Vitamin C

24. Alcohol abuse

25. Administration of bile acid sequestrants

26. Use of oral contraceptives

Questions 27–31. For each of the general anesthetics listed below, choose the associated characteristic.

    A. Oxygen administered concurrently
    B. Hepatotoxicity
    C. Rapid induction
    D. Good skeletal muscle relaxation
    E. Hallucinations during recovery

27. Thiopental

28. Ether

29. Nitrous oxide

30. Ketamine

31. Halothane

Questions 31–36. For each of the analgesic groups listed below, select the corresponding characteristic.

    A. Produce marked physiological dependence
    B. Associated with Reye's syndrome in children
    C. Overdose causes fatal hepatotoxicity
    D. Induce withdrawal in opiate-dependent persons
    E. None of the above

32. Narcotic agonist-antagonists

33. Narcotic analgesics

34. Salicylates

35. Acetaminophen

36. Nonsteroidal anti-inflammatory drugs

Questions 37–40. For each of the hypertensive agents listed below, choose the associated adverse effect.

    A. Prolonged atrioventricular conduction velocity
    B. Tachycardia
    C. Hyperkalemia
    D. Hypokalemia
    E. None of the above

37. Captopril

38. Hydralazine

39. Propranolol

40. Hydrochlorothiazide

Questions 41–45. For each of the antineoplastic agents listed below, choose the associated adverse effect.

    A. Hemorrhagic cystitis
    B. Folic acid deficiency
    C. Cardiotoxicity
    D. Neurotoxicity
    E. Almost 100% incidence of nausea and vomiting

41. Methotrexate

42. Vincristine

43. Cyclophosphamide

44. Doxorubicin

45. Cisplatin

Questions 46–49. For each of the antacids listed below, choose the associated adverse effect.

    A. Systemic alkalosis
    B. Diarrhea
    C. Hypophosphatemia
    D. Systemic acidosis
    E. None of the above

46. Magnesium hydroxide

47. Calcium carbonate

48. Sodium bicarbonate

49. Aluminum hydroxide

Questions 50–54. For each of the antibacterial agents listed below, choose the associated adverse effect.

    A. Permanent discoloration of tooth enamel
    B. Ototoxicity
    C. Disulfiram-like reaction following alcohol ingestion
    D. Hemolytic anemia in persons with G6PD deficiency
    E. Bone marrow depression

50. Moxalactam

51. Sulfinpyrazone

52. Streptomycin

53. Chloramphenicol

54. Tetracycline

ANSWERS

1. C	15. B	29. A	42. D
2. B	16. D	30. E	43. A
3. A	17. B	31. B	44. C
4. B	18. A	32. D	45. E
5. C	19. D	33. A	46. B
6. B	20. E	34. B	47. A
7. C	21. A	35. C	48. A
8. B	22. C	36. E	49. C
9. D	23. D	37. C	50. C
10. A	24. B	38. B	51. D
11. C	25. A	39. A	52. B
12. A	26. E	40. D	53. E
13. B	27. C	41. B	54. A
14. A	28. D		

7

BEHAVIORAL SCIENCES

Frank Pastore

What follows is an extensive array of facts that are garnered from the lecture series, textbooks on behavioral sciences and psychiatry, journal articles, and relevant books. This chapter is not an attempt to teach behavioral sciences, but rather it explores facts and ideas that are particularly relevant to the National Medical Boards Part I. The subject matter can be divided into five sections: (1) development, (2) understanding human behavior, (3) psychopathology, (4) the physician's role, and (5) the physician and society.

DEVELOPMENT

Human development is an incredibly complex phenomenon. It is complicated by the fact that it is constantly changing and each phase offers a world of observations. It is also an area of relatively new knowledge. Although infant development is studied by dozens of noted scientists, adult development is studied by relatively few. Not only are there many different and unique stages of development, but each stage can be studied from a variety of perspectives. Students must familiarize themselves with each of these perspectives. Take a few minutes to review the variety of stages and perspectives listed below before proceeding with the rest of the material.

The life cycle. One develops a personality not at a steady pace but rather in phases. There are periods of relative quiescence followed by marked changes and rapid growth. This is true throughout one's life.

The epigenic principle. As in embryology and psychoanalytic theory, development progresses when each phase is properly met and mastered at the proper time and in the proper sequence. Humans add a dimension of flexibility that is enormous, and in spite of not achieving certain milestones, a person has the ability to adapt in remarkable ways.

The phases. The developmental phases are as follows: (1) prenatal, (2) infancy, (3) toddlerhood, (4) preschool, (5) school age, (6) pubescence, (7) adolescence, (8) adulthood, and (9) senescence. Each phase is a complex set of challenges that involve physiological and psychological variables. In addition, each is further subdivided and can be viewed from several perspectives. These perspectives include (1) psychosexual (Freudian-psychoanalytic), (2) psychosocial (Erik Erikson), (3) cognitive (Piaget), (4) physiological, and (5) object relations (M. Mahler).

PRENATAL

The beginning of human development precedes birth. Even prior to conception, exposure to environmental toxins such as radiation may affect spermatogenesis and oogenesis (e.g., trisomy 18 is believed to be due to testicular exposure to radiation). The impact of drugs, pollutants, and infectious agents has not been fully elucidated in the development of sperm or ova. We should also realize that, in addition to biologic factors, the expectations of the parents—whether they are eager, reluctant, or otherwise—will have an impact on the offspring that eventually develops. Therefore, an individual's future development is affected by both biologic and psychological forces prior to conception.

Forces at work on the developing fetus have been more clearly demonstrated. It is certain that while in the uterus the embryo can be affected by infections such as rubella, by drugs such as heroin and alcohol, by radiation, and by systemic illness such as diabetes mellitus. Studies have demonstrated that a fetus in the last trimester is capable of vision, hearing, taste, and touch. Additional maternal factors that can affect development prior to birth include nutritional status and cigarette smoking. Mothers who are anxious may expose their fetuses to higher level of stress through increased levels of adrenal hormones or through other means. Their babies will have lower birth weight and increased activity. Genetic influences will have obvious or subtle effects on the embryo. (Conditions contributing to mental retardation are discussed under "Psychopathology—Childhood and Adolescent Disorders.")

Of historical interest, Otto Rank postulated that the process of birth itself was of extreme importance and that all anxiety in subsequent life could be traced back to the trauma of birth. This idea has not gained wide acceptance.

Birth trauma such as obstetric complications can have a profound influence on future development. The human neonate is sensitive to influences such as physical trauma and, even more importantly, hypoxia. Studies have demonstrated that in twins the birth order can affect the newborn's blood oxygen level, and there can be a correlation with subsequent IQ development.

INFANCY

Infant development can be viewed from a variety of perspectives, each of which attempts to explore a key aspect of the infant's life. Each perspective offers a partial view of the incredibly complex process of development. The six views presented constitute a simplification including physical and maturational, behavioral, psychosexual, psychosocial, cognitive, and ego maturational models. The period of infancy extends from birth to the time of toddlerhood, approximately 12 to 18 months. Physical development proceeds rapidly.

Physical development

The **brain** at birth (350 g) is 25% of its mature weight. At 6 months, it is 50% of mature value. The brain at 10 years is 100% of its mature weight.

The process of myelination in the CNS begins at 2 to 4 months in the fetus and continues for several years after birth. The number of cells within the brain increases linearly until birth and then more slowly until 6 to 12 months. Several aspects of the architecture of the CNS development need to be noted. The cortex is not as well developed in the neonate as is the spinal cord or brain stem. The inner cell layer develops more rapidly than the outer cell layer of the cortex. By 2 months there is (1) increased dendritic arborization, (2) increased vascularization, (3) increased myelination, (4) increased glial proliferation, and (5) neogenesis.

A group of reflexes are present from birth and disappear at various stages of development. Their failure to appear or persistence in time indicates possible pathology. Their demonstration clinically may be decreased by the state of alterness of the infant or other factors not related to pathology.

Steppage.   If you hold the baby upright against but a little below a horizontal surface, the baby will lift a leg as if trying to step onto the surface. This reflex disappears by 1 month.

Grasp reflex.   Objects placed in the palm cause the hand to close. This reflex usually disappears by 2 months, possibly as late as 6 months.

Moro reflex.   If the head is tipped downward (simulating falling), the arms and legs go out as if to embrace the mother. This reflex usually disappears by 3 to 4 months.

Sucking reflex.   Any object brought to the infant's mouth will elicit a brisk sucking action. This reflex disappears by 4 months (while awake).

Rooting.   If an object is placed against the perioral area, the mouth will move toward the stimulus. This reflex disappears by 4 to 7 months.

Tonic neck reflex.   If the infant's head is turned to one side, the contralateral arm goes up and the ipsilateral arm goes out like a fencer's (also called fencer's position reflex). This reflex disappears by 6 months.

Behavioral observations

In addition to possessing the inborn reflexes described above, the infant can be observed to exhibit competencies, states of alertness, and temperamental variabilities.

Temperament.   In observing infants, we note several tendencies in their behavior and interaction. Historically, people were described in terms of the four humors—for example, a melancholic (black bile) person was irritable and pessimistic. In the recent past, people were categorized on the basis of their body type (endomorphs, ectomorphs, mesomorphs). Temperament can be defined as the inborn constitutional predisposition to react to stimuli in a specific way. Infants can show varied and stable activity levels, rhythmicity, and adaptability. When infants are followed up, these temperamental characteristics are found to continue. Other aspects—distractibility, withdrawal, and persistence in tasks—are not as stable from infancy to early adulthood.

Competencies.   Infants at birth are able to look, listen, and vocalize as well as to position and orient themselves.

States.   This is a commonly repeated behavior pattern that is stable in the organism. It involves cortical and subcortical influences. Prechtl defined several major states: quiet sleep; active sleep (also called REM sleep), which may provide internal stimulation; quiet wakefulness, which provides the greatest sensory input for the infant, active wakefulness, and crying.

Psychosexual development

A full discussion of psychoanalytic theory will not be undertaken here, but elsewhere in this chapter. However, it is important to discuss some aspects of psychoanalytic theory to understand how they pertain to the development of the infant. **Freud** held that the mind could be understood by looking at the human **drives.** The drives were believed to be innate, stimulating the organism toward gratification. Some drives served physiological needs such as hunger and thirst. Others had important and complex interactions with other persons. The two dominant drives with which the human had to struggle were the sexual and the aggressive drives. The sexual drive was not used in the same sense that we commonly use it but related to the release of tension accompanied by pleasure. Freud theorized that throughout development certain areas of the body were dominant in the seeking of pleasure. The first of these places was the mouth. In infancy, the human striving was for gratification in the area of the mouth, hence the term **oral stage.** The oral stage is defined by the infant's deriving pleasure through sucking, feeding, and later through biting. Although the drive toward oral gratification initially serves the life-sustaining process of feeding, oral activity gradually becomes pleasurable in itself. Later, character traits of an oral nature could emerge. A person who was given excessive gratification during this stage or who received inadequate oral gratification could undergo a **fixation** in psychic organization. Oral characters were described as either **oral incorporative** (those who consistently seek to get from others, passively wishing to be cared for as dependent children) or **oral aggressive** (those who retain strong needs for care from others but do not feel they can obtain what they need without being grasping or hurting others in the process). Furthermore, infants that were indulged excessively were thought to acquire a lasting and inappropriate optimism that prevents them from providing for themselves as adults, as they feel certain that others will look out for them. Those who were deprived and frustrated were seen to have developed a deep-seated pessimism, becoming hostile and resentful when their needs were not met. They tend to give up easily.

Psychosocial development

Erik Erikson added an important dimension in understanding human nature. He augmented psychoanalytic theory by adding a social dimension. While Freud looked at particular zones of the body around which important drives were organized, Erikson felt there were particular times or crises during an individual's innate maturation. He defined each stage as consisting of a task that should be mastered if adequate development is to continue. Freud's stage of the oral period occurs concomitantly with Erikson's stage of **basic trust versus mistrust**. During this stage, infants gain a fundamental attitude of security in their surroundings and in themselves. The prevalent mode for this stage is incorporation. This is exemplified by the infant's comfort in developing the ability to receive and to accept. By **getting what is given** and learning to get somebody to do for them what they wish to have done, infants develop the basic groundwork for their later capacity to give to others.

Cognitive development

The Swiss psychologist **Jean Piaget** was interested in how children gain knowledge, which he called **genetic epistemology**. The developing human had innate abilities to gain knowledge. At each stage, the infant was driven by a need to master. It has been postulated that this is a basic drive—the mastery drive. He believed that at each stage the child had a basic organizational structure that existed beneath the surface behavior, which he termed a **schema**. Piaget was interested in how children think (cognition is a synonym for thinking). He discovered that children had distinctive patterns of thinking that varied according to the stage at which the child was. Piaget thought of thinking as an internalized (within the mind) action of the baby or child. The concept of schema represents "whatever is repeatable and generalizable in an action." When babies suck the breast, they are applying a cognitive structure, "the sucking schema." The breast becomes meaningful for the baby as a concept and is said to be **assimilated** into the knowledge of the infant. Through the process of assimilating various objects, the child learns. **Accommodation** is the process by which schemas are modified to fit external reality. The child's initial sucking schema is modified by the sense of touch and therefore broadens the child's repertoire.

Piaget's first stage is termed the **sensorimotor stage**. It extends from birth to 2 years. It consists of reflex actions (birth to 6 weeks) and primary circular reactions (6 weeks to 4 months). In primary circular reactions, the child progresses through the repetition of certain behaviors (sucking for example). In the process of repetition, the action is more finely tuned and feeding becomes more efficient.

In **secondary circular reactions** (4 to 8 months), infants may accidentally smack a rattle, causing a pleasant or interesting noise. They will repeat the action to gain the resultant noise. The child's will is beginning to form. He or she is beginning to see that there is a difference between internal actions and external results.

Tertiary circular reactions occur after 1 year of age and demonstrate that cognition is occurring. The behaviors are varied—for example, an object may be repetitively dropped but in different ways. The child introduces novelty as a way of exploring the properties of objects.

During the sensorimotor period, if the child is playing with a toy and it is removed, the child will not search for it. After about 1 year, the child will attempt to locate the toy. A mental representation is said to have taken place, and even though the object is out of sight, it is not out of mind. **Object permanence** refers to cognitive development. A similar term, object constancy, is an analytic term. In analytic jargon, a person will become represented by a mental image to the child. People are termed "objects," and it is understood that they are not inanimate objects but people.

Stages of ego development

Margaret Mahler focused on the development of the child's relationship with the mother and how the child gradually develops a sense of being separate from the mother. (Although we use the term *mother*, the person may not be the biologic mother but any person who fulfills the nurturing role of the mother). There are five phases in the progress to the development of an independent self-concept. Although the fifth phase, rapprochement, actually belongs to the discussion of toddlerhood, we will include it here.

In the **normal autistic phase** (birth to 1 month), the infant functions on a purely instinctual basis. There is a hypothetical stimulus barrier that together with the mother's caring for the infant's needs prevents the infant from being overwhelmed. The infant's predominant task is the establishment of some control over his or her basic physiological processes.

In the **normal symbiotic phase** (1 to 5 months), the infant gradually differentiates good or pleasurable stimuli from bad or painful ones. The infant's perception that pleasurable experiences are dependent on a source outside of the bodily self makes the transition from the autistic to the symbiotic phase. Although there is awareness of an outside source of gratification, the boundaries between the infant and the mother are not well differentiated and the two are conceived by the infant as being fused (symbiotic). One behavior that heralds the beginning of the symbiotic phase is the **social smile**. Although there is some controversy about when it begins, most authors state that between 2 and 3 months the child will respond to a human face. Actually, even drawings with two eyes will elicit the response. It indicates the attachment of the child to its caregivers.

The **differentiation phase** (5 to 9 months) is the phase during which the infant is exploring the mother's face, scanning the environment both near and far. The infant increasingly takes pleasure in the use of his or her own body, at times pushing away from the mother. Those infants with an adequate symbiotic phase will explore a stranger's face with pleasure. **Recognition memory** occurs during this phase. It is the ability to recognize a familiar object or person but to be unable to retain the mental image after the familiar object or person is removed from view. Infants in which there may have been an inadequate symbiosis will respond with discomfort. **Stranger anxiety**, which usually surfaces at 8 months of age, is evidence for the belief that infants have differentiated themselves from others and their mothers from strangers.

In the **practicing phase** (9 to 16 months), the infant crawls away from the mother, not fully aware of her whereabouts. The infant's attention focuses on inanimate objects in the environment. Greater activity occurs.

In the **rapprochement phase** (16 to 24 months), the

acquisition of upright, free locomotion and the beginnings of representational thought cause toddlers to become aware of the finality of their separateness. Toddlers constantly approach their mother, wishing to share their experiences and skills. They may on the one hand wish to expand their autonomy and on the other to stay close to their mother. There are a number of fears—fears of bodily damage (castration anxiety, covered later), fears of loss of the mother (separation anxiety), and fears of loss of the mother's love. This may help explain the toddler's increased crankiness. The toddler develops **evocative memory**, or the ability to evoke the mental image of the mother or familiar animate or inanimate object in the object's absence. At this stage, an infant or toddler will search for a toy if it is placed behind a pillow because the mental image is not erased. As in the game peek-a-boo, the infant eagerly searches for people as well.

Transitional objects are substitutes for the mother, such as a favorite doll or blanket. The child associates these familiar things with the mother's presence, and when they are removed, the child will protest loudly. Adults may make use of transitional objects in order to reduce anxiety when they bring familiar objects to a new office or to a hospital.

Maturational model

Development proceeds from birth through infancy from the cephalic (head) region downward. The first area to be developed is the eyes (oculomotor control). This is followed by head and arm movements, sitting, and trunk and hand coordination. Finally the legs, feet, fingers, and thumbs develop. The progression is from the CNS outward and downward, probably correlating with myelin formation.

TODDLERHOOD

As its name implies, toddlerhood is heralded by the ability of the child to walk. This occurs around 12 to 18 months, the average being 15 months. Toddlerhood extends to approximately 3 years of age. The toddler is growing in a number of ways.

Physical development

Although we will not explore physical development as we did for infancy, it is important to note several aspects of growth. Gains in height and weight slow down markedly. Between the ages of 2 and 5, annual increments are less than at any other time before the attainment of adulthood. Gross motor skills are increased. The toddler, having just learned to walk, begins to master aspects of running, jumping, and going up stairs. The toddler gains fine motor control, such as some skills in dressing, buttoning, drawing circles, and squares. Mastery of toilet training depends on the ability to control the sphincters. When a toddler is beginning to walk, there is not sufficient neural control over the sphincters. Not until a child can run and turn or stop is there evidence of sufficient myelinization for sphincter control. The added dimension of being verbal enough to communicate the need to use the toilet also facilitates toilet training (about 2 1/2 years). A child may void spontaneously soon after feeding time. This is termed the gastrocolic reflex. When toilet training is achieved prior to 18

months of age, it is probably the result of reinforcement of this reflex.

Psychosexual development

Freud called the first year of life the oral phase because mouthing and sucking constitute such prominent aspects of the infant's behavior. The second and third years of life were originally thought of as the **anal phase**, in which the chief concern was primarily centered on the eliminative functions. Toilet training probably now involves less parental investment of energy than it did when Freud made his observations. According to Freudian theory, conflicts during toilet training lead to a number of character traits and difficulties, including tendencies toward being stingy, overly clean, and obstinate. In addition, the obsessive-compulsive disorders are said to have their origin during this period. Freud stated, "In the second year of life the anal-erogenous zone seems to become the chief executive of all excitation which now, no matter where it originates, tends to be discharged through defecation." Tendencies toward prolonging the pleasure by retention of feces are in later life reflected in the qualities of being concerned with possessions and money. Finally, sadism is said to have its origins during this period, as do other conflicts over power.

Psychosocial development

Increasing maturation of the musculature allows the toddler to gain control of his or her body and thereby establish a sense of autonomy. Toddlers increasingly become aware of their **will**. They soon come into conflict with parental wishes. For the toddler, the struggle is self-expression or suppression. If a toddler's will is attacked, he or she will experience a feeling of shame—that of performing an unacceptable act in view of others. This will lead to an overcontrol and fear of self-expression. They will doubt their actions and require reassurance.

Cognitive development

Toddlerhood sees a transition from the sensorimotor stage to the preoperational stage. The child will continue to use circular reactions (repetitive behaviors) while mastering the inanimate items in life. A child will pile blocks on top of each other and repeat this endlessly. In the beginning of the preoperational stage, there is a shift from involvement in actions and sensations to involvement in thoughts.

It is difficult to separate the study of speech and thinking from one another, since they both develop simultaneously and clearly are intimately related. Piaget's focus, however, is particularly on thought. Several key concepts during the preoperational stage include the following:

Representational thought.   An object can be mentally recalled in its absence.

Egocentricism.   Children view themselves as the center of the universe. They cannot put themselves in someone else's place. A child asked to describe an object upside down without seeing it placed that way would be unable to shift the perspective.

Animism.   Everything that moves is alive, like cars, or trees swaying in a breeze.

Artificialism.   Everything is made for humans and by humans. The child may ask "Where do clouds come from?"

Symbolism.   Words come to represent people. As mentioned in discussing Margaret Mahler's work in the Infancy section, children use transitional objects that are symbolic representations of significant people in their lives.

Lack of conservation.   If children are shown a short beaker of water, which is then emptied into a tall beaker, they think that there is more water in the tall beaker. Even though they saw the same amount of water being poured, they cannot conceptualize that both beakers contain the same amount.

Separation-individuation

It is important to recall that during this time the child is beginning the process of separation from the mother. This was discussed in the previous section under the practicing and rapprochement phases described by Mahler.

Speech

It is believed that the babbling of infants is similar throughout the world and that any infant can learn any language. The sounds that children make stimulate them to repeat them (a circular reaction). Some linguists believe that there are six basic early words: dada, mama, nana, baba, papa, tata. Through the process of positive reinforcement by the parent, words are increasingly used and refined by the child. These words may be formed at the end of the first year. A baby can say 3 words at 12 months and 12 words by 18 months. By 3 years, the toddler may possess 500 to 900 words. In addition, there is the beginning of syntax — sentence structure.

Discipline

The period of toddlerhood is also known as the "terrible twos." The conflicts over the child's desire to explore and the possible dangers involved are a source of struggle. Several points are helpful to remember in dealing with a child's **undesirable behavior.**

1. The single most important ingredient is a warm, loving relationship between parent and child. The fear of loss of love is the parents' ally in helping the toddler gain self-control.
2. The parents should provide external control, taking care not to be too rigid or to allow too much freedom.
3. Parents should be able to express their own anger without feeling guilty. The child should not be humiliated or called names in the process.
4. One technique for gaining obedience is by temporarily withholding attention. In a social setting, the child may have to be removed or, while at home, sent to his or her room.
5. During the early phases of toddlerhood, children are highly distractible. Drawing attention to some new activity can often be effective.

Gender identity

In studies conducted on humans and other species, males seem to be more muscularly active and more prone to physical aggression. Society has strong stereotypes that affect how parents will interact with their babies. Infants who were identified as male or female and dressed accordingly were treated in stereotyped ways by parenting figures who were unaware of their true sexuality. Attributes and interactions encouraging such aggressiveness were noted when the parent thought that the infant was a boy.

Between 2 and 3 years of age, children will attempt to copy the dress and behavior of the parent of the same sex. **Biologic gender identity** refers to the anatomic and structural differences that are dependent on chromosomes, hormones, and sex organs. This may be overridden by social influences. **In studies in which there was a discrepancy between biologic factors and sex assigned at birth, the assigned sex had the major impact in the gender identity.** This was true of various conditions, including adrenal cortical hyperplasia and others. The **core gender identity** refers to how the child sees himself or herself. It is believed to be crystallized by 3 years of age.

Play

During the period of toddlerhood, there may be an opportunity for 2- and 3-year-olds to play together. If they are observed, it is noted that they only occasionally cooperate or interact. Their play is termed **parallel play** because they seem to not interact.

PRESCHOOL-AGE CHILDREN

Although toddlerhood begins at about 18 months and ends at approximately 3 years, there is an overlap with the period preceding and following it. The preschool period begins at about 3 years and continues until approximately 6 years of age. Many processes that have begun during toddlerhood, such as gender identity formation, are continued during this period.

Physical development

Between 3 and 5 years of age, there is a relatively constant but slow growth of approximately 5 pounds in weight and 2 to 3 inches in height. The child gains in fine and gross motor activities. By 4 years of age, 75% of children can button up clothing, dress without supervision, copy a circle and a cross, balance on one foot, and hop on one foot. Perhaps the most significant events that occur are in the area of psychosexual development.

Psychosexual development

Although the preschool age is ushered in by children's increased fondling of their genitals, there is some controversy about whether there is a spurt in sex hormones during this period. The increased fondling of genitals occurs in both sexes. This reflects the societal view that dominated in Freud's day. Although genital play may be seen as early as infancy, it begins in earnest by 3 years of age.

At 3 years of age, the boy's pleasure in his penis is manifested by his wanting to show if off. At some point, he may become aware that little girls do not have a penis. This may initiate the idea that his penis was lost and may produce fears that he may be castrated (emasculated). Freud considered castration anxiety to be a universal and critical aspect of all male development and that it played a major role in the oedipal transition. However, this may not be true in societies different from the Victorian era that Freud lived in. Boys reared in homes where sexual matters and genitals are taken more matter-of-factly may not show this concern.

While for a boy the phallic phase is ushered in by pride in his penis, the situation is different for the little girl. A girl may have different reactions to the observation of the genital difference between the sexes. Freud postulated that the little girl will develop **penis envy**. In a healthy family, this attitude will not be reinforced and the girl will develop with a healthy view of her sexuality. In families in which boys may be given more prestige, girls may develop an attitude of inferiority in comparison with boys. Freud believed that the wish to have a penis was replaced by the desire to have a baby. Boys have also expressed attitudes of envy, such as womb envy and breast envy. The phallic phase merges into the fourth year of life, with the oedipal conflict.

Freud termed the conflict that arose between ages 4 and 6 the **oedipal conflict**, naming it after the Greek tragedy *Oedipus Rex,* by Sophocles. This is the story of a man who, unaware of his father's identity, kills him and eventually marries a woman who, unknown to him, is his mother. In his discovery of the truth, he blinds himself. Many analysts believe that the disorders known as neuroses have their origins in the lack of resolution of this conflict. The conflict for boys can be divided into seven stages:

1. In the phallic phase, boys develop an erotic tie, as well as other need-satisfying ties, to the mother.
2. The father is seen as the boy's archrival.
3. The boy is frightened of the imagined retaliation of the father for the child's tie to the mother. The boy wants to eliminate the father and continue his incestuous tie to the mother.
4. The boy fears that his prized organ, his penis, will be cut off (castration anxiety).
5. This fear is so great that the boy gives up his longings for his mother.
6. The father helps the boy identify with him, and thereby the boy comes to believe that he will grow up and have his own wife.
7. The boy internalizes a superego (conscience).

In little girls, the analogy is similar. Rivalrous feelings and desires for possession of the father engender fears of retribution from the mother. The complex is resolved when the little girl further identifies with the mother, internalizes a superego, and delays gratification for the day when she too will have a man like her mother has. The corresponding Greek tragedy is termed *Elektra*, and the complex the **Elektra complex**. The continued attachment of the little girl for the father is stronger than that of the little boy for his mother. This is reinforced on a societal level. The Elektra complex is not as completely resolved in women as is the oedipal in men, and it is socially acceptable for women to maintain closer relationships with their fathers into adolescence.

Many children during this period have fears of bodily harm that correspond to the castration anxieties mentioned. Phobias involving mutilating monsters may be representative of the underlying anxiety of harm that these children fear from their same-sex parent rivals. The oedipal conflict is not a universally accepted phenomenon. There are cultures and societies where the attachments that occur involve siblings, where rivalries are not as intense, and where attachments are not continued. However, many analysts place great importance on this stage for the formation of a number of disorders. This is reflected in a wealth of clinical material.

Psychosocial development

Children idealize their parents. They compare and fantasize about being powerful like their parents. They have competitive feelings about sexuality and other areas. The major struggle is, will their fantasies and energy be kept alive or will they be paralyzed by guilt feelings. **The child's initiative must be encouraged while appropriate limitations are applied.** Erikson described this stage as "**initiative versus guilt**," or "I am what I will be."

Cognitive development

The preoperational stage has begun during toddlerhood and will continue to the end of the preschool stage. Piaget divides this preoperational stage into two parts, preconceptual thought and intuitive thought. The latter shows some evidence of the ability to put oneself in another perspective. The former shows that concepts are seen purely from an egocentric point.

Other developmental aspects

Fantasy.   Because of the increasing use of symbolic play, a rich fantasy life evolves and many experiences can be relived and modified through the rich fantasy life.

Self-control.   There is increased mastery and control of drives, and aggressive outbursts are far fewer.

Increased attention.   A lengthening attention span allows for the playing of table games like drawing with crayons.

Speech.   The vocabulary has grown to 2,000 words at age 5 years.

Play.   Unlike parallel play of toddlerhood there is imitation, leadership, submission, withdrawal, and sex-typed behavior. Although these aspects of play indicate interaction, the initial dialogue between two children playing is more a collective monologue. One child says something, and the other replies with little connection to the original statement.

Reality.   The child is increasingly able to differentiate fantasy from reality, although magical thoughts are very common.

Moral development.   Moral development is influenced by the resolution of the oedipal conflict with **internalization of a conscience and ego-ideal (together they are superego).** During this time, the **Talion principle** is a term used to help describe the harshness of the superego—"an eye for an eye." In addition, the stage of cognitive development is important since preschool children have a rudimentary understanding of rules. In a game that she plays, a preschooler may include a rule that she always wins. There is little appreciation of more abstract rules until the next stage of cognitive development. (Moral development also proceeds from a simple reward and punishment system to an appreciation of family, society, and national norms. Learning by imitating the parents is another manner in which morals develop.)

SCHOOL-AGE CHILDREN

Most children grow 1 to 2 feet taller and gain 25 to 30 pounds of weight between the ages of 6 and 12 years. A child of 12 is on the average 5 feet tall and weighs 65 pounds.

Psychosexual development

Freud maintained that, following the resolution of the oedipal conflict, the child's sexual interest underwent a marked repression. He termed the ages following the oedipal conflict and continuing until adolescence the **latency stage** because the sexuality was latent or dormant. Two particular defense mechanisms (discussed more thoroughly later in "Understanding Human Behavior—Analytic Concepts") that emerge during this latency period are reaction formation and sublimation. In **reaction formation**, a wish or drive or feeling is replaced with its opposite. For example, a desire to return to the soiling and messiness of the anal period finds expression in the need for a latency-age child to start each school year with an absolutely clean notebook. In **sublimation**, a forbidden wish is presented in a socially acceptable manner. The desire to suck a breast, which represents oral-stage desires, can be identified in the latency-age child as a hunger and curiosity for knowledge.

Evidence for the repression of the sexual wishes can be found in the observation that the heroes for the boys during this time—Superman and Batman, for example—have no wives or attachments to women.

Psychosocial development

According to Erikson, the child at this stage responds to the dictum, "I am what I learn." The child is rapidly gaining in extrafamilial contacts with society. This is a time of making things, collecting things, and participating. Children who are given sufficient positive feedback and who sense the value of their contributions and efforts will maintain a sense of industry, otherwise they will fear humiliation and develop a feeling of inferiority (**industry versus inferiority**).

Physical attributes

1. Around the age of 7 years, the brain has achieved 90% of its adult weight.
2. Pyramidal cells have a burst in growth and achieve their largest size.
3. Frontal lobes develop between the ages of 5 and 7 years.

Cognitive development

There is a tremendous growth in logical thinking during this time. The stage is termed the phase of **concrete operations**. Children are able to **conserve** volume, length, and area. In the previous stage, a child could not tell that there was an equal amount of water in a tall or short beaker; at this stage, the child can comprehend that the amount of a substance stays the same no matter what its presentation. A child at this stage can understand that processes are **reversible**. This has medical applications in that a child who has a specific ailment like a heart disease or ear infection can understand that the process can be reversed. Prior to this, the child may believe that this organ is damaged permanently. A child will also understand how a drawing looks from a different perspective (**decentration**). In other words, there is a decrease in egocentricity. A child of 7 can arrange things into groups and can also arrange things in serial order. Because of the ability to organize and develop hierarchies, memory is more continuous, unlike the fragmented memories of the preoperational period.

School

There are three requirements for a child to be able to attend school: (1) Impulse control must be gained. (2) Separation from the parents must be possible. (3) Anxieties must be bound. In addition, the child must learn the basic academic skills of reading, writing, and arithmetic. A school-age child must develop a more mature scale of values and morality, as well as ideas and attitudes toward social groups and institutions. Some studies indicate that males have a greater difficulty adjusting to the school setting than do females. Similarly, children of a lower social class or of a minority group also have more difficulty in adjusting. It is clear that socialization, in addition to the incorporation of fundamental knowledge, is a key goal in school.

Peer groups

Peer groups play an increasing role in the socialization process. Boys tend to exclude girls more than girls exclude boys. The reasons for this are twofold. First, boys are still threatened by the residual castration anxiety and pursue supermasculine ideals. Second, girls by this age are usually 2 to 3 inches taller and increase feelings of being overwhelmed by the female. One additional reason is the attempt to develop further independence from the mother. An additional aspect is secrecy. The secrets of the peer group in part reflect the desire to keep secret the sexual interests from the oedipal period. The secret groups have numerous rules that help further the superego. However, during the latency period, the superego has a more flexible and less harsh aspect than the oedipal stage.

Self-concept

During the school-age years, the self-concept that initially was formed within the family will be shaped by the school and peer groups. Self-concept will depend on the following factors:

1. Physical condition. Feelings of inferiority may develop in a child with poor health or defects.
2. Intelligence. Children who are either less or more intelligent may be ostracized.
3. Physical build. Skinny or obese children will take special abuse, as will unusually tall or short children.
4. Social acceptance. Personality will in part determine whether the peer group accepts or rejects the child.
5. Names or nicknames. Names may reflect ethnic or minority status and may be a source of conflict.
6. Socioeconomic status. Students outside the majority group's mean income will be the source of ridicule or jealousy.
7. Success or failure. As determined by abilities, success or failure will increase or decrease self-concept.
8. School environment. Teaching skill can have an enormous impact on students. Teachers play a role that is second only to that of the parents. Children may view their teachers as similar to their parents in many ways.

Behavioral characteristics

Many factors will affect how a child behaves socially. Parental behaviors have been correlated with the child's behavior. Warm and restrictive parents will encourage a dependent child; warm and permissive parents will encourage a responsible child. Hostile and restrictive parents will foster passive children; hostile and permissive parents will foster delinquent children.

One study demonstrated that parents who explain the reasons for restrictions and consistently set limits have children with the most advanced moral development. The use of withdrawal of love and assertion of power were less successful.

ADOLESCENCE

Adolescence is the stage of development between the ages of 11 and 20 years. Adolescence is in part a creation of the Industrial Revolution. In the past, childhood merged directly into adulthood. In many societies there is no adolescence. It is believed to occur because of the greater amounts of information and the more complex social structures that modern civilization impose on its citizens. Adolescence is also viewed by some as a period when turmoil is normal. Others disagree, indicating that many adolescents pass comfortably through their teenage years without difficulties.

Some authors indicate that to understand adolescence one must appreciate the stage immediately preceding it. Preadolescence (**pubescence**) occurs following the latency period, around 10 to 12 years of age. Many texts do not make mention of this stage. It is important to understand that the preadolescent child experiences a great deal of inner tension. Somatic complaints increase, possibly reflecting the underlying hormonal and growth changes that are beginning to take place.

Physical development

There is a marked increase in the rate of growth, **growth spurt**. It occurs earlier in girls than boys. Boys may experience the spurt from ages 10½ to 16 years. Girls may experience it from 9½ years to 14½. Puberty heralds the entry of the child into an adult sexual role. Menarche in girls begins between ages 10½ and 15 years. The age of onset of puberty is decreasing. The rate has been clocked at 3 months per decade. For boys, the age of first seminal emission and sperm production occur around age 12½ to 16½ years. Girls are 2 years more developed in this sense than boys. The age when the secondary sexual characteristics make their appearance varies. In boys, these secondary sexual characteristics include enlargement of the testes, growth of pubic hair, increase in penile size, growth of facial and axillary hair, voice change, and first ejaculation. In girls, these include the development of pubic hair, axillary hair, and breast enlargement.

Psychosexual development

Freud viewed adolescence as the stage at which the sexual energies are directed toward heterosexual love objects—the **genital stage**.

Psychosocial development

Adolescents are seen as persons trying to establish a firm sense of who they are. They are interested in their social role. The failure of this sense of identity is **identity diffusion**, in which the adolescent needs to maintain an attachment to cliques or organizations or heroes.

Cognitive development

It is estimated that 70% of adults do not achieve this stage, which Piaget called **formal operations**. There are several aspects of this higher thinking process. Persons can reflect on their thinking. An adolescent might ask herself, "Why am I thinking about this subject?" Scientific thinking or the ability to form a hypothesis occurs here. A person can understand the nature of events and that there are multiple variables in the solution of some problems. Adolescents may ask philosophical questions reflecting the enjoyment of pure thought—for example, "What is the meaning of life?" "Is there a God?" One aspect of formal thinking that returns to an earlier mode of thinking is egocentricity. Adolescents are very much preoccupied with how others see them. Although they can see from others' perspectives they are more likely to assume that others have views similar to their own.

Tasks of adolescence

Various authors point to specific tasks of adolescence in addition to those already discussed. Certainly one of the major tasks of adolescence is a second **separation-individuation** process from the parents. Others point out four tasks, elaborating on Erikson's work:

1. A social identity, in which the adolescent shifts from an egocentric point of view, becoming more independent of parents and adopting the values of society.
2. A sexual identity, in which there is the development of a meaningful relationship with an opposite-sex partner.
3. A vocational identity, in which there is an increased ability to pursue an occupation and be responsible for finances and to gain pleasure from these functions.
4. A moral identity, through which the teenager's system of values becomes clarified in religious, political, and ethical concerns.

Stages of adolescence

Early adolescence (10 to 13 years) is characterized by the following:

1. Physical changes begin.
2. Attention shifts from home to outside.
3. Sexual feelings develop.
4. Regression is used as a defense. Teenagers become sloppy (anal regression) and develop peculiar eating habits (oral regression).
5. Intimacy develops. First there may be a "normal" homosexual phase in which an intense "chumship" develops.
6. Beginnings of separation are expressed through fears of being alone, fears of the dark, and fears of death and dying and abandonment.

Middle adolescence (13 to 16 years) is characterized as follows:

1. This is the most difficult period.
2. Continued secondary sexual characteristics develop.
3. Body image concerns arise.
4. Increased genital activity takes place.
5. Arguments with parents (separation continues) are common.
6. There is increased mastery of emotions.

Late adolescence (16 to 19+ years) is characterized as follows:

1. Body image is established.
2. A love object is chosen.
3. Intense attachments are formed. Marriages occur, but 70% of these end in divorce within 2 years.
4. Sexual activity begins. Approximately 50% of girls are sexually active between 15 and 19 years. The likelihood of sexual activity is increased by higher social class, black ethnicity, and no strong religious system. This rate of premarital intercourse has increased over the past 25 years.

Adolescent rebellion

Parent-teenager conflicts are not new. Although adolescence is a relatively new social phenomenon, reports dating back to ancient Greece and describing conflicts between adults and older children demonstrate the issues of rebellion. Several reports and studies indicate that adolescent rebellion may be a myth, however. One study involving 10,000 high school boys found that 70% were proud of their parents, and 80% spent half their free time at home with their parents.

ADULTHOOD

A review of the basic material relevant to adulthood takes a different form from that of earlier development. This subject has only been written about in the past three decades. As you may recall, Freudian development stopped with the achievement of the adolescent "genital stage." Similarly, Piaget neglected cognitive development after the "formal operations" period. Several authors have begun to excavate the topic.

Bernice Neugarten developed a system by which she explored the cultural expectations and milestones of adulthood. These expectations involve three principal areas: marriage, work, and parenting. People are described in terms of being late, early, or on time for these landmarks. A person who marries in his 30s is said to be late for this event. Three aspects emerged. Milestones are varied and based on age, sex, and socioeconomic class. We have just mentioned that marriage is expected during the early adulthood period; childbearing would be considered late if the couple began in their 40s. The sex of the individual plays a part. A recent study involving the probability of women marrying after the age of 35 indicated that this was highly unlikely. A woman unmarried at 35 faces fewer prospects for marriage than a man of the same age. Depending on socioecnomic class, there is a shift of approximately 10 years for the appropriate milestones (Table 7-1).

Psychosocial development

After achieving an identity, young adults share themselves with another in a close, loving relationship. Erikson described the fusion of lustful and loving feelings with a member of the opposite sex, with whom there could be sharing of work, procreation, and recreation. The stage has been termed that of **intimacy versus isolation.**

Middle adulthood

Outside of raising children, the adult focuses on guiding the next generation or bettering society. Not having children does

Table 7-1. Milestones According to Socioeconomic Class

Age	Blue-collar, working class	Upper-class, professional
30s	Considered themselves fully adult; economic independence and responsibilities are settled	Considered themselves as young adults, with time for adjustments and explorations
40s	Considered themselves to be middle-aged	Felt mature and at peak of self-confidence
60s	Considered themselves old	50s was considered middle-aged, 70s considered old

not exclude a productive middle age. Erikson referred to this as the stage of **generativity versus self-absorption or stagnation**.

Seasons of the human life

Although Levinson was criticized because he studied only males, a companion study involving women has been undertaken. Levinson's sample size is small, 40 men of various occupations, but the studies are in depth. Levinson's group found that the life cycle should be divided into four eras, each approximately 25 years long:

1. Childhood and adolescence, birth to 22 years old
2. Early adulthood, 17 to 45 (entering the adult world at 22 to 28 and settling down at 33 to 40)
3. Middle adulthood, 40 to 65
4. Late adulthood, 60 to death

An important aspect of his work involved the description of **transitions**. These occurred between the above eras and last approximately 5 years. Transitions were times that allowed for reappraisal and new opportunities. Early adult transition, ages 17 to 22, involved moving out of the parents' house and making a preliminary step into the adult world. Midlife transition, ages 40 to 45, involved coming to terms with the past and preparing for the future, particularly mourning over lost opportunities. Late adult transition occurred between age 60 and 65 years. In addition, many adults suffered an age-30 transition crisis, in which they were dissatisfied with their present life, including marriage and work, and grappled with solutions.

Carl Rogers felt that adult life involved freedom from conflict in the mature individual. He described existential living as living fully and vitally, having the ability to retain sensitivity and openness and a high degree of enjoyment of life.

Sigmund Freud, when asked what the meaning of life was, believed it to be the ability to love and to work.

Marriage

An important aspect of adult life is marriage. Out of every two marriages, one ends in divorce. The many reasons for marriage include love, raising a family, sexual attraction, security, escaping from a bad family or life situation, pregnancy, and unconscious motivations including searching for a parent substitute or to compensate for a personal deficiency.

In a survey of 400 psychiatrists, the following observations were noted regarding marriage:

1. Living together before marriage will apparently lead to a better marriage in 55% of cases. Approximately 15% of the time it will either frequently, usually, or rarely lead to a better marriage.
2. Between 50 and 75% of people marry for love. Approximately 50% of the psychiatrists believed this was true.
3. What is the optimum age for marriage? About 50% of the psychiatrists thought that the ages of 23 to 27 for men and women were optimal.
4. Which sex has the greater degree of uncertainty about marriage? According to the psychiatrists, 81% felt that men have greater uncertainty than women. Does the high rate of divorce mean that marriage is a failing institution? This is obviously untrue since 85% of men and 75% of women who divorce before age 40 remarry within 5 years.

Divorce

The **reasons for failed marriages** involve conflicts over money, sexual satisfaction, personality differences, spouses' families, children, and many more. Many psychiatrists believe that deeper unconscious forces involving unresolved conflicts from childhood play a role. A spouse may be expected to play the role of a father or mother, and unresolved anger over unmet dependency needs, attention, and other issues may come to make the marriage a battleground. Some sociologists feel that women tolerate marital tension longer than men. One study indicates that divorced women fare better in terms of physical health than divorced men. The effects of divorce on children have been found to be disturbing. In studies involving the children of divorced parents, the preschool children felt guilty and somehow responsible for the breakup. The school-age children showed the most pervasive sadness of all. Older school-age children and adolescents were better able to cope with the divorce. Other psychiatrists indicate that adolescents may be particularly vulnerable, since the task of separation is hampered by the disintegration of the family. The numbers of children living with only one parent are increasing. It is estimated that 45% of all children born in a given year will be living with only one parent by the time they are 18.

Family

In 1972, 44% of families in the United States were nuclear families. A nuclear family consists of a mother, father, and children. Thirteen percent were single-parent families. Other family types include extended family (involving grandparents, aunts, and uncles), nontraditional families (unmarried living together), or experimental (homosexual couples). One out of every five families changes its residence each year. Meyer and Hagerty have shown that streptococcal infections occur at four times the rate in families that have experienced acute stress in the prior 2 weeks. This underlies a need to look at physical illness as a possible sign of underlying emotional conflict within the family. Increasingly, the focus of the physician needs to take into account not just the sick individual but the family in which he or she resides.

Families are the building blocks of society and serve many important functions. They provide role models for the children, allow the process of socialization, meet psychological needs of a variety of types (including the handling of emotions and defense mechanisms), meet the sexual needs of the married partners, allow for reproduction of children, aid in childhood education, and provide an economic base with which the individuals can achieve security and provide for security needs.

Women in adulthood

Several factors involving the women's adult development need special mention. In spite of the advances of the woman's movement, there is still a differential in pay. Many women are caught between the choices of career and raising a family. One study indicated that women may shy away from competition, and when compared with men they were found to be significantly less competitive. Two events may be particularly important in some women's life, but these have only partly been studied: The empty-nest syndrome and the female climacteric. In the empty-nest syndrome, there is an increase in psychological symptoms. In particular, depressive feelings accompany the children leaving the home. That women should sense a loss and go through a mourning process when confronted with this event should not be surprising. One study contradicts this, however, and it should be understood that the empty-nest syndrome is not a universal phenomenon. Similar observations surround the female climacteric. Occurring at the age of 48 years (± 5 years), the loss of reproductive ability is accompanied in some women by physical symptoms of increased irritability, hot flashes, flushing, and night sweats. Certain studies have indicated that physicians may be falsely attributing these symptoms to this period and that depressive or other syndromes are no greater in this age-group than in others.

SENIOR ADULTHOOD

Senescence and the geriatric period, or senior adulthood, is generally thought of as beginning at the age of 65. As has been already noted, a man is at his peak of physical abilities around the age of 30. After this time there is a gradual decline. Technically, therefore, aging begins after age 30 years. In the United States there currently are 25 million people over the age of 65. This represents 11% of the population. The percentage of people over the age of 65 is increasing. The fastest-growing age-group is the 85+ group. The number of men per women is approximately 70 per 100. The difference in the gender composition of this age-group is expected to continue. Psychological and social behavior and feelings are important considerations in aging. Young people may behave like "old folks," and there are many seniors who don't feel old because of their psychological approach to life.

A differentiation between the terms **life span** and **life expectancy** is important to understand. One's life span appears to be genetically encoded and is fixed, approximating 100 years, ± 15 years. On the level of cell biology, under optimum conditions cells appear to have a fixed number of divisions, and this may account for the life span of a species. Life expectancy has generally increased in modern times. Factors that have contributed to the increase include improved infant care, antibiotics, and improvements in nutrition and sanitation. The average life expectancy is now more than 70 years for a person born in the United States.

Theories of aging

Aging may be the result of a number of factors:

1. DNA theory. The body continously struggles with the repair of damaged DNA; when this fails, the body deteriorates.
2. Environmental/endogenous toxins. Certain substances that cannot be eliminated from the body gradually accumulate. The cell machinery cannot handle the buildup, and cell deterioration occurs.
3. Single organ failure. Certain systems deteriorate by 50% over the life span (kidneys, lungs, and immune system), whereas other organs (heart, intestines, and liver) decline less rapidly.
4. Autoimmune theory. One's own immune system begins to lose the ability to discriminate between the body's cells and invading cells, resulting in a gradual attack on the body's own systems. Certain diseases such as collagen vascular disease and rheumatoid arthritis may occur in older patients. Antibody titers also increase in older patients.

Changes of aging

Aging affects a person physically, psychologically, and socially. Physically, there is an accumulation of lipids, the pigment lipofuscin, and calcium within the cardiovascular system. The nervous system shows a loss of neuronal mass beginning in young adulthood. EEGs show an increased alpha rhythm, which may reflect a slowing down of central electrical activity. Certain aspects of intelligence may be affected more than others. Older patients have higher verbal IQs than performance. It is believed that their decreased performance is due to anxiety about time pressure. Reaction time is slowed in the elderly. Although some authors indicate that there is a decline in problem-solving skills, others state that there is no significant change. Certainly, prejudices regarding the aged influence one's perception. This prejudice, called ageism, may also influence society's handling of its senior adults with regard to social policy in business, health care, and planning.

Psychosocial development

In order to negotiate this phase successfully, one must have had a sense of generativity. This in turn results in the feelings of having been productive. This period allows for reflection on one's achievements and the observation of the younger generation. In the face of living a life more concerned with selfish motives, there may result a sense of pointlessness and a fear of death. Erikson described this as the stage of **integrity versus despair**.

Sexuality

The prejudices mentioned earlier also relate to the misconception that the older person is somehow asexual. This is simply not true. Certain aspects of sexuality change. The sexual response can be divided into four phases—the excitement, plateau, orgasm, and refractory periods—which we will later discuss in greater detail. In older men, the refractory period is increased. The plateau phase may not occur, but in general a man can have a more prolonged excitement and plateau phase prior to orgasm. In women, there is a correlation between sexual activity and changes in the vagina. If a woman is not sexually active, she may have an increased likelihood of atrophic vaginitis. Men and women who have enjoyed sexuality in youth usually continue to experience similar pleasure and performance in senior adulthood.

Social aspects

Women live 7.7 years longer than men and marry men 4 years older. This results in approximately 12 years of living alone. The increased social isolation is a source of emotional pain for women. For men and women, the aspect of social isolation results from a number of sources, such as the following: loss of transporation (only 50% over 65 have a car), loss of income (14% of the geriatric population are below the poverty level, and inflation affects them to a greater extent because of the fixed nature of their income), loss of support systems (many are geographically separated from their children who have moved away; the three states that have the greatest number of seniors are New York, Florida, and California), and physical illnesses.

Psychiatric problems

Although a review of specific syndromes and diseases appears in another section, it is important to state here that 50% of people in the senior adulthood group will suffer depression. This is understandable in view of the losses previously described.

Death and dying

Just as there seems to be prejudice against the aged, there is great difficulty in dealing with the patient who is facing death. This is not too difficult to understand. Underlying reasons, however, play a role that may not be recognized. Fears of being overwhelmed with feelings, fears of being helpless (particularly for physicians, who believe they must be omniscient and omnipotent), and fears of the unknown are possible reasons for avoiding this subject. Typical mistakes that physicians make in dealing with a patient with a terminal illness include the following:

1. Not offering patients an opportunity to discuss their fears and feelings.
2. Giving a concrete amount of time that the patient may have to live (physicians who tell a patient that he has 6 months at the most may be exercising their need for omnipotence, and when the patient lives beyond this time he is plagued with feelings of betrayal and a lack of trust).
3. Not recognizing the different stages of dying.
4. Not knowing when to recognize the patient's wishes versus the physician's desire for a cure.

The manner in which a person may die is also changing. In 1977, heart disease, malignant neoplasms, and cerebrovascular disease ranked as the first, second, and third major causes of death, respectively. Alzheimer's disease has replaced influenza and pneumonia as the fourth leading cause of death.

Stages of dying. Elizabeth Kübler-Ross's work on dealing with dying patients serves as a base around which to understand this topic. Although she presents these stages in an order, they may not be experienced by the patient in a sequential fashion. These stages are denial, anger, bargaining, grief, and acceptance. The stage of denial begins when patients are told that they have a fatal illness. Actually, it probably precedes this in some individuals who delay seeking help because of a fear of detection of illness. This disbelief may take the form of a patient's refusing procedures or therapy or neglecting follow-up appointments. In a reasonably healthy person, however, it soon gives way. Anger may assume immense proportions, and displacements of the anger onto the doctor, family, or God may take place. Alternatively, anger may be relatively mild. Bargaining has at its source a feeling of helplessness. The aspect of being out of control may lead the individual to pose all sorts of impossible questions or ideas like, "If only I had been a better father, this wouldn's have befallen me." Grief, depression, and mourning are terms that can be applied to the next stage, in which the impact and sadness of the impending loss are felt. There is a reliving of past experiences and relationships as dying patients in some manner attempt to break the bonds that attach them to others. Acceptance has been described as being rather subdued; others observe anxiety or even euphoria. This response most likely depends on the quality of the life, the degree of maturity of the individual, the stage of life at which they are confronted with the fatal illness, and their religious beliefs.

Informing the patient. As indicated above, the physician may be reluctant to deal with this issue for a number of psychological reasons. There is also the cultural aspect of informing a patient. The Japanese have a philosophy called "wabi-sabi," which is an unstated understanding that if the doctor says nothing about the illness the patient thus assumes the fatal nature. In the past, not informing the patient was the most common pattern of physician action. In those cases, the family may be informed of the diagnosis and terminal nature of the illness. More recently, one study revealed that 98% of physicians informed their patients and 100% would themselves want to know.

Other aspects. The criteria for death are being reevaluated in the legislatures of many states because of considerations dealing with organ donations. An older set of criteria indicating the cessation of spontaneous respiratory and cardiac function is increasingly being replaced by the use of an EEG that shows isoelectric potential along with absent reflexes, absent movements, and unresponsiveness to stimuli. The role of hospice care in dealing with terminal illness has increased. A hospice is a place where people can die with dignity. Appropriate pain management and a warm, accepting, and supportive atmosphere involving the various patient's supports allow for a more dignified departure from life.

UNDERSTANDING HUMAN BEHAVIOR

NEUROLOGICAL AND BIOCHEMICAL BASIS OF BEHAVIOR

This section reviews the various brain structures and their role in behavior, as well as the various neurotransmitter hypotheses relating to behavior and certain disease states. A growing body of experimental research demonstrates this relationship. However, the idea that underlying biologic factors affect emotions is not new. It was Hippocrates who postulated that psychiatric disturbances were due to an imbalance of the four humors. An increase in black bile caused depression, which was termed melancholia. In today's view, biologic and psychological factors, together with social factors, underlie human behavior. In some behaviors or disorders, one aspect may dominate more than others. In order to explain some of these observations, we will discuss first the limbic system.

The limbic system

The limbic system refers to the ring (limbus: ring) of tissue curving around the brain stem of higher organisms. It is one of the most primitive cortical structures and has been termed the **rhinecephalon** (rhine: nose) because of its connection to the sense of smell. The limbic system was first believed to be the seat of emotion, described by Papez in 1937. His observations of patients with rabies and their associated intense emotional discharges led him to this observation. The limbic system consists of the (1) hippocampus, (2) amygdala, (3) septal nuclei, (4) parahippocampal cortex, (5) uncus, (6) anterior thalamic nuclei, (7) mamillothalamic tract, (8) cingulate gyrus, (9) habenula, (10) subcallosal and supracallossal gyri, (11) fimbria, (12) fornix, (13) anterior commissure, (14) stria terminalis, (15) stria medullaris, (16) median forebrain bundle, and (17) diagonal band of Broca. We will review only those structures in which clear syndromes and behavioral results have been elucidated. It should be understood that this system probably does not have such clearly separated components but rather acts in a complex, interconnected fashion. Thus, emotions probably result from reverberating discharges within the limbic system together with the cerebral cortex.

Hippocampus. Stimulation produces an increased arousal and anxiety. Ablation produces recent memory loss with the prevention of new learning (Korsakoff's psychosis). This is also termed anterograde amnesia, because the memory deficit occurs after the insult to the brain.

The limbic hypothesis refers specifically to schizophrenia but may be applied to other psychological conditions as well. Since it is believed that the limbic system is a major seat of emotions, lesions or impairments in this area are important in subsequent emotional disorders. Specifically in schizophrenia, one hypothesis about the etiology relates that early cerebral hypoxia during childbirth may lead to subsequent emotional damage. This rests on the observations that the hippocampus is noted to be one of the areas of the brain most sensitive to hypoxia and seizure activity (i.e., it has low threshold to seizure activity). The hippocampus is also believed to be a predominantly inhibitory structure in the brain (whereas the amygdala is believed to be an excitatory structure). The damaged "inhibitory" center accounts for the release of behaviors seen in schizophrenia and other disorders.

Amygdala. Stimulation produces autonomic arousal (sympathetic and parasympathetic) and reactions of increased alertness, fear, or rage. A peculiar syndrome results from bilateral destruction of the amygdala, the Klüver-Bucy syndrome. this consists of loss of fear and placidity, hyperorality (the animal increasingly explores with its mouth with increased sucking), and hypersexuality.

Septal nuclei.   Animals with electrical stimulation of the septal nuclei will self-stimulate at very high rates. This area is believed to be associated with pleasurable sensations. One subject pleaded not to have electrodes removed, so pleasurable was the sensation. This structure may be involved in reward systems. Lesions have demonstrated rage in rats.

Cingulate gyrus.   Stimulation produces an arrest reaction, which is manifested by cessation of other activities and an expression of attention but responsiveness to external stimuli. Posterior cingulate stimulation produces a pleasurable affect stimulating sexual behavior.

Hypothalamus

In addition to eliciting the emotions of rage, fear, and general emotional intensity, the hypothalamus plays a role in heat regulation and control of appetite. (Ventromedial lesions stimulate appetite, whereas lesions in the lateral hypothalamus area abolish the urge to eat in experimental animals.) They also regulate the pituitary gland via the hypothalamic-neuro-hypophyseal and hypothalamic-adenohypophyseal systems through release of releasing factors and inhibitory factors.

Destruction of the **ventromedial nucleus** of the hypothalamus has reportedly produced permanently ferocious animals, and stimulation has also produced rage reactions and aggressive behavior. **Dorsomedial nucleus** stimulation has reportedly produced violent rage up to the point that the animal will attack the observer. **Posterior hypothalamus** stimulation may enhance hunting behavior, whereas lesions may produce affective blunting or sleep. **Lateral hypothalamus** stimulation may produce fear and escape behavior. Feeding and self-stimulation on stimulation have also been reported.

Anterior hypothalamus

Lesions completely abolish sexual interest in monkeys, whereas stimulation of this area and the medial forebrain bundle results in penile erection and mating behavior in monkeys. When the anterior hypothalamus is spared in animals that are castrated or oophorectomized, they will respond to sex hormones with a resumption of sexual behavior.

Frontal lobes

The frontal lobes have frequently been thought of as the seat of higher intellect. Although there has been some evidence regarding the location in specific brain regions of specific abilities (language, abstract thinking, and others), it is generally held that various brain regions are capable of a variety of functions. Deficits then are more related to a quantitative loss of brain tissue and less to the localization. Nevertheless, the **frontal lobe syndrome** has been characterized by the following signs and symptoms: Patients become apathetic and lose interest in life and the pleasures they once enjoyed; they may even be unresponsive, appearing catatonic. Witzelsucht or inappropriate joking may occur. Emotional lability occurs and is characterized by sudden crying or laughing without provocation or out of proportion to the stimulus and alternating unpredictably. Judgment is impaired, particularly social judgment as seen in public nudity, public voiding, or other evidences of impulsive behavior as in suddenly striking someone for no reason.

Hemispheric specialization

As mentioned above, the question of whether intelligence is located in the frontal lobes is part of the larger question about the nature of the cortex in terms of function. The debate about diffuse versus localized function extends back over 100 years. The discovery by Paul Broca of a patient who had a well-localized lesion in the left hemisphere and who was unable to communicate verbally (aphasia) added to the "localized" theorists. The following observations are intriguing:

1. An adult with a stroke in one hemisphere will have almost total loss of speech function, whereas a child with a stroke in one hemisphere will develop nearly normal speech.
2. Asymmetries exist in brain structure: The planum temporale is large in two-thirds of brains on the left side; the sylvian fissure is longer and more horizontal in the left hemisphere.
3. Male canaries have better-developed left hemispheres than females. No structural differences have been found anatomically in the brains of men and women, however.
4. Men generally have better spatial ability than women.
5. Girls speak earlier than boys, and women have better language skills than men. They also excel at fine hand control.
6. Men have higher incidences of dyslexia, stuttering, and delayed speech.

In patients with intractable seizures, a neurosurgical procedure severing the corpus callosum breaks the spread of seizure foci from one brain hemisphere to the other. Interestingly, this has allowed an understanding of the various hemispheric functions. Typically, if the subject is shown a picture in the right visual field only the left hemisphere receives the input. When images were directed toward the left hemisphere, subjects could recall verbally what they were. However, when the image was directed to the right hemisphere, subjects could not verbalize what they had seen although they could point to a set of cards, indicating that the brain had perceived the image. From these experiments the following specializations have been noted.

The left hemisphere serves symbolic-conceptual functions. In addition, spoken language, number skills, written language, reasoning, and scientific skills are believed to be more related to the left hemisphere, as are positive emotions. Language is more complex than just words and consists of the content, syntax, grammar, semantics, and another component—prosody—the musical quality of speech. The right hemisphere includes music awareness (a musician's brain is more developed on the right side, as demonstrated on positron emission tomography [PET]). Spatial orientations, art awareness, insight, imagination, prosody, and negative emotions are predominantly on the right side. A patient with a right cerebral lesion might speak with a flat emotional tone or might show aprosody. Another impairment is agnosia. In cases of right cerebral damage, there is a denial of an impairment.

Additional studies have been done with patients in whom one eye (one hemisphere) was shown a film in which the theme demonstrated either a positive or negative emotion. It appeared that negative emotions (sadness) corresponded with an increase in left facial activity and right brain activity, so by observing the left facial muscles, one might be more likely to detect sadness.

In patients with damage to the right cortex, there is increased likelihood of deceased sadness or anxiety, and this may account for the denial (agnosia) that accompanies right lesions. Similarly, left-sided lesions might manifest more depression, since the usual upbeat emotions may be dulled by the left-sided damage.

Parietal lobe

Parietal lobe damage may be associated with variable symptoms. Lesions of the dominant hemisphere usually produce disturbances of speech, and lesions of the nondominant hemisphere produce gnostic deficits (i.e., lack of awareness of body part or of deficits).

Aphasia is the loss of the faculty of transmission of ideas by language in any of its forms—reading, writing, speaking, or failure in the appreciation of the written, printed, or spoken word. This impairment is independent of the disease of the vocal organs or appropriate sensory organs (hearing, sight). It has been found that if one single region is insulted, other areas of the same hemisphere or opposing hemisphere may "help out." When multiple areas are compromised, however, the effect on language is more devastating.

The ability to communicate via speech is most seriously disturbed following damage to the left hemisphere in right-handed individuals. Of left-handed individuals, about 20 to 30% are right cerebral dominant for speech. Although by and large the left hemisphere is the major contributor to speech, it has been found that some recovery in certain patients suffering damage to the left side of the brain can be accounted for by the contribution of the right hemisphere. There are two main types of aphasia. In expressive aphasia (motor, or Broca's aphasia), there is little speech or the speech is slow. Great effort is required in using single words, and a telegraphic style is characteristic. The understanding of spoken language and written language is intact. There is some correlation with large anterior lesions. Fluent aphasia (Wernicke's aphasia) is found in association with large posterior lesions and is characterized by long phrases and sentences, but words are used incorrectly and in a poorly organized form. Comprehension is disturbed.

Temporal lobes

A number of conditions involve the temporal lobes. Included in the temporal lobes are the cingulate cortex, the uncus, and the hippocampus. For this reason, the temporal lobes are often implicated in memory disturbances. Lesions of the lobes have caused aphasias and memory disturbances. Patients with temporal lobe epilepsy have been reported to show hyposexuality. This form of seizure disorder is called complex partial seizures. Electrical discharges located in the temporal lobes may have peculiar effects. Patients may manifest bizarre behaviors. As with other seizures, there usually are prodromal symptoms of scintillation (sparkling lights), gustatory sensations (heartburn), or feelings of unreality. The ictal event may take the form of subjective experiences or automatic behaviors. Included among these are emotions such as severe anxiety, depersonalization, derealization, feelings of déjà vu or jamais vu, paranoid ideas, and other subjective experiences. Motor phenomena may be manifest, including simple repetitive movements such as buttoning or unbottoning a shirt, lip smacking, or speech utterances. Complicated behaviors have been attributed to these seizures; however, they are rare and poorly documented. More frequently, patients who have shown criminal or violent behavior may use their illness as an excuse to avoid the consequences of their behavior. Postictally there is a sense of disorientation and confusion. Interestingly, some patients themselves report unusual behaviors in between their seizures. This interictal behavior includes personality changes, increased aggressiveness, emotional lability, moralistic fervor, increased religiosity, and increased writing.

Apraxia is the inability to carry out a behavior in spite of having the full sensory and motor abilities that are required for that behavior. For example, a person may know that a pen is a pen, will be able to name it and manipulate it, but will not know how to use it. A gait apraxia differs from gait ataxia in that patients who are ataxic know how to walk but their balance makes it extremely difficult. In gait apraxia, their coordination is fine but they forget how to walk. In one condition, for instance (not specifically a parietal lobe disease)—normal pressure hydrocephalus (NPH)—there is the triad of urinary incontinence, dementia, and gain apraxia. Parietal lobe damage is often accompanied by a variety of apraxias including forgetting how to dress oneself or how things go together or come apart (dressing or constructional apraxias). Certain defects like the aphasias mentioned above occur predominantly in the temporal frontal area (Broca's aphasia) or temporoparietal area (Wernicke's aphasia). Three conditions—alexia (inability to read), agraphia (inability to write), and acalculia (inability to solve mathematical problems)—occur in both the temporal and parietal regions, predominantly on the left side.

Biochemistry

In addition to the structural approach to understanding behavior, underlying biochemical defects and their relation to behavior have been observed over the past three decades.

Affective disorders

Noradrenergic system.   There are many studies and clinical observations supporting the role of norepinephrine in affective disorders. It has been observed that reserpine (an antihypertensive and early antipsychotic) depletes norepinephrine and also frequently causes depression. Studies have yielded interesting but sometimes inconsistent data. In some depressed patients, there is a decreased amount of 3-methoxy, 4-hydroxyphenylglycol (MHPG) (see "Catecholamine metabolism"). Some depressed patients have been found to have decreased plasma norepinephrine and others increased norepinephrine. A fourth source indicating the role of norepinephrine in depression comes from the studies involving amphetamines. D-amphetamine has an effect on a number of neurotransmitters, perhaps chief among them norepinephrine. The effect of amphetamine on mood is to improve mood and produce at times elation along with increased levels of norepinephrine. There is also a correlation with mania (an affective illness is in some ways the reverse of depression). Norepinephrine breakdown products (MHPG) are increased in some manic patients. Amphetamine may bring out manic euphoria and initiate a full-blown attack in susceptible manic patients. A fifth source supporting the role of norepinephrine is the observation that in tuberculosis wards, when patients were treated with isoniazid, some became euphoric. Isoniazid is a monoamine oxidase (MAO) inhibitor that increases CNS norepinephrine.

The primary location of the cell bodies of those neurons rich in norepinephrine is in the locus ceruleus, a nucleus located on the upper pons. Cell bodies located elsewhere in the medulla as well as the locus ceruleus send diverse projections throughout the brain. These pathways have been ellucidated via the histochemical fluorescent technique. When treated with formaldehyde, norepinephrine granules produce a green fluorescence.

It is important to know that the rate-limiting step is tyrosine being converted to dopa (dihydroxyphenylaline) via tyrosine hydroxylase. As you can see, dopamine, another important neurotransmitter, is part of the synthetic pathway of norepinephrine (Fig. 7-1). Neurons that lack the enzyme dopamine beta-hydroxylase are noradrenergic neurons rather than dopaminergic neurons.

Norepinephrine can be converted into epinephrine. Prior to its excretion in the urine, it is metabolized by two alternative metabolic pathways (Fig. 7-2). Intracellularly, MAO converts it into dihydroxyphenylglycol (DHPG), which in turn is converted by the second important enzyme, catechol-O-methyltransferase (COMT), into MHPG. COMT is present intra- and extracellularly and is the chief means for its breakdown in the peripheral blood. COMT can act directly on norepinephrine to produce normetanephrine, another important breakdown product.

Serotonergic system.   The role of serotonin (5-hydroxytryptamine) comes from the observation of decreased breakdown products (5-hydroxyindoleacetic acid [5-HIAA]) of 5-HT in the CSF of depressed patients. Antidepressants that selectively increase CNS concentrations of 5-HT have added to the evidence of its role in depression. Cell bodies are located primarily in the raphe nuclei of the lower pons. The dorsal raphe cells project to many parts of the limbic system and

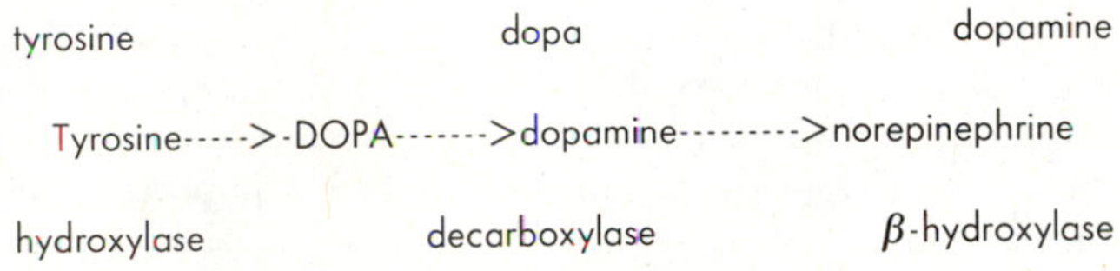

tyrosine   dopa   dopamine

Tyrosine----->-DOPA------->dopamine--------->norepinephrine

hydroxylase   decarboxylase   β-hydroxylase

Figure 7-1.   The synthesis of norepinephrine.

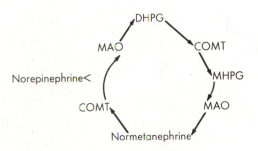

Figure 7-2.   The metabolism of norepinephrine.

cortex. Synthesis is dependent on the conversion of tryptophan via tryptophan hydroxylase to 5-hydroxytryptophan and is the rate-limiting step. 5-HT is broken down via MAO to 5-HIAA. Serotonergic systems are involved in other behavioral aspects. Serotonin has been implicated in sleep disorders, in violent behavior, and in sexual behavior.

Cholinergic system.   Evidence for the role of acetylcholine in depression comes from several observations. Workers exposed to **cholinesterase inhibitors** found in insecticides developed depressive symptoms. Centrally given physostigmine will cause an inhibited depressed picture in certain patients. As mentioned earlier, the hippocampus, which is believed to be an inhibitory brain structure, is rich in acetylcholine. Acetylcholine is the neurotransmitter that is associated with the parasympathetic system, whereas norepinephrine and epinephrine are the sympathetic neurotransmitters. On the basis of the balance of these two systems peripherally and the above observations, a **cholinergic-adrenergic balance hypothesis** has been put forward. It postulates that mood (and perhaps thought disorder) is the result of a balance between these two large neurotransmitter systems. Included in the noradrenergic system is dopamine, an important neurotransmitter. Depression then could be seen as an excess of acetylcholine or a deficiency of norepinephrine. It is interesting to note that the medications that are used in combatting psychoses are potent dopamine-blocking agents and that to alleviate their side effects anticholinergic drugs are used. Acetylcholine's role in depression is perhaps its least well understood role. It serves an enormously important function in memory. Drugs such as atropine that are used preoperatively in surgery to decrease secretions and bowel activity are potent anticholinergics. These drugs have as one of their side effects the ability to impart amnesia for the events of the surgery. The hippocampus, which is rich in acetylcholine, is the structure in the brain playing an important role in memory. Experimentally, the acetylcholinergic precursors choline and the drug **deanol** have been used to treat Alzheimer's disease and improve memory. Acetylcholine is present in higher concentrations in the brain stem. Although we are focusing on certain neurotransmitters that have been found to play a role in behavior, it should be understood that acetylcholine, norepinephrine, serotonin, and dopamine account for only a fraction of the percentage of neurotransmitters in the brain. The largest percentage is taken up by gamma-aminobutyric acid (GABA) and glycine, about which less is known.

Dopamine.   This neurotransmitter has been implicated as having a role in a number of disorders, including schizophrenia and the affective disorders. Ordinarily we think of dopamine in its role in the schizophrenic disorders. Dopamine is a precursor of norepinephrine. When schizophrenic patients are treated with the neuroleptic (antipsychotic) drugs, one of the disturbing consequences is the extrapyramidal side effects including Parkinson's disease. It has been found that these drugs block dopamine transmission and as a result cause many of the parkinsonian symptoms such as rigidity and slowness of movement. The dopamine hypothesis is implicated in the etiology of schizophrenia; the basis for this hypothesis is covered in the discussion of schizophrenia. Dopamine has been implicated in depression as well. Some patients with depression have reduced levels of homovanillic acid (HVA), the breakdown product of dopamine. This metabolite may be increased in some manic patients. Levodopa, which is used in the treatment of Parkinson's disease, can cause mania in some individuals.

Other neurotransmitters.   Doubtless there are numerous undiscovered neurotransmitters. Only recently have endogenous opioids been discovered. Termed **endorphins**, these endogenous opioid peptides may play an important role in mechanisms involving memory, pain, perception, punishment and reward, eating, and movement. The first, identified in 1975, were the pentapeptides methionine and leucine enkephalin. A larger peptide, beta-endorphin, appeared to be the parent molecule, which may be part of a larger protein beta-lipotropin.

The neurotransmitter GABA, which is present in abundance, plays a crucial role in central inhibition of impulses. GABA may act by opening the chloride channel in neurons, thus reducing excitation. Although GABA neurons are by and large believed to be short neurons, there are long projecting GABA fibers. There is now postulated a benzodiazepine endogenous substance similar to the endorphins that act on GABA to inhibit the firing of neurons. **Glycine** and **glutamic acid** are neurotransmitters of excitatory nature whose role has yet to be elucidated. The neurotransmitters norepinephrine and dopamine, although important, account for only 1 to 2% of the neurotransmitters found in the brain as a whole. Only 5 to 10% of the synapses are likely cholinergic. GABA may account for 25 to 40% of the synaptic central neurotransmission.

Memory

Memory is another area in which the biologic underpinnings are only partially understood and in which psychological factors play a role. We have already discussed how the hippocampus functions in memory and the importance of acetylcholine as a transmitter in this system. Other brain structures are also involved. Before covering these, some basic terminology regarding memory should be reviewed. Memory is believed to occur through several stages. Three aspects have been described: registration or encoding, retention, and recall. **Registration** is the ability of a subject to enter the information into the memory system. This can be tested by asking the subject to repeat words. In certain conditions such as aphasia, this may be difficult to assess. Patients may have difficulty not because their memory is faulty but because the area of the brain concerned with language expression may be impaired. Furthermore, subjects who are inattentive may not register information because their attention is focused elsewhere. Given a person who can register information, the next aspect to assess is the **retention** of the information. Certain pieces of information can be retained for the individual's lifetime, whereas others are forgotten quickly. Short- and long-term memory have been described as two different systems that people and animals use in retaining information. The amount of information in short-term memory is believed to rely on neural traces with little structural change in the nervous system, whereas long-term memory is believed to rely on alterations in the brain's neuronal structure or neurochemistry. Various experiments have been done to demonstrate the importance of early experience on memory and learning. Rosenzweig and colleagues have demonstrated that laboratory animals (rats) raised in an enriched play environment consisting of various performance tasks and novel stimuli had structurally different brains after a period of time than did rats that were raised in a more impoverished environment. In particular, rats from an enriched environment had a greater number of dendritic spines and had approximately *50% larger synaptic junctions* than did littermates from an impoverished environment. In addition, the rats from the enriched environment had heavier occipital cortices. Recently, Eric Kandel's work with *Aplysia,* a type of snail, has resulted in some interesting findings. In its natural environment, *Aplysia* will extend a gill from its respiratory chamber and will withdraw it when excited as a means of protection. The snail given repeated stimulations will eventually "learn" that the stimulus is nonthreatening and will cease the protective withdrawing. Both short- and long-term memory can be established in this species. If given a short course of training, the snail will forget its new behavior in a matter of hours or days. With somewhat longer training sessions, the behavior will be maintained for a matter of weeks. In *Aplysia,* the quantity of neurotransmitter released varies according to whether the stimulus is new or old. The amount of neurotransmitter will be greater with novel stimuli. With longer-term memory, the structure of the neuron may be changed with an increase in the number of "active zones" involved in the release of neurotransmitters.

In some studies of the brains of alcoholics, cerebral atrophy was noted and believed to be an irreversible process. One study found that there was some reversal of atrophy after a period of abstinence from alcohol. Recent memory loss is a hallmark of all severe organic brain syndromes, according to some authors. In order for memory deficits to be severe, lesions of the hippocampus should be bilateral. In addition to the hippocampus, other areas of the brain are involved. The fornix plays a role since its bilateral destruction impairs registration and **recall**. Lesions of the dorsomedian thalamic nuclei and pulvinar nuclei produce severe recent memory problems with a normal hippocampus. The mammillary bodies were thought to be the previous site of pathology in Wernicke's disease. Memory is not located in a single brain region. Pennfield demonstrated that if certain areas of the temporal lobes were stimulated memories could be evoked. If these areas were subsequently destroyed or removed, the memory would not be destroyed. It appears that the entire brain is important for retention, whereas registration may involve crucial structures listed above.

ANALYTIC CONCEPTS

The literature of psychoanalytic theory can fill an entire library. In order to become familiar with psychoanalytic concepts it is important to review Freud's work. *A General Introduction to Psychoanalysis,* a compilation of lectures now offered in paperback, was originally presented to the medical school class of the University of Vienna during the years 1915–1917. The following quote from this first lecture succinctly describes the difficulties the medical student may experience when approaching this subject and illustrates Freud's gift for writing.

First of all, there is the problem of teaching and exposition of the subject. In your medical studies you have been accustomed to use your eyes. You see the anatomical specimen, the precipitate of the chemical reaction, the contraction of the muscle as the result of the stimulation of its nerves. Later you come into contact with the patients; you learn the symptoms of disease by the evidence of your senses; the results of pathological processes can be demonstrated to you, and in many cases even the exciting causes of them in an isolated form. On the surgical side you are witnesses of the measures by which the patient is helped, and are permitted to attempt them yourselves. Even in psychiatry, demonstration of patients, of their altered expression, speech and behavior, yields a series of observations which leave a deep impression on your minds.

But in psychoanalysis, unfortunately, all this is different. In psychoanalytic treatment nothing happens but an exchange of words between the patient and the physician. The patient talks, tells of his past experiences, and presents impressions, complains, and expresses his wishes and his emotions. The physician listens, attempts to direct the patient's thought processes, reminds him, forces his attention in certain directions, gives him explanations and observes the reactions of understanding or denial thus evoked. The patient's unenlightened relatives—people of a kind to be impressed only by something visible and tangible preferably by the sort of "action" that may be seen at a cinema—never omit to express their doubts of how "Mere talk can possibly cure anybody." For they are the same people who are always convinced that the sufferings of neurotics are purely "in their own imagination." Words and magic were in the beginning one and the same thing, and even today words retain much of their magical power. By words, one can give to another the greatest happiness or bring about utter despair; by words the teacher imparts his knowledge to the student; by words the orator sweeps his audience with him and determines its judgments and decisions. Words call forth emotions and are universally the means by which we influence our fellow creatures. Therefore let us not despise the use of words in psychotherapy and let us be content if we may overhear the words which pass between the analyst and the patient.

Words were important to Freud, and through listening he became aware of a world that had hitherto been unexplored. Freud came to study psychiatry via neurology. In his work as a clinical neurologist, he saw many maladies that he was unable to treat. One such type of affliction was hysteria (which today might be diagnosed according to the *Diagnostic and Statistical Manual of Mental Disorders* [*DSM III*] as conversion disorder). In this disorder, sensory and motor problems were plentiful. In 1885 Freud arrived in Paris to study with Charcot. He began to develop ideas regarding the power of psychological forces.

Psychopathology of everyday life and topographic theory

One hint about how words belie a secret world occurs in the form of **parapraxia**, or **slips of the tongue**. People also commonly make slips of the pen, reading incorrectly and mishearing. Forgetting and misplacing are also examples of these mental errors. That there were powerful psychological forces and that they could be connected with such mundane things as saying something that one does not mean to say seem a difficult connection. When Freud began to question patients and people about these various errors, he found three patterns emerging. In the first, a speaker readily admits that an opposing thought had preceded the slip. Freud gives as an example a man who begins a meeting by saying, "A quorum is present; the meeting is closed." This same man may readily admit that the meeting was a waste of time and he wished it were over. In the second type of pattern, a person might tell you he was aware of an opposing wish but that it had not occurred to

him. Finally, a person might deny even vehemently any such opposing thought.

Forgetting is a common daily occurrence. Some people without any disease process (neither Alzheimer's disease nor any other condition affecting memory) might commonly make such errors. One person reported forgetting where she had placed a gift for her mother, a beautiful crystal figurine. She searched for hours in vain, finally recruiting her husband. They tore the house apart to no avail. When they both were totally exhausted, the woman reached between a cedar chest and the bed and produced the box in which the gift was located. She could not identify why she looked there last, nor why she might have forgotten its location and suddenly found it. The next day the mother's birthday was celebrated and was enjoyed by all. Several days later the woman was embarrassed to tell the husband that she had forgotten to give the gift after all. When this was discussed further, the woman admitted that she had liked the crystal figure very much and had wanted one for herself.

Another example of such experiences occurs with hearing. It is not uncommon for people to leave a lecture or therapy session having heard totally different points being made. In these situations, the person is **distorting** what is heard to coincide with his or her own wishes.

From these types of experiences, Freud was able to demonstrate that there are tendencies, wishes, and feelings lying outside the realm of our conscious minds. This realm we call the **unconscious**. Freud early on elaborated a theory that is called the **topographic theory**. In this theory, the mind is thought of as divided into several different realms. The first of these realms is **consciousness**. It is what occupies our attention and our mental processes from moment to moment. There is another realm that we have no awareness of and can only become aware of through special means. Thoughts or feelings that we have and that we are unaware of are in the **unconscious**. Finally, between these two **regions** there is a third region termed the **preconscious**. The preconscious is the type of awareness that we have when we say something is "on the tip of our tongue" or "in the back of our mind." We are aware that there is a thought, but we are also unable to bring it into focus. This area is extremely important in a process we will discuss below—**free association**.

It can be shown that many errors that seemingly have no apparent reason for happening have very definite logical precipitants that lie outside of our awareness. The principle that holds to these types of errors is termed **psychic determinism**. Analytic theory holds that all behavior is determined and that a large part of the motivation in behavior is unconscious. In some analytic training programs, it was customary to instruct patients in analysis to make no major changes in their lives while undergoing analysis. The patient was discouraged from marrying, divorcing, changing jobs, and making similar major changes while the analyses continued. This was because of the belief that these behaviors had to be fully examined and had as their possible motivating factor unconscious forces.

The analytic process

In the process of analysis, many behaviors occur that the analyst feels that patients should explore. Not uncommonly in analysis, patients will miss a session or be late or forget to pay their bill. When the analyst inquires into these events, patients may respond by denial or by giving some excuse such as sleeping too late or being preoccupied with other matters. This phenomenon is part of a process that is very important in analysis—**resistance**. Resistance is the force that opposes the free flow of ideas. It opposes the person's becoming aware of his or her preconscious and unconscious thoughts and feelings. Resistance may take many forms. A person's mind may go blank or may be overwhelmed with too many ideas. Patients may wish to avoid a subject and discuss some more trivial matter in its place or may suddenly become healthy and have a **flight into health**. In this situation, the patient's problems haven't truly vanished but rather have only temporarily dissipated as a form of resisting the further inquiry of the analyst.

Freud once described the entire practice of analysis in terms of understanding the operation of two principles. The first was resistance and the second was termed **transference**. The practice of psychoanalysis has many different forms. There are those who follow the early hypothesis of Freud with little revision—the Freudians. There are in addition analysts who are more concerned with personal relationships—the **interpersonalists**. In many different theoretical frameworks that use analytic techniques, the issues of resistance and transference are usually a central focus. As patients enter into analysis, the analyst discusses with them the **fundamental rule**. This is the instruction to patients to say whatever comes into their mind. It is not an easy rule to obey. Frequently a patient may think something like, "My, this seems so trivial, I won't bother telling this detail," or "My God, if my analyst hears this about me I'll get thrown in the booby hatch." As the patient proceeds to talk in analysis and follows the fundamental rule, transference will begin to develop. The patient will begin to express perceptions about the analyst. These ideas will bear little relation to the analyst, who takes care not to divulge personal information. In addition, the analyst may make use of the analytic couch, where patients lie supine and cannot view the analyst even if they wish to. The analyst, however, can see the patient's expressions and movements from this perspective. Through this procedure the patient must begin to imagine what the analyst thinks and eventually voices these ideas. The patient often attributes either unusually harsh or uncaring characteristics to the analyst. If the patient voices these ideas, the analyst will listen and eventually come to understand that these feelings or thoughts are transferred from some significant person in the patient's past. The analyst may have warm feelings for the patient, contrary to the patient's perception.

To exemplify this phenomenon, let's discuss the beginning of therapy with a hypothetical patient named Bill. Bill came to the clinic because of problems with his marriage and work, anxiety, and angry outbursts. He was seen twice weekly and spoke nonstop about his terrible living situation. Bill blamed all of his problems on his boss and his wife but could not describe any problems that arose from inside of him. Each session became alike. After a period of 2 months, he had not expressed any personal difficulties aside from those caused by these people in his life. The analyst tells him that he seems to attribute all of his problems to others and does not have any personal problems aside from these. His reaction is intense and immediate. He suddenly recalls being 8 years old and being bullied by local boys. When two in particular gang up on him, he runs home crying. His father confronts him with his crying, chastising him and telling him, "Either you go out and fight these two boys or you fight me!" He went out and fought them both. He won the fight but lost in another way—he lost his ability to trust others with his more vulnerable feelings. In the analysis he similarly thinks that if he opens up his feelings that the analyst will ridicule and chastise him like his father. His feelings toward his father are transferred or displaced onto the analyst. The phenomenon of transference occurs frequently in therapy and will be discussed in subsequent sections on the physician-patient relationship. Undoubtedly, all physicians will at some time experience this powerful phenomenon in their patients' illogical and irrational ideas about them.

Hysteria and childhood sexuality

The historical basis for Freud's understanding of the unconscious forces stems from his collaboration with **Joseph Breuer**, a prominent Viennese physician. In discussing all of these phenomena—slips, misplacing, transference, and resistance—we are speaking about the unconscious. The case on which Freud worked with Breuer and opened up the exploration of the unconscious was that of Anna O. This was the case of a young intelligent and strong-minded woman 21 years old who had a number of symptoms of unexplained etiology. Breuer had been treating her for a year in Vienna and told Freud about the case. The patient's symptoms included paralysis, vision disturbances, contractures, and diverse other motor and sensory phenomena. These symptoms could be made to disappear if the thoughts or affects that occurred at the time the symptoms formed could be brought back into consciousness. In 1895, *Studies on Hysteria* was written by Breuer and Freud. It was believed that the therapy worked because an idea had not been sufficiently discharged by way of speech. In successive cases, Freud found that ideas could be retained in the patient's mind but repressed. The repressed idea could not freely interact with other ideas, which would cause the painful idea to be modified. Freud likened the restriction of painful life events or thoughts into the unconscious to a fungus that given the light of day (reality) would not grow but in the darkness of the unconscious would grow luxuriously. A theory emerged that it was the closure of the avenues of discharge that led traumatic memories to be expressed in symbolic or somatic forms. Through the discharge of these memories and pent-up feelings, a symptom could be alleviated. This discharge was called **catharsis** and the process called **abreaction**. This is the way many lay people conceive of analysis. The Hollywood image of a psychiatrist digging into the unconscious and coming up with some terrible forgotten truth would be followed by the patient's intense emotional memory. Recall the movie *Spellbound*, in which Gregory Peck developed amnesia. As the analyst uncovered the memory of his having accidentally killed his brother, the patient was relieved of his symptom.

Freud was very interested in discovering the basic science of mental processes. He conceptualized that energic quantities were involved and that these forbidden ideas or memories could be charged with energy, and the term **cathexis** was applied. A particular idea was said to be cathected (charged with psychic energy). He spent many years attempting to develop a theoretical framework that took into account the various handlings of psychic energy. With regard to the somatic symptoms of patients in which there could be found no underlying organic etiology, this theory accounted for the symptoms by stating that the psychic energy of a traumatic event was converted into a symbolic physical event. This was termed a **conversion disorder** or **conversion neurosis**.

As Freud began to listen to a number of patients unfold their life histories to him, he found that many of these traumatic memories were sexual in nature. The **seduction hypothesis** implied that early seductions of children by adults would lead the children to develop subsequent psychopathology as adults. Freud felt that a momentous step had been taken in psychoanalysis when he challenged the truthfulness of the many seduction scenes that were being painted for him by his patients. He postulated that in childhood there were sexual feelings and ideas and that these were coloring the thoughts of his patients' recollections. He evolved the idea that it was the sexual wishes and fantasies of children that were being distorted into parental seductions. Recently, historians have begun to question Freud's revision, claiming that in reality there was an increased incidence of sexual abuse of children and Freud was actually hearing the truth. Whether this is true or not, the direction of analytic theory took a significant turn as the sexual nature of children and adults was examined.

Dream theory

This concern for the fantasy life of the patient and understanding the childhood experiences as they related to adult symptoms was a point of great magnitude in psychiatry. As the technique was elaborated, important revisions were made. Initially, Freud used **hypnosis** to allow for the patient's "talking cure." Following this, Freud attempted to persuade his patients to speak freely by urging them, even pressing on their foreheads! This was replaced by the analyst being silent and waiting for the patient to free-associate. **Free association** is the process by which a patient says whatever comes to mind, no matter how trivial or embarrassing. The patient often has many difficulties in this process. In listening to patients speak freely, Freud came to hear of their **dreams**. It became clear to Freud that, like slips of the lip or pen, dreams reflected unconscious ideas. Freud stated in his fifth lecture to students:

So dreams become the object of psychoanalytic research— another of these ordinary, under-rated occurrences, apparently of no practical value, like "errors," and sharing with them the characteristic of occurring in healthy persons. But in other respects the conditions of work are rather less favorable. Errors had only been neglected by science, people had not troubled their heads much about them, but at least it was no disgrace to occupy oneself with them. True, people said, there are many things more important but still something may possibly come of it. To occupy oneself with dreams, however, is not merely unpractical and superfluous, but positively scandalous: it carries with it the taint of the unscientific and arouses the suspicion of personal leanings towards mysticism. The idea of a medical student troubling himself about dreams when there is so much in neuropathology and psychiatry itself that is more serious— tumors as large as apples compressing the organ of the mind, hemorrhages, chronic inflammatory conditions in which the alterations in the tissues can be demonstrated under the microscope! No, dreams are far too unworthy and trivial to be objects of scientific research.

Freud's sarcasm was heavy, and dream analysis became an extremely important tool in uncovering the vast storehouse of the unconscious. Indeed, dreams are termed **the royal road to the unconscious**. It was in 1900 that *The Interpretation of Dreams* was published. Dreams are important for a number of reasons. Everyone dreams. In the early 1950s, it was found that during sleep there were two distinct stages— REM and non-REM sleep. REM referred to the rapid eye movements that occurred during this stage. On awakening the subjects, it was found that the vast majority were in the middle of a dream. Thus, dreaming occurs during REM sleep. Patients who were awakened in non-REM periods occasionally reported dreams, but they were usually much less vivid and occurred in lower percentages. Questions arose about the relation between the rapid eye movements and the dream. Was the subject attempting to use his eyes to follow the events in the dream? This question remains unanswered; in some experiments, subjects could correlate their dreaming with the eye movements. For instance, one subject reported that he was walking up a flight of stairs. The sleep observer noted that there were seven upward deviations of the eyes and this correlated with the number of steps that the subject reported in the dream. However, rapid eye movements have been reported in neonates and in subjects who have been congenitally blind.

Freud was unaware of REM sleep, and his discoveries of dreaming were important for other reasons. He found that during dreaming a subject expresses forbidden wishes and unresolved childhood conflicts. This occurs on several levels. The dream is recalled with all of the visual, auditory, and other sensory and emotional components. This material is referred to as the **manifest content**. The nature of the dream lies in the hidden meanings of the dream— the **latent content**. The dream protects the subject from the more frightening and forbidden latent content via the **dreamwork**. This usually consists of a number of defensive maneuvers, discussed later. The dream uses defense mechanisms to disguise the nature of the conflict. One such mechanism is **symbolism**. One patient reported the following dream:

I was in a study of my house drinking beers with my friends and watching TV when a lion came in. It grabbed one of my friends by the arm and started eating him. I awoke terrified.

The patient was asked to free-associate to the dream, and the material that emerged helped understand his underlying conflict. In response to asking about the lion, his immediate association was as follows:

In the study there is an ashtray that I am forbidden from using. It belongs to my father and has a picture of a lion in it. My father is like a lion when he yells at me. He is particularly angry at me now— he doesn't know how badly I've just done in school.

The dreamer is struggling with his guilt feelings about his covering up his recent failures in school, his unresolved fears of his father's anger, and his wish to disobey him. The father becomes symbolized by the lion in the dream. There are a number of mechanisms that are employed. Dreaming is an example of a process of thinking called **primary process**. In this type of thinking (which also occurs during psychoses), the subject's ability to **test reality** is diminished. Anything can happen in primary process thinking. It is illogical. Young children in their preoperational mode of thinking or even infants in their sensory-motor phase of development think like this. Cause and effect can be reversed. A person can fly, have wheels, die, and be alive in a matter of moments. A person may combine attributes of several people—have the eyes of one's mother and nose of one's brother. In primary process thinking the individual attempts to gratify instinctual wishes, usually sexual or aggressive in nature. In dreaming, there is also the intrusion of logical or **secondary process thinking**. Primary process thinking operates on the **pleasure principle**. This is the desire to gain pleasure and avoid pain. As children mature, their operating under the pleasure principle is gradually modified by the **reality principle**. This is the understanding that all things are not possible and that personal wishes and feelings have to be sacrificed at times.

Structural theory

As Freud elaborated his observations regarding dreaming and the analytic process of free association, he further detailed the topographic theory. It appeared that some sort of structure operating in the mind allowed the expression of certain ideas in the dream or in the analytic session, but not others. It was as if a "censor" were present. He eventually talked about a dream censor, which allowed for the expression of feelings. There emerged a view of the mind as containing an internal structure. This consisted of three components. The mind was divided into the **superego**, the **ego**, and the **id**. Each region had particular functions. The superego was the seat of the conscience. It was conceived of as allowing or forbidding certain impulses. As you may recall in the discussion of the development of the child, there is a particular time in life around the age of 3 to 5 or 6 years when the child struggles with feelings toward both parents. The oedipal stage and conflict are resolved with the development of the superego, or the internalized values of the parents and society. The feeling of **guilt** arises because of an attack of the superego on the person's ego.

The ego is the executive of the mind. It is that portion that is involved with various interactions with the real world. While the superego has the conscience and the ideals of the child, the ego has numerous functions. The ego functions include the following: (1) **Reality testing**. This is the ability to distinguish between inner and outer stimuli and to assess the accuracy of one's own ideas against what society believes. (2) **Judgment**. This is the ability to make decisions and carry out actions with regard to the possible consequences. (3) **Sense of reality of the world and self**. This is the sense of self-esteem and one's identity. (4) **Regulation of drives, affects, and impulses**. This is the ability to delay gratification and deal with sexual and aggressive impulses. (5) **Object relations**. When we discussed the work of Margaret Mahler and the manner in which a child gains internal mental representations during the phases of separation-individuation, we were discussing object relations. Such aspects as object constancy and the quality of these internal representations are reflected in whether we see people as predominantly good or bad. (6) **Thought processes**. This is the ability and stage of thinking, whether one can use abstract thoughts or primary process thinking. (7) **Adaptive regression**

in the service of the ego. This is the ability to relax one's defenses and regress or play. (8) **Defense mechanisms**. These are methods by which a person keeps unacceptable thoughts, feelings, or impulses away from consciousness. (Questions about defense mechanisms are frequently asked on the examination, and this subject will be discussed shortly.) An example is projection or denial. (9) **Stimulus barrier**. Each individual is sensitive to a certain level of sensory stimuli. Certain individuals need a great deal of stimuli, whereas others can be overwhelmed when two people are talking in the room at the same time. (10) **Autonomous functioning**. This refers to the ability to use one's neurological-psychological functions such as memory and motor and sensory apparatus without interference. (A person like Anna O., described above, would have obvious impairments in this ego function.) (11) **Synthesis-integration**. This consists of the ability to integrate the new knowledge into the data base and life of the individual. (12) **Mastery-competence**. One's confidence is based on the degree to which certain abilities have been mastered. Freud did not elaborate this list. It was compiled and enlarged by a group of scientists and psychiatrists who would be categorized in a school called **ego psychologists**.

The final apsect of the structural theory is the id. The id is the repository of the instinctual drives, both aggressive and sexual. It is the most primitive part of the mind, the first to develop. Animals are much closer to the id and react to their instincts in a direct fashion. Many problems that people experience arise because of their wishes conflicting with their gratification. On a theoretical level, they are the result of a battle between the various structures of the mind.

The libido theory and psychopathology

We have reviewed each of the psychosexual stages, as conceived by Freud, through which a child passes. To review, the child progresses from oral to anal to phallic levels of development. In each, the child struggles with his or her sexual pleasure from each zone. The oedipal conflict gives rise to the superego and the repression of sexual interests. There follows a period of latency, which gives way during pubescence to the genital stage of development, in which heterosexual interests are attained. This sexual drive was termed libido and, as mentioned, it could become fixated as a result of undue gratification or inhibition. In addition, the libido could return to earlier levels of development, an occurrence termed regression. A typical example is the oedipal-stage child who, on the birth of a sibling, begins to soil himself (regresses to the anal period). As can be seen, the various zones of gratification of the sexual drive or libido are diverse. The gratifications that can be derived might involve sucking, defecating, anal penetration, or genital manipulation. The fact that the libido could derive from so many different forms was described as polymorphous. If there was a failure to develop to appropriate levels of sexual expression, it was theorized that the libido was perverted. The term **polymorphously perverse** described these early libidinal or sexual interests. Psychopathology could then be conceived of as occurring in several different ways. If there was a fixation of the libido into one area, a **perversion** might ensue. Today *DSM III* would term these **paraphilias**. If the individual underwent an unsuccessful repression (not resolved) of these drives, the result would be a **neurosis**. The neurosis, which could be obsessional thoughts or phobias, in some way contained the repressed sexual wish. *DSM III* now includes the term neurosis in parenthesis beside a number of anxiety disorders and other disorders.

Anxiety and the mechanisms of defense

Anxiety is a fascinating subject. There may be an inherent aversion to studying this entity. Anxiety is referred to in a number of ways, and it is both a symptom and yet an aspect of normal life. In normal situations, however, it is unpleasant. There are other affects that are unpleasant, but under given circumstances they can be made to be pleasant. Sadness can be "sweet." People enjoy listening to sad music or watching "tearjerkers" at the movies. Even fear, which comes closest to anxiety, can be actively sought. People go to amusement parks to shriek in terror. Today's young people flock to the cinema to watch terrifying mutilations in a number of violent movies. However, anxiety is different. No one eagerly anticipates an anxiety-provoking situation such as a test or giving a speech in public. The major difference between anxiety and fear is the cause. In anxiety the cause of the pain is not known, whereas in fear there is a clear source of the pain. Otherwise, fear and anxiety are similar in that all of the autonomic, cardiovascular, and GI symptoms are alike. Freud initially thought that anxiety resulted from the damming up of sexual energies and that the sex drive (libido) was converted directly into anxiety. This theory was replaced with the **signal theory** of anxiety. According to this theory, individuals experience anxiety as a signal that their ego is about to become aware of some unacceptable thought, feeling, or impulse. The anxiety signaled the ego that the id was about to make itself known in a negative way.

A patient complained of an attack of severe anxiety. He reported this happening as he was getting into the shower. The man, although devoted to his family, had been involved in extramarital affairs in the past. He had suffered terribly from guilt and had altered this behavior. When he was asked what his thoughts were at the time of the attack, nothing could be remembered. Finally, the patient recalled that he was thinking about a phone call he had received from a rather attractive woman.

In the above case description, the patient was about to be overwhelmed by his sexual feelings and impulses toward this woman. The anxiety signaled that something was about to occur that was dangerous to him. In his therapy, he had to deal with his strong sexual feelings and how to handle them in relation to his marriage.

Anxiety may arise from a number of directions and from common conflicts in life. John Nemiah describes several basic routes that anxiety may take. The patient described above suffered from anxiety that arose from the superego. **Superego anxiety** arises when persons are afraid of their own punitive conscience. A person who slips and curses in front of an authority figure might experience this type of anxiety. If a person comes late to work and feels nervous, this type of anxiety arises. Another variety is **castration anxiety**. As was discussed in the section entitled "Psychosexual development," little boys during the phallic and oedipal stages develop increased pleasure in their penises. At the same time they wish to have sole possession of their mothers and wish their fathers

out of the picture. This wish stimulates fears of retribution on the part of the father and in particular fears of damage to their prized organ. Fears of physical mutilation during this period are relatively common. Nightmares and beliefs in monsters hacking off parts of their body are expressions of this underlying anxiety. **Separation anxiety** occurs during the period of separation-individuation described by Margaret Mahler. Here the young toddler fears that the mother might not return once she is out of sight. This subsides if the mothering figure establishes sufficient trust and the child develops object constancy. Pathological derivatives can be seen in school phobias in young children. **Id anxiety** arises from that structure of the mind that houses the drives. This type of anxiety usually is experienced when one is overwhelmed by impulses. Persons such as schizophrenic patients with poorly developed ego structures are prone to this type of anxiety.

There are many ways in which persons can defend themselves against anxiety. Some people who experience anxiety may allow it to pass. Others may reach for a drink or a cigarette or become involved in physical exercise. All of these activities defend the person from the anxiety. However, these are usually not considered defense mechanisms. A defense mechanism is a psychological device used to prevent anxiety and unacceptable ideas, feelings, and impulses from entering awareness. They are usually used unconsciously. Defenses can be erected from infancy onward. There have been attempts to categorize defenses on a developmental level. Indeed, we have already discussed the use of certain defenses at particular periods of life. For instance, we discussed the reaction formation during the anal period and the use of sublimation during the school-age period.

Denial. The person simply refuses to accept reality. This may take the form of not accepting one's own sensations, or it may reflect a person's refusal to accept irrefutable evidence. Several clinically relevant examples relate to illness. A 70-year-old woman is brought to the emergency room because of severe jaundice. The intern calls a psychiatrist because the patient refuses to be admitted, stating there is nothing wrong with her. When the psychiatrist holds up the patient's yellow hand and asks if there is anything unusual about the color of her skin, she responds no. Here the patient denies her own senses. A 55-year-old internist begins to experience severe precordial chest tightness accompanied by eructation and discomfort in his left arm. The doctor's wife insists that he go to the emergency room, but he refuses, insisting it is only "heartburn." His friend, a cardiologist, speaks with him but, despite the obvious signs, cannot convince him that he might be having a myocardial infarction. Here the person is not denying his senses but is denying the deductions and logical conclusions of his own thought processes. Many people use denial when confronted by aspects of life that are too troubling to face. This may take the form of being noncompliant with a doctor's orders, including not taking medication or not following exercises or instructions for rest.

Projection. In projection, persons attribute to others the feelings, ideas, or impulses that they themselves do not wish to face. This defense plays a major role in the paranoid patient, who usually is having trouble dealing with sexual or aggressive feelings and begins to perceive these same affects in others.

Paranoid patients may believe that others want to kill them, which is attributing to others their own murderous impulses.

Distortion.   Certain threatening perceptions or thoughts may be experienced in an altered form. Distortion occurs in very psychotic patients when they change reality into bizarre forms. A 21-year-old patient experienced some epigastric distress, which he attributed to snakes being in his stomach. The intern on call refused to perform radiological procedures, which this patient demanded. Distortion occurs in normal individuals. The game in which a group of people is asked to pass on a message from one individual to another is an example. By the end of the game, the final message bears faint resemblance to the original one. Clinically, patients may distort a few words that a physician says to them, resulting in their not taking medications as prescribed. Medical students typically distort physical sensations into the disease they are studying. A 22-year-old medical student became convinced that a muscle twitch heralded the onset of amyotrophic lateral sclerosis.

Acting out.   A person may avoid an inner feeling or idea by means of action. The significance of this action is not appreciated by the individual. Body language is perhaps the most common example. A woman who strikes a clenched fist against her chair may be unaware that she is angry at something. A young patient may forget her appointment but may be unaware of her underlying anxiety about her illness. A 32-year-old patient who usually is very responsible arrives at his session in a state of inebriation. He is unable to discuss the reasons except to explain about his business lunch. The following session, the patient talks about his impending marriage and how he thinks that it will mean the end of his having fun. Arriving drunk the previous week was an attempt to avoid his feelings about the sacrifices he was about to make; he instead demonstrated in action his underlying desire to be irresponsible. A doctor who forgets an appointment with a patient should examine this forgetfulness to find out if there are underlying feelings such as guilt for not being able to cure a case.

Repression.   A thought or feeling is kept from awareness. In the cases of hysteria that Freud worked with, this was a prominent mechanism. In these cases, what was repressed returned in a somatic symptom, but this is not necessary for the defense to be used. Repression may be directed to a single traumatic event or to a traumatic situation. A 40-year-old woman had a history of several years of alcohol abuse. During the times that she was intoxicated, she was sexually uninhibited. In the course of her analysis she became aware of a repressed traumatic situation in which she was sexually abused as a child. With the return of this repressed memory, her drinking stopped.

Suppression.   In this defense, persons actively put something out of their minds. It differs from repression in that the mind becomes aware of the thought or experience and then it is actively pushed out of awareness.

Reaction formation.   Freud described this as a brittle defense. It has been referred to during the discussion on toilet training. It occurs when one feeling or thought is replaced with its opposite. An example would be a man who treats someone in a kind manner when unconsciously he may feel hatred.

Isolation.   Here the feeling and thinking aspects of a situation are separated. Individuals may not experience one or

the other and thus may protect themselves from some unpleasant experience. This occurs commonly in physicians who may deal with experiences associated with painful feelings. A surgeon who specializes in trauma care may see the patient but not experience the frightening or painful aspects of the patient's wounds. A 50-year-old woman would come to her sessions and cry uncontrollably. She could not describe the thoughts that accompanied this affect. After some time in therapy, the session repeatedly returned to the subject of her children going away to college. She had isolated the affect from the thought of her being alone because initially it was too overpowering.

Displacement.   This is an extremely common mechanism of defense. People who act like savages on the road may be displacing anger that belongs at work or at home. Displacements are common, as illustrated by the following vignette:

A father returning home from work is in a foul mood because of an insult the boss hurled at him. His wife is a few minutes late making dinner, and he yells at her for this. In walks little Johnny, who asks his mother if he can go out and play. She in turn yells at him, reprimanding him for not realizing it is dinnertime. When Johnny sees his sister Sally playing with his toy, he flies into a rage, grabbing the toy away.

Somatization.   Physicians are well acquainted with the fact that many symptoms have no organic basis. Approximately 30% of a general practitioner's practice may be taken up with patients who are expressing their emotions through their physical complaints. Many underlying needs may be thus expressed. Typically, a person's need for attention may have only been tolerated in a family when that person became ill. Growing up in that environment might encourage a person to express the need for attention by magnifying the aches and pains of daily life. It is very important that the physician, while realizing the frequency of somatization, not attribute to the mind what may be physical in origin.

Rationalization.   Persons attribute an action or idea or feeling to some reason that is more acceptable to themselves than the actual reason. Persons may cheat on their income tax and explain that everyone does it a little. Here persons are attempting to avoid dealing with guilt and their underlying greed. A person who drinks excessively may say it's only a way to unwind that is very common. A patient who does not seek out a physician when she discovers a lump in her breast may say it's probably just a cyst or maybe it will go away.

Regression.   The person returns to an earlier level of development. A young child who begins wetting the bed when a sibling is born is one example. When people become ill, they may adapt behaviors that are in some ways regressive. They may have exaggerated complaints and act helpless and passive—more like a child than an adult. When patients become psychotic, it is believed that on a dynamic level they are returning to infantile ways of thinking in which there are magical thoughts, loss of body boundaries, and on occasion loss of the ability to verbalize.

Externalization.   This is similar to rationalization, but it is used more by antisocial personalities and is more obviously an excuse. Authors believe that externalization is common and describe it as attributing any unacceptable idea or impulse to someone else. An example would be a person feeling others are liars when he fears this about himself. It is more general than projection and requires less logic than rationalization.

Sublimination. This is considered one of the mature defenses. The unacceptable wishes or ideas or feelings are funneled into socially acceptable ones. A person who wishes to harm others may find a soldier's life rewarding, allowing him to discharge his aggressive wishes in a more socially acceptable way. Sadistic impulses may be funneled into becoming a butcher.

Humor. By making light of things, a person may avoid a great deal of anxiety or pain. Black humor is common after tragic events in some circles. A group of medical students may find themselves making an excessive number of jokes during their first days in the anatomy lab. This is an attempt to deal with the anxiety about death, about dissecting cadavers, and about their own fears of bodily damage.

These defenses can be used by practically anyone. The use of defenses is normal. They become pathological when they are used excessively or inappropriately. Certain disorders make use of particular defenses. In phobias, the original conflict is displaced onto a symbol and then avoided (a defense not discussed). The individual then avoids a conflictual part of himself. In paranoid schizophrenia, projection and distortion are used. In dissociative disorder, conversion type, the defenses of somatization, dissociation (not discussed), and repression are used.

BEHAVIORAL PSYCHOLOGY

History

Behavioral psychology shares interesting similarities with psychoanalytic theory. In both there is an attempt to explain behavior in an all-encompassing way. Psychoanalysts espousing the philosophy of **psychic determinism** have produced some conflict by insisting that behavior is due to unconscious mental forces and that it can be ultimately reduced to sexual and aggressive drives. Similarly, the followers of **B. F. Skinner** have tended to explain behavior by processes of conditioning. The elaboration of each of these systems of understanding occurred in approximately the same time frame. Beginning with **Ivan Pavlov**, studying in Russia in 1890, and B. F. Skinner, in the 1930s, there is a striking correlation with Freud's work in the 1890s and crystallizing the analytic technique in the 1930s and 1940s. The apparent conflict between psychoanalysis and behavioral psychology may have been fueled by the training of behavioralists and analysts. By and large, analysts have required an M. D. degree for training (this has changed in many areas), whereas Skinner and subsequent behavioralists have been psychologists. There is much evidence that both points of view have been valuable in understanding human behavior.

Classical conditioning

Behavioral psychology has been equated with learning theory. The primary focus is on the person's actions, although the manner in which a person thinks or feels can also be the focus of study of behavioral psychologists. The initial observations of the Russian physiologist Pavlov are well known. To review them, it is important to define certain terms: **unconditioned stimulus and response**. A subject exposed to a stimulus will have a reflexive type of response. The stimulus has as its motivating source the instinctive apparatus of the subject. Food is perhaps the most commonly used unconditioned stimulus, since all animals when hungry will respond automatically to it. In Pavlov's famous experiments, food powder would automatically produce a response (salivation) in his dogs. This is abbreviated

UCS (unconditioned stimulus) → UR (unconditioned response)

If a bell sounded whenever food was presented to the dog, the animal would soon salivate to the sound of the bell alone. The bell was the **conditioned stimulus** and the salivation was now the **conditioned response**, abbreviated

$$CS ----> CR$$

Classical conditioning can occur in many situations in life. It is one method of learning. A typical example is a common phobia, fear of dentists. Here the unconditioned stimulus may be the pain of a dentist's drill. The unconditioned response is avoidance or fear. The patient may then pair even the thought of the dentist with pain and avoid dentists inappropriately. One famous case is that of **little Albert**. In Watson's famous experiment, an 11-month-old child was shown a rat, producing no unusual response. The child was next shown a rat and at the same time was subjected to a loud, frightening noise. He became terrified. On subsequent confrontation with the rat, the child demonstrated fear.

UCS (loud frightening noise) ----> UR (fear)

CS (rat) ----> CR (fear)

By such pairings, many positive or negative associations can be learned. This may be one manner in which phobias actually develop. In the condition called agoraphobia, a person is terrified of going outside. It is believed that some of these patients have actually experienced panic attacks while outdoors. The person pairs the UCS (pain of panic attack) with being outside (CS) and then begins to believe that going outside will cause panic. This type of learning can be demonstrated to have three phases: acquisition phase, extinction phase, and spontaneous recovery phase. Figure 7-3 demonstrates that as the number of pairings is increased, there is an increase in the strength of the response. This occurs up to a point and tapers off. In the **extinction phase**, the time for extinction to occur depends on the level of previous learning. In the case of the CS of the bell eliciting the CR of salivation, if the bell is frequently presented and no UCS is presented (food), the dog begins to stop responding to the bell. It looks as if the dog has forgotten the lesson. However, if after a period of time has elapsed the dog is once again exposed to the bell, he will salivate in somewhat decreased intensity. **Spontaneous recovery** is said to have taken place. The subject in these experiments may become conditioned not only to the bell, but also to things that are similar to the bell, like loud noises. In the case of little Albert, his initial fear of white rats might be generalized to white beards or anything white. **Generalization** is the term for this process.

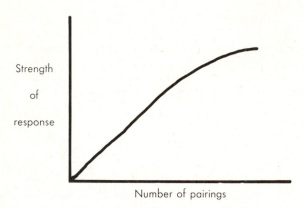

Figure 7-3. Classical conditioning. The strength of the response increases with the number of pairings.

Operant conditioning

Operant conditioning focuses the experimenter on the behavior of the individual. The individual is said to operate on the environment. The utility of this focus is that a person's behavior can be altered in more complex ways. In operant conditioning, subjects learn because of the **consequences** of their behavior. Here a new set of abbreviations signifies the behavior or response (R) and the probability of the event P(R). Different forms of operant conditioning are said to take place depending on the consequences and the probability of the event occurring.

(R) Behavior or response---->Stimulus----P(R) The probability
or   of the behavior
event   increases or
decreases

Initially, Skinner made use of an experimental chamber termed a Skinner box. The animal was allowed to roam freely, but when it accidentally pressed a lever in the course of its movement, it received a pellet of food. This was termed **positive reinforcement**. The likelihood of that event (pressing the lever) was increased. Eight forms of reinforcement are possible.

1. *Positive reinforcement.* This occurs when an action is followed by a pleasant consequence. The animal increases the behavior.
2. *Negative reinforcement.* This occurs when the animal's behavior removes a noxious stimulus. The animal is more likely to repeat this behavior. In the original Skinner box, the floor had an electric grid, and, by pressing the bar, the unpleasant shock could be reduced. Note that there is an **increase in the probability** of a behavior. Some people confuse negative reinforcement with punishment.
3. *Punishment.* When a behavior produces an unpleasant event, the probability of that behavior occurring again is decreased.
4. *Avoidance conditioning.* In this type of learning, the subject learns that by performing some behavior, painful stimuli can be avoided. In negative reinforcement the rat in the

Skinner box receives the shock and pushes the lever to reduce the shock's likelihood, but in avoidance conditioning the rat may learn that the shock will follow the flicking on of a light. When the light occurs, he anticipates the shock and presses the lever without having experienced the shock—a more advanced form of negative reinforcement.

5. *Extinction.* This is similar to extinction for classical conditioning, but here the behavior is followed by no reaction:

(R)---->No reaction---->P(R) is reduced

6. *Continuous reinforcement.* This refers to the pattern of reinforcement. Basically, every time a behavior occurs there is a reward or punishment. This is the type of learning that can easily be forgotten because once the reinforcement stops the subject associates that the reward or punishment has followed every behavior.
7. *Intermittent reinforcement.* This has been given a number of other terms— partial reinforcement, variable-ratio reinforcement, or inconsistent reinforcement. This is the type of reinforcement that occurs poorly for learning a new behavior, but once it is learned it provides the strongest edge against the behavior being lost.
8. *Delayed versus immediate reinforcement.* It is always better to have as little delay as possible between the behavior and the reinforcement.

Learning theory

Learning as a process refers to internal mental changes that are the result of experience. Four major forms of changing behavior have partly been discussed. In addition to operant conditioning, classical conditioning, and extinction, described above, a fourth form is **modeling**. Many people need only observe a model performing an activity to be able to imitate it. Imitation is involved in a number of learned phenomena including language, morals, and identifications. Verbal learning is another important method of learning.

Shaping and chaining. These are variants of operational conditioning in which the individual's behavior can be molded by successive approximations. The typical example given is teaching an animal tricks. The seal that is given a reinforcement pellet of food when it approaches a stand will increasingly approach the stand. In a step-by-step fashion, the animal is rewarded for getting on the stand, touching a set of horns, and eventually making a simple type of music. In chaining, the behaviors that are linked together are more complex than simply making a dog jump through a hoop.

Schedules of reinforcements. There are four possible arrangements in which a reinforcement can be delivered. In **fixed-ratio** reinforcement, a subject recieves a reinforcement after a certain number of behaviors. In **fixed-interval** reinforcement, there is a period of time that must elapse before the reward or punishment occurs. In this type of reinforcement, the behavior is slowest right after the reinforcement and increases in frequency close to the time of reinforcement. In **variable-ratio** reinforcement, a subject may have to press a lever up to a certain number of times, which would change. An example is a slot machine that delivers a prize with a variable number of attempts. Finally the **variable interval** delivers a reinforcement after varying periods of times.

Violent behavior and aggressive behavior

A study by Lewis of 97 juvenile offenders for violence divided up the subjects into the more and less violent groups. Significant differences could be demonstrated between the two. The more violent group had greater percentages of major and minor neurological signs and symptoms. They were much more likely to have witnessed extreme violence in the home and had greater paranoid ideation.

Violence is the strongest form of aggressive behavior. There are perhaps eight distinct types of aggression: (1) predatory (as exemplified by aggressively seeking out food or a position in the job market); (2) fear induced (when a threat is present without possibility of escape); (3) irritabiilty (this may be directed toward inanimate objects and may result from increased crowding or noxious stimuli of various sorts, (like noise); (4) territorial; (5) maternal (in protection of the young); (6) sex related (there may be increased male aggressivity in the presence of a female); (7) intermale (males will exhibit aggression within a pecking order of dominance-submission in some species); and (8) learned (by imitation or conditioning).

In studying violent behavior, we already reviewed some of the lesion experiments done with the resulting increased aggressivity. In addition, there have been a number of additional correlations. Violence is more common in the lower socioeconomic classes. Alcohol is a frequent factor in the emergence of violent behavior, as is male gender. This last point has led many investigators into performing studies on the influence of sex hormones on violence. Animals castrated at a fairly young age showed decreases in violent behavior. Testosterone plays a role in aggression but is not in itself enough of a factor. Aggressivity can be increased in certain strains of rodents by breeding, indicating a genetic component. In humans, some studies have indicated greater aggression and violence in individuals with an extra Y chromosome, XYY males.

Observations of violence have received much public attention. Whether or not watching violent TV programs or movies increases violence has been studied. In one study, the experimenter deliberately angered a group of men then showed half of them a filmed prizefight and the other half an aggression-neutral film. The students who saw the prizefight exhibited less hostility than the other students on tests administered after the film. This support for the catharsis or release of aggression by watching violence is overshadowed by the weight of evidence that indicates that viewing violence increases its expression. Preschool children shown films of aggression by an adult and observed in subsequent play demonstrated a tendency to imitate the kind of aggressive behavior seen in the film, even for mild frustrations.

From this information it can be seen that aggressive and violent behavior have a number of contributory factors— both biologic (increased incidence of neurological findings in juvenile offenders, effect of alcohol and hormones, gender, and genetic factors) and psychosocial (viewing of violence increases the expression).

Ethology

Ethology is the study of animal behavior. By undertaking a study of how other animals behave, it is hoped that aspects of human behavior can be better understood. A number of researchers have contributed valuable information to areas of study such as sexual behavior, aggression, mother-infant attachment, and emotional development. The most celebrated of these works is perhaps the Harlow monkey experiments.

Harlow performed a number of experiments testing the effects of cloth versus wire surrogate mother monkeys, examining social behavior with varying degrees of social deprivation. In studies of infant monkeys who were placed in cages and given equal access to cloth or wire surrogate mothers, the infants spent far more time climbing on and clinging to the cloth-covered models. Although the monkeys were divided into two groups and were forced to secure nourishment from the wire and cloth surrogates, even those that fed from the wire surrogate spent more time with the cloth-covered monkey. This experiment refutes the hypothesis that the basis of the attachment between mother and infant is purely the procurement of food. Originally the controversy arose because of analytic theories indicating that the instinctual drive of hunger was the motivating force in early development. The focus of the need for tactile stimulation received additional support from studies indicating that orphanage-raised infants became severely emotionally disturbed when not given tactile comforting.

In another group of experiments with young monkeys, the effect of social deprivation and maternal deprivation was noted. Young rhesus monkeys when removed from their mothers a few hours after birth were sturdier and more disease free than those remaining with their mothers. However, in spite of the controlled regimen of nurturant and physical care, achieving higher rates of survival, the baby monkeys demonstrated severe emotional disturbances. They stared fixedly into space, circled their cages in a repetitive fashion, clasped their heads in their hands or arms, rocked for long periods of time, and compulsively pinched themselves, sometimes to the point of physical trauma. When they were subsequently returned to their mothers or other peers, these severe deficits continued. These and other experiments indicate that there is a **critical period** somewhere between the third and sixth months of life during which social deprivation, particularly deprivation of the company of peers, irreversibly blights the animal's capacity for social adjustment. Harlow performed various experiments with periods of partial social isolation. He found that for shorter periods, say 60 to 90 days (equivalent to 6 months in a human), the deprivation may be reversible. Even these monkeys raised in partial isolation, when they became mothers themselves, demonstrated abnormal mothering behavior ranging from indifference to outright abuse. Further conclusions of Harlow's studies indicate that the behavior resulting from maternal deprivation could be partially (and even totally) reversed with adequate peer group exposure.

The study of human behavior takes for granted certain drives such as hunger and sexuality. Drives and instincts have been better understood by observing other animals. **Instincts** have certain basic features. They are genetic, species-specific behaviors that are not learned. Certain behaviors that have an instinctual basis are complex. Tinbergen's famous experiments on the male stickleback demonstrate these features. He observed that a certain behavior (nest building) could be elicited by certain **releasing mechanisms**, in this case the temperature of the water and the visual patterns of the appropriate environment. The instinctual behavior, termed a **fixed action pattern**, occurred in other members of the same species in the same way. The multiple complex aspects of human behavior perhaps obscure some instinctual behaviors.

One final ethologic experiment, performed by K. Lorenz, demonstrates the significance of the critical period. Shortly after hatching, goslings will become attached to their mother via a process known as **imprinting**. If the mother is not present during this time, the babies may imprint on the human observer. They will subsequently treat the human as if it were their mother. Such critical periods have also been witnessed in dogs. Puppies that are handled by humans early in life will subsequently be more trusting of humans. Other animals have also been observed to become attached to humans.

HUMAN SEXUALITY

Practically every medical specialist will be asked questions of a sexual nature. In some areas it is crucial to understand normal and abnormal sexual behavior, such as in urology, gynecology, obstetrics, family practice, pediatrics, and psychiatry. The topic is an inherently difficult one. This is reflected in a psychological game that can be played in group psychotherapy. Individuals in a group are asked to write down anonymously three things that they wouldn't want anyone to know about themselves. Invariably at least one of the items is some sexual fear, deficiency, or dissatisfaction. Masters and Johnson have reported sexual problems in a large percentage of marriages (up to 50%, according to some experts). Although we are supposedly in the midst of a sexual revolution, misinformation and apprehension abound in this area. Modern inquiry into sexual disorders and behavior gained momentum with the publication in 1890 of *Psychopathia Sexualis* by **Krafft-Ebing**. Modern studies by Kinsey and by Masters and Johnson will be discussed later. Their work has changed the focus from the cataloging of sexual disorders to an understanding of sexuality, beginning with normal anatomy and physiology.

The sex organs

The understanding of sexuality and reduction of sexual anxiety begins with proper knowledge of the terms for the sexual organs. In a survey of medical students, 60% were found to have had no prior sex education. Their knowledge was obtained largely from peers or inadequate hygiene classes in high school.

Women have no single sex organ; instead, a number of structures are involved in female sexuality. This fact and the fact that the vagina is hidden from view have made the female genitals mysterious and frightening to some males and females. Many women deal with their own confusion by referring to their sexual organs as "down there." The mystery is further compounded by the fact that only recently has there emerged evidence of an additional structure related to sexual pleasure—the **Graffenburg spot**, or G spot, on the anterior wall of the vaginal vault. The female genitalia consist of external and internal structures. The external structures, termed the **vulva**, consist of the labia major and minora, the clitoris, and the

vaginal introitus (opening). The internal genitalia consist of the vagina, cervix, uterus, and ovaries.

The male genitalia consist of the penis, testes, and scrotum. Many men feel a great deal of curiosity and insecurity about the size of their penis. Surprisingly, there are few studies on the variation in size of men's penises. There are, however, numerous quotations stating that the size of a man's penis has nothing to do with a woman's sexual gratification. Either a large or small penis can be accommodated by the vagina, which can expand to hold it via engorgement of its tissues. One of the few studies on the size of the penis was conducted by Masters and Johnson, who found in a sample of 80 men that men's penises varied from 7.5 to 11.5 cm when flaccid and gained an additional 7 to 8 cm on erection.

Sexual myths abound. Just as a man might worry without justification about the size of his penis, so might a woman worry about her vagina or breasts. Common fears include the idea that the vagina is too small or that it will be damaged by the penis. In some women, fears of insects and snakes can be traced to their fear that they will somehow get inside the vagina.

Physiology of sex

Masters and Johnson's studies on the stages of sexual response have allowed a detailed understanding of men and women's shared patterns. The four stages described are excitement, plateau, orgasm, and resolution. They occur in this order. Each stage is accompanied by various physical changes, described below (Table 7-2).

Excitement. It is interesting to note that in males and females, the state of readiness for intercourse can occur in less than a minute. In males, the **erection** of the penis occurs as the

Table 7-2. The Stages of Sexual Response

Phase	Male	Female
Excitement (minutes to hours)	Erection; scrotum tightens; nipples erect	Vaginal lubrication; nipple erection; labia minora enlarge
Plateau (30 seconds to 3 minutes)	Increased pulse, blood pressure, respirations; myotonia; testes enlarge	Increased blood pressure, pulse, respirations; labia minora change color; orgasmic platform—vagina; myotonia; sex flush of skin
Orgasm (3 to 15 seconds)	Ejaculation	Vaginal contraction; contractions of sphincters and uterus
Resolution (10–15 minutes; if no orgasm ½-1 day)	Loss of erection; autonomic return to baseline	Reduction in swelling of all structures; return to baseline in autonomic variables

venous blood engorges the corpora cavernosa. The scrotum becomes tighter and lifts slightly, along with the testes. Although nipples may become erect, this is seen more commonly in females. The female equivalent of erection is vaginal lubrication and engorgement. In the past, it was thought that the vagina became lubricated by action of the Bartholin's glands, but this is not the case. Vasocongestion (the same mechanism as in males) accounts for the lubrication of the vaginal walls. The clitoris becomes hard. Nipple erection occurs in two-thirds of women. Changes occur in the labia. There are variations between nulliparous and multiparous women. The labia minora become enlarged. The uterus (and cervix) ascend into the false pelvis. The excitement phase may last from several minutes to several hours in both sexes.

Plateau. In males, the essence of the plateau phase is the increased autonomic variables (blood pressure rises 20 to 80 mm Hg systolic, 10 to 40 mm Hg diastolic; pulse increases to 175 beats per minute; respirations increase) and increased myotonia (muscle contractions involving facial and other groups). The testes enlarge by 50%. Other changes occur as well. In females, there is similar autonomic excitation. Additionally, color changes occur in the labia minora (bright red). The breasts enlarge by 25%. The orgasmic platform, which is the lower one-third of the vagina, is in a constricted state. This allows for increased friction on the penis and also indirectly increases friction on the clitoris via the movement of the labia. The skin develops a sex flush. The plateau phase lasts 30 seconds to 3 minutes.

Orgasm. In males, ejaculation occurs, usually marked by three to four contractions and release of about 1 teaspoon of seminal fluid including 120 million sperm. Autonomic arousal is only slightly greater than in the plateau phase. In females, contractions of the vagina and uterus occur. Contractions of the sphincters of the rectum and urethra occur in both sexes. Orgasm lasts from 3 to 15 seconds in both sexes.

Resolution. The male penis loses erection and returns to its fully flaccid state in 5 to 30 minutes. Autonomic variables decrease to normal in 10 minutes. In females, autonomic variables return to normal and erectile tissue returns to its preexcitement state. In both sexes, if there is no orgasm there is a more prolonged return to baseline of swelling and autonomic variables.

In males, there is a **refractory period** that lasts from several minutes to many hours. During this time, a male cannot achieve another erection or ejaculation. Women may have rapid and multiple orgasms, there being no refractory period.

The autonomic pathways include sympathetic and parasympathetic pathways. Sympathetic nerves are responsible for ejaculation. Because of sympathetic innervation of the glands and ducts associated with ejaculation, neuronal discharge in this system results in the inability to hold back ejaculation—ejaculatory inevitability. The parasympathetic system controls erection.

Gender identity formation

A person's sense of being male or female is his or her **gender identity**. Children begin to think of themselves as male or female based on the gender assignment and rearing from birth. This identity is usually irreversible by 18 months and complete by 4½ years. An individual's sex (male or female) and sexual identity (femininity and masculinity) may not be congruent. Two terms require definition: **Core gender identity** is the self-identification of a person as being male or female. **Gender role identity** is the self-concept of being masculine or feminine. An individual may know that he is a male but feel feminine. Thus a conflict may arise between his core gender identity and his gender role identity. **Gender identity** has thus been confusingly defined to mean a combination of both gender role identity and core gender identity.

Freud postulated that a boy's sense of masculinity came from the oedipal conflict, in which he gave up his mother out of fear of castration and identified with his father. Females, on the other hand, were envious of the father's penis but later developed a desire to have the father's baby. The female's identity resulted in a sense of inadequacy and inferiority. Karen Horney, a female psychoanalyst, took exception to this and felt that little girls did not develop a sense of femininity but that it was innate. It is interesting to note that in blind children, boys born with a congenital absence of a penis and girls with a congenital absence of a vagina develop an adequate sense of their gender differences. Although the genitals play an important part in sense of masculinity or femininity, they are not crucial. So far, then, three factors have been shown to lead to a sense of gender identity: (1) the observable genitals, (2) the sex that one is reared, and (3) an innate sense ("biologic force") of one's sexual identity. (This last factor was previously presented under "Neurological and Biochemical Basis of Behavior.") In order for male rats to develop a male behavior pattern, they must be exposed to a testosterone pulse during early development. In humans, too, there is a need for a testosterone pulse during fetal development for the genitalia to develop correctly. It has been found that the fetus becomes masculinized from a basic feminine configuration. Animals in which this early androgen exposure is absent exhibit female behavior. The genitals develop during the seventh week of fetal life, male characteristics depending on the presence of fetal testosterone. Exogenously administered testosterone will also have a masculinizing effect. The fourth factor in gender identity is one's **psychological development**, which involves the resolution of any interferences in the appropriate development.

Neurological basis of sexuality

It is believed that, prior to the masculinization due to fetal testosterone, there is a fetal androgen that causes the regression of the müllerian duct system and allows the development of the wolffian duct system. Therefore, a person with an XY chromosomal pattern can be genetically both male and female but look phenotypically female if this organizing hormone (fetal androgen) is missing.

It has been postulated that certain aspects of the limbic system that occur together are concerned with basic survival functions: **feeding, fighting, self-protection (escape), and sexual behavior**. In certain experiments using electrical stimulation of various limbic structures, sexual behavior can be elicited alone or with other behaviors.

For example, in the macaque monkey, squirrel monkeys, and others, the following structures have been implicated as causing penile erections: the median forebrain bundle, fornix, anterior thalamic nuclei, mammillary body, and septum. In stimulation of the amygdala in the macaque, there resulted first oral activity then penile erections. In squirrel monkeys, stimulation in the region of the septum and amygdala elicited biting, chewing, and combat behavior.

Penile erections are noted in two other species, the Ugandan kob and the chimpanzee, during aggressive behavior. Both bruxism (chewing movements) and penile erections occur during REM sleep in humans. Many species of monkeys including green monkeys and baboons use sexual displays of the genitals in aggressive protective behavior. Even the shield of Mars in mythology is symbolic of the male phallus and war!

Sexual behavior, myths, and variations

Sexual behavior can be noted in infants. It was believed that during the Victorian era a nursemaid would calm an infant by touching its genitals, but infants can be aroused by stimulation of their genitals and may engage in such self-stimulation. Sex play begins more earnestly during the period around 3 years old. This play is normal. Parents may unnecessarily traumatize their children by reacting to this behavior with alarm or severe punishment. "Playing doctor" is part of normal sexual curiosity. When children begin to exhibit this kind of behavior, the parents need to explain what is appropriate behavior. Children may ask questions about sexual anatomy—usually the differences between males and females. Information should be given commensurate with the level of the child's understanding. At times, because of the parents' anxiety, explanations may not be given or may be overly elaborate. The following joke illustrates this point. Little Billy arrived home from school during the second grade. He asked his parents what sex was. His mother was embarrassed and said, "Your father will explain." Billy's father became very anxious and commenced a long discussion beginning with the birds and bees and discussing sexual anatomy, conception, intercourse, and birth. Billy looked bewildered and asked, "I have this form from school to fill out and it has a blank next to sex—What do I put?" "Put 'male'," Billy's father sheepishly replied.

The myths surrounding sexuality are plentiful, including those about masturbation, which is normal and harmless behavior. It not only occurs during childhood and increasingly so during adolescence, but also during adulthood—even among married men and women. Even as recently as this century, some texts have indicated that masturbation may cause insanity, hairy palms, baldness, loss of energy, and much more. There are also many myths concerning sexual intercourse during menstruation. Many people think of it as unclean or harmful, which is not the case. In primitive cultures, women were ostracized during their menstrual periods. Some studies have found that women suffer from more anxiety, depression, and irritability during the period prior to menstruation. A woman in England claimed she committed murder because of her premenstrual tension, and was acquitted. The nature of a women's orgasms has been a subject of controversy. Women can experience pleasurable sensations in the clitoral and vaginal areas. Freud and subsequent analysts maintained that the vaginal orgasm was superior to the clitoral orgasm. The work of Masters and Johnson has found this not to be true.

Sexuality can be experienced in a number of variations, which are in themselves not pathological and offer certain benefits. There is a wide variety of positions for sexual intercourse. The most well known is the male superior position, also known as the missionary position. It allows for face-to-face contact and adds in this way to the intimacy and romance of sexuality. The female superior position maintains the face-to-face contact and permits a woman to obtain more clitoral stimulation than in the male superior position. Women who have trouble achieving an orgasm may find this position helpful. Men with back injuries or other diseases that may make exertion or movement difficult may also find this position preferable. In addition to genital-genital contact, oral-genital contact may provide diversity and stimulation. In couples struggling with premature ejaculation, this may provide for a more mutually satisfying form of sexuality. In the rear entry position, the woman may kneel with her pelvis raised and her back arched. The male enters from behind her. This position may be more comfortable during pregnancy and may be preferred by some women because it allows them to directly stimulate their clitoris manually. There are numerous other positions.

Besides variations in positions, there are variations in the sex preferences of the partners. **Homosexuality** occurs as a preferred method of sexuality in 4 to 6% of males and 1 to 3% of females. The American Psychiatric Association has declassified it as a disease. In *DSM III,* a person who is distressed by his or her homosexual orientation is diagnosed as sexual disorder not otherwise specified. Homosexual experiences are common and have been reported in 40 to 50% of all males, usually occurring during childhood or adolescence. A noted psychiatrist calls this the period of **chumship** or normal homosexuality, which precedes the onset of adolescence. Most homosexuals profess no desire to become heterosexual. One subtype of homosexuality, termed **pseudohomosexuality**, has less to do with an erotic interest in the same-sex individual but rather is found in males who feel inadequate as males. They equate their low feelings of power with being like a woman and equate this with being homosexual. Their sexual activity has issues of submission and domination at its core. Finally, individuals may find themselves choosing homosexual partners simply because there are no heterosexual persons available, such as in institutions.

There is a wide range of normalcy in terms of sexual appetite. At the extremes are those individuals with no sexual drive and those with an insatiable one (satyriasis in males and nymphomania in females). Sexual drive is probably to some degree genetically determined, but psychological forces play an important role. There may as well be a reinforcing principle so that those individuals who abstain from sexual activity may find their drive decreases and those who engage in more activity may find their sexual appetite increases. Biologic forces play a role. Certainly, illness will decrease drive. Hormonal influences may increase or decrease sex drive. Testosterone administered exogenously to males who have waning sex drive in midlife has been found to increase drive in some cases. Estrogens given to females in the menopausal period similarly may increase sexual interest—particularly if accompanied by testosterone. Finally, social factors play a part in sex drive, which is modified to some degree by the expectations for conformity by the social setting and culture.

Sexual studies

The Kinsey study of male and female sexual behavior was obtained by questionnaires and interviews. The studies conducted in 1948–1953 shed new light on adult sexual behavior. Basic statistics regarding normal and abnormal sexual behavior were obtained. Among the findings was the observation that women enjoy sex more than was previously thought and are capable of more orgasms than was thought. The discovery that men have a peak in sexual activity around 18 years old and that woman peak later in adulthood is important. The work of Masters and Johnson regarding the sexual physiology and anatomy as well as response cycle has allowed a more detailed understanding of sexual behavior.

Genetic sexual disorders

Klinefelter's syndrome.   This syndrome is associated with an XXY chromosome complement. The additional X chromosome interferes with the full masculine development. The afflicted individual is phenotypically male and has small testes. The penis may be small, and breast development may occur after puberty. Various psychiatric problems may be encountered, including mental retardation, gender identity disturbances, and depressive disorders. Reproductively, these individuals tend to be sterile.

Turner's syndrome.   In this syndrome, the absence of the second chromosome (XO) prevents either masculine or full feminine development. Although the individual is phenotypically female, there is gonodal agenesis; if the gonads are present, they are poorly developed. The external genitals are those of a female. There are associated features of webbed neck, short stature, and sterility.

XYY syndrome.   There is some controversy about the features of this disorder. It is believed that these individuals have poor impulse control, and they are found in greater numbers in the prison population. They may have increased sex drive and also are tall in stature.

Testicular feminization or androgen insensitivity syndrome.   These individuals are genotypically males, XY, but phenotypically females. The target tissues (brain and fetal genital tissues) are insensitive to the androgen produced. Therefore, the external genitals are those of a female, although testes can be present but inconspicuous.

Adrenogential syndrome.   The individuals are genotypically females, XX. The adrenal glands produce excess androgens in females, resulting in the development of external genitalia that appear masculine. The genitalia show both male (penis, testes) and female (vagina, uterus) structures. The behavior of the individual will depend on the manner in which the child is raised. This is also known as a hermaphroditism (containing both male and female sexual organs).

Sexual disorders

This review will discuss disorders listed in *DSM III-R,* an updated edition. There are four major types of sexual disorders: gender identity disorders, paraphilias, sexual dysfunctions, and other sexual disorders.

Gender identity disorders.   This group is divided into two categories, those occurring during childhood and those in adulthood, termed **transsexualism.** In childhood sexual gender identity disorders, the parents, peers, and others may note that the behavior of the child is that of the opposite sex. The terms "sissies" and "tomboys" are commonly used for these individuals. The work of Green has reviewed the findings in this area. Tomboyism (masculine behavior in females) is common, whereas sissy behavior (feminine behavior in males) is not. There is little social disapproval of tomboyism but great social disapproval of sissy behavior. Subsequent development of sissies but not tomboys indicates that they may develop sexual disorders. The diagnosis of gender identity disorders of childhood rests on dress, toy preference, activity preference, roles played in fantasy games, peer-group composition, and physical mannerisms. Psychotherapy for these children focuses on alerting the child to behaviors that might lessen their having friends, attempting to alter them to some degree. Replacement of feminine games for more neutral games may be undertaken. The improvement of the father-son relationship may be pursued.

Transsexualism is a persistent sense of discomfort about one's anatomic sex and a wish to live as a member of the opposite sex. The ratio of males to females affected is 3 to 1. Transsexuals may be categorized into those who begin feeling different as early as they can remember (primary) and those who begin wishing a sex change at various times and later in development (secondary). Psychodynamics indicate that the mothers of transsexuals have themselves been denigrated for their having been born women and therefore may seek to change their son, both as a means of revenge and as an attempt to nurture the feminine aspects that were denied in herself. The transsexual boy's father was usually passive and distant. The etiology could also include biologic components—recall the importance of fetal androgen in masculinizing behavior in later life. The decision to alter sex surgically is one that is difficult. In cases in which this has been done, there have reportedly been good results. The individual is happier and usually has a good postsurgical adjustment. In those cases in which the individual is not happy, there may have been underlying psychopathology of a severe personality disorder or schizophrenia. Psychiatric evaluation clearly is an important part of the presurgical approach. Psychotherapy in altering transsexuals has had a poor success rate when the desire is long standing. Results in those cases with more recent onset are probably better. Surgical results can be quite good, and female functioning is attained, although the individual is sterile.

Paraphilias.   Paraphilias involve activities in which sexual gratification is obtained by altering key aspects of the sex drive. Freud's paper on sexuality entitled *Three Essays to the Theory of Sex* discusses the paraphilias (and ego-dystonic homosexuality, which in Freud's day was termed "inversion"). In it he describes the sex drive as being broken down into two components: the **object** (the person toward whom the sexual attraction was directed) and the **aim** toward which the instinct strives. The normal sex object was a person of the opposite sex. The normal sexual aim was the union of the genitals in the characteristic act of copulation. Either the object or the aim of the drive could be changed. So if the object were a person of the same sex, an "inversion" was said to have occurred. If the aim became a matter of looking at the person, a "perversion" was said to have occurred (voyeurism). Seven different paraphilias are noted: fetishism, transvestitism, zoophilia, pedophilia, exhibitionism, voyeurism, sexual masochism, and sexual sadism.

Fetishism. In this condition, the individual cannot achieve sexual gratification without some inanimate object, usually an article of clothing. In the example of a shoe fetish, the individual may need to ejaculate into the shoe or have a woman wear certain shoes. The fetish may serve as a transitional object with a parental figure and allay underlying separation anxiety, or there may be in the patient's history an arousing experience with a parent or family member in which the fetish was present. The sexual desire is thus displaced onto the inanimate object.

Zoophilia (bestiality). This is a rare perversion in which the object of sexual gratification is an animal. In learning about sexuality, adolescents in rural areas may engage in some form of sexual relations with animals.

Transvestitism. This disorder consists of a man's dressing in women's clothing, in fantasy or in reality. It is not reported as a disorder in women. The afflicted individual finds this behavior more arousing than any other form of sexuality. He may be secretive about it, but there are groups of transvestites who form social cliques. The male is normal biologically and may be married and participate in "macho" vocations. The transvestite does not wish to become a woman (or then would be termed transsexual). The disorder begins usually in childhood or adolescence.

Pedophilia. The adult who is sexually aroused by children prefers them to adults. The children are prepubertal. When this disorder is noted in adolescence, it must be distinguished from sexual ''play'' depending on the age of the child. The psychodynamics of this may involve fear of being emasculated by an adult woman or anger directed against women. Pedophilia may involve strangers, but the more common pattern involves family members or friends and acquaintances.

Exhibitionism. The image of the man with a raincoat exposing himself to women or children on the street is what is usually brought to mind by the term exhibitionism. However, exhibitionistic behavior can take more subtle forms. For the diagnosis of this disorder, the individual must repetitively expose his genitals to unsuspecting persons for the purpose of achieving sexual excitement. The disorder is reported in males predominantly. The psychodynamics are related to the individual's anxiety about his genitals. There is some underlying fear of castration, which is reduced by seeing the expression on the victim's face. In effect, he learns that indeed he has a penis. Undoubtedly there are many other factors at work. The individual may feel inadequate sexually and usually has a less than satisfactory sex life. His inadequacy can be reassured by this behavior. During childhood, in the preschool period the child will demonstrate his genitals as a source of pride. A tolerant parental reaction will help the child develop a healthy body image. If the behavior persists, there may be some unresolved issue. When the behavior repeatedly demonstrates itself in school, the possibility of sexual abuse may be present. In some families, the guilt about sexuality may produce such a negative reaction in the parents that this early normal genital displaying may meet with profound reprimand and shock. The underlying conflict that is produced may then be reenacted in adulthood.

Voyeurism. The individual repeatedly and preferentially chooses to watch unsuspecting people in the act of undressing or engaged in sexual activity. Voyeurism may represent a fixation during a stage of early and normal sexual curiosity. The unresolved anxiety and guilt may propel the individual (usually male) to repeat the previously traumatic experiences.

Sexual masochism. The individual preferentially chooses to be humiliated, bound, beaten, or otherwise made to suffer as a means of feeling sexual excitement.

Sexual sadism. The individual has repeatedly and intentionally inflicted psychological or physical suffering on a nonconsenting or consenting partner in order to produce sexual excitement.

Sexual sadism and masochism are neither exclusively male nor female disorders. The underlying dynamics indicate that power issues in the person's development are being directed or expressed in a sexual manner. Sadistic behavior usually indicates underlying rage that is unable to be dealt with by verbal expression or conscious resolution. In masochistic disorders, the issue may involve power conflicts in development as well as issues of guilt and punishment.

Sexual dysfunction

Sexual dysfunction comprises a group of disorders in which there is an inhibition in sexual desire or performance. In these conditions there is the need for a thorough medical evaluation, since many illnesses and drugs or medications can be at fault. If the disorder persists without an underlying organic etiology, then the diagnosis of psychosexual dysfunction of the appropriate type is made. The surgical-medical conditions described below are just a few of the many that can cause sexual dysfunction.

Systemic illness. These can include cardiac, renal, neoplastic, neurological, pulmonary, and infectious illnesses. These usually decrease the sexual desire (libido) or may interfere with the nerve or vascular supply.

Endocrine diseases. Diabetes mellitus in particular may cause 50% of males in the latter part of the illness to become impotent due to neuropathy or vascular problems. Diseases or surgery of the genital tract or related areas can also cause impotence. Certain types of prostatectomy, inflammations of the penis, or infection of the urinary tract can also produce impotence.

Medications and drugs. Antihypertensive agents probably interfere with sexuality more than any other type of drug. Thiazide diuretics are a frequent cause of impotence. Guanethidine (Ismelin), clonidine, methyldopa (Aldomet), propranolol, and reserpine all have been implicated. Antipsychotic drugs and tricyclic antidepressants may impair sexuality through their anticholinergic and sympatholytic effects. Any CNS depressant such as sedatives, alcohol, cannabis, or antihistamine may decrease libido and impair erection and ejaculation. In one clinic study, 35% of men attending an outpatient medical clinic suffered from impotence. Of that group 25% had impotence caused by medications.

Hypoactive sexual desire. This is a persistent and pervasive loss of desire not attributed to organic factors. In females, this is termed frigidity.

Inhibited sexual excitement. This is referred to as impotence or male erectile disorder (*DSM III-R*) in men and failure to lubricate in females or female sexual arousal disorder (*DSM III-R*).

Inhibited orgasm (female and male). *DSM III-R* defines inhibited (female/male) orgasm as the persistent or recurrent delay in or absence of orgasm following a normal sexual excitement phase during sexual activity. It is fairly common in women, at least in studies conducted in the 1930s to 1950s. The rate of anorgasmia in the healthy female population age 16 to 50 may be 36%. It is believed to be due to greater sexual-social prohibitions aimed at women.

Dyspareunia. In females more than in males there is the association of pain in the genitals without an underlying organic cause.

Premature ejaculation. The man ejaculates before he wishes it to occur. The physician must judge the length of time that is reasonable. A person who ejaculates after several minutes and whose partner finds sex to be mutually gratifying certainly does not qualify for this diagnosis.

Vaginismus. This refers to spasm of the outer third of the vagina that prevents successful intercourse. Once again, there is an absence of organic factors.

In the six conditions described above and others not mentioned, there are many factors that can be found to be at the root of the problem. Kaplan divides the etiologic factors into four groups: (1) here-and-now causes, (2) intrapsychic (unconscious) factors, (3) dyadic (relationship) issues, and (4) learned behavior (conditioning). The here-and-now causes include sexual anxiety, fear of performance, lack of communication about what excites the partner, and excessive need to please the partner. Intrapsychic factors are many. For example, the analytic theory postulates that premature ejaculators reveal unconscious rage against women and a desire to harm them. Similarly, unconscious memories about sexuality may be associated with guilt and anxiety. Often there can be an improvement in sexual relations when the relationship in general improves. Interpersonal conflicts regarding expression of anger, nonsexual affection, or other issues may spill over into the sexual arena. Learning theory maintains that the person may become conditioned to a disorder. For example, when a man who has excessive work pressure is occasionally impotent and anticipates failure regularly, he has conditioned himself to become automatically apprehensive and thereby nonarousable.

Therapy is directed at the underlying cause. Most often the interview will reveal a combination of the above four etiologic factors. Reducing sexual ignorance and giving permission reduces anxiety and guilt about sexuality. The opportunity to speak about sexual matters begins the process of desensitization. Therapists vary in the techniques used. Although analysts work with the individual toward understanding the unconscious sources and then working them through, sex therapists work with the couple. The use of a therapy that focuses on the couple rather than on the individual was pioneered by Masters and Johnson. The underlying communication difficulties and the possibility of one of the couple sabotaging the therapy are thus reduced. Sex therapists often work in teams. The use of opposite-sexed cotherapists reduces the likelihood that one of the partners will feel discriminated against. Initial therapy involves the couple's discussing their sex lives, interests, and related issues. The therapists may provide sexually explicit material including videotapes to reduce guilt and anxiety and stimulate arousal. The next aspect of therapy will be directed to the underlying problem.

For impotence, the couple is instructed to undergo a series of nondemanding sexual experiences termed **sensate focus**. In this technique, the couple is instructed to avoid intercourse but to become more familiar with the pleasure induced by erotic, sensual touching. By becoming more aware of the erotic pleasures aroused, the man's natural ability to have an erection will be stimulated. The couple is taught that a man cannot "will" an erection but that it occurs when he loses himself in the pleasure of the encounter. By gently caressing the body, after a time including the genitals, full erections can be maintained. The couple is encouraged to use fantasies in becoming aroused. Communicating what is pleasurable increases arousal. By reducing what is termed **spectatoring**, the individuals stop the process of looking at themselves perform and instead become participants. Another technique is to encourage selfishness in pursuing one's pleasure with one's partner.

In cases of premature ejaculation, several techniques have been described to be very successful. In many of these therapies, the male is directed toward being stimulated either extravaginally (Seman's on-off method) or vaginally (Masters and Johnson's squeeze technique). The stimulation is carried to the feeling of impending ejaculation. At that time, it is either stopped or the partner squeezes the penis just below the rim of the glans. The stimulation is started again after the feeling of impending ejaculation subsides. In Dr. Semans' work, the patients were cured after just a few sessions and subsequently regained their ability to control their ejaculation. Masters and Johnson report a 98% cure rate. Techniques that have attempted to decrease the amount of stimulation by the use of anesthetic creams or condoms have not been very successful.

In inhibited sexual arousal of females (frigidity), the techniques that are employed are similar to those for impotence in men. The sensate focus experience with women suffering from frigidity can elicit feelings of arousal. This is gradually expanded to include genital touching. Genital touching is practiced gently; sometimes oils or creams increase the pleasure. In vaginismus, in which spasms of the outer third of the vagina occur, the female is instructed to insert her fingers after some sensual touching or fantasy time. By gradually introducing larger diameters (first a single finger, then two, etc.) the woman eventually tolerates the penis.

HUMAN SLEEP AND SLEEP DISORDERS

This section will describe the structure and physiology of normal sleep and sleep that is disturbed. The advances in this area have been steady over the past dozen years. There is currently a new classification system for sleep disorders, and many sleep disorder centers are now found at university settings for the study and alleviation of sleep problems. In addition, new pharmacologic means have made the treatment of sleep problems less complicated.

Sleep research predates the 20th century. However, the work of **Nathaniel Kleitman** in the United States heralded the modern era. He was interested in the slow, rolling eye movements that occurred during sleep onset and decided to study eye movements throughout the night. Together with his graduate student **Eugene Aserinsky**, he documented findings that were a breakthrough in understanding sleep physiology. When **William Dement** joined the research group as a sophomore medical student, more correlations regarding eye movement and sleep were noted, producing today's view of sleep stages.

Sleep structure

Sleep is divided into two types, REM and non-REM. Each has a different EEG pattern, physiology and mental events.

REM sleep is also called desynchronized or delta sleep because of the EEG pattern. Other names include fast, active, or paradoxical sleep because the EEG pattern and behavior resemble those in the awake state. The waves are low amplitude and fast, just like an awake recording. REM sleep has a regular periodicity of every 90 minutes. REM sleep can be further divided into two components, tonic and phasic. During the tonic period, there is decreased peripheral blood flow, increased cerebral blood flow, and increased brain temperature (indicating heightened CNS activity). Thermoregulation is decreased in the body with hypotonia of the upper airway muscles and intercostals. There is near paralysis of the gravity muscles. Phasic activity includes irregular breathing and apnea, the characteristic rapid eye movements, muscle twitches, and variable increases in the heart rate and blood pressure.

During REM sleep, the **mental activity** is that of dreaming. Dreams can be recorded during non-REM periods, however they are less vivid and briefer. The dream activity in itself is a complex phenomenon. There are competing theories about the underlying mechanisms of dreaming. Freud believed that the dream was a biologic mechanism that functioned to keep the person asleep. His most famous book, *The Interpretation of Dreams,* is today part of the foundation of psychoanalysis. The various dreams that are reported in this work demonstrate the various mechanisms by which dreamers defend themselves from unresolved issues extending back to their earlier development. In his book he describes the incorporation of daily residue, which may take the form of the **manifest content**, or the images and experiences as they occur in the dream. There is believed to lie below this a **latent content**, or hidden meaning of a dream, which demonstrates the wishes, fears, and conflicts of the individual. To properly interpret a dream, the analyst has to have a full understanding of the patient's life and the patient's associations to the dream material. Recently theories in opposition to this have been put forth. In the **activation-synthesis hypothesis**, the brain dreams as a consequence of activation of its various parts. That is to say, the dream is a synthesis of the brain's responding to internal stimulation, such as from nuclei of the oculomotor system. Another theory of dreaming is that it represents an attempt of the brain to integrate current memories into long-term storage by connecting them with historically relevant experiences in the past. The longer that one waits after a REM period ends, the greater the likelihood that the dreamer will forget the dream. Eight minutes after termination of a REM period without awakening, it is unlikely that a dreamer will recall the dream.

Non-REM sleep is also called slow-wave sleep, orthodox or synchronized sleep (S-state sleep), or quiet sleep because of the characteristic wave pattern and behavioral correlates. Non-REM sleep can be divided into three stages. In stage 1, there is a gradual loss of consciousness. College students with their eyes taped open could only partly respond to images presented to them. The EEG pattern shows theta waves (waves of from 3 to 7 cycles per second [cps]). This period usually lasts around 5 minutes. It is followed by stage 2. The characteristic waveform during this stage is sleep spindles and K complexes, the former representing packets of 12 to 14 cps waves of around 1 second duration. The K complexes are slow negative EEG deflections with positive components. If awakened during this stage, the subject may report thoughts about the day's activities of brief duration. Stages 3 and 4 have been combined into a single stage, delta sleep. This is named after the slow delta waves, which are from 1/2 to 2 cps. These are high-amplitude waves of 75 μV. When at least 20% of the EEG shows delta waves, delta sleep is said to be present. Delta-wave sleep is also called the deepest sleep because it takes the greatest amount of stimulation to awaken the sleeper. Physiologically, the brain and body show the lowest amount of functioning with decreases in the blood pressure, heart rate, and respiratory rate. The brain temperature and cerebral blood flow both decrease.

Sleep architecture

The time between when the person's head hits the pillow until the first stage of sleep is termed **sleep latency**. The time for the appearance of the first REM period is termed **REM latency**. As we fall asleep, we progress from wakefulness to stage 1 sleep, then gradually deeper into stage 2, and finally delta sleep. Delta sleep tends to occur predominantly at the beginning of the sleep cycle. As stated before, after approximately 90 minutes we experience the first REM period, with its characteristic EEG and eye movements. Throughout the night, we awaken many times. Seven or so awakenings of brief (a minute or so) duration are considered normal. The first REM period is relatively brief, but as the night progresses the REM period increases in length. Near the time of awakening, it may last around 30 to 60 minutes.

Sleep and aging

Total sleep is greatest during infancy (around 18 hours) and lessens until adulthood with two major decreases around 4 years old and during adolescence. At that time it reaches its adult average level of 7.5 hours. Sleep is said to deteriorate with age. This means that as we age there are an increased number of awakenings and a decrease in delta sleep. Delta sleep is believed by some to be needed for restful sleep. Certain sleep disorders such as night terrors occur more in childhood when there is a greater amount of delta sleep and decrease as the individual ages and delta sleep duration shortens. Sleep latency, the time in bed before sleep ensues, increases as we get older. Although there are correlations between sleep difficulties and aging, it should be understood that there is a good deal of individual variation. There are individuals who sleep only 3 hours a night and those who sleep 11 hours. The proper amount of sleep is the amount that an individual needs to feel refreshed and function well the following day. Various studies have attempted to correlate sleep needs with temperamental variables. Short sleepers tended to be more outgoing, and longer sleepers tended to be worriers. Those who slept much more or less than the average had higher mortality rates!

Neurochemical mechanisms of sleep

The underlying mechanisms regulating sleep are complex and incompletely understood. Several facts imply a series of discrete interacting systems. If REM sleep is deprived, there will be a rebound increase in it, implying a self-regulating system. The fact that rebound will occur for non-REM sleep implicates such a system here as well. The fact that REM and non-REM alternate with a regular rhythm also implies a regulating model.

The mechanisms of sleep involve many systems. The first hypothesis, set forth by Bremer in the 1930s, basically stated that the brain stem waked the cortex. His experiments involving cats showed that a lesion between the medulla and the pons produced little effect on the sleep-wake cycle, but a lesion in the midbrain made the animal permanently drowsy (showing slow-wave sleep). The structure of the ascending reticular activating system was thought to be responsible for awakening the animal; when it was not stimulated, the animal fell asleep passively.

Experiments by other researchers found that specific lesions in such areas as the thalamus in cats or the raphe nuclei could either cause an animal to fall asleep or prevent an animal from falling asleep. Therefore sleep could also be an active process.

Some evidence about specific sites involved in sleep phases has been found to be contradictory. Destruction of the dorsal raphe nuclei resulted in insomnia, which disappeared with administration of serotonin (the dorsal raphe nuclei are rich in serotonin). The paradox was found in the locus ceruleus. When this center was destroyed, cats had trouble with REM sleep. It was therefore postulated that the locus ceruleus induces REM sleep. Other researchers postulate that the locus ceruleus (with the dorsal raphe nuclei) turns REM off.

So far three areas of the brain have been described as being involved in sleep: the reticular activating system (passive hypothesis), the dorsal raphe nuclei, and locus ceruleus nuclei. In addition, it has been found that each person's sleep rhythm is regulated by an internal clock called the circadian clock. This is probably the suprachiasmatic nuclei of the hypothalamus. Individuals removed from all time cues will settle into a period of sleep and activity of 25 hours, not 24. People use cues of alarm clocks or morning sun to adjust their internal clocks.

The sensory system can arouse an individual sufficiently to disturb sleep. Certain peptides such as delta-sleep-inducing peptide (DSIP) or an S factor, which promotes sleep in rabbits, have been isolated. It is clear that the mechanisms of sleep are multiple and interact in a specific manner.

Classification of sleep disorders

The Association of Sleep Disorder Centers has devised a classification scheme that comprises four major groups. The most common disorders will be discussed with both their new and old terminology. The four major groups are (1) disorders in initiating and maintaining sleep (DIMS), (2) disorders of excessive somnolence (DOES), (3) disorders of the sleep-wake cycle, and (4) parasomnias. In general, patients who have insomnia may either have trouble falling asleep or staying asleep. Younger persons usually have trouble in initiating sleep, whereas older individuals have trouble staying asleep and may have early morning awakening. The individual without sleep difficulty usually has a sleep latency of 18 minutes. Those with insomnia have a sleep latency averaging 54 minutes.

DIMS. These are referred to in the old terminology as the insomnias. It is essential to realize that insomnia is not a symptom but a group of disorders. When confronted with a patient who has difficulty in sleeping, the appropriate question to ask is, "What is the correct diagnosis?" There are nine different diagnoses:

1. Psychophysiologic
2. Psychiatric
3. Drug and alcohol related
4. Sleep-induced respiratory impairment (sleep apneas)
5. Sleep-related myoclonus and restless legs
6. Medical, toxic, and environmental
7. Childhood onset
8. Other DIMS
9. No DIMS

Insomnia is a common problem, and one-third of the U.S. population is affected. Approximately 2% of the population will receive a prescription for this problem. Psychophysiologic sleep disorders are of three types: acute (several days), short term (several weeks), or long term ($>$ 3 weeks).

Chronic insomniacs account for 5% of the clients of sleep disorders centers. These individuals can fall into at least two groups. Certain individuals show increased muscle tension and are fidgety. Instead of being aware of the source of their anxiety, they "somatasize" their anxiety. Therapy can be geared to helping them become more aware of their feelings and the underlying reasons and working out their conflicts. Another group becomes conditioned to external cues to stay awake instead of fall asleep. Such individuals use their bedroom for many other activities such as reading, eating, paying bills, talking on the telephone, etc. They have broken the natural conditioning that associates the bed with sleep. Eliminating those activities from the bedroom can be very helpful.

The second large group of DIMS are those associated with psychiatric disorders. In the next section, we will briefly discuss the various psychiatric diagnoses. For now it is important to realize that many different psychiatric problems may manifest themselves in difficulties in falling asleep or maintaining sleep. Anxiety disorders, schizophrenia, and personality disorders all have been represented. The most important is affective disorders. It has been postualted that sleep problems are very common in depression and that one aspect, REM latency, may be a biologic marker for depression. Many patients who are depressed will have onset of REM in 50 minutes or less, instead of taking the customary 90 minutes to begin their first REM period. In addition, the REM periods are more intensive and longer. These patients responded to the tricyclic antidepressants, which decrease REM sleep. In addition, it has been postulated that depression is caused by abnormalities in two key neurotransmitters: norepinephrine (the major neurotransmitter of the locus ceruleus) and serotonin, both of which are implicated in the biologic mechanisms of sleep. Finally, in some countries depressed patients are treated by sleep (especially REM) deprivation.

Although many people may drink alcohol to induce sleep, alcohol is not an effective hypnotic because it tends to cause more fragmented sleep. Other drugs that interfere with sleep include thyroid medications, asthma medications, contraceptives, any stimulant medications, MAO inhibitors, and the tricyclic antidepressant imipramine.

Sleep apnea may present either with DIMS but more commonly finds the sufferer complaining of excessive tiredness (DOES). Patients suffering with sleep apnea have the following symptoms: loud snoring, obesity, night sweats, blackouts, and serious morning headaches. There are three types of sleep apneas: central, obstructive, and mixed. In central sleep apnea, the brain suddenly fails to cause the diaphragm to move and there is subsequently no air movement. In obstruction, there is some physical abnormality or enlargement partially occluding the airway. Individuals with micrognathia (small jaw), enlarged tonsils, or unusual oropharyngeal anatomy may present in this way. The telltale snoring sound is an attempt to overcome the obstruction. In mixed types, both features are present. This condition is more common in men than women in a 30-to-1 ratio. The treatment in cases of obesity is weight loss. If the patient does not lose weight or there is no surgically removable obstruction, then tracheostomy will yield a dramatic improvement.

Nocturnal myoclonus and restless legs syndrome are best reported by a bed partner. In these two conditions, sleepers are constantly awakened by their own leg movements. In nocturnal myoclonus, involuntary leg twitches involving the anterior tibialis muscle occur at 30- to 40-second intervals. When an episode occurs, it may last 5 minutes to several hours. It occurs only while the patient is asleep and may be unilateral or bilateral. In contrast, restless legs syndrome also occurs when the individual is awake. An uncomfortable sensation is felt in the calves, thighs, and feet—usually bilaterally. The sensation is relieved by movement. The causes are unknown, but it is associated with iron deficiency, neuropathies, pregnancy, and cancer. Usually there is no pathology. There is a familial incidence in a number of patients.

Practically any **medical condition** can disrupt the normal sleep cycle. Some disrupt sleep because of the pain they cause. This is found most commonly in surgical conditions. In medical conditions in which sleep is commonly compromised, we find congestive heart failure and pulmonary conditions. The treatment should be directed toward the underlying condition. Pain medication and hypnotics need to be used with caution because of possible compromised renal, hepatic, and respiratory function.

DOES.   There is an overlap of DIMS and DOES in that some conditions in which the patient presents with complaints of being excessively tired are identical to those in which the patient presents complaining of trouble sleeping. They are classified according to which is the prominent complaint. It is logical that an individual who has trouble sleeping during the night will feel tired the next day! There are certain conditions, however, that only manifest themselves as excessive sleepiness.

Sleep disorder centers see more cases of excess sleepiness than insomnia. After ruling out medical conditions or depression, the next two most common causes of DOES are sleep apena and narcolepsy. **Narcolepsy** is a condition of excessive daytime drowziness associated with abnormal REM sleep manifestations. The person may experience sudden unexplained feelings of weakness. There may be **cataplexy**, which is the sudden loss of muscle tone with the patient collapsing to the ground. In addition, **sleep paralysis** may occur. This is a condition in which the person is awake but unable to move any muscles. On falling asleep, a person may experience vivid hallucinations termed **hypnogogic hallucinations**. If an EEG is conducted in a sleep laboratory, the sufferer, on falling asleep, immediately enters into a REM period. The condition can be extremely problematic for the individual, causing difficulties at work and increased accidents. The treatment includes the judicious use of stimulants such as amphetamine or methylphenidate.

Drugs that may cause excess sedation include minor tranquilizers, antihistamines, antidepressants, antipsychotics, antihypertensives, long-acting hypnotics, and withdrawal of stimulants. Medical conditions that can also cause excess sleepiness include encephalitis, anemia, endocrine disturbances, and neoplasms. A full medical workup is necessary to rule out these and other conditions.

The disorders of the sleep-wake schedule.   **Chronobiology** is the study of the natural rhythms that occur in all living things. The regularity of much animal behavior depends on environmental cues. The stickleback's sexual nest-building behavior was mentioned in reference to water temperature. Other animal behaviors are regulated by internal clocks, which use the environment for cues. We have already mentioned that in humans there is a regular oscillation in activity and sleep patterns. If an individual is removed from all time cues by being placed in a room without windows and insulated against sound, we can study the rhythm of sleep and wakefulness that will ensue. As mentioned, most people will not keep their regular 24-hour schedule but will settle into a schedule that will vary between 24 and 28 hours. Some may stay awake for 20 hours then sleep for 8 hours on a regular basis.

It is noted that there are a number of autonomic and endocrine variables that also oscillate during the day. Body temperature is coupled to the sleep cycle so that a person has the lowest temperature during sleep and a temperature rise during the morning. By placing a person in an environment free of time cues, the two rhythms become uncoupled, with temperature maintaining a circadian (24-hour) cycle and sleep and activity gradually lengthening.

The sleep-wake schedule disorders may have enormous importance. There are two types: transient and persistent. The transient varieties are seen when people change time zones. In **jet lag**, a person feels tired during the daytime and awake during the night when moving from New York to California. The internal clock has not adjusted to the new external clock. Another more dangerous situation occurs in shift work in individuals such as nurses, police officers, and factory workers, who may suddenly shift from a daytime set of hours to a nighttime set. The individual usually reports feeling tired and irritable in the new work routine. Studies of industrial accidents have found that accidents increase when workers have recently shifted to new hours. For instance, it was found that at Three Mile Island the nuclear disaster occurred when the engineers had been shifting their tours of duty. These engineers made serious judgment errors in that they overrode computer warnings on three separate occasions, resulting in the release of radioactive material. Some participants in shift work may have persistent difficulties in sleeping. Another disorder of persistent sleep-wake schedules is found in certain individuals whose sleep phase is shifted either ahead or behind the rest of the population. They experience increased fatigue in the evening; however, if they can follow their own rhythm their disorder disappears. Unfortunately, those individuals must conform to a regular work schedule, as others do. A form of therapy called **chronotherapy** will enable them to reschedule their wayward clocks.

Parasomnias.   The parasomnias are a heterogeneous collection of problems that may be found in adults and children. These disorders may represent problems in being aroused from sleep, such as in **somnambulism** and **night terrors** (pavor nocturnus). These are more common in children, occur more in delta sleep, and occur early in the night. While they are occurring, affected individuals are difficult to arouse. The events are poorly recalled by the individual.

Night terrors are extremely frightening to the parents and child and may precipitate an emergency room visit. The child suddenly begins screaming in a terrified, blood-curdling manner. This occurs without precipitant while sleeping. The child does not respond to the parents' attempts to provide comfort or reassurance. Children between the ages of 4 and 10 are most often affected, but night terrors may occur earlier or persist into adulthood. Night terrors can be distinguished from nightmares by the fact that they occur during delta sleep (nightmares occur during REM sleep), the person cannot recall any dream material (the nightmare sufferer recalls vivid nightmares), and the person cannot be aroused from the state (nightmare victims can be aroused).

Somnambulism is a disorder that occurs during delta sleep. The individual may be capable of walking around the house or even leaving it. It usually begins in childhood and is usually outgrown by the teenage years. Some studies have found evidence of other psychopathology in adults who suffer from this—usually neurosis or personality disorder.

Enuresis is a not uncommon condition. Approximately 10% of girls and 15% of boys suffer from this during childhood. It is first important to distinguish if urinary continence was ever achieved. If so this type of enuresis is considered secondary— the more common type. When urinary continence was never achieved, the diagnosis of primary enuresis warrants a thorough investigation of the underlying anatomic or physiological lesion, which may involve the nervous system or the GU system. Secondary enuresis may be the result of family stress, and the physician should obtain a family history. Particular factors that may exacerbate enuresis are parental strife, the birth of siblings, school difficulties, and even sexual abuse. Children who wet their beds until age 3 years are considered normal, as opposed to those who still wet their bed at 4 years. Enuresis follows a family pattern, and approximately 70% of all enuretics have a first-degree relative who is or has been enuretic at some time. Enuretics in recent studies have been found to urinate at all sleep stages, not just delta sleep, although previous reports attributed this to difficulty in being aroused. Enuresis is not highly correlated with psychiatric disorders, although there has been a tendency to categorize it as such. There are two principal treatment methods now used. The first is the pad and bell method. In this treatment, the bed is outfitted with a device that rings a bell when the pad becomes wet. The aroused individual becomes conditioned to the sense of impending urination and increases sphincter pressure. The cure rate for this method is between 50 and 100%, depending on the study. It is postulated that this is a form of classical conditioning, although aversion conditioning is also a factor. In addition to the bell and pad method, medications are used. Imipramine has been found to be an effective treatment. However, it eliminates bed-wetting totally in only 30% of children, and the symptoms resume when the medication is withdrawn.

Treatment of sleep disorders

The decision whether or not to use sleep medication has to be arrived at by the physician and patient. There are certain contraindications to the use of **hypnotics**: a history of abusing drugs or alcohol, respiratory impairment, and sleep apnea. The barbiturates have practically ceased being used as hypnotics, except intravenously in surgical uses or narcosynthesis (truth serum used in certain disorders). Today the benzodiazepines are the drugs of choice when temporary treatment of insomnia is needed. The student should recall that there are limited REM-suppressant effects from these medications; however, they do appear to suppress delta sleep. Longer-acting agents like flurazepam (Dalmane) have half-lives that may be 40 to 100 hours. The problem that this causes is morning "hangover" or sedation. Two new shorter-acting agents, **triazolam** (half-life of 3 to 4 hours) and **temazepam** (half-life 8 to 12 hours) can reduce this difficulty.

Brief sleep loss for several days is not harmful to most people. Sleep deprivation experiments have shown that total and prolonged sleep deprivation will result in fatigue, irritability, paranoid ideation, and misinterpretation of stimuli. Previous reports indicated that, with REM deprivation or sleep deprivation, psychoses would invariably supervene. This has not been demonstrated subsequently. For this reason, simple reassurance that a natural return to sleep will occur in a few days is not bad advice in many cases. The following factors have been found to disturb sleep: (1) either excess noise or quiet, depending on what the individual is accustomed to, (2) temperatures that are too high, (3) use of stimulants such as tobacco or caffeine, and (4) the chronic use of hypnotics. **Good sleep hygiene** requires regular daily exercise and a light bedtime snack. It was originally believed that milk was particularly good because it was rich in tryptophan, the precursor to serotonin, which is thought to promote sleep induction. However, studies have shown that there is no increase in serum tryptophan levels after drinking a glass of milk. Eating may release endogenous gut opiodes, which may produce a feeling of well-being and induce sufficient relaxation to help the individual fall asleep. A regular arousal time is another good sleep hygiene technique. It has been found that the single greatest influence on one's circadian clock is a regular arousal time. Sleep is also aided by not trying too hard to fall asleep. The harder one tries to sleep, the greater is the CNS arousal, which ultimately destroys sleep. Becoming involved in a nonstimulating activity such as reading or busying oneself if one cannot sleep will allow the natural mechanisms to take over after a time.

PSYCHOLOGICAL TESTING

In this section we will review the aspects of psychological testing, which consists of a group of tests that gather information about specific aspects of the person's life. There are perhaps a thousand different psychological tests. Each aspect of human behavior, thinking, or feeling can be approached using quantitative means of evaluation. Standardized tests that are valid (measure what they intend to measure) and reliable (can be reproduced by different users of the test) can be developed for assessing everything from anxiety levels to suicidal potential. You will probably never encounter these tests. **Structured nonprojective tests** such as IQ tests are considered a general measurement of intelligence. The definition of intelligence is "the power of reasoning and understanding; the ability to meet situations successfully, particularly new situations." Intelligence can be broken down into three categories: (1) abstract, referring to the ability to handle abstract ideas and symbols; (2) mechanical, referring to the capacity to understand and manage technical mechanisms; and (3) social, the ability to understand and manage human relations and social affairs. The **Stanford-Binet** IQ test defines IQ as the ratio of mental age as measured by their test to chronological age ($IQ = $ mental age/chronological age $\times$ 100). The current IQ tests use a standard with the mean by convention being 100 points and the standard deviation being 15 points.

Intelligence tests such as the Stanford-Binet make use of a

Intelligence tests such as the Stanford-Binet make use of a number of objects, cards, pictures, and miniature house items. These tests are administered individually. Various studies have found that IQ tends to be steady over time, but upward or downward shifts by as much as 50 points can occur. The Stanford-Binet has been replaced in part by the Wechsler Intelligence Scale for Children (**WISC**). In adults, the corresponding examination is the Wechsler Adult Intelligence Scale (**WAIS**). This examination studies two broad areas: verbal ability and nonverbal ability. The verbal part uses subtests for information, comprehension, and vocabulary. The nonverbal portion tests such items as block design (the ability to copy a two-dimensional pattern with blocks). Together the two scores yield a full score. There has been much controversy about IQ tests as being culturally biased. To some degree this is true. IQ tests ask questions that may reflect a lower score, depending on one's cultural values. This is particularly important because IQ tests have been used in comparing different cultural groups and making inferences regarding genetic components of intelligence. This was reflected most horribly in the Nazi doctrine of racial superiority. It has been shown that giving a disadvantaged child an enriched education can increase his or her scores on intelligence tests. The scales have been interpreted as follows: IQ $>$ 130 $=$ very superior, 120 to 130 $=$ superior, 100 to 110 $=$ bright normal, 90 to 100 $=$ normal/average, and

$<$ 70 $=$ retardation. What are the uses of the intelligence test? There are several. First, it gives us an overall impression of the person's ability to achieve academically. Next, it helps in terms of assessing the type of psychopathology that is present. It can help highlight difficulties in abstracting that reflect both organic brain syndromes and schizophrenia. It can help demonstrate problems in judgment as seen in the above conditions but also in severe personality disorders. It is not diagnostic for these conditions but adds more information to the overall picture.

Another important test is the Minnesota Multiphasic Personality Inventory (**MMPI**). This is a nonprojective test that can be administered without an examiner being present. The individual answers a set of questions. These questions test for various personality traits. Among the scales that are used are the hypochondriasis scale, depression scale, paranoia scale, and others. From the data, the psychologist can make an assessment about the personality disorder or traits that the individual has. This type of test is most useful in outpatient clinics, where personality disorders might more likely be encountered.

The next group of tests are the **projective tests**. In these, individuals must respond to relatively vague stimuli and in so doing reveal part of their inner world. Perhaps the most famous of these tests is the **Rorschach test**, also known as the inkblot test. The subject is given a series of 10 cards with various designs on them. Some have color and others are black and white. They are given in a standardized way with limited directions. The examiner makes a verbatim record of the patient's responses, along with the time it takes to react and the time spent on each card. Responses are then scored as to whether the individual focuses in on one detail or on the whole design. Important information can be inferred from the patient's associations about humans and whether there is action in the associations. The Rorschach response can be helpful in diagnoses and dynamics. Patients who have difficulty with reality testing will at times respond bizarrely to the cards. Some people have stated that this is a very useful test for diagnosing borderline personality disorder (see below).

Another projective test is the Thematic Apperception test (**TAT**). In this test, the patient is asked to comment on a variety of cards. Each card depicts people with various expressions and in different settings. For example, there is one card of a young woman on the edge of a sofa looking over her shoulder at an older man, who may have surprised her. It is assumed that patients identify with one of the figures in the card and express through a made-up story their own feelings, wishes, and fears. In this manner, it may be possible for individuals to express concerns that otherwise might be defended against.

The human figure drawing test, also termed the draw-a-person test (**DAP**), is a type of projective test that may give information about the person's self-concept and body image. The examiner simply asks the patients to draw a person on a blank piece of paper. Questions about the person might then be asked to further understand patients' underlying feelings about themselves or significant others.

The **Bender gestalt test** is a visuomotor coordination test used to screen for signs of organic impairment of cerebral functioning. The test consists of a series of nine figures presented one at a time to the patient. The patient must copy them down. The figures are simple geometric forms or combinations of dots, such as shown in Figure 7-4.

In copying these figures, the patient who is organically impaired will show problems in angulation, distortions, omissions, or repetitiveness. The Bender gestalt test cannot be performed by a child before the age of 3. By 10 to 12 years of age, the child should reasonably be able to copy the figures.

PSYCHOPATHOLOGY

CHILDHOOD AND ADOLESCENT DISORDERS

The following section will attempt to summarize a variety of disorders of childhood and adolescence. The review will follow chronological age.

Infancy

The child is born with a genetic endowment into a definite family with a definite socioeconomic situation. The infant will be subject to all of the biologic agents that can affect adults, such as viral and bacterial infections and toxic environmental problems. These will be acted on by the nature of the parents' nurturing behavior. We will not go into detail about all the medical-surgical conditions that can affect early human behavior but will highlight some.

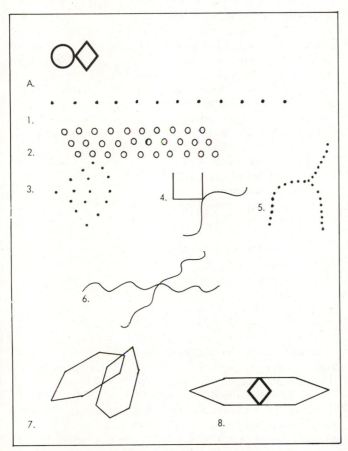

Figure 7-4. Test figures from the Bender visual motor Gestalt test of a normal man age 34 to 40 years.

Mental retardation.   Certain inborn genetic problems will affect intellectual development. The old classification of mental retardation listed the most profoundly retarded as "idiots" and those somewhat higher in intellect as "imbeciles." Those who were most intelligent were termed "feebleminded." Today the classification has used less pejorative terms and has been divided as follows: profound, $IQ < 25$; severe, IQ 25 to 40; moderate, IQ 40 to 55; mild, IQ 55 to 70.

Mental retardation has various etiologic components. Approximately 50% of cases have no known cause. The remaining 50% can be caused by genetic problems (25%) or environmental problems (25%), fetal alcohol syndrome for example. Early assessment by Apgar score will not correlate well with intelligence. It is estimated that 3% of the U.S. population is mentally retarded. The majority of the cases (>85%) are mild to borderline types.

Trisomy 21 (Down's syndrome, mongolism) is one genetic cause of retardation. Patients have moderate to severe retardation. The risk of producing an afflicted child is greater in middle-aged mothers. The number of cases is about 1 in 700 in the general population but 1 in 100 in middle-aged mothers. This is one of the indications for amniocentesis.

Other trisomy conditions include trisomies 5, 13, 18, and 22, which are associated with retardation and a host of stigmata. Persons with sex chromosome abnormalities may have retardation, but conditions like **Turner's** and **Klinefelter's** syndromes usually are associated with normal intelligence.

An unusual disease, **Crouzon's syndrome** or **craniosynostosis**, has recently been prominent in the news because of a markedly increased incidence in one area of one of the western states, suggesting a discrete environmental factor. In this disorder, retardation results because the skull closes prematurely and the growing brain is not permitted to develop.

Many factors can affect the developing fetus and result in retardation: prematurity, viral infections of the mother, maternal smoking, alcohol or drug use, diabetes mellitus, obstetric complications, and others.

Psychogenic factors and disorders.   Even in a presumably normal and biologically healthy child, the influence of early emotional factors can be enormous. The recent work of T. B. Brazelton has shown the importance of mother-child "fit." In observing films of mothers and infants, it can be noted that there is a sort of ballet or dance that is going on. The mother takes cues from the child, and the child from the mother. The infant, when overstimulated, will turn away. In a normal interaction, there is a reciprocal response in the mother. Mothers who struggle with fears of rejection may cause overstimulation and may not respond to the infant's signals for disengagement. Problems in early infant development, including sleeping or eating difficulties, may be traced in some mother-infant dyads to a poor interaction. It is not just the behavior of the mother that influences the infant but the fit that is important. A certain infant may be relatively docile and, if paired with a very aggressive mother, may not develop as well, manifesting problems. By studying the interaction, problems in the fit can be ascertained.

That the mother plays a crucial role in the development of the infant and child has been shown most powerfully by Renee Spitz. In his observations of infants raised in a nursery and a foundling home, powerful facts emerged. When infants were separated from their mothers, the infants developed psychopathology. The setting for the study was at a nursery and a foundling home. The nursery was used as a penal institution for delinquent girls. The foundling home housed children of married women who were unable to support their families. They paid the home to provide care and some services. These settings demonstrated different things. In the nursery, the children were deprived of their mothers around 6 to 8 months of age. This separation lasted 3 to 4 months. The infants became emotionally withdrawn, lost weight, and had insomnia. Intellectual functions declined. The initial weepiness was replaced by rigidity of facial expression, and the children would scream when a stranger came near (**anaclitic depression**). If the mother returned after a separation of 3 to 4 months, these symptoms would begin to resolve; if the separation lasted 5 to 6 months, however, the behavior worsened.

In the face of total maternal deprivation, the symptoms became worse. A condition termed **marasmus** ensued, in which the child was totally passive, demonstrated severe retardation, and had trouble sitting and walking. A number of these children developed such severe pathology that a third of them died. The environment was clean and hygienic. The infants had received adequate nutrition, but the key to their problems was the lack of adequate human interaction.

Infantile autism. In this condition, the child has the prominent symptom of being unresponsive to other people. The child acts as though people are inanimate things to be used. Kanner's initial description also included the aspects of the child's resistance to change and insistence on repetition. Children with this condition may take great time in observing a rotating wheel or repeatedly opening and closing a toy box. In addition, they have highly disturbed or sometimes absent communication. The disorder is diagnosed when the symptoms begin during the first 30 months of life. Certain studies found that there is a greater incidence in children who were exposed to German measles (rubella) or who had phenylketonuria. Initially, it was thought that the parents caused this condition by being extremely cold and uncaring. Subsequent investigations have not substantiated this. The treatment of autistic children was with psychotherapy, which is now being used less frequently. Children now are more commonly being treated with educational models in an attempt to improve communication and behavioral techniques to reduce their temper tantrums and need for sameness. Occasionally the use of medications has been helpful; however, this is not the mainstay of treatment. The prognosis varies but may be guarded. Those cases in which there is little communication have shown the more difficult course. It has been reported that only one in six makes an adequate social adjustment.

Failure to thrive. This term is used to describe a group of disorders characterized by problems in physical and mental development during infancy. The etiologic factors include congenital abnormalities, infectious diseases, and a host of medical-surgical conditions. Interestingly, there are situations where the difficulty can be traced to poor maternal care. Studies from a variety of institutes have demonstrated that an environment that is low in nurturing emotional care will result in infants that have inadequate weight gain and/or growth failure.

Childhood

A large number of behavior disorders can occur during childhood. For certain areas, a very basic familiarity with certain conditions is needed—practically only a definition or so—whereas in others more depth is needed. The conditions that will be discussed include (1) childhood-onset pervasive developmental disorder, (2) specific developmental disorder (dyslexia in particular), (3) attention deficit disorder with and without hyperactivity, (4) conduct disorder (juvenile delinquency), (5) anxiety disorders of childhood (particularly school phobia), (6) eating disorder (particularly pica-anorexia nervosa), (7) stereotyped movement disorder (particularly Gilles de la Tourette's), and (8) stuttering.

Childhood-onset pervasive developmental disorder. Affected children demonstrate sustained impairment in social relationships and have difficulty in appropriate affective responsivity. The onset is after 30 months of age. The student should be aware that the problem is found in a variety of behaviors, as opposed to specific developmental disorders (see below). Examples of the behaviors include self-mutilation such as biting oneself, peculiarities in movement, and abnormalities in speech such as monotonous voice. This disorder is extremely rare.

Specific developmental disorders. The disorders that are discussed here include specific defects in a number of areas. Reading, arithmetic, language, articulation, and spelling each can have particular difficulties. Reading is perhaps the most studied aspect. The reading disorder is also termed **dyslexia**. It is a common disorder in which the individual is significantly below level in reading skills as ascertained by standardized individually administered tests. The child's chronological age should be between 8 and 13 years to determine the significance of the discrepancy. A lag of 1 year behind the school group is considered significant. Reading difficulties that are severe are frequently associated with psychiatric problems. Rutter's extensive evaluation has described many of the important facets of dyslexia. Dyslexia is found in males more than in females, in the ratio of 3 to 1, and is present in the general population with a prevalence rate of 4 to 8%. The task of reading involves the following parameters:

1. The ability to discriminate curved from straight lines, such as "u" and "v", and left from right, such as "b" and "d."
2. The ability to translate from one sense (vision to hearing) to another.
3. The ability to understand the meaning of the written material.
4. Motivation.
5. Intelligence (as measured by IQ).
6. Opportunities (family, culture).

Many studies have tried to ascertain correlates of reading ability. Speech is positively correlated. At one time it was thought that the problem lay in visuospatial problems or lack of coordinated eye movements. This hypothesis has not received wide support. Although there is a slight correlation with left-handedness, this is not considered an important factor. Signs of brain damage such as in persons with epilepsy or cerebral palsy are positively correlated. Low socioeconomic status and large families are also correlated with poor reading ability. There is a strong correlation between temperament and reading, concentration being very important. If the reading problem occurs later in education, it probably represents not a reading difficulty but rather a motivation problem.

The World Federation of Neurology defines dyslexia as "a disorder manifested by difficulty in learning to read despite conventional instruction, adequate intelligence, and sociocultural opportunity." It is dependent on fundamental cognitive disabilities, which are frequently of constitutional origin. Attempts to subclassify it have not yet been successful. Studies that have focused in on whether the chief problem lies in constructional problems (right brain function) or language problems (left brain function) have favored a language problem deficit.

Treatment attempts offering perceptual training have not been generally successful. Psychotherapy directed at issues of self-esteem and conduct have been only partly successful. Social learning techniques using behavioral therapy have had good results, but outcome is short-term and continuous reinforcement is needed. The use of medications such as methylphenidate (Ritalin) has not been very successful. Parental involvement, having affected children read to the parents, has been helpful. It probably is effective because of the increased reading practice and the value that the parents place on it.

Attention deficit hyperactivity disorder. This is an area where there is much disagreement about terminology and diagnosis. The term attention deficit disorder (ADD, overactivity, hyperactivity) has only recently been used with the development of *DSM III-R* and recently further modified to attention deficit hyperactivity disorder (AHAD). In the past, the term minimal brain dysfunction (MBD) included a large number of these cases. It was assumed that the child's difficulties in attention and hyperactivity were the result of some subtle neurological disorder possibly stemming from birth trauma or hypoxia. The disorder became the center of controversy, with mothers claiming that their children were responding to food additives such as dyes and preservatives. The Feingold diet was supposed to eliminate such substances as red dye and a host of other products and resulted in decreased activity and improved concentration in some children. Current research does not favor such observations, but the subject is not closed. Researchers and clinicians have not reached a consensus about the exact nature of the illness. *DSM III-R* defines ADHD as having eight of the following: often fidgets, difficulty remaining seated, easily distracted, difficulty awaiting turns in games, blurts out answers before the question is completed, difficulty following through with instructions, difficulty in sustaining attention in tasks, shifts from one activity to another, talks excessively, interrupts others, does not seem to listen to what others are saying, loses things, engages in physically dangerous activities. It is not uncommon, affecting 3% of the population. The ratio of males to females is 10 to 1. The onset is after age 3, and peak years of diagnosis are 8 to 10. The difficulty with the attention aspect of this disorder is that it is hard to define. Attention is a complex process that involves many different cognitive functions such as the ability to resist distractions, the ability to register information, and the ability to focus on specific stimuli. The **etiology** is undetermined. Abnormalities in EEG and neurophysiologic functions exist but are slight. Genetic influences and parental influences are also postulated and in certain cases can be demonstrated. ADHD can persist

into adulthood. It often stops before adolescence, and occasionally it shows only minimal problems, with impulsivity or low frustration tolerance in an adult.

The **treatment** of ADHD has centered on medication. Stimulants such as methylphenidate or Pemoline (Cylert) and amphetamine (Dexedrine) have been drugs of choice. There is an overwhelming amount of evidence that these stimulants reduce hyperactive behavior in children. Medicated hyperactive children also show lower error rates on psychological tests of attention and improvement on the WISC. Side effects such as sleeplessness, appetite loss, and head and abdominal pains have been reported. The major differences in drugs include the fact that methylphenidate and amphetamines have shorter duration of action and need to be taken several times daily. Pemoline may take 2 to 3 weeks to become effective but can give more continuous levels throughout the day. Beside medication, behavioral therapy and psychotherapy have been used and are effective. The problem of treating this condition with medications is that it is unknown whether these drugs improve classroom learning. Another condition that may occur with the medication and that has not been fully discounted is state-dependent learning, a curious phenomenon that has been noted with barbiturates and alcohol and may exist with stimulant use. Persons who learn a task of certain facts while under the influence of a substance may not be able to recall the knowledge or skill when the substance is not present in their system. Once the substance is reintroduced, the learned material is recalled. The learning depends on the state of the CNS with regard to chemical milieu. Further studies need to be conducted in this area.

Conduct disorders. This is a fairly common problem that also consists of a diversity of behaviors. The disturbed conduct includes such behaviors as running away, stealing, fighting, truancy, and lying. It is differentiated into group type (those that occur in a group setting), solitary aggressive, and undifferentiated. An older and more common term used by the legal system, "juvenile delinquency," has been applied to some of the most severe of these disorders. In general, these problems beginning in childhood and occurring with increased frequency in adolescence involve a young person's behaving in socially deviant ways so as to break social rules or violate the rights of others. The epidemiology of juvenile delinquency reviewed by Adolph Christ notes the following: There has been an increased rate of serious crime including rape, murder, and armed robbery. These have increased threefold. The peak age is 16. Male offenders outnumber females 5 to 1. There are higher rates in lower socioeconomic groups. There is an increased incidence in broken homes. This last point is interesting in that those homes in which the father has died or the mother is working do not have increased rates. In those homes where the mother has died, the rates of delinquency for girls has increased. There is an increased incidence in homes where discipline is inadequate. Particular types of conduct disorder may have underlying causes. Stealing has been associated with the feeling of being unloved and has been termed comfort stealing when it occurs in otherwise well-socialized boys and girls. Some parents unwittingly condone inappropriate behavior. Such parents have what is termed a **superego lacunae**—a space or deficit in their sense of right and wrong, possibly limited to one area. Anna Freud pointed out that aggression in youth may be caused by a large number factors, including biologic problems with impulse control, parental neglect, unstable relationships at home, and fear of feminine strivings in adolescent males. A need to be caught in a criminal act may be an expression of guilt.

Treatment has been the most problematic area. When the conduct disorder is mild and does not involve aggressive acts, psychotherapy and group therapy may be effective. The more serious cases of conduct disorder are difficult to treat. The treatment of juvenile delinquency (which accounts for those worst cases of conduct disorder) has been wrought with failure. Incarceration may only lead these youths to become more skilled criminals. Many adolescents with a conduct disorder suffer from the less serious types of conduct disorder and go on to adjust reasonably well to adult life.

Anxiety disorders. Anxiety may take many forms during childhood and adolescence. One form involves trouble leaving the parental home, particularly going to school (school phobia). *DSM III-R* calls this not a true phobia but rather separation anxiety disorder. A child so afflicted may have stomachaches or other hypochondriacal or somatic complaints in order to avoid leaving home and going to school. The problem may occasionally manifest itself at nighttime, and the child may have difficulty going to sleep, suffering exaggerated fears of monsters or the dark. The underlying cause may be an overly intense attachment to the mother. Other cases may reflect fears of leaving home because of physical violence or abuse at home or fears of parental divorce. Treatment is via psychotherapy, marital therapy, or family therapy. The use of minor tranquilizers may occasionally be of benefit.

Eating disorder (pica). Pica is the eating of nonnutritive substance such as dirt, paint chips, hair, etc. The major danger in this relatively rare disorder is the possibility of suffering lead poisoning by eating lead-based paint chips. Although it was thought that this disorder was the result of an underlying mineral deficiency, it is more likely attributed to an absent or inattentive mother.

Stereotyped movement disorder. Involuntary repetitive, rapid, purposeless motor movements are described as tics. They need to be differentiated from motor movements associated with neurological conditions such as Sydenham's chorea or other neurological movement disorders. They usually represent a childhood reaction to stress. Prevalence for transient tics has been reported to be quite high during childhood, with a rate of 12 to 24%. The movements may involve blinking of the eyes or facial muscles. Gilles de la Tourette's syndrome involves tics with involuntary vocalizations, which are usually grunts but may include curse words. Although its cause was originally thought to be psychogenic, today it is increasingly believed to be neurological. Treatment with haloperidol (Haldol) has been effective in many individuals. Behavioral therapy is sometimes an effective technique, particularly with children concurrently suffering with retardation.

Stuttering. This disorder typically begins between the ages of 2 and 4 years. This is the time when the child's language development is progressing rapidly. The sentence structure becomes complex. At this age, children usually repress sexual and aggressive drives, and a new baby frequently enters the family. Sibling rivalry has been postulated by many to be the cause of this disorder. Others have postulated the cause to be anxiety about separation from the mother or other emotional trauma that occurs during the time of language acquisition. The prognosis is usually good, with 50 to 80% of children outgrowing it. In more persistent cases, behavior therapy has been used. In the younger stutterer, the parents may reinforce fluent speech with increased attention. In older stutterers, a program of systematic desensitization may be tried.

Child abuse and incest. Following Kempe and colleagues' landmark paper "The Battered Child Syndrome," physicians have become more aware of this problem. The battered child syndrome represents more than the failure-to-thrive syndrome already discussed. In child abuse, willful physical damage is done to the child. Children may be beaten with electric cords or receive broken bones by being thrown down stairs. Only a small percentage of abusive parents are psychotic, and the majority are parents who themselves were abused. The defense mechanism of identification with the aggressor may be the salient psychodynamic in such parents. In many states, it is now mandatory that all physicians, nurses, and medical students report such incidents. Sexual abuse is a variant of this situation. Father-daughter incest is the most common. When there are stepparents, the stepfather may be involved. Rarely does incest occur between mother and son. When incestuous activity is discovered, it has often been revealed that the mother has knowingly or unknowingly contributed to its occurrence. Treatment of this condition often involves a combination of individual therapy for the victim, the parents and family, and marital therapy offered conjointly where resources permit. The tendency to react with immediate withdrawal of the child from the family many times has not helped the troubled youngster. Epidemiologically both sexual and child abuse have been found in all socioeconomic levels and does not appear to be strongly correlated with social class. Although prevalence figures are not well known, it is believed to be not uncommon.

Adolescence

Many of the conditions that are reported to occur during the period of childhood can also occur during adolescence. As has been mentioned, delinquency in particular increases during the teenage years. Adolescence is also the beginning of the time when more severe disorders begin to become apparent. Schizophrenia has been reported to be a disorder that begins during late adolescence and early adulthood. In the past, manic-depressive illness was thought to affect only adults, but there is increasing evidence of its beginning during adolescence. The important conditions that occur during this period include (1) anorexia nervosa, (2) bulimia, (3) adolescent suicide, and (4) teenage pregnancy.

Anorexia nervosa. This condition begins during adolescence, when the patient has a problem dealing with the idea of bodily maturation. It is marked by a fear of sexuality together with certain underlying conflicts, including marked separation anxiety and a perfectionistic attitude toward school work, boyfriends, and friendships. The disorder is preponderantly found in girls, although there are male anorexia sufferers as well. These teenagers do not rebel as the usual teenager does; instead they become involved in a power struggle around food exclusively. The definition of anorexia according to *DSM III-R* requires that the sufferer refuse to maintain body weight over a minimal normal weight for age and height set at 15% of minimal normal weight. In addition, there is a disturbed body image—the patient feels that she is fat in spite of evidence to the contrary. There is a preoccupation with food, an intense fear of becoming fat, and no underlying medical disorder to explain the weight loss. The patient may engage in physical exercise to excess. Physical changes include cessation of menses. Sometimes amenorrhea may precede the onset of anorexia, leading to the belief that in some individuals this is a hypothalamic disorder. Family studies have shown that the family is overcontrolling, rigid, and overprotective and that they suppress verbalization of emotion. The theory that sufferers are overdependent and closely bound to the mother has been put forth. Underweight is also reinforced by the media. A study of the weight of young women chosen for Playboy centerfold photographs found that many came close to the 25% below ideal body weight postulated for anorexics. The prognosis is thought to be poor if the victim shows a severe weight loss at presentation, is past adolescence at onset, has a history of vomiting and laxative abuse, and has a poor premorbid social adjustment.

The current **treatment** makes use of both psychoanalytic psychotherapy and behavioral techniques. In severe cases, hospitalization may be necessary, particularly because approximately 10% of cases may succumb to metabolic abnormalities associated with the severely malnourished state. The approach is to reinforce positive behaviors and punish inappropriate behaviors (e.g., food is not eaten or is secretly disposed of) by isolating the patient or removing privileges. Psychotherapy also deals with the unrealistic perfectionistic beliefs and attachment to the patient's mother. There is a good prognosis in 40% of cases.

Bulimia nervosa. In this condition there are recurrent episodes of consumption of high-calorie foods with termination of a binge by vomiting, sleep, or self-inflicted pain. Patients can become exceptionally skilled at vomiting and can vomit by just "willing" it. Eating is done in a secretive and inconspicuous manner. The individual is frequently attempting to lose weight and shows wide fluctuations in weight. Patients with this disorder are frequently depressed and impulsive and may abuse drugs or alcohol. Many of these patients (>40%) use laxatives in an attempt to lose weight or abuse diet pills or diuretics. Once again, there seems to be a constellation of family symptoms that contributes to this condition. Families with a bulimic patient are found to have a higher incidence of depression and alcoholism. The family overvalues dieting and thinness. In some cases, the child who is premordibly obese is pressured by the family to be thin at a time when this is not physically possible. Bulimia is associated with obesity, which is defined as being from 30% above ideal body weight (mild) to 100% above ideal body weight (morbid obesity). Among people who are obese, 25% have a severe binge eating problem and 50% have a moderate problem. Frequent vomiting causes metabolic and other medical consequences: reflux esophagitis, dental caries (from the hydrochloric acid), hypokalemia (from the loss of chloride), cardiac arrest (due to low potassium), and hair loss. **Treatment** involves the use of psychotherapy. The use of antidepressants has met with some success as well. Several recent findings indicate that more males are afflicted than was previously thought. Recent work has also revealed a new affective disorder called **seasonal affective disorder**. In this disorder, patients become depressed during the winter months. Their depression is associated with binge eating and weight gain.

Adolescent suicide. There has been an unexplained increase in the number of suicides among adolescents. Suicide is the second leading cause of death among teenagers, automobile accidents being the first. It is believed that some of these accidents were intended or were unconsciously motivated suicides. Girls attempt suicide 20 times more frequently than boys, and teenage boys are more successful (10 times greater actual suicides than females). One theory put forward states that there may be increased competition among adolescents because of their greater percentage in the population. They may respond to this competition by feeling overwhelmed and hopeless about the future. Among adolescents who have attempted or contemplated suicide, 84% have an unwanted stepparent, 72% have one or both natural parents absent from the home, and 62% have both parents working.

Teenage pregnancy. This is a serious problem in the United States. The birthrates for women of this age are among the highest for advanced countries. Approximately 10% of adolescent girls becomes pregnant, and the percent is higher in lower socioeconomic groups and in the nonwhite community. Complications of pregnancy are greater among teenagers, with increased maternal death rates, toxemia, and other disorders. Teenage mothers are also poorer mothers in that they may have inadequate nutrition, lack parenting skills, drop out of high school, and have repeated unwanted pregnancies.

ADULT DISORDERS

The psychopathology questions on the Behavioral Sciences section of the boards, although fewer than those in Part II, are nonetheless quite extensive. Students are expected to have a detailed understanding of the signs and symptoms of various major psychiatric disorders and to understand the etiology, prevalence, and various methods of therapy for these disorders. There is some overlap, in that the questions in pharmacology may be repeated here. This review will cover the various syndromes in as expedient a manner as possible. The disorders discussed include schizophrenia, affective disorders, personality disorders, organic mental disorders, and anxiety disorders.

Schizophrenia

Schizophrenia is many times misunderstood by patients and their families as meaning "split personality." This confusion arises from their knowing that the prefix "schiz" means split. In the context of this disease, it has another meaning—"fragmented." Thus, schizophrenia is a disorder characterized by fragmentation of mental processes. Around the turn of the century **Emil Kraepelin** is referred to this disorder as **dementia praecox**, an early onset dementia, so named because many of the patients who were hospitalized began to show deterioration in their intellectual functioning. Today it is understood that schizophrenia is very different from dementia. In dementia there is a problem with memory and other cognitive functions, which are preserved in schizophrenia. The tragedy of this illness is that the onset occurs early (praecox) in adulthood. The diagnosis of this disorder has rested on the recognition of characteristic signs and symptoms. After Kraepelin, Eugene Bleuler coined the term schizophrenia and described the disorder on the basis of **four A's**: affect, autism, associations, and ambivalence. These signs will be described in more detail later.

The diagnostic criteria for schizophrenia have now been more elaborately detailed in *DSM III-R*. The criteria involve the patient's meeting a lengthy set of problems, with major headings A through F. A general understanding of these signs and symptoms is mandatory. The characteristic features are (1) delusions, (2) hallucinations, and (3) disordered thinking. A **delusion** is a belief that is fixed and contrary to reality. Many people have beliefs that are not shared by others—for example, some people believe and others do not believe in the existence of God. What makes a person's belief a delusion is the social context. On this basis, in the USSR political dissidents are considered delusional. In our country, problems arise when we define as delusional someone who believes that they are possessed by the devil. In the 16th century, they would not have been so considered. Today some religious groups maintain that such possessions are common, whereas psychiatrists who study the full picture of the signs and symptoms believe that a "possessed" person is instead mentally ill. This can at times present problems in people belonging to certain religious groups. The delusions that a patient with schizophrenia suffers from are more often than not bizarre. **Bizarre delusions** have no possible basis in fact. A common bizarre delusion in schizophrenics is the belief that their mind is being controlled by radio waves, radiation, sinister beings, poisons, or other means. patients may also believe that their bodies, emotions, and willpower are being controlled. These delusions have been termed thought broadcasting, thought insertion, made feelings, and made will. Although they were at one time considered pathognomonic for schizophrenia, this has not been accepted to date. Besides bizarre delusions, patients suffer from somatic delusions (e.g., a patient believes that he has snakes in his stomach), grandiose delusions (a patient believes he is Napoleon or Einstein), and nihilistic delusions (a patient believes that the world is ending or that everything is dead). Delusions can occur in other disorders as well. They are found in Alzheimer's disease, manic-depressive disorder, and other disorders discussed below.

Hallucinations are perceptions in which there is no source of sensory stimulation. This distinguishes them from **illusions**, in which a person has a perception that is a gross distortion of some actual sensory stimulation. For example, if a person sees a man standing alongside a deserted road, this is a hallucination if no man is there. However, if there is a stop sign or some other source of sensory stimulation, it is an illusion. Hallucinations are thought of as being a more severe form of problem in testing reality. Hallucinations in schizophrenia are predominantly auditory (although visual hallucinations occur in 10% of schizophrenics). The auditory hallucinations are usually one or more voices speaking more than one word on several occasions. They frequently speak in a derogatory way about the patient. One of the more common auditory hallucinations in men is that of hearing a voice calling them a homosexual, or for women that of hearing voices calling them a prostitute. Hallucinations can also be olfactory. Smells without sources of stimulation can be a sign of a frontal lobe tumor. If accompanied by seizures, they may be termed **uncinate fits** because of the lesion's position near the uncus. Tactile hallucinations involve the perception of touch. Most commonly they are not seen in schizophrenia but rather in delirium tremens (see below). Although many patients with schizophrenia have hallucinations, many others do not.

Disorders of thinking are a third type of symptom found in schizophrenia. The patient may have **thought blocking**. In this symptom, patients may stop speaking in midsentence because their thoughts suddenly stopped. Another problem in thinking is **loosening of associations**. An adult will normally communicate in a logical and coherent fashion. One thought will follow another with a reason. In loosening of associations, the patient will say several things that have no connection. For example, "I was walking down the block, if you can that is, try to climb this building it is July." Sometimes a thought will begin and the patient will follow it off on a tangent, losing the original thought—**tangential thinking**. Eventual return to the point is termed **circumstantial thinking**. In all of these deviations, the form or stream of thinking is disturbed. These are also called **formal thought disorders**. If there are hallucinations or delusions, we speak about abnormalities in the content not the form of thinking.

Any of the three—delusions, hallucinations, or thought disorders—may be present. One at least must be present at some time during the illness to confirm the diagnosis, and more than one is often present. They signify a cardinal feature of schizophrenia—that is, a break with reality.

There are additional features crucial to diagnosing this disorder. There must be a deterioration in functioning. It may occur in school, at work, or socially. It is common for parents of schizophrenics to come to the hospital with an adolescent and complain, "Johnny isn't the same anymore. He's not able to do what he used to!" Since this illness frequently has its onset in young adulthood, the break may come during high school or college.

Some symptoms may precede the acute symptoms such as hallucinations, in which case they are called prodromal. If they follow the acute symptoms they are called residual. Among the prodromal or residual symptoms are illusions, social isolation, poor personal hygiene, strange speech patterns, magical or superstitious thinking, flat affect, and bizarre behavior such as talking to oneself in public or assuming peculiar postures.

The symptoms termed acute (hallucinations, delusions, or disordered thinking) and those termed prodromal or residual must combined have a duration of at least 6 months. If they are less than that, a different diagnosis termed **schizophreniform psychosis** is used. There usually is no stressor to the onset of schizophrenia. If there is an overwhelming stressor, then the disorder may be termed **brief reactive psychoses**. The term psychosis is used in these disorders and is defined as a disorder in which there is a defect in one's contact with reality.

Schizophrenia may not be diagnosed without first being certain there is no physical cause. Use of drugs such as amphetamine, angel dust, LSD, and others may mimic it. In addition, a large number of conditions including brain tumors, collagen vascular diseases, cerebral infections, metabolic diseases, and others may mimic this disorder.

There are five subtypes of schizophrenia. These include catatonic, paranoid, undifferentiated, residual, and disorganized. In the **catatonic** type, there is mutism with strange postures. The patient may demonstrate waxy flexibility (if the examiner raises the patient's arm above his head, it remains there for a period of time). In the **paranoid** type, patients are extremely distrustful and often refuse to answer questions for fear that what they say may be used against them. The **disorganized** type is characterized by a child-like silliness with marked loosening of associations. This was formerly called hebephrenic schizophrenia. **Undifferentiated** is applied when none of the other pictures predominates. In the **residual** type, the patient is free of acute symptoms and demonstrates the residual symptoms already mentioned.

Epidemiology. Frequently it is erroneously stated that the incidence of schizophrenia is approximately 1%. Actually, this is the lifetime prevalence of the disease. This is to say that 1 out of 100 Americans will have had schizophrenia at some time in their lives. The incidence is around 0.05%. Sex ratio is equal in males and females. It is more common in lower socioeconomic groups and in large cities. Jews are less likely to have the disease than Christians. Blacks and Hispanics are more likely to have it than whites. It is found more commonly in persons with birthdays during the months of March and April.

Genetics. In the general population, the risk of developing schizophrenia is 1%. In first-degree relatives, the risk is 15%. If two parents are affected, the risk is 40%. Monozygotic twins have a concordance rate of 40 to 60%. This last point has been used to strengthen both biologic and psychological theories for schizophrenia. If the disorder were genetic, the concordance rate would be 100%. There are two genetic theories: (1) a single gene with variable penetrance and (2) a polygeneic inheritance (believed to be the mechanism in diabetes mellitus). Adoption studies indicate that if a child of a schizophrenic is adopted by a normal parent, he or she maintains the same risk (10 to 15%). Children of normal parents adopted by schizophrenic parents do not have increased rates of the disorder.

Etiology. The cause is unknown. A number of theories have been put forth. A combined biopsychosocial model attempts to describe this illness as resulting from multiple factors. The term **biopsychosocial** has become standard, reflecting the diverse possible causes of this illness.

Biologic factors. Many biologic theories have attempted to explain this disorder. None is satisfactory. Among the most common is the **dopamine theory**, which postulates an excess activity in the dopaminergic system of the brain. It is based on the observation that amphetamines increase central dopamine and cause psychoses in some individuals. Secondly, the antipsychotic agents block dopamine receptors and ameliorate symptoms. Other neurotransmitters have been implicated— namely, norepinephrine, GABA, serotonin, and others. There are many other theories implicating viral agents, food sensitivities, and neurophysiological abnormalities. CT and PET scans have shown some patients with this disorder to have increased ventricular size and decreased blood flow and brain activity in the frontal lobes.

Psychological factors. These factors are supported through the psychoanalytic investigations of patients with this and related disorders. Some theories indicate that early conflicts between mother and infant can predispose to this disorder.

Sociocultural factors. There is an increased risk of schizophrenia in those who have recently changed their home countries. Schizophrenia is more common in lower socioeconomic groups, indicating that the stresses of this life-style increase the likelihood of the illness. Those who develop the illness in developing countries fare better than those in industrialized nations. This is believed to be due to greater social support and less stress in these nations.

Course and prognosis. The course of this illness is variable. Kraepelin described it in simplistic terms, but it is useful to think that about one-third will deteriorate. The actual picture is more complex, with many variations including a shift-like pattern, in which there is a partial recovery with some underlying deficits. Patients have made full recoveries after years of illness, but this is more rare. The prognostic variables have been contested. Factors associated with good premorbid social and occupational functioning with good affect have been the most favorable. Those who show blunting of affect with a gradual onset and no social activity have a poor prognosis.

Treatment. It has been suggested that the treatment of schizophrenia without medication risks being considered malpractice. Although this has not been tested, for legal purposes there is good reason to place medication as a cornerstone in the treatment of these disorders. The introduction of the **antipsychotic** drugs, also known as **neuroleptics**, resulted in the rapid decrease in the number of patients who were in state hospitals. Patients who formerly were unable to be free of their symptoms found improvement in many aspects favorable. The two most commonly used antipsychotics are **chlorpromazine** (Thorazine) and **haloperidol** (Haldol). These drugs differ in significant ways (Table 7-3). Chlorpromazine is given in higher doses (less potent) and is more sedating. Haloperidol is a high-potency (low-dosage) medication with low sedation but high extrapyramidal side effects.

Patients with schizophrenia will have a variety of symptoms, as described. Those symptoms more likely to respond to medication include hallucinations, agitation, combatativeness, hostility, impaired sociability, hyperactivity, and tension. The symptoms less likely to respond include impaired insight, judgment, memory, and chronic delusions.

There are many possible **side effects** of neuroleptics. The most important are the four distinct extrapyramidal reactions. **Pseudoparkinsonism** is characterized by bradykinesia (slow movements), muscle rigidity (cogwheel or lead-pipe feeling in extremity movements), pill-rolling tremor, and mask-like facies. **Akathisia**, also known as restless legs syndrome, is an uncomfortable feeling with the inability to sit still. **Acute**

Table 7-3. A Comparison of Chlorpromazine and Haloperidol

	Chlorpromazine	Haloperidol
Potency	Low	High
Sedation	High	Low
Extrapyramidal	Low	High
Hypotension	High	Low
ECG changes	Low	Low

dystonia is a sudden uncontrolled spasm of various muscle groups, including the neck, face, and eye muscles. **Tardive dyskinesia** is a late-onset disorder caused by long-term treatment with antipsychotics. Repetitive movements of the tongue and mouth are characteristic. The arms and legs may also have choreoathetoid movements. All four side effects are believed to involve the extrapyramidal system between the substantia nigra and the corpus striatum (nigrostriatal system). Pseudoparkinsonism and acute dystonias are the easiest to treat with antiparkinsonian agents such as benztropine (Cogentin) or trihexyphenidyl (Artane). Akathisia, although not very serious, is difficult to treat but may respond to decreased doses or use of sedatives. Tardive dyskinesia may be irreversible in 30% of cases; middle-aged and older women seem to develop this in greater numbers.

In addition to the extrapyramidal side effects listed, the antipsychotic agents also can cause **hypotension**. This is usually orthostatic (in response to a person's rising from a supine position). How does this occur? The neuroleptics work by blockage of various systems. They block the dopamine receptors, and this is believed to be the cause of their therapeutic action and of their extrapyramidal side effects. They also block alpha-adrenergic neurons, thus causing hypotension. Finally, they interfere with the cholinergic neurotransmitter system and cause central and peripheral anticholinergic side effects.

The anticholinergic symptoms may occur with neuroleptics, with the antiparkinsonism agents (Cogentin), and with the antidepressants. The symptoms include dry mouth, dry mucous membranes, pupillary dilatation (mydriasis), decreased bowel activity, increased heart rate, inability to void urine, increased temperature, and possibly even organic brain syndrome (to be discussed).

There are multiple therapeutic interventions using **psychotherapy**. Supportive psychotherapy, helping the patient with reality testing, increasing feelings of self-esteem, and increasing sense of security all are important in treating the patient. Recently, the use of family therapy and psychoeducation have helped patients and families understand the nature of the disorder.

Affective disorders

There are many types of affective disorders: (1) major depressive episode, (2) manic-depressive disorder (bipolar disease), (3) dysthymic disorder (depressive neurosis), (4) cyclothymic disorder, and (5) organic affective disorder.

Major depressive disorder.   Severe depression is a common disorder, with a lifetime risk of 10 to 15% of the population. It is 2 to 3 times more common in women. The symptoms include decreased or increased sleep and appetite, decreased energy and enthusiasm, guilt feelings, decreased concentration, suicidal ideas, and an all-pervasive sadness. Duration must be at least 2 weeks to warrant the *DSM III-R* diagnosis. The etiology includes biologic aspects (formerly termed endogenous depression) or psychological forces (formerly termed exogenous depression). This terminology has certain drawbacks. It is clear that there are a variety of factors in the cause of this illness. Biologically, it has been found that patients treated with the antihypertensive reserpine suffer depression, leading to the

belief that norepinephrine or serotonin is involved in depression. This was strengthened by the observation that some of the antidepressants have an effect on the neurotransmitter balance in the brain, often increasing either serotonin or norepinephrine or both. In addition to the biologic theories, a number of psychological theories have been applied in treatment.

Patients who retroflex rage, who have unusually harsh superegos, or who have learned to think in pessimistic ways can have their depression eliminated by psychotherapy. Among the antidepressants that have been effective, two are particularly important— **imipramine** and **amitriptyline**. The antidepressants have their effect in 2 to 3 weeks, once the appropriate dosage is reached. Absorption patterns vary, and the recent introduction of blood level determinations of antidepressants has made their use more effective. With the exception of nortriptyline, all other antidepressants seem to have increased effectiveness with increased dosage. The dosage is limited by the **side effects**, which can be very serious: ECG changes leading to arrhythmias, anticholinergic side effects, orthostatic hypotension, and increased anxiety, agitation, and psychosis in predisposed individuals. The antidepressants described above are termed tricyclic because of their structure and have been found to be effective in approximately 60% of cases. Another group of antidepressants, the **MAO inhibitors**, work by blocking the enzyme MAO, which normally breaks down the neurotransmitter norepinephrine. It also increases dopamine and serotonin. This is in contrast to the method of action of the tricyclic compounds, which increase neurotransmission by down-regulatory beta-adrenergic presynaptic nerve terminals. The most serious side effect of the MAO inhibitors is the potential for hypertensive crisis if the patient eats foods such as cheddar cheese that contain tyramine. The danger with both types of antidepressants (tricyclic and MAO inhibitors) is that the lethal dose and therapeutic dose are not far apart, making an overdose a very serious consideration.

Manic-depressive illness.   Persons with this affective disorder suffer alternating episodes of depression with mania. Mania is characterized by distractibility and increased self-esteem (grandiose delusions such as being Christ or God). The patient's thoughts are racing, they exhibit flight of ideas, their speech is rapid and pressured, and they engage in activities that are reckless and include hypersexuality, reckless spending, speeding, and dangerous hobbies. They sleep little. Their mood, which is the most prominent symptom, may be either elated, euphoric, or irritable. The lifetime prevalence or risk of this disorder varies, around 1%. It is considered by many to be less common than schizophrenia, however. Its course is variable, and a person may experience recurrent episodes of mood swings. The onset usually is before 30 years of age; however, an increased onset during adolescence has been observed. Mania has been postulated to have its etiology rooted in biologic and psychological grounds. Recently, the tendency to think of it as a biologic disorder has been increased. This is because of the higher concordance rates in monozygotic twins (approaching 90% in some studies), the greater familial incidence, the greater efficacy of lithium for mania than neuroleptics for schizophrenia, and the observation of certain genetic patterns (an X-linked dominant pattern of inheritance; in others, an autosomal pattern of abnormal lithium membrane transport in red blood cells). Psychologically mania has been described as a reaction to depression and an attempt to avoid overwhelming depressive feelings.

Treatment includes a trial of lithium carbonate. First used as a salt substitute, it was soon noted to have mood-affecting properties. Lithium is a salt that has toxic effects in close range to its therapeutic effect, so *blood levels must be carefully monitored. Therapeutic levels are between 0.8 and 1.5 mEq/L.* Lithium has helped prevent relapse of depressive and manic episodes and helps in the treatment of the acute manic episode. It is also of some (although limited) help in the depressive phase alone. Usually, however, the acute mania requires initial treatment with an antipsychotic. Lithium is effective in approximately 70% of cases. When it is ineffective, carbamazepine (Tegretol) has been found to be helpful. The toxic effects of lithium are potentially serious. These include GI disturbances such as diarrhea, vomiting, and nausea; muscle twitches and fasciculations; dryness of the mouth; polyuria and polydipsia; tremulousness of the hands; ataxia; confusion; and seizures. The treatment of manic-depressive persons is important because risk of suicide is increased in this affliction.

Dysthymic disorder. This is also called depressive neurosis and is similar to a major depressive episode except that the symptoms are less intense and the duration is 2 years. In general, it has been described as a depressive condition in which psychological issues may be a prominent factor. Unconsciously there may be an excess of guilt or an inability to accept a previous loss. Freud's paper on mourning and melancholia talked about an identification with the lost person and a turning inward of anger at the lost person, resulting in self-condemnation and suicidal ideas. The treatment involves psychotherapy and/or pharamcotherapy. Studies that have focused on the use of both psycho- and pharmacotherapy have found a slight advantage to using both. Some studies indicate that pharmacotherapy is as effective as psychotherapy, and others that psychotherapy has certain benefits. This issue is not settled.

Cyclothymic disorder. This is similar to manic-depressive disorder except that the level of intensity of the pathology is less. This disorder was previously described as a personality disorder, but because of genetic and family studies it has been placed with the affective disorders. The manic episode is usually mild and has been described as hypomanic. These patients may respond to lithium, antidepressants, and psychotherapy. Further studies need to be conducted. Certain patients who have had recurrent hypomanic periods alternating with major depressions have been described as a bipolar type II and are distinguished from cyclothymic patients.

Organic mood disorder. This is perhaps one of the most important because it is often overlooked. Many patients present to an internist with vague somatic complaints and fatigue. The internist may miss such cases of somatic depression (also called masked depression). The psychiatrist, on the other hand, may fail to recognize depression with an underlying organic cause. When there clearly is a drug or illness responsible for the depression or mania, the term organic mood disorder is applied. Many drugs can cause depression. The antihypertensives methyldopa (Aldomet), propranolol (Inderal), reserpine, clonidine, and the thiazide diuretics have been implicated. Oral contraceptives and a wide variety of other drugs can cause

depression. Amphetamines and cocaine may elicit manic reactions. Many physical illnesses may present with depressive symptoms. Cancer, hypothyroidism, Addison's disease, collagen vascular disease, diabetes mellitus, any infection, anemia, and many physical illnesses may first make themselves apparent with depression. In addition, many patients experience significant depression following a serious illness. It has been recommended that patients who are discharged from a coronary care unit be told that they may experience a depressive episode. Any sedative agent such as **diazepam** (Valium) or an antipsychotic or barbiturate may cause depression.

Personality disorders

People may be said to act in a repetitive manner. Feelings, behaviors, or thoughts all may be expressed or experienced in a way that is repeated and characteristic. When specific repeated aspects of the personality cause conflict for the individual, then a personality disorder is said to exist. Patients with personality disorders usually do not recognize their problem but rather have difficulty in relationships with others, either in marriage, work, or school. As an example, a person may feel good about being strong minded. The spouse, on the other hand, complains about the stubborn attitude. The number of aspects of a personality are potentially limitless. *DSM III-R,* however, divides all of human personality disorders into 12 different types. It is important to have a working knowledge of the various personality disorders, discussed in the paragraphs that follow.

Paranoid. Paranoid persons are characteristically suspicious of others and mistrust them. They expect trickery, are hypersensitive to criticism, and have a limited degree of emotional warmth.

Schizoid. Schizoid individuals are loners. They do not feel discomfort about being alone, but prefer it. They are also emotionally cold. There is nothing otherwise that is noticeably odd about these persons.

Schizotypal. Affected persons suffer symptoms similar to those of schizophrenia, except their contact with reality is much better. If the individual has psychotic symptoms such as hallucinations, delusions, or thought disorders, they are usually brief, mild, or well controlled. These patients therefore can have brief psychoses. They are described in general as being odd or eccentric, having many magical beliefs, and participating in fringe groups such as religious cults.

Histrionic. This disorder is more common in women. The person craves the attention of others and attempts to draw others' attention by self-dramatization and excess emotion. They are usually seductive. Their relationships with others show them to be emotionally shallow and selfish. They may manipulate others with threats of suicide.

Narcissistic. These patients crave the attention of others. They are in addition vain and self-important. They may have grandiose fantasies about themselves. They tend to either idealize others or devalue them.

Antisocial. This is perhaps the most difficult to treat. The person is chronically violating the rights of others. Besides becoming involved in criminal acts such as assault and robbery, these individuals do not take responsibility for their children, spouses, financial burdens, or any social obligation.

They may be charming and suave, only to use this talent to manipulate and use others.

Borderline. The term borderline implies that these patients exist on the border of psychoses or schizophrenia. The patient suffers from intense and disturbed relationships and has an unstable personality with recurrent lapses into psychosis. The patient may suffer from severe anger and depression. There frequently are manipulative suicide attempts, including wrist cutting and overdoses. Feelings of abandonment are frequent.

Avoidant. This is the wallflower who is too shy to make friends but secretly craves to be cared for.

Dependent. This persons is clinging and wants others to make their life's decisions.

Compulsive. On coronary care units, this is the type A personality. The patient is rigid and emotionally repressed, except for anger. They are frequently impatient and irritated at others' lack of performance. These patients may become professionals and can be workaholics.

Passive-aggressive. These patients drive others crazy by constant dawdling, procrastination, and forgetting important events. They are unable to see the underlying motivation, which involves anger at others.

Organic mental disorders

In this group of disorders, the patient suffers from symptoms or demonstrates signs that can be shown to be caused by specific organic impairments. The demonstration of an organic basis can be either from physical, laboratory, or radiological findings or from the patient's history. The syndromes that are most commonly involved include those discussed in the paragraphs that follow.

Delirium. This is an extremely important group of disorders in which the patient has a sudden onset of impaired attention to the environment. The patient must also demonstrate two of the following: **speech incoherence, sleep-wake reversal** (up at night, drowsy during daytime), **psychomotor agitation** to retardation, and **visual hallucinations** (olfactory, tactile, or auditory may also occur but less frequently). It usually indicates severe process and may be interpreted as a harbinger of death unless the underlying cause is detected. Hypoxia, hypoglycemia, electrolyte abnormalities, infectious meningitis, hypertensive encephalopathy, intracranial hemorrhages, and acute poisonings or withdrawal from alcohol or sedatives are among the most serious causes. The characteristic feature also includes **memory impairment** and **disorientation**.

Dementia. This group of disorders in the recent past was thought to be irreversible. It has been shown that, although this is the case in the majority of patients, a number of dementias may be treatable and to some degree reversed. The disorder is insidious in onset (subtle). There is a progressive loss of intellectual functions such as the ability to use abstract reasoning, to use judgment, and to be able to dress oneself or perform activities (apraxias). The hallmark, however, is **memory impairment**. Dementia may be caused by a number of diseases. **Alzheimer's disease**, or senile dementia, is perhaps the most common, occurring in 40 to 60% of the cases. This disease is progressive, irreversible, untreatable, and fatal. The disease typically starts between 50 and 60 years of age and involves progressive memory loss. Characteristic pathological findings on autopsy include neurofibrillary tangles and senile plaques in the frontal and temporal lobes (and diffusely throughout the brain).

Another type of dementia that is reversible is **normal pressure hydrocephalus** (NPH), which includes the triad of ataxia, dementia, and urinary incontinence. It may account for 10% of cases in some studies. Repeated small strokes may also cause dementia and can be slowed by appropriate medical management. In this disorder, known as **multi-infarct dementia**, there is a stepwise progression of memory loss accompanied by asymmetric lesions of either cortex. Consequently there also are motor weakness and sensory findings, which improve in time.

Wernicke-Korsakoff's syndrome. There are two aspects to this disorder, both caused by the dietary deficiency of vitamin B_1 (thiamine). The Wernicke's aspect involves a triad of ataxia, ophthalmoplegia (usually involving a weakness of the sixth cranial nerve), and dementia. The Korsakoff's syndrome refers to the memory disturbance, which is profound and may involve **confabulation**. This is demonstrated by patients who create fictional stories to cover up for their severe memory disturbance. This ailment commonly afflicts chronic alcoholics.

Anxiety disorders

This is a group of eight disorders previously referred to as neuroses. There is an increasing amount of information about the underlying biology of this group of disorders. The term neurosis indicates that in the past it was thought that these disorders were caused by the presence of unconscious conflicts, a belief still largely held today as well. The causes of anxiety disorders include a wide variety of organic factors. Substances such as cocaine, amphetamines, marijuana, over-the-counter diet pills containing phenylpropanolamine, caffeine, and tobacco all can provoke severe anxiety in certain individuals. Cardiac conditions such as angina pectoris, mitral value prolapse, and cardiac arrhythmias may present with anxiety. Endocrine disorders such as hyperthyroidism, hypoparathyroidism, Cushing's disease, hypoglycemia, and pheochromocytoma all may present with anxiety. Neurological disorders such as brain tumors and temporal lobe epilepsy may also demonstrate this problem.

Panic disorder with agoraphobia. Persons with agoraphobia have a fear of being out in public or at home alone. This fear is a phobia—it is irrational. Victims know that it is reasonable, yet they are unable to help themselves. Some believe that it is more common in housewives and that they become locked into the home setting. Others point out that there is a high association between this disorder and panic attackes. They postulate that if patients were out in public alone and experienced a severe overwhelming and unprovoked attack of anxiety, this experience was so painful that they began to restrict their activity. Patients with agoraphobia may be dependent personalities. Treatment includes psychotherapy, group therapy, tricyclic antidepressants and MAO inhibitors, and anxiolytics such as diazepam.

Panic disorder without agoraphobia. The patient has recurrent, unprovoked, sudden, overwhelming panic. Symptoms include tachycardia, hyperventilation, syncope, fear of dying or going insane, tingling of extremities, and others. A large number of these individuals have a sensitivity to sodium lactate, which when infused by IV will provoke an attack (in normal persons this IV infusion does not have such an effect to such a degree).

Generalized anxiety disorder.   In this disorder, the individual has a relatively persistent feeling of anxiety. There are signs of increased autonomic activity, including increased heart rate, respirations, and blood pressure. Afflicted persons may show jitteriness and excessive movement of the extremities. There is an emotional uneasiness, worrying, and fearful rumination about the events in life. The person may startle easily. Therapy involves both psychotherapy and pharmacotherapy. Benzodiazepines such as valium have been very successful. The problem with medication is that it may interfere with the psychotherapeutic task of working out the patient's conflicts.

Simple phobia.   Most people probably have some phobias. The most common phobias involve (1) fear of storms and (2) fear of animals. People may fear anything from snails to dust. There are a number of competing theories about phobias. The analytic theory holds that the phobia is a displacement of some forbidden impulse onto a symbol. The classic case was little Hans, who had a fear of horses that could be traced to his fear of his competitive feelings with his father. Learning theory holds that people may have anxiety erupt in a setting in which the fear is associated with one aspect of the environment. The patient comes to be conditioned to the object and thus begins to avoid it. In this case, therapy is directed toward desensitizing the individual to the frightening symbol or situation. In analytic theory, patients must first understand the nature of the displacement and then gradually face the feared thing with the therapist's help.

Social phobia.   Here what is feared is an activity in a social setting. The activity may be speaking, eating, or using public toilets. Speaker's phobia is relatively common, although incidence figures are not available. Fear of performance in public may be found in actors and actresses or musicians. Psychotherapy aimed at understanding the underlying conflict may reveal that there is a repressed exhibitionistic wish. Pharmacotherapy with the use of propranolol, a beta-blocker, has been shown to be helpful for reducing the hand tremor, tachycardia, and shakiness of voice.

Obsessive compulsive disorder.   In this group of disorders, the individual is forced to repeat an activity such as checking a door or has a recurrent thought that cannot be voluntarily suppressed. In the former instance, we speak of compulsions; in the latter, obsessions. Therapy involves psychotherapy, behavior therapy, and pharmacotherapy. The medication clomipramine (a relative of imipramine) is effective in 60% of patients. The underlying psychological issue may involve a desire to be messy, with the patient using reaction formation and checking things to be certain they are clean.

Posttraumatic stress disorder.   In this disorder, which became more intensively studied following the Vietnam war, the individual has repeated flashbacks of a traumatic event, which usually was life threatening. In addition, these patients suffer from recurrent nightmares and recollections of the event. They may misidentify current relationships in terms of the past event and be easily startled by loud noises or quick movements. In addition to combat, violent crimes such as rape may elicit this reaction, as may natural disasters. Therapy is directed toward a rapid assessment near the scene of the disaster. The patient is encouraged to have an abreaction (to relive the experience and release the pent-up emotions). Sometimes narcosynthesis, or the uncovering of repressed feelings by use of IV short-acting barbiturates, will help the therapist use this material for the victim to learn about the fears.

ALCOHOL AND SUBSTANCE ABUSE

Alcoholism

Alcoholism is a tremendous health problem that is widely overlooked by physicians. Perhaps 50% of alcoholics seen by doctors go undiagnosed. Estimates are that 5 to 10% of the adult population is afflicted with alcoholism. It is the fourth leading health problem, preceded by cardiovascular disease, lung disease, and cancer.

There are several patterns of alcoholism: (1) regular daily excessive drinking, (2) regular heavy drinking on weekends only, and (3) long periods of sobriety interspersed with binges that last weeks or months.

Genetic and familial studies indicate that biologic factors probably play a part. Sons of alcoholic fathers who are adopted by nonalcoholic parents have a threefold greater rate of alcoholism than the general population. There is a fourfold increased risk of a first-degree relative's developing alcoholism.

The detection of alcoholism is not easy, because patients often use a tremendous degree of denial. One approach that has been useful is the **CAGE questions**: (C) Have you ever considered **cutting down** the amount of alcohol consumption? (A) Are others **annoyed** by your drinking? (G) Have you ever felt **guilty** about your drinking or its results? (E) Have you ever taken an **eye-opener** (morning drink)? A positive response to one question is suggestive of alcoholism.

Alcoholism may consist of a pattern of alcohol abuse, as described above. In addition, there may develop tolerance (higher doses/amounts are needed for the same effect) or withdrawal symptoms. In that case, alcohol dependence is said to exist. In alcohol withdrawal, there are potential fatal consequences. **Delirium tremens** is a type of delirium that may occur several hours to 10 days after cessation of drinking. The patient shows signs of autonomic hyperactivity, tremulousness of the extremities, diaphoresis, and signs of delirium. The peak onset is 3 to 4 days after the patient's last drink. There is an approximate mortality of 10%. Treatment consists of large doses of chlordiazepoxide (Librium) given early in the treatment. Additionally, thiamine (vitamin B_1) is given because of the possibility of Wernicke's disease.

Alcohol may affect various organ systems, including the GI tract (gastritis, esophageal varices, ulcers), nervous system (peripheral neuropathies, cerebellar degeneration), heptic (cirrhosis), cardiovascular (cardiomyopathy), endocrine (increased estrogen in males secondary to liver degeneration, with consequent testicular atrophy and female breast development). The **fetal alcohol syndrome** may occur in infants of mothers who consume ethanol during pregnancy. It is associated with characteristics such as short palpebral fissures and a diminished philtrum, possibly a lower IQ, and diminished birth weight.

The treatment of alcoholism is a complex task. First there is a need for detoxification in those patients who have developed physical dependence. By taking progressively smaller doses of chlordiazepoxide(Librium), the patient is gradually freed from withdrawal symptoms. The next aspect of treatment is the most difficult. Abstinence may be maintained by an emphasis on regular attendance at an alcoholism support group. Alcoholics Anonymous is the single most effective treatment group for alcoholics. It is now generally believed that an alcoholic cannot return to social drinking and that total abstinence is mandatory. Alcoholics Anonymous meetings provide the necessary reinforcement and social support that will help patients avoid relapses. The use of psychotherapy in patients suffering from alcoholism can also be beneficial. It should be noted that 70% of alcoholics have no other psychiatric diagnoses. Some people feel that there may be an alcoholic personality. This has not been definitely established. Another useful approach is the use of disulfiram (Antabuse). This medication can cause an extremely unpleasant reaction if alcohol is consumed concurrently. The reaction includes nausea, vomiting, headaches, and anxiety. Potentially serious reactions can occur as well.

Other substance abuse

There has been an increase in media attention to drug abuse— particularly to **cocaine** abuse. Indications are that the amount of abuse has escalated as well. In 1982, it was estimated that there were 4.2 million regular users of cocaine in the United States. The average age of the cocaine user was 30 years, males outnumbered females 2 to 1, and it appeared to be abused by predominantly white, college-educated people. Cocaine is classified as a stimulant, although it has been incorrectly referred to in the past as a narcotic. It has specific medical uses, predominantly in ophthalmology as a local anesthetic with some vasoconstrictive properties that reduce the likelihood of bleeding. It acts by increasing the release of noradrenalin from the presynaptic vesicles. Its actions are principally sympathomimetic, with increases in vital signs, pupillary dilation, and increased GI motility. There are many potential dangers of cocaine use. First, it is addictive— more addictive than narcotics. Cocaine, as is true of all street drugs, is usually cut with other drugs. Thus it is impossible to know the true amount of drug that is being consumed. Several celebrities recently died accidentally from accidental overdosage as a result of this. Cocaine can cause a brief psychosis that usually remits in 24 hours. It can produce a "crash" when a chronic user discontinues use. This crash usually appears as a depressive episode, and suicide becomes a danger. Chronic use may also impair the users' judgment, with an inflated sense of their own potential. Users frequently run into financial problems, interpersonal problems, and vocational difficulties. The average addict uses 6 g/week at a cost of $100/g. Treatment for cocaine addiction follows similar guidelines to alcoholism, with the need for support groups, confrontation, and at times hospitalization. There is no withdrawal delirium as in sedative-hypnotic/alcohol abusers.

Marijuana is a drug that has been used across cultures and for centuries. The active component is tetrahydrocannibinol (THC). Marijuana has been called one of the "gateway" drugs because it is believed that users may go on to more dangerous drugs such as cocaine or heroin. Physical signs of marijuana intoxication include increased pulse rate, dry mouth, and conjunctival erythema. There are no pupillary changes. There is an impairment in short-term memory and difficulty in attention. A withdrawal syndrome is characterized by irritability, nausea, vomiting, diarrhea, and sleep disturbances. Two major difficulties associated with marijuana use are an amotivational syndrome and the precipitation of psychoses in predisposed individuals. The amotivation syndrome may be particularly destructive for adolescents. It has also been reported in adults who have used marijuana for years. It is believed to be one of the unrecognized aggravating factors in many young chronic schizophrenics as well.

Angel dust, known chemically as phencyclidine, is considered a hallucinogen by many. In some areas its use has reached epidemic proportions. It is frequently added to marijuana to produce what is called "super pot." Originally marketed as an anesthetic, it was removed from the market because of its serious adverse reactions, which included psychotic disorder. In mild doses, it causes euphoria and a feeling of detachment from the body. It causes signs of autonomic hyperactivity like the stimulants, but causes miosis (stimulants such as cocaine and amphetamines cause mydriasis). Angel dust has also received a reputation for causing extreme combatativeness and violent behavior in certain individuals. The psychotic symptoms may be alleviated by haloperidol, symptoms of agitation by diazepam. Other hallucinogens such as LSD, mescaline, and peyote are more well known for causing marked visual hallucinations and illusions.

MDMA, or **ecstasy**, is a recently developed "designer" drug. It has been touted by some psychiatrists as increasing the amount of therapeutic insight in patients. It was legally obtained until the past year. Because of its novelty, the drug was not recognized by the regulating state and federal agencies and thus could be purchased openly in bars or elsewhere as a nondrug. It causes dryness of the mouth, sweating of palms, and tachycardia. In many it induced a transient state of euphoria. Users can get panic reactions similar to those suffered by marijuana users. The greatest danger at this point appears to be in its preparation by basement chemists. In California, a number of illicit laboratories produced a variant of MDMA that caused an irreversible destruction of the substantia nigra and permanent Parkinson's disease in young people.

SOMATOFORM DISORDERS

Because a variety of disorders may present with physical complaints, it is extremely important for physicians to be certain that there is no underlying organic cause. In one study, it was found that 30% of patients who were written off as having psychosomatic symptoms could be found after several years to have organic lesions that had previously been undetectable. This is important for two reasons. First, many of these patients probably have underlying psychological factors responsible for their complaints. Second, organic cause is being overlooked in a sizable number of cases. For this reason, even when suspecting one of the somatoform disorders, never completely rule out physical causes! There are five particular somatoform disorders according to *DSM III-R*. These are somatization disorder, conversion disorder, somatoform pain, hypochondriasis, and dysmorphic disorder.

In **somatization disorder**, also known as Briquet's syndrome, the patient has multiple physical complaints affecting a variety of organ systems. The patient, typically female, complains of headaches, menstrual irregularities, fainting spells, GI symptoms, vague neurological symptoms, and more. The most common complaints are fatigue, weakness, blurred vision, and pain. Sometimes these patients will have had many surgical procedures without significant findings or results. Referral to a skilled psychotherapist is in order. The patient is then usually treated rather with supportive psychotherapy, not by ignoring the physical complaints.

In **conversion disorder** there is usually a loss of physical functioning. This loss of functioning appears to be related to events in the person's life in a temporal manner. The patient is said to have primary and secondary gain. In **primary gain**, an underlying conflict is relieved by its expression in a bodily symptom. In **secondary gain**, the patient usually receives attention and special consideration from the family for being "sick." For example, a medical student suddenly developed paralysis of the right arm. A full medical-surgical and neurological workup with nerve conduction velocities, radiographic investigation, CT scan, and electromyographic examination revealed nothing. The patient's symptom spontaneously resolved after an important examination. The patient was not voluntarily or secretly avoiding the exam. In this student's case, the primary gain was the alleviation of the test-taking anxiety. The secondary gain was the attention of the classmates and family who provided support. Conversion occurs because an unconscious drive, feeling, thought, or impulse is converted into a symbolic physical symptom. Some authorities feel that conversion reactions are common and may be a major reason for referral to a general practitioner's office. Patients who use conversion reactions usually select an organ or anatomic location that is determined by its meaning and associations. For example, a person who may refer his problems to a leg paralysis may in the course of psychotherapy reveal that his mother's leg was damaged in an automobile accident. The leg takes on an association to his mother and becomes significant in the person's unconscious. Another aspect of conversion disorder is **la belle indifférence**. This refers to the seeming apathy that patients have over their symptom. This can be encountered with organic lesions as well but is a hint of underlying conversion disorder. Treatment of these patients is aimed at uncovering the unconscious meaning and gradually working through the traumatic memories, experiences, forbidden ideas, or impulses. Sometimes placebo medications can work miracles in these patients. In nations that are not industrialized, there seems to be a greater incidence—the more psychologically sophisticated the nation, the less conversion may be used. In one such nation, a medical emergency room routinely would give saline injections to treat the numerous cases of conversion paralysis that appeared there, yielding excellent results.

Somatoform pain is present when there is pain in the absence of demonstrable organic pathology or the pain is exaggerated in comparison with the level of pathology. These patients usually deny emotional factors in their lives. At first they idealize their doctors and then devalue them.

Hypochondriasis is the persistent focusing of attention on some believed illness. A particular sign or symptom is usually either manufactured or magnified. Many people have daily aches and pains from the bumping around that is part of life. A hypochondriac will exaggerate these symptoms to a great degree. These patients frequently "doctor shop" in an attempt to establish a diagnosis. In all of the conditions discussed above, it is best not to attempt to confront patients with the psychological nature of their problems. Instead, an attempt to use various modalities, to some degree accepting the physical nature, will lead to a therapeutic alliance. This in turn will allow for the discussion of relevant dynamic issues. Many possible dynamic issues have been found in these disorders. For example, in psychogenic pain there may be an underlying guilt complex related to either sexual feelings or some experience in the patient's life. In conversion disorder, an underlying dynamic may be the patient's fear of aggressive impulses. The number of possible underlying or unconscious issues is astounding. In addition, there are social factors. Persons of certain cultures, such as the Italians or Jews, may be more demonstrative in their pain experiences than, say, the English.

In **dysmorphic disorder**, a patient has an exaggerated sense of some physical defect like his nose being too large.

PSYCHOSOMATIC DISORDERS

A number of medical-surgical illnesses have physical and psychological underpinnings. Among them are asthma, essential hypertension, dermatitis, peptic ulcer, rheumatoid arthritis, and ulcerative colitis. These disorders may be brought out by general stress or by specific emotional issues. In coronary artery disease, there is an association with the type A personality. Studies have shown that psychotherapy directed at reducing the characteristics of irritation, annoyance, and anger have reduced patients' reinfarction rates. In patients with asthma, underlying conflicts may involve difficulty with separation. Peptic ulcer patients have been described as unusually pseudo-independent and high achievers. They are unable to express their dependency needs directly and must assume the sick role as a means of doing this. Arthritis sufferers have responses on Rorschach cards of knights in armor, arthropods, and other images having a tough exoskeleton and a soft and frighteningly vulnerable inner core. Although such theories are certainly not held by all, there have been reports of good results with psychotherapy in certain cases.

STRESS AND STRESS REDUCTION

One final key aspect to understanding disordered behavior is the concept of stress. Stress is a force that is deleterious to living organisms. Some view stress not as deleterious but rather a part of life—something that represents a change or a demand. Such a concept indicates that a person needs a certain degree of stress in life to maintain optimum performance. Walter Cannon in the early 20th century felt that there was a "dynamic equilibrium" that the animal attempts to maintain in the face of threat of change. This concept of **homeostasis** is important in understanding stress, for when homeostasis is disrupted, disease can begin. When confronted with stress, physiological reactions include (1) increased alertness, (2) increased muscle tension, (3) autonomic hyperactivity (sympathetic over parasympathetic), (4) hormonal changes (increased growth hormone, thyroid hormones, cortisol, and decreased sex steroids and insulin), and (5) catecholamines predominant over indoleamines (serotonin) in the CNS. This initial set of reactions is considered the **alarm** phase. If an organism is exposed to continuous major stress, a **general adaptational syndrome** occurs, as was noted by Hans Seyle. The body responds with an alarm phase, mounts resistance, and finally reaches the exhaustion phase. A number of factors mediate how a person handles stress—first, the nature of the person. Some individuals thrive on intense stimulation. They perceive a change as something exciting to be mastered. For such an individual, there are few deleterious results from the stress. Thus, personality type is one aspect. The meaning of the experience to the individual is important. For one person, a job promotion can be a welcome thing and for another a worrisome burden. The duration of the stress is more important than the intensity of the stress. There needs to be rest and recuperation. Holmes and Rahe in 1967 devised a social readjustment rating scale, which tallied 43 items and their relative importance as stressors in an individual's life. The most important stressors were found to be (1) death of spouse, (2) divorce, (3) marital separation, (4) jail term, and (5) death of close family member. It has been noted that, with the possible exception of drug abuse, in the psychiatric syndromes that have been studied (neurosis, depression, schizophrenia, and alcohol abuse) there is a relationship of stressful life events to onset of the illness. The relationship extends to physical illness as well. One study of a huge sample of men found that those men who lost their spouse while in their 60s versus men who had not lost their spouse had a fivefold increase in heart attacks and cancer. For women, however, the loss of their husband did not increase their rate of illness as much. Social support systems are therefore considered extremely important in reducing stress.

Stress probably plays a part in many if not most diseases. There are some in which its role is primary. Headaches of the muscle tension type, ulcerative colitis, irritable bowel syndrome, and asthma are but a few. How then can stress be reduced? Manipulating the environment by changing jobs or neighborhoods may be appropriate in some cases but in others it is either impractical or not relevant. Development of social support groups is one important method of reducing stress. Occasionally, we are under stress because our belief system alerts us to nonexistent or unconscious dangers. There is some evidence that, in industrialized societies, expectations are too high, leading to chronic frustration. In these cases, psychotherapy may help in dealing with the underlying conflicts. Additionally, biofeedback techniques allow the stressed person to focus directly on such factors as muscle tension, heart rate, temperature, and respiratory rate to bring about a lowering of the stress response. Repeated exposure to such learning experiences possibly hastens the relaxation process.

THE PHYSICIAN'S ROLE

THE PHYSICIAN-PATIENT RELATIONSHIP

Many integral and interactive factors can affect the relationship between a doctor and a patient. At least three sets of variables affect the interaction. First, there are those "intrapsychic" factors related to the physician's basic training, personality, family upbringing, strengths, and weaknesses. Second, there are those factors that the patient contributes—upbringing (including culture), medical myths, personality, education, strengths, and weaknesses. Additionally, there is the disease itself. How the patient responds to it, experiences it, and copes with it all depend on the preceding factors and innate aspects of the disease itself. Finally, there is the mixture of these two unique persons—the chemistry that in each case is special, with all of its strengths and failings.

The physician

Physicians have historically been trained under a paternalistic pattern of delivering health care. Their teachers were never wrong. There was a rigid pecking order with students at the bottom followed by interns and residents. The physician was all knowing and all powerful. This pattern exists to some degree today, but on the whole has been combined and in some contexts replaced by a model of **humanism** or humanistic medicine. In humanism, the patient is seen as a person first and as a patient second. In the paternalistic model, patients were more passive and the physician did not have to explain things or have a great deal of interaction with them except to instruct them on the proper limitations of activities and how to take medications. In the humanistic model, the patient is more active. This in part may be the result of some increase in the level of education of the general population. Through the media, books, and families, people have become more knowledgeable about diseases. The patient today wishes to be informed of the proper diagnosis, prognosis, treatment alternatives, medication names, side effects, adverse reactions, and more. Because of the increased number of malpractice cases, the general population has become more suspicious of physicians. Physicians are no longer held in such great esteem. Today's physician must understand this. Through the use of explanations, physicians are more likely to inform their patients and their families of the nature of the illness. For the physicians's part, this has meant an increased amount of communication. From a number of studies, it has been demonstrated that there is less malpractice among physicians who communicate with patients. Physicians can better communicate with their patients by following the guidelines listed here.

1. Allow adequate time. The hectic pace of providing medical care does not always allow sufficient time for becoming acquainted with the patient, but knowing the patient as a person is crucial to developing an alliance.
2. Provide nontechnical explanations. The student and resident are immersed in a field that has its own language. Explanations are often inadvertently given in complex jargon that the patient cannot understand. The physician must therefore speak plainly.
3. Ask if there are questions and if the patient understands.
4. Explain procedures, tests, and medications. It is helpful to supply the patient with graphic education pamphlets.
5. Be attuned to the patient's emotional response. Fear, sadness, and other feelings may block understanding.

The patient

The person who is being examined is a complex, emotional being. There are many different ways in which she or he might relate. A patient who overtly cooperates may covertly undermine therapy. Noncompliance with medication is a common vexing problem for physicians. One study examined the contents of the wastebaskets of a medical outpatient department and found there a sizable percentage of the clinic doctor's prescriptions. Some studies have found medication noncompliance of about 50%. There are many reasons for this. Psychologically, denial of the illness is a commonly encountered problem. Similar to this is minimizing. Other dynamic considerations include a masochistic or self-destructive tendency in some people, an underlying conflict with authority in which the act of noncompliance is seen as a defeat of the authority figure, and depression and feeling that all is hopeless. In addition to psychological factors, social factors play a part. In certain ethnic communities, belief in folk medicine may take priority over organized medicine. Lack of understanding of the instructions, inability to read a prescription, and lack of money to purchase the medication all may contribute to noncompliance. Multiple doses may be forgotten, and for this reason compliance is more likely to be achieved with single doses or long-acting injections.

A physical or emotional illness puts enormous strain on a person. There may be an intensification of the defense mechanisms that the patient has used to a lesser extent in dealing with life. A person who customarily uses intellectualization as a way of dealing with anxiety may find this defense heightened. The use of the defense may take on a pathological quality. Generally there is a regression in response to illness. This regression is characterized by an increase in passivity, demandingness, self-centered behavior, and feelings of vulnerability, helplessness, and inadequacy. As a result of these forces, the patient may react in a variety of ways. Patients who are **angry** may in part be reacting to the loss of autonomy and the fear of bodily damage. Physicians must not take their anger personally but seek reasons for its presence. Sometimes all that is necessary is listening, other times the environment may have to be manipulated. Changing rooms, substituting medications, and a variety of other decisions may have to be addressed. At Massachussetts General Hospital, patients who have had a myocardial infarction are told they may expect to feel **depressed** on returning home. This advice helps them understand this as a normal part of dealing with the losses that the heart attack may have provoked. When addressing this issue in patients, the danger of suicide must be taken into account. **Anxiety** may result from a number of factors. Fantasies about the illness and feelings of one's body being damaged may reach exaggerated proportions. Sometimes, providing the patient with a healthy dose of reality by discussing a realistic prognosis and the difficulties experienced with the illness helps a patient reduce tension. Anxiety is increased when the patient feels **helpless**. Suggest activities that the patient may engage in to regain a sense of some control. For example, patients with postsurgical conditions may be encouraged to use "blow bottles." This is recommended not just for the prevention of atelectasis but also to increase the sense of activity and mastery over illness. Some patients have an unusually harsh superego and blame themselves for the illness and think of it as a retribution for wrongs they have done. Uncovering these feelings of **guilt**, providing reassurance, and arranging for religious counseling in the person's faith can reduce inappropriate guilt and speed recovery.

Doctor-patient chemistry

In ideal situations, the patient and doctor like each other and respect each other. There will be cooperation in achieving a common goal— the alleviation of the individual's suffering. Unfortunately, all too often this is not achieved. The most common reason for failure is the physician's lack of empathy and the patient's transference reactions. Empathy is the ability to put oneself in another's shoes. This is particularly difficult to do with patients, since their shoes are frequently filled with pain, fear, sadness, and feelings of helplessness, inadequacy, and vulnerability. Empathy can fail when the patient is particularly angry and the doctor reacts defensively. Patients who feel hopeless may stimulate in the doctor feelings of being a failure. Physicians can best manage these difficulties by trying to understand why they are having difficulty empathizing. The reason may often be **countertransference**. The concepts of transference and countertransference are analytic terms that have previously been described. In respect to the doctor-patient relationship, they are particularly important to understand. Transference and countertransference are displacements from earlier or other relationships on to the doctor and patient, respectively. The patient's transference to the doctor may be that of a parent who was not available or was unusually critical, punitive, or physically abusive. For example, an oncology patient may complain that her doctor is uncaring and cold. The oncologist may not have that impression. By recognizing that it might be transferential, he might say, "I care about you and how you do. Is there someone else who is treating you (has treated you) this way?" The physician may then find that a nurse, a technician, or even another physician may have handled the patient brusquely in the rush of the hospital workday. The physician is subject to the same difficulty, in this case termed countertransference. For example, a student physician began to interview a patient and suddenly stopped short, indicating that she was through. Later on she explained that she had a strong negative reaction to the patient, who reminded her of her own mother.

INTERVIEWING AND MENTAL STATUS EXAMINATION

Obtaining information from a patient can be done in a number of ways. An interview is more than just a means of obtaining information, however. It is a crucial component in the patient's recovery. For this reason, it is reasonable to think of interviewing from several models. In the medical model, emphasis is placed on **closed-ended questions**. These are questions that receive finite quantitative information. "Does your arm have numbness or tingling?" "Have you ever vomited blood before?" "How much?" Such questions will reveal information and associations within the physician's mind. This in turn will provoke new thoughts and new questions. Bedside diagnostic manuals speak of the "P, Q, R, S, T" approach to various symptoms. The **provoking** and **palliative** aspects of a symptom, the nature and **quality** of the symptom, the **radiation** of an anatomic pain, the **severity** and temporal aspects can all be elicited. This is found in the portion of the interview that is termed the review of systems. **Open-ended questions**, on the other hand, show us how the patient thinks and help us gain a broad view of the patient's problems. "What brought you into the hospital?" "Describe what that was like." "Tell me more." All are directed at obtaining the patient's impression. In general, patients have different styles of communication. Some patients who are very talkative may need more closed-ended questions to keep the interviewer from being overwhelmed with information. Others who may be uncommunicative may need more open-ended questions to get them going. A good interview integrates both.

It is important to know at the outset why you are interviewing the patient. An interview for an insurance company is very different from one in which there is the beginning of a therapeutic relationship. When physicians commence the interview, they should be aware of their **goals**. The goal often is to establish a diagnosis. Such diagnostic interviews contain a high number of closed-ended questions and an approach that attempts to elicit yes-or-no responses to particular symptoms. In psychiatry, there is also the need for understanding why the illness began, from a psychological and sociological perspective. Questions then attempt to assess the present problems through previous experiences. The ability to empathize and put yourself in the patient's place enables the interviewer to see the situation in your mind's eye and ask appropriate questions.

Certain techniques may be needed in given situations. **Confrontation** is an important technique that addresses the patient's denial in such illnesses as alcoholism or addresses the patient's attempt to evade the truth in such cases as malingering or antisocial personality disorder. **Silence** is a technical aid that the interviewer must keep in mind. Keeping silent generates a certain degree of anxiety in the patient, frequently prompting the patient to reveal information. Extended silence can hamper communication, however. The interviewer must make use of **nonverbal communication**. Patients who exhibit closing posture (crossing the arms and legs) may be moving away from important feelings. Any facial expression that connotes an emotion should be asked about. "You smiled when I mentioned your husband—why is that?" Emotions thus portrayed frequently indicate underlying factors that may yield the diagnosis or the dynamics of a case. Patients who keep looking over their shoulder might be assumed to be paranoid, but only by asking can one's suspicions be confirmed. In one such case, a patient was asked the reason for his frequent backward glances. It turned out that this patient had posttraumatic stress disorder and began to discuss how since his combat experience he can never sit without his back to a wall.

One crucial aspect of a psychiatric interview is the **mental status examination**, a systematic appraisal of the patient's psychological state. Observation is the first step, and a person's behavior and appearance are noted and questions addressed. Behavior has in psychiatry been termed **psychomotor activity**, referring to the amount and nature of activity. For example, some patients with depression have decreased psychomotor activity. Others with an agitated depression may have increased psychomotor activity with hand-wringing behavior.

Speech is assessed and its rate and quality noted. The presence of pressured speech connotes anxiety or even mania.

Sparse speech may indicate depression, catatonic schizophrenia, or paranoid feelings. Dysarthria refers to speech that is garbled, including slurred speech, a tipoff to substance abuse. Scanning speech is found in cerebellar disorders. The level of consciousness usually describes a person's alertness. It may include a person's ability to be oriented to person, place, and time. Difficulties such as disorientation are found in organic brain syndromes like delirium and dementia.

Mood and affect are assessed next. Mood is a pervasive sustained emotion that colors one's perception of the world. Typical moods are depressed, anxious, euphoric, and suspicious. Affect is the immediate observable emotion. A person with a depressed mood may initially manifest a happy affect, but it is overshadowed by the predominant mood. Affect traditionally has also been used to describe the range of emotions. A person with schizophrenia is said to have a flat, blunted, or inappropriate affect. A manic-depressive in the manic phase will show labile affect.

Thinking consists of two components: stream or form of thinking and content of thinking. The stream or form is the manner in which the thoughts are put together. As previously described, loosening of associations is seen in schizophrenia. The content of thought includes obsessions, delusions, and ideas of reference. The latter is illustrated by a patient who inappropriately attributes a person's comment as directed toward herself. A patient who thinks that the gas station attendant is touching his tie to signify that he wants the patient to get only a half tank of gas is an example of an idea of reference. An idea of influence is the belief that others' through various means are influencing a person's feelings, actions, or thoughts. These may be loosely held beliefs or may reach the proportions of a delusion. They are not in themselves delusions unless they are unshakable and not based in reality.

Also included in the mental status exam are assessment of memory, intelligence, and insight. Several specific cognitive functions—namely, the ability to concentrate and use abstract reasoning—are ascertained by specific types of questions. To understand the person's ability to concentrate is important. Concentration is impaired in patients with depression, mania, and various organic brain syndromes including delirium and dementia. The best test of this is serial 7s. The person is asked to subtract backward from 100 by 7s. The examiner does not help the patient or encourage, other than to give the initial instructions. If this is too difficult a task, subtracting backward from 21 by 3s can be used. Patients with impairments in this ability will falter and attempt to avoid this test. Abstract reasoning is best measured by asking proverbs. Patients with schizophrenia and organic brain syndrome will respond with concrete or bizarre answers to simple proverbs.

TREATMENT MODALITIES

The approach to treating various problems of living and psychopathological states can be taken from three, albeit not exclusive, modalities: psychotherapy, pharmacotherapy, and somatic therapy.

Psychotherapy

The types of psychotherapy are too numerous to review at length here. In general, therapy can be individual, group, marital/couple, or family oriented. Individual therapy can be insight oriented or supportive. In **insight-oriented therapy**, individuals attempt to change their pathological relationships, feelings, or thought patterns by becoming aware of the forces in their development that brought them about. Insight-oriented psychotherapy often makes use of analytic concepts. Psychoanalysis is a type of insight-oriented psychotherapy that involves two or more sessions per week and a focus on therapy of transference, resistance, and dreams. There are many types of psychoanalytic analysts, from classic Freudian to interpersonal. In **supportive psychotherapy**, the focus is on understanding one's present rather one's past and on improving the already existing defense systems. This type of therapy is often used in more difficult illnesses such as schizophrenia. Psychoanalysis is more often used in the mild neuroses and personality disorders. **Group therapy** can involve a variety of techniques, from primal scream, to transactional analysis, to gestalt groups. The focus on groups is the individual in the context of his or her current relationships in the group. Insight may be used and is connected to the person's interactions within the group setting. In marital therapy and family therapy, the focus is not on a "sick" patient but rather on an ill couple or family relationship. The focus is away from individual psychopathology and toward the system. For example, a family may come into therapy because of a teenager who runs away. It might soon become apparent that the nature of the adolescent's behavior is rooted in the marital difficulties of the parents. A family therapist might then focus on how the family interactions affect each member. The parental discord can be discussed in terms of how it induces anxiety or anger in the house.

How does change occur? There are a number of ways. Insight, as mentioned above, is a process by which persons understand their current difficulties in terms of previous experiences. The unconscious is made conscious, and individuals can then use this information. For example, a medical student may have difficulty with nursing supervisors. During the course of therapy, she learns that they remind her of an overbearing mother. With this new information, she is more likely to approach them with more curiosity and care and perhaps change her interaction. In addition to providing insight, psychotherapy also works by helping the patient to release pent-up feelings (also called catharsis), check out reality, model after the therapist, learn to master certain feelings, and experience a healthier relationship with the therapist and with significant others.

Studies on the efficiency of psychotherapy have shown that many different types of psychotherapy are effective. Although some studies indicate that psychotherapy may not be effective and others fail to show differences between types, most psychiatrists practice some form of psychotherapy. Clearly there is need for more studies in this area.

Pharmacotherapy

Pharmacotherapy is an effective mode of therapy using various psychoactive substances. The number of drugs can be classified into several different groups based on their clinical use or chemical profiles. These include the major tranquilizers (also called antipsychotics and neuroleptics), antimanic drugs, antidepressants (including tricyclics and MAO inhibitors),

psychostimulants, and minor tranquilizers (also called sedative-hypnotics).

These various medications have been discussed as they arose in each section of psychopathology. The use of psychopharmacologic agents together with psychotherapy is an area under current investigation. Current research indicates that there is some benefit from the cocomitant use of the two modalities.

Somatic therapies (Electroconvulsive therapy)

Electroconvulsive therapy (ECT), or "shock" therapy as it is called in lay terms, is a highly effective and safe form of therapy for the treatment of depression. People have exaggerated and irrational fears based on a number of sources. First and foremost is the history of the procedure itself. When first used on a large scale in the 1930s this procedure was crude and potentially dangerous. At that time, patients were not given muscle relaxants and sedation was minimal. The grand mal seizures that were produced could cause bone fractures, cardiac disturbances, and muscle damage. Witnessing such procedures was horrifying. Today this image is kept alive by detractors of psychiatry who demonstrate it in the movies and television. ECT provides the most effective and quickest means of relieving depression and has fewer side effects than other forms of therapy. The number of treatments required varies, but most depressions are cleared in 5 to 10 treatments. Sessions are usually given three times weekly on alternate days. The major treatment indication is major depression. Dysthymic disorder and other types of depression are not effectively treated in this manner. With selected patients, substantial rates of improvement are found in 80 to 90% of cases. ECT can be given to patients with complex medical problems. It is safer than antidepressant medications in cardiac patients. It can safely be given to women who are pregnant. There are two areas of caution. First, it is contraindicated when there is the possibility of CNS masses. Second, patients who do have cardiac problems may have an added strain on this system because of the seizure, but this is minimized by careful collaboration with a cardiologist. One possible adverse reaction to this procedure is amnesia. Patients who are treated with ECT have reported some memory difficulties, which have been found to be diffuse and usually mild. For this reason, alternate electrode placement has been tried. In bilateral electrode placement, the metal disks are placed on a line midway between the external canthus of the eye and the tragus of the ear (in the temporofrontal lobe area) on each side of the head. In unilateral treatment, the electrodes are placed on an area to the right of the vertex and the right standard placement. It is believed that by passing a current through the nondominant hemisphere, such memory difficulties are almost entirely avoided.

Other forms of therapy

Although psychotherapy, pharmacotherapy, and somatic therapy occupy the bulk of a psychiatrist's practice, there are alternate forms of therapy that are used with increasing popularity. Hypnosis, behavioral therapy, and biofeedback all have been substantiated to be effective in a variety of settings. In **hypnosis**, the subject's unconscious is reached by a series of relaxation techniques, and suggested thoughts exert an effect once the person regains consciousness. **Hypnosis** has reportedly been successful in the treatment of phobias, smoking, and obesity. **Behavioral therapy** uses a series of positive and negative reinforcers and can be used for a wide variety of conditions. Although originally used mostly for institutionalized patients as a way of altering specific behavioral problems, it has become more widely used and can be helpful in the treatment of depression, schizophrenia, obsessions, phobias, and addictive problems. **Biofeedback** has also become more of a standard in the treatment of conditions such as anxiety disorders, psychophysiological disorders such as headaches, irritable bowel syndrome, colitis, hypertension, and others. It has been reimbursed under many insurance policies.

THE PHYSICIAN AND SOCIETY

A number of aspects of the behavioral sciences reflect human interactions on a larger scale. These are not applied solely to the study of human behavior but pertain to the other basic sciences and clinical sciences as well. For the purposes of study, there are six areas: epidemiology, health-care delivery systems, socioeconomic variables, transcultural issues, statistics and research designs, and forensic psychiatry. These will be discussed from the viewpoint of understanding basic definitions and concepts in a review fashion.

EPIDEMIOLOGY

Epidemiology is the study of health conditions in the population. There are many aspects to this field. Epidemiologists study the nature of diseases including the **etiology**: the distribution of disease in the population, including sex, age, ethnicity, and any variable that can distinguish one group from another. Epidemiology also studies the determinants of the disease and what causes it to spread. The number of diseases that are covered include all that are known. They can be of infectious or noninfectious nature.

In studying a disease, certain terms are commonly used. The **frequency** of a disease, whether it is common or rare, is reflected in the terms incidence and prevalence. **Incidence** is the number of new cases occurring within a specific time period. The incidence rate is the number of new cases divided by the size of the population at risk. The **prevalence** is the number of cases of a disease present during the time of the study. (It includes those at the beginning of the study as well as those added during the study period.) Patients are at risk for a disease if they have certain **risk factors**. Risk factors are characteristics of an individual that increase the chances of illness being contracted. In the Framingham study, many of the risk factors for heart disease were demonstrated. Hypertension, smoking, and type A personality were found to be risk factors for coronary artery disease (there are other risk factors as well). The National Institutes of Mental Health (NIMH) Epidemiologic Catchment Area Program (ECA) is a study that is distinguished by its sample size of 20,000 total subjects. In addition, it used a detailed diagnostic interview schedule to define mental illness in *DSM III* terms. Finally, it attempted to link epidemiologic and health service use data. The three sites include New Haven, Baltimore, and St. Louis. In this study,

lifetime prevalence rates for 15 different psychiatric disorders were obtained. These were schizophrenia/schizophreniform disease, 2.0%; substance use disorders (including alcohol and others), 15%; major depressive epidose, 6%; mania, 1%; anxiety/somatoform disorders, 10%; personality disorder, 2%; and any disorder covered, 29%. The age-group with the highest rates for most disorders was found to be the young adults (25 to 44 years). The disorders that were most prominent in men were antisocial personality and alcohol abuse. Disorders that were most common in women were depressive episodes and phobias. Rates of mental illness were found to be higher in those who were not college educated and in those living in inner-city environments. Of all the adults in the population in the study areas, 6% sought help for mental health reasons during a 6-month period.

SOCIOECONOMIC VARIABLES

In the 1950s, two researchers, August **Hollingshead** and Frederick **Redlich**, undertook the study of social class and mental illness in New Haven. A group of approximately 2,000 individuals who were under psychiatric care were studied. In comparing the relationship between social class and illness, it was found that those in the lower social classes suffered from more psychiatric conditions than did those in upper classes. It was also found in this study that those in the upper classes received treatment more on an outpatient basis and the poorer classes were more often found in hospitals. Even when rates of initial hospitalization were compared (which should come closer to reflecting the actual incidence of disorder), there was greater mental illness in the lower classes. In the Midtown Study, 1,600 people were randomly selected in the age range of 20 to 59 years. Questionnaires were given. Symptoms were much more evident in the lowest social class, where nearly half were impaired. The study also demonstrated that there was social mobility with those showing a downward drift in social classes when they were suffering from mental illness. Those individuals with mental illness were thought to "drift downward" from upper to lower classes because of their illness, thus the larger number of patients in lower socioeconomic classes was not felt to be due exclusively to the greater stress and deprivation of the lower classes.

Another study conducted in the mid-1930s demonstrated that among 35,000 admissions to state and private mental hospitals, there were patterns of social distribution. Faris and Dunham found that the highest rates of mental disorders were in the center of the city and in low socioeconomic groups. This led them to the hypothesis that social isolation from normal social contacts and a lack of a stable environment were factors leading to mental illness. Two studies demonstrate that urban living versus rural environment is *not* associated with higher rates of mental illness.

HEALTH-CARE DELIVERY SYSTEMS

Issues of medical care and how it is received and distributed in the population are of a great importance for physicians. Given all the medical information that doctors must possess, it would be gratifying if they could use it to help people. Unfortunately, the delivery system is often based on political issues. Federal, state, city, county, and other agencies play a major part in how services are delivered. Income, social status, and other factors must be taken into account. In the 1960s, as part of the "Great Society" program, Medicare and Medicaid were established. In 1984 the daily cost was $1 billion. Currently, nearly $400 billion yearly is spent on medical care. The reasons for the high cost are multiple. Chief among these is the high cost of medical technology, its development and technical support staff. Another factor is that the population is growing older, increasing the burden of chronic diseases. As mentioned in the section on senescence, the largest-growing segment of the population is the over-75 group. The elderly currently comprise 11% of the population but consume 30% of its health resources. An additional factor in increased cost is better survival from birth of the handicapped and those with prematurity and congenital problems. The impact on health care is seen in terms of the use of hospitals. Hospitals are the single most costly aspect of health care, accounting for 50% of the total expenditures (while physician costs are 18%). One final source of increased expenditures is nursing homes, which house 5% of those 65 and older and 20% of those 85 and older.

Health care is paid for by a variety of means—in **Medicare**, those over 65 years old. Recipients of medicare must be disabled. Medicare has two parts, A and B. A covers the hospital bills and B covers medical bills. (However, not everyone has part B. Those who do not must pay $100 per year, which is deducted from the social security check.) Medicare covers the nursing home if this is needed after hospitalization. **Medicaid** is a payment system that is set up to serve the poor. It pays a fixed amount of money to hospitals and physicians for inpatient and outpatient treatment. For example, Medicaid pays $30 for 35 minutes of psychotherapy with a psychiatrist. It is estimated that between 60 and 80% of the population has some form of insurance to pay their medical bills. Those from a lower income level and those working in small industries and family businesses usually are uninsured. Nonwhites are 50% more likely to be uninsured than whites. Almost all insurance policies cover hospitalization for medical or surgical reasons. **Major medical** policies also include outpatient services. Only 70% or so of insurance policies have major medical coverage. Insurance policies can differ in the degree to which a person receives money for ancillary services such as dentistry, medications, or optical needs. These are termed riders. Insurance policies usually include a **deductible**, which is a certain amount of money that must be paid by the patient before the insurance will pay (customarily, $100 to $200). Another method of insurance involves copayment, which means that the patient must pay a certain percentage of the bill. Typically this is after the deductible and amounts to 20% on average. Some policies have an indemnity, which means that they will pay a fixed amount of money and no more for a given procedure— the patient is responsible for the rest.

There are a variety of types of medical arrangements for the delivery of care. In the past, physicians were by and large independent practitioners. This has gradually been integrated with other forms. For example, group medical practice (physicians operating in a group of three or more) now is the arrangement for around 30% of physicians. A Health Maintenance organization (HMO) is a prepaid multispecialty group practice. A person in an HMO has all health needs provided by the HMO. HMOs have been able to keep costs of medical care down because there is a decreased rate of referrals and the HMO is run on a for-profit basis. If it keeps utilization down, it makes a profit. Although there is no increase in mortality when using an HMO, the question of quality of care has not been settled. An Individual Practice Association (IPA) is a type of HMO (50% of HMOs are IPAs) in which physicians may remain in their office while they administer care. They are paid a fixed amount of money per visit. Hospitalizations and referrals must be approved by the IPA.

Health-care costs have risen progressively over the past 10 years. In comparison to other living expenses, the health-care dollar has increased out of proportion. Today health care costs 10% of the gross national product (GNP). The federal government has paid the largest share, with 29% of the total health bill. State and local governments account for 11%, private insurance for 27%, and consumers paying out of pocket account for 32%. Only 1% is paid for by philanthropic foundations. One attempt to cut the cost has been the introduction of diagnosis-related groups (DRGs), a method of limiting the amount that Medicaid and Medicare will reimburse a hospital for a given condition. The government will pay only the average cost for a given condition. If a hospital can discharge a patient sooner, it will pocket the profit. If it takes longer, the hospital will shoulder the loss. Another way that the government can reduce inefficient hospital practices is to make payment tied to occupancy rates. Hospitals usually have to have a 80% occupancy rate in order to receive full reimbursement. The occupancy rate is the percentage of beds filled.

CULTURAL PSYCHIATRY

Culture can be defined as the pattern of behavior of human groups transmitted by symbols, embodied in artifacts, and passed down by tradition. Culture can be seen as related to etiology in that certain child-rearing practices, stressful roles, and cultural changes can affect individuals' mental well-being. Culture can also affect how a mental illness is expressed. There are certain culture-bound syndromes that are not found in other societies. Such a condition is **amok**, found in Southeast Asia and Malaysia. In this disorder, a person goes on a killing rampage. The assaults may last for minutes, hours, or days, until the individual is killed or restrained. **Latah**, a syndrome found in Alaska and Siberia, consists of echolalia (repeating one's words back), coprolalia (cursing), and mimicry. **Koro**, found among the Chinese, is a deep panic with a belief that one's penis is going to retract inside the abdomen and that death will ensue. Cultural psychiatry has added to understanding the nature of the family in our culture. In the United States, the nuclear family is the basic paradigm for families. It has been shown that for normal individuals in such a family, the social network involves about 25 individuals, whereas for neurotics it contains about 15, and for psychotics about 7.

CULTURAL FACTORS

Cultural psychiatry has had profound impact on psychoanalytic thinking. Although it was believed that the oedipal conflict was a universal phenomenon, it has been shown that this is not the case. In some societies, the family dynamics involve complex relationships. Freud also postulated that the male was superior to the female in society because he possessed a penis. Margaret Mead reported some societies in which women were the dominant sex and others in which neither dominated.

The understanding of cultural aspects of psychiatry has relevance because many people in our society believe in some culturally biased aspect of health care. For example, among the Puerto Rican population there may be a belief in **espiritismo**. Among black Americans **root work** and other beliefs can be found. Patients may resist medical treatment and secretly follow their faith healers. Inquiring about this may set the stage for an ingegration of modern medicine with the individual's cultural belief.

STATISTICS

Certain basic concepts are expected to be known regarding statistics. The importance of this area lies in the critical reading of scientific papers in medicine. Statistics that describe a particular group, for example the average grade on a test, are called **descriptive statistics**. **Inferential statistics** take information about a particular group and apply it to a population larger than the original group studied. Several basic concepts described the **central tendency** of a group. This is an attempt to summarize a large amount of data into a description of the entire group. Three different measures are important. The **mean** is the sum of all the scores divided by the number of scores. This score is affected by extremes. The **median** is the middle score, where 50% of the scores are higher and 50% are lower than this score. The **mode** is the most frequently occurring score. This can give us an indication of how most of the students in a groups did.

A description of the **range** or **variance** of scores tells us the lowest to highest scores obtained. Another measure of variation that is used widely in statistics in the **standard deviation**. The standard deviation is usually symbolized as S. As an example of obtaining the standard deviation, imagine the scores obtained in a group as 1, 3, 4, 5, 7. The mean score would be 4. To obtain the standard deviation, we must find the deviation of each of the raw scores from the mean. For the number 1 the deviation is 3, for the number 3 the deviation is 1, etc. The next step is to square each of the deviations. For the deviation 3 the square is 9, for the deviation 1 the square is 1, etc. In the third step, we add up these squared deviations and then divide by N. Finally we take the square root of this final number. This is symbolized in the formula

$$S = \sqrt{\frac{(X_1 - \overline{X})^2 + (X_2 - \overline{X})^2 + \text{etc.}}{N}}$$

In this example, the standard deviation is 2. N is the total number of scores, and X_1 represents the first raw score. $\overline{X}$ is the mean of the sample. The use of standard deviations is important because it gives us some basic language for understanding how groups perform. The pictorial representation that is most helpful in this regard is the **distribution curve**. Most natural phenomena distribute themselves in a normal distribution curve. There are many ways in which a distribution curve can be arranged depending on the data. A normal distribution curve is symmetrical. *The mean, median, and mode all are the same number*. The curve may also have variations in the peak and the degree of asymmetry. Graphs that are flattened are called platykurtic; those that are peaked are leptokurtic. Similarly, they can be skewed to the right or left, as shown in Figure 7-5. In a normal curve (see Fig. 7-5), 68% of all of the cases will be one standard deviation above and one standard deviation below the mean. In addition, 95% of the cases will fall within two standard deviations below and above the mean. Another way of analyzing data is to look at how the variables are correlated. Variables can be positively correlated (also called direct correlation), negatively correlated (also called inverse correlation), or not correlated (Fig. 7-6).

The fact that variables may be directly related does not prove that they are related as cause and effect. This is especially true for psychological variables, where the cause often has multiple determinants. In comparing variables, experimenters are concerned with whether the data are meaningful. Several different tests can be done to determine whether data comparing an experimental and control group are significant. One test that is used is the **t-test**, or Student's t-test. In this test, two means are compared, and if the control mean is far enough apart from the experimental mean, the two groups are statistically different. The null hypothesis is a statement that the two means are equal to each other and that the results are not significant. Most experiments attempt to disprove the null hypothesis. Another more frequently used description of data is the alpha coefficient. The L-level, or **level of significance**, is given in decimal form. A level of significance of 0.01 means that 1 in 100 times the experimental results can be obtained as a result of chance or sampling error. The most common level of significance of data is 0.05, meaning that 5 times in 100 the data can be obtained by chance. When the level of significance is greater than this, the experimental results are questionable.

FORENSIC PSYCHIATRY

The field of forensic psychiatry is quite vast. The interface of psychiatry and the law can be found in areas involving the legal aspects of doing antibody testing for acquired immunodeficiency syndrome (AIDS), the competency of patients to refuse treatment, issues of malpractice, divorce, and child custody. For our purposes, the following areas will be covered: (1) competence to stand trial, (2) insanity defense, (3) ability to make a will, (4) guardianship of children in divorce, and (5) civil rights of committed patients.

Being found **competent to stand trial** is different from being found competent of committing a crime, the latter being addressed under the insanity defense issue (see below). Prior to a patient's facing a trial, it must be assessed whether or not the patient has an understanding of the charges at the time of the trial. In addition, persons must be able to participate in their own defense. The difficulty in such situations is that if there is a question of patients' competence to stand trial, they must be examined by a court-ordered psychiatrist. If the psychiatrist finds a patient incompetent, the patient may be held for treatment for an indeterminant amount of time until able to stand trial. In this way, certain patients' freedoms may be deprived. This procedure may be invoked far more often than the insanity defense.

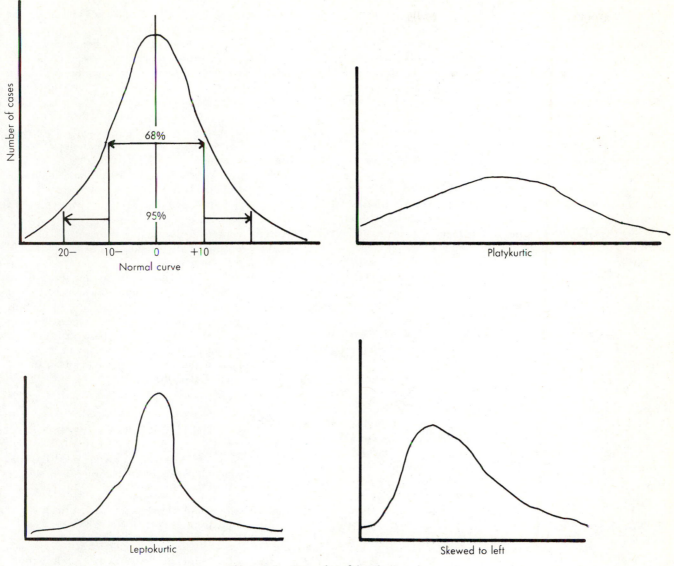

Figure 7-5.   Examples of distribution curves.

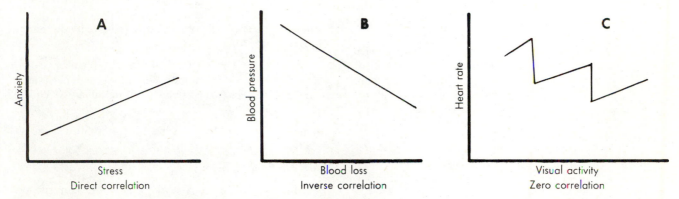

Figure 7-6.   How variables are correlated. (*A*) **Direct correlation.** (*B*) Inverse or negative correlation. (*C*) Zero correlation.

The **insanity defense** recently gained national attention with the trial of John Hinkley, who attempted to assassinate President Reagan. In criminal law, the principle of mens rea (guilty mind) was maintained—that is, persons who did not possess an intention or thoughts about their crime could not be found guilty. This defense is most clearly posited under the M'Naghten Rule (1843), which states that it must be clearly proved that *at the time of the act, the accused must have labored under such a defect of reason from diseases of the mind so as to not know the nature and quality of the act or, if he did know, then to not know that what he was doing was wrong.* Because of certain dissatisfactions with this rule, several alternative rules were formulated. The case of *Durham* v. *United States* found that the accused was not guilty by reason of insanity if . . ". . . his unlawful act was the *product of mental disease or defect*." The American Law Institute (ALI) rule attempted to incorporate the fact that persons could know that what they were doing was wrong but that they might not be able to control the impulse. In the ALI rule, a person is not responsible for a criminal act if at the time of the act the conduct was the result of mental disease or defect or he lacked substantial capacity either to appreciate the criminality of his conduct or to conform his conduct to the requirements of the law." This implied knowing that it was wrong and ability to control one's behavior. Hinkley was acquitted because, although he knew what he was doing, he could not control the impulse.

Testamentary capacity is not the ability to give testimony but rather the ability to make a will. There are three requirements for a person to make a will. He must realize without prompting the nature of the act of making the will. He must know the extent of his property (and possessions) and must realize the natural objects of his bounty and their claims on him (those who may be rightly entitled to his possessions or whom he desires to receive his possessions).

In **guardianship** cases, a historical shift has occurred. In the past, the father was felt to be the head of the family and to have "property rights" of the children. Recently the "tender-age doctrine" has allowed that the mother has the ability to provide the needed nurturant care. In today's legal system, the court decides the placement of the child based on the best interests of the child.

One of the most unusual aspects of the medical subspecialty called psychiatry is that physicians find themselves with the power to prevent people from having certain freedoms and rights. The process of **commitment** varies from state to state. Commitment can be based on a patient's dangerousness or on his or her having a mental disease that can be improved with treatment but that the patient is denying. A mental patient admitted on standard commitment papers is not denied civil rights. He or she can petition the court for a trial to be released. Patients who are then judged "insane" by a judicial action are thereby rendered incompetent and are deprived of certain civil rights. They may lose the right to buy or sell property, sign legal papers, practice a profession in which they possess a license (like medicine), and many other civil rights.

SUICIDE

Perhaps suicide is the one area of the behavioral sciences that has been the most extensively studied. The U.S. rate of suicide is 12 per 100,000—about the same as in other nations. Of the many statistics that have been collected on suicide, the following are among the most important:

1. Males *commit* suicide 4 times more often than females.
2. Females *attempt* suicide much more often than males.
3. Attempted suicide is 10 times more common than actual suicide.
4. The most common method of suicide for men is with guns and for women with poisons.
5. Increasing age, white race, and social isolation are generally associated with an increased incidence of suicide.
6. Suicide is not limited to lower classes but is highest in lower and upper classes.
7. There is an increased risk for those with previous treatment for emotional disorders.
8. Current depressive disorder, alcoholism, or physical health problems predispose to suicide.

The evaluation of a potentially suicidal patient is one that demands great care. Many factors besides those listed above must be considered. The patients' interest in getting help, their ability to control themselves, and the presence of support systems such as caring families are involved in the decision to treat such patients inside or outside of the hospital. The use of pharmacotherapy combined with psychotherapy is certainly an important approach. In the most severe cases, patients should be hospitalized and ECT performed.

BIBLIOGRAPHY

Aserinsky E, Kleitman N: Regularly occurring periods of eye motility and concomitant phenomena during sleep. Science 118:273–274, 1953.

Bemporad JR (ed): Child Development in Normality and Psychopathology. Brunner/Mazel, New York, 1980.

Brazelton TB: Neonatal assessment. *In* Greenspan SI, Pollack GM (eds): The Course of Life: Psychoanalytic Contributions Toward Understanding Personality Development. Vol I. Infancy and Early Childhood. National Institute of Mental Health, Washington, DC, 1980.

Brazelton TB, Koslowski B, Main M: Origins of reciprocity. *In* Lewis M, Rosenblum L (eds): Mother-Infant Interaction. John Wiley & Sons, New York, 1974.

Brill AA (ed): The Basic Writings of Sigmund Freud. Random House, New York, 1938.

Christ AE: Conduct disorder and the problem of juvenile delinquency. *In* Simons RC (ed): Understanding Human Behavior in Health and Illness, 3rd ed. Williams & Wilkins, Baltimore, 1985.

Dement WC: Some Must Watch While Others Must Sleep. WH Freeman, San Francisco, 1974.

Faris (see Sadock, below).

Fenichel O: The Psychoanalytic Theory of Neurosis. WW Norton, New York, 1945.

Freud A: Nondelinquent disturbances of conduct. *In* Rutter M, Hersov L (eds): Child and Adolescent Psychiatry—A Modern Approach. Blackwell Scientific Publications, Oxford, 1985.

Freud S: The Interpretation of Dreams. Macmillan, New York, 1914.

Freud S: Introductory Lectures to Psychoanalysis. Boni and Liveright, New York, 1920.

Freud S: Collected Papers, IV, V. Basic Books, New York, 1959.

Friedrich EV: Schizophrenic disorders. *In* Scully JH (ed): Psychiatry. Harwal, Media, PA, 1985.

Goldfried MR, Davidson GC: Clinical Behavior Therapy. Holt, Rinehart & Winston, New York, 1976.

Green R (ed): Human Sexuality: A Health Practitioner's Text. Williams & Wilkins, Baltimore, 1975.

Harlow FH, Harlow MK: Love in infant monkeys. Sci Am 200 (6):68, 1959.

Harlow FH, Harlow MK: Social deprivation in monkeys. Sci Am 207(5):136, 1962.

Hollingshead (see Sadock, below).

Holmes TM, Rahe RM: The Social Readjustment Rating Scale. J Psychosom Res 11:213, 1967.

Horney K: New Ways in Psychoanalysis. WW Norton, New York, 1939.

Kandel ER: From metapsychology to molecular biology: Exploration into the nature of anxiety. Am J Psychiatry 140(10):1277, 1983.

Kaplan HS: The New Sex Therapy. Brunner/Mazel, New York, 1974.

Kempe CH, Silverman FN, Steele BF, Droegemuller W, Silver HK: The battered child syndrome. JAMA 181:17, 1962.

Kinsey AC, Pomeroy WB, Martin CE, Gebhard PM: Sexual Behavior in the Human Male. WB Saunders, Philadelphia, 1948.

Kinsey AC, Pomeroy WB, Martin CE, Gebhard PM: Sexual Behavior in the Human Female. WB Saunders, Philadelphia, 1953.

Kraft-Ebing R von: Psychopathia Sexualis. FA Davis, Philadelphia, 1983.

Kübler-Ross E: On Death and Dying. Macmillan, New York, 1969.

Levinson DJ et al: The Seasons of a Man's Life. Alfred A Knopf, New York, 1978.

Lewis (see Pincus, below).

Lorenz KZ: Evolution and Modification of Behavior. University of Chicago Press, Chicago, 1965.

Mahler M, Pine F, Bergman A: The Psychological Birth of the Infant. Basic Books, New York, 1975.

Meyer RJ, Hagerty R: Streptococcal infections in families. Pediatrics 29:539, 1962.

Mullahy P: Oedipus Myth and Complex. Grove Press, New York, 1948.

Nash E, Stoch B, Harper G: Human Behavior. David Philip, Cape Town, 1984.

Nemiah JC: Comprehensive Textbook of Psychiatry, 2nd ed. Williams & Wilkins, New York, 1975.

Pennfield (see Restar, below).

Pincus JH, Tucker GJ: Behavioral Neurology, 3rd ed. Oxford University Press, New York, 1985, p. 79.

Prechtl (see Brazelton, above).

Restar R: The Brain. Bantam Books, New York, 1984.

Risch SC, Kalin NM, Murphy DL: Pharmacological challenge strategies: Implications for neurochemical mechanisms in affective disorders and treatment approaches. J Clin Psychopharmacol 1(4):239, 1981.

Rosenzweig MR, Bennett EL, Diamond MC: Brain changes in response to experience Sci Am 226(2):22, 1972.

Rutter M: Infantile autism and other pervasive developmental disorders. *In* Rutter M, Hersov L (eds): Child and Adolescent Psychiatry—A Modern Approach. Blackwell Scientific Publications, Oxford, 1985.

Semans JM: Premature ejaculation: A new approach. South Med J 49:353, 1956.

Sadock BJ, Kaplan MI, Freedman AM, Sussman N: Psychiatry in the urban setting. *In* Freedman AM, Kaplan MI, Sadock BJ: Comprehensive Textbook of Psychiatry. Williams & Wilkins, Baltimore, 1975.

Spitz RA: The First of Life. International Universities Press, New York, 1956.

Tinbergen N: The Study of Instinct. Clarendon Press, Oxford, 1951.

SAMPLE QUESTIONS

DIRECTIONS: Each question below contains five suggested answers. Choose the one best response to each question.

1. A patient is hallucinating, believes that others are talking about her, and complains that some outside force is causing her to commit acts. She is most likely suffering from

    A. schizophrenia
    B. major depressive episode
    C. schizotypal personality disorder
    D. organic brain syndrome
    E. none of the above

2. A common side effect of the antipsychotic drugs is

A. ECG changes
B. neuroleptic malignant syndrome
C. extrapyramidal manifestations
D. hepatotoxicity
E. aplastic anemia

3. The number of new cases of a particular disease is the

A. incidence
B. prevalence
C. group at risk
D. initial cohort
E. proband

4. There is an increased likelihood of hypertensive crisis with the use of which of the following psychotropic medications?

A. Neuroleptics
B. Tricyclic antidepressants
C. MAO inhibitors
D. Benzodiazepines
E. Lithium carbonate

5. All of the following observations concerning the endorphins are true EXCEPT that they

A. may play a part in pain and memory
B. are pentapeptides
C. function by altering cell membranes
D. are short-lived substances
E. may be part of a larger β-lipoprotein

6. All of the following structures have been found to be involved in memory EXCEPT the

A. hippocampus
B. fornix
C. pulvinar nuclei
D. dorsomedian thalamic nuclei
E. globus pallidus

7. During the school-age period, cognitive development is characterized by all of the following abilities EXCEPT

A. the use of reverse logic
B. conservation of volume, length, and area
C. grouping objects
D. arranging serial order
E. seeing things from other perspectives

DIRECTIONS: Each question below contains four suggested answers of which **one** or **more** is correct. Choose the answer:

A if **1, 2, and 3** are correct
B if **1 and 3** are correct
C if **2 and 4** are correct
D if **4** is correct
E if **1, 2, 3, and 4** are correct

8. Which of the following statements concerning the children of divorced parents are true?

1. Adolescents generally fare better than preschool children
2. Preschool and school-age children show the greatest difficulty
3. Parents underestimate the impact on children
4. In therapy, children reveal guilt about the divorce

9. Functions that have been shown to occur primarily in the left hemisphere include

1. spoken language
2. mathematical skills
3. reasoning
4. spatial skills

10. Which of the following statements correctly describe supportive psychotherapy?

1. The therapist probes the patient's past
2. Dreams are a focus of attention
3. It makes use of negative transference
4. Issues of self-esteem are addressed

11. Which of the following statements correctly describe a toddler's development?

1. Development is completed by 18 months of age
2. Neural control of the sphincters is achieved by age 18 months
3. Gains in height and weight approximate those in infancy
4. The cognitive stage may remain the same until age 5 years

12. A 3-year-old is capable of

1. Recalling an object in its absence
2. Using words to represent people or things
3. Assuming that machines have feelings
4. Playing with another 3-year-old without constant supervision

13. Freud's topographic theory includes which of the following components?

1. Ego
2. Superego
3. Paraconscious
4. Preconscious

14. Which of the following defense mechanisms play a key part in the latency period?

    1. Sublimation
    2. Projection
    3. Reaction formation
    4. Displacement

15. Which of the following are true statements about dyslexia?

    1. It is more common in boys than girls
    2. It is a common disorder
    3. Other psychiatric problems are often related
    4. It is found in equal numbers in all socioeconomic groups

16. Which of the following are considered adequate treatment for attention deficit hyperactivity disorder?

    1. Individual psychotherapy
    2. Thioridazine
    3. Methylphenidate
    4. Amphetamine

17. Which of the following are true statements regarding juvenile delinquency?

    1. There has been an increase in serious crimes
    2. They represent a small proportion of conduct disorders
    3. There are higher rates in lower socioeconomic groups
    4. They are positively associated with broken homes

18. The limbic system consists of the

    1. hippocampus
    2. amygdala
    3. septal nuclei
    4. hypothalamus

19. Essential elements in the analytic process include

    1. transference
    2. dream interpretation
    3. resistance
    4. the analytic couch

20. Which of the following statements about dreams are true?

    1. They are an excellent means of understanding the patient's unconscious
    2. They occur only during REM sleep
    3. They make use of symbolism
    4. Their visual imagery demonstrates their latent content

21. Patients with compulsive personality disorder are characterized as being

    1. anxious
    2. unusually passive
    3. at increased risk of heart disease
    4. prone to substance abuse

22. Narcosynthesis can be helpful in treating

    1. conversion disorder
    2. posttraumatic stress disorder
    3. psychogenic amnesia
    4. agoraphobia

23. Which of the following changes occur in the sleep of elderly persons?

    1. Delta sleep decreases
    2. REM sleep decreases
    3. Time awake in bed increases
    4. Sleep disturbances increase

DIRECTIONS: The groups of questions below consist of lettered choices followed by several numbered items. For each numbered item select the **one** lettered choice with which it is **most** closely associated. Each lettered choice may be used once, more than one, or not at all.

Questions 24–27. For each description below, choose the type of reinforcement that is being described.

    A. Continuous reinforcement
    B. Intermittent reinforcement
    C. Delayed reinforcement
    D. Immediate reinforcement
    E. Retrograde reinforcement

24. A young dyslexic patient is learning to discriminate certain letters. After each correct discrimination, his teacher compliments him

25. The type of reinforcement that is most difficult to extinguish

26. Intervening variables or events may confuse the subject about what behavior is being reinforced

27. The ratio of the reinforcement pattern is varied or the rate of reinforcement is varied

Questions 28–30. For each of the following descriptions of infant behavior, choose the principle that is at work.

    A. Recognition memory
    B. Evocative memory
    C. Transitional object
    D. Object constancy
    E. Differentiation phase

28. An infant is hungry but is able to delay gratification of being fed

29. An infant calms down when a favorite doll is placed near him

30. An infant can separate from her mother without undue anxiety

Questions 31–33. For each of the toddler behaviors described below, choose the principle that is at work.

  A. Autonomy versus shame and doubt
  B. Preoperational thinking
  C. Concrete operations
  D. Artificialism
  E. Parallel play

31. A toddler is flying in a jet. Shortly after take-off he observes that the buildings and autos are becoming progressively smaller. He inquires of his father, "Why are the cars shrinking?"

32. While on the airplane the child notices another youngster who has a coloring book. He begins to wriggle in his seat and eventually frees himself to walk toward the other child.

33. The first child is now escorted back to his seat with some protest. Unable to have his way, he establishes eye contact with the other child and begins to draw in his own book.

Questions 34–38. For each of the developmental descriptors below, choose the age period with which it is most closely associated.

  A. Infancy
  B. Toddlerhood
  C. Preschool
  D. School age
  E. Adolescence

34. Latency

35. Oedipal period

36. Concrete operations

37. Industry versus inferiority

38. Genital stage

Questions 39–43. For each of the diagnostic tests described below, choose the correct name.

  A. WAIS
  B. WISC
  C. TAT
  D. MMPI
  E. Rorschach

39. A projective test in which the examiner might be concerned about a patient's response to color

40. Might help to determine if depression is part of a characterological problem

41. Adults will probably receive the same score as they did when they were children

42. Helpful in determining the degree of organicity in adults

43. Replaced the Stanford-Binet

Questions 44–48. For each manifestation of chromosomal abnormality described below, choose the corresponding syndrome.

  A. Klinefelter's syndrome
  B. Testicular feminization
  C. Turner's syndrome
  D. Adrenogenital syndrome
  E. XYY chromosome

44. Male phenotype, underdeveloped genitals

45. Female phenotype, XY chromosomal pattern

46. Impulsivity, tall stature

47. Both male and female genitalia present

48. Normal XX chromosomal pattern

ANSWERS

1. A		25. B	
2. C		26. C	
3. A		27. B	
4. C		28. B	
5. C		29. C	
6. E		30. D	
7. A		31. B	
8. E (all)		32. A	
9. A (1,2,3)		33. E	
10. D (4)		34. D	
11. D (4)		35. C	
12. E (all)		36. D	
13. D (4)		37. D	
14. B (1,3)		38. E	
15. A (1,2,3)		39. E	
16. B (1,3)		40. D	
17. E (all)		41. A	
18. A (1,2,3)		42. A	
19. B (1,3)		43. B	
20. B (1,3)		44. A	
21. B (1,3)		45. B	
22. A (1,2,3)		46. E	
23. E (all)		47. D	
24. A		48. D	

INDEX